ATLAS OF DIAGNOSTIC IMAGING
of dogs and cats

Massimo Vignoli
John Graham

ATLAS OF DIAGNOSTIC IMAGING
of dogs and cats

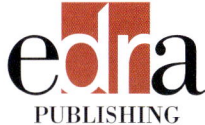

Massimo Vignoli, John Graham – Atlas of diagnostic imaging of dogs and cats
©2022 Edra Publishing US LLC – All rights reserved
ISBN: 978-1-957260-20-4
eISBN: 978-1-957260-30-3

Book Publishing Manager: **Costanza Smeraldi, Edra S.p.A.**
Paper, Printing and Binding Manager: **Paolo Ficicchia, Edra S.p.A.**
Cover: **Gaetano Altamura, Edra S.p.A.**
Layout: **T&T Studio, Milano, Italy**
Copyediting: **Mercedes González Fernández de Castro – Science & Health Publications**

The rights of translation, electronic storage, reproduction or total or partial adaptation by any means (including microfilms and photostatic copies), are reserved for all countries. No part of this publication may be reproduced, stored in a retrieval system, or transmitted in any form or by any means, electronic, mechanical, photocopying, recording or otherwise, without permission in writing from the Publisher.

Knowledge and best practice in this field are constantly changing: As new research and experience broaden our knowledge, changes in practice, treatment, and drug therapy may become necessary or appropriate. Readers are advised to check the most current information provided (i) or procedures featured or (ii) by the manufacturer of each product to be administered, to verify the recommended dose or formula, the method and duration of administration, and contraindications. It is the responsibility of the practitioners, relying on their own experience and knowledge of the patient, to make diagnoses, to determine dosages and the best treatment for each individual patient, and to take all appropriate safety precautions. To the fullest extent of the law, neither the Publisher nor the Editors assume any liability for any injury and/or damage to persons or property arising out of or related to any use of the material contained in this book.

This publication contains the author's opinions and is intended to provide precise and accurate information.

The processing of the texts, even if taken care of with scrupulous attention, cannot entail specific responsibilities for the author and/or the publisher for any errors or inaccuracies.

The Publisher has made every effort to obtain and cite the exact sources of the illustrations. If in some cases he has not been able to find the right holders, he is available to remedy any inadvertent omissions or errors in the references cited. All registered trademarks mentioned belong to their legitimate owners.

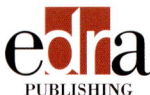

Edra Publishing US LLC
3309 Northlake Boulevard,
Suite 203, Palm Beach Gardens,
FL, 33403
EIN: 844113980

info@edrapublishing.com
www.edrapublishing.com

Printed by "Graphicscalve S.p.A.", Costa di Mezzate – Bergamo (Italy)

Editors

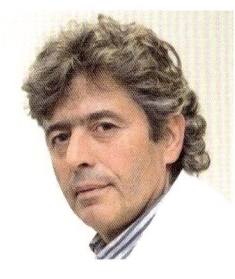

Massimo Vignoli DMV, DScM, PhD, SRV, DECVDI

Graduated at the University of Bologna. Specialist in veterinary radiology at the University of Torino. Residency program in diagnostic imaging at University of Zuerich and the university of Torino. Travel Award and Resident Prize at the EAVDI/ECVDI European Congress, Murcia 2002, with the project "CT-guided biopsy in the skeleton". Diplomate of the European College of Diagnostic Imaging (DECVDI). Author and coauthor in 239 scientific studies, 114 of them in scientific journals. Coeditor and/or coauthor of the books "Radiology of the dog and cat" (Poletto Editore, 2005), "Veterinary Computed Tomography" edited by Tobias Schwarz and Jimmy Saunders (Wiley-Blackwell, 2011) and "Manual of first aid and traumatology in small animals" edited by Fabio Viganò, (Elsevier, 2013).
President of the Italian Society of Veterinary Diagnostic Imaging (SVIDI) from 2001 to 2004. Coordinator for diagnostic imaging of the Post University school, SCIVAC, Cremona, from 2005 to 2010. Adjunct professor at the University of Naples from 2007 to 2009. Lecturer at the School of Specialization in Clinic and Pathology for Pet Animals from 2007 to 2008, Master of Oncology and Master of Diagnostic Imaging (2008 to date) at the University of Pisa. Lecturer at the Master of Diagnostic Imaging, University of Camerino from 2010 to 2013. He obtained the Academic degree of Doctor in Veterinary Sciences (PhD) at the University of Ghent, 2010. Since December 2015 he is Professor at the University of Teramo, and consultant for the Veterinary Clinic Pet Care in Bologna, Italy.
His fields of interest are radiology, ultrasound, CEUS, computed tomography, and interventional radiology.
Graduated also in Sports Science in November 2018 with the thesis: "Correlation between vision training and batting in baseball".

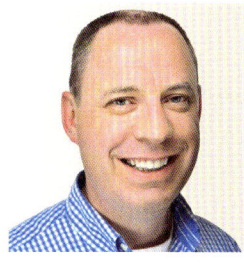

John Graham MVB, MSc, DVR, MRCVS, DECVDI, DACVR

John Graham graduated from the Faculty of Veterinary Medicine of University College in Dublin, Ireland. He worked for five years in mixed animal and small animal practice in the United Kingdom. He then completed a residency program in diagnostic imaging in the Department of Clinical Radiology of the Swedish University of Agricultural Sciences, Uppsala, Sweden. He was a visiting lecturer in veterinary radiology at the School of the Veterinary Medicine, Onderstepoort, South Africa. He joined the faculty at the College of Veterinary Medicine, University of Florida, working there until 2003. He has worked in private referral practice in the USA and Canada. He now works as a radiologist for Idexx Telemedicine. He is a diplomate of the American College of Veterinary Radiology and of the European College of Veterinary Diagnostic Imaging. He has spoken at national and international meetings, coauthored many scientific papers and contributed to and written several textbooks. He is interested in all facets of small animal diagnostic imaging. In his spare time, Dr. Graham enjoys road and mountain biking, skiing, reading, cooking and travel.

Contributors

Ryan B. Appleby DVM, DACVR
Ontario Veterinary College, University of Guelph
Guelph, Canada

Mylène Auger DMV, DACVR
AnImages
Montréal, Québec, Canada

Chiara Bergamino DVM, DECVDI, DVMS, MRCVS
Veterinary Radiologist
VetCT Ltd
Cambridge, United Kingdom

Juliette Besso DEDV, DECVDI
Consultant itinérant en Imagerie
Paris, France

Susanne Boroffka DVM, PhD, DECVDI
Specialistische Dierenkliniek Utrecht
Utrecht, The Netherlands

Carolina Carlsson Nilemo DVM, DECVDI
Section of Diagnostic Imaging,
SLU University Animal Hospital (UDS)
Uppsala, Sweden

Serena Crosara DVM, PhD, DECVIM-CA (Cardiology)
Department of Veterinary Sciences, University of Parma
Parma, Italy

Ruth Dennis MA, VetMB, DVR, DECVDI, FRCVS
Dick White Referrals
Six Mile Bottom, Cambridge, United Kingdom

Alessandra Destri DVM, MRCVS, DECVDI
Southern Counties Veterinary Specialists
Ringwood, United Kingdom

Pamela Di Donato DVM, PhD, MRCVS, DECVDI
Ospedale Veterinario Portoni Rossi
Zola Predosa (Bologna), Italy
Antech Imaging Services
Foutain Valley, California (USA)

Lorrie Gaschen DVM, PhD, Dr.med.vet, DECVDI
School of Veterinary Medicine, Louisiana State University
Baton Rouge, Louisiana (USA)

Ingrid Gielen MSc, DVM, PhD
Department of Medical Imaging
and Small Animal Orthopaedics, Ghent University
Merelbeke, Belgium
Department of Radiology and Radiation Hygiene
Faculty of Veterinary Medicine, University of Belgrade
Belgrade, Serbia

Robson F. Giglio MV, MS, PhD, DACVR
Small Animal Medicine and Surgery Department,
College of Veterinary Medicine, University of Georgia
Athens, Georgia (USA)

L. Abbigail Granger DVM, DACVR
School of Veterinary Medicine, Louisiana State University
Baton Rouge, Louisiana (USA)

Gert ter Haar DVM, MRCVS, DECVS
Specialistische Dierenkliniek Utrecht
Utrecht, The Netherlands

Hock Gan Heng DVM, MVS, MS, DACVR, DECVDI
VetCT Specialists Ltd
Orlando, Florida (USA)

Séamus Hoey MVB, DACVR, ECVDI, MRCVS
School of Veterinary Medicine,
University College Dublin
Belfield, Ireland

Jessica Ingman DVM, DECVDI
Section of Diagnostic Imaging,
SLU University Animal Hospital (UDS)
Uppsala, Sweden

Chee Kin Lim DVM, BVSc(Hons), MMedVet (Diag Im),
FMCVS (Vet Imaging), DECVDI
VetCT Specialists Ltd
Orlando, Florida (USA)

Contributors

Angela J. Marolf DVM, DACVR
College of Veterinary Medicine and Biomedical Sciences,
Colorado State University,
Fort Collins, Colorado (USA)

Chiara Mattei DVM, DECVDI
Ospedale Veterinario Portoni Rossi
Zola Predosa (Bologna), Italy

Hester McAllister MVB, DVR, DECVDI
School of Veterinary Medicine, University College Dublin
Belfield, Ireland

Ehren M. McLarty DVM, DACVR
School of Veterinary Medicine, University of California
Davis, California (USA)

Barbara Posch CertVDI, DECVDI
VetCT Teleradiology Consultant
Salzburg, Austria

Antonella Puggioni Dr. Vet Med, VDI, DECVDI
School of Veterinary Medicine, University College Dublin
Belfield, Ireland

Nathalie Rademacher DVR, DACVR, DECVDI
School of Veterinary Medicine, Louisiana State University
Baton Rouge, Louisiana (USA)

Marco Russo DVM, PhD, MRCVS
Department of Veterinary Medicine and Animal Sciences,
University of Naples "Federico II"
Naples, Italy

Rick F. Sánchez BSciBiol, DVM, CertVOphthal, DECVO, FHEA
Specialistische Dierenkliniek Utrecht
Utrecht, The Netherlands

Daniela Schweizer Prof. Dr. med. vet., DECVDI
Division of Clinical Radiologie, Vetsuisse Faculty,
University of Bern
Bern, Switzerland

Cliona Skelly MVB, PhD, DVR, DECVDI
School of Veterinary Medicine, University College Dublin
Belfield, Ireland

Swan Specchi DMV, DACVR
Ospedale Veterinario Portoni Rossi
Zola Predosa (Bologna), Italy
Antech Imaging Services
Foutain Valley, California (USA)

Margret S. Thompson DVM, DACVR
College of Veterinary Medicine, Cornell University
Ithaca, New York (USA)

Christopher R. Tollefson DVM, MS, DACVR
College of Veterinary Medicine, Cornell University
Ithaca, New York (USA)

Margareta Uhlhorn DVM, DECVDI
Section of Diagnostic Imaging,
SLU University Animal Hospital (UDS)
Uppsala, Sweden

Henri van Bree Prof. DVM, PhD, DECVS, DECVDI
Department of Medical Imaging
and Small Animal Orthopaedics, Ghent University
Merelbeke, Belgium

Federico Vilaplana Grosso LV, DECVDI, DACVR
College of Veterinary Medicine, University of Florida
Gainesville, Florida (USA)

Micaela Zarelli DVM, DECVDI, MRCVS
Antech Imaging Services
Fountain Valley, California (USA)

Foreword

Diagnostic imaging is a key component in the care of companion animal patients. In recent decades the available imaging modalities have expanded from conventional radiography to include ultrasonography, computed tomography and magnetic resonance imaging and all are employed on a daily basis in both general and specialty veterinary practice. The transition from film screen radiography to digital radiography has transformed the veterinary practice by making diagnostic radiography quicker, easier and cheaper, and facilitates rapid transmission, sharing and interpretation of images.

This textbook is intended to provide a broad overview of diagnostic imaging of companion animals for students and general practitioners. Interpretation of diagnostic images is a visual science and our goal was to incorporate as many images as possible in the textbook. Images are presented throughout the textbook to illustrate normal anatomy, species differences, anatomic variation and common pathology. Radiography remains the most commonly employed diagnostic imaging modality in both general practice and specialty practice, and the textbook provides a thorough review of the use of this imaging modality for all body systems. As ultrasound is now widely employed in general practice, this imaging modality is also covered in detail, particularly where it complements diagnostic radiography. Computed tomography and magnetic resonance imaging are also discussed to show how these imaging modalities can supplement radiography and ultrasonography and where they are superior. In addition to the images included in the textbook, there are also linked online video files which more clearly show normal physiologic function and dynamic pathology. We hope that this textbook will provide a comprehensive reference to assist practitioners in interpreting diagnostic images of their patients.

Massimo Vignoli
John Graham

Table of contents

SECTION I — General introduction

CHAPTER 1 Diagnostic imaging — 1
Daniela Schweizer

SECTION II — Appendicular skeleton

CHAPTER 2 Normal bones and joints — 19
John Graham and Massimo Vignoli

CHAPTER 3 Appendicular skeleton: radiology and techniques — 27
Nathalie Rademacher

CHAPTER 4 Fundamental bone and joint alterations — 33
Nathalie Rademacher

CHAPTER 5 Fractures — 41
Cliona Skelly and Hester McAllister

CHAPTER 6 Skeletal diseases of unknown etiology — 51
Robson F. Giglio and Federico R. Vilaplana Grosso

CHAPTER 7 Elbow dysplasia — 61
Massimo Vignoli

CHAPTER 8 Hip dysplasia — 69
Ingrid Gielen and Henri van Bree

CHAPTER 9 Osteochondrosis — 79
Ingrid Gielen and Henri van Bree

XI

CHAPTER 10	**Other congenital developmental and hereditary diseases**	91

Séamus Hoey and Antonella Puggioni

CHAPTER 11	**Metabolic bone diseases**	105

Alessandra Destri

CHAPTER 12	**Soft tissues**	115

Barbara Posch, Antonella Puggioni and Massimo Vignoli

SECTION III — Axial skeleton

CHAPTER 13	**Diseases of the skull**	133

Federico R. Vilaplana Grosso and Robson F. Giglio

CHAPTER 14	**Brachycephalic obstructive airway syndrome**	163

Susanne Boroffka and Gert ter Haar

CHAPTER 15	**Eye and orbit**	171

Susanne Boroffka and Rick F. Sánchez

CHAPTER 16	**Vertebral column**	183

Ruth Dennis

SECTION IV — Thorax

CHAPTER 17	**Thoracic wall, diaphragm, and pleura**	219

Chee Kin Lim and Hock Gan Heng

CHAPTER 18	**Mediastinum**	241

Ehren M. McLarty

CHAPTER 19	**Congenital and acquired cardiac diseases**	267

L. Abbigail Granger and Serena Crosara

CHAPTER 20	**Lung: anatomy, techniques, and interpretation principles**	315

John P. Graham and Juliette Besso

CHAPTER 21	**Trachea**	339

Chiara Mattei

CHAPTER 22	**Infectious pulmonary disease**	**349**
	John P. Graham	

CHAPTER 23	**Pulmonary infiltrations**	**363**
	Margareta Uhlhorn, Carolina Carlsson Nilemo and Jessica Ingman	

SECTION V — Abdomen

CHAPTER 24	**Abdominal cavity and retroperitoneal space**	**399**
	Christopher R. Tollefson	

CHAPTER 25	**Gastrointestinal contrast studies**	**415**
	Lorrie Gaschen	

CHAPTER 26	**The stomach**	**437**
	Lorrie Gaschen	

CHAPTER 27	**The small intestine**	**451**
	Lorrie Gaschen	

CHAPTER 28	**The large intestine**	**469**
	Lorrie Gaschen	

CHAPTER 29	**Normal liver and hepatic parenchymal disease**	**481**
	Mylène Auger	

CHAPTER 30	**Biliary system**	**499**
	Pamela Di Donato and Swan Specchi	

CHAPTER 31	**Portosystemic shunts**	**517**
	Lorrie Gaschen	

CHAPTER 32	**Pancreas**	**525**
	Angela J. Marolf	

CHAPTER 33	**Spleen and lymph nodes**	**535**
	Margret S. Thompson	

CHAPTER 34	**Urinary tract contrast studies: technique and normal appearance**	**547**
	Micaela Zarelli and Chiara Bergamino	

CHAPTER **35** **Kidneys and ureters** 555
Ryan B. Appleby

CHAPTER **36** **Urinary bladder and urethra** 577
Ryan B. Appleby

CHAPTER **37** **Prostate, testicles, ovaries, and uterus** 599
Marco Russo and Massimo Vignoli

SECTION VI Interventional radiology

CHAPTER **38** **Interventional radiology** 617
Massimo Vignoli

Abbreviations

AHDS	Acute hemorrhagic diarrhea syndrome		**EHBDO**	Extrahepatic biliary duct obstruction
AHNPE	Acute hydrated nucleus pulposus extrusion		**FCE**	Fibrocartilaginous emboli
AKPKD	Autosomal dominant polycystic kidney disease		**FCP**	Fragmented coronoid process
ANCNPE	Acute non-compressive nucleus pulposus extrusion		**FE**	Flexor enthesopathy
aPTT	Activated partial thromboplastin time		**FeLV**	Feline leukemia virus
ARDS	Acute respiratory distress syndrome		**FIC**	Feline idiopathic cystitis
ASD	Atrial septal defect		**FIV**	Feline immunodeficiency virus
BAS	Brachycephalic airway syndrome		**FLUTD**	Feline lower urinary tract disease
BPH	Benign prostatic hyperplasia		**FOD**	Focus-object distance
CaCL	Caudal cruciate ligament		**FORL**	Feline odontoclastic resorptive lesions
CBD	Common bile duct		**GBM**	Gallbladder mucocele
CC	Choledochal cyst		**GI**	Gastrointestinal
CCL	Cranial cruciate ligament		**GT**	Gastrocnemius tendon
CCT	Common calcaneal tendon		**HCT**	Hematocrit
CEH	Cystic endometrial hyperplasia		**HD**	Hip dysplasia
CES	Cauda equina syndrome		**HHCT**	Helical hydro computed tomography
CEUS	Contrast-enhanced ultrasound		**HIF**	Humeral intracondylar fissure
CFHO	Circumferential femoral head osteophyte		**HO**	Hypertrophic osteopathy
CMC	Carboxymethylcellulose		**HOD**	Hypertrophic osteodystrophy
CMO	Craniomandibular osteopathy		**HV**	Hepatic vein
CrCLD	Cranial cruciate ligament disease		**ICCJ**	Ileocecocolic junction
CSF	Cerebrospinal fluid		**IEWG**	International Elbow Working Group
CT	Common tendon		**IOHC**	Incomplete ossification of the humeral condyle
CT	Computed tomography		**IVU**	Intravenous urography
CTA	Computed tomographic arthrography		**kVp**	Kilovoltage peak
DAR	Dorsal acetabular rim		**LLR**	Left lateral recumbency
DCM	Dilated cardiomyopathy		**mAs**	Milliampere-seconds
DEH	Dysplasia epiphysealis hemimelica		**MCPD**	Medial coronoid process disease
DI	Distraction index		**MCE**	Multiple cartilaginous exostosis
DISH	Disseminated idiopathic skeletal hyperostosis		**MD**	Mitral dysplasia
DJD	Degenerative joint disease		**MED**	Multiple epiphyseal dysplasia
DLPMO	Dorsolateral-plantaromedial oblique		**MLO**	Multilobular osteochondroma
DLS	Dorsolateral subluxation		**MPA**	Main pulmonary artery
DLSS	Degenerative lumbosacral stenosis		**MPR**	Multiplanar reconstruction
DTM	Dorsal tracheal membrane		**mpr**	Multiplanar-reformatting
DV	Dorsoventral		**MRI**	Magnetic resonance imaging

NDBS	Non-gravity dependent biliary sludge	**SDFT**	Superficial digital flexor tendon
NMV	Net magnetic vector	**STIR**	Short tau inversion recovery
NSH	Nutritional secondary hyperparathyroidism	**T1W**	T1-weighted
OA	Osteoarthritis	**T2W**	T2-weighted
OAAM	Occipitoatlantoaxial malformation	**TAPSE**	Tricuspid annular plane systolic excursion
OC	Osteochondrosis	**TCB**	Tissue core biopsy
OCD	Osteochondritis dissecans	**TD**	Tracheal diameter
OFD	Object-to-film distance	**TD**	Tricuspid dysplasia
OSD	Oculoskeletal dysplasia	**TD:TI**	Tracheal luminal diameter/thoracic inlet distance ratio
OSPT	One-stage prothrombin time	**TE**	Time to echo
PDA	Patent ductus arteriosus	**TGC**	Time gain compensation
PDW	Proton density-weighted	**TI**	Thoracic inlet
PE	Pericardial effusion	**TMJ**	Temporomandibular joint
PG	Pressure gradient	**ToF**	Tetralogy of Fallot
PHPV	Persistent hyperplastic primary vitreous	**TPO**	Triple pelvic osteotomy
PHTVL	Persistent hyperplastic tunica vasculosa lentis	**TR**	Time of repetition
PNST	Peripheral nerve sheath tumor	**TT/3R**	Tracheal luminal diameter/width of the proximal third of the third rib ratio
PL	Patellar luxation		
PPDH	Peritoneal pericardial diaphragmatic hernia	**UAP**	Ulnar anconeal process
PRAA	Persistent right aortic arch	**US**	Ultrasonography or ultrasound
PS	Pulmonic stenosis	**VD**	Ventrodorsal
RCC	Retained cartilage core	**VLAS**	Vertebral left atrial size
RCB	Radial carpal bone	**VRA**	Vascular ring anomaly
RLAD	Radiographic left atrial dimension	**VSD**	Ventricular septal defect
RLR	Right lateral recumbency	**WHWT**	West Highland White Terrier
SAD	Spinal arachnoid diverticula	**WL**	Window level
SAS	Subaortic stenosis	**WW**	Window width
SSC	Squamous cell carcinoma		

SECTION I
GENERAL INTRODUCTION

CHAPTER 1

Diagnostic imaging

Daniela Schweizer

> **KEY POINTS**
>
> - A veterinarian should request only those imaging examinations that will have an impact on diagnosis, treatment, and/or prognosis.
> - Basic knowledge about the physical principles of the modalities is mandatory to understand the advantages and disadvantages of each modality. This plays a key role in deciding which imaging study will answer the clinical question.
> - Electromagnetic waves that might cause ionization of biological tissues are considered harmful to the patient and the personnel exposed. Radiography and computed tomography cause ionization, and their use is regulated and should be based on the principles of justification, limitation, and optimization.
> - Image quality is influenced by spatial resolution, contrast resolution, blurring, and signal-to-noise ratio; however, high image quality is not equivalent to diagnostic quality.
> - Both visual inspection and interpretation are the keys to interpreting an imaging study.
> - Pitfalls during image interpretation occur due to search errors, detection errors, and recognition errors.

Brief introduction to the different modalities

Advances in technology have made diagnostic imaging an invaluable tool in solving clinical problems in veterinary medicine. The wide availability of different imaging modalities carries the risk of forgoing the process of creating a coherent problem list based on the clinical complaint, the medical history, and the clinical examination of our patients. However, a coherent problem list is essential to select the right imaging test and to ask the right questions to be answered by imaging. Veterinarians must not only weigh the risks and benefits of a particular study for an individual patient but also consider the impact of clinical decision-making on the patient, even if the diagnostic test is readily available. A veterinarian should request only those examinations that will have an impact on diagnosis, treatment, and/or prognosis. In addition to providing a diagnosis and establishing a prognosis, veterinarians must often consider cost efficiency, depending on the financial means of the pet owners. Considerations before performing imaging studies:

- Avoid ordering tests when the results will not impact patient care.
- Review tests previously performed to answer current questions.

- Order the best test to maximize quality, efficiency, and cost-effectiveness.
- Prepare your patient to maximize diagnostic information and avoid repeat studies, e.g., fasting prior to elective abdominal ultrasonography.

Choice of modality is a very important part of the diagnostic approach. To know which modality is the right one to answer the clinical question, one must be aware of the advantages and limitations of each modality. Many of the advantages and limitations are inherent to their physical principles.

Radiography

A radiograph is a two-dimensional projection of a three-dimensional object and reflects differences in X-ray attenuation by different body tissues.

What is an X-ray?

X-rays are a type of electromagnetic radiation of extremely short wavelength and high frequency, with wavelengths ranging from about 10^{-8} to 10^{-12} meters and corresponding frequencies from about 10^{16} to 10^{20} hertz (Hz). In comparison to other electromagnetic waves such as visible light, X-rays have a shorter wavelength and carry more energy in the form of photons. The photons react with the matter as if they were particles and are able to ionize tissue. Therefore, X-rays are considered as ionizing radiation (**fig. 1.1**).

Where do X-rays come from?

X-rays are produced within the X-ray tube by energy conversion: the tube encloses a vacuum and contains two electrodes: the anode with a positive charge and the cathode with a negative charge (**fig. 1.2A**). The cathode produces and emits electrons that cross the high voltage between the cathode and anode. The tube current (mA) determines the number of electrons accelerated towards the anode and the tube voltage (kV) determines how much the electrons are accelerated towards the anode. At the anode, the electrons are suddenly decelerated due to the positive charge of the anode and interact with the anode material at the focal track. By interacting with the anode material, approximately 99% of the electron energy is converted into heat, and only 1% is converted into X-ray photons. The emitted X-ray photons carry different amounts of energy, creating an X-ray spectrum (**fig. 1.2B**). The tube voltage (kV) sets the peak energy of the beam spectrum. Very low energy X-rays are removed from the X-ray beam by physical filters before reaching the patient; this is desirable as lower energy X-rays have a high probability of attenuation within the patient before reaching the detector and contribute to the patient dose but not the image.

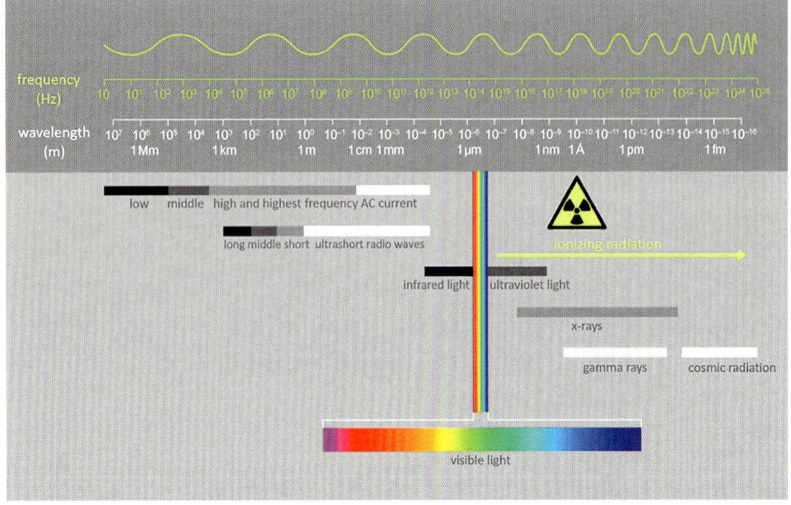

Fig. 1.1 Spectrum of electromagnetic waves showing the frequency and wavelength. The higher the frequency and the shorter the wavelength, the more energy is transported. If the energy is high enough to cause ionization of tissues, the electromagnetic waves are considered as ionizing radiation. © Vetsuisse-Fakultäten Bern und Zürich.

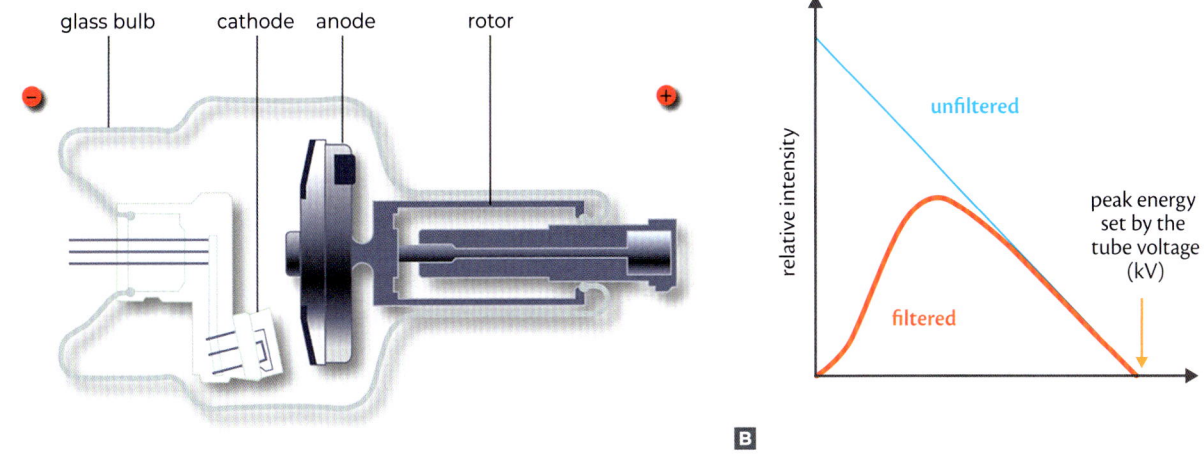

Fig. 1.2 (**A**) The X-ray tube is a glass cylinder containing a positively charged cathode and a negatively charged anode. The cathode produces and emits electrons that are accelerated within the vacuum toward the anode. By interaction with the anode material, X-ray photons are produced. (**B**) X-ray spectrum showing the different energy levels of X-rays produced in relation and their relative intensity. The tube voltage (kV) sets the peak energy of the beam spectrum on the x-axis. Very low energy X-rays are removed from the beam by physical filters before reaching the patient. © Vetsuisse-Fakultäten Bern und Zürich.

What happens if X-rays hit an object?

When X-rays in the energy range of diagnostic X-rays (40-120 kV) interact with matter, two interactions of the X-rays are responsible for the resulting image: (1) the photoelectric effect, which results in complete energy absorption within the matter, and (2) Compton scatter.

If a photoelectric effect happens, the entire kinetic energy of the incident photon is transferred to the electron. As a result, the electron is ejected, and the photon is absorbed (**fig. 1.3A**). This exchange of energy from the photon to the electron can only happen if the energy of the incident photon is equal to or slightly higher than the binding energy of the electrons of the inner shells of the atom. The likelihood of a photoelectric effect is much higher with low energy photons of less than 100 kV and in matter with a high atomic number, such as bone (atomic number of calcium = 20), iodine, barium, or lead. As a result of the photoelectric absorption, the photons are removed from the X-ray beam and will not propagate to the detector system. The differences in absorption between adjacent tissues will result in contrast on the image.

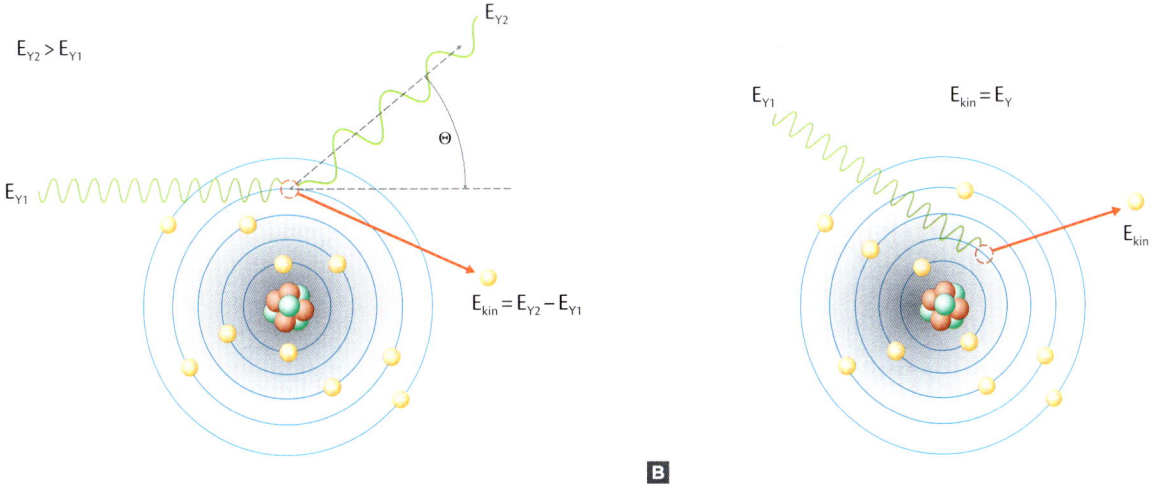

Fig. 1.3 (**A**) The photoelectric effect is a complete transfer of the kinetic energy of the incident photon to the electron, resulting in the absorption of the photon. (**B**) Compton scattering occurs if only part of the kinetic of the photon is transmitted to the electron, and the photon will change its direction. © Vetsuisse-Fakultäten Bern und Zürich.

If a photon interacts with electrons of the outer shell, only part of their kinetic energy is transmitted to the electron (**fig. 1.3 B**). As a result of the partial loss of energy, the photon will change its direction, i.e., scattered. This so-called Compton scattering happens if the energy of the incident photon is much higher than the binding energy of the electrons of an atom. It is the predominant effect for photons >100 kV. This process can happen several times within the matter, whereby the higher the physical density, the higher the electron density and, therefore, the likelihood of interactions. Alternatively, the photon will pass through the object without further interaction and hit a detector system (film-screen system, CR plate, or digital detector). The more often a photon undergoes a Compton effect, the stronger the attenuation of photons received by the detector.

How is the image created?

Behind the object, an imaging system (either conventional intensifying screens and film or a digital detector) reacts with the remaining, possibly attenuated X-rays that were not absorbed. The more photons hit the imaging system, the more film blackening occurs (**fig. 1.4**). Conventional screen film combinations use silver halogenic crystals within the film emulsion that undergo chemical reduction by photons. Whereas they respond approximately linearly in the mid exposure range, the response at each end of the spectrum is very non-linear. Therefore, both underexposure and overexposure result in low contrast areas on the image: while underexposure results in insufficient film blackening, overexposure causes excessive blackening (**fig. 1.5**). Digital radiography uses either a storage phosphor plate (computed radiography, CR), which is read by a laser after the exposure, or by converting the incident X-ray directly into an electrical signal (direct digital radiography, DR). These detectors are made from scintillators (i.e., materials that release light photons via fluorescence following excitation by X-ray photons). The current generation of commercial detectors is made from rare earth ceramic materials. The light photons are converted to electrical signal in photodiodes. This electrical signal is digitized.

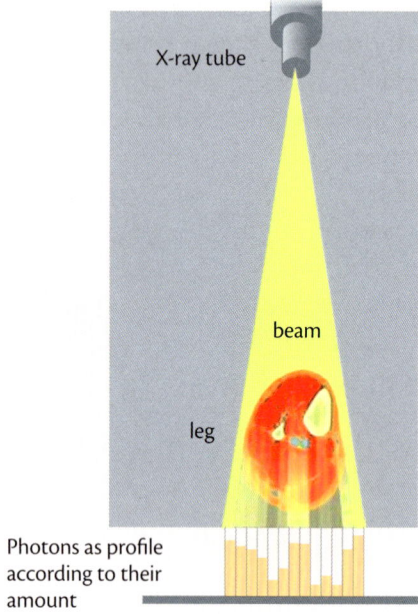

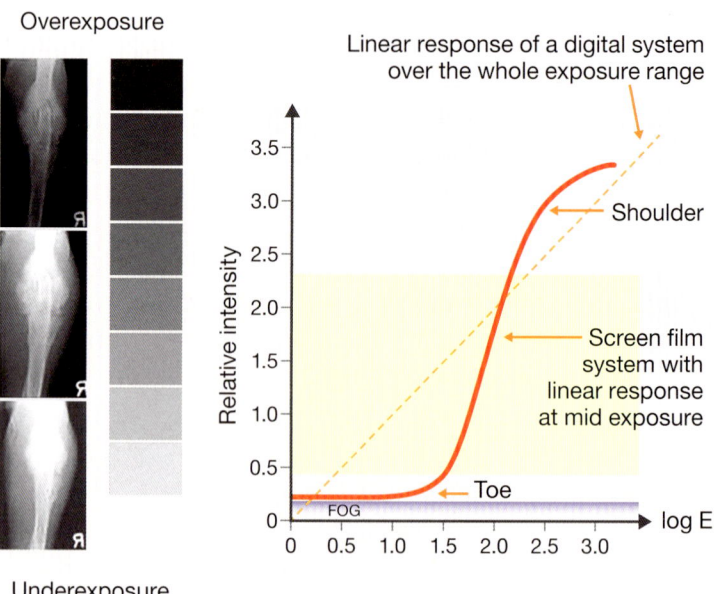

Fig. 1.4 An object (distal limb with bones and muscles) within the X-ray beam. Different tissues cause different attenuation of the X-ray beam, depending on the thickness and composition. The more photons hit the imaging system, the more film blackening will occur. © Vetsuisse-Fakultäten Bern und Zürich.

Fig. 1.5 Relationship between exposure and optical density (film blackening): the response of a screen film combination is non-linear at underexposure and overexposure; only in the mid exposure range it responds linearly. An advantage of a digital system compared to a screen film system is that they have a linear relationship between optical density and exposure (orange dotted line). © Vetsuisse-Fakultäten Bern und Zürich.

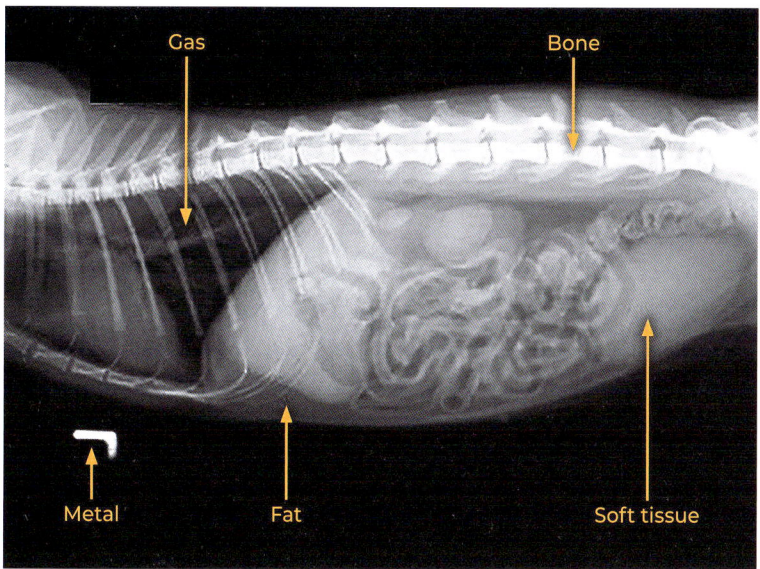

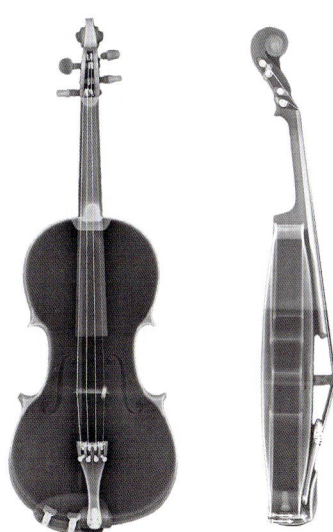

Fig. 1.6 On radiography, five opacities can be differentiated: gas, fat, soft tissue (same as water), mineral (or bone), and metal, with the latter one being the one with the most absorption/attenuation and resulting in the least film blackening. © Vetsuisse-Fakultäten Bern und Zürich.

Fig. 1.7 Orthogonal radiographs of a viola. The shape, arrangement, and exact localization of the different components can only be assessed by looking at both radiographs. © Vetsuisse-Fakultäten Bern und Zürich.

Both CR and DR have a linear relationship between optical density and exposure and therefore are not restricted in the same way as film/screen radiography. However, if a radiograph is underexposed, only a few photons hit the detector system, resulting in a grainy radiograph.

The higher the attenuation, the fewer photons hit the imaging system. Areas on the image that are brighter indicate, therefore, tissues with more attenuation or absorption. Such an area is called opacity. Darker areas on the image are called radiolucencies and represent tissues with lower attenuation/absorption. Since both absorption by photoeffect and attenuation by Compton scatter contribute to the attenuation of an X-ray beam, we can summarize that attenuation is dependent on the atomic number (Z) of the tissue, its physical density, and on the thickness of the object. In projection radiography, we are able to differentiate between five opacities: gas, fat, soft tissue (same as water), mineral (or bone), and metal, with the latter one being the one with most absorption/attenuation and resulting in the least film blackening (**fig. 1.6**). The relative opacities of various substances and tissues will determine the ability of plain films to differentiate between them. For example, blood, muscle, and liver will have an almost identical opacity, as will most solid or fluid-filled organs and tissue masses. The muscular heart filled with blood will appear homogeneous soft tissue opaque relative to the air-filled lungs on both sides of it.

Since every point of the image represents the attenuation of all tissues the X-ray beam passed through, the resulting image of attenuation is a summation image with superimposition of different anatomic structures. Only two orthogonal views allow localization of individual structures and abnormalities. A single radiograph will not be able to precisely locate a lesion (**fig. 1.7**).

Computed tomography

As in radiography, a computed tomography (CT) image shows differences in X-ray attenuation by body tissues; however, it is a cross-sectional image, and superimposition does not play a role.

What is the difference of CT compared to radiography?

While in radiography the X-ray tube is stationary, in CT it rotates 360° around the object, creating projections at all angles by using a thinly collimated X-ray beam (1-10 mm). Moreover, the detectors of the CT scanner do not produce an image: opposed to the tube, a detector composed of scintillation

SECTION I   GENERAL INTRODUCTION

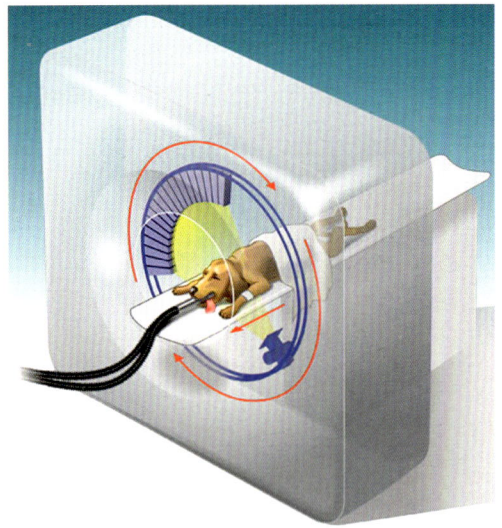

Fig. 1.8 In CT, the X-ray tube rotates 360° around the patient (red arrows), creating projections at all angles by using a thinly collimated X-ray beam (1-10 mm). Opposed to the tube, a detector composed of scintillation crystals quantifies the X-ray transmission through tissues. © Vetsuisse-Fakultäten Bern und Zürich.

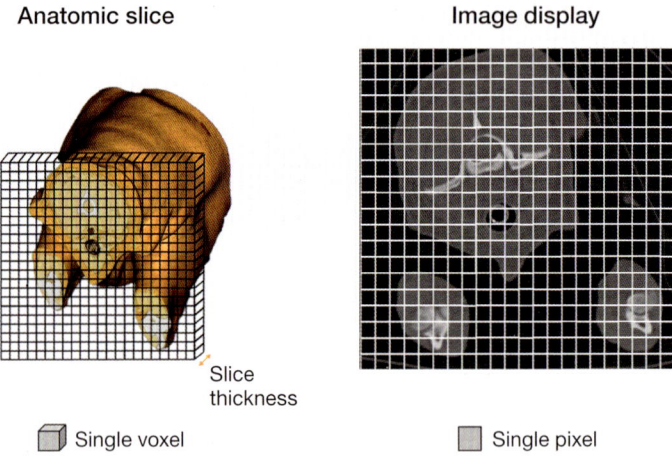

Fig. 1.9 Images are acquired as slices with a certain slice thickness. Each volume element (voxel) of the object is assigned to a specific X-ray attenuation value of each pixel on the resulting cross-sectional digital image. © Vetsuisse-Fakultäten Bern und Zürich.

crystals quantifies the X-ray transmission through tissues for each of these projections (**fig. 1.8**). This allows a sophisticated computer algorithm to geometrically reconstruct the data for each volume element (voxel) of the object and to assign a specific X-ray attenuation value to every pixel on the resulting cross-sectional digital image (**fig. 1.9**).

How does a CT work?

On modern CT scanners, the X-ray tube and detector are mounted opposite one another in a rotating gantry. The detector array consists of a series of rows of detector elements aligned axially to the patient. Nowadays, there are typically 16-320 detector rows and 800-1000 detector elements in each detector row. During a CT acquisition, some or all the detector rows may be active. In order to scan the required anatomy, the patient is positioned on a table and moved through the gantry. During axial scanning, the gantry makes one revolution around the stationary patient while projection data is acquired, followed by an incremental table movement, and this is repeated until the entire desired anatomy is imaged. During helical scanning, the scanner continuously acquires projection data as the patient table moves through the gantry. Helical scanning allows a volume scan to be acquired much faster. In addition, helical scanning allows the reconstruction of axial images at overlapping intervals. The scan pitch is defined as the table movement during one tube rotation divided by the nominal X-ray beam width. Typical ranges of pitches are 0.7-1.4, although modern specialized scanners allow a pitch of 0.1-3.2. During dynamic scanning, the scanner continuously acquires projection data at one patient table position. This allows the selected patient anatomy, e.g., the heart, to be scanned over a period.

What are we actually seeing on a CT image?

The CT image is a two-dimensional attenuation map of the cross section through the patient. The slice thickness of the image corresponds to the thickness of the voxel. The typical display image in CT is composed of 512 rows, each of 512 pixels, i.e., a square matrix of 512 × 512 = 262,144 pixels. Each point in the map is assigned to a linear attenuation coefficient. The calculated attenuation values depend on the properties of the tissue, namely its electron density, which is related to the atomic number and physical density of the tissue. The attenuation value is not dependent on the thickness of the object. To form an image, the attenuation values are converted into CT numbers.

CT numbers are also known as Hounsfield Units (HU) to honor Sir Godfrey Hounsfield, a Nobel prize winner in 1979 for his work in the field of computed tomography: the Hounsfield Units for air and water were set to −1000 for air and 0 for water by definition. All other CT numbers relate to the linear attenuation coefficient of water:

- Air = −1000 HU
- Lung = −500 HU
- Fat = 120 to −60 HU
- Water = 0 HU
- Muscle = +10 to +40 HU
- White matter = +20 to +30 HU
- Grey matter = +37 to +45 HU
- Liver = +40 to +60 HU
- Cancellous bone = +700 HU
- Compact bone = +1000 HU

The CT numbers are displayed as gray values; by convention, the gray scale assigns higher CT numbers to lighter shades of gray, whereas lower CT numbers are represented by darker shades (**fig. 1.10**). In an ideal world, the image would be displayed with different shades of gray for each CT number. However, an image with an 8-bit depth contains only 256 shades of gray. Even more limiting, the human eye can differentiate fewer than 40 shades. Therefore, a gray scale is used where a certain range of CT numbers is assigned to a shade of gray.

The amount of CT numbers assigned to each level of gray is determined by the window width. By increasing the window width, more CT numbers are assigned to one shade of gray. On the contrary, a narrow window width results in fewer CT numbers assigned to a certain gray level. For example, a window width of 2000 HU could mean that the gray scale ranges from −1000 HU to +1000 HU, and a window width of 100 HU could mean that the gray scale only ranges from 0 HU to +100 HU. A narrow window width, therefore, results in a much faster transition from black to white. All CT numbers below the window are displayed as black, whereas all CT numbers above are displayed as white. The window level determines the CT number in the middle of the window and is chosen according to the anatomy. For the evaluation of the lung, which consists mainly of gas (−1000 HU), the window level is set to around −500. For the evaluation of abdominal organs, the level is set to around 50 HU.

What is meant by a filter, kernel, or algorithm?

The reconstruction kernel, also referred to as "filter" or "algorithm," is a mathematical method applied to the raw data to increase image quality. A soft convolution kernel acts as a low pass algorithm; it smoothes edges and reduces the image noise, while a sharp convolution kernel equal

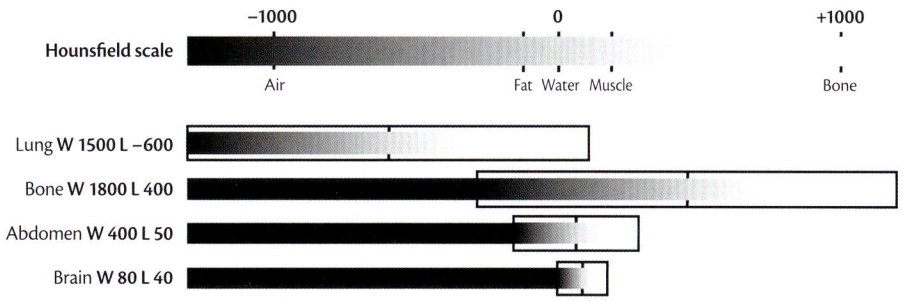

Fig. 1.10 By definition, the CT number, also known as the Hounsfield unit of air, is −1000 for air, 0 for water, and around +1000 for bone. The gray scale assigns higher CT numbers to lighter shades of gray, whereas lower CT numbers are represented by darker shades. The amount of CT numbers assigned to each level of gray is determined by the window width (W). Using a large window width, more CT numbers are assigned to one shade of gray, while, in a narrow window, only a few CT numbers are assigned to a certain gray level. A narrow window width, therefore, results in a shorter transition from black to white. All CT numbers below the window are displayed as black, whereas all CT numbers above the window are displayed as white. The window level (L) determines the CT number in the middle of the window and is chosen according to the anatomy. For the evaluation of the lung, which consists mainly of gas (−1000 HU), the window level is set to around −500. For the evaluation of abdominal organs, the level is set to around 50 HU. © Vetsuisse-Fakultäten Bern und Zürich.

to a high pass filter enhances edges but increases the image noise. Sharp convolution kernels are applied to tissues with inherently high CT contrast, such as bone or lung. Conversely, soft tissue kernels are applied to tissues with inherently lower contrast, such as the brain or liver. As most anatomic regions include tissues with both high and low inherent contrast, it is often desirable to create at least two data sets utilizing at least two different convolution kernels (**fig. 1.11**). These kernels can be applied to raw data of one acquisition, but the number of images that need to be transmitted, stored, and reviewed is increased.

What are the advantages of CT compared to radiographs?

The resulting CT image has two significant advantages compared to radiography: first, by creating a cross-sectional image, the superimposition of structures is eliminated. Second, the thinly collimated X-ray beam eliminates scatter and increases the sensitivity of CT to subtle differences in X-ray attenuation by at least a factor of 10.

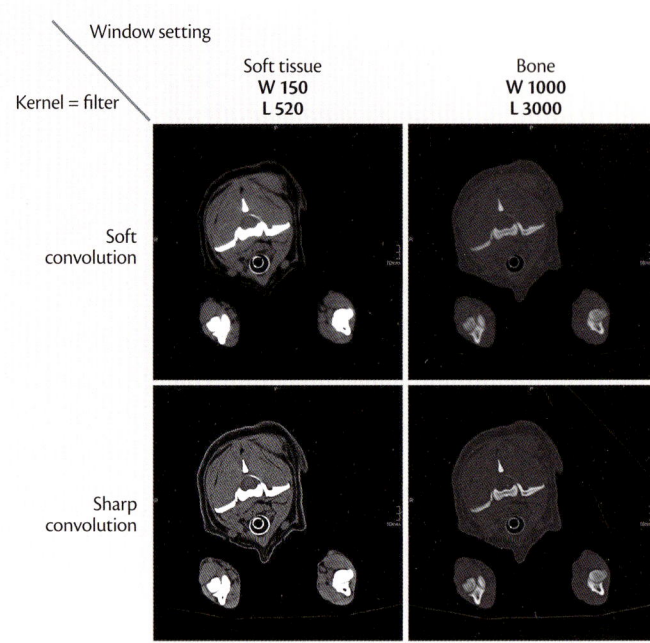

Fig. 1.11 CT images, including the neck and both elbows of a dog displayed in different kernels and window settings. Note the difference in visibility and sharpness of bone and soft tissue structures in the different settings. © Vetsuisse-Fakultäten Bern und Zürich.

Magnetic resonance imaging

Magnetic resonance imaging (MRI) uses magnetic fields and electromagnetic waves in the frequency range of radio waves to visualize body tissues based on hydrogen protons. As the energy transmitted to the body by the radiofrequency waves is not causing ionization of tissues, the method is non-ionizing and considered as non-invasive.

What is the fundamental concept of MRI?

Atoms with an odd number of protons such as hydrogen (1H) are spinning around their own axis. A spinning charge generates a small magnetic field. If such a moving charge is brought into a strong static magnetic field (such as the MR scanner), it aligns along the main magnetic field, either parallel or antiparallel. A slightly higher number of protons orient themselves parallel to the magnetic field, causing a net magnetization within the tissue.

In addition to the alignment of nuclei, the external magnetic field causes a tumbling of the protons around the static magnetic field, like a spinning top. The tumbling is named precession and happens at a resonant frequency ω that is directly proportional to the strength of the magnetic field B_0 (in Tesla). Furthermore, ω depends on the gyromagnetic ratio γ, a constant unique to every atom: $\omega_0 = \gamma B_0$. For hydrogen protons, γ is equal to 42.56 MHz per Tesla. In a 1.5T scanner, the resonant frequency of hydrogen protons is consequently 63.84 MHz. If a radio wave of exactly the same frequency as the proton's resonant frequency is applied, the energy of the radio wave is transmitted to the protons, and they become excited. This phenomenon of energy transfer is called resonance phenomenon, giving the method its name (**fig. 1.12**).

What happens after excitation?

As an effect of excitation, more protons flip from the parallel to the antiparallel status, which requires slightly more energy. As result, the magnetization vector flips perpendicular to the static magnetic field into the so-called transverse plane. The angle alpha towards the transverse plane is a function of the strength and duration of the RF pulse. If equal amounts of protons are aligned parallel and antiparallel, the angle is 90°. At the same time, the transmitted energy from the RF pulse allows the excited protons to synchronize their tumbling and their magnetic fields to point in the same direction at one point in time. At this stage, they are considered to be in-phase, and a transverse magnetization vector occurs. This transverse component of the rotating electromagnetic field induces a current that is measured (**fig. 1.12F**). The transverse magnetization is, however, not stable. After the RF pulse is turned off, the in-phase precession decays because of proton-proton interactions. This dephasing process is called transverse relaxation and follows an exponential function with a time constant T2 (T2 relaxation time).

During the decay of the transverse magnetization, the spins reorient themselves along the main magnetic field of the scanner. This reorientation process is called longitudinal relaxation and reoccurs with a time constant T1 (T1 relaxation time). T1 and T2 values are tissue-specific and enable MRI to differentiate between the different types of tissues when using properly designed MRI pulse sequences.

What is the signal in MRI reflecting?

In order to gain information about the biochemical properties of a tissue, sequences with different sequence parameters are used: one important parameter is the time of repetition, TR. It is the time in between two excitations, i.e., two RF pulses. If the TR of a sequence is long, protons within all tissues will be back to their original energy status (parallel alignment) before they undergo a new excitation. This will apply to homogenous tissues with a long T1 relaxation time. Differences in T1 relaxation time will then be neglected. If TR is short, the signal will strongly be influenced by the T1 relaxation time of the tissue. Another important parameter influencing the signal is the time to echo, TE. It is the time interval between the excitation and the recording of the signal. If the TE of a sequence is long, the

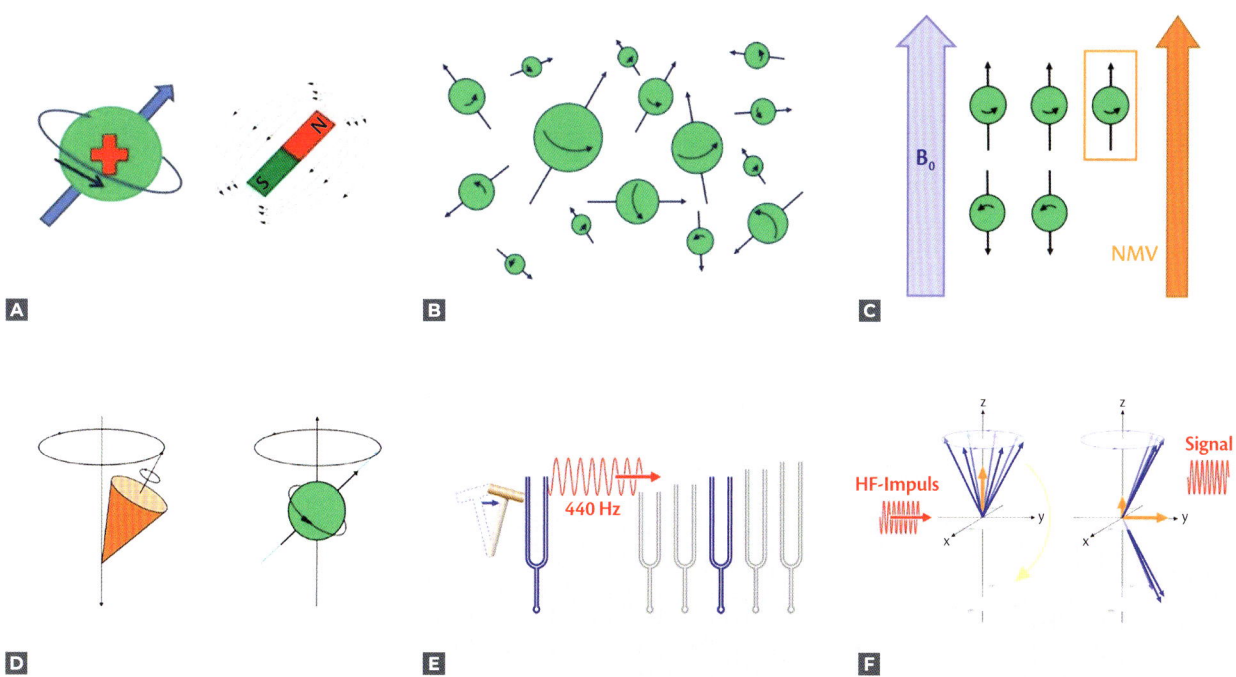

Fig. 1.12 Resonance phenomenon in MRI. (**A**) A positively charged particle such as a proton spins around its own axis. The moving charge induces a small magnetic field. (**B**) Random distribution of protons within the tissue. (**C**) In an external magnetic field B_0, the protons align along the main magnetic field, either parallel or antiparallel. A small excess of protons aligns parallel creating a net magnetic vector (NMV) in the direction of the main magnetic field. (**D**) In the external magnetic field similar to a spinning top, the protons rotate around the static magnetic field. This motion is called precession and happens at a specific precessional frequency. (**E**, **F**) Comparable to a tuning fork, the protons absorb energy of an external radiofrequency pulse that has the same frequency as the resonant frequency. © Vetsuisse-Fakultäten Bern und Zürich.

signal will be stronger for tissues, where hydrogen protons stay in phase for a longer period, such as pure water, whereas a mixture of water and proteins will result in faster dephasing leading to less signal. TE and TR can be chosen by the operator and allow different weightings of sequences, a weighting towards the longitudinal magnetization (T1-weighted sequence) or weighting towards the transverse magnetization (T2-weighting). Based on the signal of tissues on T1-weighted and T2-weighted images, one can conclude about the biochemical properties of the tissue. Therefore, different sequences of one area of interest must be acquired and should be evaluated simultaneously.

Other sequences exist that focus on certain properties such as disturbances of the homogeneity of the magnetic field due to, e.g., metallic substances like a T2* gradient echo sequence. Such a sequence can be used to detect hemorrhage. Diffusion-weighted sequences focus on the diffusivity of hydrogen protons within the tissue (diffusion-weighted images).

An MR scanner contains a primary magnet producing a very strong static magnetic field (B_0). A 1.5 T scanner (1 T = 10,000 G), for example, has a field strength that is 30,000 times stronger than the Earth's magnetic field. Besides the main magnet, there are additional coils inside the magnet: shimming coils are used to shape the magnetic field and increase the homogeneity of the magnetic field. Gradient coils temporarily change the magnetic field along any direction for spatial localization of the recorded signal. The coils send radiofrequency pulses into the subject for excitation, and receiver coils act as an antenna to measure the current flow resulting from transverse magnetization. By applying magnetic field gradients along spatial dimensions on top of the static magnetic field, the information for each slice is accumulated within the so-called dimensional k space. Fourier analysis transforms the k space data into an image with pixels of different gray values.

Nowadays, clinical MRI is based on the excitation of hydrogen protons, but theoretically, all nuclei with an odd number of protons are magnetically excitable, such as sodium (11 Na), phosphor (15 P), or fluorine (19 F). Hydrogen protons are ideally suited for MRI because they are abundant in body tissues; water is the largest source of protons in the body, followed by fat.

Ultrasound

Ultrasound (US) is a real-time cross-sectional imaging technique where returning echoes from pulses of ultra-high frequency sound are recorded.

Sound waves

Unlike the above-described modalities, the technique of ultrasound imaging is based on acoustic waves. Acoustic waves are a type of mechanical waves where the energy is transmitted by compression and decompression of matter. Therefore, acoustic waves can only propagate within a medium and cannot transmit their energy in a vacuum. The acoustic waves are generated within the transducer, which contains a piezoelectric crystal. If an electric current is applied to the piezoelectric crystal, the crystal expands, resulting in a mechanical wave. As electromagnetic waves, ultrasound waves are characterized by their frequency and wavelength: $f = c/\lambda$.

The speed of sound within soft tissues is approximately 1540 m/s. In diagnostic ultrasound, frequencies between 2-20 MHz, and the wavelength is approximately 1-0.1 mm in tissue.

The frequency of ultrasound waves is too high to be detected by a human ear.

Ultrasonic waves propagate longitudinally and straight within the medium until they are reflected, refracted, diffracted, or absorbed (**fig. 1.13**).

Interaction of sound waves

▍ **Reflection** Reflection occurs mainly at interfaces between two media with different acoustic impedance. The acoustic impedance Z of the tissue describes the resistance to sound propagation and is dependent on the density ρ (rho) of a medium and the sound wave velocity c in the corresponding medium: $Z = \rho c$.

If an ultrasonic wave hits an interface between two media with different acoustic impedance, part of the wave is reflected and travels back to the transducer as an echo; the other part penetrates deeper into the tissue. The amount of reflection (echo) depends on the difference in acoustic impedance of the two media. The greater the difference between the two media, the stronger the reflection of the ultrasound waves and the brighter the image. For example, a muscle-fat interface causes only about 1% of the ultrasound waves to be reflected, whereas almost total reflection occurs at a muscle-air interface. This explains why the transducer must be coupled to surfaces by means of gel or water: to avoid reflection by air.

▌**Refraction** Depending on the properties of tissues, the ultrasound waves propagate slight differences in sound velocity. When an ultrasound wave passes from one tissue to another, the frequency of the ultrasound wave remains unchanged while the wavelength changes. This leads to a change in direction of the wave propagation, which is called refraction. The angle of refraction is determined by the change in the speed of sound and depends on the angle of incidence. If the angle of incidence to the boundary surface is exactly 90° and the speed of sound in both media is the same, no refraction occurs.

▌**Diffraction** Tissues with marked differences in impedance to the surrounding tissues act as obstacles

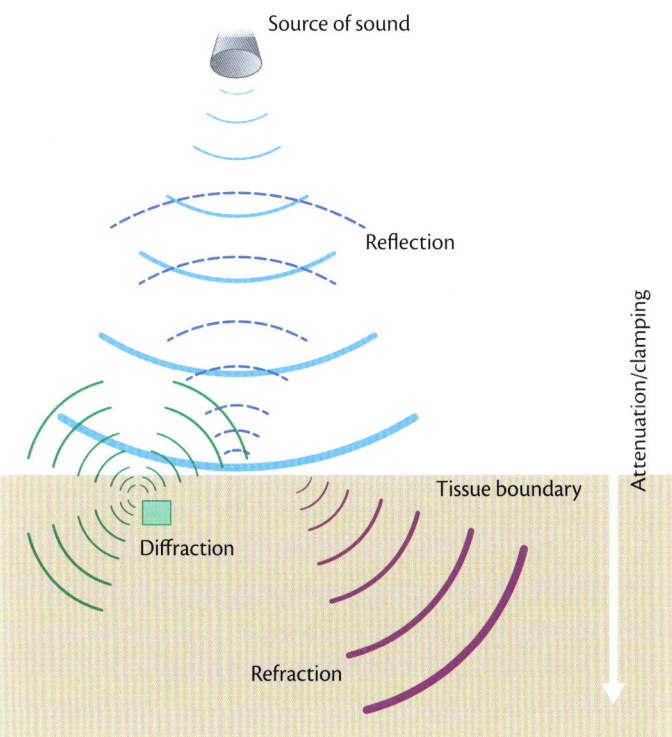

Fig. 1.13 Principle interactions of sound waves with matter: ultrasound waves propagate longitudinally and straight within a medium until they are reflected, refracted, diffracted, or absorbed. All interactions result in attenuation (damping) of the original pulse. Only ultrasound waves that are reflected back to the ultrasound probe act as an echo and contribute to the resulting image. © Vetsuisse-Fakultäten Bern und Zürich.

and prevent sound waves from propagating in a straight line. The sound waves are consequently diffracted. Whether sound waves are diffracted or reflected by obstacles depends on their wavelength. Due to complicated interference of the waves, which will not be explained in more detail here, diffraction occurs when the wavelength is larger than the obstacle itself or larger than a hole in an obstacle. The amount of diffraction increases with greater wavelengths.

▌**Scatter** Every interaction that leads to an oblique direction of the propagation of the ultrasound waves is considered as scatter. Both reflection and diffraction contribute to scatter. Specular scattering occurs when the structure is much larger than the ultrasound wavelength, resulting in reflection. Diffuse scattering occurs when the structure is much smaller than the ultrasound wavelength, and the incident wave is scattered equally in all directions. Diffractive scattering occurs when the size of the structure is less than or about a wavelength, and the amount of scattered energy is different for different scattering directions. The sonographic image of an organ with its specific echotexture is actually the result of scatter that returns to the transducer as echoes.

Absorption

If particles in a tissue are small enough, they will move as a single entity and propagate the energy of the sound wave. If large molecules are present, the vibration becomes chaotic without proper propagation but transformation of energy into heat.

Each of these interactions results in an attenuation (damping) of the original pulse. Only ultrasound waves that are reflected back to the ultrasound probe generate an echo and contribute to the resulting image. The attenuation depends on the frequency of the ultrasonic waves: attenuation [dB] = depth [cm] × frequency [MHz]. With increasing frequency, the attenuation increases, and thus the penetration in tissue decreases. In soft tissues, there is an almost linear relationship between the frequency of the ultrasound wave and the attenuation (dB/cm). As a rule of thumb, the loss is 0.5 dB per cm and per MHz (0.5 dB/cm/MHz). Attenuation or attenuation losses can be compensated to a certain extent by time-controlled or depth-dependent amplification (TGC = time gain compensation). The amplitudes of echoes from tissue boundaries that are close to the transducer are reduced; signals from more distant reflectors, on the other hand, are progressively amplified.

The transducer, with its piezoelectric crystal, does not only act as a transmitter of sound waves but as a sensor for returning echoes too. The distance of the reflector to the ultrasound transducer is calculated according to the speed of sound within soft tissues of 1540 m/s. As such, the location of a returning echo is calculated as a function of the speed of sound and the time between sending and receiving. Eventually, a line is built up underneath each crystal, and all lines result in a two-dimensional image. This image represents a slice, and by moving the transducer and scanning in different planes, a complete evaluation of the three-dimensional anatomy is performed.

One of the advantages of ultrasound is that images are acquired in real-time, and therefore movement such as intestinal peristalsis and cardiac contractions can be observed. One image line can be observed over time in motion mode (M-mode).

If ultrasound waves hit a moving reflector, the frequency of the ultrasound wave is changed. If the reflector is moving away from the transducer and in the same direction as the acoustic wave, the frequency is decreased; if the reflector moves towards the acoustic wave, the frequency is increased. The frequency shift, the so-called Doppler phenomenon, is detected by the transducer and according to the positive or negative shift of the frequency displayed on the image. The Doppler signal enables that moving blood can be displayed with colors on a B-mode image, usually showing blood moving away from the transducer in blue and blood flowing towards the transducer in red. If the sound wave hits the reflector at a 90° angle, no change of frequency occurs, and no Doppler signal is recorded.

Radiation protection in veterinary diagnostic imaging

Modalities that might cause ionization of biological tissues are considered harmful to the patient and the personnel exposed. In veterinary medicine, the exposure to our patients, the animals, is not regulated, and any harm is presumed to be outweighed by the diagnostic information acquired. However, as veterinarians, we should not harm our patients and, just as importantly, protect all personnel involved in the acquisition of images.

What are ionization and ionizing radiation?

The process in which an electron is given enough energy to break away from an atom is called ionization. This process results in the formation of two charged particles: the molecule with a net positive charge and the free electron with a negative charge. Each ionization releases energy that is absorbed by the material surrounding the ionized atom. In fact, the energy from one ionization is more than enough energy to disrupt the chemical bond between two carbon atoms. X-rays have very high frequencies (in the range of 100 billion hertz) and very short wavelengths (1 million millionths of a meter). X-rays, which are at the upper end of the electromagnetic spectrum, are therefore considered as ionizing radiation (**fig. 1.1**).

How can ionizing radiation damage biological tissues?

When ionizing radiation hits biological tissues, physical, chemical, and biological effects occur in the cell. A distinction is made between two effects of radiation on cells: a direct effect, i.e., ionizing radiation directly damages DNA, and the indirect effect, i.e., the radiation effect on water. Since cells consist largely of water, the most important reaction is water radiolysis resulting in the formation of free radicals and peroxides (H_2O_2). Concerning radiography in medicine, it is almost exclusively the indirect effect that plays a role. The resulting radicals can react with biomolecules (proteins, membranes, DNA) and thus damage cellular structures and function. Damage might occur in somatic cells but also in germ cells that can transmit damage to the offspring.

What is the relation between dose and effect?

There are two effects of an absorbed radiation dose: a deterministic effect and a stochastic effect. For deterministic effects, a threshold dose exists below which no pathological changes occur. For deterministic effects, the severity of the damage increases with the dose once the threshold is exceeded. Examples are radiation syndrome, erythema of the skin, edema, or cataract. Concerning diagnostic radiology, such effects should never occur but could potentially happen after 20 or more CT scans or extensive fluoroscopic interventions.

For diagnostic imaging, the stochastic effect is of greater importance (stochastic = random, following the laws of probability). Stochastic effects can occur at any dose and there is no threshold, but the probability of stochastic effects increases with increasing dose. This implies that damage could occur even with a small radiation dose and a risk of damage cannot be ruled out even for the smallest doses. Stochastic effects include the induction of cancer if body cells are affected. If germ cells are affected, genetic damage can be transmitted to the offspring. Because of their long latency period, they are also known as late damage. Most solid tumors in humans only appear after an average latency period of about 25 years. Leukemias, on the other hand, can manifest only a few years after irradiation. Their mean latency period is 5-8 years, and their incidence falls back to normal population levels about 20 years after exposure. However, cancer incidence is influenced by so many factors that it is not possible (at present) to distinguish cancer induction by ionizing radiation from other causes. Because every dose, no matter how small it is, has a biological effect, the International Commission on Radiological Protection (ICRP) uses the following principles for all controllable exposure situations: justification, limitation, and optimization.

▌ **Justification** No unnecessary use of radiation is permitted, which means that the advantages of the exposure must outweigh the disadvantages. If no benefit can be expected from a study, then it must not be conducted. Furthermore, non-ionizing imaging tests should be used where feasible and if the diagnostic utility is similar. If radiation exposure is unavoidable, care must be taken to ensure that the exposure achieves a diagnostic quality study, that there is as little radiation exposure as possible to personnel, and that no harm is caused to the patient.

▌ **Limitation** Each individual must be protected against risks that are too great, through the application of individual radiation dose limits set by national law. In order to calculate the risk of cancer or late damage in general, the effectiveness of the type of radiation and the sensitivity of the tissues with regard to cancer induction must be taken into account. For this reason, the absorbed dose in Gray (Gy; 1 Gy corresponds to the absorption of 1 Joule/kg) is multiplied by a radiation-specific weighting factor WR and given as equivalent dose H in Sievert (Sv). The weighting factor for X-rays is 1; therefore, the absorbed dose equals the equivalent dose in radiography and CT. The sensitivity of the various organs is taken into account by multiplying the equivalent dose by the organ-specific weighting factor WT resulting in the effective dose E (in Sv). If X-rays are for example exclusively applied to the lung, the absorbed dose is multiplied by WR = 1 and by a tissue-specific factor for the lung, WT = 0.12. The weighting factors of all organs sum up to 1, which corresponds to irradiation of the whole body. If a radiation dose of X-ray photons is applied to a whole body, the absorbed dose D in Gy is equal to the effective dose in Sv. The effective dose allows the direct calculation of the cancer risk, which is based on epidemiological studies from experience (atomic bomb victims from Hiroshima and Nagasaki). Calculated over the lifetime, a risk factor of 5% per Sv is assumed for the total population but there are uncertainties regarding the accuracy, and one is far away from the precision of physical measurement or a physically precisely determinable quantity. However, no data on mutation induction are available in the dose range below 0.1 Sv. In humans, despite extensive studies, no statistically significant increase in the mutation rate due to diagnostic and occupational exposure has been demonstrated to date. In order to assess the genetic risk to the offspring from ionizing radiation, it is, therefore, necessary to refer to data from animal studies (especially in mice). In the case of germ cell changes, it is basically not possible to distinguish between radiation-induced and spontaneously occurring mutations. Only statistical analyses allow limited conclusions to be drawn about the radiation risk.

▎ **Optimization** This process is intended for application to those situations that have been deemed to be justified. It means "the likelihood of incurring exposures, the number of people exposed, and the magnitude of their individual doses" should all be kept As Low As Reasonably Achievable (known as ALARA principle, or more common in UK: As Low As Reasonably Practicable [ALARP]). The principle takes medical, economic, and societal factors into account and implies that the highest possible image quality should be achieved with the lowest possible dose.

Exposure of personnel

Do you remember the Compton effect as an interaction of X-rays with matter? It is responsible for the scatter radiation, which is responsible for the main source of exposure to the personnel. A large part of it originates in the patient itself. To keep exposure of the personnel as low as possible, the following principles of radiation protection should be applied:

▎ **Shielding** All personnel in the X-ray room during an examination should use protective clothing or choose a location behind protective barriers. However, protective clothing does not provide sufficient protection against radiation from the primary beam and is only intended to protect against scatter radiation.

▎ **Collimation** The smaller the exposure field the less scatter radiation arises from the animal body. This reduces the overall exposure for personnel within the room. In addition, the risk of getting one's hands caught in the primary radiation is reduced. Care should be taken to set the field as small as possible (radiation protection) but as large as necessary for diagnosis.

▎ **Keep distance** Increasing distance reduces dose effectively. Distance can be as simple as stepping away one step from the patient if feasible.

Imaging quality assurance

Assessment of image quality in medicine is subjective in many ways and high image quality is not the equivalent to diagnostic quality. In general, factors influencing image quality are spatial resolution, contrast resolution, blurring, and signal-to-noise ratio.

Spatial resolution

Spatial resolution is the imaging system's ability to distinguish between closely spaced high-contrast objects, such as the two sets of lines shown above (in line pairs/mm). For all digital images, it is primarily determined by the pixel size and matrix (number of pixels per edge length). The smaller the pixels (or the higher the matrix with constant field of view), the better the spatial resolution.

Contrast resolution

Contrast resolution in radiology refers to the ability of an imaging system to distinguish between differences in gray values, no matter if they arose due to differences in attenuation, absorption, or reflection of X-ray photons or ultrasound waves or transmission of radiofrequency energy in MRI.

The inherent contrast resolution of a digital image is given by the number of possible pixel values and is defined as the number of bits per pixel value: an 8-bit system can show $2^8 = 256$ gray values as opposed to a 12-bit system, which shows $2^{12} = 4096$ gray values. A system with a low number of gray values is considered as a high contrast system. However, if the 12-bit system can clearly show two near-by gray value intensities, the system will have a high contrast resolution. An image with a high number of gray values has a large dynamic range.

SNR and CNR are not completely independent of each other: each point within an image must exceed a certain perception threshold in order to be recognized. The perception threshold depends on the quality of the object, i.e., its size, contrast, and blur. Object size and object contrast influence each other. Very small details with high contrast (e.g., pulmonary osteomas with mineral opacity) are still visible, while larger structures with low contrast may fall below the perception threshold (e.g., small pulmonary metastases that are soft tissue opaque).

Blurring

Blurring means that an object point is not depicted as a dot, but as a larger or smaller circle that is not clearly defined. Image blur or sharpness is closely related to spatial resolution. In medical imaging, there are three main causes of blurring: geometric blur (radiography), motion blurring, and inherent blurring related to the imaging system (detector blur).

▎ **Geometric blur** Ideally, an X-ray tube produces X-rays from a point source. Actually, the focal spot has a two-dimensional extent at X-rays arising from each end of this circle. As a result, the edges of an object are blurred on the image by the so-called penumbra (Latin word for semi-shade). The larger the object-to-film distance (OFD), the larger the penumbra. Geometric blurring is therefore a function of the focal spot size. To minimize geometric blur, the smallest possible OFD at the largest possible focus-object distance (FOD) and a small focal spot size are required (**fig. 1.14**). The effects of OFD on geometric blur can be easily demonstrated by the shadow of your hand on a wall: as the distance of the hand from the wall increases, the contours of the shadow become more blurred.

▎ **Motion blur** Every voluntary and involuntary movement of the patient or the recording system during image acquisition results in motion blur. Organ movements, e.g., of the heart and lungs and the gastrointestinal tract are considered involuntary patient movements. Motion blur can be reduced by shortening the exposure time. In veterinary medicine, sedation and anesthesia of a patient are a measure to reduce voluntary motion blur and are especially recommended for skeletal images. This enables correct positioning and reduces the radiation exposure to the personnel.

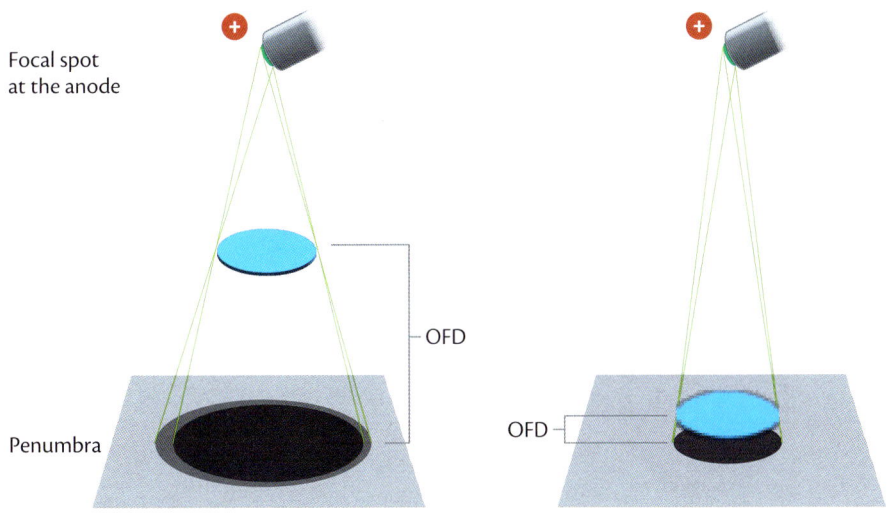

Fig. 1.14 Geometric blurring occurs due to two-dimensional extent of the focal spot resulting in blurring of object margins, the so-called penumbra. Minimization of geometric blur is achieved with the smallest possible OFD and the largest possible focus-object distance. © Vetsuisse-Fakultäten Bern und Zürich.

▌**Signal-to-noise ratio** The signal-to-noise ratio compares the level of the desired signal to the level of background noise. Noise signals have nothing to do with the object being imaged and can often not be actively reduced on an image. The higher the signal noise becomes less important. If we think about X-ray photons on the image receiver system as a signal, at a low-dose rate, noise is particularly prominent. With an increasing dose rate, the signal increases due to the higher number of photons, and therefore the SNR is increased. The signal-to-noise ratio can be illustrated by a box containing small objects: only after a certain number of photons reached the box, the outlines of the objects become visible. The more photons fall into the box, the clearer its outline will be (high SNR) (**fig. 1.15**).

Concerning digital images, the signal is related to the pixel/voxel size: the larger the pixel, the more signal can be collected per time. For illustration, imagine a small and a large box: more photons will reach and fall into the larger box compared to the small box (smaller pixel). This explains how spatial resolution and SNR influence each other: the smaller the pixel, the higher the spatial resolution, but the lower the signal, if collected within a fixed time.

Concerning radiography, scatter is an important source of noise. While Compton scatter is contributing to the difference in attenuation between tissues, it also reduces the contrast between different tissues. The amount of Compton scatter increases with increasing thickness of the object, increasing beam size, and increasing tube voltage. To reduce scatter, the beam field should be collimated as small as possible. Using an anti-scatter grid is recommended for objects thicker than 10 cm. It must be kept in mind that using a grid requires an increase in exposure and therefore radiation to the personnel is increased.

Artifacts

There are various image artifacts in medical images that are not seen in natural images. Artifacts can generally be categorized as hardware-related and patient-related artifacts. The hardware-related artifacts are associated with the technology of the imaging system.

Concerning radiography, artifacts due to the motion of the patients are common. In CT common artifacts are linked to strong attenuating objects that result in beam hardening and streaks. In MRI, B_0 field inhomogeneity is responsible for many artifacts while in ultrasound, strong reflectors or reflection by gas are leading to artifacts. Such artifacts are even helpful to characterize the tissues. For further details, please refer to textbooks of the different modalities.

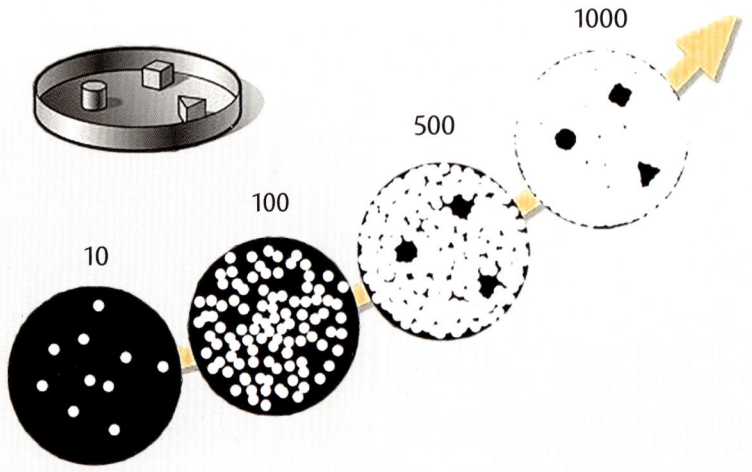

Fig. 1.15 Signal-to-noise ratio illustrated by a box containing small objects: only after a certain number of photons reach the box the outlines of the objects become visible. The more photons fall into the box, the clearer the outlines will be (high SNR). © Vetsuisse-Fakultäten Bern und Zürich.

Imaging interpretation and pitfalls

Diagnostic quality

Before starting the actual interpretation of an imaging study, the diagnostic quality should be assessed:

- Are all desired anatomical structures depicted within the study?
- Are there any technical limitations? Is the positioning of the patient correct? Could suboptimal positioning such as obliquity or rotation influence the interpretation?
- Are there any artifacts present?
- Is the study complete? Can the clinical question be answered?
- In case of follow-up examinations: were the images taken under the same conditions as the previous study to ensure that images are comparable?

In conclusion, there is a difference between image quality, i.e., how "pretty" images look, and image information, i.e., how well one can make a diagnosis from the image. While a certain level of image quality is necessary to establish a diagnosis, we can often make a diagnosis on images despite noise, artifacts, and poor resolution. As noted above, we must perform exams at a point, which balances image quality with harm to the patient/personnel.

Image interpretation

Basically, image analysis involves two processes: visual inspection and interpretation.

- **Viewing conditions** According to convention, projection radiographs are viewed as the observer looks at the patient, placing the patient's right side to his own left side. The cranial or rostral aspect of the patient is on the left side of the screen. Looking at lateral views of limbs, the dorsal/cranial aspect is projected on the left side as well as the lateral aspect on dorsopalmar/dorsoplantar and craniocaudal views, respectively.

It is recommended to read radiographs under conditions where one can concentrate to focus on the image and interpretation. In order to be able to see every part and all the important features of an image, optimal viewing conditions are necessary. In general, it is recommended that the ambient lighting match the brightness of your screen, which is stated to be 20-40 lux.

- **Detection of abnormalities** The first task in the analysis of an image is the detection of an abnormality. This has primary importance because all following steps rely on detection efficacy. To detect a potentially significant finding requires knowledge of normal anatomy. A systematic approach is recommended to limit the possibility of overlooking abnormalities. What type of systematic approach seems of minor importance and images can be read "line by line", "centripetal or centrifugal" (from outside to inside or vice versa), or organ-centered. Especially for cross-sectional images, identification of abnormalities seems higher when scrolling through the series while looking at a certain region or organ system in contrast to scanning one entire slice after the other.

- **Description of radiographic findings** The next step is the characterizing of a lesion as a specific type; the diagnostic features of a lesion include location, size, shape, border delineation, and, depending on the modality, opacity (radiographs), attenuation (CT), signal intensity (MRI) or echogenicity (ultrasound). Furthermore, a pattern of distribution such as focal, multifocal, or diffuse and bilateral symmetric or asymmetric as well as the presence of a mass effect or volume loss, association to organs, or other abnormalities characterize lesions and specify them.

- **Radiological diagnosis** A thorough characterization allows concluding on a radiological diagnosis, summarizing the findings. For example, after describing a bone lesion by its location, periosteal reactions, type of lysis, and transition zone you should be able to conclude the diagnosis of a monostotic aggressive or bone lesion, according to its features.

▌Interpretation The final step is to provide a helpful list of differential diagnoses; helpful in the sense that it does not contain a list of all possible differentials, but that the differential diagnosis is prioritized in the light of the patient's signalment, history, and clinical findings, as well as your own experience and subjective assessment. This list of differentials is supposed to guide you to the next diagnostic steps or to establish prognosis and treatment options.

Pitfalls in image interpretation

Every of the above-mentioned step carries the risk of errors. Being aware of these errors might help to prevent them.

▌Search error This type of error occurs when the observer never fixates on the lesion and the lesion is just missed, see also detection of abnormalities.

▌Recognition error A recognition error happens if the observer fixates on the target, but for a duration shorter than the threshold dwell time needed to recognize the lesion and results in a failure to identify the finding as abnormal. The threshold for lesion detection depends on the imaging modality and ranges from 500 to 1000 ms. Both search and recognition errors are considered as perceptual errors.

▌Decision-making error Decision-making errors occur when a lesion has been identified and fixed for an extended period of more than one second, but the observer does not attribute appropriate significance to the lesion, e.g, dismissing a lesion as an artifact or over-diagnosing an anatomical variant as pathology.

References

1. McKean SC, Ross JJ, Dressler DD, Brotman DJ, Ginsberg JS (editors). Principles and Practice of Hospital Medicine. New York, McGraw-Hill, 2012.
2. Bushberg JT, Seibert JA, Leidholdt EM, Boon JM (editors). The Essential Physics of Medical Imaging 3rd edition. Philadelphia, Wolters Kluwer, 2012.
3. Curry TS, Dowdey JE, Murry RC (editors). Christensen's Physics of Diagnostic Radiology 4th edition. Lea & Febiger, 1990.
4. Jacobson FL, McKean SC. Introduction to radiology. In McKean SC, Ross JJ, Dressler DD, Brotman DJ, Ginsberg JS (editors). Principles and Practice of Hospital Medicine. New York, McGraw-Hill, 2012.
5. Romans LE. Physics and instrumentation. In Romans LE (editor). Computed Tomography for Technologists. Philadelphia, Wolters Kluwer, 2019, p 8.
6. Schofield R, King L, Tayal U, Castellano I, Stirrup J, Pontana F, et al. Image reconstruction: Part 1 - Understanding filtered back projection, noise and image acquisition. *J Cardiovasc Comput Tomogr* 14:219-225, 2020.
7. Shannoun F, Blettner M, Schmidberger H, Zeeb H. Radiation protection in diagnostic radiology. *Dtsch Arztebl Int* 105:41-46, 2008.
8. Agency IAE. Radiation protection and safety in veterinary medicine. 1400 Vienna, Austria: Vienna International Centre, 2021.
9. Degnan AJ, Ghobadi EH, Hardy P, Krupinski E, Scali EP, Stratchko L, et al. Perceptual and interpretive error in diagnostic radiology - Causes and potential solutions. *Acad Radiol* 26:833-845, 2019.
10. Itri JN, Tappouni RR, McEachern RO, Pesch AJ, Patel SH. Fundamentals of diagnostic error in imaging. *Radiographics* 38:1845-1865, 2018.
11. Lee CS, Nagy PG, Weaver SJ, Newman-Toker DE. Cognitive and system factors contributing to diagnostic errors in radiology. *AJR Am J Roentgenol* 201:611-617, 2013.

SECTION II

APPENDICULAR SKELETON

CHAPTER 2

Normal bones and joints

John Graham and Massimo Vignoli

> **KEY POINTS**
>
> - The mineral content of bone means it is ideally suited to radiographic assessment.
> - Two orthogonal projections are the minimum requirement for assessing most bone structures.
> - Incomplete mineralization in juvenile patients can obscure injury and make interpretation challenging.
> - Radiographs of the contralateral limb or a control subject may help distinguish normal anatomic variation from pathology.
> - Radiographic remodeling from injury may take 3 to 5 days to become evident in juvenile patients and over 10 days in mature patients.

Radiography of the skeleton

Bone is in many ways the ideal structure for assessment by radiographs, and the first radiographic image ever obtained was of a human hand. The mineral content of bone ensures good radiographic contrast with surrounding soft tissues and shows the internal structure. Survey radiographs are the first-line diagnostic choice to evaluate patients for skeletal disease, skeletal trauma, and skeletal manifestations of systemic disease. For most body parts, two orthogonal projections, such as mediolateral and craniocaudal radiographs, are the minimum requirement. Oblique images may be needed to assess complex joints such as the carpus and tarsus. Radiographs of long bones should include the joints at the proximal and distal extents (**fig. 2.1**). Radiographs of the joints should be centered on the joint itself and include the adjacent long bones (**figs. 2.2** and **2.3**). Unless there is a clinical contraindication, sedation or anesthesia are recommended for most patients to assist in obtaining consistent diagnostic positioning. Radiographs of the contralateral limb, a healthy sibling, or a normal age-matched cat or dog of the same breed can be very helpful in distinguishing pathology from normal variation in immature patients. It is important to remember that bone is a living, dynamic structure constantly undergoing remodeling by osteoblasts and osteoclasts. This is more obvious in juvenile patients when an insult to the bone may result in radiographically visible changes within 3 to 5 days. In mature patients, remodeling changes may take up to 10 to 14 days to become visible on radiographs. It is recommended that the reader acquire an atlas of normal radiographic anatomy to assist in interpretation.

SECTION II APPENDICULAR SKELETON

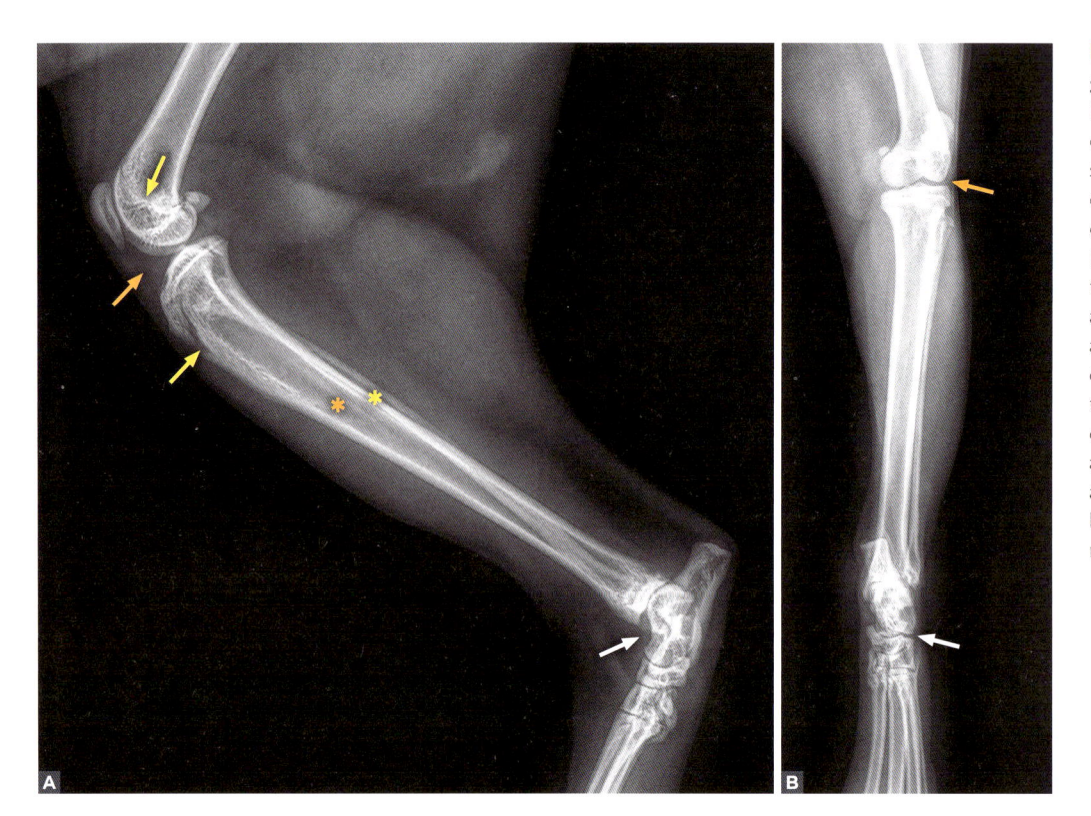

Fig. 2.1 Normal radiographic study of the right hind leg of a 14-month-old spayed female British shorthair cat. Radiographs of long bones should include the joints at the proximal and distal extents, in this case, the stifle (orange arrows) and tarsus (white arrows). The growth plates of the distal femur and the tibial tuberosity are incompletely closed (yellow arrows). The tibial (orange asterisk) and fibular (yellow asterisk) diaphyses are normal.

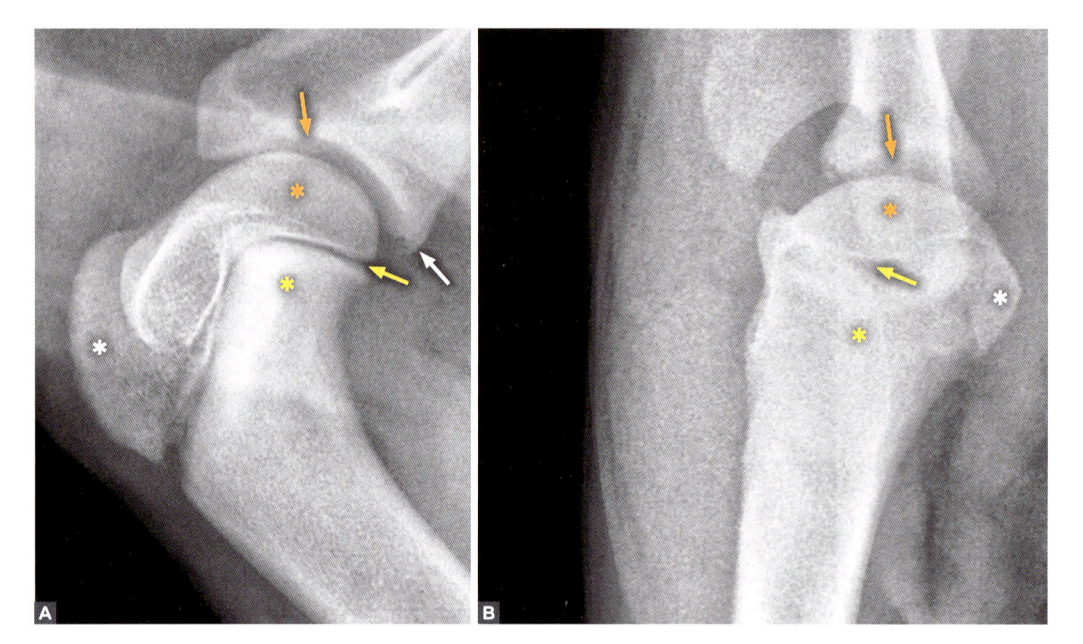

Fig. 2.2 Mediolateral and caudocranial projections of a normal shoulder of a five-month-old female mixed breed dog. Radiographs show the glenoid cavity (orange arrows), humeral head or proximal epiphysis (orange asterisks), physis (yellow arrows), and proximal metaphysis (yellow asterisks). There is incomplete ossification of the caudal margin of the glenoid (white arrow). The cranioproximal margin of the greater tubercle of the humerus is indistinct from incomplete ossification (white asterisks).

Ultrasound of the skeleton is used for the assessment of skeletal disease. Ultrasound is reflected at the bone surface and can assess bone margins for proliferation or lysis. Ultrasound is more helpful in the evaluation of the soft tissues of the musculoskeletal system, such as tendons, ligaments, muscles, joint capsules, and effusions or articular cartilage (**figs. 2.4** and **2.5**).

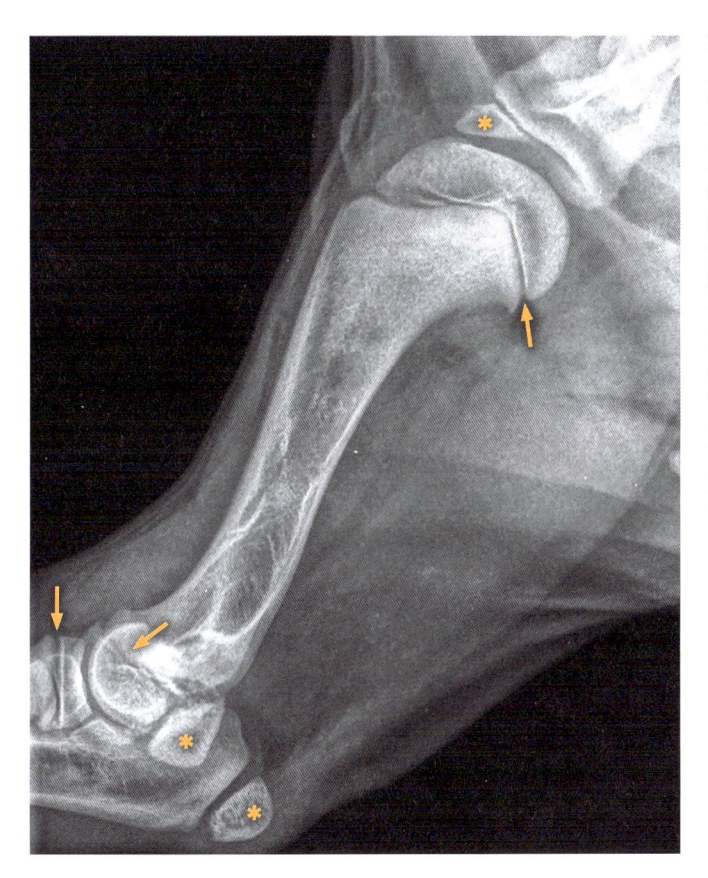

Fig. 2.3 Mediolateral radiograph of the humerus of a four-month-old Mastiff with a history of intermittent lameness. The radiograph is normal and shows features of a juvenile skeleton with incomplete mineralization. Open growth plates are visible in the proximal humerus, distal humerus, and proximal radius (arrows). There are separate ossification centers of the supraglenoid tubercle, medial epicondyle of the humerus, and olecranon (asterisks), separated from the adjacent bones by a radiolucent growth plate. The proximal humeral epiphysis is completely mineralized, but there is no visible mineralization of the greater tubercle of the proximal humerus.

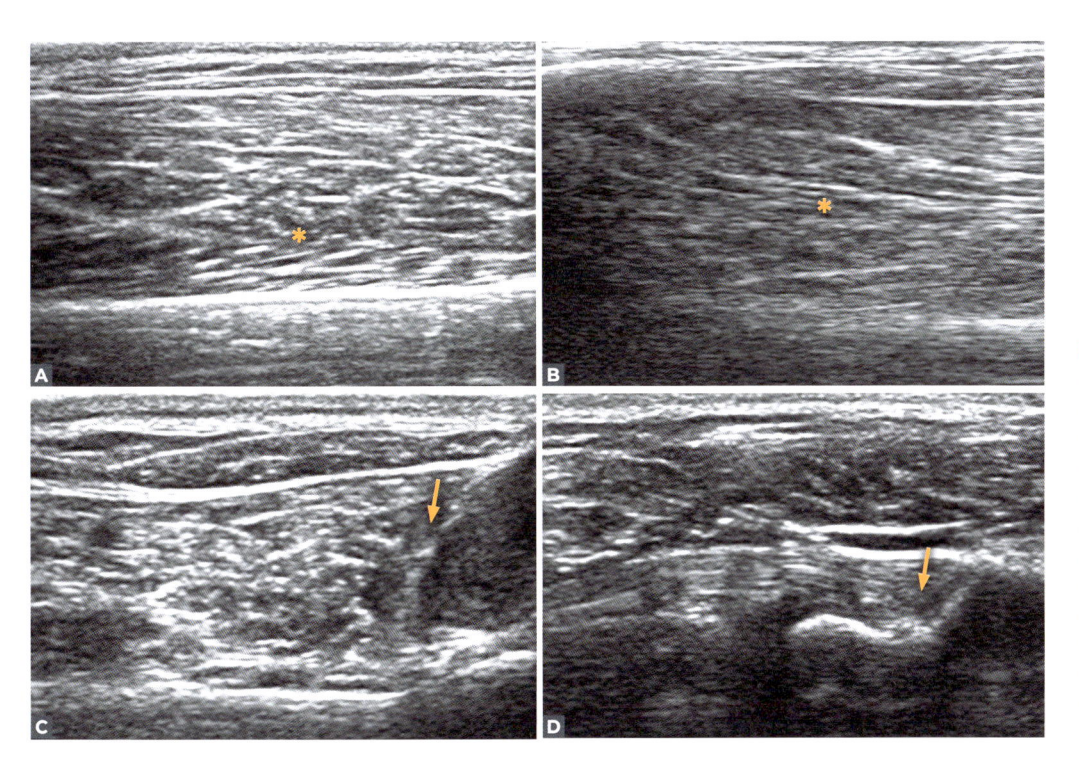

Fig. 2.4 A five-year-old spayed female mixed breed dog. The images show a normal supraspinatus muscle (asterisks) (**A**) and its tendon at the insertion on the greater tubercle (arrow) of the humerus (**B**). The normal infraspinatus muscle (**C**) (asterisk) and its tendon (**D**) at the site of insertion on the greater tubercle (arrow), just distal to the most proximal point.

SECTION II APPENDICULAR SKELETON

Fig. 2.5 Ultrasound of the shoulder joint of a dog. The image shows the biceps tendon of the origin (orange arrows) at the supraglenoid process of the scapula (asterisk). A small amount of fluid is visible deep in the tendon in the joint capsule and tendon sheath (white arrows).

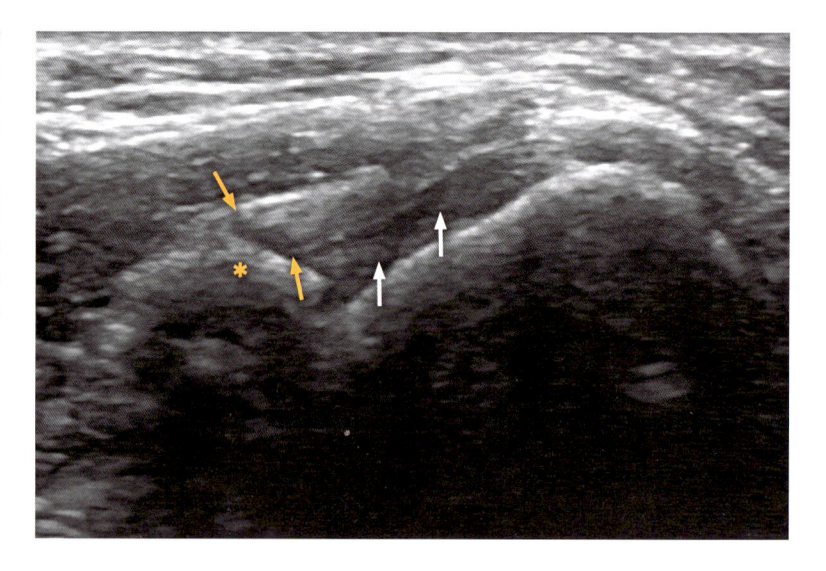

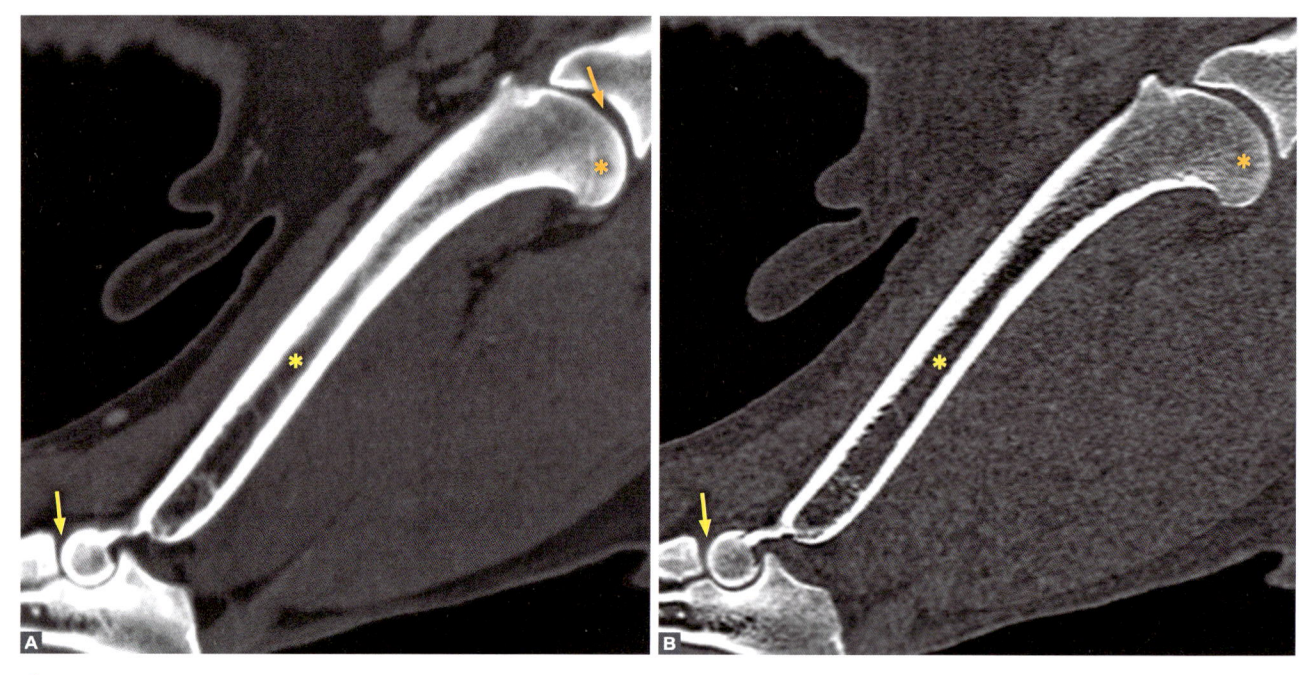

Fig. 2.6 Computed tomography sagittal plane reconstruction of a normal humerus in soft tissue window (**A**) and bone window (**B**) of a three-year-old spayed female Samoyed. Shoulder joint (orange arrows), elbow joints (yellow arrows), epiphyses (orange asterisks), and diaphyses (yellow asterisks) are shown. Note the honeycomb-like trabecular bone within the epiphyses and metaphyses.

Computed tomography (CT), as it uses X-rays, is superbly adapted to imaging bone, with superior contrast to radiographs and the capacity for detailed imaging of internal bone structure. Images acquired in thin slices can be reprocessed in multiplanar reconstructions (MPR) to highlight specific structures (**figs. 2.6-2.9**). MRI is slightly less suitable for imaging bone pathology, as it depends upon the water content of tissue, which is limited in normal bone. MRI is the imaging modality of choice for evaluating the soft tissue structures of the skeleton, particularly intra-articular structures, because of its excellent contrast resolution and capacity to acquire images in any plane (**fig. 2.10**).

CHAPTER **2** Normal bones and joints

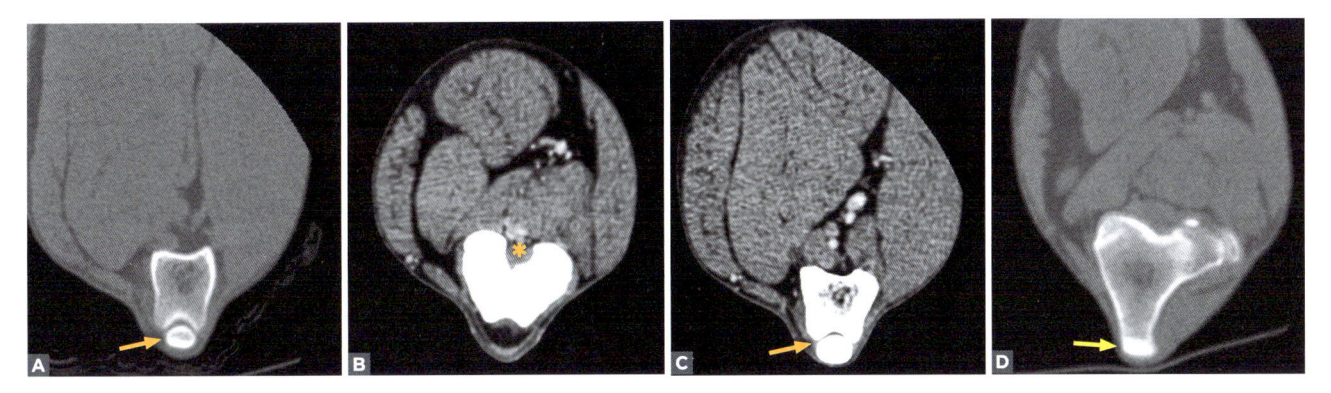

Fig. 2.7 Computed tomography images of a normal knee of an adult male Dobermann. Bone (**A**) and soft tissue (**B**) windows at the level of the femoral trochlea and patella (orange arrows). Distal to it (**C**), the intercondyloid fossa with the origin of the cruciate ligaments (asterisk) is visible. (**D**) Shows the tibial crest, the insertion site of the patellar (quadriceps) tendon (yellow arrow).

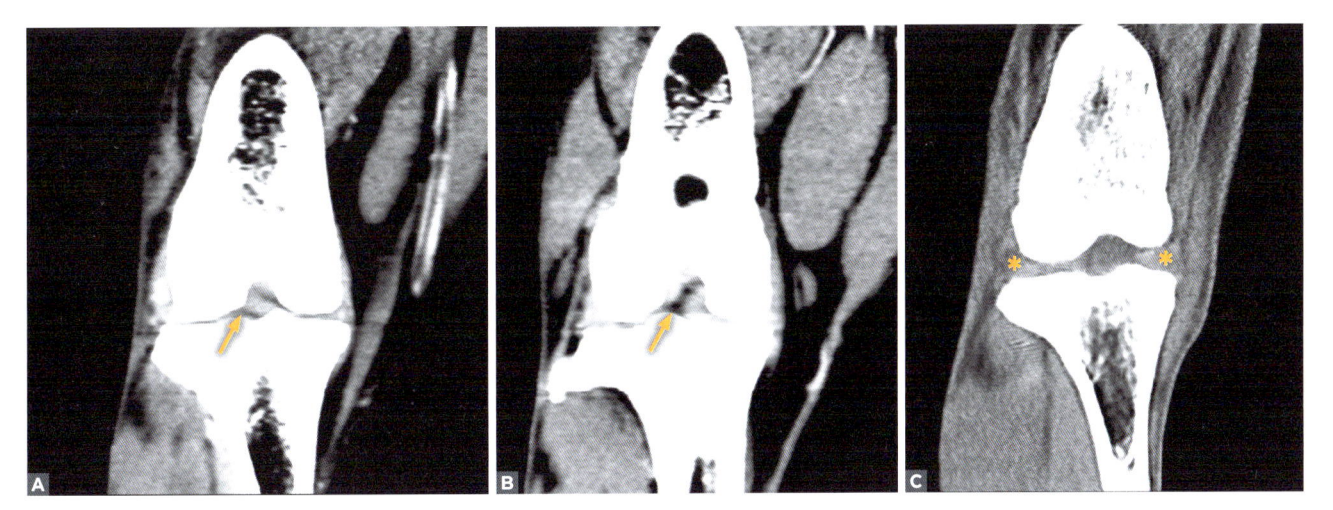

Fig. 2.8 Multiplanar dorsal reconstructions of the knee of the same dog as in fig. 2.7 in soft tissue window. Cranial (**A**) and caudal (**B**) cruciate ligaments are well visible (arrows), as well as the menisci (**C**) (asterisks).

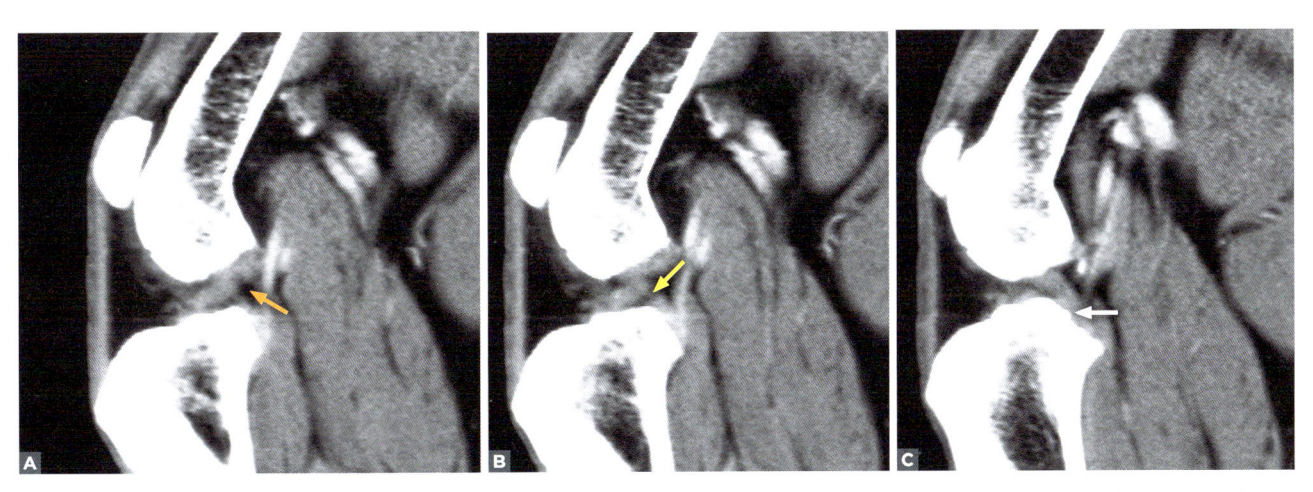

Fig. 2.9 Same dog as in fig. 2.7 in a soft tissue window sagittal reconstruction. (**A**) The cranial cruciate (orange arrow) ligament, (**B**) the crossing (yellow arrow) of the ligaments, and (**C**) the caudal cruciate (white arrow) ligament are clearly visible.

SECTION II APPENDICULAR SKELETON

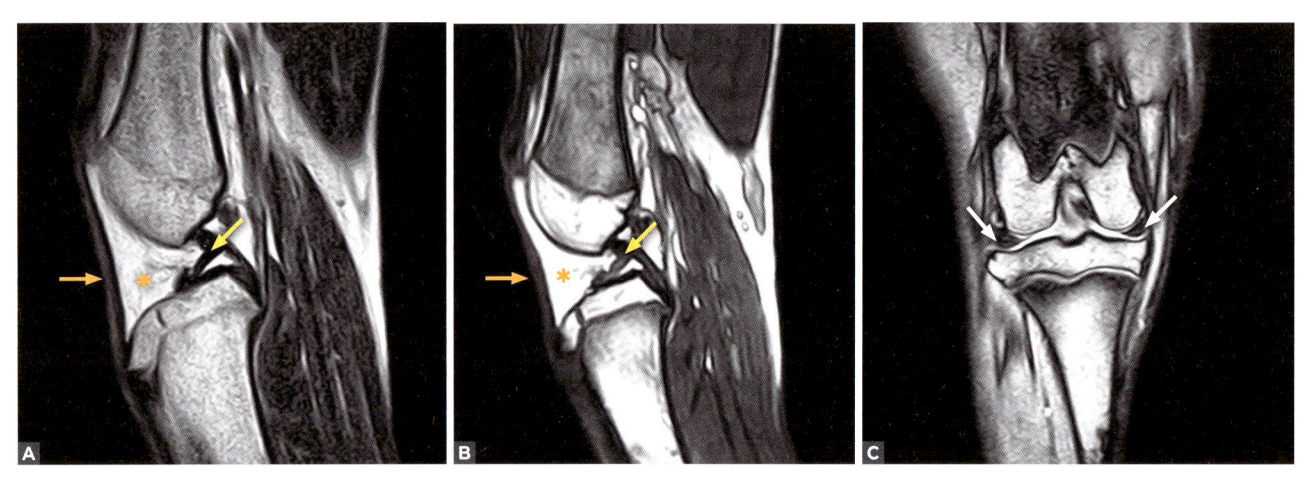

Fig. 2.10 MRI of a normal stifle joint of a dog in sagittal T2 and 3D HYCE, and in dorsal high-resolution gradient echo. The patellar (quadriceps) tendon (orange arrows), infrapatellar fat (asterisks), cranial and caudal cruciate ligaments (yellow arrows), and menisci (white arrows) can be seen. The contrast between soft tissue structures is superior to that in CT images (fig. 2.8), and MRI is preferred for assessing tendons and ligaments.

The juvenile skeleton

In the fetal and juvenile dog or cat, bone develops either by endochondral or intramembranous ossification. In the case of endochondral ossification, the bone develops from mineralization and ossification of cartilage at the growth plates or physes. This is how the vertebrae and all tubular long bones in the skeleton are formed. The growth plates are interposed between the epiphysis and metaphysis, which is the site where the bone grows in length. The epiphyses are the components of the long bones which form the articular surfaces of joints. There are also separate ossification centers, termed apophyses, in many long bones at the site of origin or insertion of larger tendons and ligaments. In contrast, flat bones, such as those of the skull, scapula, or pelvis, and cuboidal bones, such as those of the carpus and tarsus, are formed by intramembranous ossification in which mineralization occurs within a fibrous connective tissue precursor of the bone without formation of cartilage. The pelvis and skull are formed by the fusion of several flat bones originating from discrete ossification centers. Incomplete ossification and fusion of multiple osseous components can make the assessment of these structures in neonatal and juvenile patients quite challenging. Apophyses are also present in some of the flat bones, such as the supraglenoid tubercle of the scapula, which is the origin of the biceps brachii muscle.

In neonatal patients, the diaphyses of long bones are partly mineralized and visible on radiographs, but the epiphyses of many long bones, cuboidal bones, apophyses, and sesamoid bones are comprised entirely of soft tissue and thus not visible on radiographs. The earliest sign of mineralization is the appearance of a small ovoid region of mineralization roughly in the center of the soft tissue precursor of the bone. Incompletely mineralized structures usually have a ragged, poorly defined margin that should not be mistaken for pathology. Complete mineralization of these ossification centers is usually present by 4 months of age. The physes or growth plates appear as a radiolucent band interposed between the epiphysis and metaphysis and are comprised of cartilage. Ossification of the cartilage occurs at the metaphyseal aspect and results in longitudinal growth of the bone. The bone is relatively wider at the metaphysis than in the diaphysis, and as the bone grows in length, osteoclastic activity at the outer cortical margin reduces the diameter. The effect of this osteoclastic remodeling is to make the outer cortical margin of the metaphysis unsharp or indistinct, and this is referred to as the cut back zone. The growth plates of the long bones close at varying times, and all are closed at maturity. Growth plate closure in normal dogs depends upon the overall body size and growth plate location, i.e., skeletal maturity occurs at 5-6 months of age in small breeds and about 11-13 months in giant breeds (**table 2.1**). The long bone growth plates close between 5 and 13 months of age. The apophyses of the iliac crests often remain open up to 5 years of age in normal dogs. After growth plate closure, a radio-opaque band may persist at the site, sometimes referred to as a physeal scar. Closure of the long bone growth plates in normal cats may be delayed by neutering before or at the time of puberty, and open long bone growth plates may be seen in normal patients up to 2-3 years of age. For skeletally immature patients, it is often helpful to obtain radiographs of the contralateral limb to determine if the appearance represents normal variation or pathology. Similarly, if there is suspicion of systemic disease affecting the skeleton or developmental skeletal disease such as dwarfism, radiographs of a normal sibling or an age-matched individual of the same breed may be very helpful for the characterization of lesions.

Sesamoid bones are bones formed within tendons to ensure free movement of the tendon where it passes over an angular osseous structure. The largest sesamoid bone in the body is the patella, located in the tendon of insertion of the quadriceps femoris muscle. There are also large sesamoid bones in the tendons of origin of the gastrocnemius muscles, positioned at the caudal proximal aspect of the femoral condyles. Paired sesamoid bones are present at the distal aspect of the interosseous muscle in the distal metacarpus and metatarsus. There are also small, round sesamoid bones at the dorsal aspect of the metacarpophalangeal and metatarsophalangeal joints, which should not be

Table 2.1 Age at the appearance and fusion or closure of the ossification center/physes of the main bones of the appendicular skeleton

Structure	Location	Age at the appearance of the ossification center	Age at fusion or closure
Radius	Proximal epiphysis/growth plate	1-2 weeks	10-13 months
	Distal epiphysis/growth plate	2-3 weeks	6-8 months
	Proximal epiphysis/growth plate	3-5 weeks	6-11 months
	Distal epiphysis/growth plate	2-4 weeks	8-12 months
Ulna	Distal epiphysis/growth plate	8 weeks	8-12 months
Pelvis	Pubis	Birth	4-6 months
	Ilium	Birth	4-6 months
	Ischium	Birth	4-6 months
	Os acetabulum	7 weeks	5 months
	Symphysis pubis		Up to 5 years
	Iliac crest	4 months	1-5 years
Femur	Proximal epiphysis (head)/growth plate	2 weeks	7-11 months
	Distal epiphysis/growth plate	2-3 weeks	8-11 months
Tibia	Proximal epiphysis/growth plate	3 weeks	6-12 months
	Distal epiphysis/growth plate	3 weeks	8-11 months
	Tuberosity	8 weeks	6-8 months to epiphysis
Fibula	Proximal epiphysis/growth plate	9 weeks	8-12 months
	Distal epiphysis/growth plate	2-7 weeks	7-11 months

mistaken for chip fractures. There is an inconsistent sesamoid bone in the tendon of origin of the ulnaris lateralis muscle at the lateral aspect of the elbow joint in larger dogs.

The adult skeleton

In skeletally mature cats and dogs, the cortices of the long bones show uniform mineralization with marked contrast to the soft tissues. The subchondral bone adjacent to the articular surface is usually more opaque, as this is a component of the bone that bears a substantial load. The margin of the subchondral bone at the joint space should be smooth and well-defined. For most joints, the contour of the articular surface of the subchondral bone will mirror that of the subchondral bone of the facing bone of the joint. In most synovial joints with normal congruency, the subchondral bone of the articular surfaces conforms to and matches each other. For example, the glenoid of the scapula has a concave margin that matches the convex contour of the humeral head. An exception to this is the normal stifle joint, where cartilaginous menisci are interposed between the condyles of the distal femur and condyles of the tibial plateau. The visibility of the joint space is dependent upon the X-ray beam being centered at the joint space and oriented parallel to the joint space, and there may be an artifactual narrowing of the joint space when the X-ray beam is centered away from the joint or the joint positioned obliquely. Joint spaces may appear quite wide in juvenile patients from incomplete ossification of the epiphyses and cuboidal bones. Joint space widening should be assessed with caution in small animals, as radiographs are rarely acquired with the patient bearing weight, and traction on the limb to ensure diagnostic positioning may result in some widening of the joint space. The trabecular bone within the epiphysis and metaphysis should have a well-defined fine honeycomb appearance, blending with the cortices. The cortices of the diaphyses of the long bones have uniform dense radiopacity. The thickness of the cortices will vary depending upon the load placed on the bone and the diameter. For example, the cortices of the humerus are slightly thinner in the proximal diaphysis than in the distal diaphysis. For most long bones, fine trabecular bone is visible within the bone at the metaphyses, while the medullary cavity in the diaphysis is usually devoid of detail. The blood supply to long bones is delivered via the nutrient artery. This passes through the cortex of the diaphysis, appearing as an oblique line usually more visible on one projection.

References

1. Thrall DE, Robertson, ID (editors). Atlas of normal radiographic anatomy and anatomic variance in the dog and cat. St Louis, Elsevier, 2011.

2. Ticer JW (editor). Radiographic techniques in small animals. Philadelphia, WB Saunders, 1975.

CHAPTER 3

Appendicular skeleton: radiology and techniques

Nathalie Rademacher

> **KEY POINTS**
>
> ▎ Sedation or anesthesia should be used for optimal image quality, particularly the positioning of appendicular skeletal radiographs.
> ▎ Collimation to the joint or long bones of the area of interest is recommended to eliminate distortion and minimize scatter radiation.
> ▎ Two orthogonal views are the minimum examination for any region of the appendicular skeleton.
> ▎ Additional specific projections can be acquired depending on the suspected disease process.
> ▎ Advanced imaging such as ultrasound, MRI, or CT may be needed especially for soft tissues, and since normal radiographs do not out completely exclude pathology.

Radiographs are the primary imaging tool for the assessment of the appendicular skeleton in cats and dogs. However, it is important to note that normal radiographs do not rule out all disease processes. Indications for radiographic examination for any region of the appendicular skeleton include, but are not limited to:

▎ Trauma.
▎ Congenital defects.
▎ Developmental diseases.
▎ Metabolic diseases.
▎ Inflammatory diseases.
▎ Infectious diseases.
▎ Neoplastic diseases.

Radiographic views should be performed in sedated or anesthetized dogs and cats to avoid motion unsharpness (**fig. 3.1**) and for radiation protection by reducing exposure of the personnel since manual restraint can be avoided, thus reducing the number of retakes (**fig. 3.2**). Furthermore, correct positioning is more easily and consistently obtained when radiographs are acquired with sedation or anesthesia, which is critical for diagnosis.

Exposures with high kVp and low mAs techniques should be chosen as there is good inherent contrast in bone, and motion artifact is minimized by the shortest possible exposure time. The technique selected should result in good radiographic contrast which will allow assessment of both the bones and soft tissues and adequate penetration of bone to show tra-

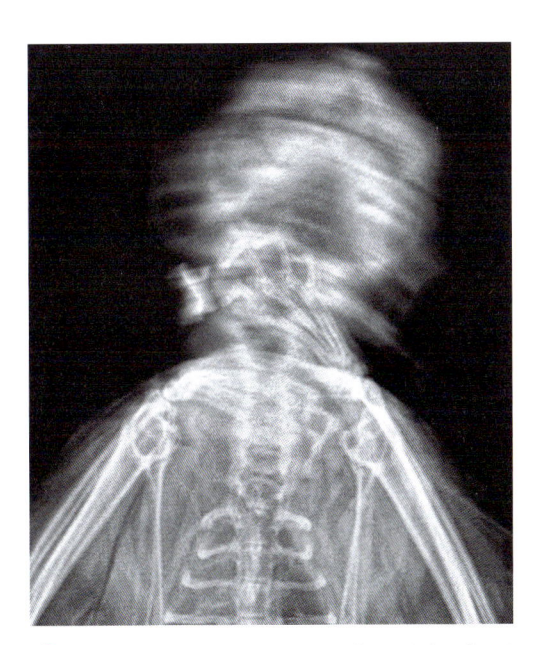

Fig. 3.1 Dorsoventral radiograph of a cat's head and neck. Patient movement results in severe unsharpness, and the image is nondiagnostic.

SECTION II APPENDICULAR SKELETON

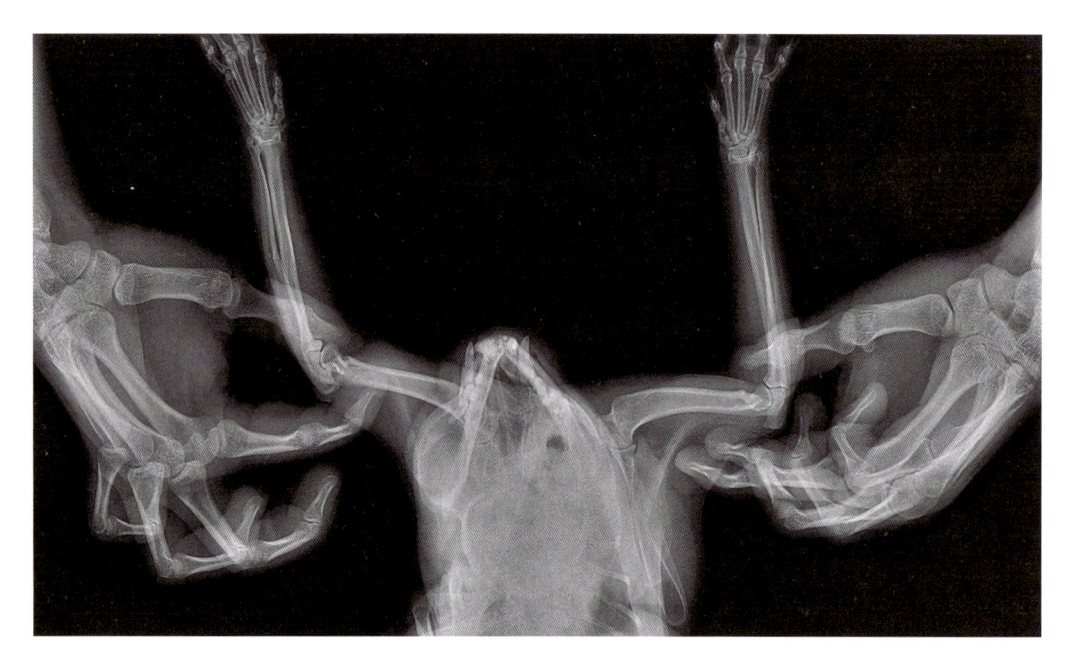

Fig. 3.2 Ventrodorsal radiograph of a cat obtained to assess both front legs. The patient was not sedated, and unprotected hands and wrists are exposed to the primary beam, which is a serious violation of radiation safety rules. Compounding this error, the image is nondiagnostic.

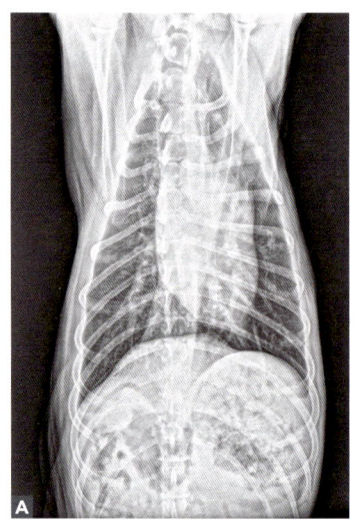

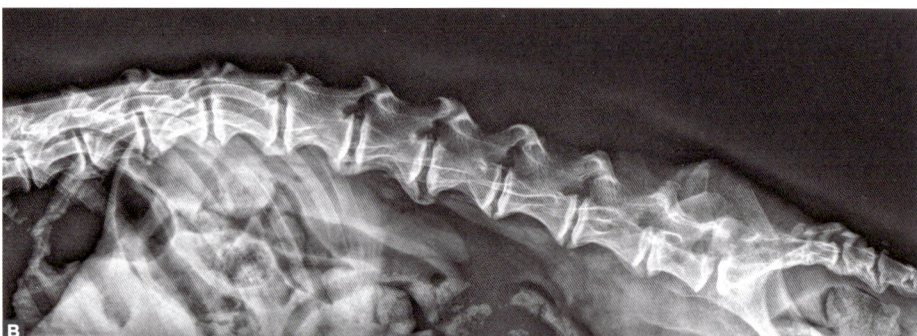

Fig. 3.3 (**A**) Underexposed ventrodorsal radiograph of the thorax of a dog resulting in decreased contrast and with the included skeletal structures appearing homogeneously white. (**B**) Lateral radiographs of the lumbar spine with moderate to severe overexposure including soft tissues, lung parenchyma, and retroperitoneal space. Planking artifact is also present.

becular detail.[1] Both under- and overexposure should be avoided: underexposure will present bones as homogeneous white structures with no visible internal detail (**fig. 3.3A**), while overexposure will reduce the visibility of the soft tissue structures (**fig. 3.3B**).

Two orthogonal views (mediolateral and craniocaudal/caudocranial or dorsopalmar/dorsoplantar) are the minimum requirement for the evaluation of any region of the appendicular skeleton.[1,2] Several radiographs of the limb should be made, centered, and collimated to a specific region of interest in the limb rather than trying to image the entire limb in a single image, which will cause distortion and hinder diagnosis. Radiographs of the joints should include approximately one-third of the long bones proximal and distal to the joint (**fig. 3.4**). Radiographs of the long bones should include the proximal and distal joints (**fig. 3.5**). Additional radiographic views may be needed to demonstrate some abnormalities. These include:[1]

- Comparison radiographs.
- Oblique radiographs.
- Tangential or skyline radiographs.

- Stressed or compressed radiographs including traction or torsion/rotation radiographs.
- Weight-bearing radiographs.
- Serial (over time) radiographs.

Radiographs of the contralateral limb are especially helpful in immature patients to diagnose subtle abnormalities of the growth plates and epiphyses by comparison to the normal limb (**fig. 3.6**). However, it must be kept in mind that many developmental and systemic diseases will result in symmetrical changes, and radiographs of a normal sibling may be more helpful for comparison. In mature animals, comparison radiographs are usually not indicated unless needed to differentiate normal anatomic variation from pathology or to confirm a subtle or equivocal lesion (**fig. 3.7**). Oblique radiographs project different aspects of a joint or region and maximize the

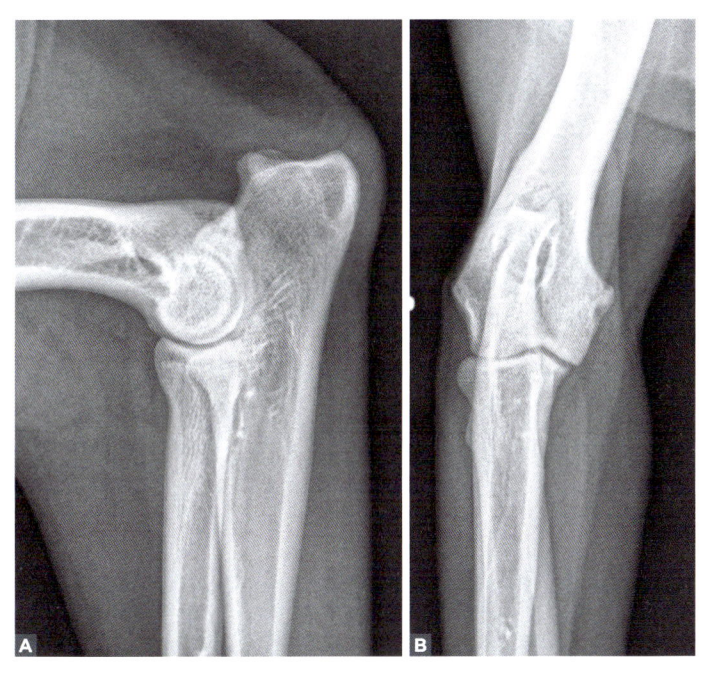

Fig. 3.4 Orthogonal mediolateral (**A**) and craniocaudal (**B**) radiographs of a normal canine left elbow to show how centering at the joint shows the joint space more clearly without distortion.

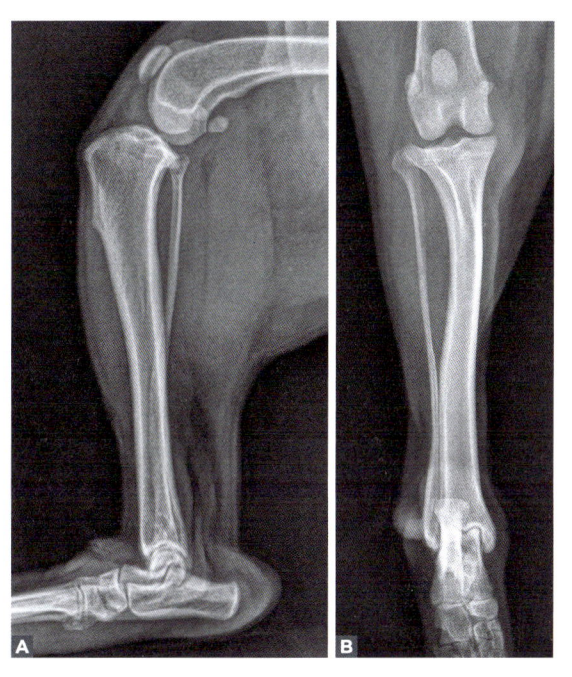

Fig. 3.5 Orthogonal mediolateral (**A**) and craniocaudal (**B**) radiographs of the right crus of a dog for surgical planning to represent an example of radiography of long bones centered and collimated to include the proximal and distal joints.

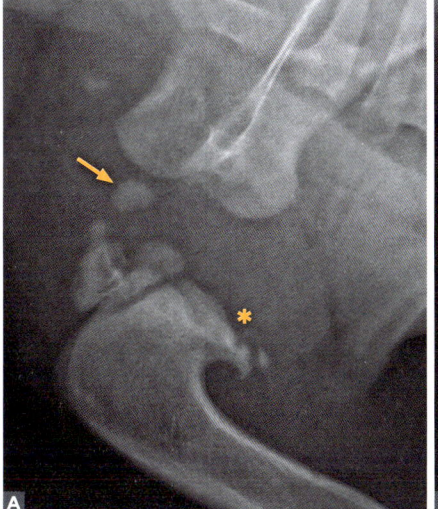

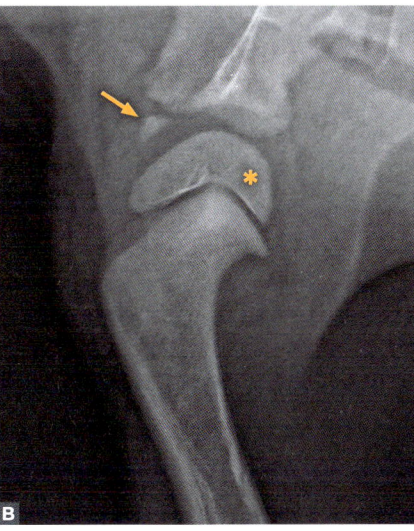

Fig. 3.6 Mediolateral radiographs of the abnormal right shoulder and normal left shoulder in a three-month-old dog with chronic right forelimb lameness. There is partial nonuniform mineralization of the most cranial aspect of the proximal epiphysis, which comprises several irregularly shaped fragments while there is no visible mineralization of the caudal two-thirds (asterisk). The proximal metaphysis has an undulating irregular contour. The apophysis of the supraglenoid tubercle is displaced caudally and distally and has less distinct margins than in the normal limb (arrows). The changes are unilateral which excludes systemic disease or an abnormality of endochondral ossification and are most likely secondary to traumatic injury as a neonate. *Arrows*, supraglenoid tubercle; *star*, humeral head epiphysis.

SECTION II APPENDICULAR SKELETON

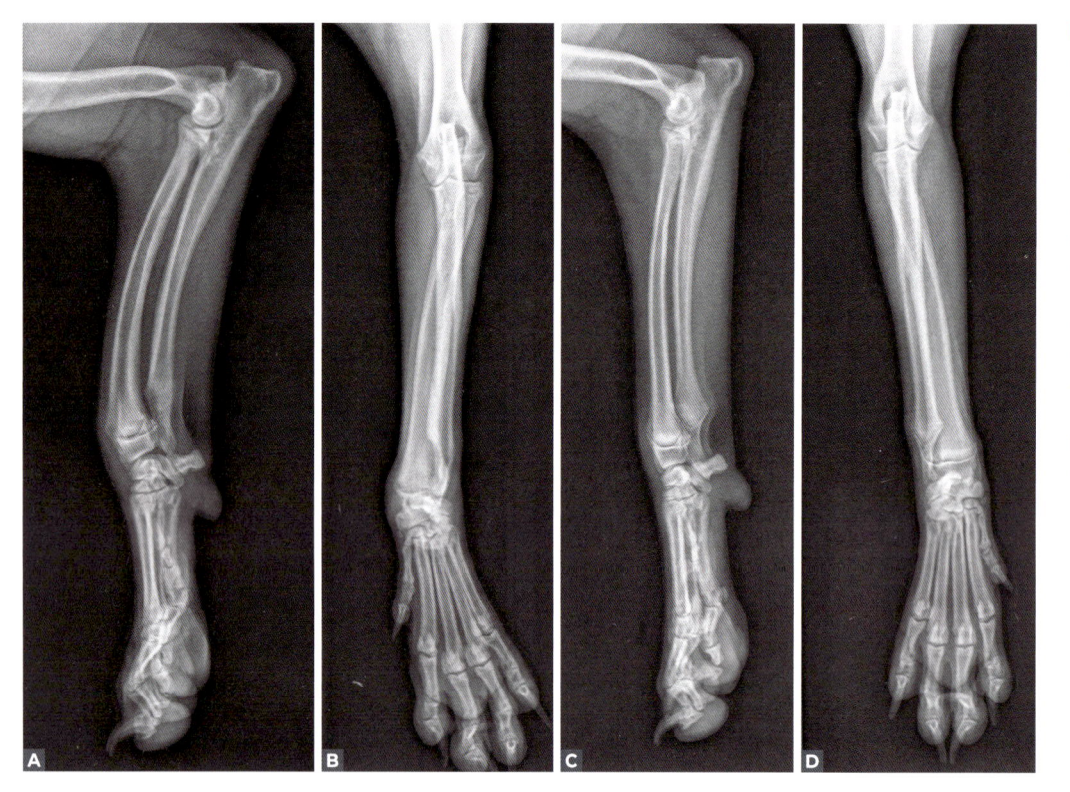

Fig. 3.7 Mediolateral and craniocaudal radiographs of the left antebrachium and extremity (**A-B**) of a nine-month-old spayed female Fox Terrier with chronic left forelimb lameness due to premature closure of the left distal ulnar physis resulting in a shortening of the ulna and secondary cranial bowing of the radius and valgus deviation of the carpus and foot. (**C-D**) Comparison radiographs of the normal right limb.

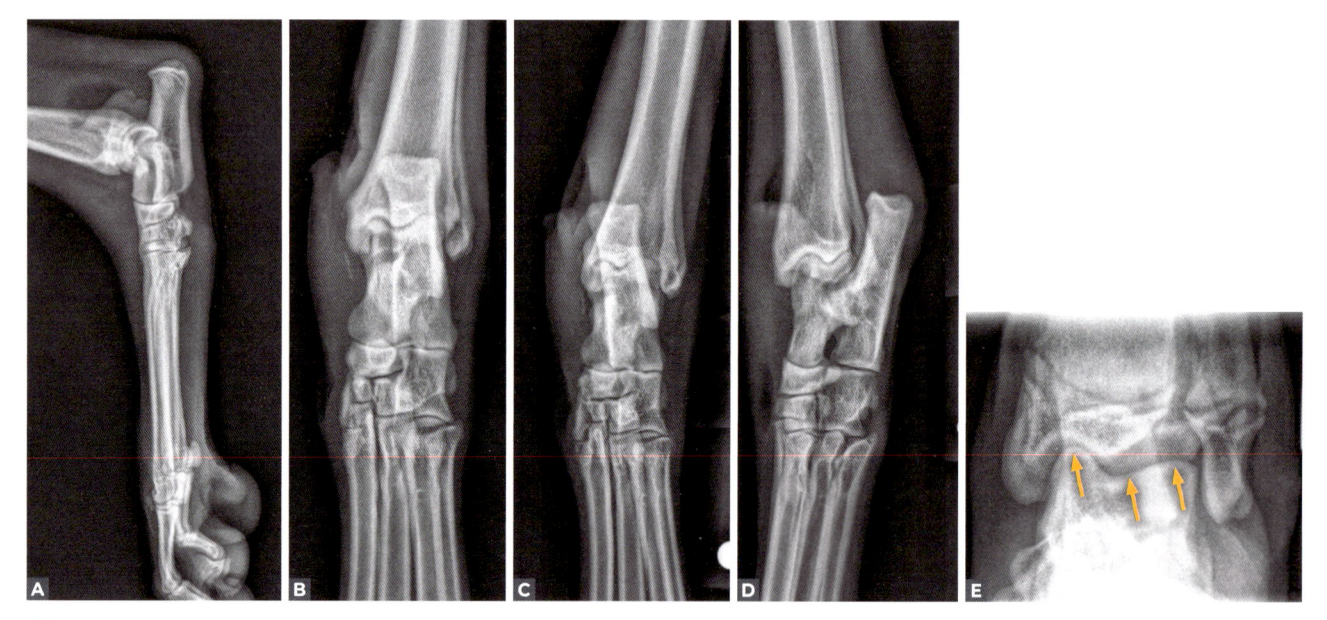

Fig. 3.8 (**A**, **D**) A complete set of views of the tarsus of a one-year-old spayed female Dane mix with suspicion of having been hit by a car and lameness located to the tarsus comprising (**A**) mediolateral, (**B**) dorsoplantar, (**C**) dorsomedio-450 plantarolateral oblique (DMPLO) and (**D**) dorsolateral-450 plantaromedial oblique (DLPMO) views. A moderate amount of soft tissue swelling surrounds the right tarsus. At the most proximal aspect of this swelling at the plantaromedial aspect there is an irregularly shaped, smoothly marginated cutaneous defect. Thin linear to pinpoint, well-defined mineral fragments are present in the soft tissue at the medial aspect of the talocrural joint in the region of the medial collateral ligament, at the proximal aspect of the medial malleolus of the tibia, and just distal to the medial malleolus. The soft tissue swelling is consistent with contusion and edema and the defect with a laceration. The small mineral fragments could represent avulsed bone or road debris in a wound or on the skin. Medial and lateral instability of the right talocrural joint with suspect medial collateral ligament avulsion or injury (partial or complete tear) was diagnosed by physical examination. (**E**) A flexed dorsoplantar radiograph of the left tarsus of a young dog to highlight the trochlear ridges (arrows) of the talus without superimposition of the calcaneus, used in cases of suspected osteochondritis dissecans of the talus, particularly the lateral trochlear ridge. For this projection, the dog is positioned in dorsal recumbency with the metatarsus and digits pointed to the ceiling and the beam centered at the talocrural joint space. The image is normal.

chances of projecting an edge lesion tangentially, especially in a complex joint (**fig. 3.8**).[3] The entrance point of the primary X-ray beam is typically moved 30 to 45 degrees medial (**fig. 3.8C**) or 30 to 45 degrees lateral (**fig. 3.8D**) to the entrance point used for a craniocaudal (dorsopalmar, dorsoplantar) view. Specific projections may be used to reduce superimposition when assessing complex joints, such as a flexed dorsoplantar projection of the tarsus which shows the trochlear rides of the talus without superimposition of the calcaneus (**fig. 3.8E**). Tangential or skyline radiographs (**fig. 3.8E**) (e.g., cranioproximo-craniodistal radiographs) are lesion-oriented views usually used for imaging the anatomy such as the bicipital groove of the humerus or the patellar groove of the femur and patella, e.g., in cases of sagittal patellar fractures (**fig. 3.9**).

Stress radiographs are defined as radiographs obtained with the application of a controlled force upon a joint to show and assess the severity of instability, subluxation, or luxation not apparent on standard projections (**fig. 3.10**).[4] Stress radiographs require general anesthesia to eliminate pain and ensure consistent positioning. They are made by stabilizing the limb proximal and distal to the joint

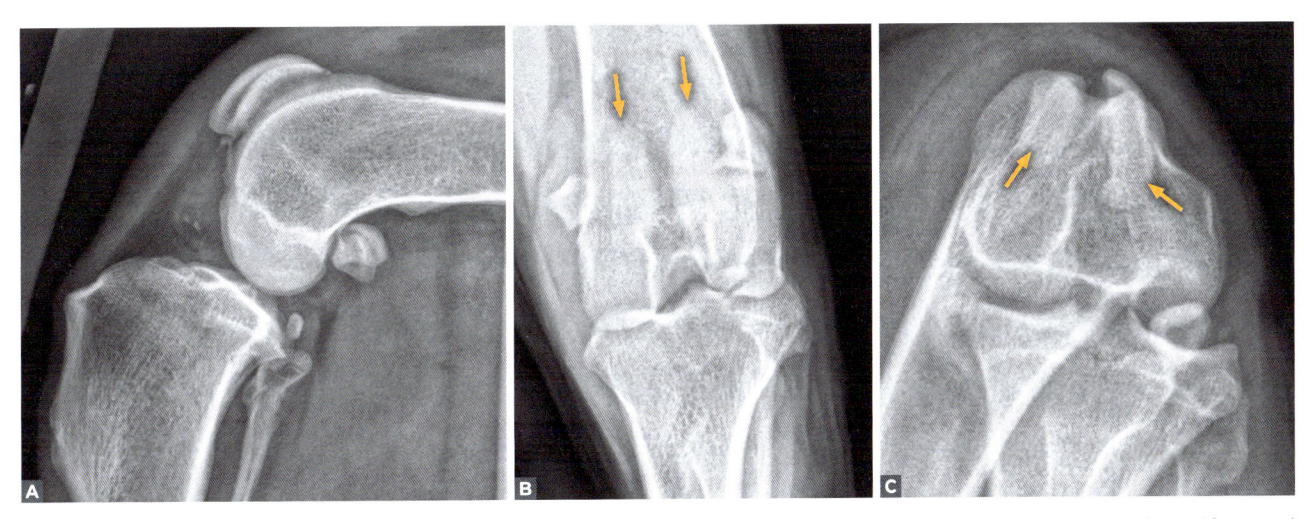

Fig. 3.9 (**A**) Mediolateral and (**B**) caudocranial radiographs of the left stifle and (**C**) a cranioproximal-craniodistal skyline view of the left distal femur and patella in a seven-year-old neutered male Doberman with acute left hind lameness after playing outside. There is intra-articular effusion in the left femorotibial joint, causing cranial displacement of the infrapatellar fat pad. There are several small, well-defined osseous fragments located at the base of the patella and within the femorotibial joint space. A complete, sagittal fracture of the left patella with sharp fracture margins can be seen superimposed on the distal femur on the caudocranial radiograph (arrows). The fracture fragments are displaced medially and laterally, exacerbated by flexion on skyline projection.

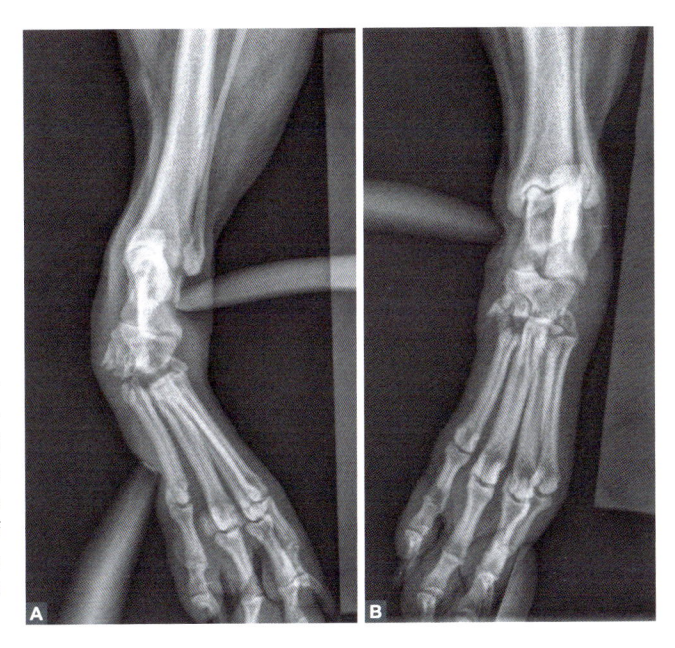

Fig. 3.10 Dorsoplantar radiographs of the left tarsus and foot with lateral (**A**) and medial (**B**) stress applied to the foot. The patient is a four-year-old spayed female Shih Tzu with lameness after jumping off the couch and with comminuted articular fractures of the distal row of the tarsal bones and head of the second metatarsal. Stress is applied with a wooden spoon to force the foot laterally (**A**) resulting in widening of the medial aspect of the tarsometatarsal joint and lateral subluxation of the metatarsals due to rupture of medial collateral ligaments and joint capsule. Stress applied to force the foot medial (**B**) shows no instability of the tarsal joints.

SECTION II APPENDICULAR SKELETON

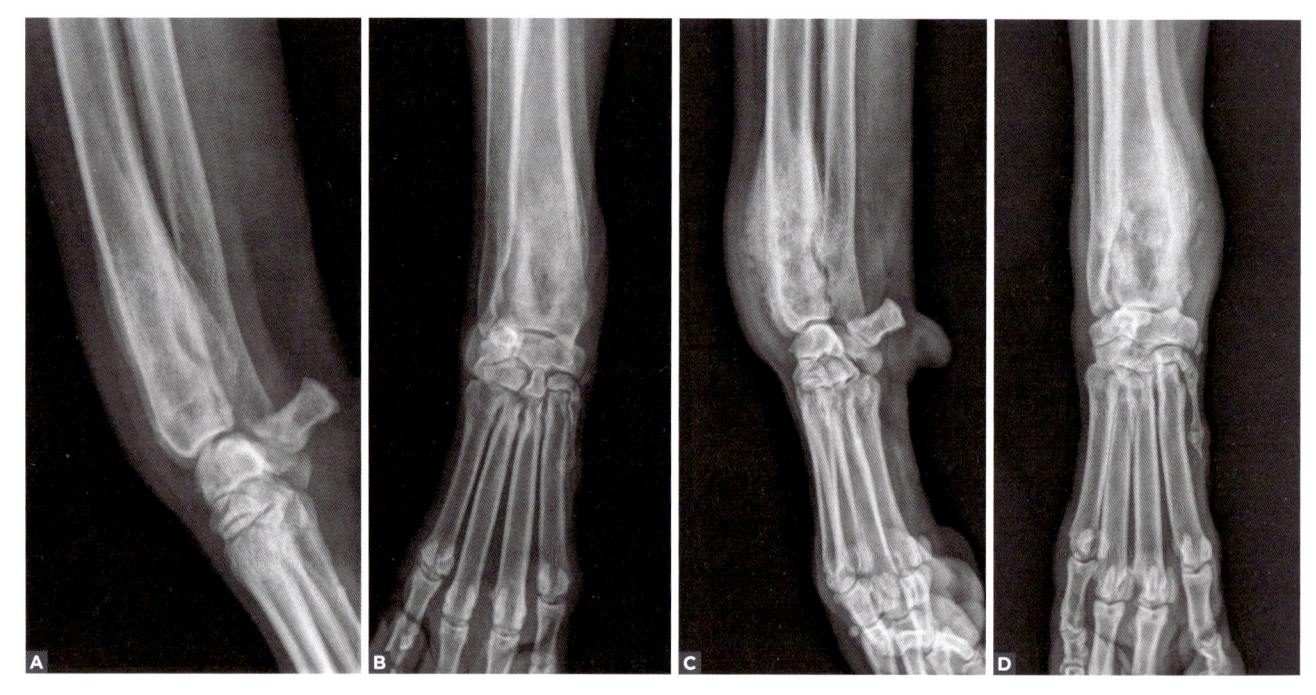

Fig. 3.11 (**A**) Mediolateral and (**B**) dorsopalmar radiographs of the right carpus of a seven-year-old neutered male Mastiff with chronic lameness due to suspected osteosarcoma. There is lysis of the trabecular bone in the medullary cavity of the distal radial metaphysis and epiphysis, seen on the dorsopalmar projection. Small foci of lysis are also visible in the medial cortex of the distal radius. There is periosteal new bone with nonuniform mineralization and smooth well-defined margins on the cranial, medial, and caudal cortices of the distal radial metaphysis and adjacent diaphysis. The lesion has an indistinct but relatively short transition to normal bone. Based on the lesion appearance, location, and patient signalment, osteosarcoma is the most likely diagnosis. Mild broad-based soft tissue swelling is noted along the cranial and medial aspects of the distal radius. Fine-needle aspirations were non-diagnostic. Mediolateral (**C**) and dorsopalmar (**D**) recheck radiographs of the right carpus obtained two months later show more severe circumferential soft tissue swelling of the right distal antebrachium. There is progressive new bone formation which shows relatively uniform mineralization but now has irregular poorly defined margins. There is progressive moth-eaten to permeative lysis within the medullary cavity. The lesion was confirmed as osteosarcoma by repeat fine-needle aspiration and cytology.

and applying force typically with wooden or plastic spoons to demonstrate joint laxity. Comparison stress radiographs with the normal side can be obtained if it is not certain that the extent of joint movement is pathological.[1] Compression or distraction radiographs are mainly used to confirm laxity of the coxofemoral joints for early diagnosis of hip dysplasia, such as PennHip® radiographs.[5] Serial radiographic examinations are also very useful in the investigation of orthopedic disease to assess the progression of remodeling over time, evaluate treatment response, and detect lesions not evident on initial images (**fig. 3.11**).[1,2] They are mostly used in the evaluation of fracture healing.

References

1. Muhlbauer MC, Kneller SK. Radiography of the Dog and Cat: Guide to Making and Interpreting Radiographs. New York, Wiley-Blackwell, 2013.
2. Baines E. Clinically significant developmental radiological changes in the skeletally immature dog: 1. Long bones. *In Practice* 28:188-199, 2006.
3. Thrall DE. Principles of Radiographic Interpretation of the Appendicular Skeleton. In Thrall DE (editor). Textbook of Veterinary Diagnostic Radiology 7th edition. St. Louis, Elsevier, 2018, pp 334-347.
4. Farrow C. Stress radiography: applications in small animal practice. *J Am Vet Med Assoc* 181:777-784, 1982.
5. Reagan JK. Canine Hip Dysplasia Screening Within the United States: Pennsylvania Hip Improvement Program and Orthopedic Foundation for Animals Hip/Elbow Database. *Vet Clin North Am Small Anim Pract* 47:795-805, 2017.
6. Kim SE, Lewis DD, Pozzi A. Effect of tibial plateau leveling osteotomy on femorotibial subluxation: in vivo analysis during standing. *Vet Surg* 41:465-470, 2012.

CHAPTER 4

Fundamental bone and joint alterations

Nathalie Rademacher

> **KEY POINTS**
>
> ▎ Degenerative joint disease (DJD) is the most common diagnosed orthopedic disorder.
> ▎ Radiographic DJD changes are non-specific and do not correlate with pain and clinical severity of lameness.
> ▎ Radiographically, primary bone neoplasms, metastatic neoplastic bone lesions, and osteomyelitis result in an aggressive bone lesion.
> ▎ In endemic areas, oligostotic bone lesions might be associated with fungal osteomyelitis.
> ▎ Histopathology is required for a definitive diagnosis.
> ▎ Benign neoplasms are uncommon.

Degenerative joint disease

Degenerative joint disease (DJD) or osteoarthrosis (OA) is the most commonly diagnosed joint disease in veterinary medicine and is a slowly progressive, irreversible degenerative disease of synovial joints characterized by pain, disability, cartilage destruction, synovitis, and bone remodeling.[1] Older dogs are usually affected; however, it is estimated that 20% of dogs one year of age or older are affected.[2] The weight-bearing joints of medium-sized to large dogs are most often affected, although it can involve any synovial joint in any dog and cat. The most frequent locations are the coxofemoral (**fig. 4.1A**), shoulder, and stifle joints. Underlying causes are numerous and include normal force on an abnormal joint (e.g., OCD, elbow [**figs. 4.1B** and **4.1B**] or hip dysplasia) or abnormal forces on a normal joint (e.g., trauma, joint instability, epiphyseal aseptic necrosis).[2]

Fig. 4.1 (**A**) Extended ventrodorsal radiographs of the pelvis of a seven-year-old, neutered male German Shepherd dog with bilateral subluxation of the coxofemoral joints with severe osteoarthrosis and severe muscle atrophy secondary to bilateral hip dysplasia. Mediolateral (**B**) and craniocaudal (**C**) radiographs of the right elbow of an eight-year-old neutered male English Bulldog with lameness associated with multiple legs. Severe degenerative changes are noted due to severe elbow osteoarthrosis, present in both elbows in this patient.

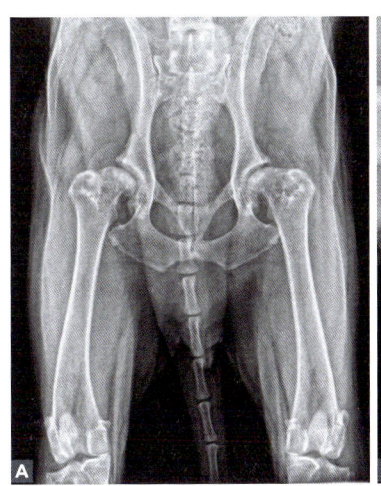

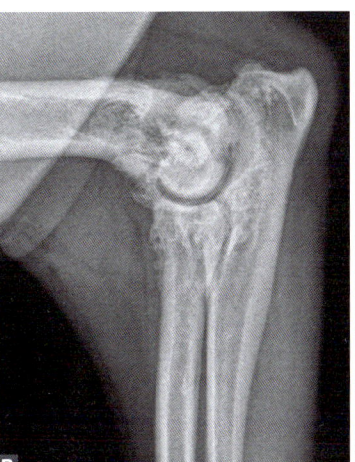

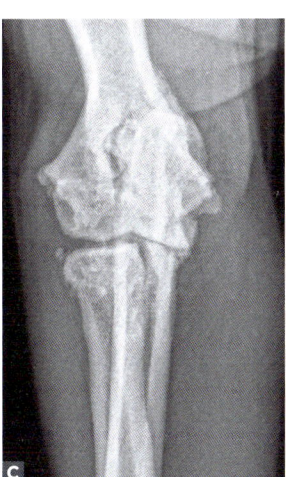

Radiographic signs develop later than the structural changes associated with DJD, and clinical signs do not correlate well with radiographic signs. Additionally, most radiographic signs of joint disease are nonspecific. Also, patients with progressive joint disease may have different signs when examined during different phases of the disease. Sound knowledge of joint pathophysiologic characteristics is as important in the diagnosis of joint disease as the ability to make and interpret radiographs of joints. Radiographic signs of DJD[3] include:

- Joint swelling.
- Decreased subchondral bone opacity.
- Increased subchondral bone opacity.
- Subchondral osseous cyst-like lesions.
- Perichondral bony proliferation (osteophytes).
- Enthesophytes.
- Mineralization of periarticular soft tissues.
- Intra-articular calcified bodies.
- Joint luxation, subluxation, or incongruency.
- Joint malformation.

Osteophytes consist of cartilage and later become radiographically visible when they become ossified. They are seen as bony outgrowths at the periphery of the articular cartilage. Enthesophytes are bony proliferations at the level of the joint capsule, ligaments, tendons, or fascia insertion into the bone.

General radiographic principles for evaluation of aggressive bone lesions

Radiographic abnormalities of bones and joints are usually divided into non-aggressive (trauma, degenerative changes) and aggressive lesions (neoplasia, osteomyelitis) based on radiographic findings. Various disease processes can have overlapping radiographic findings, and cytology or histopathology is almost always needed for a definitive diagnosis. Radiographic aggressive bone lesions result either from neoplastic or infectious causes and radiographic signs are listed here:[4]

- Soft tissue swelling can be either articular, periarticular, or superficial.
- Number of bones involved can be monostotic, oligostotic, or polyostotic.
- Location of the lesion might be metaphyseal, diaphyseal, or centered on a joint.
- Periosteal new bone formation can be the result of neoplasia, infection, trauma, or septic arthritis and can elevate the periosteum and form various patterns of periosteal reaction.
- Considerable overlap with different disease processes and different periosteal reactions has been reported.[5] Smooth periosteal reaction is primarily seen with benign, slow processes such as a healing fracture[5] and is a uniformly opaque single layer of new bone formation (**fig. 4.2A**). Lamellar periosteal reactions are multiple layers of bone concentrically layered like an onion skin appearance (**fig. 4.2B**). Spiculated periosteal reaction is the result of a rapid underlying process preventing the formation of new bone under the raised periosteum and is often subdivided into a columnar or palisading periosteal reaction that is radiographically seen as vertically oriented columns of new bone oriented perpendicular to the cortex (**fig. 4.2C**), whereas in sunburst periosteal reaction it radiates in a divergent pattern (**fig. 4.2 D**), and amorphous being irregular and disorganized (**fig. 4.2E**).[5]
- Lysis is differentiated into geographic, moth-eaten, or permeative lysis, indicating the progressive degree of aggressiveness. Geographic lysis is radiographically seen as a single, large, relatively well-defined region of bone loss (**fig. 4.3A**), whereas moth-eaten lysis is represented as multiple medium to small foci of bone loss (**fig. 4.3B**), and permeative lysis is seen as multiple pinpoint foci of bone loss (**fig. 4.3C**).[6]

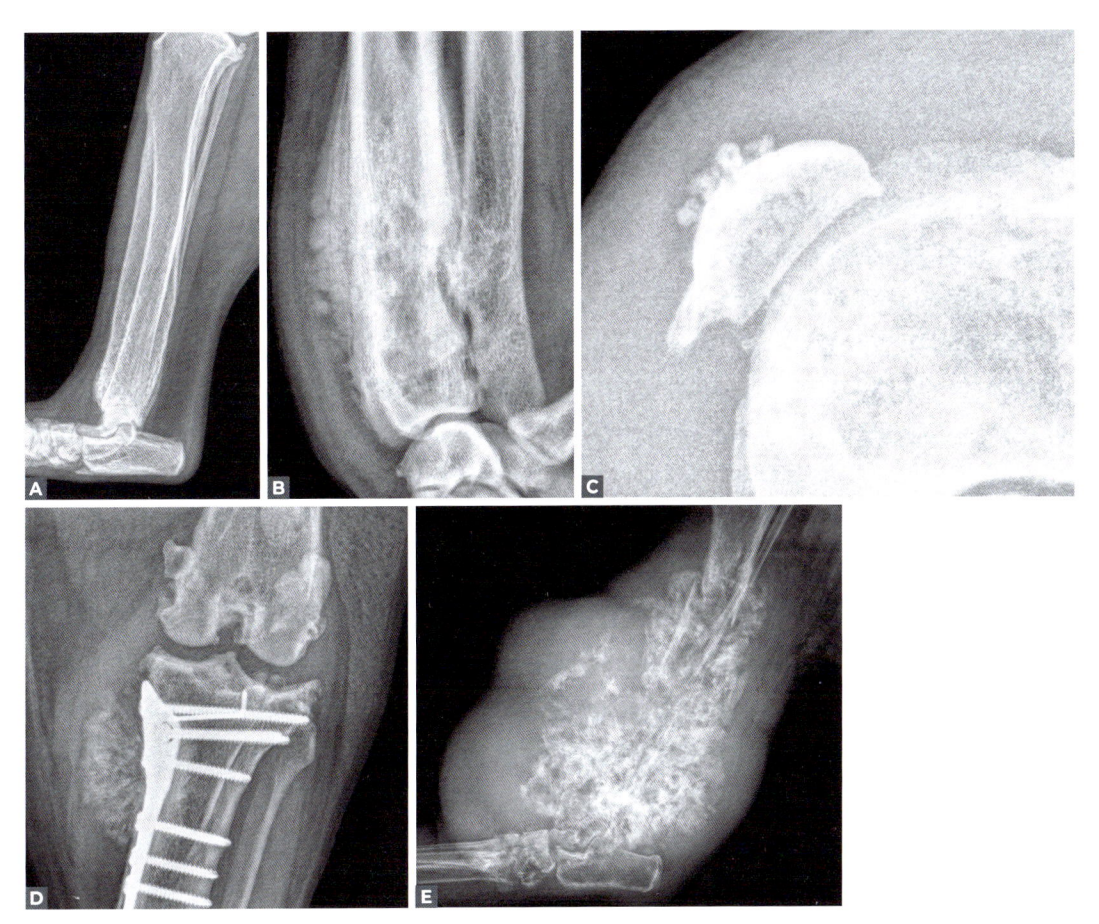

CHAPTER **4** Fundamental bone and joint alterations

Fig. 4.2 (A) A smooth, uniformly opaque single layer of new bone formation is noted along the tibial diaphysis in this five-year-old spayed female Siberian Husky with hypertrophic osteopathy due to a mediastinal histiocytic sarcoma. (B) Note the faint multiple concentric layers of bone in this male neutered seven-year-old Mastiff with lamellar periosteal reaction at the right cranio-distal radius due to osteosarcoma. (C) Note the vertically oriented columns of new bone oriented perpendicular to the patella cortex representing spiculated periosteal reaction of the left stifle in this seven-year-old male Mastiff diagnosed with histiocytic sarcoma. (D) Note the divergent pattern representing sunburst periosteal new bone formation medial along the proximal tibia in this Rottweiler with confirmed implant-associated osteosarcoma. (E) Note the highly disorganized and irregular new bone formation in this four-year-old spayed female Rottweiler consistent with amorphous periosteal reaction due to osteosarcoma.

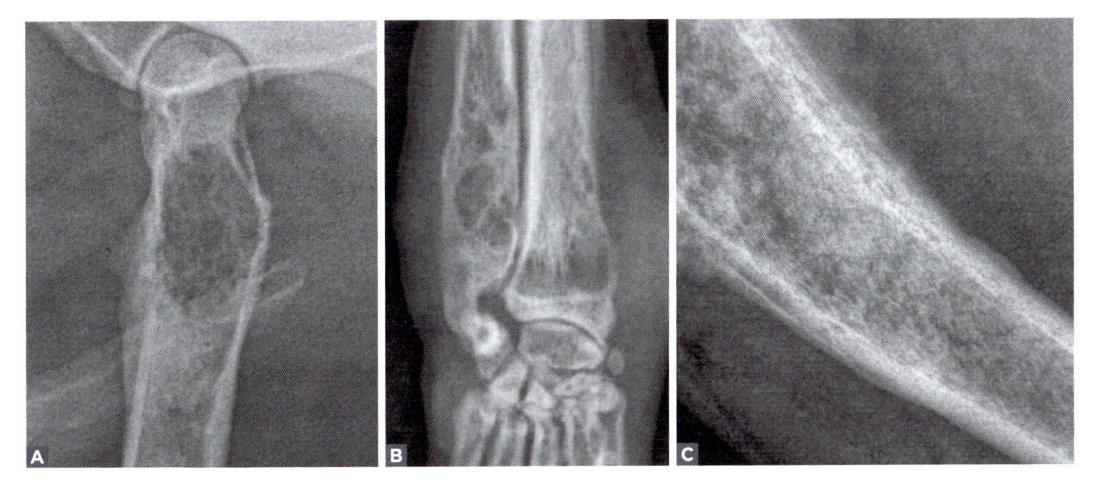

Fig. 4.3 (A) Geographic lytic lesion seen as a well-defined, slightly irregularly marginated radiolucency noted in the right proximal femur on the mediolateral radiograph of a three-year-old male Labrador Retriever with confirmed osteosarcoma. (B) Craniocaudal radiograph of the right carpus in an adult spayed female Domestic medium hair cat with confirmed histoplasmosis. Note the moth-eaten lysis of the distal ulna and radius seen as multiple small to medium-sized areas of bone loss. (C) Multiple faint pinpoint foci of bone loss representing permeative lysis are noted in the right humerus of an eight-year-old intact male Irish Setter with confirmed osteosarcoma at this location.

SECTION II APPENDICULAR SKELETON

▎A long zone of transition is characterized by an incomplete or poorly defined demarcation of the lesion to normal bone within the medullary cavity.

Bone neoplasia

Osteosarcoma is the most common primary malignant bone tumor in dogs and cats and represents more than 80% in dogs and 70% in cats of primary neoplasms originating from the skeleton,[7] followed by chondrosarcomas, fibrosarcoma, and hemangiosarcoma. Large and giant breed dogs (mainly German Shepherds, Rottweilers, Doberman Pinschers, Irish Setters and Boxers, Saint Bernards, Great Danes, Golden, and Labrador Retrievers)[7,8] are overrepresented with a bimodal age distribution (with peak incidence at 1-2 years and 7-9 years of age)[9] and in cats older than ten years. Osteosarcoma can occur anywhere in the skeleton but most commonly in the metaphyses of the distal radius (**fig. 4.4**), proximal humerus (**fig. 4.5**), distal femur and proximal and distal tibia in dogs.[9] The distal radius is associated with a lower rate of metastasis, while localization at the proximal humerus, distal femur, or proximal tibia has a high metastasis rate and increased mortality.[10] In cats, the hindlimbs seem to be more affected, and the lesion appears to be more lytic. Unlike dogs, osteosarcomas in cats are locally invasive but slow to metastasize, with an overall incidence of metastatic rate less than 10%. Appendicular osteosarcomas may be primarily lytic, primarily productive, or most commonly mixed, with lytic and productive features. Primary bone tumors typically affect a single metaphysis of a long bone and may extend into the epiphysis or diaphysis or adjacent bone joints. The occurrence of implant-associated osteosarcoma is extremely low (0.0008%).[11] Benign bone tumors such as osteoma, osteochondroma, and bone cysts are uncommon.[7]

Metastatic bone tumors arise more commonly from carcinomas than sarcomas,[12] and mammary and pulmonary neoplasms are a common source of bone metastasis[13] and can be found either in axial or appendicular skeleton (**fig. 4.6**).

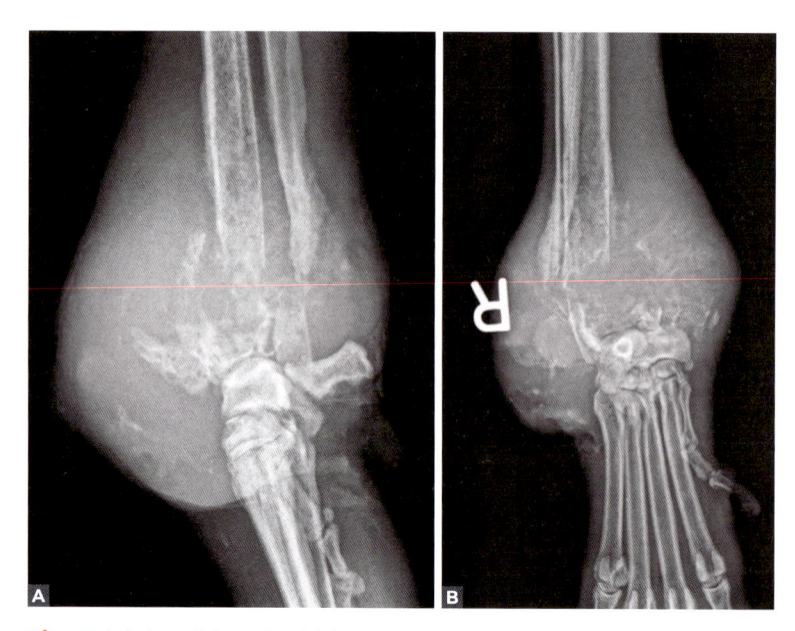

Fig. 4.4 (**A**) Mediolateral and (**B**) craniocaudal radiographs of the right distal radius of an eight-year-old intact male Irish Setter. Severe soft swelling, cortical destruction, permeative lysis, and irregular periosteal new bone formation of the distal metaphysis of the right radius are present with a pathologic fracture of the distal radius and ulna with craniomedial displacement. This dog was diagnosed with osteosarcoma.

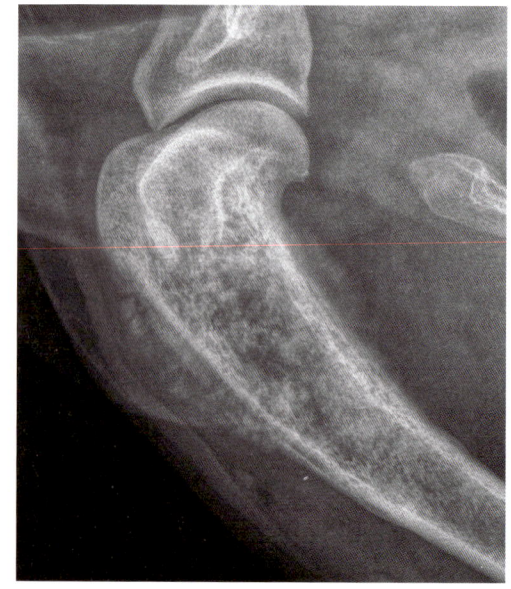

Fig. 4.5 Mediolateral radiograph of the right humerus of a nine-year-old spayed female Rottweiler with moth-eaten lysis, cortical thinning, and palisading new bone formation of the proximal metaphysis of the right humerus due to confirmed osteosarcoma.

CHAPTER **4** Fundamental bone and joint alterations

Radiographic appearance can vary from bone lysis to new bone formation changes, and all the intermediates between these two extremes include soft tissue swelling, cortical destruction, periosteal reaction, a long zone of transition characterized by an incomplete or poorly defined demarcation of the lesion to normal bone within the medullary cavity and lysis of the cortex and or medulla.[4, 7] Neoplasia (primary bone tumors, metastasis) and fungal or bacterial osteomyelitis both result in radiographic aggressive bone lesions and require biopsy and histopathology for a definitive diagnosis. Additional findings such as the number of bones involved (monostotic, oligostotic, polyostotic), location (metaphyseal, diaphyseal), signalment, history, physical and laboratory findings as well as geographic location can help prioritize (**table 4.1**) for differential diagnoses. Pathologic fractures can occur without abnormal or overt trauma due to weakening of the bone (**fig. 4.4**). Radiographs remain the main imaging modality in veterinary medicine for bone neoplasia evaluation; however, CT and MRI are more and more used in veterinary medicine.[7] CT allows evaluation of bone destruction and sclerosis anatomically, which is particularly useful for axial sites. MRI can assess the tumor extent and its relationship with the surrounding structures, which is particularly interesting for axial sites, given the proximity of the vertebral canal.

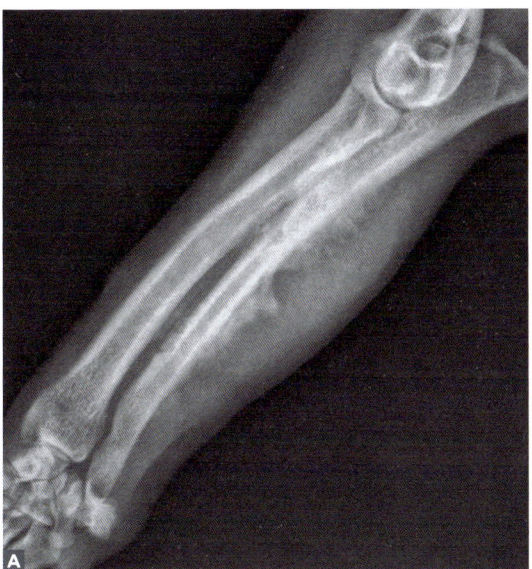

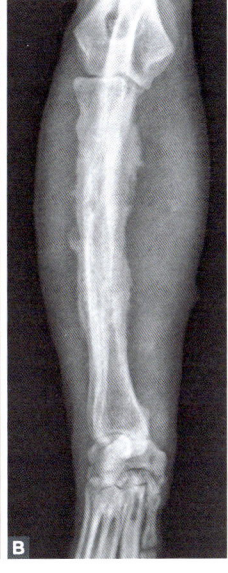

Fig. 4.6 (**A**) Mediolateral and (**B**) craniocaudal radiograph of the right radius and ulna of a 14-year-old male Shih Tzu with confirmed metastatic carcinoma. Note the irregular, partially palisading periosteal reaction with minimal cortical destruction with a long zone of transition along the ulnar diaphysis.

Subungual tumors versus subungual infections

The digit is also a location where radiographic differentiation between infectious and neoplastic bone lesions is impossible. The most common canine subungual tumor is squamous cell carcinoma (**fig. 4.7**), commonly occurring in large breed dogs with black hair coats, followed by melanomas.[14] Inflammatory conditions of the digit are also common. Digital tumors typically involve a single digit. A syndrome of metastasis of pulmonary tumors to multiple digits has been identified in cats[15] (so-called "lung digit syndrome") (**fig. 4.8**).

Table 4.1 Summary of radiographic features for differentiation of aggressive bone lesions.			
Bone pathology	**Location**	**Mono-or polyostotic**	**Age**
Primary bone tumor	Metaphysis	Monostotic	Bimodal
Metastatic	Metaphysis or diaphysis	Polyostotic	Old
Multifocal tumors	Anywhere	Polyostotic	Old
Fungal osteomyelitis	Diaphysis	Mono-, oligostotic	Young to middle age
Bacterial osteomyelitis, hematogenous	Metaphysis	Polyostotic	Young
Bacterial osteomyelitis, penetrating trauma	Anywhere	Monostotic or adjacent bones	Any

SECTION II APPENDICULAR SKELETON

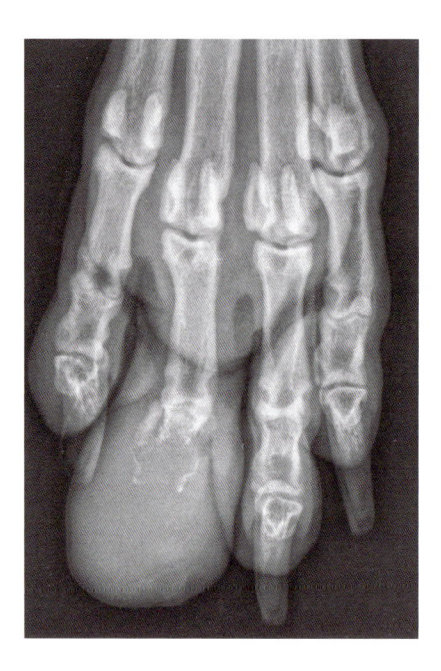

Fig. 4.7 Dorsopalmar radiograph of the right front foot of a 16-year-old neutered male Rottweiler with a confirmed subungual melanoma affecting the fourth digit with absent P3 and aggressive bone lesion of the distal portion of P2 of the same digit with associated severe soft tissue swelling.

Fig. 4.8 (**A**) Mediolateral radiograph of the left hind foot and (**B**) plantarodorsal view of the right hind foot of a nine-year-old spayed female cat with a two-month history of swollen and ulcerated digits on the right front and bilateral hind feet. Polyostotic aggressive bone lesions affecting P3 of all digits of the left hind and third digit on the right hindlimb are noted in this cat, consistent with metastatic carcinoma. (**C**) Ventrodorsal thoracic view of the same cat as figs. 4.8A and 4.8B. A well-defined, smooth to irregularly marginated cavitary mass within the left caudal lung lobe at the level of the left caudal lobar bronchus is present. This is consistent with primary lung neoplasia, and bronchial carcinoma is confirmed.

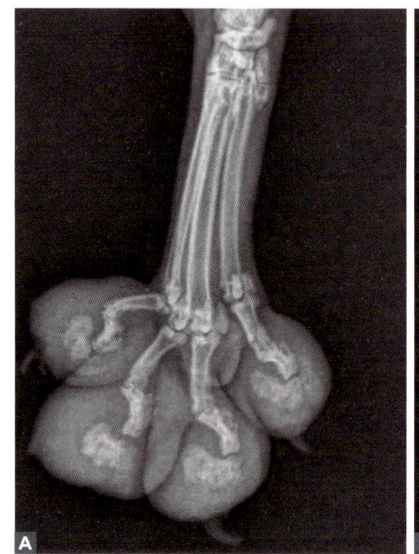

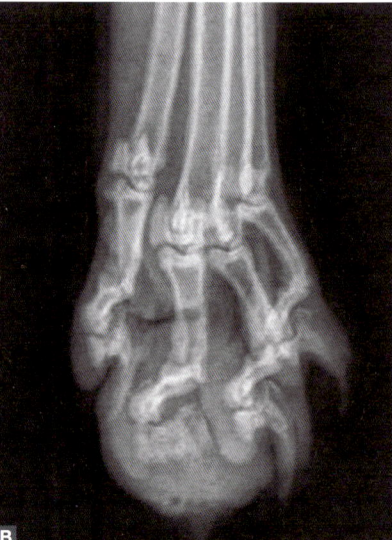

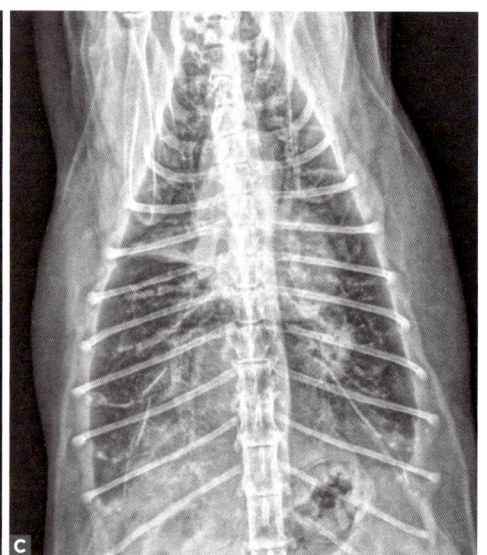

Osteomyelitis

Osteomyelitis, the inflammation of bone and bone marrow, might be either of exogenous or hematogenous origin and might be caused by bacterial or fungal organisms, with both resulting in radiographic aggressive bone lesions.[16] Bacterial infections typically result from exogenous causes such as a penetrating injury from an open fracture and after a car accident (78%), a bite wound (17%), ascending infection due to pododermatitis (5%), or surgery (**fig. 4.9**) and, less commonly, from hematogenous spread.[17,18] One study reported that exogenous osteomyelitis is more frequently caused by a single microorganism in 59% of cases with a predominance of Gram-positive bacteria, most frequently *Staphylococcus* spp., followed by *Streptococcus* spp., *Escherichia coli*, other enteric bacteria, and anaerobic bacteria.[16] Most lesions from bacterial osteomyelitis will have a periosteal reaction that is less aggressive than with a neoplastic lesion. Periosteal reactions with osteomyelitis often have a palisading or columnar appearance, but columnar periosteal reactions can sometimes

CHAPTER 4 Fundamental bone and joint alterations

be found with neoplastic bone lesions as well. Hematogenous bacterial osteomyelitis lesions are usually polyostotic and occur in young dogs and therefore are not typical for neoplastic disease. Sampling and microbiologic testing should always be performed before the initiation of any treatment.

Fungal osteomyelitis should be considered when polyostotic aggressive bone lesions are present. Typically, large breed young adults are affected, generally of hematogenous origin, and are most commonly identified in geographic endemic areas, such as the Midwest/Mississippi valley and Eastern USA and Canada (blastomycosis) and the desert southwest (coccidioidomycosis) regions of the United States (fig. 4.10). However, cases may be seen in non-endemic regions when infected dogs are relocated or become infected when traveling, and a complete travel history should be obtained. Dogs with osteomyelitis caused by *Coccidioides* spp. were younger and weighed less compared to dogs with osteosarcoma in a recently published study with axial lesions and nonadjacent polyostotic disease more common, but the radiographic appearance did not differ between osteomyelitis and osteosarcoma.[19] Fungal osteomyelitis in cats is rare, with the most commonly reported being histoplasmosis[20] (fig. 4.11) with a high prevalence in the Midwest and

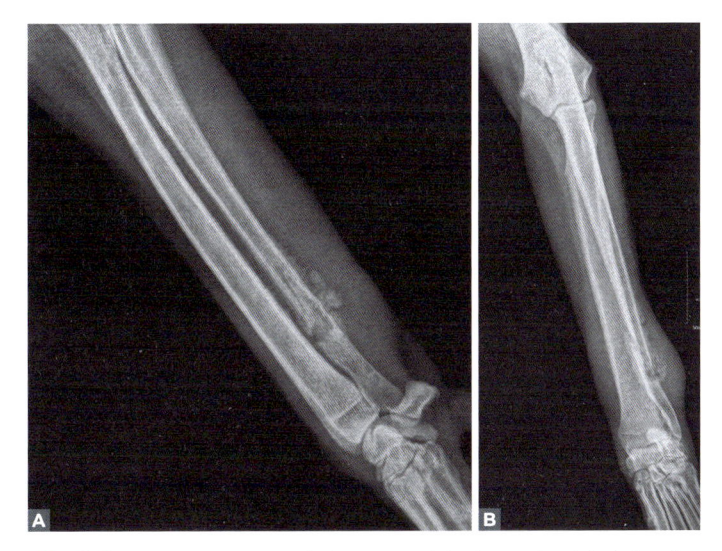

Fig. 4.9 (A) Mediolateral and (B) craniocaudal radiographs of the left radius and ulna of a ten-year-old neutered male Weimaraner that was bitten 10 days before and ran into a wheelbarrow after. Note the large focal soft tissue swelling of the distal ulna with amorphous periosteal reaction and focal cortical destruction due to the reported bite wound. This was confirmed as bacterial osteomyelitis.

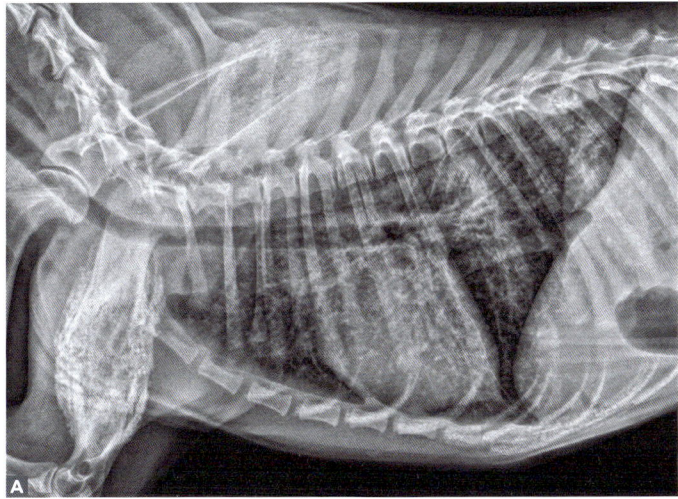

Fig. 4.10 (A) Left lateral and (B) ventrodorsal views of the thorax of a seven-month-old intact male Pitbull with polyostotic aggressive bone lesions of the left humerus, left scapula, right ulna, and multiple ribs with miliary nodular pulmonary pattern and sternal lymphadenopathy confirmed due to coccidioidomycosis.

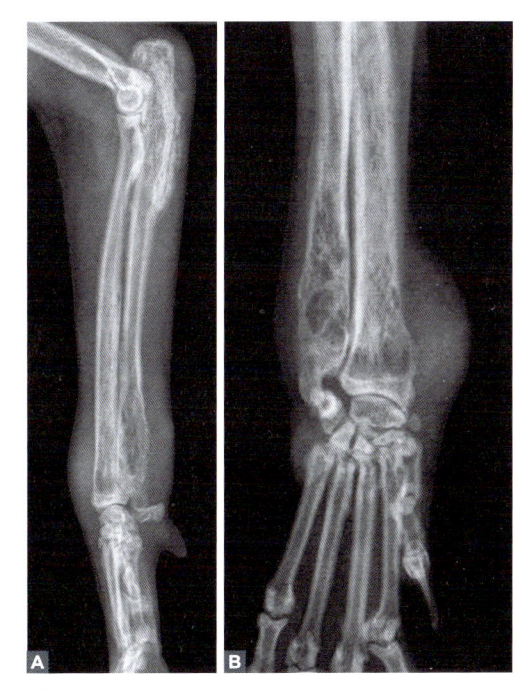

Fig. 4.11 (A) Mediolateral radiograph of the right radius and ulna and (B) craniocaudal radiograph of the right carpus in a female spayed Domestic medium hair cat of unknown age with confirmed fungal osteomyelitis due to histoplasmosis affecting the distal radius and ulna as well as the proximal ulna.

South of the US, with inflammatory arthritis a common presentation.[20] However, over the past 20 years, the incidence of opportunistic fungal infection has increased substantially in dogs receiving multiagent immunosuppressive therapy, with a recent study showing an incidence of 6.5% in dogs being treated for immune-mediated disease.[21]

References

1. McLaughlin R. Management of chronic osteoarthritic pain. *Vet Clin North Am Small Anim Pract* 30:933-949, ix, 2000.
2. Johnston SA. Osteoarthritis. *Vet Clin North Am Small Anim Pract* 27:699-723, 1997.
3. Allan G, Davies S. Radiographic signs of joint disease in dogs and cats. In Thrall DE (editor). Textbook of Veterinary Diagnostic Radiology 7th edition. St. Louis, Elsevier, 2016, pp 403-433.
4. Thrall DE. Principles of radiographic interpretation of the appendicular skeleton. In Thrall DE (editor). Textbook of Veterinary Diagnostic Radiology 7th edition. St. Louis, Elsevier, 2016, pp 334-347.
5. Rana RS, Wu JS, Eisenberg RL. Periosteal reaction. *AJR Am J Roentgenol* 193:W259-272, 2009.
6. Thrall DE. Radiographic features of bone tumors and bone infections in dogs and cats. In Thrall DE (editor). Textbook of Veterinary Diagnostic Radiology 7th edition. St. Louis, Elsevier, 2016, pp 390-402.
7. Vanel M, Blond L, Vanel D. Imaging of primary bone tumors in veterinary medicine: which differences? *Eur J Radiol* 82:2129-2139, 2013.
8. Szewczyk M, Lechowski R, Zabielska K. What do we know about canine osteosarcoma treatment? Review. *Vet Res Commun* 39:61-67, 2015.
9. Guim TN, Bianchi MV, De Lorenzo C, Gouvea AS, Gerardi DG, Driemeier D, et al. Relationship between clinicopathological features and prognosis in appendicular osteosarcoma in dogs. *J Comp Pathol* 180:91-99, 2020.
10. Schmidt AF, Nielen M, Klungel OH, Hoes AW, de Boer A, Groenwold RH, et al. Prognostic factors of early metastasis and mortality in dogs with appendicular osteosarcoma after receiving surgery: an individual patient data meta-analysis. *Prev Vet Med* 112:414-422, 2013.
11. Arthur EG, Arthur GL, Keeler MR, Bryan JN. Risk of osteosarcoma in dogs after open fracture fixation. *Vet Surg* 45:30-35, 2016.
12. Cooley DM, Waters DJ. Skeletal metastasis as the initial clinical manifestation of metastatic carcinoma in 19 dogs. *J Vet Intern Med* 12:288-293, 1998.
13. Trost ME, Inkelmann MA, Galiza GJ, Silva TM, Kommers GD. Occurrence of tumours metastatic to bones and multicentric tumours with skeletal involvement in dogs. *J Comp Pathol* 150:8-17, 2014.
14. Grassinger JM, Floren A, Muller T, Cerezo-Echevarria A, Beitzinger C, Conrad D, et al. Digital lesions in dogs: A statistical breed analysis of 2912 cases. *Vet Sci* 8:136, 2021.
15. Gottfried SD, Popovitch CA, Goldschmidt MH, Schelling C. Metastatic digital carcinoma in the cat: a retrospective study of 36 cats (1992-1998). *J Am Anim Hosp Assoc* 36:501-509, 2000.
16. Siqueira EG, Rahal SC, Ribeiro MG, Paes AC, Listoni FP, Vassalo FG. Exogenous bacterial osteomyelitis in 52 dogs: a retrospective study of etiology and in vitro antimicrobial susceptibility profile (2000-2013). *Vet Q* 34:201-204, 2014.
17. Gieling F, Peters S, Erichsen C, Richards RG, Zeiter S, Moriarty TF. Bacterial osteomyelitis in veterinary orthopaedics: pathophysiology, clinical presentation and advances in treatment across multiple species. *Vet J* 250:44-54, 2019.
18. Rabillard M, Souchu L, Niebauer GW, Gauthier O. Haematogenous osteomyelitis: clinical presentation and outcome in three dogs. *Vet Comp Orthop Traumatol* 24:146-150, 2011.
19. Shaver SL, Foy DS, Carter TD. Clinical features, treatment, and outcome of dogs with Coccidioides osteomyelitis. *J Am Vet Med Assoc* 260:63-70, 2021.
20. Fielder SE, Meinkoth JH, Rizzi TE, Hanzlicek AS, Hallman RM. Feline histoplasmosis presenting with bone and joint involvement: clinical and diagnostic findings in 25 cats. *J Feline Med Surg* 21:887-892, 2019.
21. Dedeaux A, Grooters A, Wakamatsu-Utsuki N, Taboada J. Opportunistic fungal infections in small animals. *J Am Anim Hosp Assoc* 54:327-337, 2018.

CHAPTER 5

Fractures

Cliona Skelly and Hester McAllister

KEY POINTS

- Standard positioning and good quality images are paramount for identification of fractures and especially for subtle lesions.
- Oblique, positional or tangential projections may be necessary.
- Complex joints may need computed tomography (CT) to fully evaluate the full extent of the problem.
- Physeal injuries may cause abnormal growth and development of limbs.
- Fracture healing is not visible on radiographs for 7-10 days after injury.
- Pathological fractures should be suspected if there is no history of trauma.

A fracture is a discontinuity of bone disrupting its normal integrity when a direct or indirect force is applied, that is greater than the bone's inherent strength. The majority of fractures in dogs and cats are a result of blunt force trauma. However, underlying disease processes, such as osteopenia, osteomyelitis or neoplasia can undermine the strength of the bone and result in pathological fractures due to a reduced or even negligible causative force. Stress or fatigue fractures can also occur as result of repetitive stress and are primarily seen in racing or working dogs.

When describing fractures, the anatomical location, the degree of separation, displacement, angulation, rotation, foreshortening and the fragmentation should be noted. In long bone fractures, the position and orientation of the distal fragment is reported relative to the proximal fragment.

Fracture classification

Fractures may be classified in different ways and usually more than one classifying term is needed for complete description (**fig. 5.1**). The broadest generic classification[1] is whether the fracture is a closed (simple) fracture, in which the skin remains intact, or an open (compound) fracture, when the skin at the site of fracture is breached. Gas in the soft tissues adjacent to a fracture may obscure or mimic fracture lines.

Incomplete fractures are usually seen in long bones that are immature or demineralized. The bone in a partial or incomplete fracture remains in one piece as only one cortex is disrupted. They can be subdivided into greenstick fractures, where the cortical disruption occurs on the convex side of the diaphysis, torus (or buckle) fractures that have concave sided cortical disruption, with both types resulting in abnormal diaphyseal curvature.

Fig. 5.1 Types of fracture diagram: (**A**) transverse, (**B**) oblique, (**C**) spiral, (**D**) comminuted, (**E**) incomplete, (**F**) segmental.

Fig. 5.2 Salter-Harris classification: normal physis and Salter-Harris fracture types.

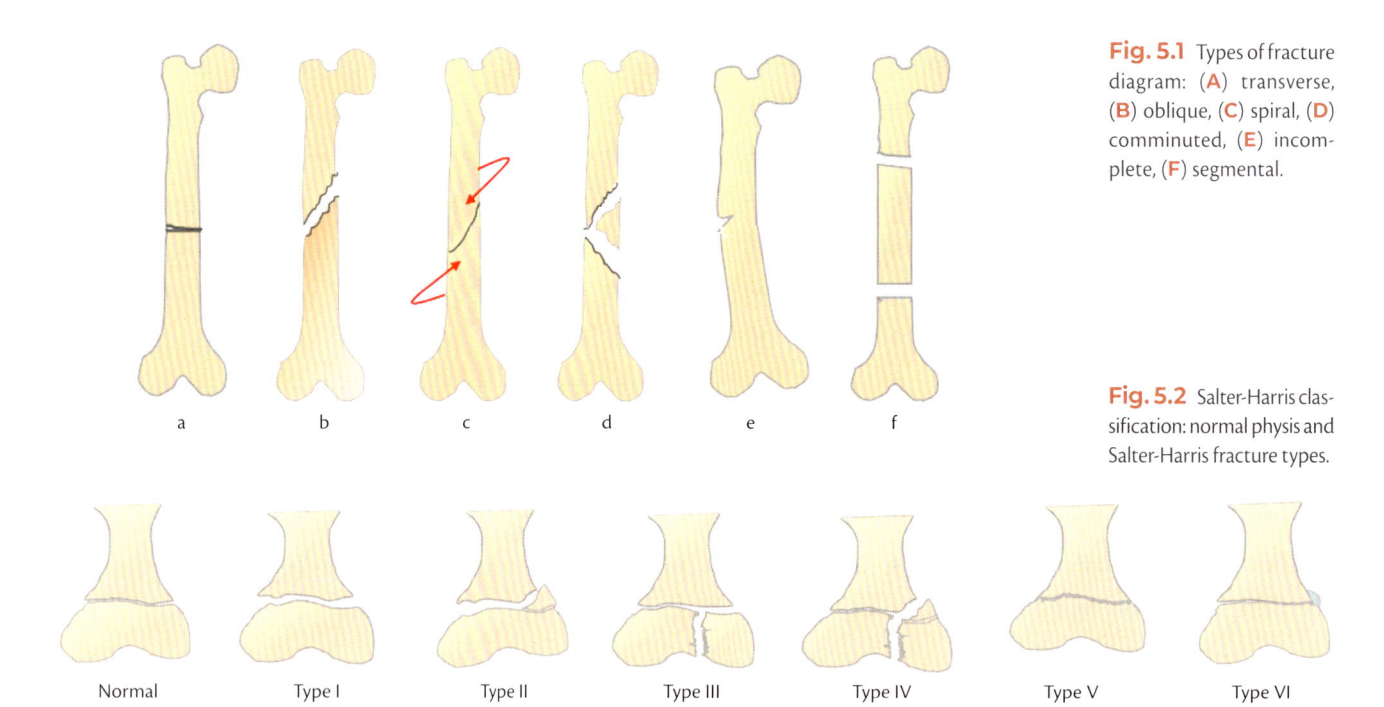

"Folding" fractures are incomplete fractures where one cortex folds or crumples in on itself, and are associated with skeletal demineralization due to nutritional secondary hyperparathyroidism.

For complete fractures, the number of bone fragments is a classifying descriptor as well as the angle of the fracture. Fracture lines are termed transverse if oriented perpendicular to the long axis of the bone or oblique when the fracture line is oriented at an angle to the long axis. The position of the distal or caudal fragment or fragments in relation to the proximal or cranial fracture segment is used to describe the fracture displacement.

A segmental fracture has two or more fracture lines within the same bone with a sizeable, separated, usually cylindrical interposed fragment. A comminuted fracture has three or more fracture fragments. The term "multiple" is used when fracture lines do not connect within the same bone. In young animals, fractures through or adjacent to a growth plate are classified under the Salter-Harris System,[2] (**fig. 5.2**). Physeal fractures may disrupt normal endochondral ossification and result in premature closure or asynchronous growth of the physis with subsequent angular limb deformities (**fig. 5.3**).

Other fracture types include impacted or compression fractures, when fracture fragments are driven vertically into each other and cause an increased opacity of the cortex or medulla. Slab fractures are vertical fractures through the cuboidal bones of the carpus and tarsus and are invariably articular (**fig. 5.4**). Chip fractures usually occur at the bone margin adjacent to a joint. Avulsion fractures are fractures that occur at the site of insertion of tendons or ligaments and occur as a result of their abnormal pulling action (**fig. 5.5**). Monteggia fractures occur through the proximal ulna with an associated luxation of the radial head (**fig. 5.6**).

Stressed radiographic views are often useful to demonstrate joint stability as a result of periarticular fractures (**fig. 5.7**). Shearing type fractures may result in complete traumatic amputation of bone fragments (**fig. 5.8**).

It is important to differentiate radiolucent fracture lines from normal bone structures and anatomical variants. Anatomical confounders include open and closing physes, nutrient foramina, fascial planes and Mach lines,[3,4] which are optical illusions caused by superimposing bones creating radiolucent lines mimicking fractures (**fig. 5.9**). Mach lines must be differentiated from true fissure fractures (**fig. 5.10**).

CHAPTER 5 Fractures

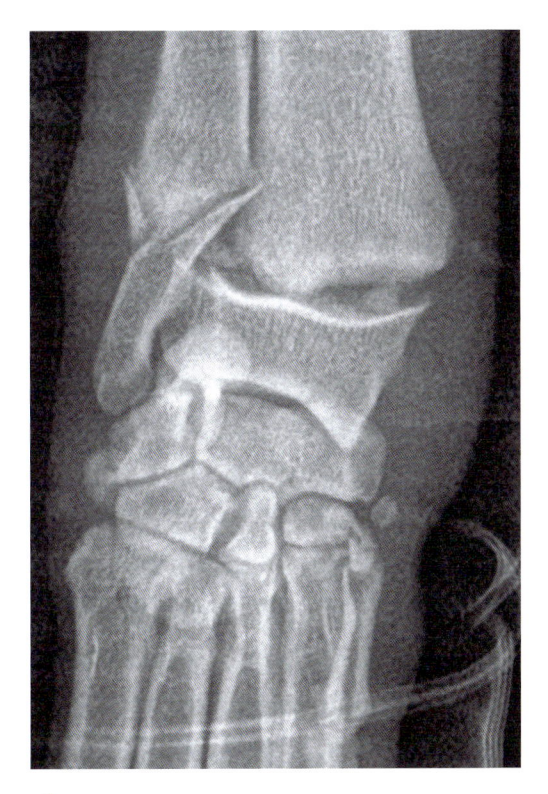

Fig. 5.3 Craniocaudal projection of the distal antebrachium of a nine-month-old Labrador Retriever. Physeal separation with lateral displacement of the distal radial epiphysis– type 1 Salter-Harris. Narrowing of the lateral half of the distal ulnar physis due to impaction– type V Salter-Harris.

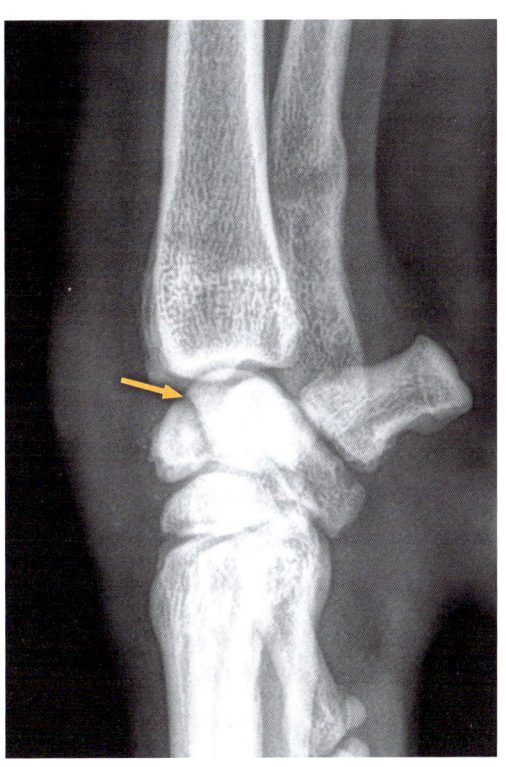

Fig. 5.4 Mediolateral projection of the carpus of a seven-year-old English Springer Spaniel. Minimally displaced slab fracture through the intermedioradial carpal bone (IRCB) extending vertically from the antebrachiocarpal to the intercarpal joint (arrow). There is an associated soft tissue swelling, IRCB sclerosis and osteophytosis primarily of the IRCB and accessory carpal bones. Fracture of radial carpal bone.

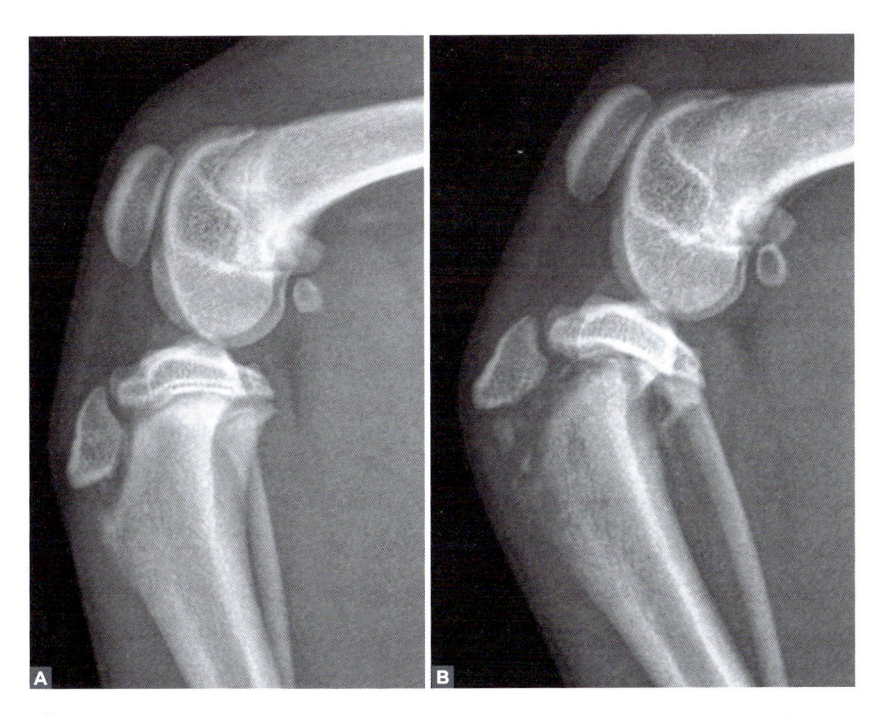

Fig. 5.5 Mediolateral studies of the stifle joints of a six-month-old Miniature Schnauzer. (**A**) Normal right stifle joint for comparison. (**B**) Left stifle; the tibial tuberosity is avulsed from the tibia and has been distracted proximally. It remains attached to the proximal tibial epiphysis, which is displaced caudally with two triangular attached metaphyseal fractures evident immediately caudal to the proximal tibial diaphysis. Type 2 Salter-Harris fracture.

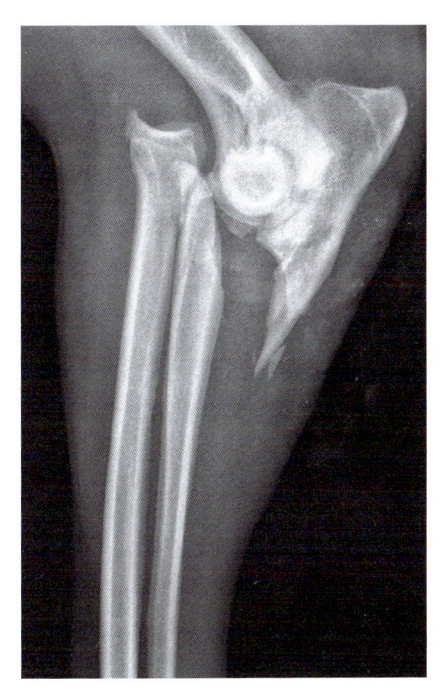

Fig. 5.6 Mediolateral projection of the antebrachium of a four-year-old Old English Sheepdog. An articular, vertically orientated, oblique fracture through the proximal ulnar diaphysis. The distal ulnar fragment is cranioproximally displaced as is the luxated radial head. This is a Monteggia fracture.

43

SECTION II APPENDICULAR SKELETON

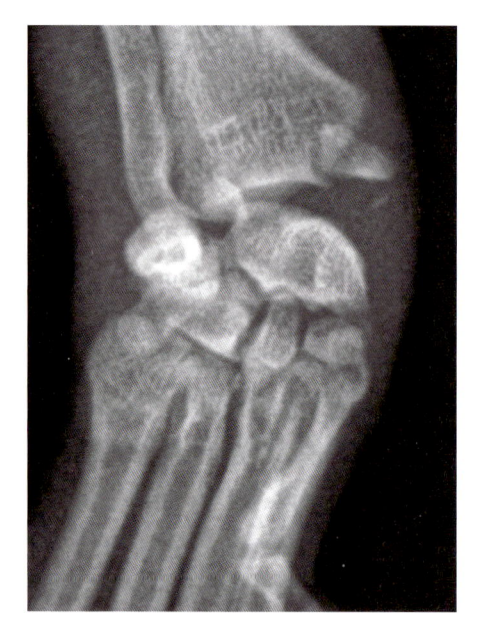

Fig. 5.7 Dorsopalmar projection of the carpus of a four-year-old Chihuahua with lateral stress applied to the metacarpal region. Widening of the antebrachiocarpal joint medially with an avulsed triangular fracture fragment off the distomedial aspect of the radius at the site of attachment of the medial collateral ligament. The ensuing joint instability evident on the stressed view was inapparent on the standard dorsopalmar projection. Fracture of the styloid process of the radius.

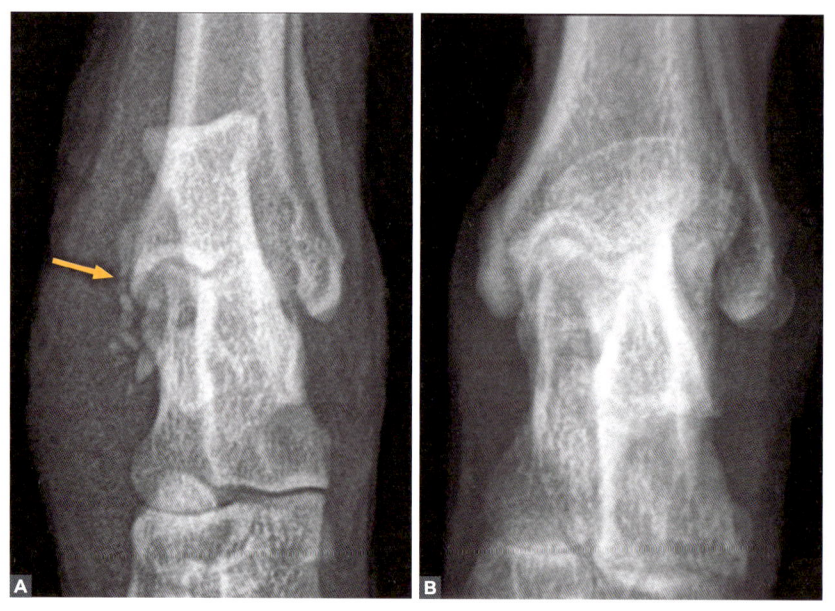

Fig. 5.8 Dorsoplantar projections of the right and left tarsii of a two-year-old Cockerpoo that was involved in a road traffic accident. (**A**) The medial malleolus of the right tibia is completely absent and there is extensive soft tissue swelling (arrow). This type of injury results in joint instability and stressed views should be considered. (**B**) Normal dorsoplantar projection of the left tarsus for comparison. Fracture of medial malleolus of the right tibia.

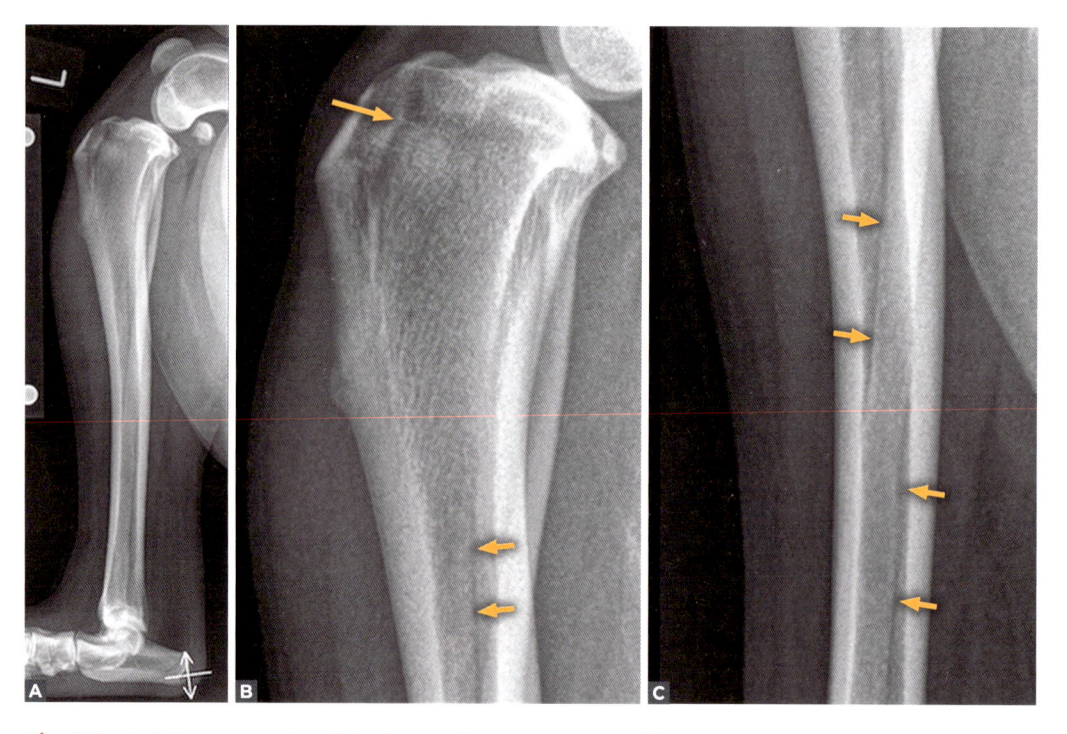

Fig. 5.9 Mediolateral projection of the tibia and fibula of a four-year-old female Labrador Retriever (**A**) with magnified proximal (**B**) and mid-diaphyseal (**C**) inserts. (**B**) The nutrient foramen is visible as a vertical radiolucent line in the proximal tibial diaphysis and should not be mistaken for a fissure fracture (orange arrows). The remnant of the physis of the tibial tuberosity is also present (white arrow). (**C**) Radiolucent lines are present where the fibula diagonally crosses the tibial diaphysis. These are "Mach lines" which are artefactual and may be mistaken for pathology (orange arrows).

44

CHAPTER 5 Fractures

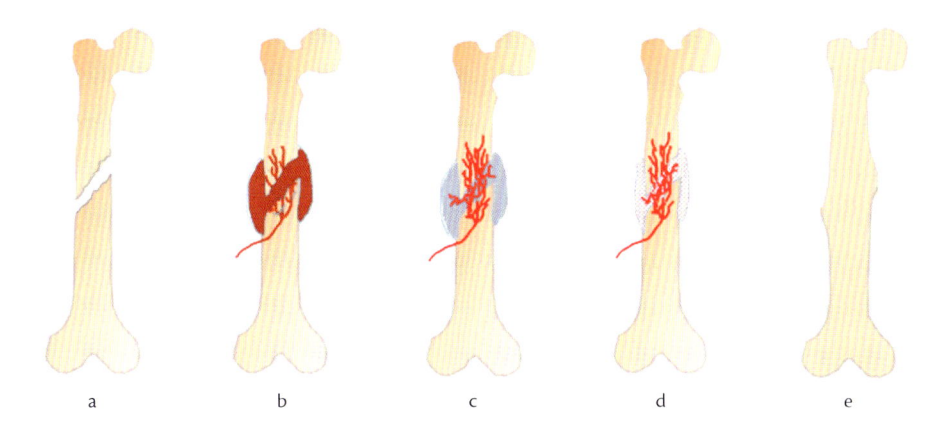

Fig. 5.11 Diagrammatic representation of the stages of fracture healing.

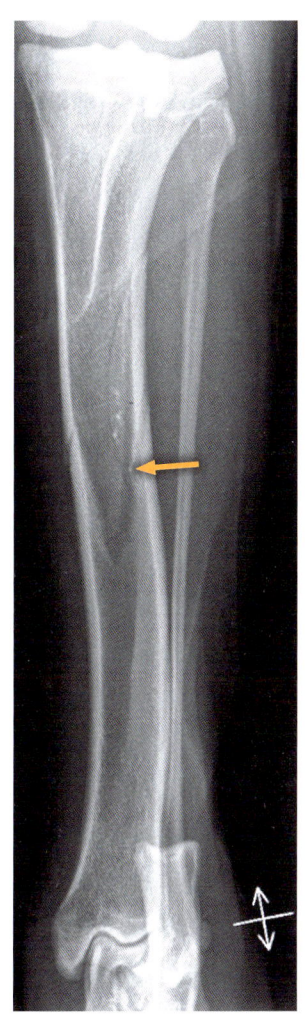

Fig. 5.10 Craniocaudal projection of the tibia and fibula of a two-year-old Neapolitan Mastiff. Obliquely orientated radiolucent fissures are visible through the medial cortex distally and lateral cortex proximally with an interlinking large V-shaped defect through the medullary cavity (arrow). Displacement is minimal. The fibula is intact. Multiple fissure fractures through the mid-diaphysis of the tibia.

Fracture healing

A number of factors affect fracture healing; these include the type, location, blood supply and degree of contamination of the fracture site, in addition to the fracture fixation method and the stability of the fracture fragments. The age of the animal and the presence of concurrent systemic disease also need consideration.

Fracture healing may be either primary or secondary in nature and is dependent on the degree of stability. Primary healing occurs when the fracture site is bridged with osseous tissue (intramembranous ossification) without callus formation and occurs with anatomical reduction and internal fixation of the fracture.

Most fractures heal by secondary healing (endochondral ossification) producing an unstructured callus which subsequently remodels. There are four, often overlapping stages of healing (**fig. 5.11**).

- Hematoma formation (1-5 days).
- Formation of fibrocartilaginous callus (5-11 days).
- Bony callus formation (11-28 days).
- Remodeling of bone (day 18+).

Radiological signs of healing take at least 7-10 days to be visible.

Fracture complications

Fracture complications occur when the normal healing time frame is compromised (delayed or non-union), when the united fragments are malaligned (malunion) or if the bone becomes infected.

In delayed union, there is evidence of bone healing but at a slower rate than expected. This is a subjective assessment. These fractures usually heal if given sufficient time and if any deficiency in support or fixation is corrected.

Non-union of fractures occurs when there is no progression of bone healing activity over an extended period and pseudoarthrosis may result. Non-unions can be viable or non-viable.

Viable non-unions occur due to fracture instability, resulting in exuberant callus formation with round flared fracture ends, giving a so called "elephant foot" appearance (**fig. 5.12**). Internal fixation of the fracture is required to promote healing.

45

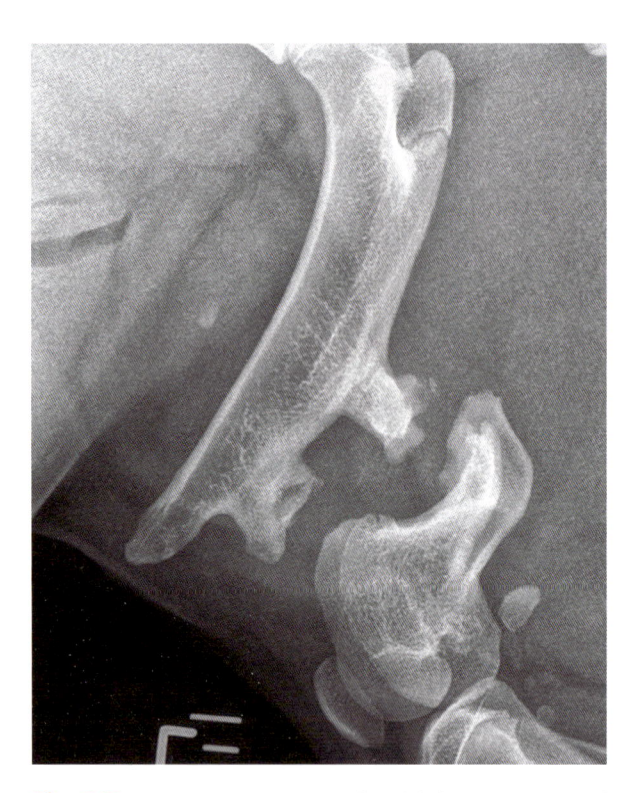

Fig. 5.12 Mediolateral projection of the left femoral diaphysis of a one-year-old Lurcher. Non-union of a chronic, simple diaphyseal fracture with caudoproximal displacement of the distal fragment. The separated fracture ends flair with flanges of new bone that are smooth, rounded with no active callus formation. This appearance is sometimes described as an "elephant foot" callus.

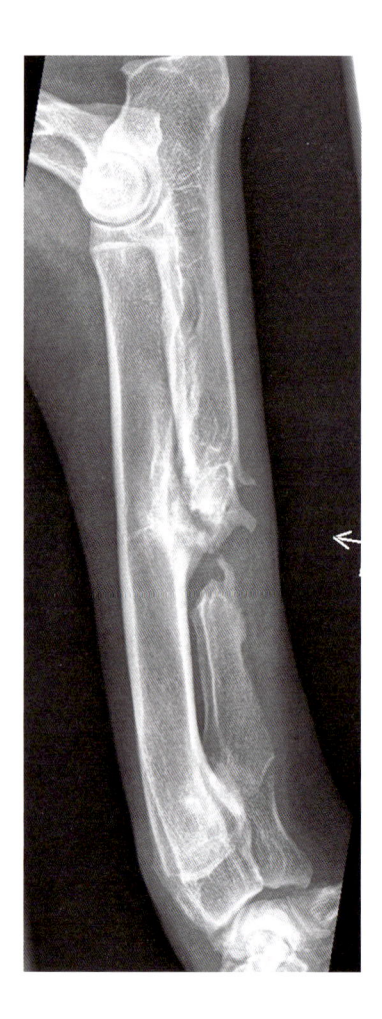

Fig. 5.13 Mediolateral projection of the right radius and ulna of a nine-month-old Weimaraner. The mid diaphyseal radiolucent deficit of the ulna has rounded, tapering fracture ends with smooth spicules of bone. Proliferative new bone on the caudal cortex of the closely apposed mid-radial diaphysis is uniting with the proximal ulnar fragment indicating early synostosis formation. Non-union and synostosis.

Non-union is considered non-viable when there is little or no callus formation over a prolonged period. Atrophic non-union has no callus formation with tapering separated fracture ends. If the gap between the fracture ends is considerable, callus formation is unable to bridge the defect, and is therefore termed a defect non-union fracture (**fig. 5.13**). Compromised blood supply is the primary cause of non-viable non-unions, and if a separated bone fragment is also present at the fracture site, this is termed a necrotic non-union.

A malunion is a healed fracture with an abnormal bone conformation. Malunions can occur due to difficulties in fracture fixation especially in complicated and/or comminuted fractures, substandard fixation technique or asynchronous growth in immature animals.

Malalignment may result in secondary complications due to abnormal bone/joint stresses. Fragments of adjacent fractured bones may conjoin when healing resulting in a synostosis (**fig. 5.14**).

Fracture of the femoral neck may be inapparent on a standard ventrodorsal projection but it can be more apparent on a flexed "frog leg" view or vice versa (**fig. 5.15**).

Osteomyelitis at the fracture site may occur in open fractures or as a sequel of surgical treatment. Radiological features include excessive callus production, active, aggressive periosteal reaction extending beyond the immediate fracture site and soft tissue swelling. The resulting osteolysis may loosen implants. Systemic disease, such as juvenile osteomyelitis, may also result in fractures of the affected bone (**fig. 5.16**). A separated bone fragment may form a sequestrum if it is isolated from its blood supply. Radiographically, it retains its original bone opacity, lies within a radiolucent cavity which is surrounded by a zone of sclerotic bone which is termed the involucrum (**fig. 5.17**). Pathological fractures may occur in cases of osteopenia or in neoplastic bone (**fig. 5.18**).

CHAPTER 5 Fractures

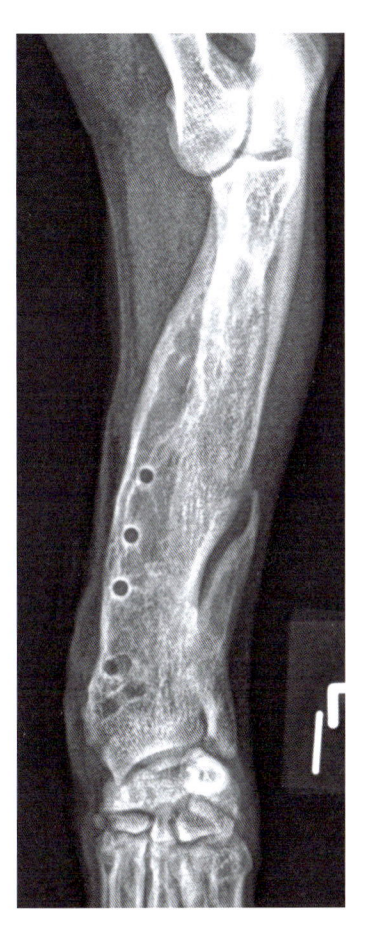

Fig. 5.14 Craniocaudal projection of the left radius and ulna of a 14-year-old Pyrenean Sheepdog. There are several round, radiolucent screw holes in the distal radius following implant removal of surgically stabilized diaphyseal fractures. The proximal ulnar fracture fragment has completely united with the healed radial fracture resulting in a synostosis. There is a non-union of the elongated and tapering proximal margin of the distal ulnar fragment. Non-union and synostosis.

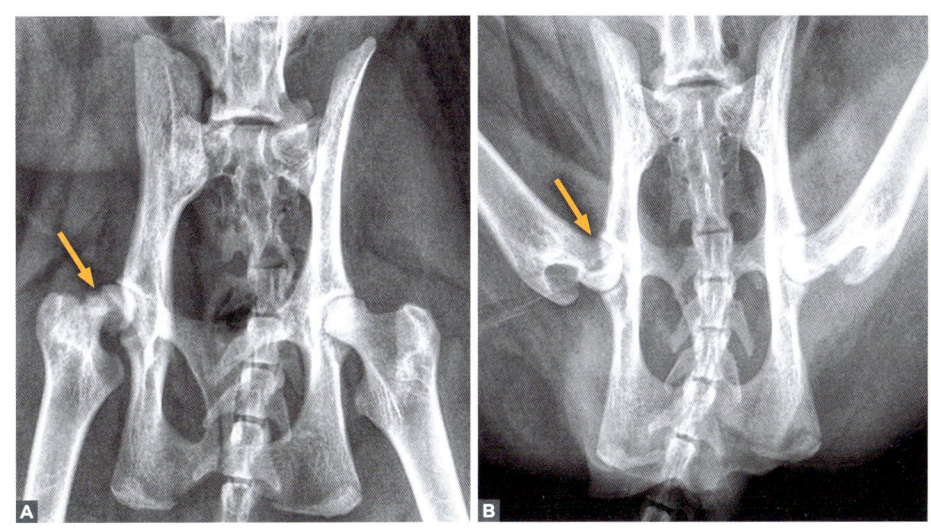

Fig. 5.15 Extended (**A**) and frog leg (**B**) ventrodorsal projections of a three-year-old male Maine Coon cat. There is a fracture through the right femoral neck at the site of the closed physis (arrows). The separation is clear on the extended view and barely perceptible on the "frog leg" or flexed projection. Both projections are advisable for assessment of femoral neck injuries. Fracture of the femoral neck.

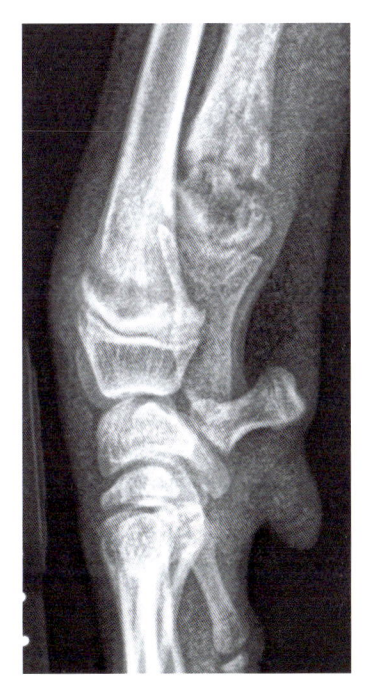

Fig. 5.16 Mediolateral projection of the distal antebrachium of a four-month-old Border Collie with confirmed multicentric juvenile osteomyelitis. There is marked demineralization of the metaphyseal regions of the radius and ulna with cortical disruption of the cranial and caudal ulnar cortices with minimal displacement. Pathological, non-displaced fracture of the distal ulna.

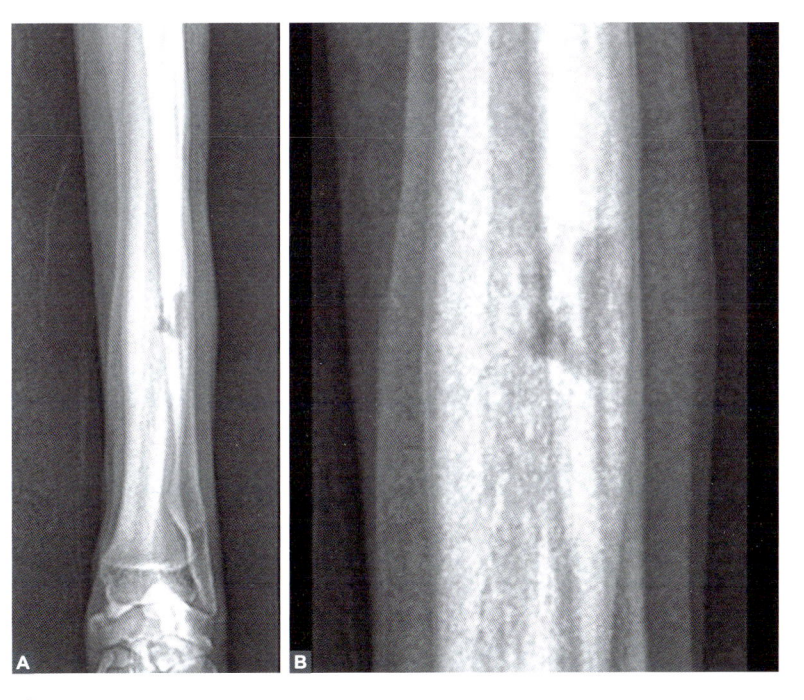

Fig. 5.17 Craniocaudal projections of the antebrachium of a ten-month-old Whippet. A circumscribed, focal radiolucent zone is visible in the distal third of the mid diaphysis of the ulna (**A**) with magnified insert of the region (**B**). The rectangular cortical fracture fragment is devoid of vascular supply and lies within a radiolucent cavity. This fragment is a sequestrum.

SECTION II APPENDICULAR SKELETON

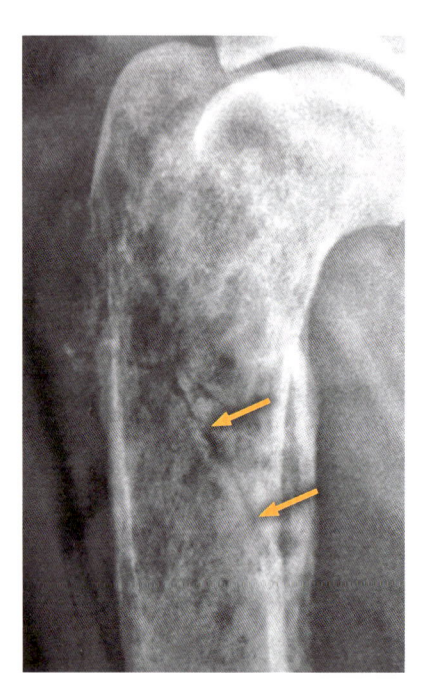

Fig. 5.18 Mediolateral projection of the proximal humerus of an eight-year-old Akita. An incomplete, oblique, minimally displaced, fissure fracture of the proximal humerus has disrupted the cranial cortex proximally with a laminar periosteal reaction of the caudal cortex (arrows). Multiple focal radiolucencies in the proximal humeral diaphysis gives a moth-eaten appearance. Pathological fracture of the proximal humerus secondary to neoplastic disease.

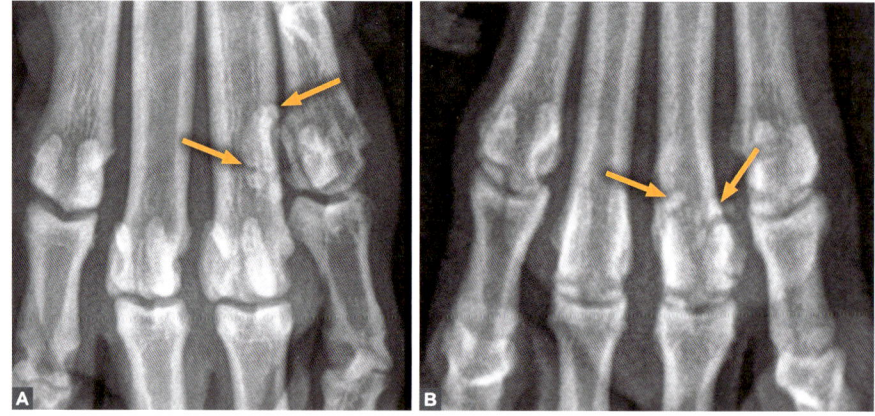

Fig. 5.19 Dorsopalmar projections of the metacarpophalangeal joints of a four-year-old Rottweiler (**A**) and a six-year-old crossbred collie (**B**). (**A**) The second palmar sesamoid has four separate parts that are smooth and rounded (arrows). Bipartite sesamoids occur in the second and/or seventh palmar sesamoid bones and are usually clinically insignificant and should not be mistaken for fractures. Bipartite sesamoids. (**B**) Multiple fragmentation of the fifth and sixth sesamoid bones. The fragments are sharply defined indicating they are of recent origin (arrows). Fractured sesamoids.

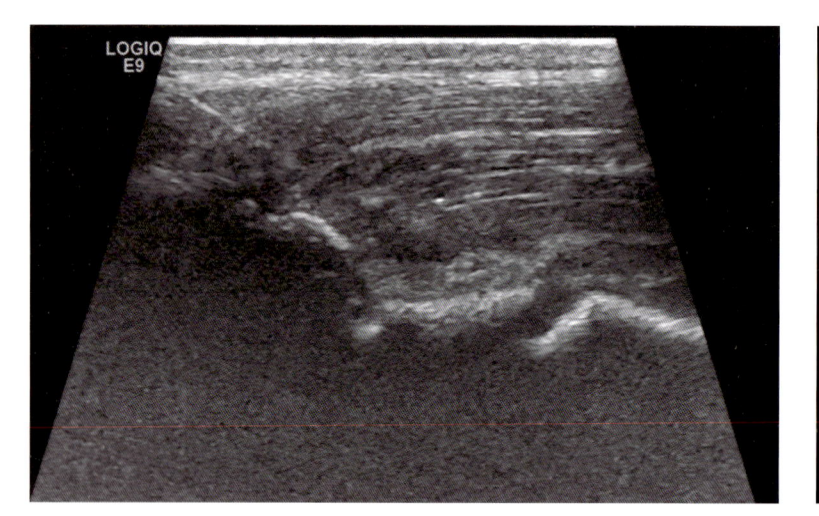

Fig. 5.20 Sagittal ultrasound image of the humeral diaphysis of a 2.5-year-old-male American Pit Bull dog with a mid-diaphyseal fracture and a discharging sinus tract. The undulating hyperechoic line of the cortex with distal acoustic shadowing is disrupted centrally at the site of the fracture. A thin linear hyperechoic needle is visible at the top left-hand corner of the image and extends obliquely to the area of cortical disruption to aspirate the area for culture and sensitivity. Cortical bone defect with needle placement for a fine-needle aspirate.

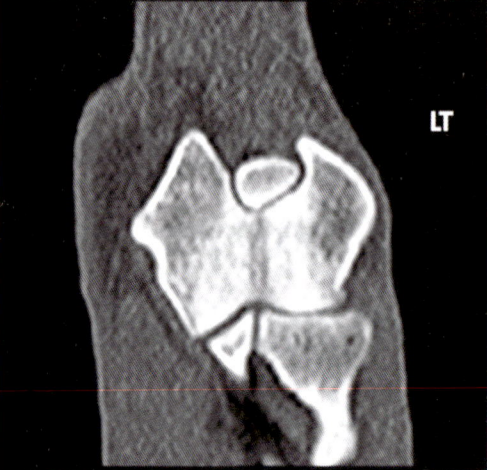

Fig. 5.21 Dorsal CT plane of the elbow of an adult 11-year-old English Springer. There is a vertical line through the center of the humeral condyle extending from the supratrochlear foramen to the joint with sclerosis in the adjacent bone. This type of non-displaced fracture of the humeral condyle is often not visible on radiographs. Fractured humeral condyle.

The second and seventh palmar sesamoids are occasionally bipartite or multipartite as an anatomical variant. This is seen more often in Greyhounds and Rottweilers and must not be confused with true fractures where the fragments are sharp and well defined (**fig. 5.19**).[5]

Other imaging modalities

Ultrasonography is occasionally used to show early callus formation which is not radiographically apparent (**fig. 5.20**).[6]

Computed tomography is used for complex joints such as the carpus, tarsus or elbow, as the superimposed bones can make accurate assessment and identification of fractures difficult (**fig. 5.21**).

References

1. Brinker WO, Olmstead ML, Sumner Smith, et al. Classification of fractures in small animals. In Brinker WO, Olmstead ML, Sumner-Smith G, Prieur WD (editors). Manual of internal fixation in small animals 2nd edition, Berlin, 1998, Springer pp 267-270.
2. Salter RB, Harris WR. Injuries involving the epiphyseal plate. *J Bone Joint Surg Am* 45:587-622, 1963.
3. Papageorges M, Sande RD. The Mach Phenomenon. *Vet Radiol Ultrasound* 31:274-280, 1990.
4. Papageorges M, How the Mach Phenomenon and shape affect the radiographic appearance of skeletal structures. *Vet Radiol Ultrasound* 32: 191-195, 1991.
5. Weinstein JM, Mongil CM, Smith GK. Orthopedic conditions of the Rottweiler. Part 1 *Compendium of Continuing Education Practice Veterinarian (Small Animal)* 17:813-830, 1995.
6. Risselada M, Kramer M, de Rooster H, et al. Ultrasonographic and radiographic assessment of uncomplicated secondary fracture healing of long bones in dogs and cats. *Vet Surg* 34:99-107, 2005.

CHAPTER 6

Skeletal diseases of unknown etiology

Robson F. Giglio and Federico R. Vilaplana Grosso

> **KEY POINTS**
>
> - Panosteitis produces self-limiting diaphyseal trabecular bone sclerosis in young dogs.
> - Shifting leg lameness is a classic clinical feature of panosteitis.
> - Hypertrophic osteodystrophy occurs in the metaphyses of long bones of young dogs.
> - Hypertrophic osteodystrophy is initially a mixed osteolytic and osteoproliferative process, and when chronic it is osteoproliferative.
> - Hypertrophic osteopathy produces diffuse palisading diaphyseal periosteal proliferation in older dogs.
> - Hypertrophic osteopathy is secondary to an inciting factor, either neoplastic or inflammatory in the thorax or abdomen.
> - The most common site of occurrence of retained cartilage core is the distal metaphysis of the ulna.
> - Retained cartilage core may produce growth impairment of the affected long bone and angular limb deformity.
> - Multiple cartilaginous exostosis is characterized by the presence of multiple benign and expansile osseous lesions affecting the appendicular and axial skeleton.
> - Craniomandibular osteopathy produces an irregular osseous proliferation of the mandible and ventral bones of the calvarium, and terrier breeds are overrepresented.

This chapter encompasses several skeletal diseases of unknown etiology. These diseases are not related to each other. Each of these diseases has a typical signalment and characteristic distribution of lesions. Almost all of these diseases are polyostotic. Knowledge of these features is paramount to diagnose these diseases. Some of these diseases have osteolytic and osteoproliferative features which may appear aggressive. In almost all cases, the combination of signalment, history, and clinical and imaging findings are sufficient to make a diagnosis. Biopsy may be required for lesions with an atypical presentation.

Panosteitis

Panosteitis, also known as eosinophilic panosteitis or enostosis, is a self-limiting disease that affects bones of large and giants dog breeds, such as German Shepherds, Labrador Retrievers, Golden Retrievers, Doberman Pinchers, Rottweilers, Bernese Mountain dogs, and Saint Bernards. Basset

SECTION II APPENDICULAR SKELETON

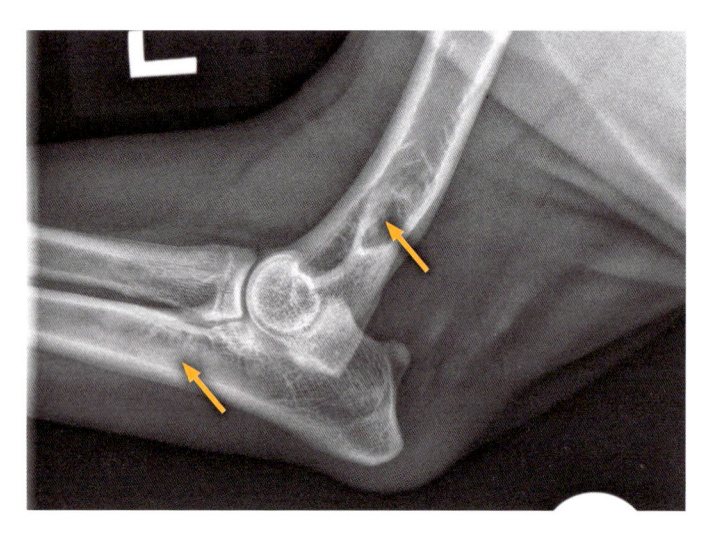

Fig. 6.1 Mediolateral projection of the left elbow of a seven-month-old male Golden Retriever. Radiographic signs of early panosteitis. There are multifocal regions of ill-defined increased trabecular bone opacity in the distal humerus and proximal ulna (arrows).

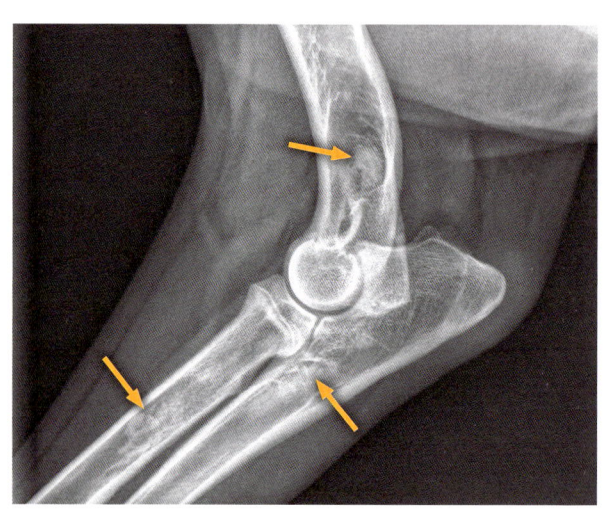

Fig. 6.2 Mediolateral projection of the right elbow of an eight-month-old male German Shepherd dog. Multifocal regions of ill- and well-defined increased trabecular bone opacity are present in the distal humerus and proximal radius and ulna (arrows), compatible with subacute to early chronic panosteitis.

Hounds and Dachshunds are also affected. Although of unknown etiology, some authors speculate that excessively high dietary protein or calcium could produce increased intraosseous pressure due to vascular proliferation and local bone formation adjacent to the nutrient foramina. This disease affects young dogs (from around 5 to 18 months of age), and it has a predisposition for the diaphyses of long bones, near their nutrient foramina. Males are more often affected than females. Affected animals demonstrate acute lameness and osseous pain. Systemic signs, such as fever, hyporexia, and lethargy may also be present. A common clinical feature of this disease is shifting leg lameness, as sequential lesions affect different long bones at different time points. The most commonly affected bones are the humerus, radius, ulna, femur, and tibia.[1,2]

The radiographic signs will depend upon the stage of the disease. In acute cases, we may see focal ill-defined diaphyseal sclerosis with a mildly accentuated trabecular pattern (**fig. 6.1**). In subacute to early chronic cases, there are multifocal and well-defined sclerotic lesions in the medullary cavity (**figs. 6.2** and **6.3**). Adjacent smooth well defined periosteal new bone may be seen in more severe cases (**fig. 6.4**). This is the stage of the disease where the radiographic changes are more pronounced. In late chronic cases, the medullary bone changes may disappear; however, the adjacent periosteum may appear mildly rough. Obvious radiographic lesions are chronic and may be inactive. The severity of the clinical signs and the severity of the radiographic findings do not correlate well. These osseous changes are more evident on computed tomography (CT) as there is no superimposition of structures (**fig. 6.5**). The differential diagnosis for these findings of increased trabecular bone opacity with or without adjacent periosteal proliferation includes bone infarction, infection, or neoplasia. Given that panosteitis occurs in younger dogs, neoplasia would be a less likely differential for the patients with this signalment. These differentials for aggressive osseous changes should be greater consideration if the patient's lameness and osseous pain persist or worsen.[1,2]

Hypertrophic osteodystrophy

Also known as metaphyseal osteopathy, this is also a disease that mainly occurs in young (from approximately three to eight months of age), large and giant breed dogs, such as Great Danes, Weimaraners, German Shepherds, Boxers, Chesapeake Bay Retrievers, and Irish Setters. Few case reports

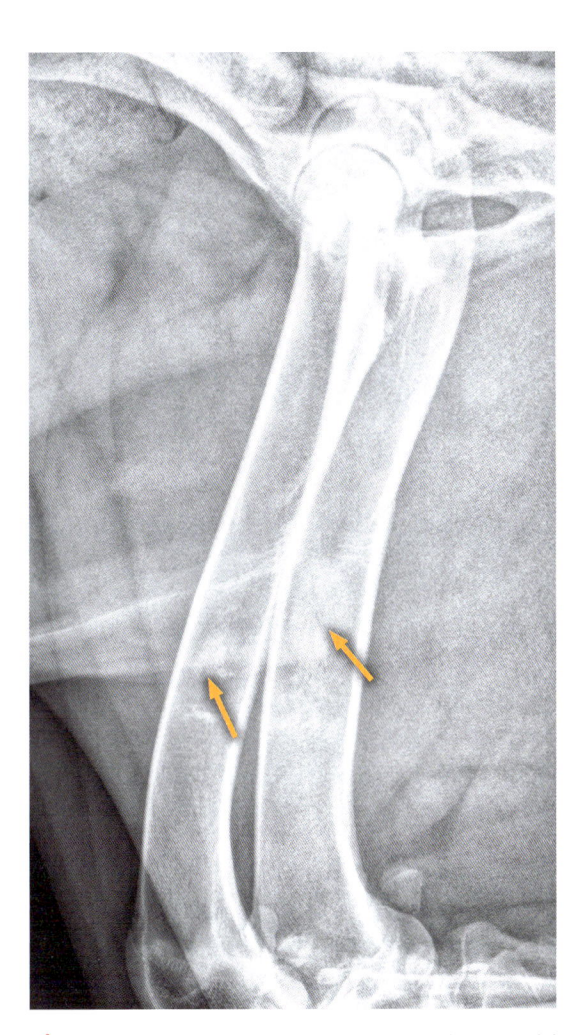

CHAPTER **6** Skeletal diseases of unknown etiology

Fig. 6.3 Cropped right lateral projection of the caudal abdomen of an eight-month-old male German Shepherd dog. Multifocal region of ill- and well-defined increased trabecular bone opacity are present in the mid diaphysis of the femurs (arrows), compatible with subacute to early chronic panosteitis.

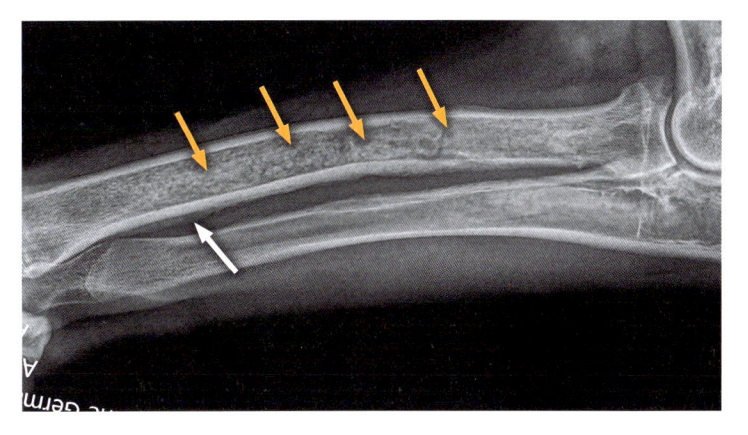

Fig. 6.4 Cropped mediolateral projection of the right antebrachium of an 11-month-old male German Shepherd dog. Radiographic signs of chronic panosteitis. There are multifocal and patchy regions of increased trabecular bone opacity of the radius (orange arrows) with adjacent periosteal proliferation along the caudodistal radial diaphysis (white arrow) are present.

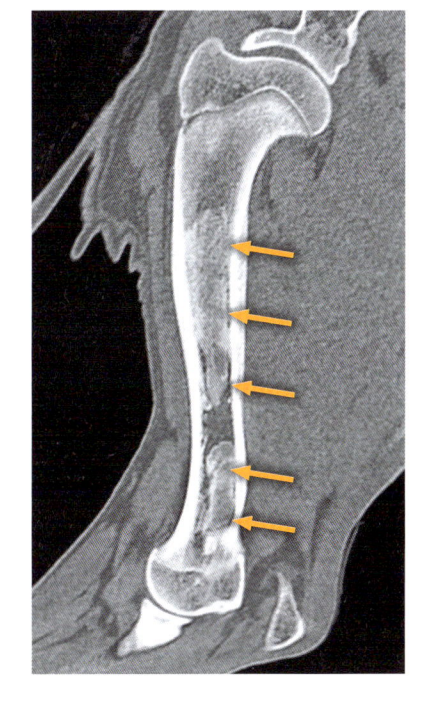

Fig. 6.5 Sagittal CT reconstruction in bone window of the left humerus of a seven-month-old male German Shepherd dog. Multifocal and well-defined fusiform to oval regions of increased osseous attenuation are seen along the humeral diaphysis (arrows) compatible with panosteitis.

of hypertrophic osteodystrophy (HOD) in cats were published. It is usually a self-limiting disease, although, in severe cases, it may produce angular limb deformities. Its etiology remains unknown, speculated causes including vaccination protocols, canine distemper virus, *Escherichia coli* infection, over-supplementation of vitamins and minerals, hypovitaminosis C, and vascular anomalies. Besides lameness, there may also be systemic signs, including fever, lethargy, generalized pain, and diarrhea. This disease is polyostotic and occurs at the metaphyses of long bones. It is more commonly located at the distal metaphyses of the radius, ulna, and tibia, although all long bones can be affected. The physes and epiphyses are not affected by this process. These lesions are bilaterally symmetrical and have two distinct radiographic appearances based on the disease's progression. In the early stage, there is irregularly marginated, linear osteolytic lesion in the metaphysis parallel to the physis (**figs. 6.6** and **6.7**). This lytic metaphyseal area is sometimes described as "double physeal sign". There is metaphyseal sclerosis in more chronic cases. Mineralization occurs in the soft tissues adjacent to the metaphysis, appearing as a cuff or band around the bone. This mineralization is incorporated into the cortex in chronic cases, resulting is widening and sclerosis of the metaphyses (**fig. 6.8**). The main differential diagnosis for these lesions is hematogenous infectious metaphysitis, which is seldom symmetrical, affecting a single site or several random sites.[1,3,4]

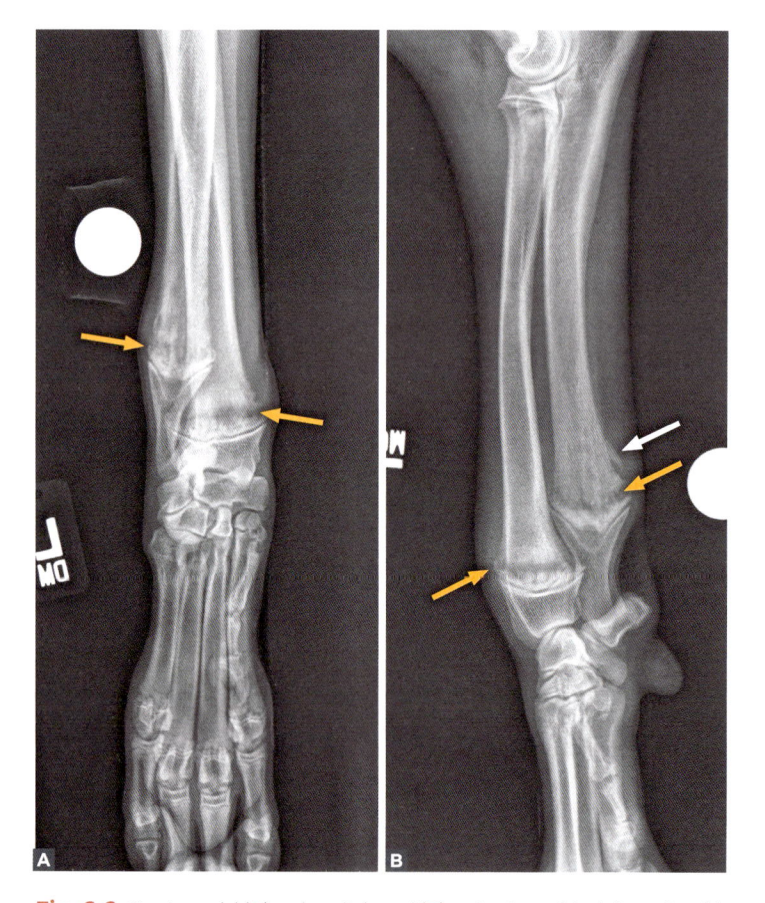

Fig. 6.6 Craniocaudal (**A**) and mediolateral (**B**) projections of the left antebrachium of a six-month-old male Great Dane. Centered on the distal metaphysis of the radius and ulna, there is an irregularly margined and elongated area of osteolysis with abundant surrounded sclerosis (orange arrows), representing subacute hypertrophic osteodystrophy. There is also a mild periosteal proliferation of the caudal aspect of the distal ulnar metaphysis (white arrow).

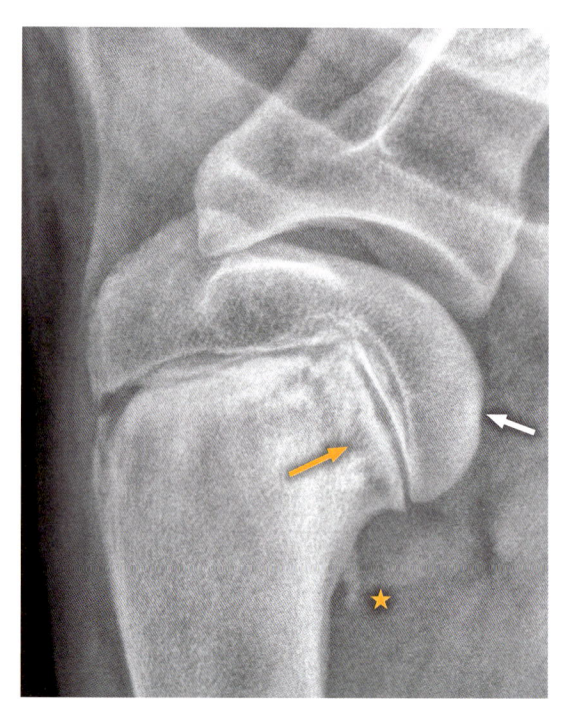

Fig. 6.7 Mediolateral projection of the right shoulder of a six-month-old male Great Dane. Centered on the proximal metaphysis of the humerus, there is an irregularly margined and elongated area of osteolysis with abundant surrounded sclerosis (orange arrows). There is also mild periosteal proliferation of the caudal aspect of the humeral metaphysis (star). These changes are compatible with subacute hypertrophic osteodystrophy. In addition, there is mild flattening of the caudal aspect of the humeral head with adjacent subchondral bone sclerosis (white arrow), representing osteochondrosis.

Hypertrophic osteopathy

Also known as Marie's disease, hypertrophic osteopathy (HO) is a polyostotic disease that mainly affects the diaphyseal region of the long bones, at first affecting the bones of the distal limb such as phalanges, metacarpus, metatarsus, carpus, and tarsus, progressing proximally. These lesions are often bilaterally symmetrical and affect older dogs (usually more than 8.5 years old) with no breed predisposition. Few case reports of HO in cats were published. Clinical signs included lethargy, hyporexia, lameness, and reluctance to walk. Radiographic features of HO include circumferential palisading periosteal proliferation in multiple bones, with associated substantial adjacent soft tissue swelling (**fig. 6.9**). HO is an osteoproliferative disease with no osteolytic component. The pathophysiology has not been fully elucidated. These lesions are secondary to primary lesion in the thorax or, less often, the abdomen. Reported causes include primary or metastatic neoplasia in the thorax, (**fig. 6.10**), heartworm or *Spirocerca lupi* infestations, fungal pneumonia, intrathoracic foreign body, and aortic thromboembolism and abdominal neoplasia, especially of the genitourinary tract and liver. Thoracic and abdominal radiographs are recommended to identify the primary lesion. If the inciting factor is removed, gradually, there may be complete or partial resolution of the HO changes.[5,6]

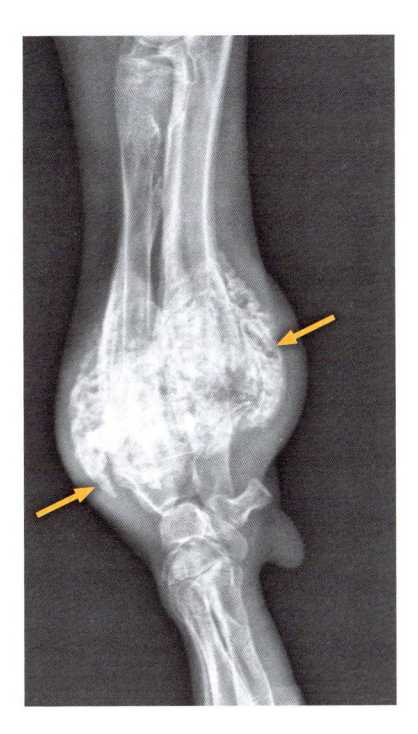

CHAPTER 6 Skeletal diseases of unknown etiology

Fig. 6.8 Mediolateral projection of the right antebrachium of a five-month-old male Weimaraner with severe chronic hypertrophic osteodystrophy. Centered on the distal radial and ulnar metaphyses, there is exuberant and circumferential solid and minimally irregular and flocculated periosteal proliferation (arrows).

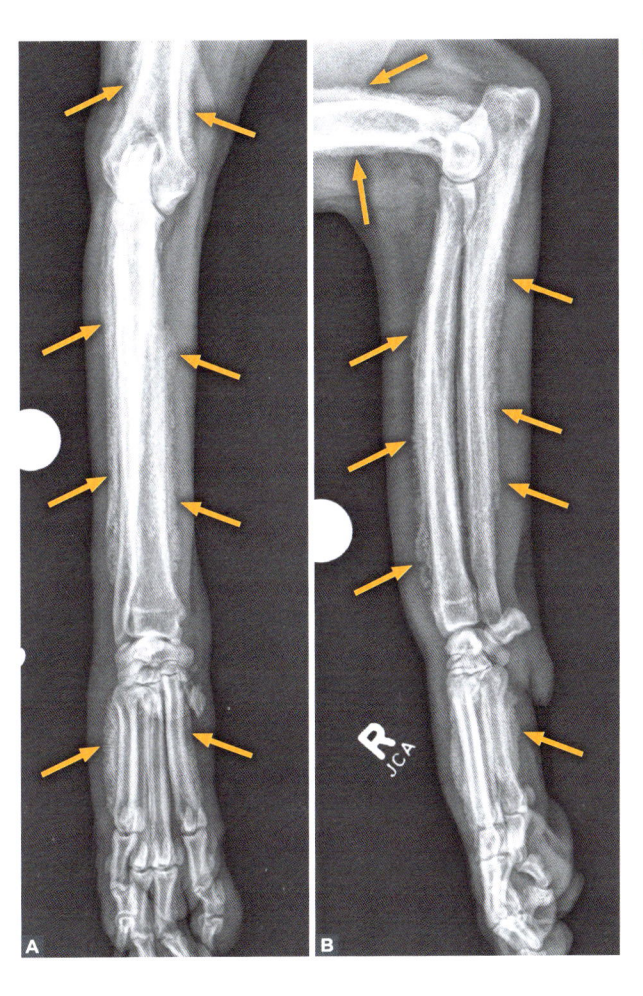

Fig. 6.9 Craniocaudal (A) and mediolateral projections (B) of the left antebrachium and manus of a nine-year-old neutered male Boxer with hypertrophic osteopathy. There is exuberant, circumferential, mainly diaphyseal palisading periosteal proliferation in all the bones included in the collimation (arrows), with associated soft tissue swelling.

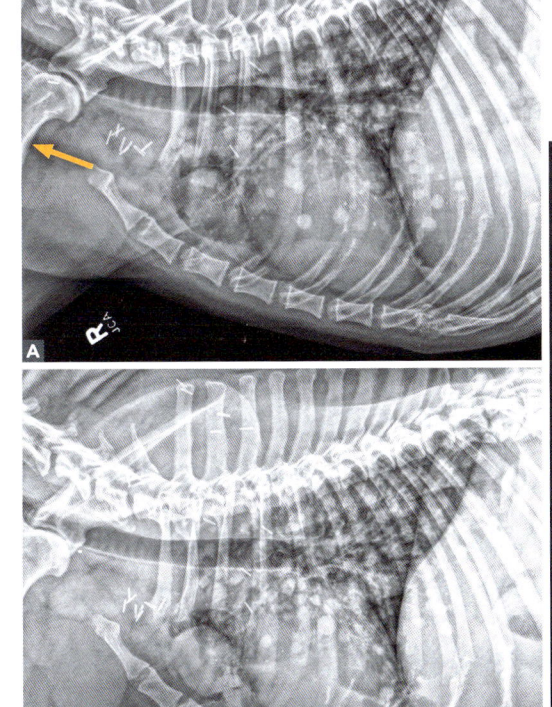

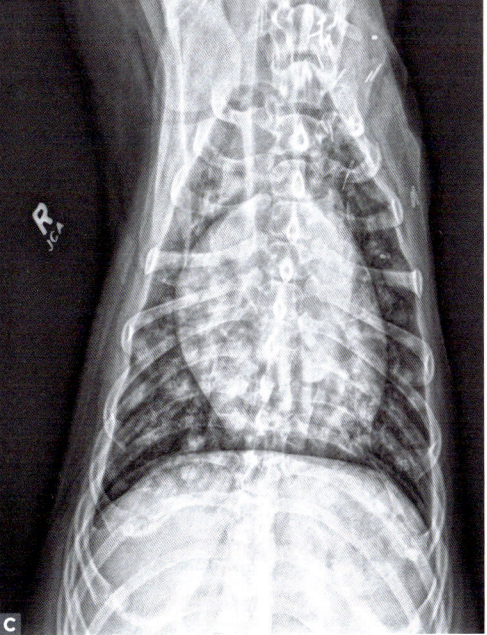

Fig. 6.10 Right lateral (A), left lateral (B), and ventrodorsal (C) projections of the thorax of a nine-year-old neutered male Boxer with hypertrophic osteopathy. There are multiple various-sized pulmonary nodules, compatible with metastasis of the previously excised soft tissue sarcoma of the left thoracic limb (prior to limb amputation). Note the subtle palisading periosteal proliferation is present along the caudal humeral diaphysis (arrow).

SECTION II APPENDICULAR SKELETON

Retained cartilage core

Retained cartilage core (RCC) occurs in immature large and giant breed dogs. This disease is caused by the lack of proper endochondral ossification originating from an active physis of a long bone, and the etiology is unknown. The most common location of the RCC is the distal ulnar metaphysis, and less often, in the lateral aspect of the distal femoral physis. The lesion may cause impairment of the lengthening of the affected bone. In the antebrachium, asymmetrical growth of the radius and ulna causes elbow joint incongruency and angular limb deformity. Most cases are mild and clinically insignificant. The main radiographic feature of RCC is the presence of a conical lucency surrounded by various degrees of sclerosis within the metaphysis, with a direct extension of the growth plate (**fig. 6.11**). In severe cases of RCC of the distal ulna, we may see radius curvus, short ulna, elbow incongruency, carpal valgus, and evidence of degenerative changes in the elbow and antebrachiocarpal joints.[7]

Incomplete ossification of the humeral condyle

The humeral condyle comprises the capitulum (lateral portion), which mainly articulates with the radial head, and the trochlea (medial portion). In immature dogs, there is a sagittal accessory growth line between the capitulum and the trochlea, contiguous with the distal physis of the humerus. This accessory growth line is fused by approximately at three months of age. Incomplete fusion weakens the condyle, predisposing to articular condylar humeral fractures. Incomplete ossification of the humeral condyle (IOHC) is more prevalent in spaniel and chondrodystrophic breeds, such as bulldog breeds, and crosses and some large breed dogs, such as Rottweilers and German Shepherd dogs, and is more common in males. This disease is frequently bilateral, and patients with condylar humeral fractures should get a CT

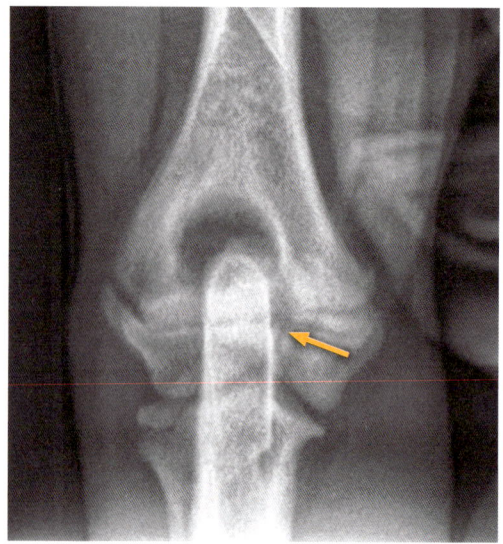

Fig. 6.12 Craniocaudal projection of the right elbow of a five-month-old female French Bulldog. A small, vertically oriented, lucent line is present between the humeral trochlea and capitulum (arrow), representing an incomplete ossification of the humeral condyle, which is partially superimposed over the proximal ulna.

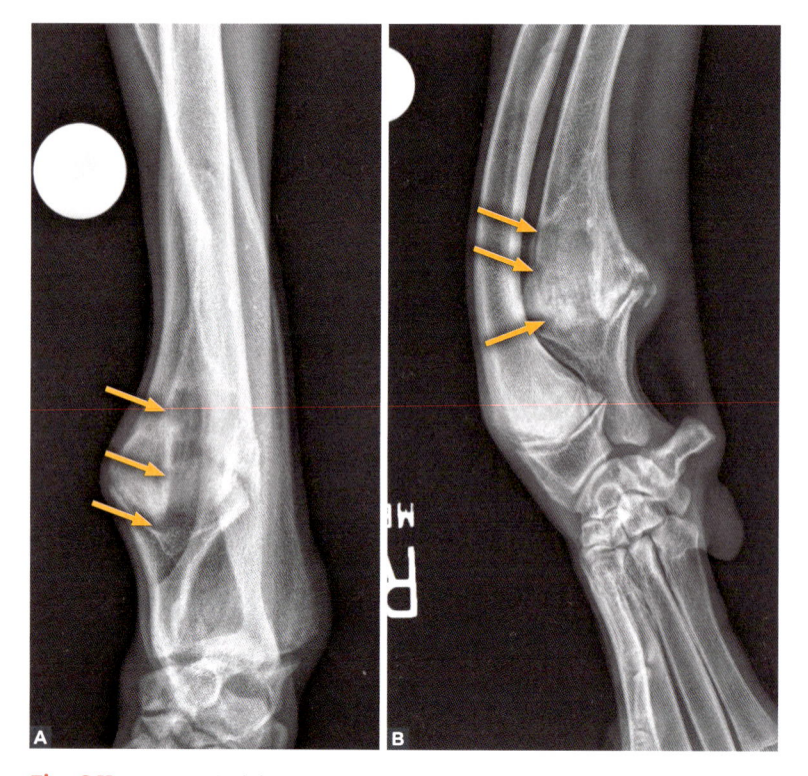

Fig. 6.11 Craniocaudal (**A**) and mediolateral (**B**) projections of the right antebrachium of a six-month-old female Irish Wolfhound. Extending from the distal physis of the ulna to the distal metaphysis, there is a rounded to elongated lucent area surrounding by mild sclerosis (arrows). These findings are compatible with retained cartilaginous core of the distal ulna physis.

CHAPTER **6** Skeletal diseases of unknown etiology

or radiographs of the contralateral elbow to look for evidence of IOHC. If identified, prophylactic surgical procedures should be considered. Radiographic signs of IOHC include a sagittal lucent line between the humeral trochlea and capitulum extending from the articular surface to the distal humeral physes (or physeal scar) with adjacent sclerosis (**figs. 6.12** and **6.13**). Due to the normal superimposition of this central region of the humeral condyle with the olecranon of the ulna, supinated oblique craniocaudal projections should be performed to evaluate the central region of the humeral condyle with less ulnar superimposition, but radiographic diagnosis is challenging.[8] CT is more sensitive and preferred if available.

Multiple cartilaginous exostoses

Multiple cartilaginous exostoses (MCE) is an exuberant multifocal area of benign osseous and cartilaginous proliferation caused by a non-regulated proliferation of cartilaginous islands, which may occur in both the appendicular and axial skeleton. When there is only a singular lesion, it is called osteochondroma. This benign osseous proliferation usually ceases growth after the dog reaches maturity; however, they commonly keep growing after osseous maturity in cats. There is no specific breed predilection. These proliferative lesions are usually not clinically significant, although it may produce clinical signs if it causes compression and deviation of important structures, most notably spinal cord compression in cases of vertebral MCE. This disease can undergo malignant transformation with the benign osseous masses turn into osteosarcoma and chondrosarcomas. Radiographically, MCE is characterized by multifocal, various-sized, distinct, poorly and irregularly marginated, heterogeneously mineralized osseous nodules and masses seen more frequently in ribs, vertebral spinal processes and multifocal locations of the appendicular skeleton, causing variable degrees of cortical erosion/expansion (**figs. 6.14** and **6.15**).[3,9]

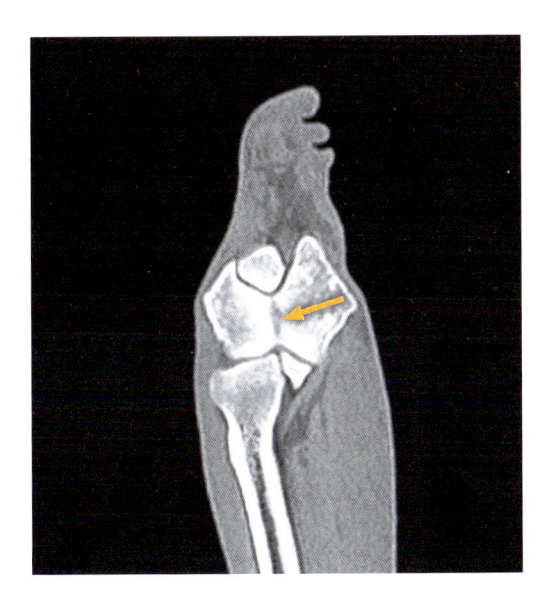

Fig. 6.13 Dorsal plane reconstruction in bone window of the right elbow of a six-year-old neutered male Weimaraner. There is a faint, vertically oriented, hypoattenuating line between the humeral trochlea and capitulum (arrow) surrounded by sclerosis which corresponds to an incomplete ossification of the humeral condyle.

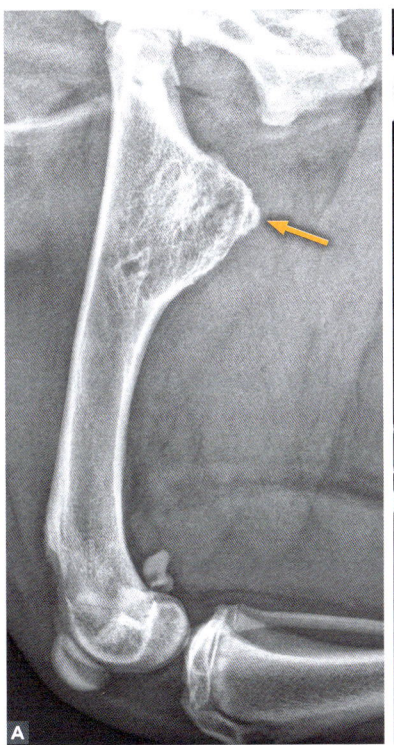

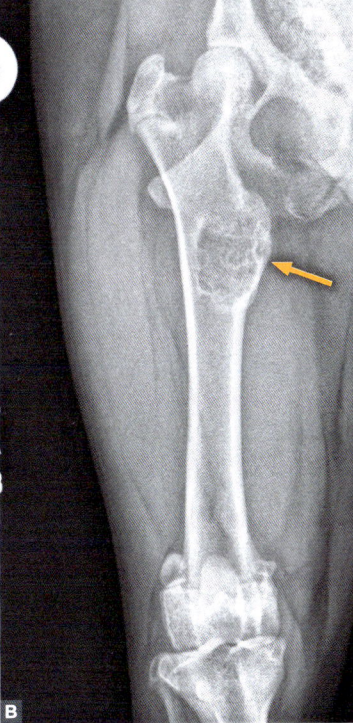

Fig. 6.14 Mediolateral (**A**) and craniocaudal (**B**) projections of the right femur of a ten-month-old neutered male Labrador Retriever. An expansile osseous lesion is present in the caudomedial aspect of the proximal femoral diaphysis (arrows), compatible with osteochondroma/multiple cartilaginous exostoses.

SECTION II APPENDICULAR SKELETON

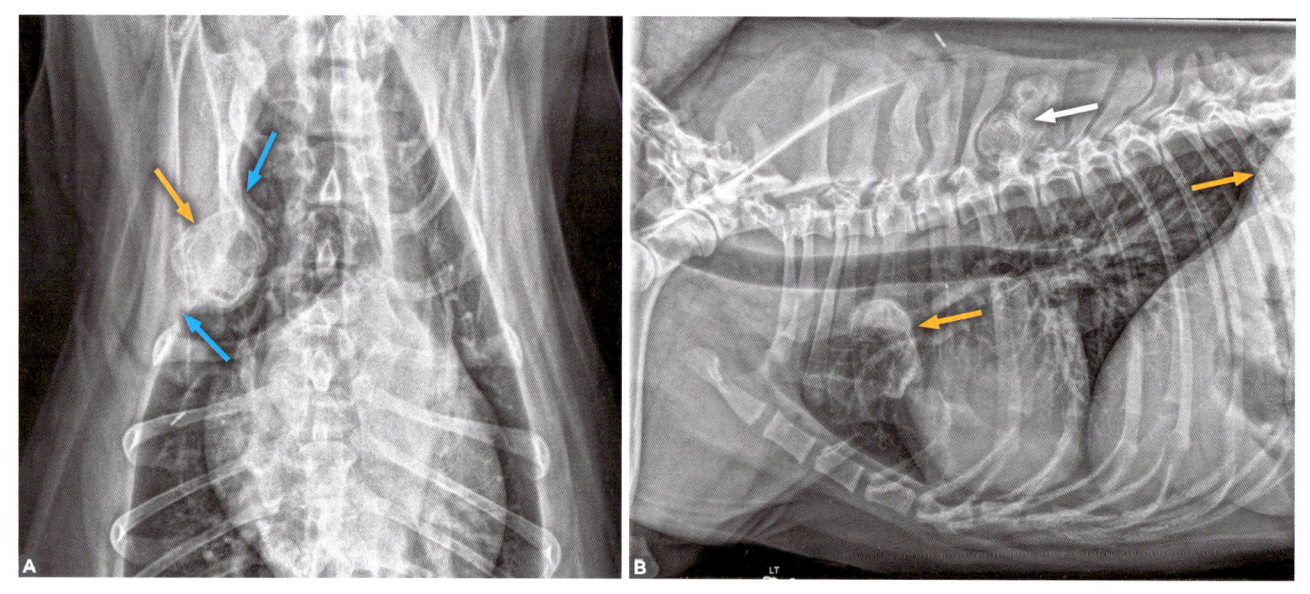

Fig. 6.15 Cropped ventrodorsal (**A**) and left lateral (**B**) projections of the thorax of a ten month old neutered male Labrador Retriever. Expansile osseous lesions are present in some of the ribs (orange arrows) and mid-thoracic spinous processes (white arrow), compatible with multiple cartilaginous exostoses. In addition, on the ventrodorsal projection, this expansile rib lesion is causing an extrapleural sign (blue arrows).

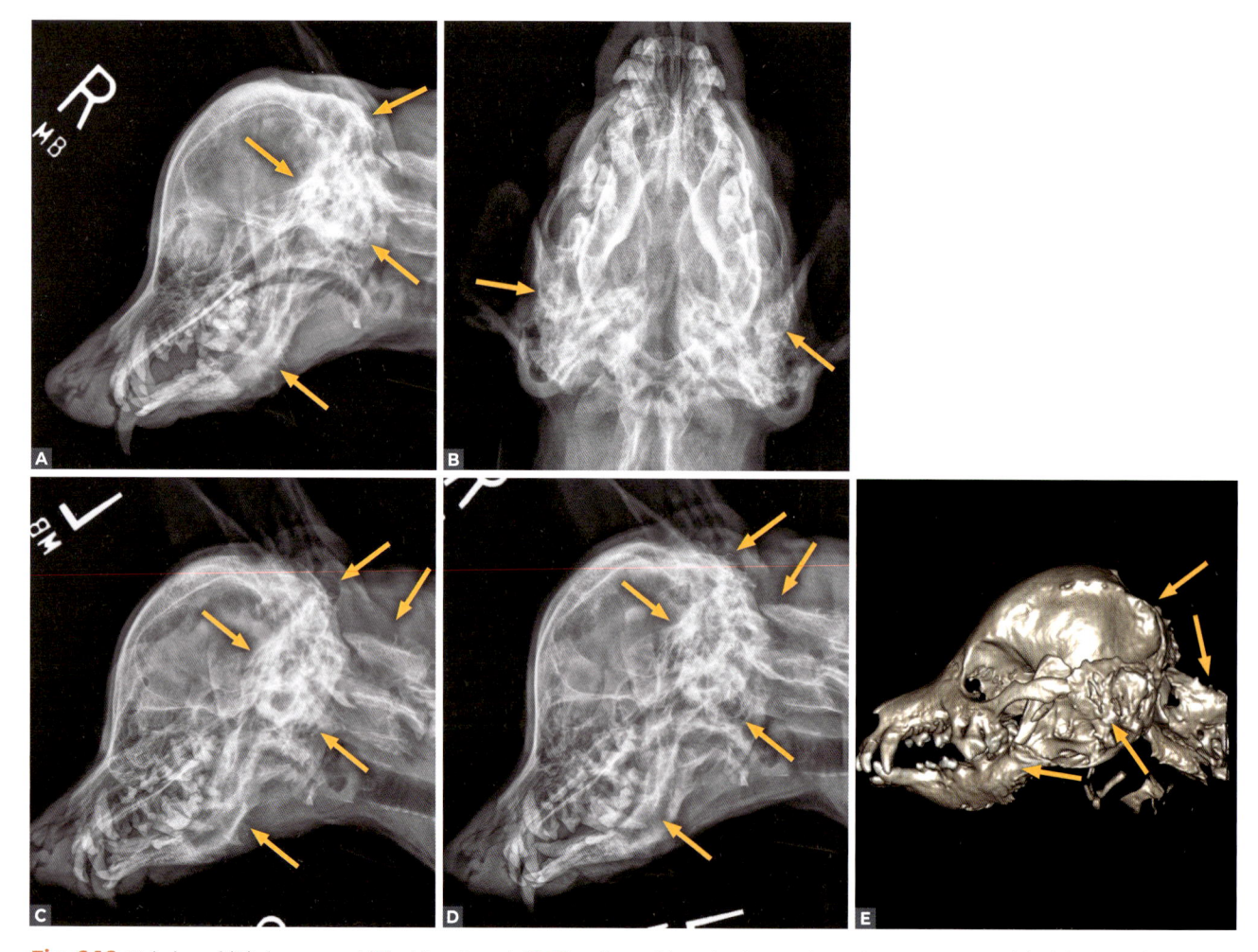

Fig. 6.16 Right lateral (**A**), dorsoventral (**B**), oblique laterals (**C**, **D**), radiographic projections, and a 3D CT reconstruction (**E**) of the skull of a two-year-old female West Highland White Terrier. There is bilateral, multifocal, exuberant, irregular, and interrupted osseous proliferation along the ventral margin of the mandibles, temporal and occipital region of the skull, and atlas and axis (arrows), characterizing a severe case of craniomandibular osteopathy.

Craniomandibular osteopathy

Craniomandibular osteopathy (CMO) is a proliferative polyostotic disease that primarily affects the mandible and calvarial bone. This disease is more common in young (3-12 months old) terrier breeds, most notably in West Highland White Terrier (WHWT), Cairn Terrier, and Scottish Terrier and sporadically in breeds such as Bullmastiff and Labrador Retriever. It was demonstrated to be a recessive autosomal inherent in WHWT and of complex inheritance in Deutsch Drahthaar dogs. In mild cases, CMO can be a self-limited disease with minimal mandibular and calvarial osseous remodeling. The main clinical features of this disease include difficult in prehension, mastication and to open the mouth, mandibular swelling and pain, and fever. The prognosis is guarded when exuberant osseous proliferation occurs around the temporomandibular joints, causing ankylosis of the joint. In more severe cases, the exuberant osseous remodeling may persist, causing clinical signs after the patient reaches maturity. On radiographs, there is usually symmetrically bilateral irregular and interrupted osseous proliferation affecting the mandibles, temporal, and occipital bones, most commonly (**fig. 6.16**).[3,10]

References

1. Demko J, McLaughlin R. Developmental orthopedic disease. *Vet Clin North Am Small Anim Pract* 35:1111-1135, 2005.
2. Muir P, Dubielzig RR, Johnson KA. Panosteitis. *Comp Cont Educ Pract Vet* 18:29-33, 1996.
3. Alexander JW. Selected skeletal dysplasias: craniomandibular osteopathy, multiple cartilaginous exostoses, and hypertrophic osteodystrophy. *Vet Clin North Am Small Anim Pract* 13:55-70, 1983.
4. Harrus S, Waner T, Aizenberg I, Safra N, Mosenco A, Radoshitsky M, Bark H. Development of hypertrophic osteodystrophy and antibody response in a litter of vaccinated Weimaraner puppies. *J Small Anim Pract* 43:27-31, 2002.
5. Cetinkaya MA, Yardimci B, Yardimci C. Hypertrophic osteopathy in a dog associated with intra-thoracic lesions: a case report and a review. *Vet Med* 56:595-601, 2011.
6. Headley SA, Ribeiro EA, Santos GJVGD, Bettini CM, Junior EM. Canine hypertrophic osteopathy associated with extra-thoracic lesions. *Cienc Rural* 35:941-944, 2005.
7. Carrig CB. Growth abnormalities of the canine radius and ulna. *Vet Clin North Am Small Anim Pract* 13:91-115, 1983.
8. Marcellin-Little DJ, DeYoung DJ, Ferris KK, Berry CM. Incomplete ossification of the humeral condyle in spaniels. *Vet Surg* 23:475-87, 1994.
9. Jacobson LS, Kirberger RM. Canine multiple cartilaginous exostoses: unusual manifestations and a review of the literature. *J Am Anim Hosp Assoc* 32:45-51, 1996.
10. Vagt J, Distl O. Complex segregation analysis of craniomandibular osteopathy in Deutsch Drahthaar dogs. *Vet J* 231:30-32, 2018.

CHAPTER 7

Elbow dysplasia

Massimo Vignoli

KEY POINTS

- Elbow dysplasia is a hereditary polygenic disease that involves medium to large breed dogs during skeletal development.
- Associated primary conditions can be found.
- Specific radiographic views have been reported by the IEWG.
- Radiography is limiting for a diagnosis, especially for FCP/MCPD.
- Primary disease not always visible, secondary changes like osteoarthritis are more commonly seen.
- For definitive diagnosis CT is recommended when radiographs are not definitive, especially for FCP/MCPD.

Elbow dysplasia is a hereditary polygenic disease that occurs during skeletal development.[1] The factors involved in the development of this pathology are the asynchronous growth of the radius and ulna compared to the normal elbow (**fig. 7.1** and **fig. 7.2**) and the development of an ulnar notch too small in circumference to contain the humeral trochlea, thus creating joint incongruity.[2] The main conditions of elbow dysplasia are fragmentation of the medial ulnar coronoid process (FCP)/medial coronoid process disease (MCPD), non-union of the ulnar anconeal process (UAP), osteochondrosis/osteochondritis dissecans of the medial humeral condyle or humeral trochlea (OC/OCD). These conditions lead to osteoarthritis, the severity of which is quantified by measuring

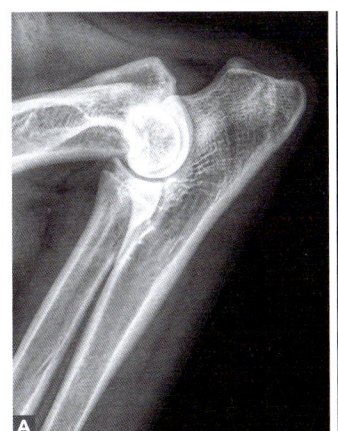

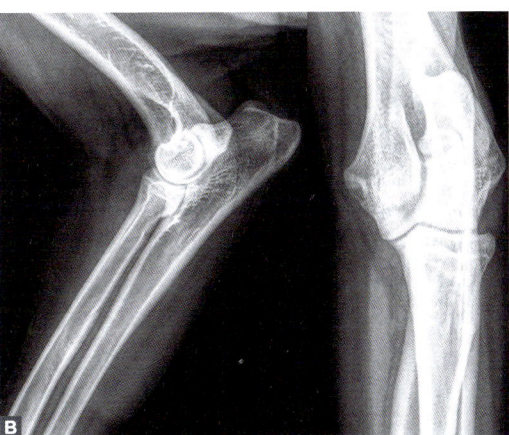

Fig. 7.1 (**A**) Mediolateral flexed and extended and (**B**) craniocaudal projection showing a normal elbow.

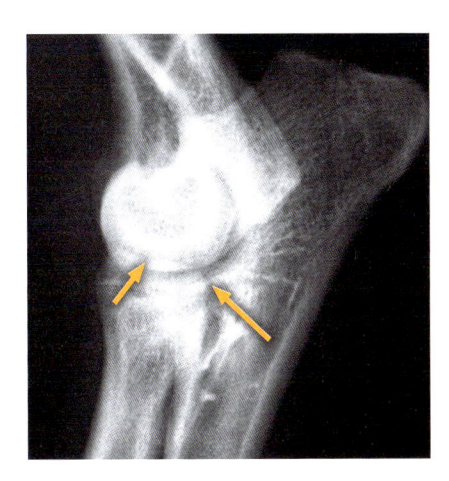

Fig. 7.2 An eight-month-old dog with asynchronous radio-ulnar growth (arrows).

the length of the osteophytes and classified as: grade 0 – normal elbow; grade 1 – mild arthrosis: ulnar sclerosis or step ≥2 mm between radius and ulna or osteophytes <2 mm; grade 2 – moderate arthrosis: osteophytes of 2-5 mm; grade 3 – severe osteoarthritis: osteophytes >5 mm and/or primary visible lesion such as FCP, OCD, UAP.[3] Flexor tendon enthesopathy can be concomitant with other lesions.[4] Dysplasia of the elbow usually occurs bilaterally, and one or two or more conditions can be detected together.

The International Elbow Working Group (IEWG) has established precise rules to standardize research: at least one mediolateral projection flexed at 40° for each elbow is required and a mediolateral in neutral position is strongly recommended, approximately 110° and a craniocaudal with 15° of pronation.[5] The most affected are medium to large breed dogs, some of them with prevalence of specific lesions, such as Rottweiler (FCP), Bernese Mountain dog (MCPD), Golden Retriever (MCPD, OCD), German Shepherd (MCPD, UAP), and Labrador Retriever (MCPD, OCD).

The clinical signs are lameness and a painful elbow on manipulation, with progressive worsening as osteoarthritis worsens.

Ununited anconeal process

The anconeal process of the ulna is present in some breeds as separate center of ossification, which usually fuses with the ulna between four and five months of age. It has been suggested that the cause of UAP is an incongruous growth of the radius and the ulna, causing abnormal pressure on the anconeal process.[6] A flexed mediolateral view of the elbow joint is required. This view displaces the medial epicondylar physis away from the anconeous process, avoiding a possible overlap of this radiolucent line with the anconeal process, and therefore leading to an incorrect diagnosis. The radiographic signs are: radiolucent line of separation between the anconeal process and the ulna; the line can be sharp or irregular with sclerosis of the edges. Periarticular osteophyte formation is present in more advance cases (**fig. 7.3**).

Fragmented coronoid process/medial coronoid process disease

The FCP/MCPD has been reported as the most common developmental anomaly affecting the elbow joint of the dog. It affects mainly medium and large breed dogs, with higher incidence in dogs. Neutral mediolateral and craniocaudal pronated view are recommended, with the latter reported to be the most sensitive view.[5] The radiographic signs can vary from a well-defined mineralized fragment medially to elbow joint, to an irregular or round and blunted coronoid process better visible in mediolateral view, or not visible at all, especially if the X-ray beam do not strike the lesion parallel or the fragment is undisplaced (**figs. 7.4** and **7.5**).

Periarticular osteophyte formations are visible as a consequence of the condition, first seen in the ulnar notch and on the anconeal process. Because the underdevelopment of the trochlear notch places the medial coronoid process (MCP) above the head of the radius, the high-lying MCP can damage the opposing articular cartilage of the humeral condyle resulting in an abrasion called "kissing lesions" (**fig. 7.6**).

Computed tomography (CT) is considered superior to radiology for the evaluation of the FCP/MCPD,[7,8] and it is now routinely used for the study of the elbow in dogs; in addition, it has been reported to be the gold standard to study radio-ulnar incongruity.[9] Technically the CT study should be

CHAPTER **7** Elbow dysplasia

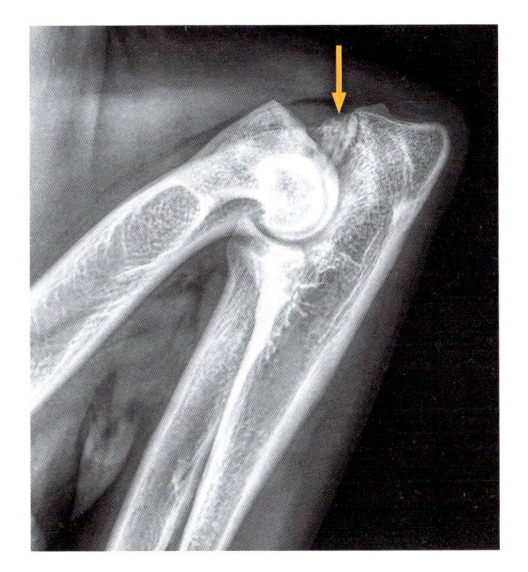

Fig. 7.3 Mediolateral projection of the elbow of a two-year-old female Abruzzese Shepherd dog with UAP. A radiolucent line of separation between the anconeal process and the ulna is visible, with bone sclerosis at the ulnar edges, as well as an osteophyte formation on the anconeal process (arrow).

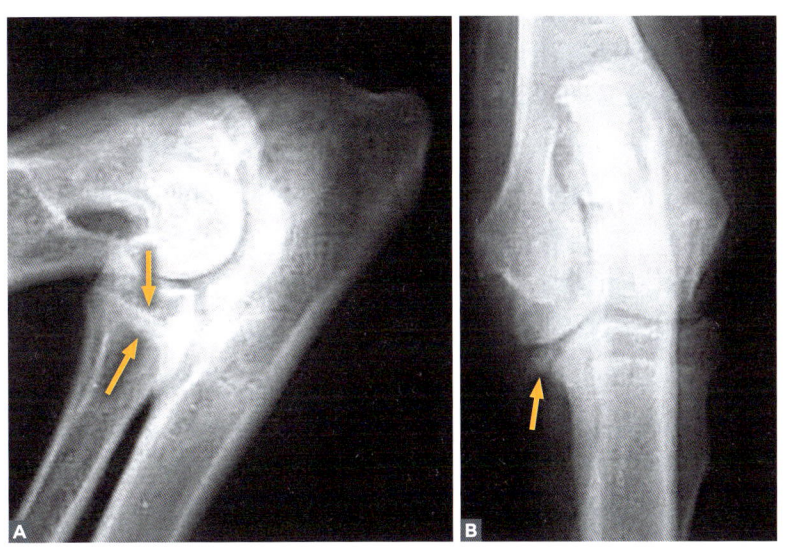

Fig. 7.4 A two-year-old male Labrador Retriever. In both flexed mediolateral (**A**) and craniocaudal (**B**) projections a well-defined fragment is visible at the medial ulnar coronoid process (arrows). Ulnar notch sclerosis and periarticular osteophyte formations on the anconeal process and radius head are visible, consistent with osteoarthritis.

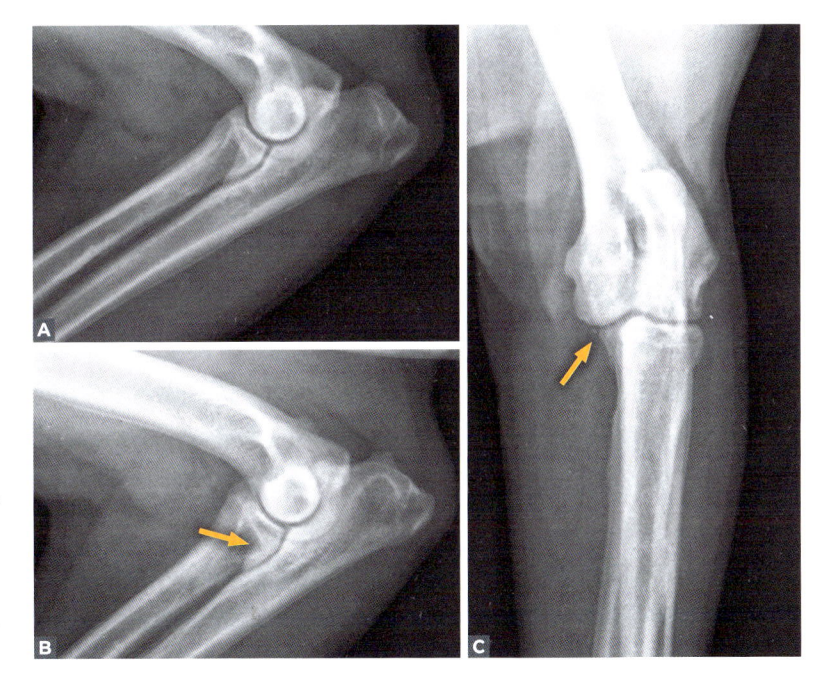

Fig. 7.5 A two-year-old female Labrador Retriever. Comparison between the mediolateral projection of the right normal (**A**) and left elbow affected by FCP (**B**) shows an irregular and truncated coronoid process in (**B**), while in (**A**) it appears well formed. The pronated craniocaudal projection of the left elbow (**C**) highlights a small fragment.

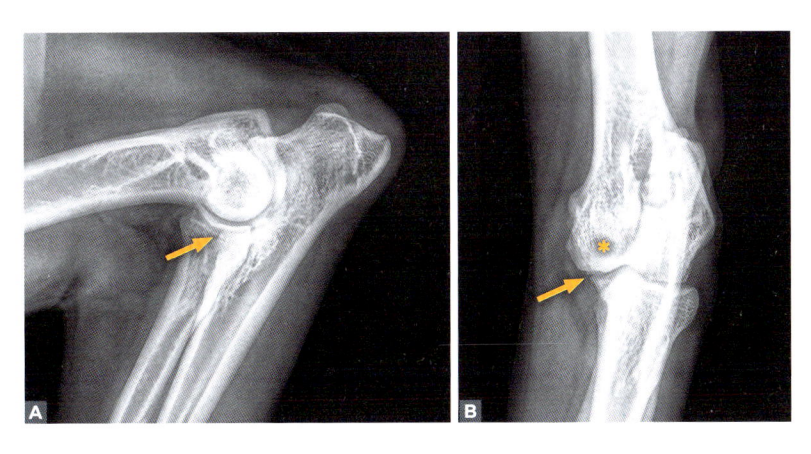

Fig. 7.6 A two-year-old male Border Collie. On the mediolateral projection (**A**) an irregularly shaped MCP is visible (arrows). The craniocaudal pronated view shows a «kissing lesion», consisting of a flattened and irregular medial humeral condyle border, with subchondral sclerosis (asterisk).

SECTION II APPENDICULAR SKELETON

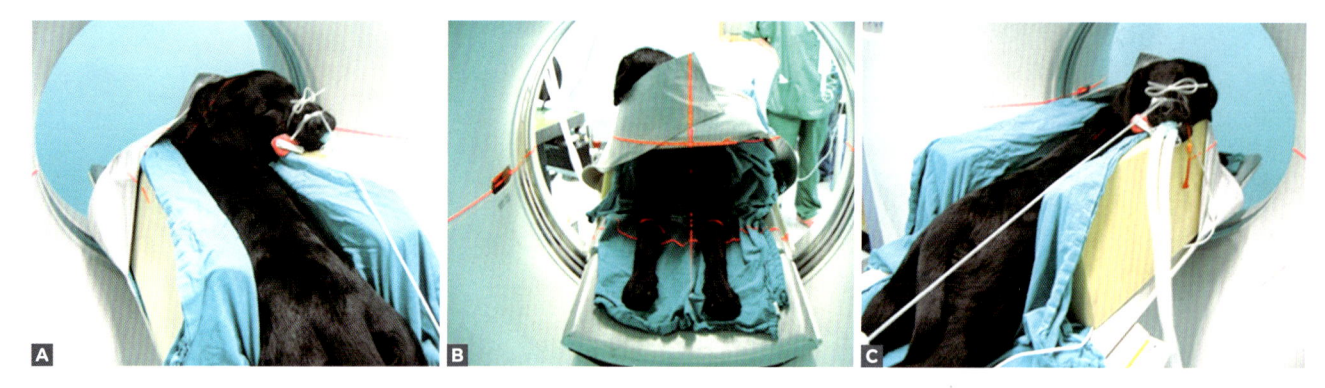

Fig. 7.7 The images (**A-C**) show one of the possible positions for the study of the elbows in CT, with the head rotated sideways and backwards, maintained by a rope. Other positions include lateral or dorsal decubitus with extended forelegs, with the aim of avoiding overlapping between head/neck and elbows, which causes streak artifacts.

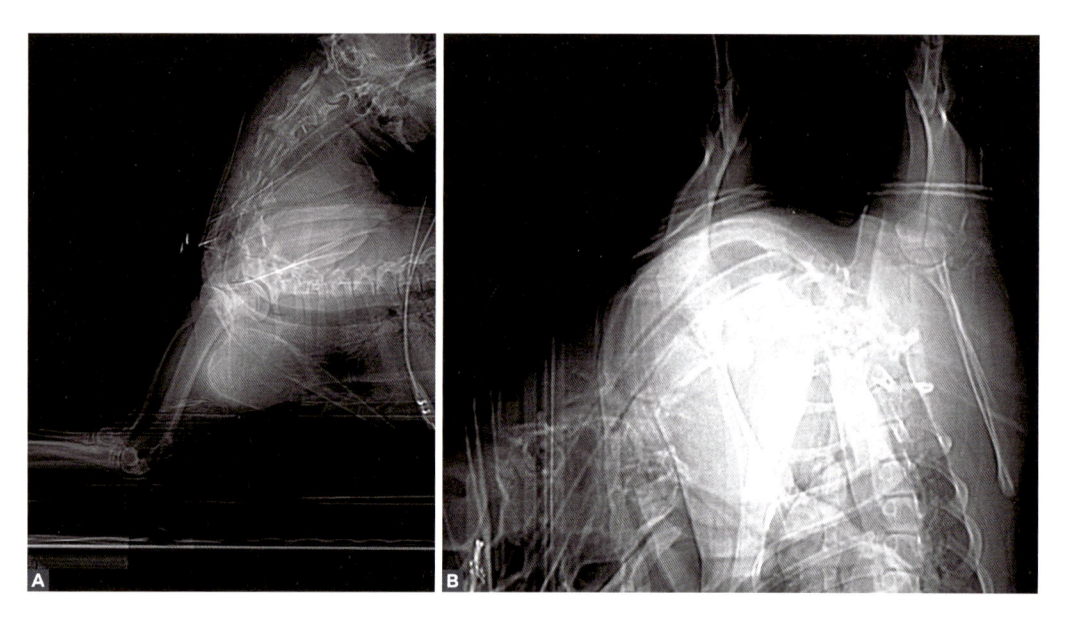

Fig. 7.8 Same dog as in fig. 7.7 before. The images show the scout views, where it is possible to verify that despite the rotation of the head and neck, the trachea does not undergo any narrowing.

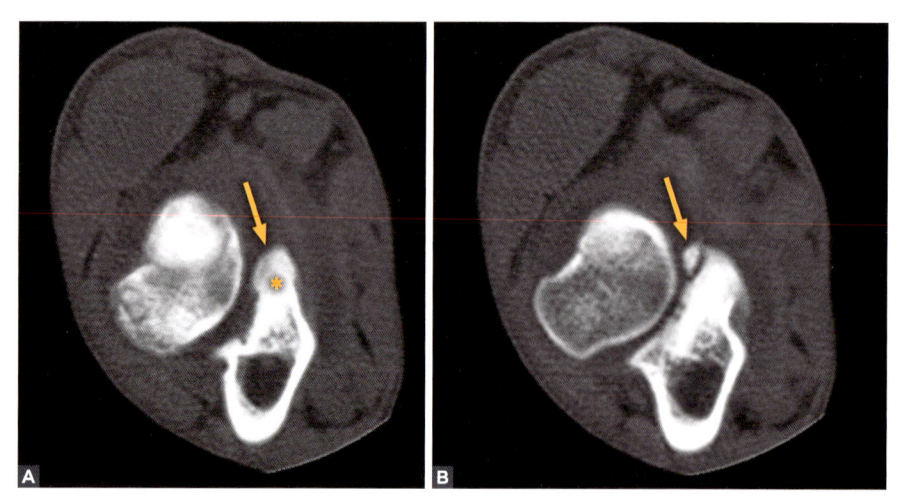

Fig. 7.9 A one-year-old male Bernese Mountain dog. The CT images with bone window show a severe osteophyte formation (arrow) (**A**) on the MCP (arrow), with bone sclerosis (asterisk), and a fragmented MCP (**B**) (arrow).

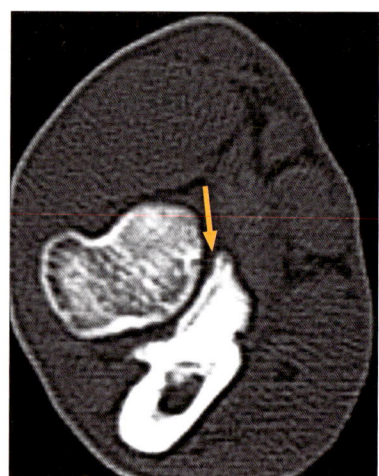

Fig. 7.10 A nine-month-old male Labrador Retriever. The transverse CT image of the elbow with bone window, shows a misshapen MCP, with an osteophyte formation (arrow), and bone sclerosis without any fragment, leading to a diagnosis of MCPD and osteoarthritis.

CHAPTER 7 Elbow dysplasia

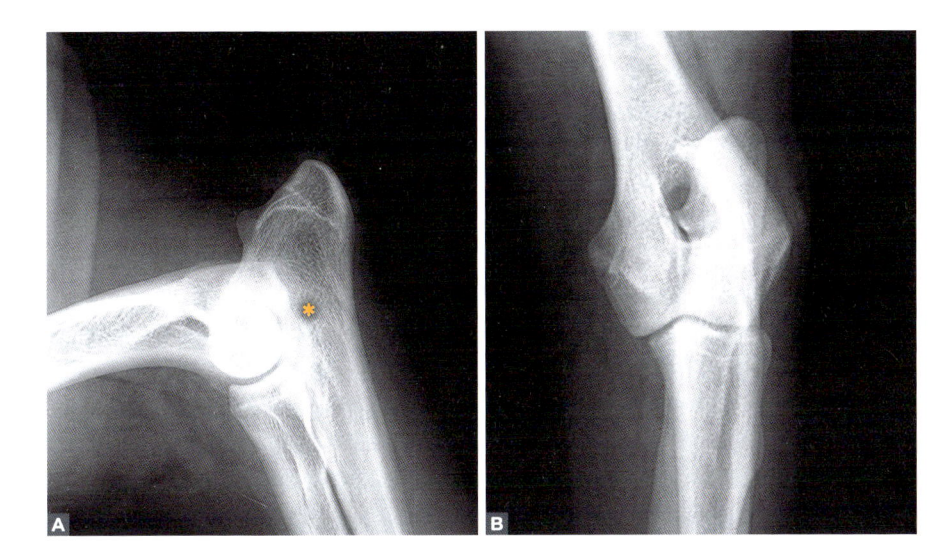

Fig. 7.11 An 18-month-old male Bouvier Des Flandres. Mediolateral and craniocaudal pronated radiographic views show mild sclerosis of the ulnar notch (asterisk), with no clear sings of other condition.

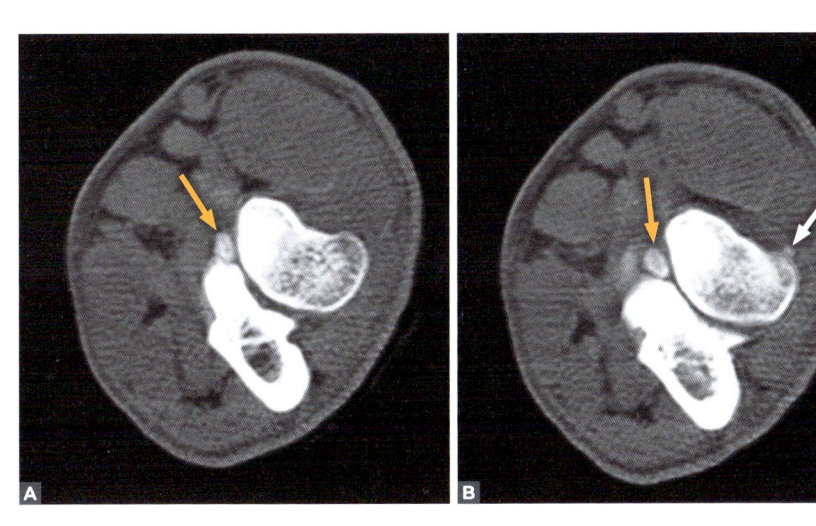

Fig. 7.12 Same dog as in fig. 7.10. The CT study clearly shows a rather big undisplaced fragment of the MCP (orange arrows) (**A-B**), with bone sclerosis. In addition, a round mineralization on the supinator muscle tendon or lateral collateral ligament (white arrow) (**B**), without any clinical relevance.

taken with 1 mm slice thickness,[10] and attention should be paid to positioning, with head and neck displaced from the superimposition of the elbows, in order to avoid streak artifacts (**figs. 7.7-7.12**).

Flexor enthesopathy

Flexor enthesopathy (FE) has been described as a cause of elbow pain in medium and large breed dogs and has been characterized radiographically as irregular margination of the medial humeral epicondyle with adjacent calcified bodies or a spur. The disease has been classified as primary if occurs alone with a prevalence of 6%, or concomitant with other elbow conditions with a prevalence of 34%.[4] Flexed mediolateral and craniocaudal pronated views allow to see the lesion. Radiographic signs are irregular margination of the medial humeral epicondyle, enthesophyte formations, calcified body in the elbow, osteophyte formations when osteoarthritis is present. Radiographic characteristics did not differ between primary and concomitant flexor enthesopathy groups. Radiography can be considered a first screening method for detection of flexor enthesopathy, but in case no other lesions are visible, CT can be useful to exclude other conditions, especially FCP (**fig. 7.13**). In some cases, a multifocal mineralization of the tendon can mimic a FCP lesion on pronated radiographic projection (**fig. 7.14**).

SECTION II APPENDICULAR SKELETON

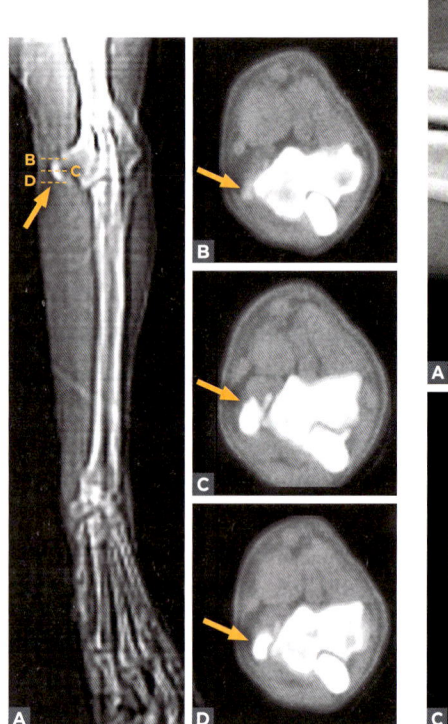

Fig. 7.13 A six-year-old male Cavalier King Charles Spaniel. On a radiographic craniocaudal image of the elbow, with artifacts because it is a CT scout projection, and three consecutive CT slices at the level of the medial humeral epicondyle highlight an irregular margination of the medial humeral epicondyle, enthesophyte formations, and a calcified body (arrows).

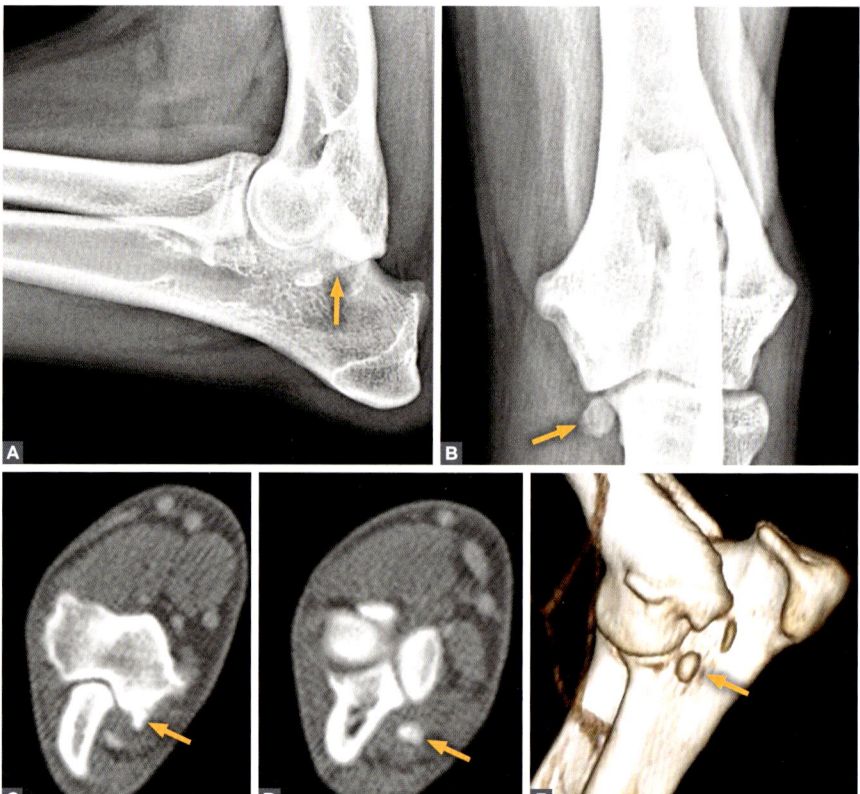

Fig. 7.14 A two-year-old mixed breed dog with mild to moderate recurrent lameness. On radiographic mediolateral projection (**A**) a mineralization is visible (arrow) at the insertion of the flexor tendons, corresponding to the bone fragment visible in CT (**C**). However, on craniocaudal pronated radiographic projection (**B**) a second mineralization is visible (arrow), mimicking a FCP lesion. The CT in transverse view (**D**) and volume rendering (**E**) clearly shows that the mineralization is still in the tendons.

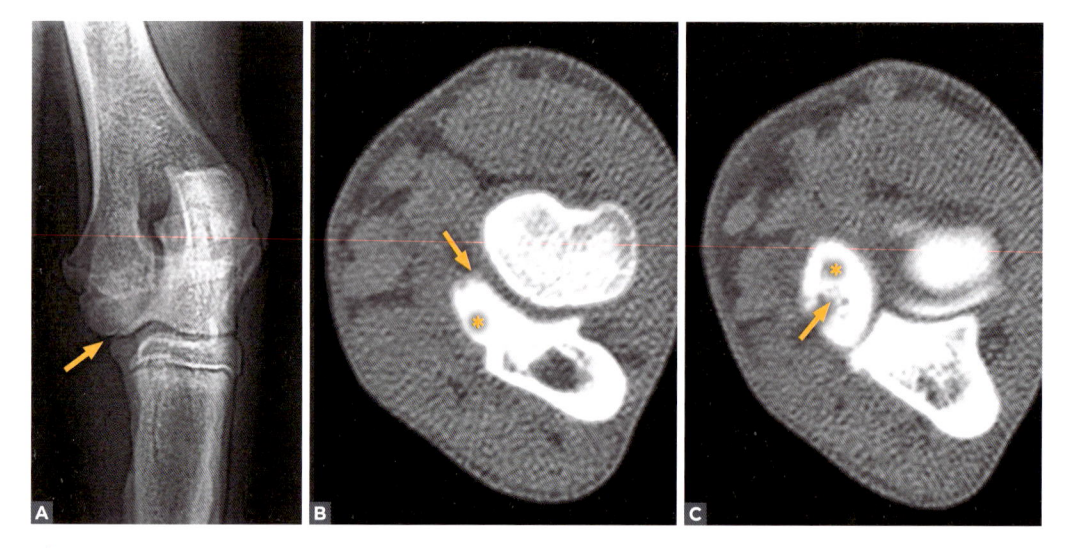

Fig. 7.15 A six-month-old Labrador Retriever, with moderate lameness clinically localized in the elbows. Craniocaudal pronated radiographic view (**A**) shows flattening of the medial aspect of the humeral condyle (arrow) with barely visible radiolucent area in the medial condyle. The MCP might be abnormally shaped, but no fragment is visible. The transverse CT images shows an irregularly shaped MCP, with a very small fragment and an osteophyte formation (arrow) with bone sclerosis (asterisk) (**B**); the medial humeral condyle appears to be affected by multiple radiolucent punctate areas (arrow) surrounded by bone sclerosis (asterisk) (**C**), typical of an OC lesion.

Osteochondrosis/osteochondritis dissecans

Osteochondrosis/osteochondritis dissecans of the humeral trochlea is a primary pathology of the epiphyseal cartilage, consequent to a disturbance of the endochondral ossification process. Mediolateral, craniocaudal, and eventually craniocaudal oblique views are suggested for the diagnosis. Radiographic signs are: flattening of the humeral condyle, semicircular subchondral defect, widening of the joint space, subchondral sclerosis, a calcified cartilaginous flap, and secondary degenerative joint disease. However, OCD sometimes it is not as easy to evaluate radiographically as the FCP. In those cases, CT can be helpful (**fig. 7.15**). The multiplanar reconstruction can be useful to better display the pathological condition (**fig. 7.16**).

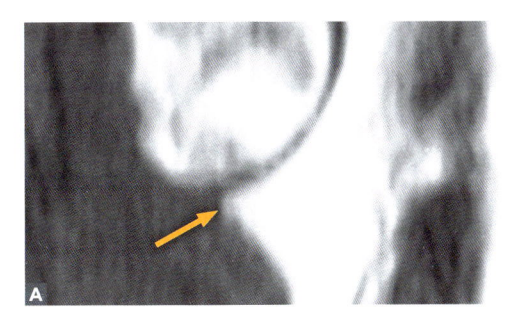

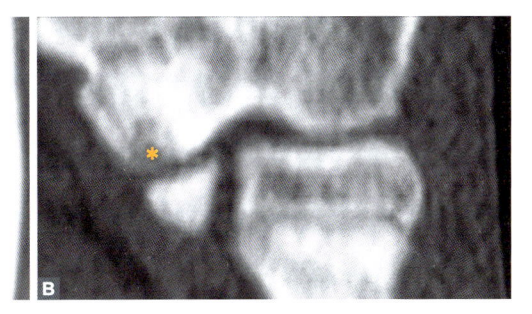

Fig. 7.16 Same dog as in fig. 7.14. The MPR shows a very small fragment of the MCP (arrow), and a round hypoattenuating area in the medial humeral condyle, surrounded by bone sclerosis, typical of an OC lesion (asterisk).

References

1. Audell L. Heredity of elbow dysplasia: Can elbow dysplasia be controlled by judicious breeding? *AAHA Scientific Proceedings* 730-733, 1990.
2. Olsson SE. General and etiologic factors in canine osteochondrosis. *Vet Quart* 9:268-278, 1987.
3. Ohlerth S, Tellhelm B, Amort K, Ondreka N. Explanation of the IEWG grading system. *IEWG Proceedings* 14-16, 2016.
4. de Bakker E, Saunders J, Gielen I, van Bree H, Coppieters E, Van Ryssen B. Radiographic findings of the medial humeral epicondyle in 200 canine elbow joints. *Vet Comp Orthop Traumatol* 25:359-365, 2012.
5. Wosar MA, Lewis DD, Neuwirth L, Parker RB, Spencer CP, Kubilis PS, Stubbs WP, Murphy ST, Shiroma JT, Stallings JT, Bertrand SG. Radiographic evaluation of elbow joints before and after surgery in dogs with possible fragmented medial coronoid process. *J Am Vet Med Assoc* 214:52-58, 1999.
6. Sjöström L. Ununited anconeal process in the dog. *Vet Clin North Am Small Anim Pract* 28:75-86, 1998.
7. Rau FC, Wigger A, Tellhelm B, Zwick M, Klumpp S, Neumann A, Oltersdorf B, Amort K, Failing K, Kramer M. Radiographic evaluation of elbow joints before and after surgery in dogs with possible fragmented medial coronoid process. *J Am Vet Med Assoc* 214:52-58, 1999.
8. Villamonte-Chevalier A, van Bree H, Broeckx B, Dingemanse W, Soler M, Van Ryssen B, Gielen I. Assessment of medial coronoid disease in 180 canine lame elbow joints: a sensitivity and specificity comparison of radiographic, computed tomographic and arthroscopic findings. *BMC Vet Res* 11:243, 2015.
9. Samoy Y, Van Ryssen B, Gielen I, Walschot N, van Bree H. Review of the literature: elbow incongruity in the dog. *Vet Comp Orthop Traumatol* 19:1-8, 2006.
10. Zweifel RT, Di Donato P, Hartmann A, Kramer M, von Pückler KH. Improved computed tomography accuracy with a 1-mm versus 2- or 3-mm slice thickness for the detection of medial coronoid disease in dogs. *Vet Comp Orthop Traumatol* 33:45-50, 2020.
11. Tyrrell D, Beck C. Survey of the use of radiography vs. ultrasonography in the investigation of gastrointestinal foreign bodies in small animals. *Vet Radiol Ultrasound* 47:404-408, 2006.

CHAPTER 8

Hip dysplasia

Ingrid Gielen and Henri van Bree

> **KEY POINTS**
>
> - Hip dysplasia (HD) is an important hereditary orthopedic condition. It is not a congenital condition because affected dogs are born with morphologically normal hips.
> - Although many imaging modalities such as radiography, computed tomography (CT), ultrasound (US), magnetic resonance imaging (MRI) and arthroscopy can be used in the assessment of canine patients with hip dysplasia, the ventrodorsal, hip-extended radiograph is the most used radiographic projection for evaluating canine hips.
> - The lack of accurate evaluation of subluxation and the relatively low inter- and intraobserver agreement seen when used as a screening tool complicates the incidence of false-negative evaluations.
> - Distraction-stress radiography techniques are used to better estimate the degree of subluxation of the hip joint.
> - Ultrasound imaging has been described in the dog to detect joint laxity with mixed results. Disadvantages of this technique include inability to evaluate acetabular morphology after approximately eight weeks of age in dogs and subjectivity of the evaluation and scoring systems.
> - Computed tomography (CT) is not used routinely for the evaluation of canine hips. In our clinic CT is mainly used to evaluate acetabular rim damage which is an important criterion when triple pelvic osteotomy (TPO) is considered. It is also valuable to detect degenerative changes at an early stage.
> - Magnetic resonance imaging (MRI) is infrequently used for the evaluation of canine hip dysplasia. Associated inflammation within the thigh muscles and also joint effusion can be evaluated.
> - Arthroscopy is more invasive than diagnostic imaging techniques but it enables to evaluate the hip joint. It can detect joint and cartilage damage before the onset of radiographic signs of osteoarthritis.

Hip dysplasia (HD) is an important hereditary orthopedic condition, often seen in large or giant breed dogs, although it can occur in smaller breeds and cats as well. The disease affects male and female dogs equally. HD is not a congenital condition because affected dogs are born with morphologically normal hips. The hip joint is a ball and socket joint and in affected dogs, the soft tissues that normally stabilize the hip joint become lax within the first few weeks of life. This laxity of the joint is followed by degenerative joint disease (DJD) or osteoarthritis (OA), which is the body's attempt to stabilize the laxity of the loose hip joint. Many affected dogs have dysplasia on both hips. Several factors lead to the development of hip dysplasia in dogs, beginning with genetics. Factors such as excessive growth rate, types of exercise, and improper weight and nutrition may enforce this genetic predisposition.[1] In the detection of hip dysplasia there are two issues: there is the clinical patient where the early diagnosis is important to determine an adequate treatment. Secondly, there is the screening for breeding purposes and these animals are mostly without clinical symptoms.

Canine hip dysplasia affects both young and old dogs. Often, young dogs will show a sudden onset of hindlimb lameness. The sudden onset of clinical signs is thought to be associated with microfractures of the socket, as this area is overloaded with pressure due to chronic abnormal load bearing due to laxity from the displaced joint. As the animal reaches maturity (12-18 months old) these fractures heal, usually resulting in improvement of the clinical signs symptoms of the condition subsiding. Most dysplastic dogs between 12 and 14 months of age walk and run soundly and are free of significant pain.

Older dogs show all the classical signs of osteoarthrosis and/or degenerative osteoarthritis. There is lameness after heavy exercise, a waddling gait, and difficulty rising after laying down and pain when handling the hips. The signs may come on suddenly, or can have a gradual one could notice a gradual decline in usual activity.[2]

Although clinical signs and palpable joint laxity may indicate hip dysplasia, diagnostic imaging is the principal method to diagnose hip dysplasia in the patient. Many imaging modalities such as radiography, computed tomography (CT), ultrasound (US), magnetic resonance imaging (MRI) and minimally invasive surgical procedures, such as arthroscopy, can be used in the assessment of canine patients with hip dysplasia. Hip radiographs performed under general anesthesia are the preferred method for diagnosing hip dysplasia. The most reported techniques include hip-extended radiography, Norberg angle, distraction-stress radiographs, measurement of the Norberg angle, and occasionally, the less used dorsal acetabular rim (DAR) view. A properly positioned hip-extended radiograph is useful as a screening tool for hip dysplasia and for detection of osteoarthritis but may not adequately demonstrate the degree of hip laxity. Distraction radiographic methods such as the PennHIP™ method allow for an objective measurement improved detection of laxity.[3]

The ventrodorsal, hip-extended radiograph is the most used radiographic projection for evaluating canine hips. Proper positioning of the extended hip view for this view often requires heavy sedation and/or general anesthesia and is achieved by placing the animal in dorsal recumbency, extending the hindlimbs caudally with parallel and slightly internally rotated femurs. A properly positioned radiograph should include a symmetric pelvis, parallel and fully extended femurs, and patellas that are centered within the femoral trochlea (**fig. 8.1**). This radiographic position is one of the most often used by screening organizations such as the Orthopaedic Foundation for Animals (OFA), Fédération Cynologique Internationale, and the British Veterinary Association/Kennel Club. Common errors in positioning include obliquity of the pelvic radiograph, failure to fully extend the limbs, and inadequate internal rotation of the femurs (**fig. 8.2**). Radiographic evidence of osteoarthrosis of the coxofemoral joint includes femoral periarticular osteophyte formation of the femoral head, neck, and craniolateral acetabular rim, subchondral sclerosis, subchondral sclerosis of the craniodorsal acetabulum, osteophytes along the acetabular margin, and joint remodeling (**fig. 8.3**). The caudal curvilinear enthesiophytosis at the insertion of the joint capsule (CCO, or Morgan line) and circumferential femoral head osteophytosis (CFHO) (**fig. 8.3**) represent two radiographic features that have been reported to be early osteoarthrosis that predict later development of more characteristic signs of osteoarthritis.[4] In the absence of radiographic signs of osteoarthritis, joint subluxation on the hip-extended radiograph is considered diagnostic for hip dysplasia. The degree of subluxation can be subjectively evaluated or objectively quantified using quantitative methods such as the Norberg angle and femoral overlap (% coverage). However, the hip-extended radiograph may mask joint subluxation by tightening the joint capsule as the limbs are extended and forcing the femoral

CHAPTER 8 Hip dysplasia

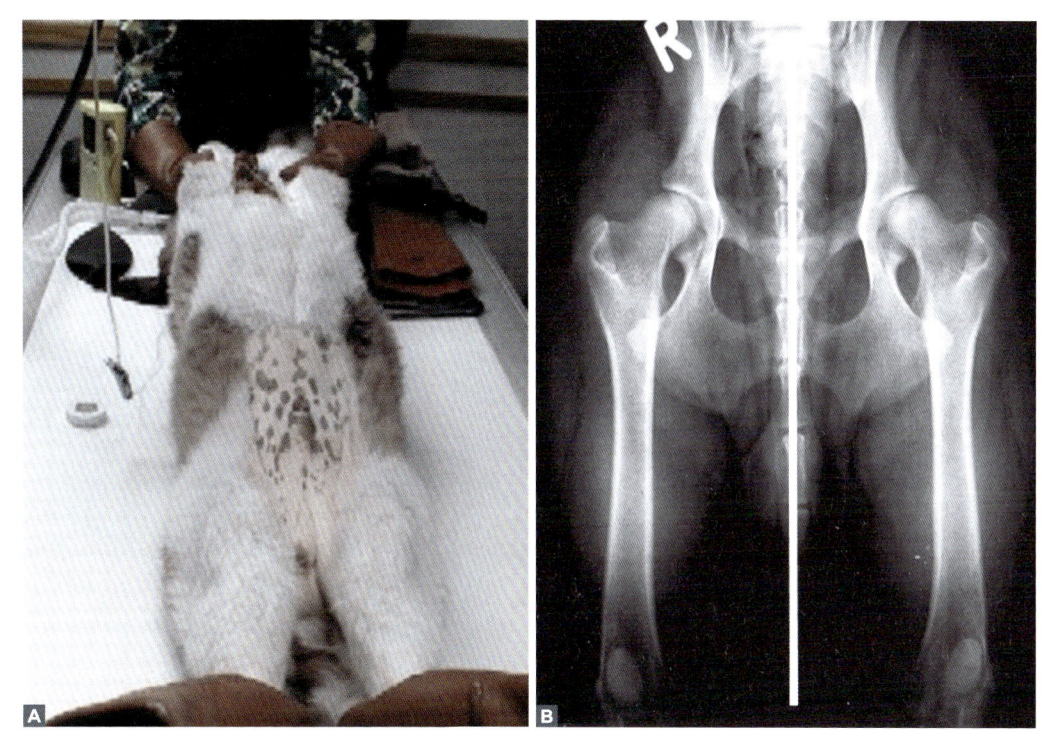

Fig. 8.1 (**A**) A properly positioned dog includes a symmetric pelvis, parallel and fully extended femurs, and patellas that are centered within the femoral trochlea. The femurs are internally rotated to achieve proper positioning of the patellas. (**B**) The result of a properly positioned radiograph: the pelvis is completely symmetric; the right half should be the mirror image of the left half.

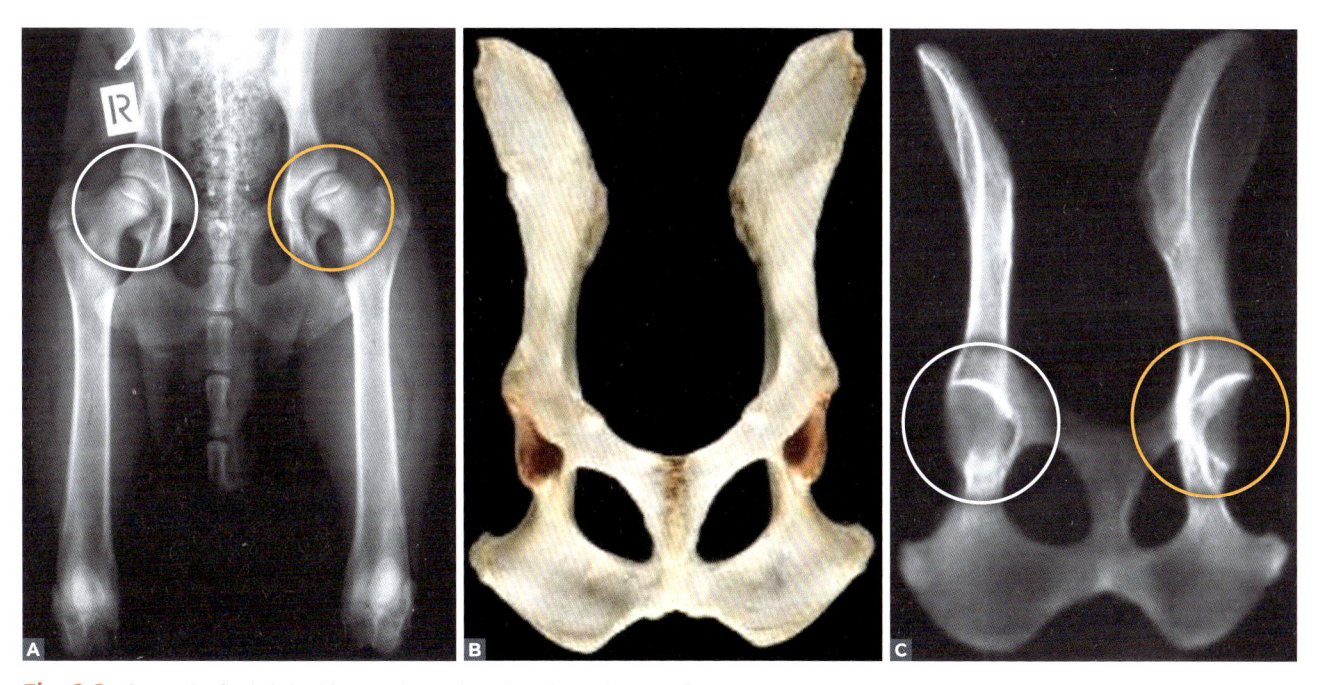

Fig. 8.2 The result of a slightly oblique radiograph making the evaluation of the acetabular depth and joint congruity problematic. (**A**) Extended hip view of a normal dog with an asymmetrically positioned pelvis. The pelvis in (**B**) is symmetric and has normal acetabulae. (**C**) The radiograph of the pelvic specimen is oblique to show how the depth of the acetabula is altered due to geometric distortion. The acetabulae are not symmetric in this radiograph: the right one (white circle) is deeper than the left one (orange circle). The left acetabula artifactually appears shallow compared to the right side (**B**, **C**). The specimen (**B**) used for the radiograph in (**C**) has normal acetabulae.

SECTION II APPENDICULAR SKELETON

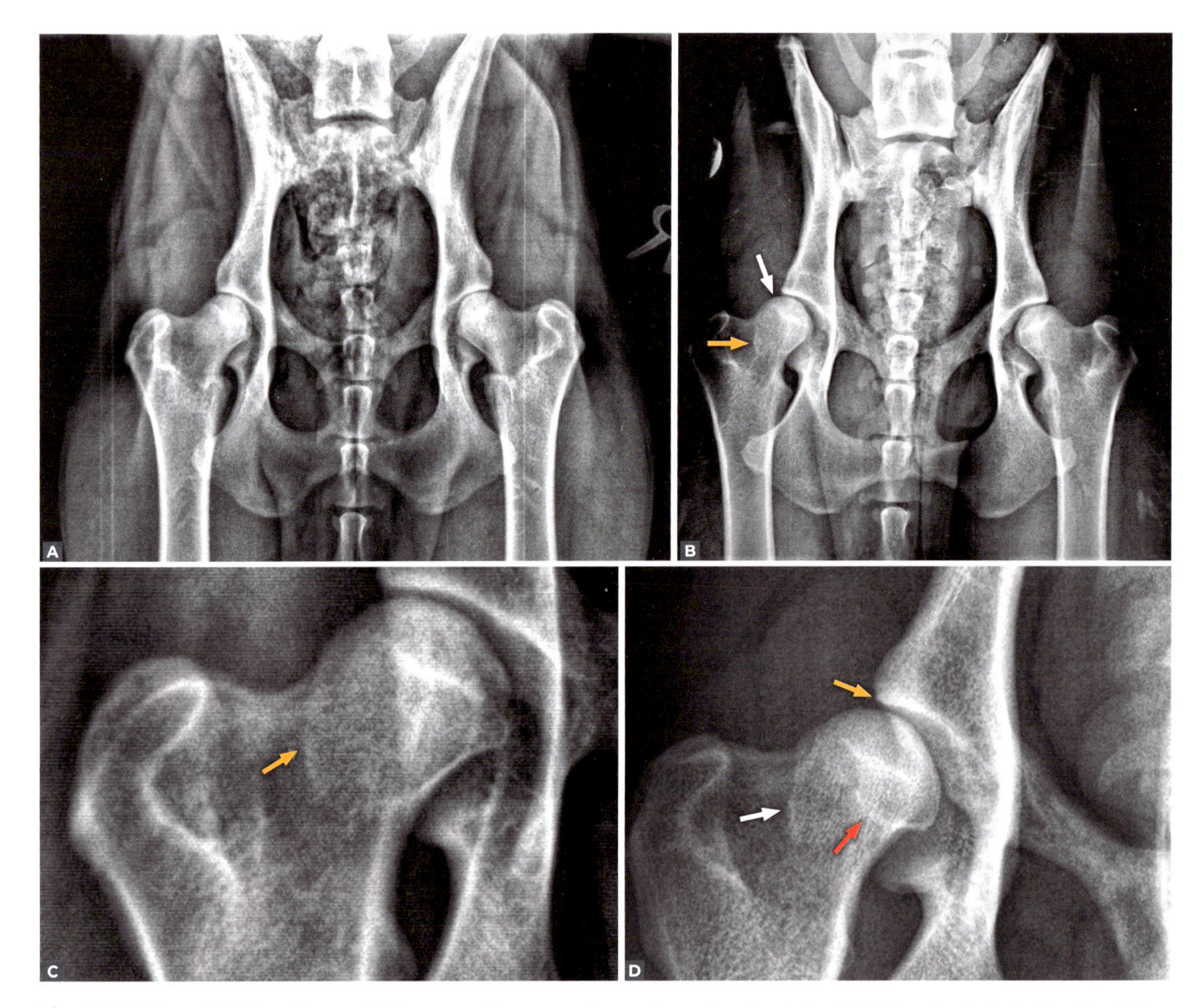

Fig. 8.3 (**A**) Normal hip joint with a parallel joint space without any evidence of osteophytosis or laxity. (**B**) A bilaterally dysplastic hip with a shallow acetabulum and incongruent joint space. There is subchondral sclerosis of the craniodorsal acetabulum (white arrow) and a caudal curvilinear enthesophyte at the capsule attachment (Morgan line) (orange arrow) representing early signs of osteoarthrosis. (**C**) A hip joint with a deep acetabulum but a faint Morgan line is already visible. (**D**) A dysplastic hip with a shallow acetabulum and a short joint space. A Morgan line (white arrow), as well as a circumferential femoral head osteophyte (CFHO) formation (red arrow) and subchondral sclerosis of the craniodorsal acetabulum (orange arrow) are visible.

heads to sit more deeply within the acetabula. The relatively low interobserver and intraobserver agreement seen when used as a screening tool further complicates the incidence of false-negative evaluations and the low reliability within and between experienced observers increases errors in the screening process and surgical decision making.

Diagnostic techniques for hip dysplasia

Norberg angle

The Norberg angle is calculated by measuring the angle between a line that connects the center of the femoral head between the left and the right hip and a line that connects the center of the femoral head with the lateral tip of the cranial acetabular rim. A larger angle indicates a deeper acetabulum and more congruent hips, whereas smaller angles are consistent with increasing degrees of subluxation. A Norberg angle greater than 105° is generally considered to be normal. Slight rotation of the pelvis on the radiograph will substantially affect both the Norberg angle and the femoral overlap, causing the congruency of one hip joint to be overestimated, with underestimation of the contralateral hip joint. Furthermore, the use of a strict reference value for the Norberg angle is not appropriate because a value consistent with dysplastic hips can vary between breeds.[5]

Dorsal acetabular rim view

The DAR (dorsal acetabular rim) view was first described by Slocum and Devine in 1990. This radiographic view is used to evaluate the dorsal aspect of the acetabular rim, which is the area of the acetabulum that receives much of the stress concentration with subluxation of the femoral head during ambulation. The DAR view achieves an unobstructed view of the dorsal acetabular rim from a cranial to caudal perspective. Correct radiographic positioning results in superimposition of the iliac wings, iliac body, acetabulum, and tuber ischii, with an unobstructed view of the dorsal acetabular rim. The DAR view is reportedly useful to document the degree of degenerative joint damage as the acetabular rim progresses from sharply pointed in the normal dog to more rounded and blunt with joint damage.[6] However, the DAR radiographic view is not widely used because diagnostic quality images can be difficult to obtain. Acetabular rim damage can be more easily evaluated by using computed tomography (CT) avoiding all superimposition.

Distraction-stress radiography techniques

Distraction-stress radiography techniques are used to better estimate the degree of passive laxity of the coxofemoral joint.[7,8] The distraction stress radiography methods most used include the University of Pennsylvania Hip Improvement Program (PennHIP), dorsolateral subluxation measurement (DLS), and the Flüuckiger subluxation index. The PennHIP method of radiography is performed in a heavily sedated or anesthetized animal. Three radiographic projections are obtained: a standard hip-extended radiograph, a neutral stance-phase compression radiograph, and a neutral distraction radiograph. For the distraction radiograph, a fulcrum device is placed between the proximal femurs, and adduction results in hip subluxation in abnormal dogs. From the distraction radiograph, a distraction index (DI) can be calculated as the degree of femoral head subluxation from the acetabulum (**fig. 8.4**). A DI score of 0 equates to no subluxation, whereas a DI score of 1 equates to a fully luxated joint. A PennHIP distraction index of >0.3 in dogs older than 16 weeks of age is generally considered to indicate an increased risk of future osteoarthritis development.[8]

Ultrasound imaging of human neonates has been used since 1980 as a screening tool for hip dysplasia in at-risk patients. A similar technique has also been described in the dog to detect joint laxity with mixed results. Disadvantages of the technique include inability to evaluate acetabular morphology after approximately eight weeks of age in dogs because of femoral head ossification, subjectivity of the evaluation and scoring systems, and the lack of normal reference values. Results of one study suggest that static and dynamic ultrasonography of hip joints in puppies between 16 and 49 days of age is technically feasible but cannot be recommended for detecting puppies that will develop canine hip dysplasia between the ages of 12 and 24 months (**fig. 8.5**).[9]

Furthermore, the clinical utility of ultrasound is highly operator-dependent. For these reasons, ultrasound is not routinely used for diagnosing or screening canine patients for hip dysplasia.

Computed tomography

Computed tomography (CT), although nowadays available in veterinary medicine, is not used routinely for the evaluation of canine hips. CT provides accurate and easy evaluation of coxofemoral joint indices while the animal is positioned in a weight-bearing position, which may be a better indicator of the degree of functional laxity. Various CT hip indices have been proposed and compared

SECTION II APPENDICULAR SKELETON

A Distraction index (DI) = d/r

B Compression index = 0

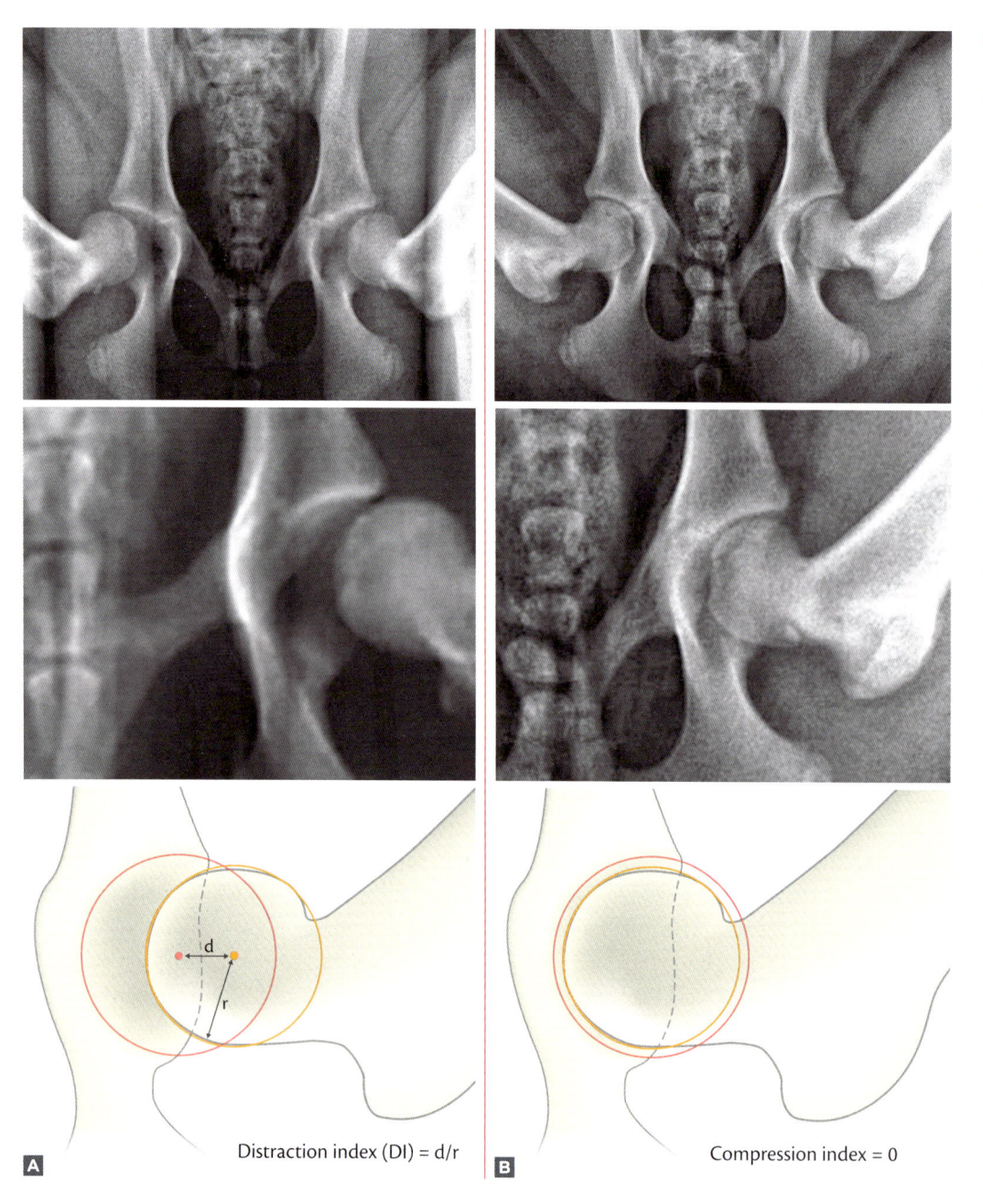

Fig. 8.4 A radiograph was taken with the dog heavily sedated or anesthetized and positioned in dorsal recumbency. First a flexed pelvic limb compression view was taken (**A**) and then a distraction view with a distraction device placed between the thighs (**B**). Afterwards the canine DI (distraction index) was calculated considering d/r. *d*: distance between the center of the femoral head and center of acetabulum; *r*: radius of the femoral head. (**A**) Represents the compression view and (**B**) the distraction view showing hip laxity due to hip dysplasia.

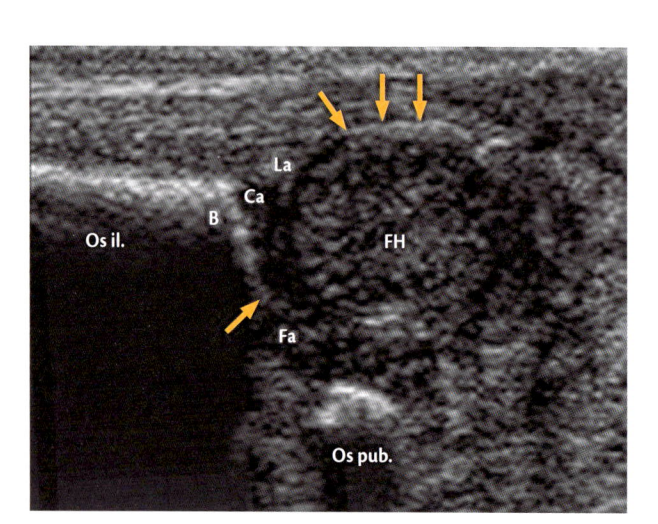

Fig. 8.5 Ultrasound image of a very young dog being assessed for hip dysplasia. *Os il.*, os ilium; *FH*, femoral head; *La*, labrum acetabulare; *B*, bone edge; *Ca*, cartilage; *Os pub.*, os pubis; *Fa*, fossa acetabulare. Courtesy of Prof. Martin Kramer, Gießen University, Gießen, Germany.

with PennHIP and OFA conformation scores but the normal reference ranges for these CT values and the ability to use these in clinical situations requires further investigation.[2,10] In our clinic CT can be mainly used to evaluate acetabular rim damage which is an important criterion when triple pelvic osteotomy (TPO) is considered (**fig. 8.6**). CT is also anecdotally valuable for the detection of degenerative changes at an early stage.

Magnetic resonance imaging

Magnetic resonance imaging (MRI) has not been established for assessment of hip dysplasia in dogs. Although more and more access to conventional MRI is possible also in veterinary medicine, it is infrequently used for the evaluation of canine hip dysplasia and bone disorders in general. On the other hand, MRI is an excellent imaging modality for the evaluation of soft tissues, ligamentous structures, joint capsule, and the subchondral bone (**fig. 8.7**).[3] In hip dysplasia, associated inflammation within the thigh muscles and joint effusion can be evaluated (**fig. 8.7**). Nevertheless, factors such as cost, examination time, required expertise, and need for general anesthesia preclude its use in canine patients for the evaluation of hip dysplasia.

Arthroscopy

Although arthroscopy is more invasive than diagnostic imaging techniques, it enables the evaluation of the hip joint and can detect joint and cartilage damage before the onset of radiographic signs of osteoarthritis (**fig. 8.8**). It has been demonstrated that approximately 50% of dogs without radiographic signs of DJD have moderate to severe cartilage lesions identified arthroscopically. Therefore, arthroscopy can be used as a diagnostic tool for improved assessment of the status of the hip point before surgical interventions are carried out.[11]

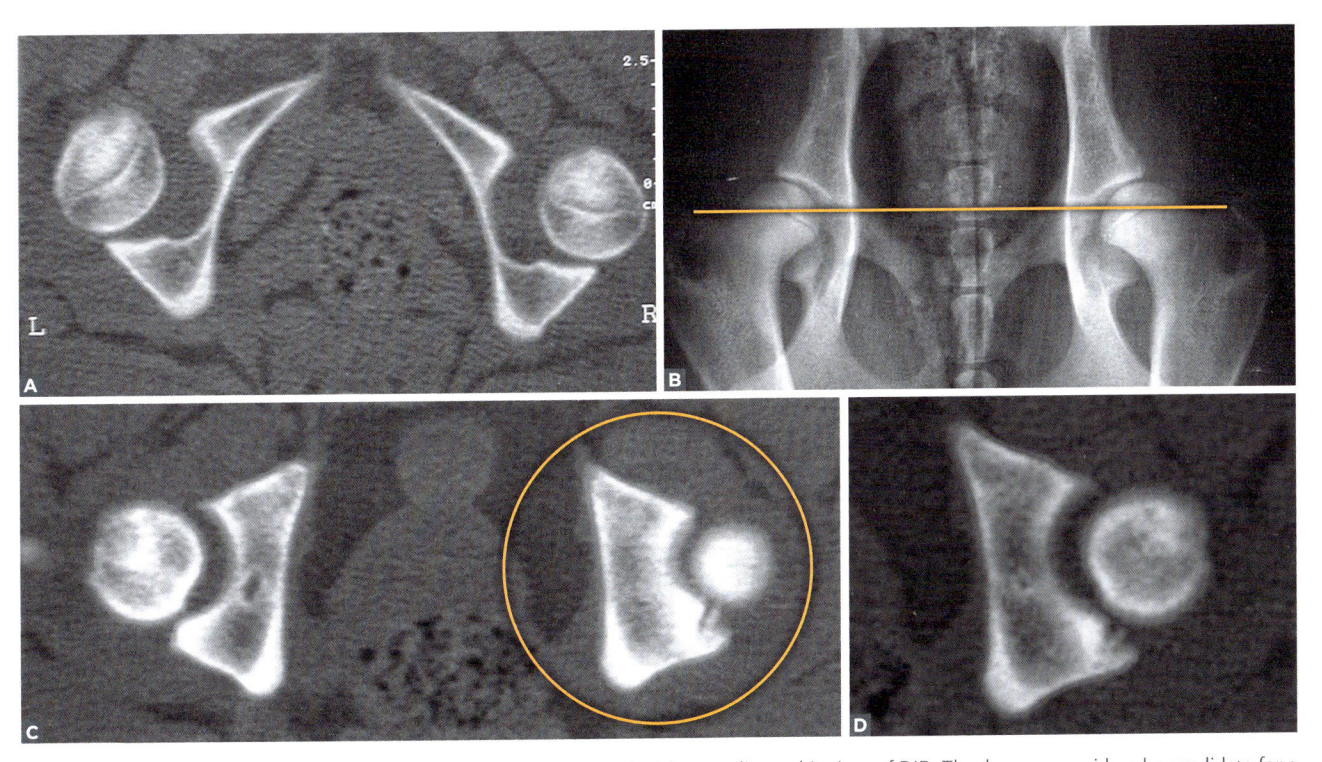

Fig. 8.6 (**A**) CT image of a six-month-old dog with hip dysplasia and without radiographic signs of DJD. The dog was considered a candidate for a triple pelvic osteotomy and therefore the dorsal rim was being assessed for pathology (**C-D**). (**B**) An image of a non-damaged dorsal rim to compare. The dorsal rim of the acetabulum shows fragmentation (**C-D**) and therefore was rejected for surgery.

SECTION II APPENDICULAR SKELETON

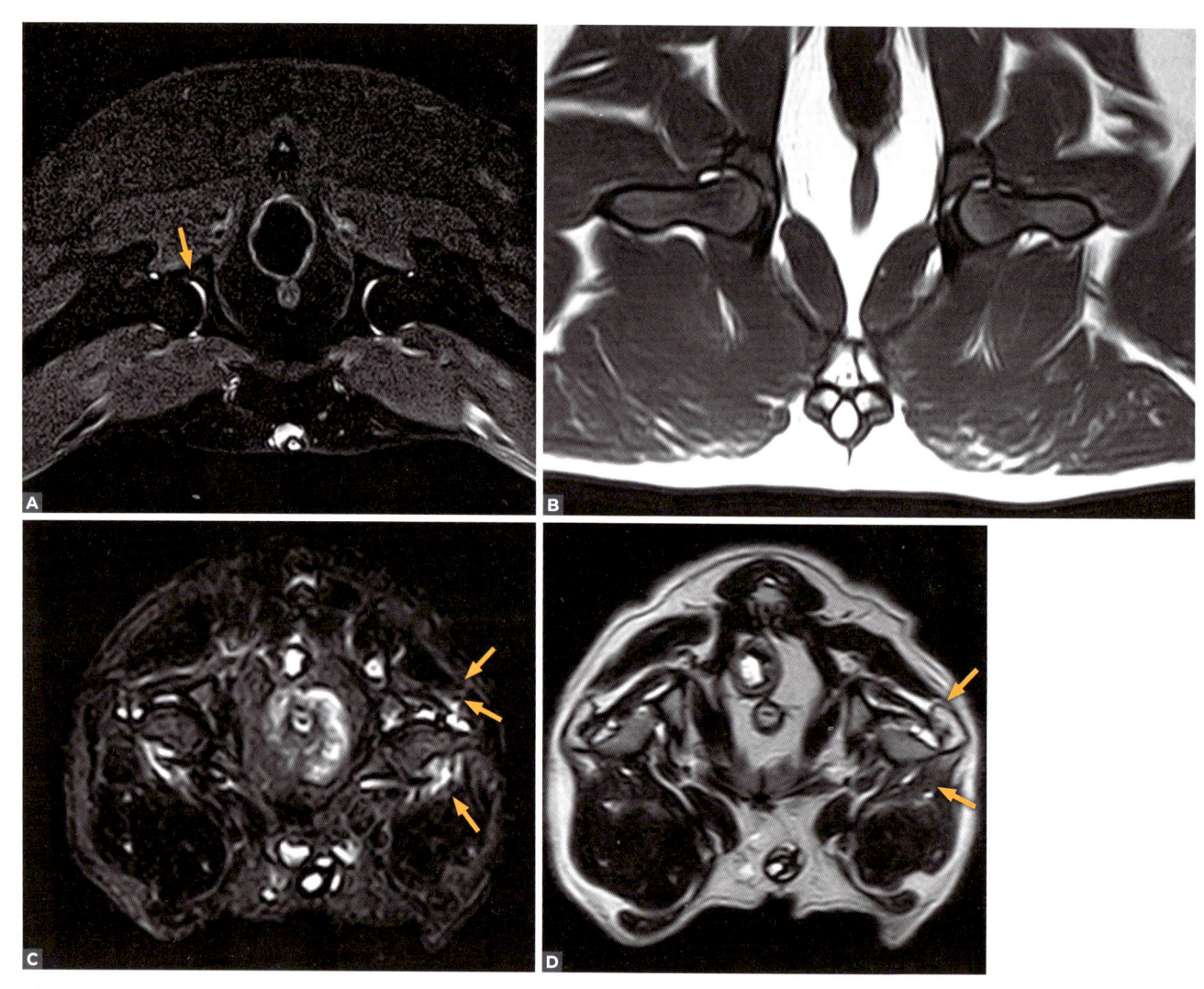

Fig. 8.7 MRI images of a normal (**A-B**) and dysplastic (**C-D**) hip joint. (**A**) Transverse T2W fat suppressed image showing the synovial fluid as a hyperintense structure (arrow). The osseous structures are hypointense and the muscles have a moderate intensity. (**B**) Dorsal T2W image showing the osseous anatomy of the hips and normal surrounding musculature. (**C**) Transverse STIR image of dysplastic hip joint. Muscle atrophy of the left upper thigh is present as well as fluid distention the left hip joint (arrows). (**D**) Transverse T2W image of the same joint as (**C**) where the anatomical structures can be seen in more detail. Muscle atrophy and the inflammation within the surrounding muscles (arrows) are visible.

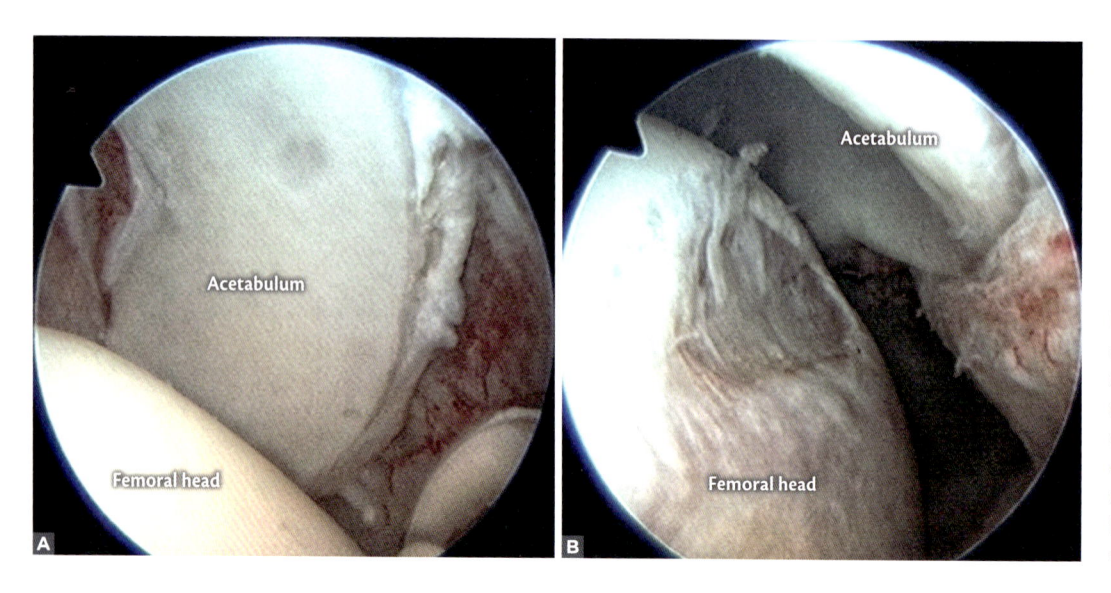

Fig. 8.8 An arthroscopic image of a normal (**A**) and dysplastic (**B**) hip. The acetabular edge and femoral head can be evaluated. The dysplastic hip has cartilage damage due to the wear and tear.

76

References

1. Broeckx BJG, Verhoeven G, Coopman F, Van Haeringen W, Bosmans T, et al. The effects of positioning, reason for screening and the referring veterinarian on prevalence estimates of canine hip dysplasia. *Vet J* 201:378-384, 2014.
2. Schachner ER, Lopez MJ. Diagnosis, prevention, and management of canine hip dysplasia: a review. *Vet Med (Auckl)* 6:181-192, 2015.
3. Ginja MM, Ferreira AJ, Jesus SS, Melo-Pinto P, Bulas-Cruz J, Orden MA, San-Roman F, Llorens-Pena MP, Gonzalo-Orden JM. Comparison of clinical, radiographic, computed tomographic and magnetic resonance imaging methods for early prediction of canine hip laxity and dysplasia. *Vet Radiol Ultrasound* 50:135-143, 2009.
4. Szabo SD, Biery DN, Lawler DF, Shofer FS, Powers MY, Kealy RD, Smith GK. Evaluation of a circumferential femoral head osteophyte as an early indicator of osteoarthritis characteristic of canine hip dysplasia in dogs *J Am Vet Med Assoc* 231:889-892, 2007.
5. Janssens L, De Ridder M, Verhoeven G, Gielen I, van Bree H. Comparing Norberg angle, linear femoral overlap and surface femoral overlap in radiographic assessment of the canine hip joint. *J Small Anim Pract* 55:135-138, 2014.
6. Slocum B, Devine TM. Dorsal acetabular rim radiographic view for evaluation of the canine hip *J Am Anim Hosp Assoc* 26:289-296, 1990.
7. Smith GK, Biery DN, Gregor TP. New concepts of coxofemoral joint stability and the development of a clinical stress-radiographic method for quantitating hip joint laxity in the dog. *J Am Vet Med Assoc* 196:59-70, 1990.
8. Santana A, Alves-Pimenta S, Martins J, Colaço B, Ginja M. Comparison of two distraction devices for assessment of passive hip laxity in dogs. *Front Vet Sci* 7:491, 2020.
9. Fischer A, Flöck A, Tellhelm B, Failing K, Kramer M, Thiel C. Static and dynamic ultrasonography for the early diagnosis of canine hip dysplasia. *J Small Anim Pract* 51:582-588, 2010.
10. Farese JP, Todhunter RJ, Lust G, Williams AJ, Dykes NL. Dorsolateral subluxation of hip joints in dogs measured in a weight-bearing position with radiography and computed tomography. *Vet Surg* 27:393-405, 1998.
11. Ulfelder EH, Hudson CC, Beale BS. Correlation of distraction index with arthroscopic findings in juvenile dogs with hip dysplasia. *Vet Surg* 48:1050-1057, 2019.

CHAPTER 9

Osteochondrosis

Ingrid Gielen and Henri van Bree

KEY POINTS

- Osteochondrosis (OC) is a developmental disorder marked by abnormal endochondral ossification of epiphyseal cartilage in joints.
- Osteochondritis dissecans (OCD) is the form of OC in which the articular cartilage is fissured and forms a cartilage flap.
- In dogs, one of the most common predilection sites of OC is the caudal humeral head.
- In all radiographic techniques, OC is noticed as a radiolucent roundish area surrounded by a sclerotic rim.
- A positive contrast arthrogram can be helpful in identifying lesions when the cartilage flap has not mineralized; additionally, the differentiation between unattached and attached cartilage flaps and osteochondral fragments can be noticed.
- Computed tomography (CT) is helpful in detecting early lesions and in imaging small joints, like the elbow and tarsal joints.

Osteochondrosis (OC) is an abnormality of endochondral ossification in which the articular cartilage of the epiphysis fails to form subchondral bone. The articular cartilage is thickened, and because it is subject to movement and stress, it is prone to tearing, especially in the areas that bear the most weight, such as the caudal aspect of the humeral head. Repeated trauma can cause a flap of cartilage detached from the underlying bone, which is termed osteochondritis dissecans (OCD). Because of the tear, the joint fluid can come in direct contact with the underlying epiphyseal bone, which causes inflammation and pain. Usually, the dog will experience lameness at this point. As long as the cartilaginous flap remains attached the lesion will not heal, and lameness will persist. In the shoulder joint, once the flap has been released or been removed surgically, the defect in the articular cartilage is filled in with fibrocartilage, a type of "scar" cartilage. Complications may arise when cartilaginous fragments, referred to as "joint mice" become entrapped in the bicipital tendon sheath, causing synovitis, adhesions and pain.[1,2] In approximately one third of the cases of OC, the disease is bilateral. Occasionally, it is present in several different joints in the same individual. It is seen twice as often in males as in females. This developmental disease occurs in rapidly growing medium-to-giant breed dogs, typically between 6 and 9 months of age, but can occur as late as 12 months or older. Currently, the shoulder joint is still the most common site, being affected in 74% of the cases. The elbow joint is affected in 11%, the talocrural joint in 9%, and the stifle joint in 4% of the cases.[2]

In most cases, radiology is still the first screening tool used. Ultrasound (US), computed tomography (CT), and magnetic resonance imaging (MRI) are also of value in the detection of specific and discrete OC lesions.

Radiography is an excellent technique for bone structure imaging, being readily available, inexpensive, quick, and has excellent spatial resolution and image contrast. The major limitation is the superimposition of complex three-dimensional anatomy in a two-dimensional image, which may obscure lesions. This is especially an issue in smaller complicated joints such as the elbow and talocrural joints.[2]

Ultrasonographic examination of joints requires substantial experience and a standardized examination procedure. In most joints, even small amounts of fluid accumulation (hypo- to anechoic) can be easily demonstrated in the joint pouches. The subchondral bone is visible as a hyperechoic band overlying the bone, which completely blocks ultrasound transmission creating a complete acoustic shadow. The cartilage can be examined for thickness and integrity. Synovial proliferation can be evaluated as well.[3,4]

Superior soft tissue contrast resolution and absence of superimposition are the major advantages of CT over conventional radiography. CT greatly facilitates examining complex joint structures such as the elbow, tarsus and carpus. Another advantage is that high resolution thin CT images can be reformatted in multiple anatomic planes. CT can distinguish far smaller changes in X-ray attenuation by tissues than radiography. This feature, the capacity to adjust the gray scale of the digital image, and the elimination of overlying structures, means CT is superior for detection of subtle new bone production and lysis than conventional radiography.[2]

MRI is ideal for assessing the soft tissue components of a joint, but is also valuable for assessing cartilage and bone pathology. With this technique, multiplanar images are readily obtained and differentiation between different structures and pathologic processes is possible by using different sequences. MRI is especially sensitive to bone marrow alterations (bone bruising). The visualization of normal and abnormal cartilage is difficult in the dog because the articular cartilage in dogs is very thin.[4] The intravenous injection of contrast agents can be useful in the detection of inflammatory processes.

The shoulder joint

In the shoulder, OC lesions can be detected radiographically in most cases. These lesions manifest as a flattening at the caudal area of the humeral head.

Shoulder osteochondrosis is often bilateral and radiographs of both joints should be obtained in all affected patients.

Early lesions may appear as subtle flattening of the subchondral bone at the caudal aspect of the humeral head. With larger lesions, there may be more extensive flattening or a concave defect in the subchondral bone. In some cases, a flap may be visible if there is partial mineralization of the flap. This is uncommon, and radiographs cannot distinguish osteochondrosis from osteochondritis dissecans in most patients. Slightly pronated supinated mediolateral radiographs may be needed to identify small lesions. Periarticular osteophytes from secondary degenerative joint disease may be present in chronic cases. Positive contrast arthrography provides a limited assessment of the joint space and capsule, but is most useful to determine if the articular cartilage is intact, fissured or has formed a flap. Contrast arthrography can locate non-mineralized intra-articular osteochondral fragments, especially within the synovial sheath of the biceps brachii, which cause synovitis, adhesions and relatively more severe clinical signs (**figs. 9.1** and **9.2**).[4,6]

US can be utilized in the shoulder joint for the assessment of OC lesions. For this examination, a high frequency linear transducer (7.5-15 MHz) is utilized, and the patient might need to be anesthetized.[3] The humeral head is seen as a hyperechoic curvilinear interface with a complete acoustic shadow, and the cartilage as a thin overlying anechoic layer. The subchondral defect has irregular margins, and the presence of second hyperechoic lines at the bottom of the subchondral defect seen on US is a reliable sign for the presence of a flap (**fig. 9.3**).[3,4]

In rare cases CT may be preferred, such as OC of the glenoid cavity, and in cases with a very small OC lesion of the humeral head that is not confirmed on radiographs[7] (**fig. 9.4**). In CT contrast ar-

CHAPTER 9 Osteochondrosis

Fig. 9.1 A six-month-old Border Collie. (A) Mediolateral view of a small OC lesion involving the caudal aspect of the humeral head (arrow). (B) Mediolateral view of a positive contrast arthrogram of an OC lesion. Thick cartilage is covering the subchondral defect. There is no contrast medium visible underneath the cartilage and no flap is seen (arrow).

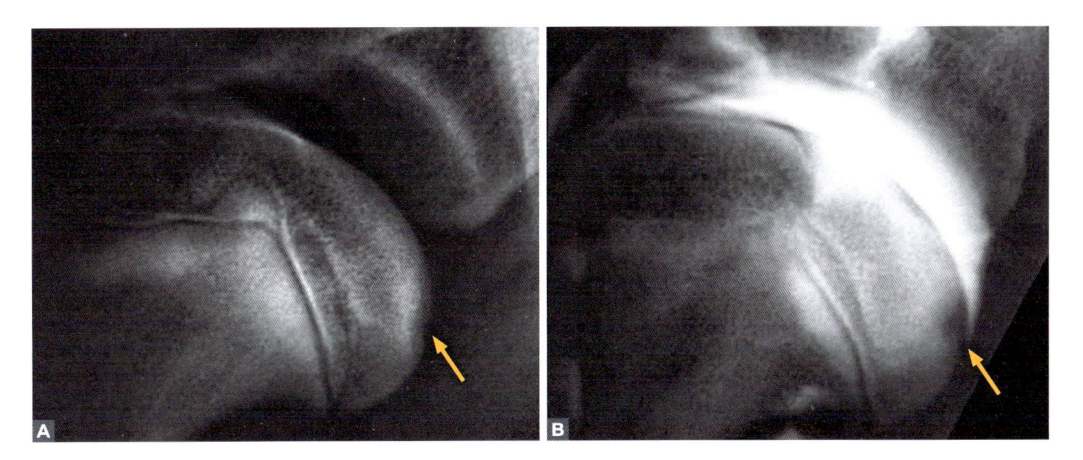

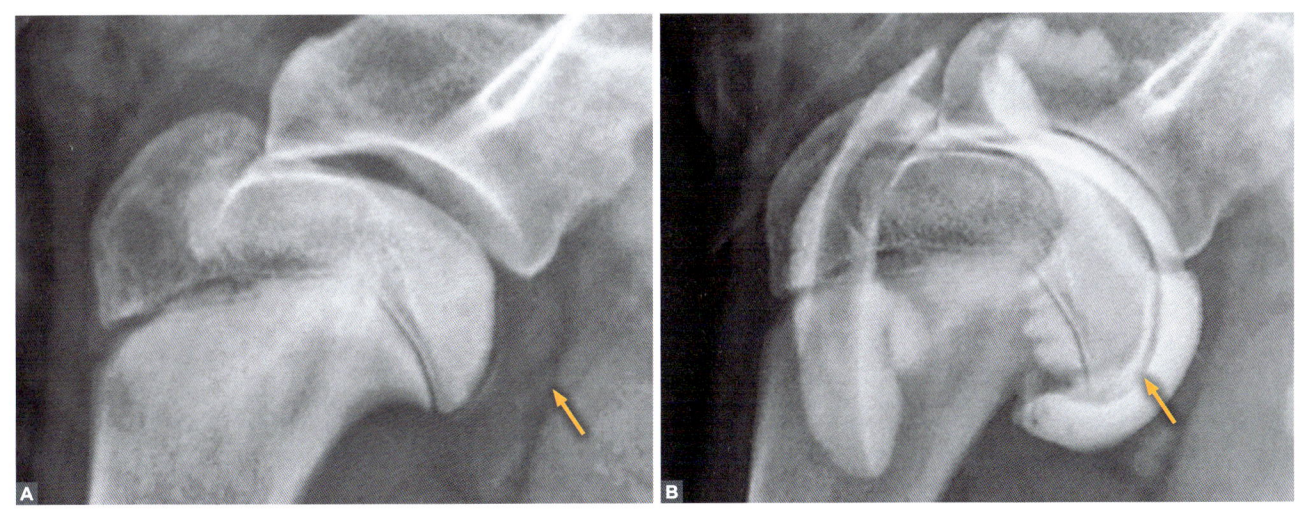

Fig. 9.2 (A) Mediolateral view: a thin mineralized cartilage flap is visible lying parallel to the flattened subchondral bone of the caudal humeral head (arrow). (B) The corresponding arthrogram shows contrast medium between the flap and bone, confirming OCD rather than OC (arrow).

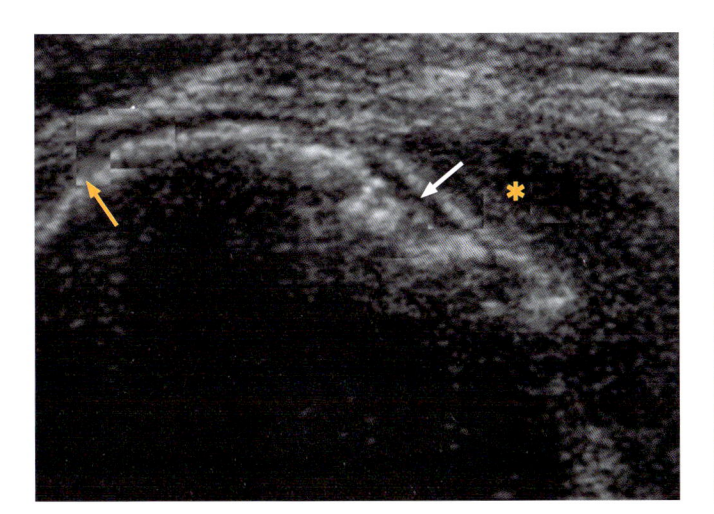

Fig. 9.3 Longitudinal ultrasound image of the caudal humeral head with a clinical OCD lesion. The normal articular cartilage (orange arrow) is noticed as hypoechoic on top of the hyperechoic subchondral bone of the humeral head. There is visible joint fluid (asterisk). The hyperechoic line represents the detached flap (white arrow).

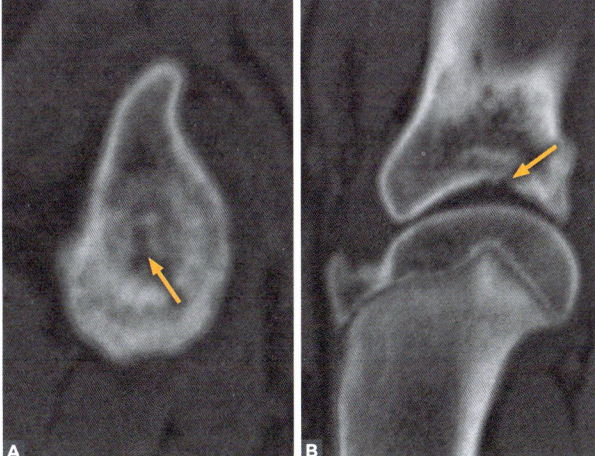

Fig. 9.4 A seven-month-old female Flatcoated Retriever. (A) Transverse and sagittal reconstructed (B) CT images of the shoulder joint. In the central part of the glenoid cavity, a hypoattenuating lesion of the subchondral bone is present, surrounded by a sclerotic band (arrows). The location is uncommon, but imaging features are characteristic of an OC lesion.

SECTION II APPENDICULAR SKELETON

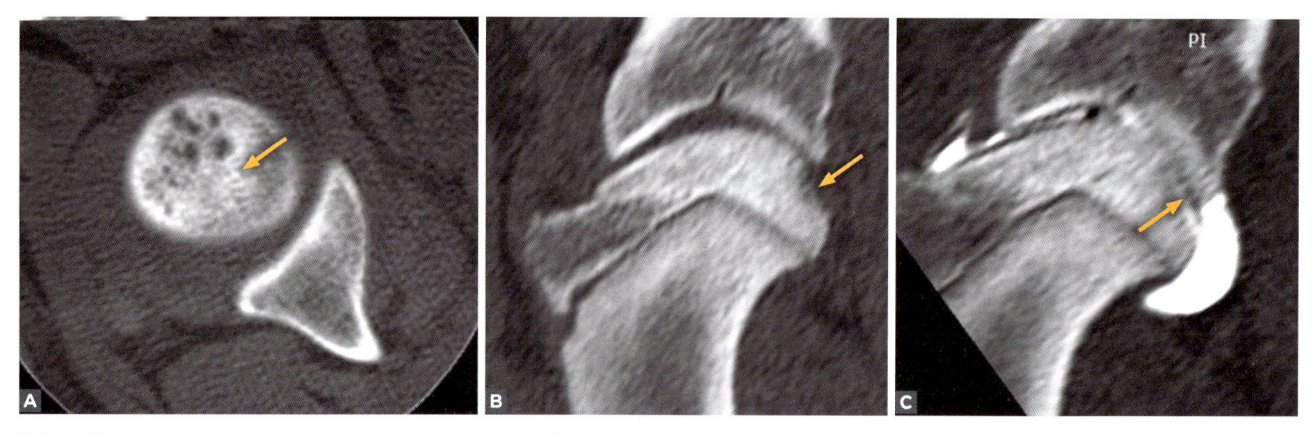

Fig. 9.5 A six-month-old Tibetan Mastiff. (**A**) Transverse and sagittal reconstructed and (**B**) sagittal reconstructed after intra-articular contrast administration (**C**) CT images. Radiolucent roundish areas surrounded by sclerosis are present at the caudal part of the humeral head (arrows). The contrast arthrogram shows contrast deep to the cartilage flap (arrow in image **C**).

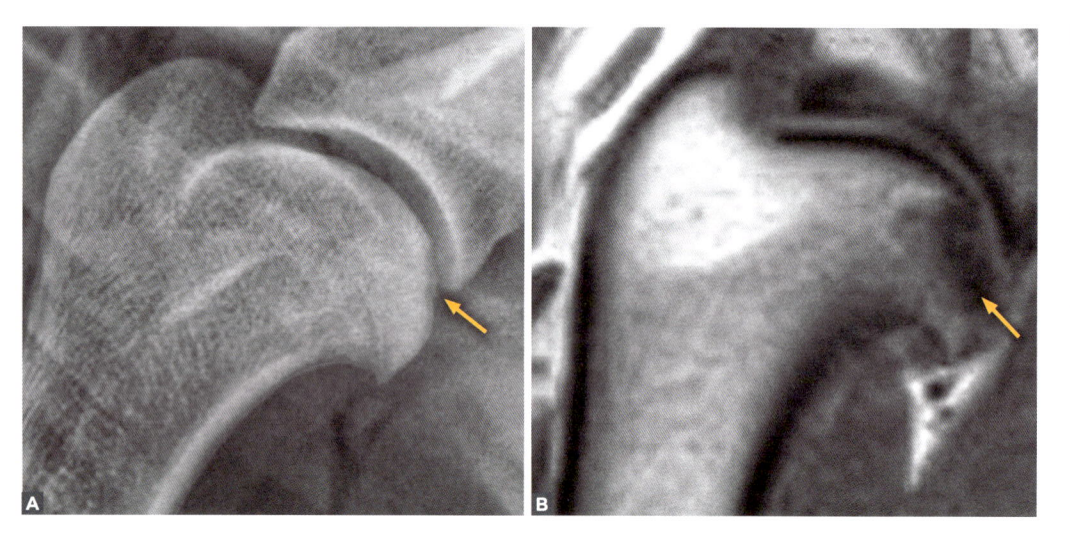

Fig. 9.6 A 1,5-year-old Labrador Retriever. (**A**) Mediolateral view and corresponding MRI image, low field (**B**) of an OCD lesion. The radiograph shows the shallow broad concave defect of the caudal part of the humeral head and a mineralized flap (arrow). On MRI the extent and severity of subchondral bone involvement is better appreciated (arrow). Although a defect of the caudal humeral head is detected, the flap is not demonstrated.

thrography, water soluble, non-ionic, iodinated contrast medium is injected intra-articularly and the CT examination is repeated. This is a useful technique providing superior sensitivity in the evaluation of intra-articular ligaments, articular cartilage of the humeral head and biceps tendon.[8] The contrast medium delineates the margins of the synovial and cartilaginous structures (**fig. 9.5**).

MRI allows the evaluation of normal and abnormal articular cartilage, although the optimal sequencing for the detection of canine cartilage lesions is still undefined.[1,4] The visualization of cartilage and its lesions is difficult in the dog, probably because articular cartilage in dogs is very thin (**fig. 9.6**). The intravenous injection of gadolinium-containing contrast agents can demonstrate subchondral inflammatory lesions in cases of OCD.

The elbow joint

OC of the elbow joint affects the trochlea of the humeral condyle and is best detected on the cranial 15° lateral-caudomedial oblique radiographic view and usually appears as a shallow concave defect or surrounded by sclerosis (**fig. 9.7**).[9] Usually, there is adjacent sclerosis of the subchondral bone surrounding the radiolucency.[9] It is important to distinguish between OC lesions and "kissing" lesions, due to lesions of the humeral condyle secondary to fragmentation of the medial humeral

epicondyle. "Kissing" lesions appear as shallow defects in the subchondral bone similar to OC lesions but are located at the medial margin of the trochlea where OC lesions are usually at the center.[10]
On CT, elbow OC lesions are often more extensive than expected from radiographs (**fig. 9.8**). With CT, a clear distinction between "kissing" lesions and real OC lesions of the medial humeral condyle is made more readily, especially as this modality is superior for assessing the medial coronoid process. On transverse images, OC shows the typical features, radiolucency with a sclerotic rim. On frontal plane reconstructed images, concavity or flattening of the trochlea, subchondral lucencies and sclerosis are present. "Kissing" lesions on CT are presented as focal sclerotic lesions without radiolucency, in most cases combined with degenerative changes (**fig. 9.9**).

Elbow MRI is not routinely used. OC lesions are noticed as a different subchondral signal and flattening of the medial humeral condyle (**fig. 9.10**). Small cartilage lesions are difficult to pick up because the canine cartilage is very thin.[10]

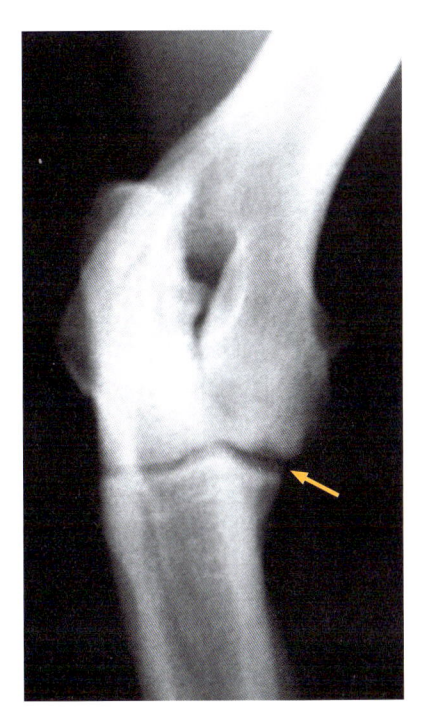

Fig. 9.7 A 15-month-old female Golden Retriever. The cranial 15° lateral caudomedial, 15° oblique projection shows a well-defined concave defect in the subchondral bone at the distal border of the trochlea of the humeral condyle caused by an OC lesion (arrow).

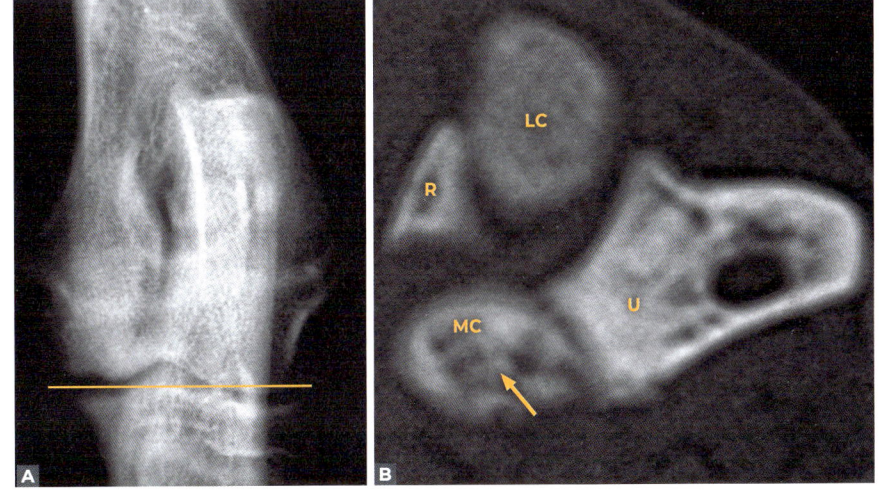

Fig. 9.8 The cranial 15° lateral caudomedial, oblique radiographic view shows flattening and a broad subchondral defect affecting the medial half of the trochlea of the humeral condyle, representing an OCD lesion (arrow). On the corresponding transverse CT image at the level of the humeroradial joint space (**B**), the extent of the OC lesion is better appreciated (arrow) with numerous poorly defined round radiolucent foci in the subchondral bone (arrow). *LC*, lateral humeral condyle; *MC*, medial humeral condyle; *R*, radius; *U*, ulna.

Fig. 9.9 (**A**) Transverse CT images of an OCD defect at the medial humeral condyle and the appearance of "kissing" lesions at the medial humeral condyle (**B**). The typical pattern of an OCD lesion is noticed (orange arrow). "Kissing" lesions appear as a stripe-like aspect at the medial humeral condyle and are associated with a lot of new bone formation (white arrow).

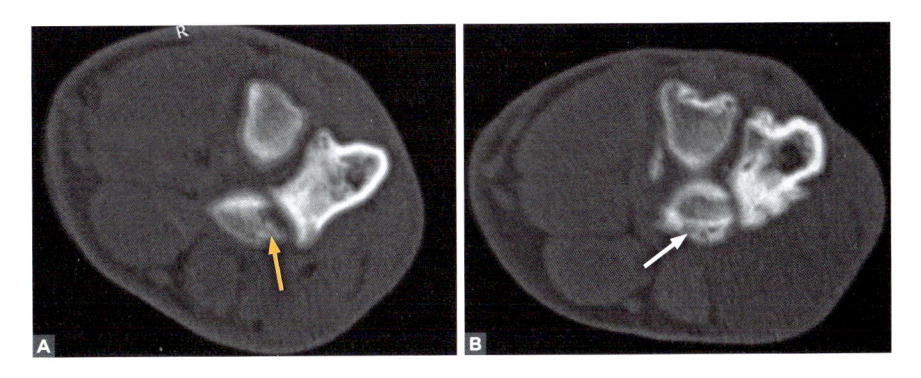

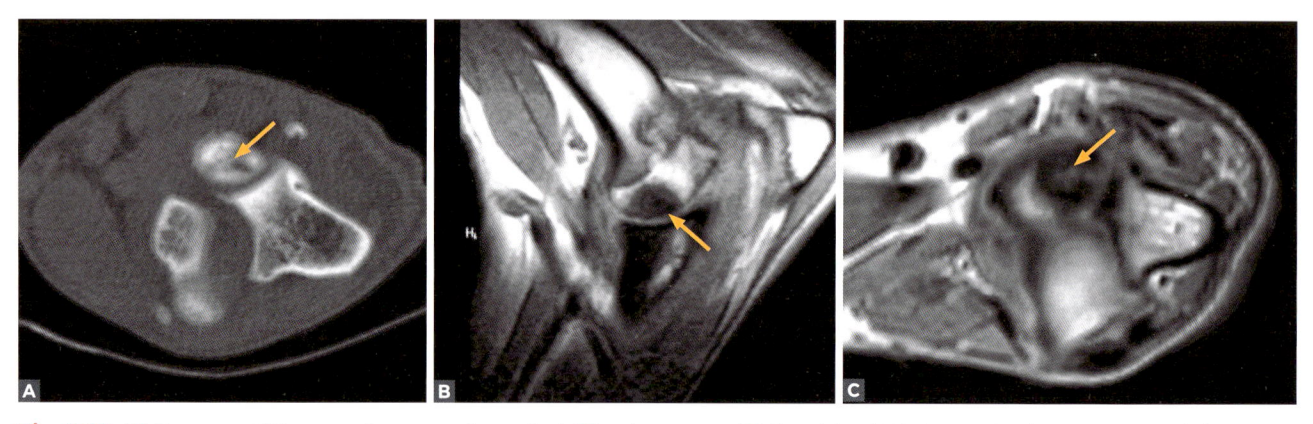

Fig. 9.10 (**A**) Transverse CT image and corresponding sagittal (**B**) and transverse (**C**) T2 weighted MRI images. On the CT image a radiolucent area surrounded by sclerosis is present at the trochlea of the humeral condyle. The MRI images show an abnormal and diffuse low signal intensity consistent with necrotic bone (arrows).

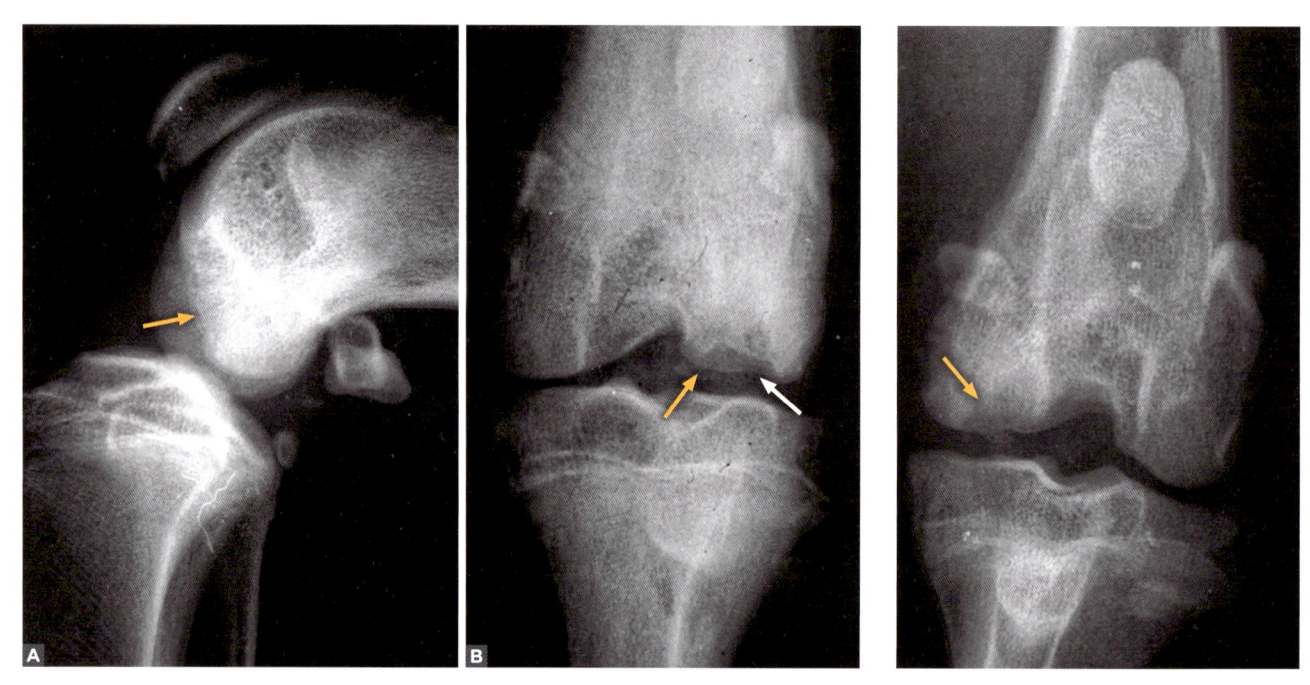

Fig. 9.11 (**A**) Lateral and (**B**) craniocaudal radiographs of the left stifle of a 1,5-year-old male Boxer with OCD. The lateral femoral condyle has an abnormal undulating contour with a parallel mineralized flap on the lateral view (orange arrow). The craniocaudal view shows a mineralized flap (orange arrow) and a large defect spanning almost the entire width of the lateral femoral condyle (white arrow).

Fig. 9.12 The craniocaudal view shows the flattening, a radiolucent defect and adjacent small osteochondral fragments at the distal and axial margins of the medial femoral condyle (arrow).

The stifle joint

In the stifle joint, radiographic changes of OC/OCD are noted as flattening or concave defects on the medial femoral condyle or the medial aspect of the lateral femoral condyle, sclerosis surrounding the defect, fragments, and secondary degenerative joint disease (**figs. 9.11** and **9.12**). Standard mediolateral and craniocaudal or caudocranial views need to be obtained. Caution is advised not to confuse the fossa of the long digital extensor tendon for an OCD lesion.[11] The lateral condyle is more frequently affected than the medial femoral condyle.[12] As in other joints, OC is often bilateral in the stifle, and it is advisable to take radiographs from both joints.[1]

Ultrasound can assess joint effusion, thickening of the capsule and defects in the cartilage. Cartilage defects in the femoral condyle associated with OCD have irregular borders with pronounced contractions. Irregular delineation and hyperechoic lines at the bottom of the subchondral defect can be noticed (**fig. 9.13**). It is known that with ultrasound, not all areas in the joint are accessible.[11] CT in stifle OCD is more sensitive to detect OC lesions than radiography (**fig. 9.14**). The severity and extent of the lesion is better defined on CT images, which is important for the prognosis. In CT contrast arthrography, the articular cartilage is identified as a hypodense area between the bone and contrast-filled joint space (**fig. 9.15**).[11]

Fig 9.13 (**A**) Craniocaudal radiograph of a stifle and corresponding transverse CT image at the level of the distal femur (**B**) of a nine-month-old Newfoundland. The CT image clearly shows a lucent defect in the lateral condyle with surrounding sclerosis (yellow arrow). This OCD lesion is not clearly visible on the radiograph (white arrow). A small fragment within the joint is also present (orange arrow).

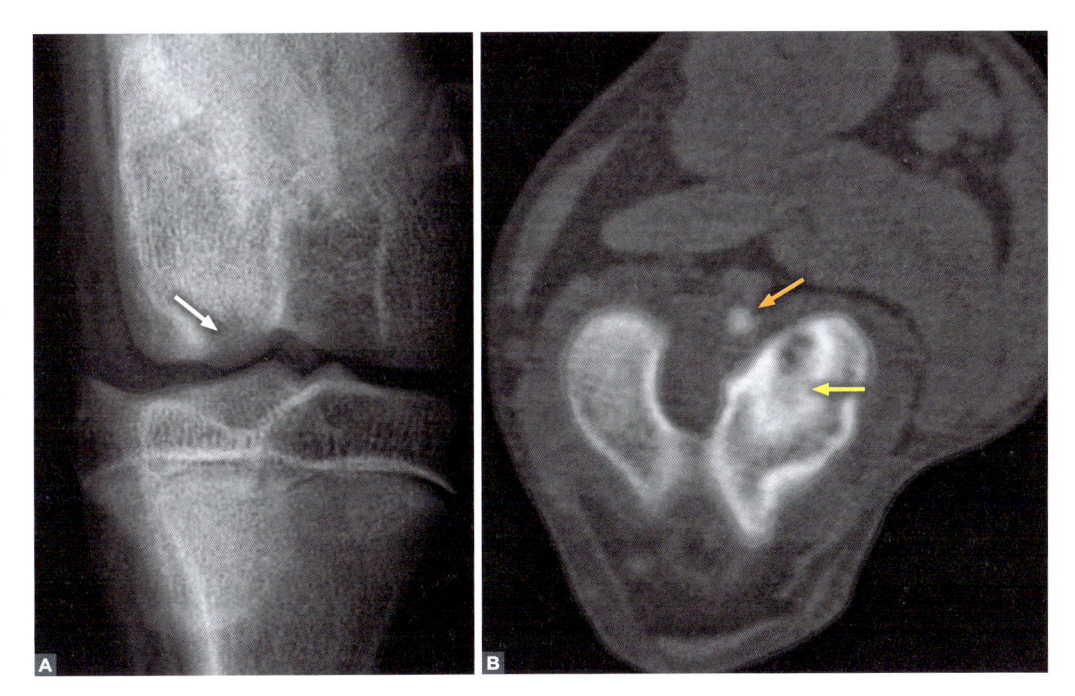

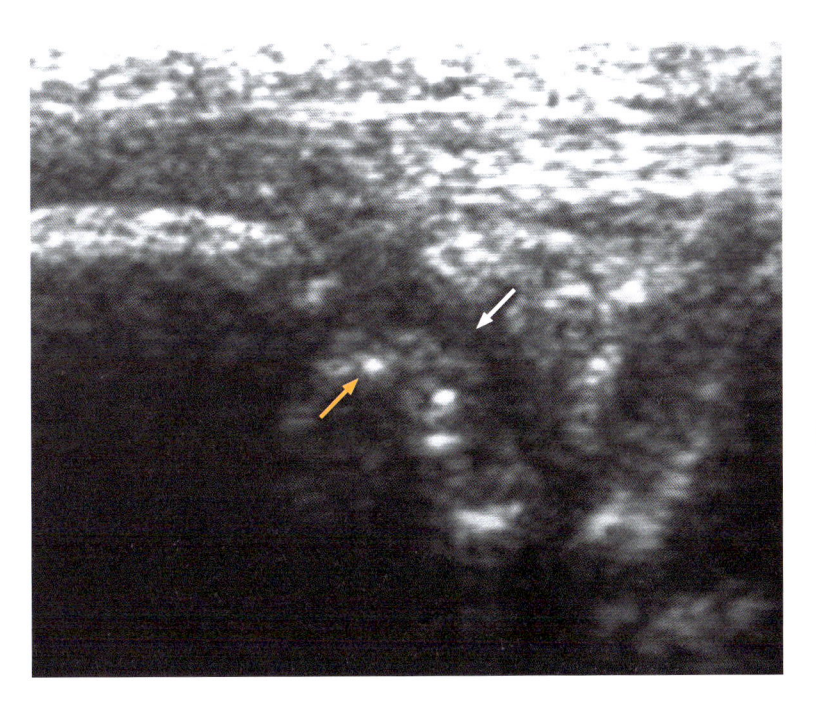

Fig. 9.14 Longitudinal ultrasound image representing OCD at the medial femoral condyle. The orange arrow points at the thickened and irregular hyperechoic subchondral bone. Joint fluid is present (white arrow).

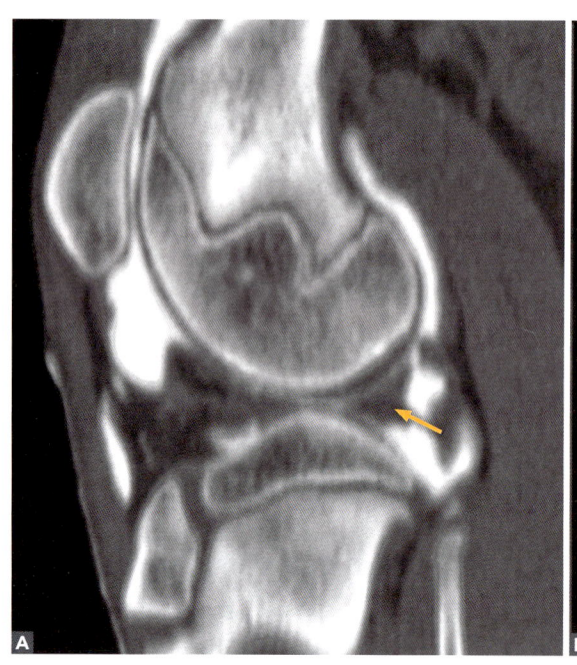

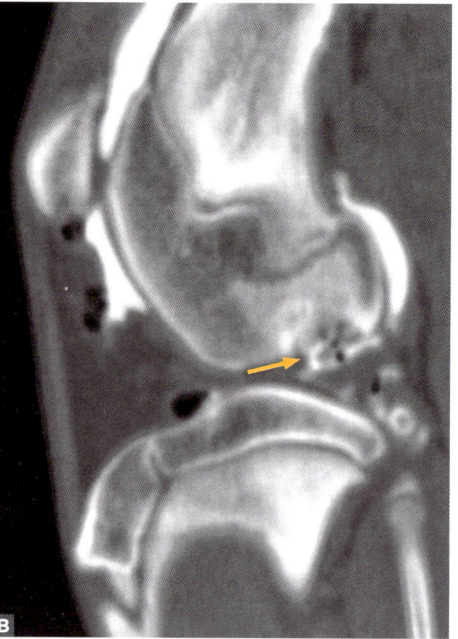

Fig. 9.15 CT contrast arthrogram, sagittal reconstructed images at the level of the lateral femoral condyle of a four-month-old Boxer with an OC lesion (**A**) and an OCD lesion in a Bull Terrier (**B**). (**A**) The contrast medium is delineating the thickened articular cartilage, but no flap can be demonstrated (arrow). (**B**) Contrast medium is present in the subchondral defect and underneath the cartilage flap (arrow). Numerous small gas bubbles are present within the joint and adjacent tissues from injection into the joint.

The talocrural joint

OC of the talocrural joint affects the medial and lateral trochlear ridges of the talus and the medial trochlear ridge of the talus accounts for 85% of cases. The first radiographic sign of OC of the medial trochlear ridge is widening of the medial talocrural joint space. When an OC lesion of the lateral trochlear ridge causes similar changes but are partly or completely obscured by the superimposition of the calcaneus on the dorsoplantar projection. Many OC/OCD lesions are missed on radiographs, even if the proposed views including the fully extended and fully flexed mediolateral, the dorsoplantar, the plantaromedial-dorsolateral and plantarolateral-dorsomedial, and a flexed dorsoplantar skyline view are taken. When limited to two standard views, the fully extended and the dorsoplantar, 72% of lateral trochlear ridge lesions can be missed.[13] Information regarding the exact location, number and size of the fragments is minimal and determining the extent of joint surface involvement is in most instances not possible on radiographs (**fig. 9.16**). Ultrasound can be helpful in visualizing some of these structures; however, the cartilage of the trochlear ridges is very thin in dogs and a significant part of the trochlear ridges is obscured by the tibia (**fig. 9.17**).[14]

In talocrural OCD, CT allows assessing the exact location, extent of the OC lesion, the size and number of associated fragments and is superior to arthroscopy to assess the entire articular surface (**figs. 9.18** and **9.19**). CT is superior in the diagnosis of lateral trochlear ridge lesions. It helps in treatment planning, particularly when using minimally invasive treatment techniques. CT contrast arthrography in tarsal OC seems promising in evaluating fragment stability in the tarsal joint (**fig. 9.20**). MRI investigations can reveal the OC lesion, the joint incongruity, and the inflammatory soft tissue proliferation (**fig. 9.21**).

CHAPTER **9** Osteochondrosis

Fig. 9.16 (**A**) Plantarodorsal view of a medial tarsocrural OCD. Notice the soft tissue distension and the enlarged joint space and associated osteochondral fragment (arrow). (**B**) Plantaromedial-dorsolateral oblique projection of a lateral tarsocrural OCD. Notice the defect in the lateral ridge and the fragment (arrow).

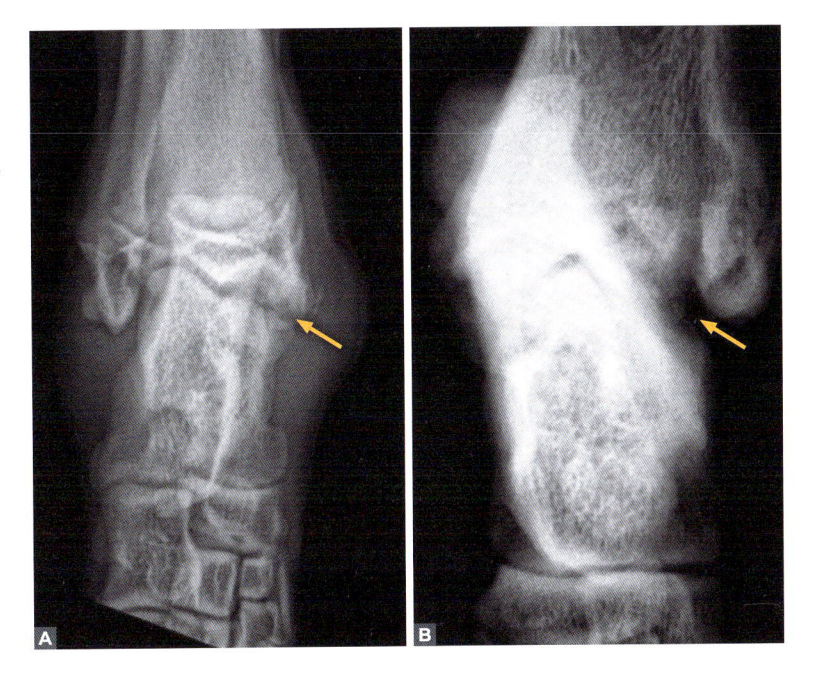

Fig. 9.17 A 14-month-old Golden Retriever. Longitudinal ultrasound image of the tarsus in extension at the level of the medial ridge of the talus. An OC lesion is present, hyperechoic irregular subchondral bone is noticed (arrow).

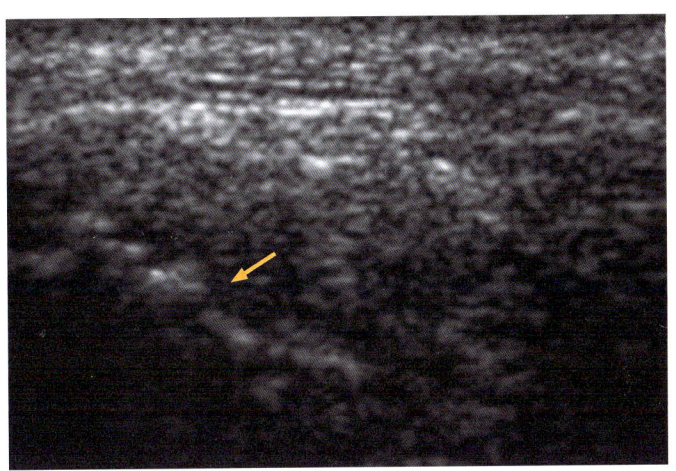

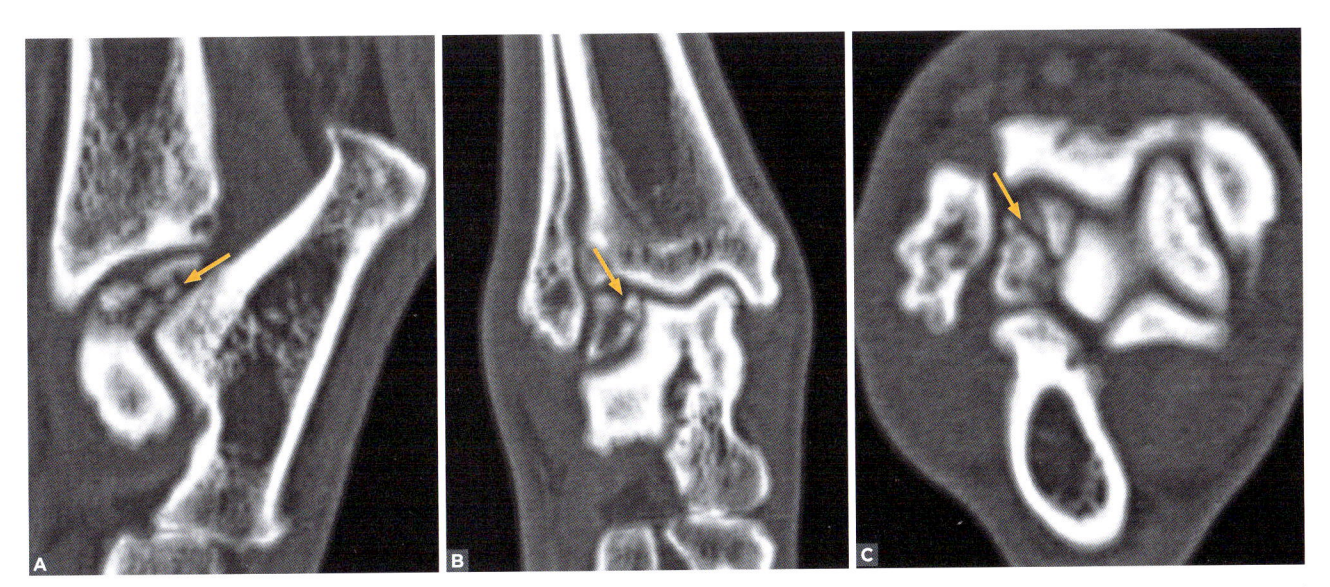

Fig. 9.18 An 11-month-old male Rottweiler. (**A**) Sagittal and (**B**) dorsal reconstructed images of the tarsal joint, and transverse view at the level of the trochlear ridges (**C**) of a lateral trochlear ridge OCD lesion of a talus. Multiple detached fragments are present on the proximal half of the lateral trochlear ridge (arrows).

87

SECTION II APPENDICULAR SKELETON

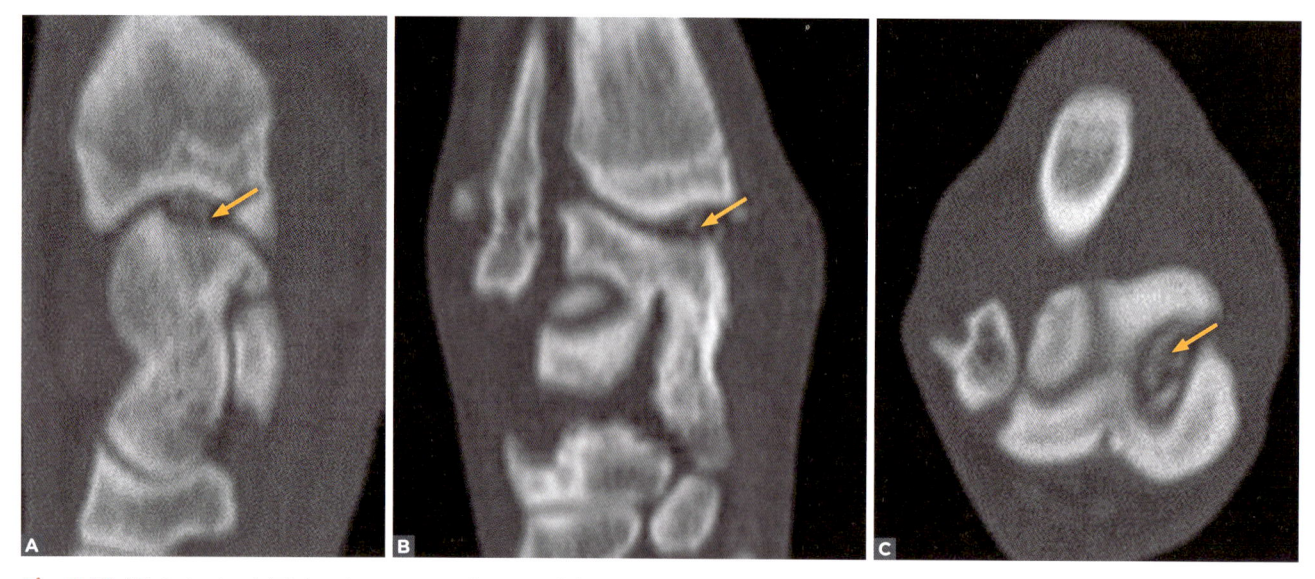

Fig. 9.19 (**A**) Sagittal and (**B**) dorsal reconstructed images of the tarsal joint and transverse view at the level of the trochlear ridges (**C**) of a medial trochlear ridge OCD lesion. Two detached fragments are present in the proximal part of the medial trochlear ridge of the talus (arrows).

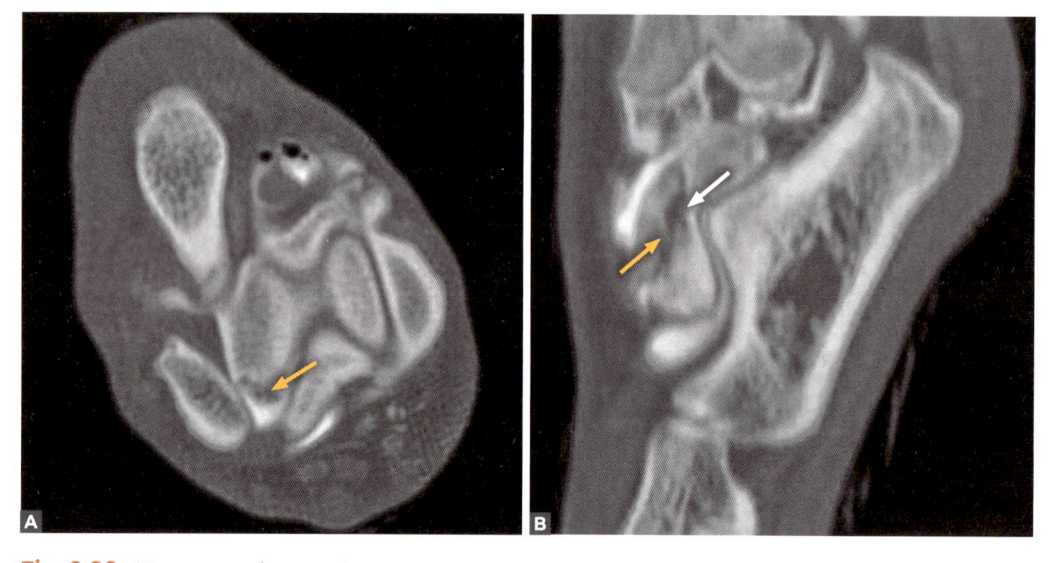

Fig. 9.20 CT contrast arthrogram images, transverse (**A**) and sagittal reconstructed (**B**) of the tarsal joint of a Bull Mastiff. At the lateral talar ridge, a large fragment is present in the dorsal part (orange arrows). There is no contrast noticed underneath the fragment. The fragment seems to be stable and attached probably with fibrous tissue (white arrow).

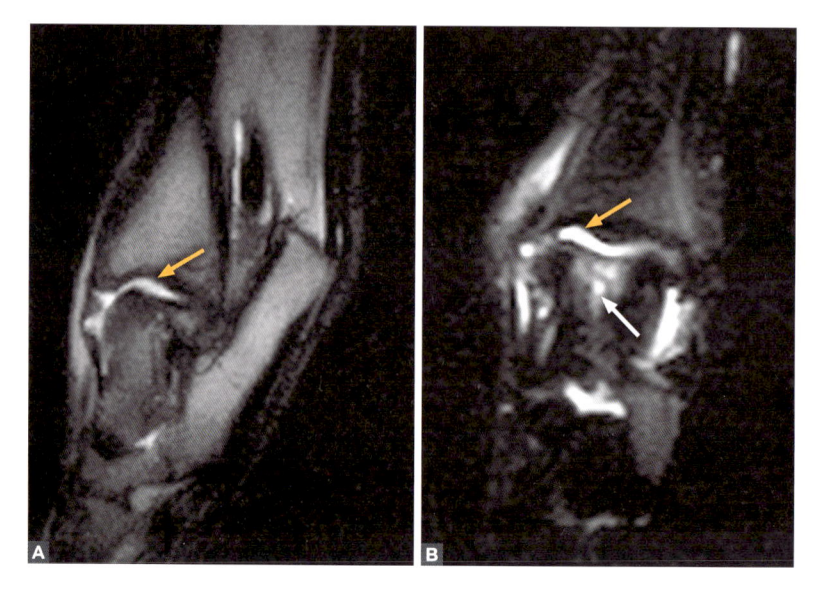

Fig. 9.21 (**A**) Sagittal and (**B**) dorsal MRI images showing flattening of the medial talar ridge and an enlarged joint space with joint effusion (orange arrows). Subchondral bone marrow edema is present in the medio-central part of the talus (white arrow).

References

1. Kippenes H, Johnston G. Diagnostic imaging of osteochondrosis. *Vet Clin North Am Small Anim Pract* 28:137-160, 1998.
2. Gielen I. Diagnostic imaging of osteochondrosis in the dog. World Small Animal Veterinary Association Scientific Proceedings 335-337, 2014.
3. Vandevelde B, Van Ryssen B, Saunders JH, Kramer M, van Bree H. Comparison of the ultrasonographic appearance of osteochondrosis lesions in the canine shoulder with radiography, arthrography, and arthroscopy. *Vet Radiol Ultrasound* 47:174-184, 2006.
4. Wall CR, Cook C, Cook JL. Diagnostic sensitivity of radiography, ultrasonography, and magnetic resonance imaging for detecting shoulder osteochondrosis/osteochondritis dissecans in dogs. *Vet Radiol Ultrasound* 56:3-11, 2015.
5. Peremans K, Cornelissen B, Van Den Bossche B, Audenaert K, Wiele C. A review of small animal imaging planar and pinhole spect gamma camera imaging. *Vet Radiol Ultrasound* 46:162-170, 2005.
6. van Bree H. Comparison of diagnostic accuracy of positive-contrast arthrography and arthrotomy in evaluation of osteochondrosis lesions in the scapulohumeral joint in dogs. *J Am Vet Med Assoc* 203:84-88, 1993.
7. Lande R, Reese SL, Cuddy LC, Berry CR, Pozzi A. Prevalence of computed tomographic subchondral bone lesions in the scapulohumeral joint of 32 immature dogs with thoracic limb lameness. *Vet Radiol Ultrasound* 55:23-28, 2014.
8. Eivers CR, Corzo-Menéndez N, Austwick SH, Thomson DG, Gibson SM, Handel I, Tobias Schwarz T. Computed tomographic arthrography is a useful adjunct to survey computed tomography and arthroscopic evaluation of the canine shoulder joint. *Vet Radiol Ultrasound* 59:535-544, 2018.
9. Chanoit G, Singhani, Denis J. Marcellin-Little, DJ, Osborne JA. Comparison of five radiographic views for assessment of the medial aspect of the humeral condyle in dogs with osteochondritis dissecans. *Am J Vet Res* 71:780-783, 2010.
10. Cook CR, Cook JL. Diagnostic imaging of canine elbow dysplasia: A review. *Vet Surg* 38:173-184, 2009.
11. Marino DJ, Loughin CA. Diagnostic imaging of the canine stifle: A review. *Vet Surg* 39:284-295, 2010.
12. Comerford J. The stifle joint. In Kirberger RM, McEvoy FJ (editors). BSAVA Manual of Canine and Feline Musculoskeletal Imaging 2nd edition. Wiley Blackwell, 2016, pp 135-149.
13. Gielen I, Van Ryssen B, van Bree H. Computerized tomography compared with radiography in the diagnosis of lateral trochlear ridge talar osteochondritis dissecans in dogs. *Vet Comp Orthop Traumatol* 18:77-81, 2005.
14. Liuti T, Saunders J, Gielen I, De Rycke L, Coopman F, van Bree H. Ultrasound approach to the canine distal tibia and trochlear ridges of the talus. *Vet Radiol Ultrasound* 48:361-367, 2007.
15. Gielen I, van Bree H, Van Ryssen B, De Clercq T, De Rooster H. Radiographic, computed tomographic and arthroscopic findings in 23 dogs with osteochondrosis of the tarsocrural joint. *Vet Rec* 150:442-447, 2002.

CHAPTER 10

Other congenital developmental and hereditary diseases

Séamus Hoey and Antonella Puggioni

> **KEY POINTS**
>
> ▌ Multiple congenital and hereditary diseases can affect juvenile patients.
> ▌ A genetic predisposition has been suggested for osteochondrodysplasia, humeral intracondylar fissure, avascular femoral head necrosis, patellar luxation, congenital hypothyroidism, and slipped capital femoral epiphysis.
> ▌ Specific details of the pathogenesis of some of these diseases are not fully understood.
> ▌ Multiple bones or limbs are usually affected.
> ▌ Radiography is in most cases sufficient to provide a diagnosis for these conditions, however special views might be needed.
> ▌ Computed tomography can be useful in providing information about concurrent disorders.

Osteochondrodysplasia

Osteochondrodysplasia describes abnormal cartilage and bone development, which can be an inherited condition in dogs. In several breeds these abnormalities in development are considered normal for the breed.[1-5] Achondroplasia is considered normal in Bulldogs, Boston Terriers and Pekingese. Hypochondrodysplasia is considered normal in Dachshunds and Beagles. In the cat, purebred and crossbred Scottish Fold cats are most affected by osteochondrodysplasia.[6,7] Patients can present with delayed or absent development of the long bones, with resultant shortened limbs and angular limb deformities, seen in Labrador Retrievers, Alaskan Malamutes and other breeds (**figs. 10.1** and **10.2**). In some cases, multiple joints may be affected in multiple epiphyseal dysplasia (MED) where the epiphyses of the long bones, vertebrae, cuboidal bones and apophyses are incompletely ossified. In Labrador Retriever, Samoyed and Northern Inuit dogs an oculoskeletal dysplasia with ocular defects such as cataracts, vitreal and retinal changes combined with skeletal deformities including short limbed dwarfism, elbow and hip dysplasia has been described.

Osteochondromatosis

Osteochondromatosis can be divided into multiple cartilaginous exostoses and synovial osteochondromatosis.
An osteochondroma is a benign proliferative condition where cartilaginous topped osseous projections extend from the bone margins. Multiple sites are commonly affected, named multiple cartilaginous

SECTION II APPENDICULAR SKELETON

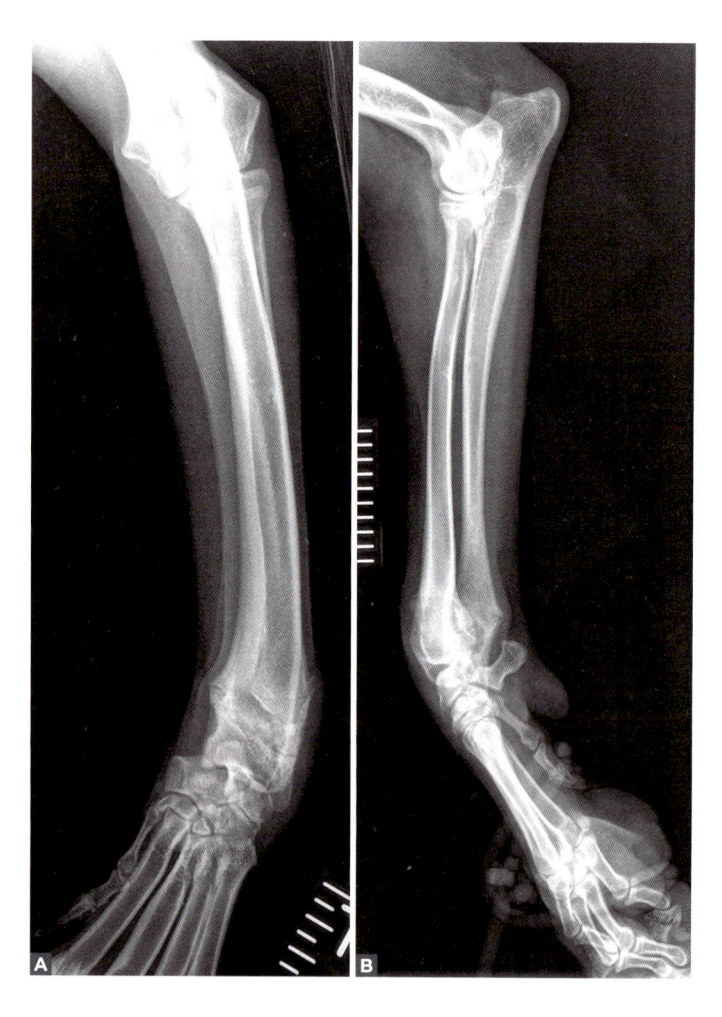

Fig. 10.1 Craniocaudal and mediolateral views of the antebrachium of a one-year-old male Setter cross, presented for angular limb deformity. Moderate medial deviation (varus) of the distal limb, centered at the irregularly shaped and increased opacity of the distal radial epiphyses. Mild medial subluxation of the antebrachiocarpal joint.

Fig. 10.2 Caudocranial and mediolateral views of both antebrachia of a ten-month-old male castrated Dachshund presented for angular limb deformity. Moderate flaring and widening of the distal ulnar metaphysis. Mild cranial bowing of the radius centered at the distal diaphysis of the radius. Moderate widening of the humeroulnar joint bilaterally.

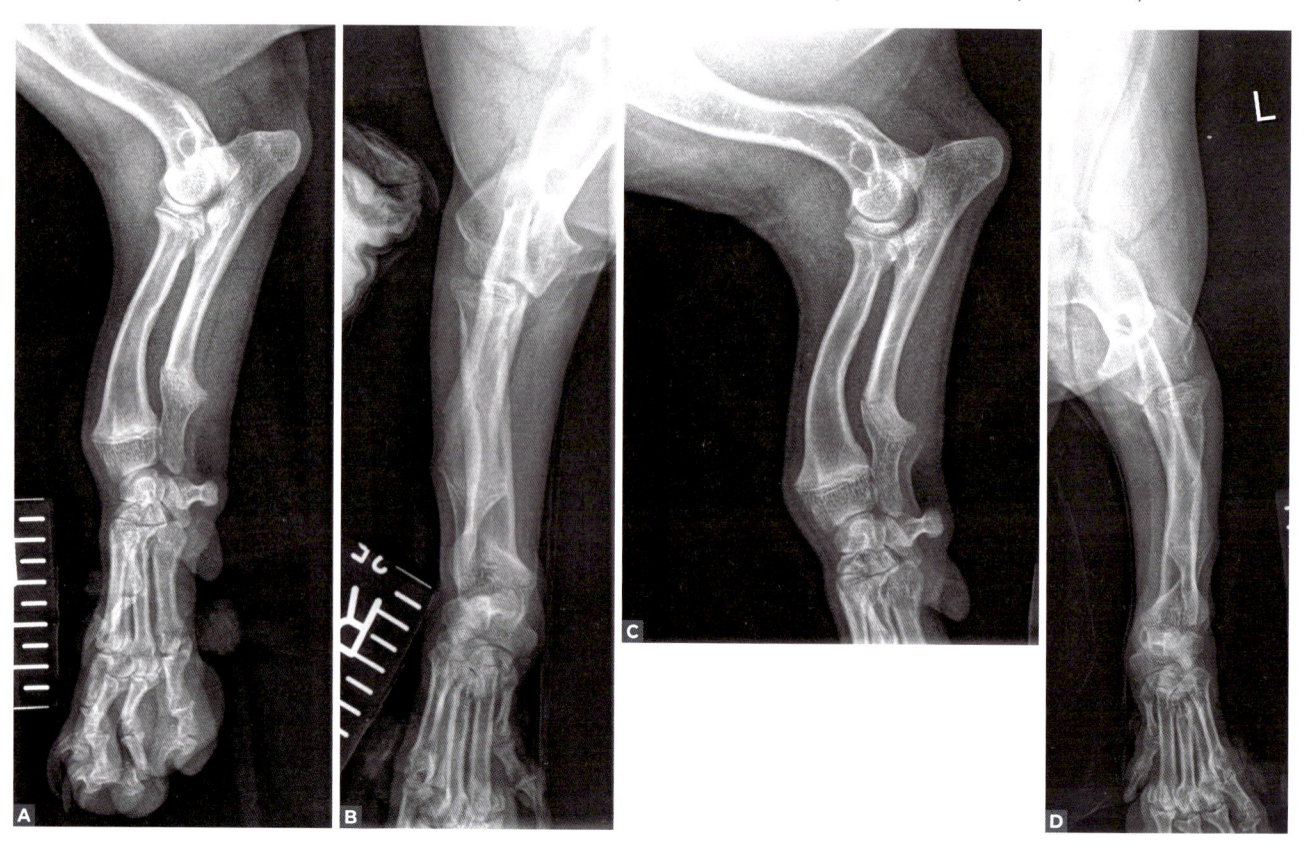

92

CHAPTER 10 Other congenital developmental and hereditary diseases

exostoses. The etiology remains unclear, but it is suggested that chondrocytes displaced from the physis may produce smooth areas of cartilage and bone perpendicular to the physis. The vertebrae, ribs and long bones are most frequently affected (**fig. 10.3**). The lesions develop until skeletal maturity and are generally incidental, non-clinically relevant findings.

Synovial osteochondromatosis, also called synovial chondrometaplasia, is characterized by intra-articular production of cartilage nodules (chondromas), which may be free floating in the joint. Chondromas may ultimately ossify forming osteochondromas which attach to the synovia (**fig. 10.4**). Osteochondromatosis has been described within joints, and to a lesser extent within tendon sheaths and bursae.[8] These smooth rounded mineralized bodies, also called "joint mice" may be incidental or cause clinical signs through mechanical trauma (**figs. 10.5-10.7**). Osteochondromatosis without a predisposing abnormality is primary synovial osteochondromas.[9-12] They can also be seen associated with degenerative joint disease and are thus considered secondary synovial osteochondromas. There have been reports of malignant transformation of osteochondromas to osteosarcoma or chondrosarcoma, which differ from osteochondromatosis by enlarging after skeletal maturation.[13]

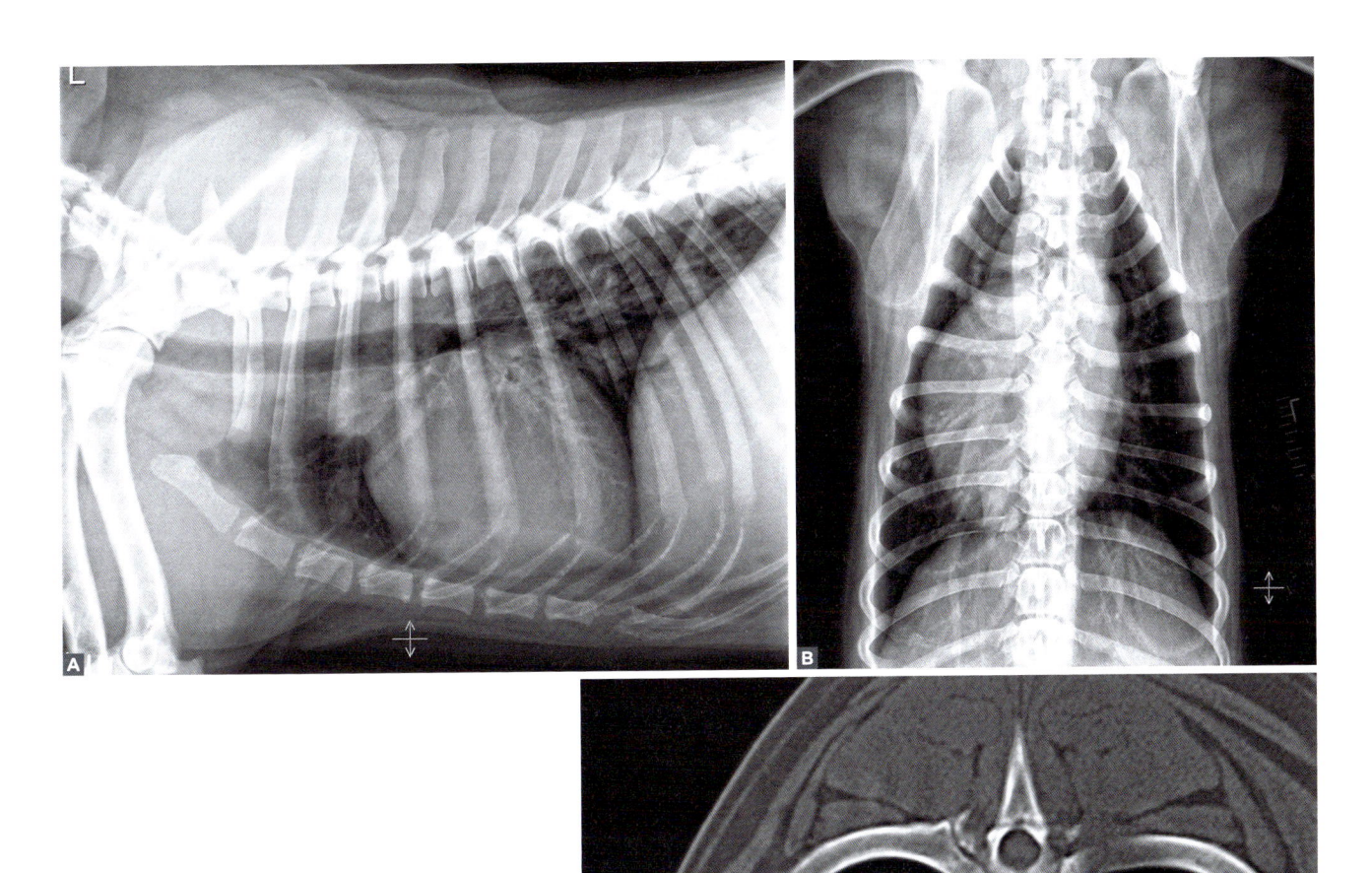

Fig. 10.3 Left lateral and dorsoventral thoracic views of a nine-year-old male Golden Retriever presented for epistaxis. Smoothly marginated mineral opacity at the proximal margin of the seventh rib. Transverse computed tomographic image in bone window showing a smoothly marginated mildly heterogeneous mineral attenuation at the dorsolateral margin of the right seventh rib, with no adjacent soft tissue swelling.

SECTION II APPENDICULAR SKELETON

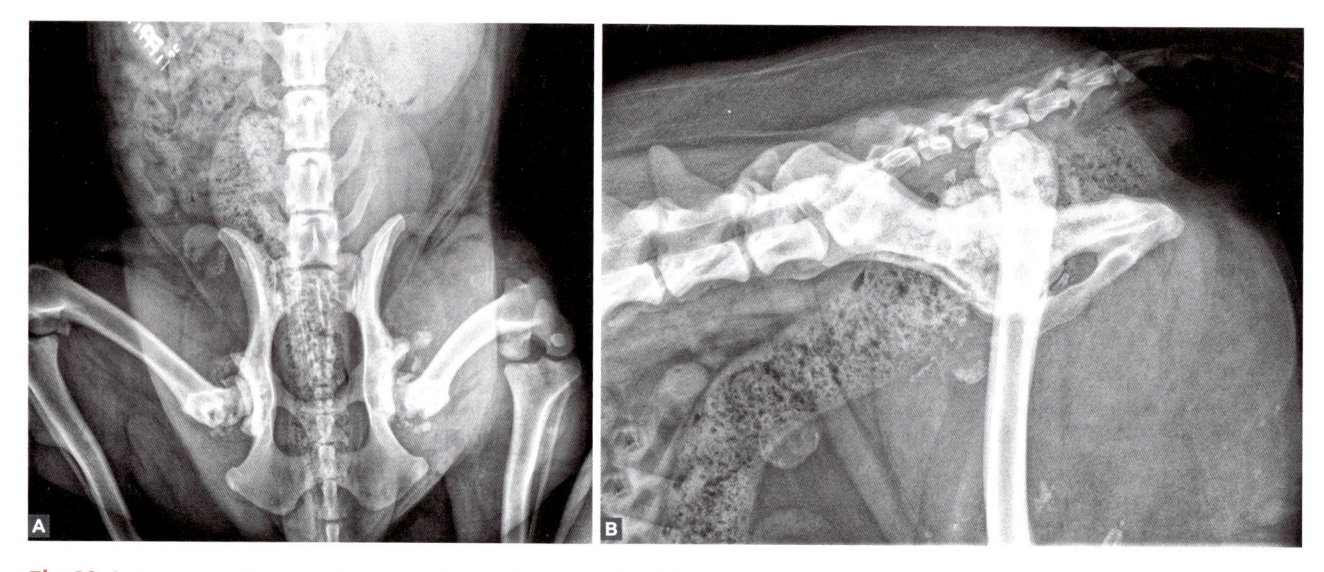

Fig. 10.4 Ventrodorsal frog-leg and right lateral views of the pelvis of an eight-year-old male castrated German Shepherd and Labrador Retriever cross. Dorsal subluxation of the left coxofemoral joint. Bilateral multiple mineral opacities within the coxofemoral joints, mildly heterogeneous and somewhat poorly defined.

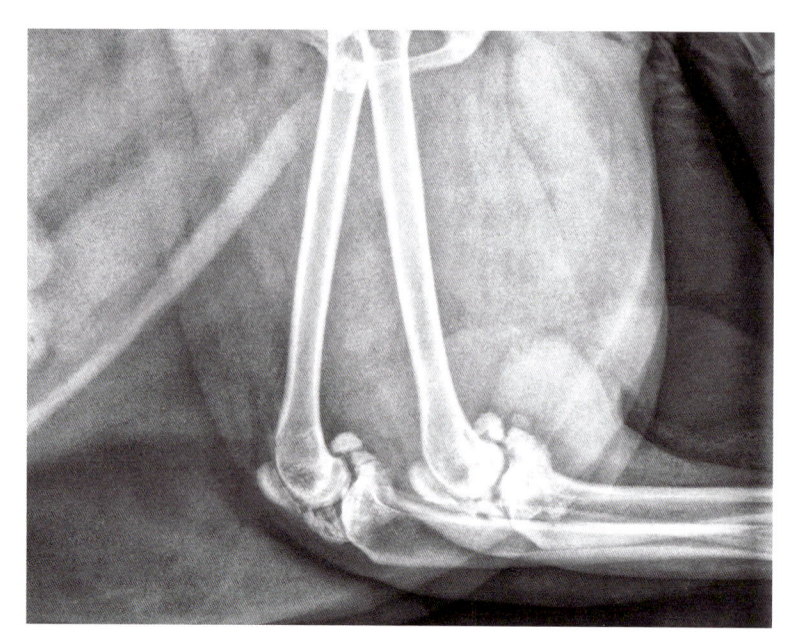

Fig. 10.5 Laterolateral view of the stifles of a 14-year-old spayed female Domestic shorthair cat presented with vomiting. Multifocal well defined mineral opacities superimposing bilaterally the femorotibial joints, consistent with meniscal mineralization and intra-articular mineralization.

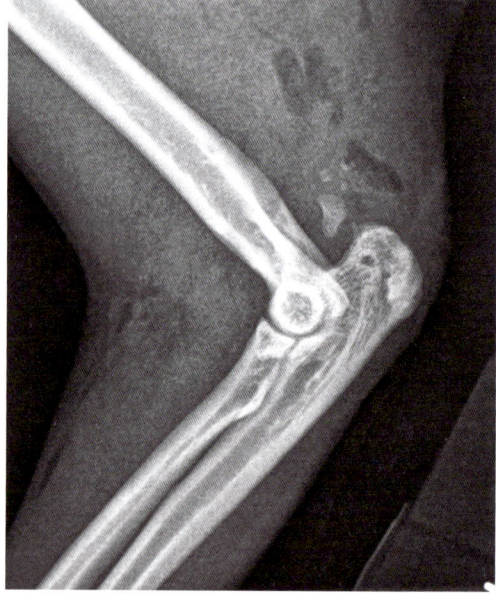

Fig. 10.6 Mediolateral view of the right elbow of a seven-year-old male castrated Domestic shorthair cat, presented with right forelimb lameness. Multiple mineral opacities superimpose the soft tissues cranial to the right ulnar olecranon.

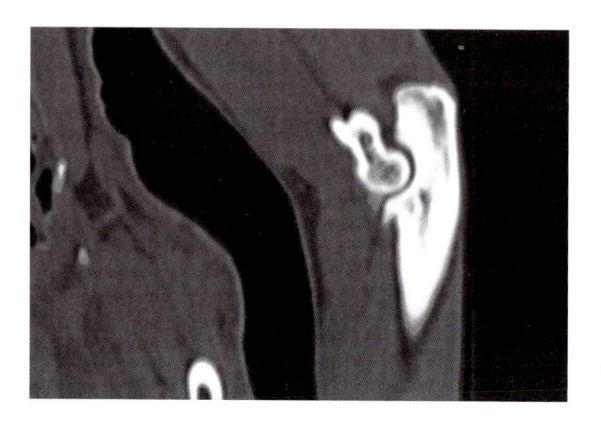

Fig. 10.7 Computed tomographic sagittal reformat in bone window of the same cat of fig. 10.6 showing a mineral attenuating structure craniodistal to the right humeral condyle.

Humeral intracondylar fissure

Humeral intracondylar fissure (HIF), previously known as incomplete ossification of the humeral condyle (IOHC), involves a discontinuity in the mid-sagittal plane of the humeral condyle. The Cocker Spaniel has been described in the UK as being overrepresented.[14-16] The etiology has been suggested to be due to failure of the medial and lateral centers of ossification of the humeral condyle to fuse, or that the fissure represents a stress fracture. In general, patients present as adult dogs, but HIF has been described in dogs as young as four months of age. Radiography can be used to assess fissure formation, with craniocaudal or 15° craniomedial-caudolateral oblique view required to identify the fissure (**fig. 10.8**).

This is made more difficult by the superimposition of the ulna and the resultant artefactual Mach line, and survey radiographic diagnosis is quite challenging. Mild new bone formation can be sometimes identified along the lateral aspect of the distal humeral metaphysis and lateral epicondyle, associated with stress remodeling. Computed tomography is the preferred diagnostic imaging modality, with the absence of superimposition and the ability to evaluate the cortical and spongiosa bone of the humeral condyle (**figs. 10.9** and **10.10**).[17,18]

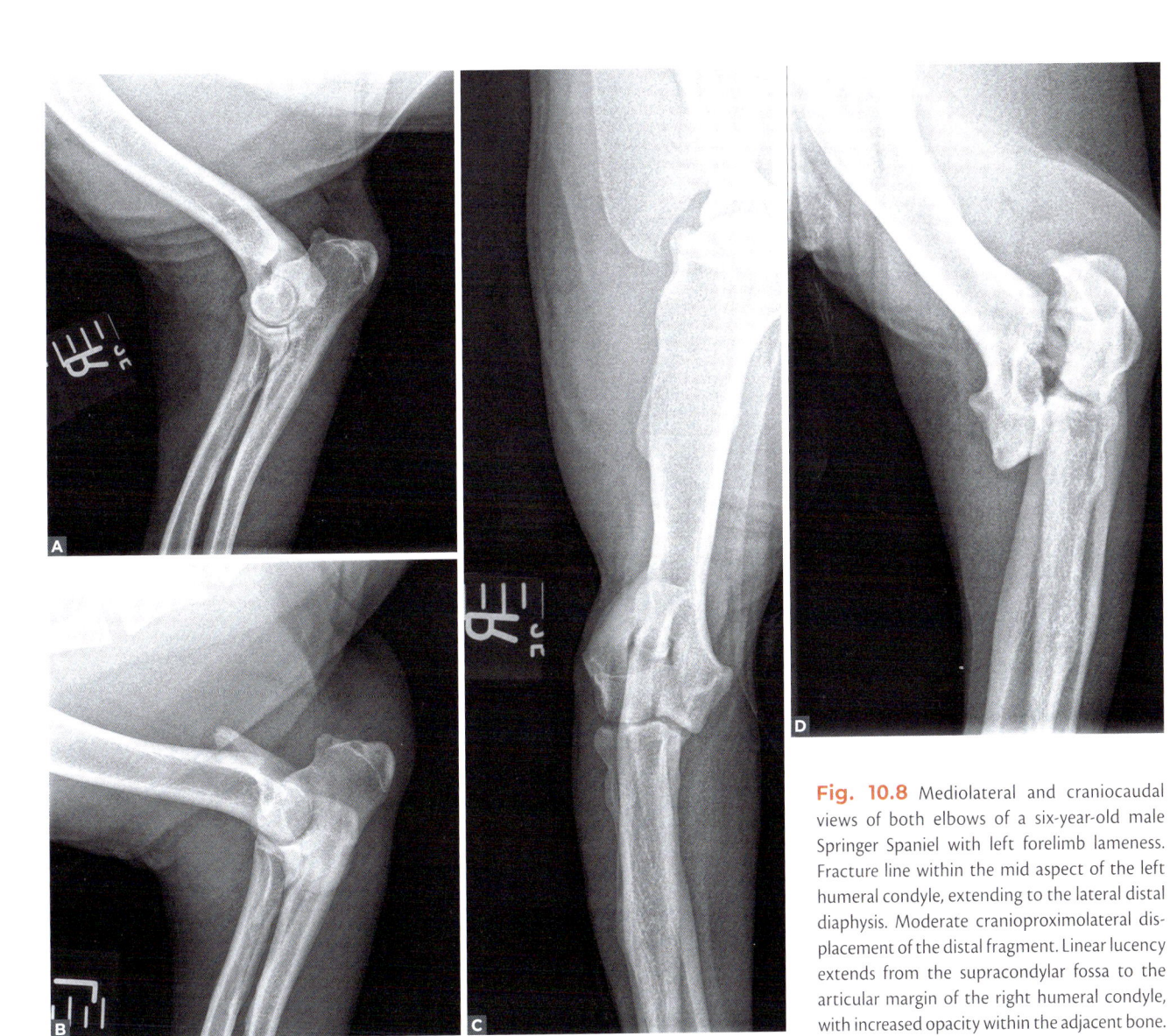

Fig. 10.8 Mediolateral and craniocaudal views of both elbows of a six-year-old male Springer Spaniel with left forelimb lameness. Fracture line within the mid aspect of the left humeral condyle, extending to the lateral distal diaphysis. Moderate cranioproximolateral displacement of the distal fragment. Linear lucency extends from the supracondylar fossa to the articular margin of the right humeral condyle, with increased opacity within the adjacent bone.

Congenital elbow luxation

Congenital luxation of the elbow is a rare condition in dogs and very rare in the cat.[20-26] Clinical signs may show in patients up to four months old and may be unilateral or bilateral. Three types are recognized: type 1 is humeroradial luxation, type 2 is humeroulnar and type 3 is a combination of humeroradial and humeroulnar. Type 1 is most commonly reported in large breed dogs and may include carpal valgus and a disruption of the radioulnar joint. Type 2 occurs most commonly in small breed dogs. It is important to distinguish congenital elbow luxation from traumatic elbow luxation and from developmental elbow luxation caused by asynchronous growth of the radius and ulna, most commonly the premature closure of the distal ulnar physis (**figs. 10.11-10.13**).

Incomplete ossification of the radial carpal bone

The radial carpal bone (also called the radiointermediate carpal bone) has three ossification centers, the *os semilunare* (representing the intermediate carpal bone), the *os scaphoideum* (representing

Fig. 10.9 Transverse and dorsal reformat computed tomographic image of the right elbow of a two-year-old female Springer Spaniel with bilateral forelimb lameness. Hypoattenuating line extends from the supracondylar fossa to the articular margin. Moderate hyperattenuation surrounds the hypoattenuating line.

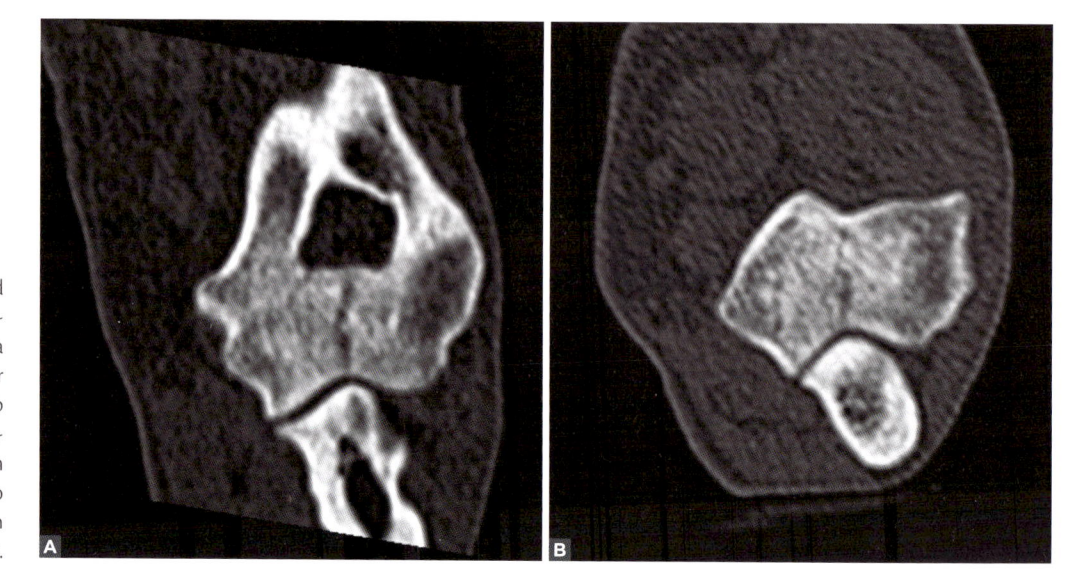

Fig. 10.10 Dorsal and transverse reformat images in bone window of a six-year-old male Springer Spaniel with left forelimb lameness. Linear hypoattenuation extending from the supracondylar fossa to the articular margin, with adjacent hyperattenuation.

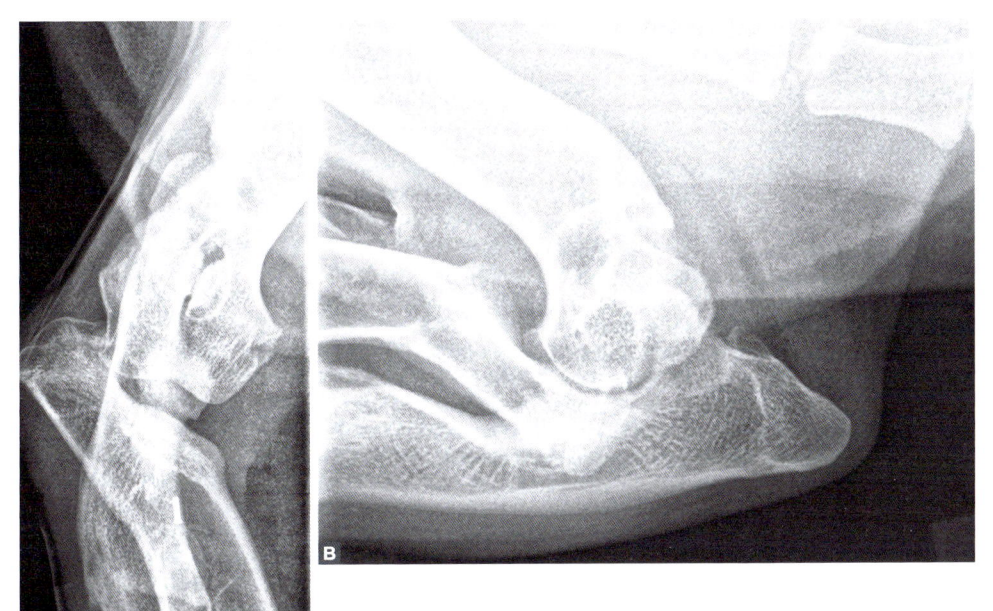

CHAPTER 10 Other congenital developmental and hereditary diseases

Fig. 10.11 Caudocranial and mediolateral views of the right elbow of a one-year-old female spayed Basset Hound presented with right forelimb angular limb deformity. Moderate caudolateral displacement of the radial head in relation to the humeral condyle. Moderate craniolateral bowing of the radius centered at the proximal diaphysis of the radius.

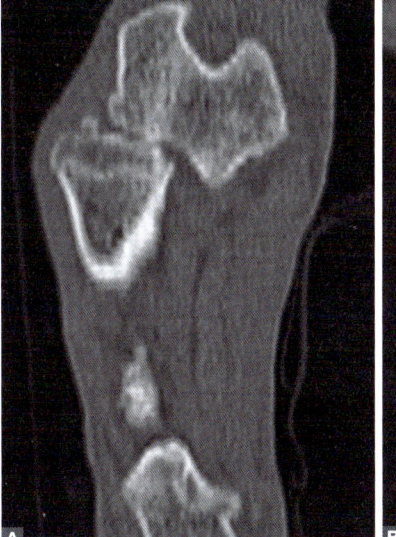

Fig. 10.12 Computed tomographic dorsal and sagittal reformat images in bone window of the same dog as in fig. 10.11. Lateral displacement of the radial head in relation to the humeral condyle. Moderate widening of the humeroulnar joint space.

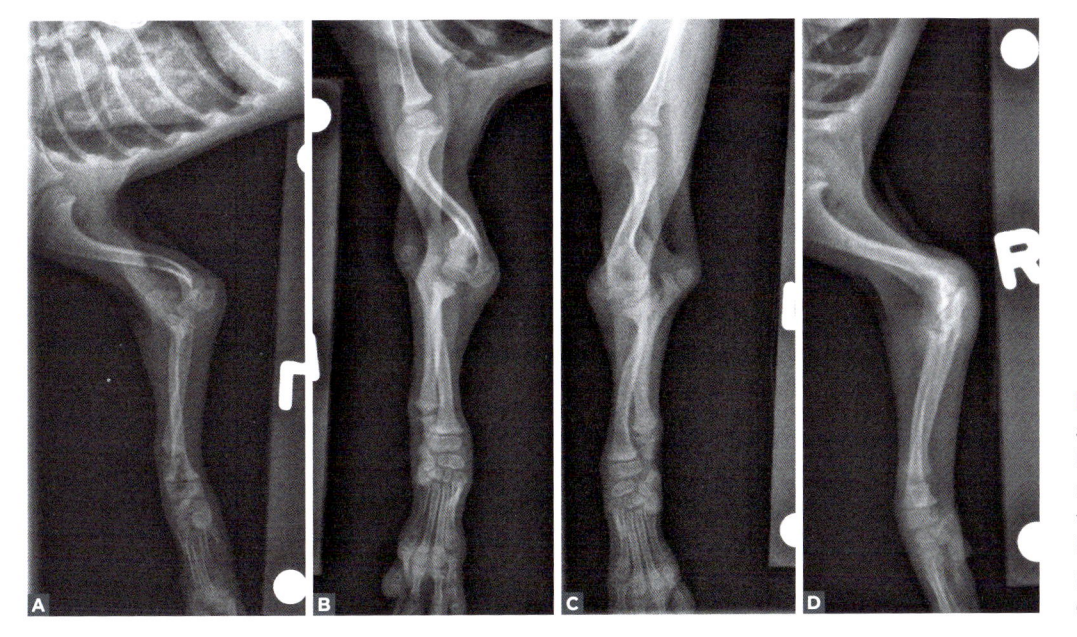

Fig. 10.13 Mediolateral and caudocranial views of both elbow joints of a two-month-old male Havanese with bilateral forelimb lameness. Marked cranio-proximolateral subluxation of the radius and ulna.

97

the radial carpal bone) and the *os centrale* (between the two). These centers fuse at three to four months of age. The lines of interface between these ossification centers are frequently identified as fracture planes in the radial carpal bone (**figs. 10.14** and **10.15**). It is suggested that areas of weakness associated with incomplete fusion predispose to fracture under intense or repeated stresses.[27-30]

Avascular femoral head necrosis

Avascular femoral head necrosis is often referred to as Legg-Calvé-Perthes disease, the name of the corresponding human condition. The disease typically affects young dogs of small and toy breeds,

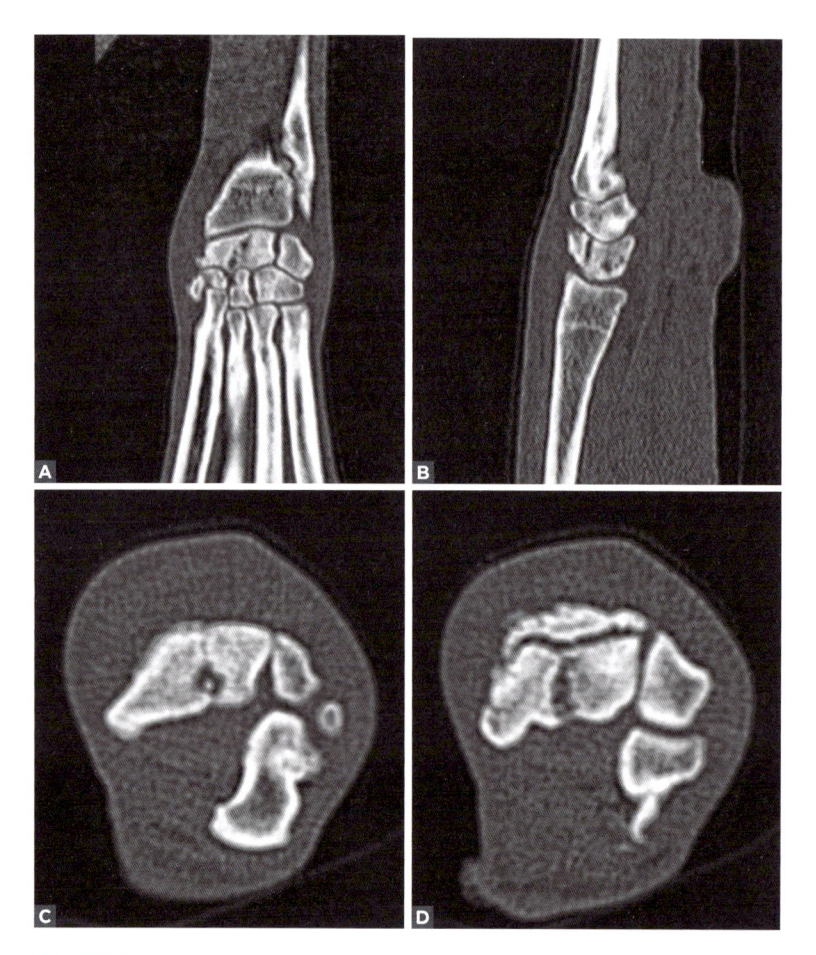

Fig. 10.14 Dorsal, sagittal and transverse images of the left carpus in bone window of a two-year-old male Boxer presented with carpal swelling. Hypoattenuating line at the mid aspect of the radial carpal bone, extending in a sagittal plane from proximolateral to distomedial direction. A communicating linear hypoattenuation at the dorsal margin of the radial carpal bone in a dorsal plane.

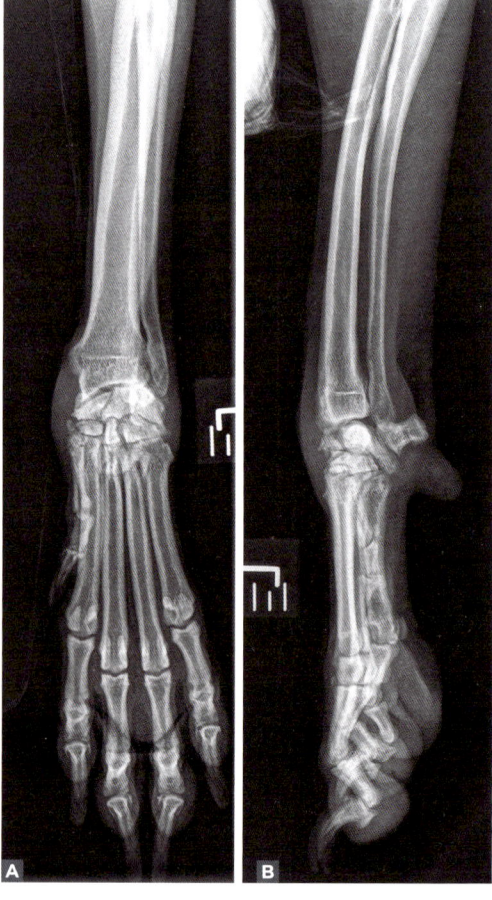

Fig. 10.15 Dorsopalmar and mediolateral views of the left carpus of a six-year-old female Springer Spaniel presented with left forelimb lameness. Linear lucency in the left radial carpal bone extending in a proximolateral to distomedial direction, with mild dorsodistolateral displacement of the lateral fragment. Several mineral fragments are at the dorsal aspect of the left radial carpal bone.

with no sex prevalence. A cascade of events starting with compromised vascular supply and ischemic necrosis of the subchondral bone of femoral capital epiphysis is at the basis of the pathogenesis and of the radiographic appearance of the condition.[31]

A genetic predisposition due to an autosomic recessive gene has been considered for breeds such as Yorkshire Terriers, West Highland White Terriers and toy Poodles; but cases have been described in Pugs, Pomeranians, Cairn Terriers, Lhasa Apsos and crossbreds.

The disease can occur bilaterally in up to 16.5% of cases. Affected dogs can be asymptomatic or present with lameness from very subtle to non-weight bearing; on clinical examination pain is present on palpation of the hip, with atrophy of the regional muscles.

Recommended radiographic projections include extended and frog leg ventrodorsal views. Radiographic changes evolve with the disease and are more conspicuous in late stages; they include a variable degree of remodeling and deformity of the femoral head, which might become smaller and irregular/squared in shape; thickening/erosion of the femoral neck; areas of subchondral radiolucency; fracture/fragmentation/collapse of the femoral head in late stages; osteophytosis/remodeling of the acetabulum which can become shallow (**figs. 10.16** and **10.17**).[32] Radiography is considered insensitive to diagnosing early stages of the disease and computed radiography and magnetic resonance have been described as better techniques for a more prompt diagnosis. MRI findings include an inhomogeneous low intensity signal in T1, inhomogeneous low-to-high signal in T2 and inhomogeneous contrast enhancement of the femoral head and neck.[33]

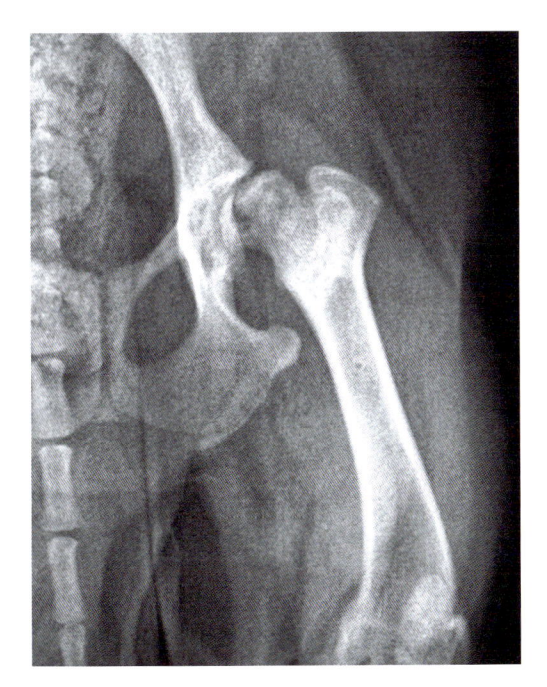

Fig. 10.16 Detail of the ventrodorsal extended view of the pelvis of a ten-month-old West Highland White Terrier presented for a lameness of five weeks duration. The femoral head is misshapen and flattened; the opacity is heterogeneous due to presence of irregular areas of lucency. The acetabulum is shallow. The dog was treated with a femoral head ostectomy.

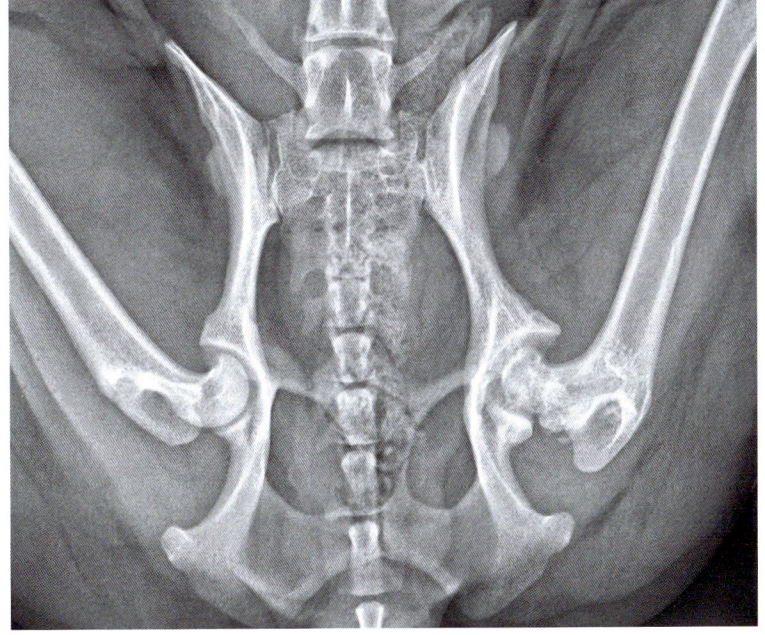

Fig. 10.17 Ventrodorsal frog-leg view of the pelvis of a one-year-old Cocker Spaniel with avascular femoral head necrosis. The femoral head is remodeled, irregular in shape and heterogeneous in opacity. The acetabulum is also markedly widened and remodeled due to the presence of large osteophytes on the cranial effective acetabular rim and caudal acetabular rim. Image courtesy of Dr. Tiziana Liuti from the Royal (Dick) School of Veterinary Studies, The University of Edinburgh.

Slipped femoral capital epiphysis and femoral physeal dysplasia in cats

Femoral physeal dysplasia is a condition of adolescent/young adult cats that leads clinically to physeal separation of the femoral head epiphysis in absence of trauma; it is considered comparable to slipped capital femoral epiphysis in humans. Siamese breed, excessive weight and neutering at a very young age have been suggested as predisposing factors; however, these theories have been recently questioned.[34] A compromised vascular supply and alteration of the insulin metabolism have been proposed amongst other causes as triggers for the pathogenesis of this condition, whereby disorganized physes remain open and are histologically characterized by a thickened layer of very irregularly organized clusters of chondrocytes separated by abundant matrix.

Affected cats present with acute, severe lameness not associated with trauma, and pain on palpation and compression of the coxofemoral/trochanteric region. The condition can be uni- or bilateral.

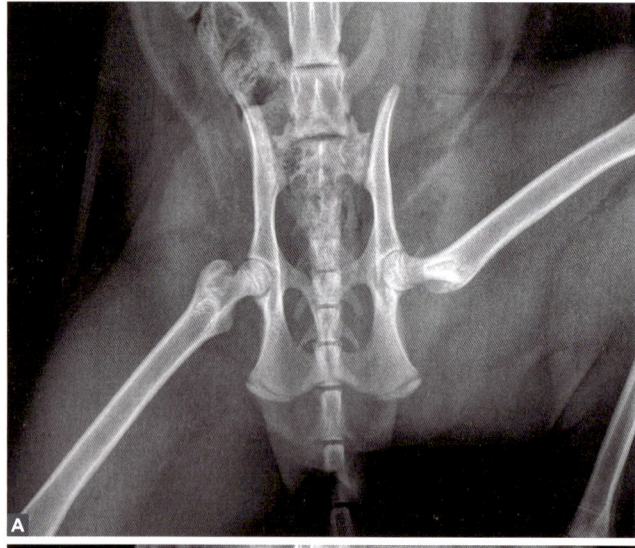

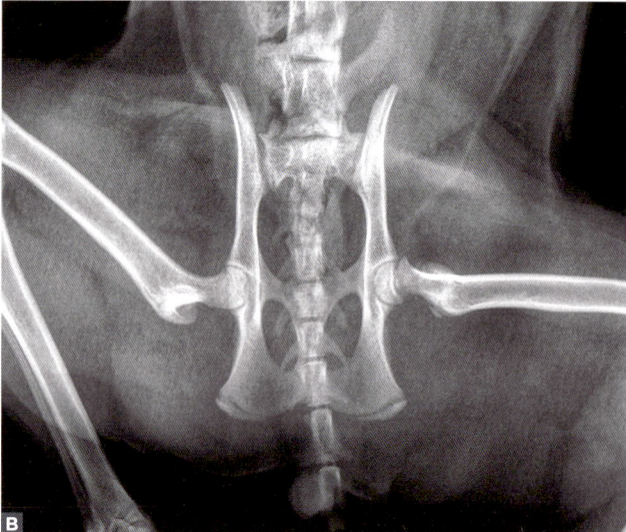

Fig. 10.18 Ventrodorsal views of the pelvis of an eight-month-old Domestic shorthair cat. The cat was poorly sedated; descending colon was on the right side. The separation of the epiphysis on the left femur could only be seen after repositioning of the leg.

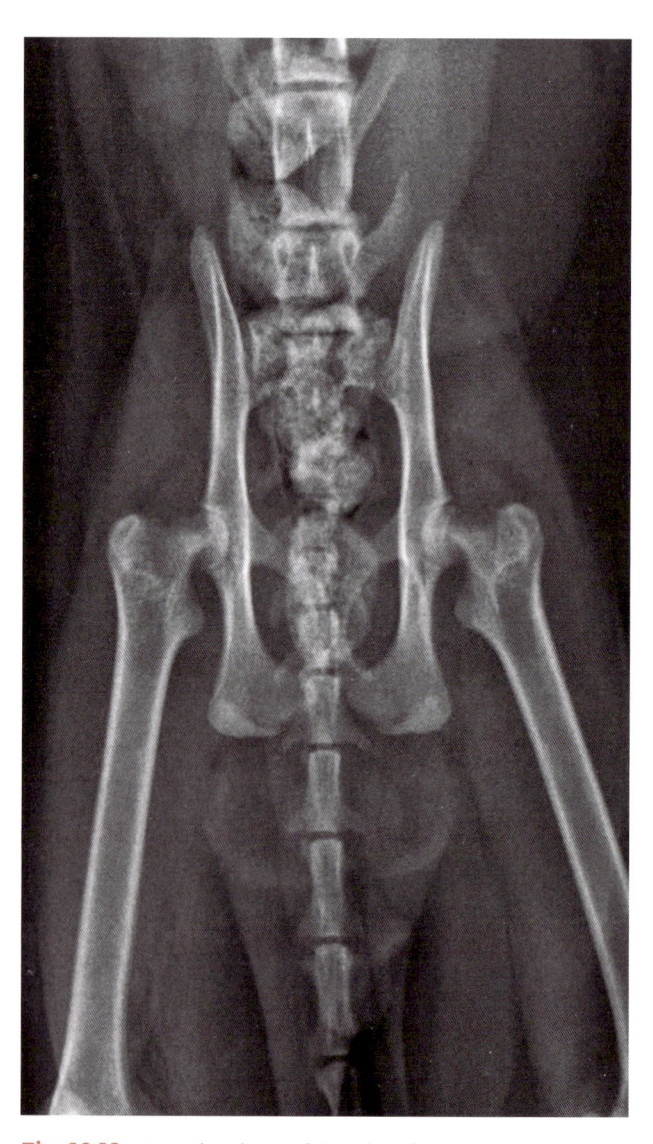

Fig. 10.19 Ventrodorsal view of the pelvis of a two-year-old Domestic shorthair cat presented for "inability to jump". The "apple core" appearance of both femoral necks is a typical feature of chronic slipped capital femoral epiphysis with secondary bone resorption.

A standard radiographic ventrodorsal view of the pelvis with extension of the hindlimbs is occasionally not adequate to show early lesions with minimal displacement; a ventrodorsal frog-leg projection with or without abduction of the affected leg has been suggested to provide better visualization of the separation. Ideally, both views should be obtained (**figs. 10.18** and **10.19**).

The radiographic finding is a Salter-Harris type I fracture of the femoral capital epiphysis, which often remains lodged within the acetabulum while the femur is mildly cranio-dorsally displaced. Chronic lesions are characterized by a more extensive resorption and remodeling of the femoral neck, creating in some cases an "apple core" outline (**fig. 10.19**). The physes of other long bones might still be open in these cats.

Recently it has been suggested that CT might show early signs of the condition, namely irregular areas of resorption in the metaphyseal region of the proximal femur.[35] The use of CT as a screening tool is, however, still debatable.

Patellar luxation

The medial, or less commonly lateral, displacement of the patella outside the homonymous sulcus in the distal femur is listed amongst the most common causes of lameness in small animals, affecting mostly dogs and in lower percentages cats. Female, neutered dogs seem to be predisposed. The literature is inconsistent in whether the dog's size correlates with the side of the luxation; however, the highest caseload is represented by small breed dogs with medial patellar luxation, while lateral luxation has historically been associated with larger breeds such as Labrador Retrievers.[36-38]

Patellar luxation (PL) can be congenital/developmental or acquired (traumatic). Congenital PL might be secondary to alterations in the alignment of the so-called "quadriceps system or mechanism" which includes the quadriceps muscles, patella and patellar tendon/ligament, trochlear groove (or sulcus) and tibial tuberosity. PL can therefore be associated with congenital malformations such as tibial varus, valgus or torsion, femoral sulcus dysplasia, etc.

Congenital PL might not become clinically patent until the dog is two or three years of age.

Clinically there are four grades of PL of increased severity: from grade I where the patella can be manually luxated, but returns into position immediately when released, to grade IV where the patella is permanently luxated and cannot be manually repositioned.

A radiographic study of the stifle usually shows luxation only in more severe cases but is more useful to assess the overall conformation of the hindlimb. The suggested radiographic projections are a caudocranial view of the hindlimb (**fig. 10.20**) or a ventrodorsal view of the pelvis including both extended hindlimbs; a medio-lateral view (**fig. 10.20B**) and a craniodistal-cranioproximal oblique-skyline view (**fig. 10.20C**). The radiographic appearance of patellar luxation varies depending upon the clinical grade:

- On the caudal-cranial view the patella can be in a usual position equidistant from the condyles on the midline of the distal femur (grade I), or it can have various degrees of medial (or lateral) displacement and appear superimposed to one of the condyles or to the soft tissues medial (or lateral) to them (grade IV).
- On the medio-lateral view the patella can be in its usual position cranial to the femoral groove or appear partially concealed because superimposed to the condylar region.
- A dysplastic or flattened patellar trochlea may be seen on a skyline view of the distal femur.

CT might provide further information on the overall alignment of the affected limb when concurrent deformities are present, as well as supplying evidence on the shape of the trochlear groove (**fig. 10.21**).

SECTION II APPENDICULAR SKELETON

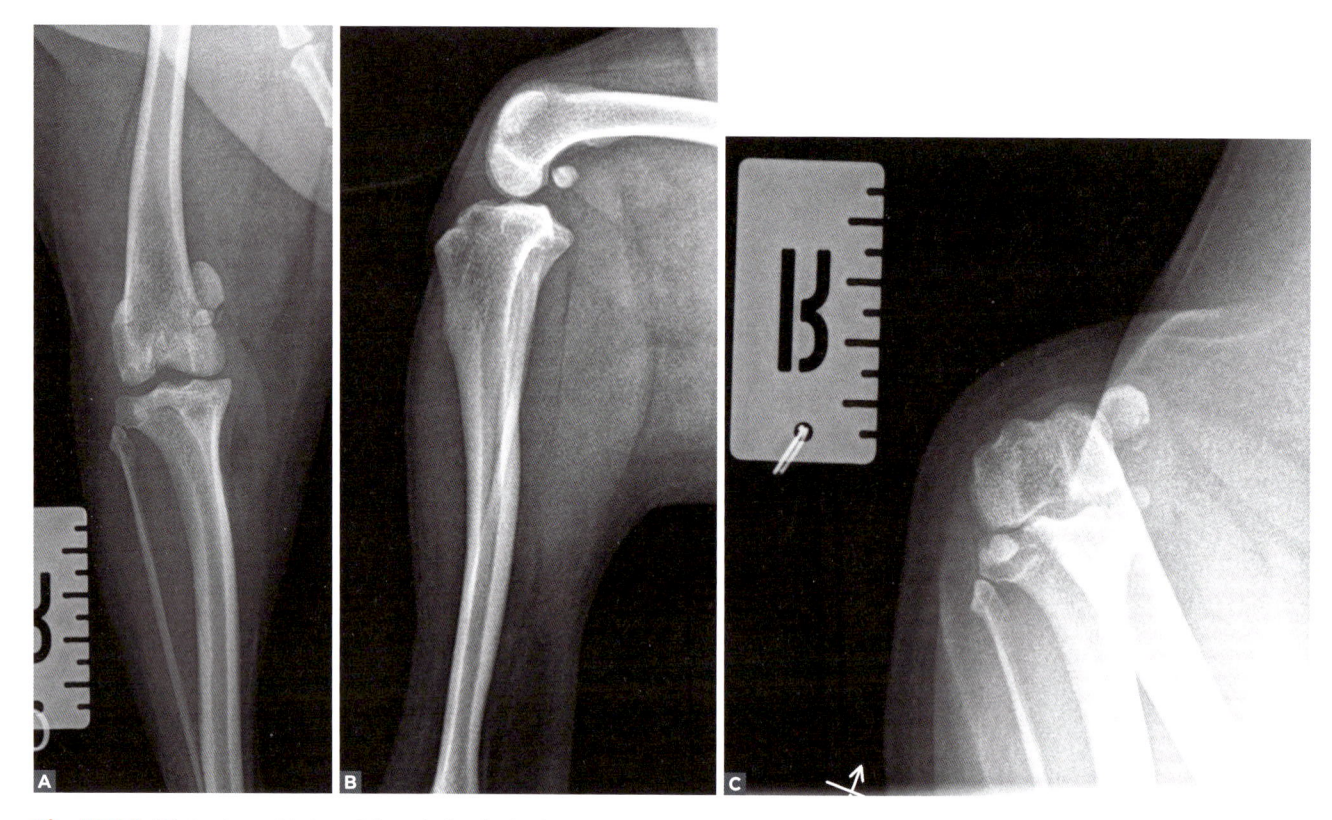

Fig. 10.20 (A) Caudocranial view of the right hindlimb of a three-year-old Cavachon with grade IV patellar luxation. The patella is severely displaced medially. The tibial crest is also located in a more medial position. (B) Mediolateral view of the right hindlimb of the same dog in (A). The patella is not visible in its position cranial to the distal femur, but it can be seen superimposed on the femoral trochlear ridges. (C) Skyline view of the same dog in (A) and (B). The patella is completely displaced outside of the trochlear groove in a position medial to the medial femoral condyle. The trochlear groove is mildly shallow.

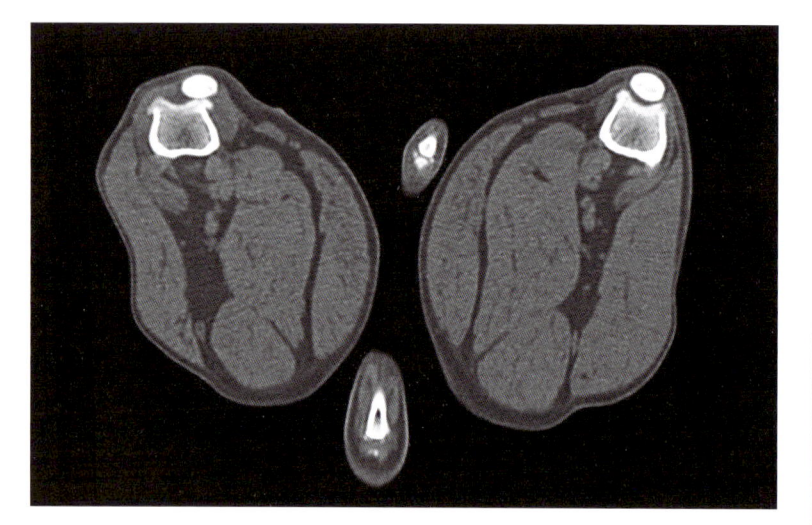

Fig. 10.21 Computed tomography image of the stifles of a two-year-old Irish Terrier presented for sudden non-weight bearing right hind lameness and diagnosed with a grade III patellar luxation at the referring veterinarian. The trochlear groove on the right femur is flattened and shallow compared to the contralateral leg. Both trochlear ridges are flattened and the medial ridge is sclerotic. The patella is moderately displaced medially.

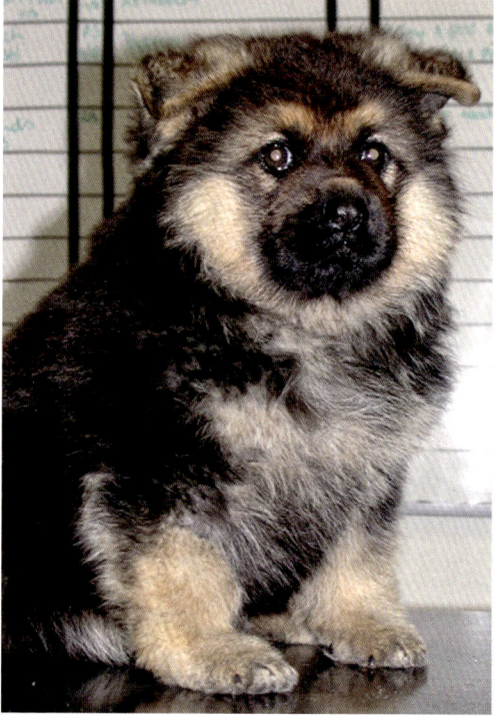

Fig. 10.22 Photograph of a German Shepherd puppy diagnosed with pituitary dwarfism and congenital hypothyroidism. Image courtesy of Prof. Carmel Mooney, University College Dublin.

Congenital hypothyroidism

Congenital hypothyroidism is an uncommon endocrine condition reported in young dogs and cats and characterized by skeletal deformities, stunted growth, macroglossia and mental impairment (**fig. 10.22**). It can affect dogs and cats.[39-44] The reduced production of the hormones thyroxine (T_4) and triiodothyronine (T_3) associated with the disorder can be secondary to aplasia, dysplasia or dysgenesis of the thyroid gland or errors in the biosynthesis of the thyroid hormones (dyshormonogenesis). A genetic/familial component has been suggested for hypothyroidism associated with goiter in certain dog breeds (Fox Terriers, Tenterfield Terriers).

Although the final diagnosis requires blood tests to confirm decreased plasma levels of the thyroid hormone and thyroid stimulating hormone concentrations, radiology can help define a list of differential diagnoses.

Radiographic findings in the appendicular skeleton are consistent with disproportionate dwarfism, but are not specific for hypothyroidism and include:

- Delayed physeal closure.
- Delayed ossification of the epiphyses that appear irregular and fragmented.
- Thickening of the long bone cortices (more often radius and ulna).
- Overall shortened/deformed long bones.
- Angular limb deformities such as carpus valgus can be present.

Radiographic findings in the axial skeleton include a short and flat skull and shortened vertebral bodies. Fracture of the vertebral epiphyses leading to tetraparesis has been described in a four-year-old Affenpischer.

References

1. Rorvik AM, Teige J, Ottesen N, Lingaas F. Clinical, radiographic, and pathologic abnormalities in dogs with multiple epiphyseal dysplasia: 19 cases (1991-2005). *J Am Vet Med Assoc* 233:600-606, 2008.
2. Fox S. Bone and joint disorders. In Schaer M, Gaschen F (editors). Clinical medicine of the dog and cat 3rd edition, Boca Raton, FL, 2016, Taylor & Francis Group, pp 637-680.
3. De Simone A, Gernone F, Ricciardi M. Imaging diagnosis-bilateral abnormal ossification of the supraglenoid tubercle and cranial glenoid cavity in an English Setter. *Vet Radiol Ultrasound* 54:159-163, 2013.
4. Sebbag L, Riggs A, Carnevale J. Oculo-skeletal dysplasia in five Labrador Retrievers. *Vet Ophthalmol* 23:386-393, 2020.
5. Smit JJ, Temwitchitr J, Brocks BA, Nikkels PG, Hazewinkel HA, Leegwater PA. Evaluation of candidate genes as a cause of chondrodysplasia in Labrador Retrievers. *Vet J* 187:269-271, 2011.
6. Malik R, Allan GS, Howlett CR, Thompson DE, James G, McWhirter C, et al. Osteochondrodysplasia in Scottish Fold cats. *Aust Vet J* 77:85-92, 1999.
7. Takanosu M, Hattori Y. Osteochondrodysplasia in Scottish Fold cross-breed cats. *J Vet Med Sci* 82:1769-1772, 2020.
8. Cross JR, Tromblee TC, Miller JM. What is your diagnosis? Osteochondroma, extraskeletal osteosarcoma, or tumor calcinosis. *J Am Vet Med Assoc* 230:1807-1808, 2007.
9. Franch J, Font J, Ramis A, Lafuente P, Fontecha P, Cairo J. Multiple cartilaginous exostosis in a Golden Retriever cross-bred puppy. Clinical, radiographic and backscattered scanning microscopy findings. *Vet Comp Orthop Traumatol* 18:189-193, 2005.
10. Smith TJ, Baltzer WI, Lohr C, Stieger-Vanegas SM. Primary synovial osteochondromatosis of the stifle in an English Mastiff. *Vet Comp Orthop Traumatol* 25:160-166, 2012.
11. Tas O, De Cock H, Lemmens P, Pool RR. Synovial osteochondromatosis and sclerosing osteosarcoma in a cat. *Vet Comp Orthop Traumatol* 26:160-164, 2013.
12. Ricker Z, Vinayahak A, Kerwin S. What is your diagnosis? Multiple cartilaginous exostoses. *J Am Vet Med Assoc* 229:1085-1086, 2006.
13. Aeffner F, Weeren R, Morrison S, Grundmann IN, Weisbrode SE. Synovial osteochondromatosis with malignant transformation to chondrosarcoma in a dog. *Vet Pathol* 49:1036-1039, 2012.
14. Moores AP, Agthe P, Schaafsma IA. Prevalence of incomplete ossification of the humeral condyle and other abnormalities of the elbow in English Springer Spaniels. *Vet Comp Orthop Traumatol* 25:211-216, 2012.
15. Moores AP, Moores AL. The natural history of humeral intracondylar fissure: an observational study of 30 dogs. *J Small Anim Pract* 58:337-341, 2017.
16. Moores AP. Humeral intracondylar fissure in dogs. *Vet Clin North Am Small Anim Pract* 51:421-437, 2021.
17. Carrera I, Hammond GJ, Sullivan M. Computed tomographic features of incomplete ossification of the canine humeral condyle. *Vet Surg* 37:226-231, 2008.
18. Farrell M, Trevail T, Marshall W, Yeadon R, Carmichael S. Computed tomographic documentation of the natural progression of humeral intracondylar fissure in a cocker spaniel. *Vet Surg* 40:966-971, 2011.

19. Piola V, Posch B, Radke H, Telintelo G, Herrtage ME. Magnetic resonance imaging features of canine incomplete humeral condyle ossification. *Vet Radiol Ultrasound* 53:560-565, 2012.
20. Heidenreich DC, Fourie Y, Barreau P. Presumptive congenital radial head sub-luxation in a shih tzu: successful management by radial head ostectomy. *J Small Anim Pract* 56:626-629, 2015.
21. DeCamp CE, Johnston SA, Déjardin LM, Schaefer SL. The elbow joint. In DeCamp CE, Johnston SA, Déjardin LM, Schafer SL (editors). Brinker, Piermattei and Flo's Handbook of Small Animal Orthopedics and Fracture Repair 5th edition, Saint Louis, 2015, Elsevier Saunders, pp 327- 365.
22. McDonell HL. Unilateral congenital elbow luxation in a Cavalier King Charles Spaniel. *Can Vet J* 45:941-943, 2004.
23. Milton JL, Horne RD, Bartels JE, Henderson RA. Congenital elbow luxation in the dog. *J Am Vet Med Assoc* 175:572-582, 1979.
24. Milton JL, Montgomery RD. Congenital elbow dislocations. *Vet Clin North Am Small Anim Pract* 17:873-888, 1987.
25. Valastro C, Di Bello A, Crovace A. Congenital elbow subluxation in a cat. *Vet Radiol Ultrasound* 46:63-64, 2005.
26. Kene ROC, Lee R, Bennett D. The radiological features of congenital elbow luxation/subluxation in the dog. *J Small Anim Pract* 23:621-630, 1982.
27. Tomlin JL, Pead MJ, Langley-Hobbs SJ, Muir P. Radial carpal bone fracture in dogs. *J Am Anim Hosp Assoc* 37:173-178, 2001.
28. Li A, Bennett D, Gibbs C, Carmichael S, Gibson N, Owen M, et al. Radial carpal bone fractures in 15 dogs. *J Small Anim Pract* 41:74-79, 2000.
29. Gnudi G, Mortellaro CM, Bertoni G, Martini FM, Cantoni AM, Di Giancamillo M, Vignoli M. Radial carpal bone fracture in 13 dogs. *Vet Comp Orthop Traumatol* 16:178-183, 2018.
30. Ferguson JF. What was your diagnosis? *J Small Anim Pract* 39:406-406, 1998.
31. Cardoso CB, Rahal SC, Mamprim MJ, Oliveira HS, Merlchert A, Coris JGF, et al. Avascular Necrosis of the Femoral Head in Dogs - Retrospective Study. *Acta Sci Vet* 46:5, 2018.
32. Thak MA, Yoon HY, Jeong SW. Early stage Legg-Calve-Perthes disease in a dog: clinical, surgical, radiological, computed tomography and histological findings. *Journal of Veterinary Clinics* 30:366-370, 2013.
33. Bowlus RA, Armbrust LJ, Biller DS, Hoskinson JJ, Kuroki K, Mosier DA. Magnetic resonance imaging of the femoral head of normal dogs and dogs with avascular necrosis. *Vet Radiol Ultrasound* 49:7-12, 2008.
34. Grayton J, Allen P, Biller D. Case report: proximal femoral physeal dysplasia in a cat and a review of the literature. *Israel J Vet Med* 69:40-44, 2014.
35. Degórska B, Sapierzyński R, Jurka P, Śliwińska MK, Kowalczyk L, Galanty M, et al. Comparison of usefulness of different diagnostic procedures in slipped capital femoral epiphysis in cats. *Medycyna Weterynaryjna* 73:637-641, 2017.
36. Di Dona F, Della Valle G, Fatone G. Patellar luxation in dogs. *Vet Med (Auckl)* 9:23-32, 2018.
37. Gibbons SE, Macias C, Tonzing MA, Pinchbeck GL, McKee WM. Patellar luxation in 70 large breed dogs. *J Small Anim Pract* 47:3-9, 2006.
38. Kalff S, Butterworth SJ, Miller A, Keeley B, Baines S, McKee WM. Lateral patellar luxation in dogs: a retrospective study of 65 dogs. *Vet Comp Orthop Traumatol* 27:130-134, 2014.
39. Bojanic K, Acke E, Jones BR. Congenital hypothyroidism of dogs and cats: a review. *N Z Vet J* 59:115-122, 2011.
40. Mooney CT. Canine hypothyroidism: a review of aetiology and diagnosis. *N Z Vet J* 59:105-114, 2011.
41. Lim CK, Rosa CT, de Witt Y, Schoeman JP. Congenital hypothyroidism and concurrent renal insufficiency in a kitten. *J S Afr Vet Assoc* 85:1144, 2014.
42. Dodgson SE, Day R, Fyfe JC. Congenital hypothyroidism with goiter in Tenterfield terriers. *J Vet Intern Med* 26:1350-1357, 2012.
43. Greco DS. Diagnosis of congenital and adult-onset hypothyroidism in cats. *Clin Tech Small Anim Pract* 21:40-44, 2006.
44. Lieb AS, Grooters AM, Tyler JW, Partington BP, Pechman RD. Tetraparesis due to vertebral physeal fracture in an adult dog with congenital hypothyroidism. *J Small Anim Pract* 38:364-367, 1997.

CHAPTER 11

Metabolic bone diseases

Alessandra Destri

KEY POINTS

- Metabolic bone diseases occur due to failure of bone maturation or abnormal bone metabolism.
- They may be congenital or acquired.
- They most often cause osteopenia, which is diffuse loss of bone mineral content.
- Radiographic changes are usually bilateral and symmetrical.

Metabolic bone diseases or osteodystrophies are caused by a failure of normal bone maturation or abnormal metabolism in mature bone, usually secondary to deficiencies or imbalances of vitamin D, calcium or phosphorus.

All metabolic bone disorders result in generalized skeletal changes which are usually bilateral and symmetrical. Although most of the skeleton is affected, overt radiographic changes may be more obvious in specific regions, e.g., the skull in renal secondary hyperparathyroidism. Radiographs are quite insensitive in detection of bone mineral loss and changes will not be evident unless at least 70% of the mineral content is depleted.

Renal secondary hyperparathyroidism

The renal form of hyperparathyroidism occurs secondary to impaired renal function and inability of the kidneys to excrete phosphorus, which cause calcium phosphorus imbalance.

This disease can present both in young animals with renal dysplasia or in adult animals with chronic renal disease.[2]

The diagnosis is based on clinical signs, radiographic findings, serum chemistry and urinalysis confirmation of renal failure.

The bones most commonly affected are the dental alveolar bones and the cancellous bones of the maxilla and mandible with loss of the lamina dura around the teeth and decreased bone opacity which is usually most severe in the skull. The teeth retain normal opacity and the characteristic radiographic feature is the appearance of floating teeth with marked reduced opacity of the facial bones (**figs. 11.1-11.3**). On physical examination the mandible and maxilla may be soft and pliable, hence the common name "rubber jaw".

Generalized decreased bone opacity and pathologic fractures of the long bones occur later.

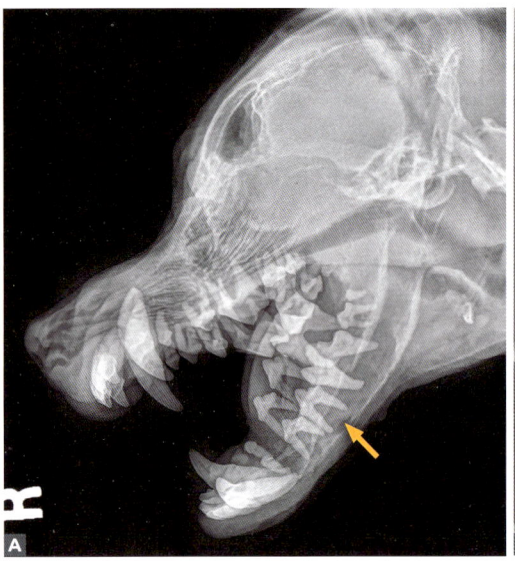

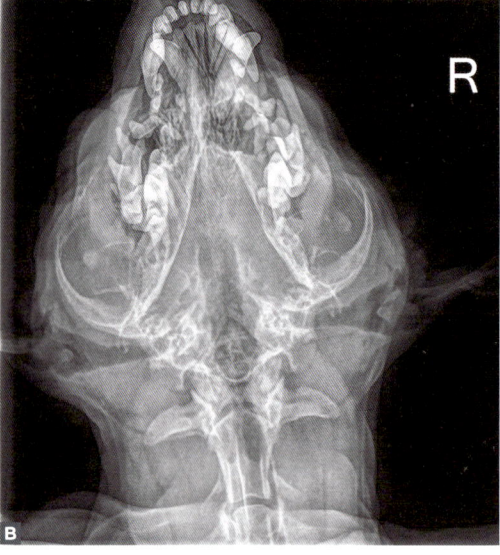

Fig. 11.1 Right lateral and dorsoventral radiographs of the skull of an eight-year-old mixed breed dog with renal secondary hyperparathyroidism. The radiographs demonstrate generalized demineralization of bone, loss of trabecular bone pattern, thinning and expansion of the mandibles and replacement of the lamina dura and alveolar crestal bone with soft tissue radiopacity, giving the appearance of the teeth "floating" (arrow).

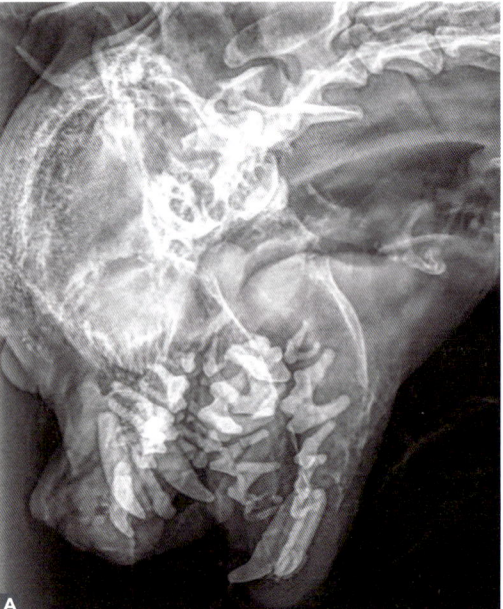

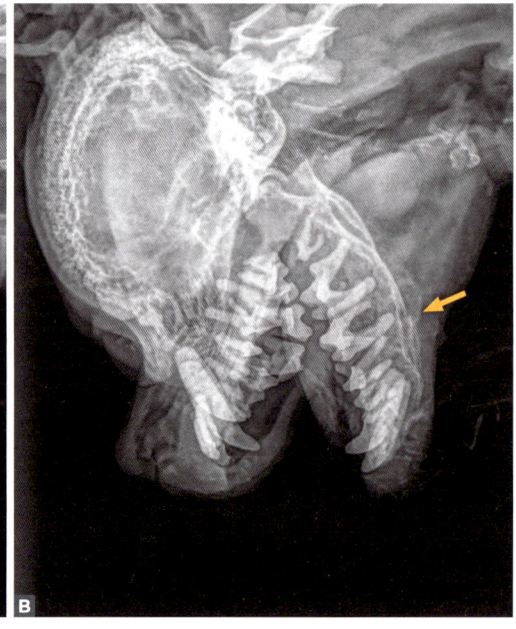

Fig. 11.2 Lateral radiographs of the skull of a nine-year-old Shih Tzu with chronic renal failure and renal secondary hyperparathyroidism. There is generalized skull demineralization with granular appearance of the frontal bones and loss of trabecular bone pattern, thinning and expansion of the mandibles (arrow).

In young animals, with higher skeletal metabolic rates, proliferative lesions of the mandible and maxilla have been reported, whereas generalized osteodystrophy and rubber jaw are more commonly observed in older dogs.[3,4]

Nutritional secondary hyperparathyroidism

Nutritional skeletal diseases were more common in small animals before general availability of commercial diets. The most common is nutritional secondary hyperparathyroidism (NSH).[5] NSH appears in animals fed with diets that are deficient in calcium or have an excess in phosphorus, such as cats and dogs that are fed only with meat. The disease affects mainly young animals due to their active bone metabolism. The inadequate uptake of dietary calcium increases intestinal absorption

CHAPTER 11 Metabolic bone diseases

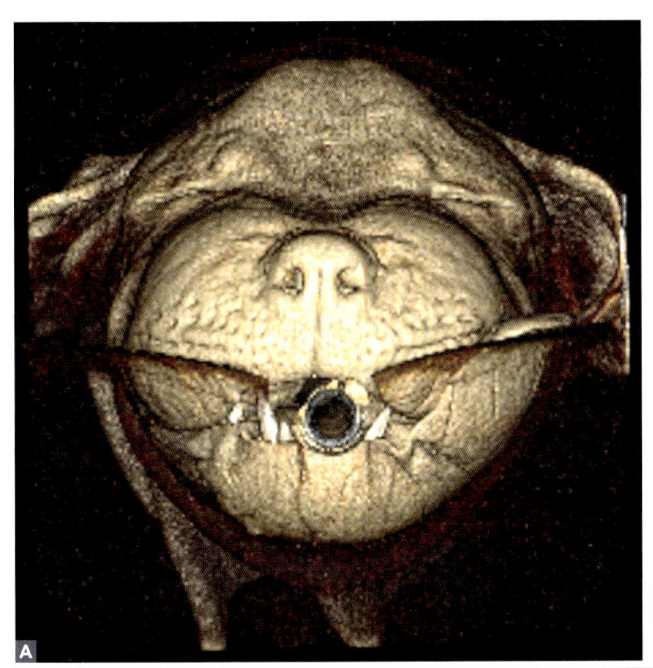

Fig. 11.3 (**A**) A nine-month-old female Rottweiler, presented for further investigation of symmetric facial swelling, dental displacement and ulceration, quiet and subdued status. Volume rendering CT image of the head of the dog highlighting the soft tissues (WW 650 HU, WL 500 HU); notice the bilateral, symmetrical swelling of the head at the level of the maxilla. (**B**) CT images of the head in the transverse plane with bone reconstruction algorithm and bone window (a, WW 4000 HU, WL 700 HU) and with soft tissue reconstruction algorithm and soft tissue window (b, WW 350 HU, WL 50 HU) at the level of tooth 108. There is marked, bilateral and symmetrical swelling and minimal amorphous mineralization of the maxillary bones, which are protruding within the nasal cavities axially and deforming the contour of the head abaxially. The maxillary and mandibular bones are poorly mineralized. (**C**) Volume rendering CT images of the head of the dog, highlighting the skeleton (WW 80 HU, WL 850 HU) on laterolateral (left) and dorsoventral (right) views. The maxillae are markedly hypoattenuating and the teeth are "floating". The rostral part of the frontal bones, presphenoid bone and mandibular rami have a punctuate appearance due to lack of mineralization. Courtesy of Dr. Jeremy Mortier, DVM, CEAV (IM), CES (CP), CPS (HE), DipECVDI, FHEA MRCVS, University of Liverpool. From: Barczak E, O'Connell E, Mortier JR. Clinical, CT and ultrasonographic features of renal secondary hyperparathyroidism in a juvenile dog. *Vet Rec Case Reports* 8:1-6, 2020.

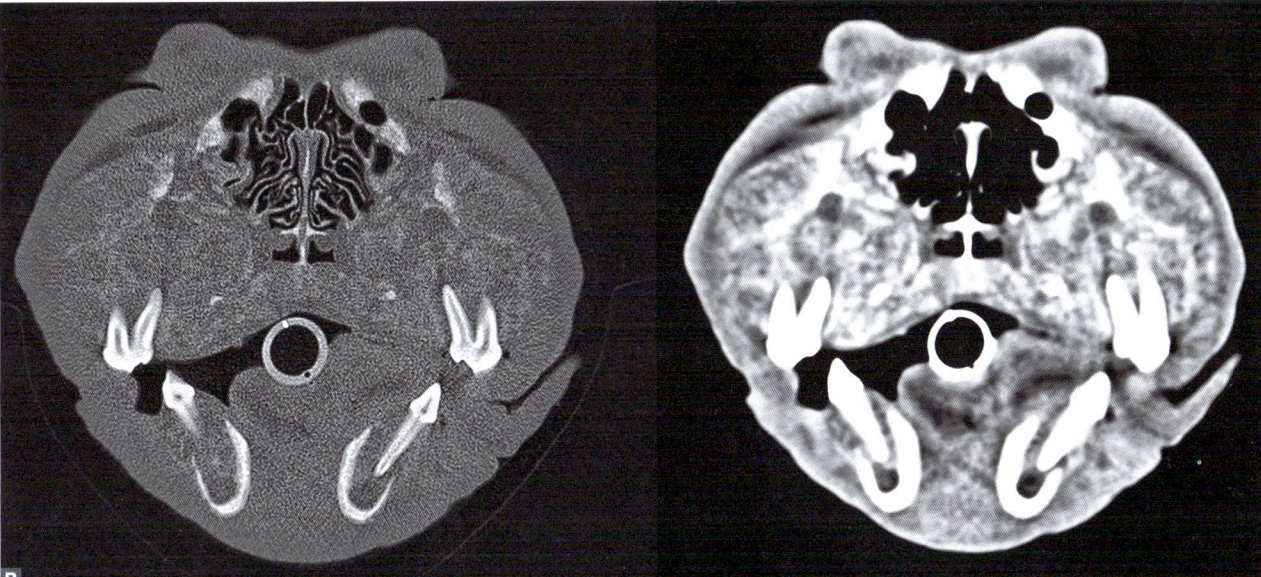

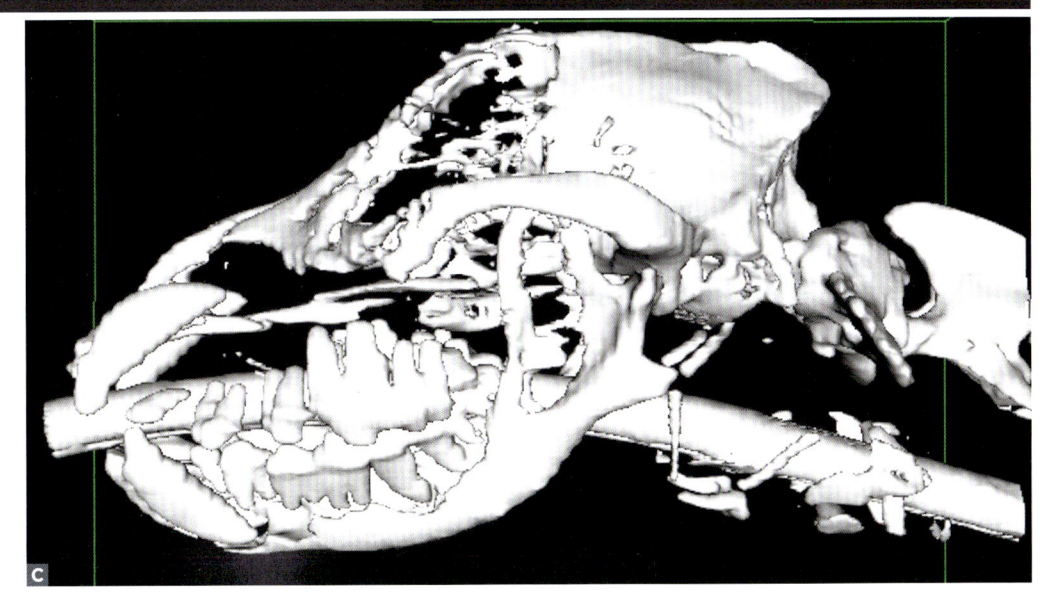

and decreases renal excretion of calcium, ultimately this imbalance causes increased mobilization of calcium from bone which leads to the observed radiographic signs.[6,7]

Typical radiographic findings in NSH include a generalized decrease in bone opacity, thin bone cortices and coarse diaphyseal and metaphyseal trabeculation.

The extremely weakening of the bones leads to folding fractures and bone deformities affecting both the appendicular and the axial skeleton. In contrast to renal hyperparathyroidism, long bones and vertebrae are more severely affected (**fig. 11.5**). In chronic severe cases the bones of the skull are involved too, with alveolar bone and lamina dura resorption giving the appearance of floating teeth (**fig. 11.4**).

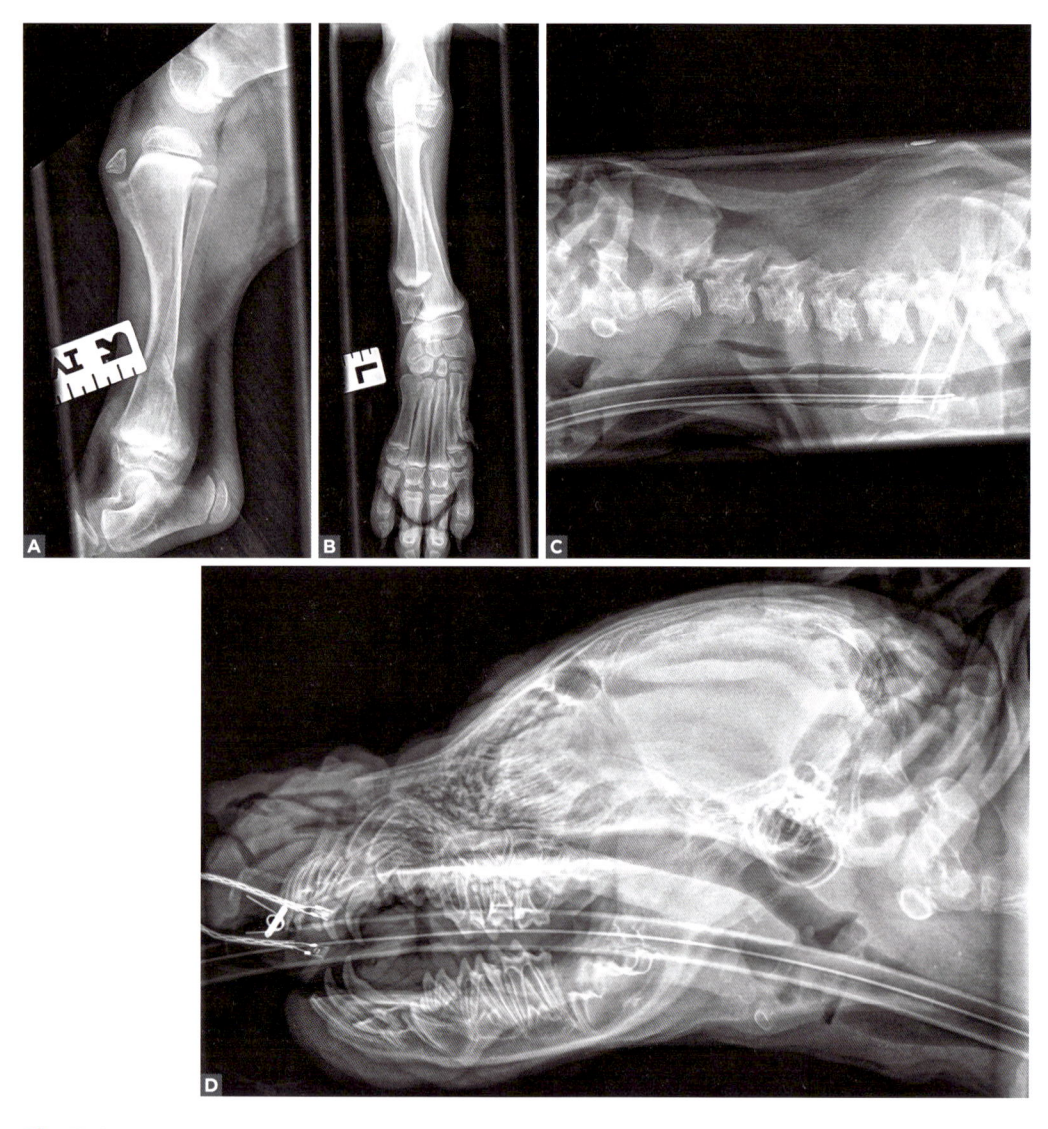

Fig. 11.4 (**A**) Mediolateral radiographs of the tibia, (**B**) craniocaudal radiographs of the elbow and antebrachium, and (**C**) lateral radiograph of the cervical spine of a two-month-old Great Dane puppy fed with a home-made diet composed of meat, rice and vegetables. The bone opacity is diffusely decreased and the bone cortices are thin. There is a folding fracture of the distal caudolateral cortex of the tibia. The cervical vertebrae have a stippled, osteopenic appearance but the epiphyses are visible and appear normally developed. The diagnosis is nutritional secondary hyperparathyroidism. (**D**) Lateral radiograph of the head of the same patient above, showing a diffuse osteopenic appearance of the skull with poorly defined margination of the frontal and parietal bone and poor mineralization of the mandible and maxilla. The dental elements appear to be floating. The calvarial bones are less affected, with a radiopacity that is almost within normal limits.

Fig. 11.5 Whole body (**A**), mediolateral of the front (**B**) and hindlimb (**C**) radiographs of a two-month-old puppy with nutritional secondary hyperparathyroidism. There is diffuse decreased opacity of the bones with numeirous folding fractures of the humeri, radi, femuri and tibiae. There is widening of the physes and flaring of the metaphysis. The carpal and tarsal bone are poorly ossified and developed.

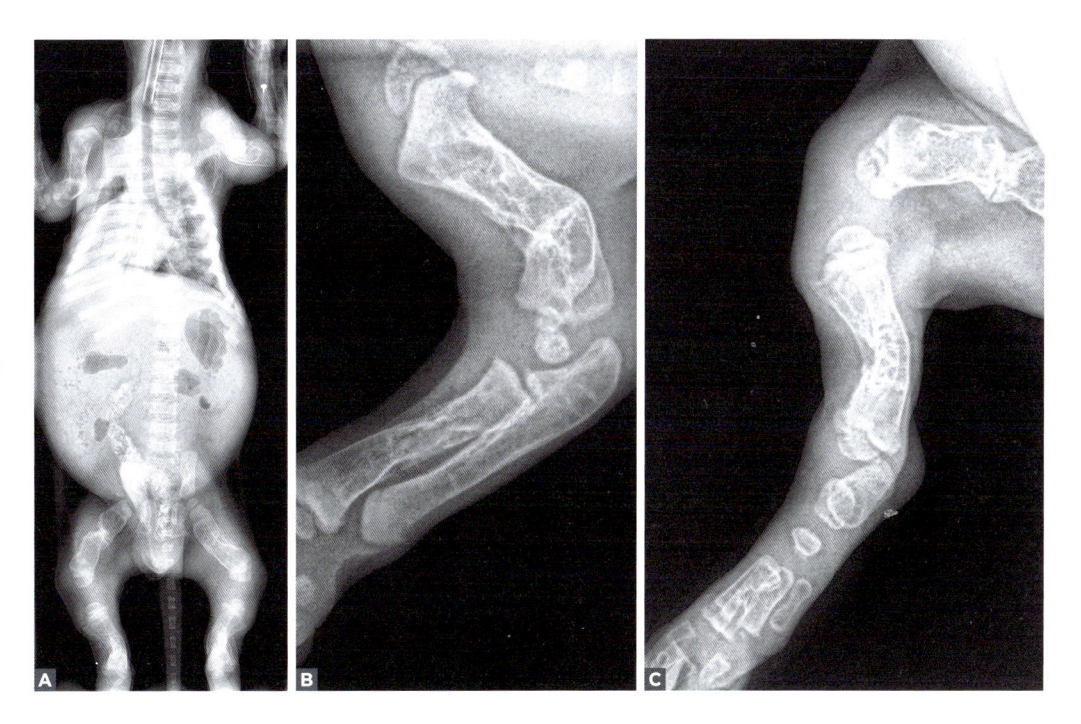

Mucopolysaccharidosis

Mucopolysaccharidoses are a range of inherited conditions in which the body is unable to properly breakdown mucopolysaccharides, long chains sugar molecules found throughout the body. As a result, these mucopolysaccharides accumulate in cells leading to multisystemic disorders.
Several types of the diseases have been reported, most commonly leading to skeletal and ocular abnormalities (except type III).
Type I, VI and VII have been reported in cats, with type VI being common in Siamese cats.
In dogs, the type VII has been observed in mixed breeds and German Shepherds.
Clinical signs vary from impaired growth, weakness, difficulties walking and corneal opacification. Radiographic signs are evident both in the axial and appendicular skeleton and are characterized by heterogenous opacity with granular appearance of the epiphyses (epiphyseal dysplasia), irregular and fragmented vertebral endplates leading to short vertebrae, which assume a cuboid shape, and increased intervertebral distance.
The diaphyses are thickened and skull changes are present such as shortened nasal conchae, aplasia and hypoplasia of the frontal and sphenoid sinuses, shortened incisive and maxillary bones.[8]

Congenital hypothyroidism

Congenital hypothyroidism is a rare disease of dogs and cats caused by thyroid dysgenesis (aplasia or hypoplasia) or serum transport abnormalities of thyroid hormones. Clinical signs are hypothermia, lethargy, kyphosis, delayed dental eruption, thickened skin, and dry hair coats. Affected individuals are disproportionate dwarfs with short broad skulls and mandibles, short limbs and long neck and trunk. Radiographic signs include reduced epiphyseal appearance, retarded epiphyseal growth and reduced long bone growth resulting in disproportionate dwarfism. The radiographic changes are more evident in the proximal tibia and humeral and femoral condyles. As in mucopolysaccharidosis, the retarded epiphyseal growth produces shortening of the vertebrae (**figs. 11.6-11.9**). Degenerative changes may appear later on in the disease.

SECTION II APPENDICULAR SKELETON

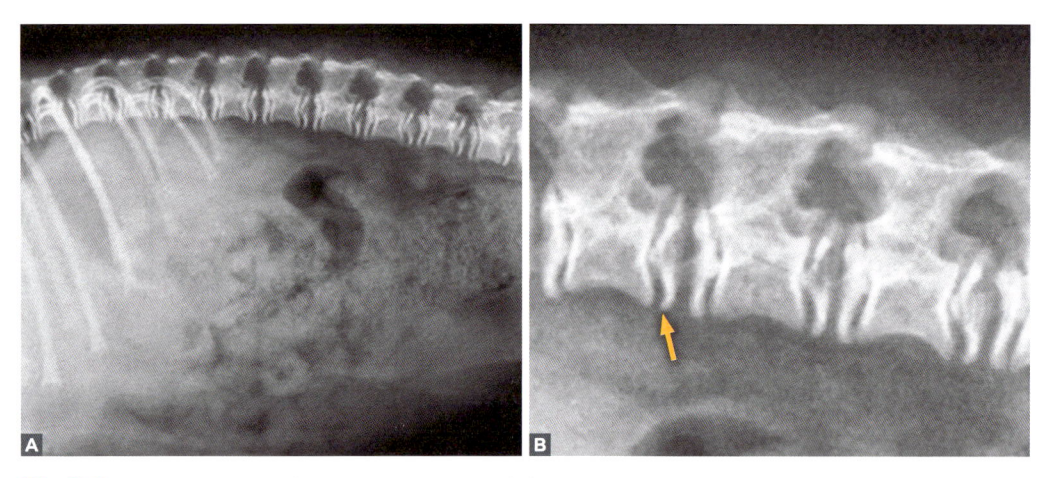

Fig. 11.6 Lateral radiographs of the thoracolumbar spine (**A**) and zoomed detail of the lumbar spine (**B**) of a four-year-old Miniature Poodle presented with back pain and subsequently diagnosed with congenital hypothyroidism. The vertebral bodies had the radiographic appearance of that of a four-month-old dog with both cranial and caudal physes still open. The endplates have a concave margin adjacent to the disc space and are incompletely mineralized (arrow).

Fig. 11.7 (**A**) Right lateral and dorsoventral (**B**) radiographs of a five-month-old cat with hypothyroidism. All physes are still open, which is normal for this age, but the vertebral epiphyses are thin and incompletely mineralized. The femoral condyles are incompletely developed and have a granular appearance. The proximal tibial physes are smaller than normal. There is severe constipation due to the presence of malformation and narrowing of the pelvic canal. Courtesy of Dr. Elisabeth Domínguez, PhD, Dip. ECVDI.

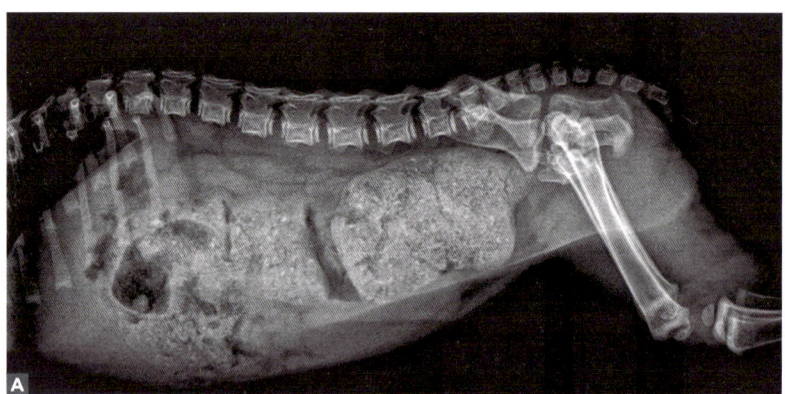

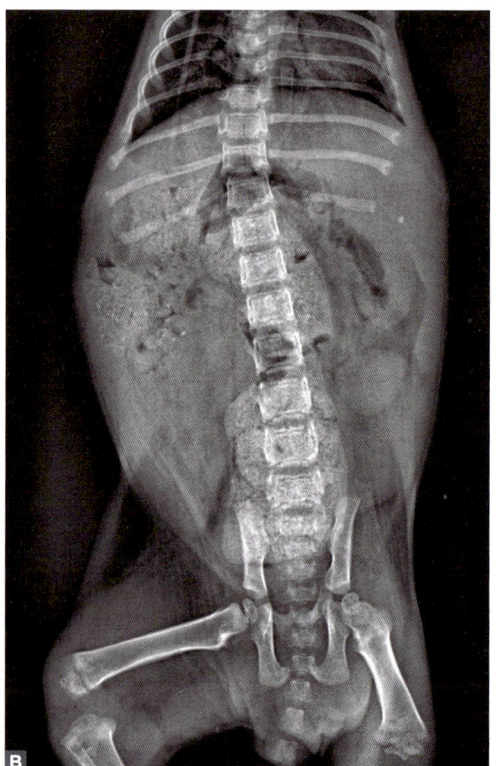

CHAPTER **11** Metabolic bone diseases

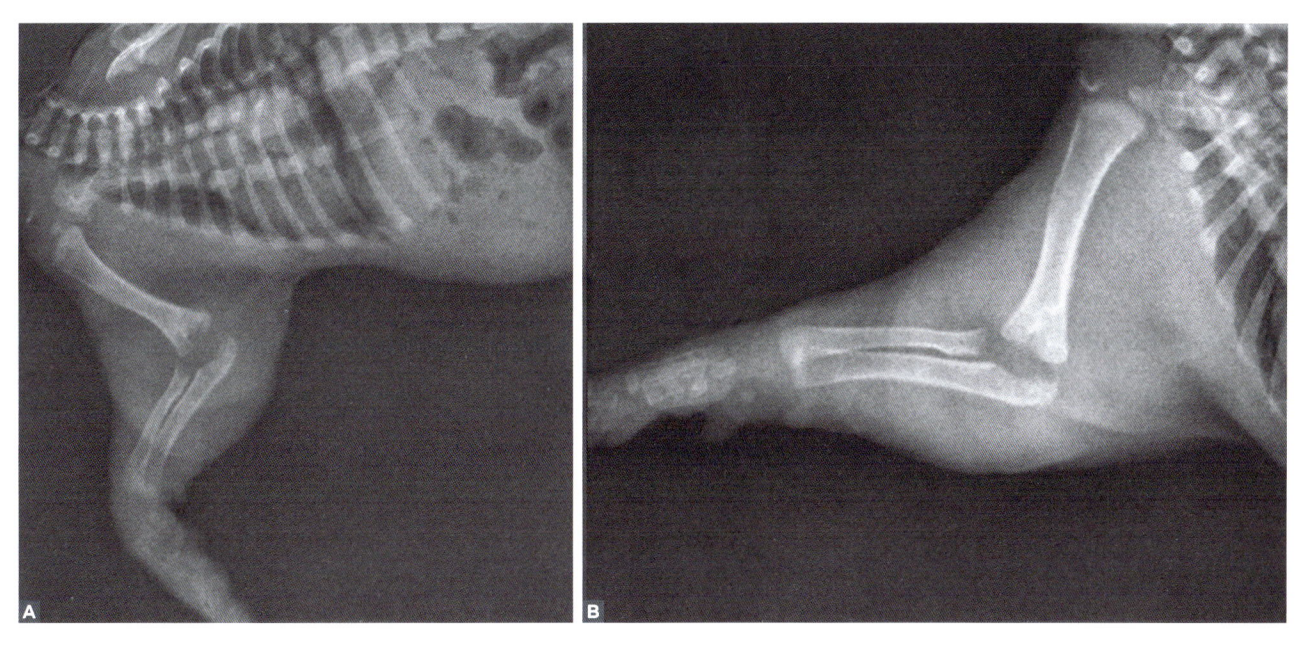

Fig. 11.8 Mediolateral radiographs of the elbows of a five-month-old puppy with epiphyseal dysplasia. The humeral heads and condyles and the radial and ulnar physes are incompletely developed. The vertebral physes are also not visualized, resulting in short vertebrae. Epiphyseal dysplasia is a radiographic feature of both mucopolysaccharidosis and congenital hypothyroidism, that ultimately result in a disproportionate dwarfism with short limbs and skull and long neck and trunk. Courtesy of Dr. Maurizio Longo, PhD, Dip. ECVDI.

Fig. 11.9 Left lateral and dorsoventral radiographs of a six-month-old German Shepherd puppy with epiphyseal dysplasia. Note the almost complete absence of the epiphyses of the long bones and vertebral endplates and the poor ossification of the carpal and tarsal bones. The degree of skeletal development is far less than expected for a patient that should be close to skeletal maturity. These radiographic features could also represent hypothyroidism and mucopolysaccharidosis. Courtesy of Dr. Maurizio Longo, PhD, DECVDI.

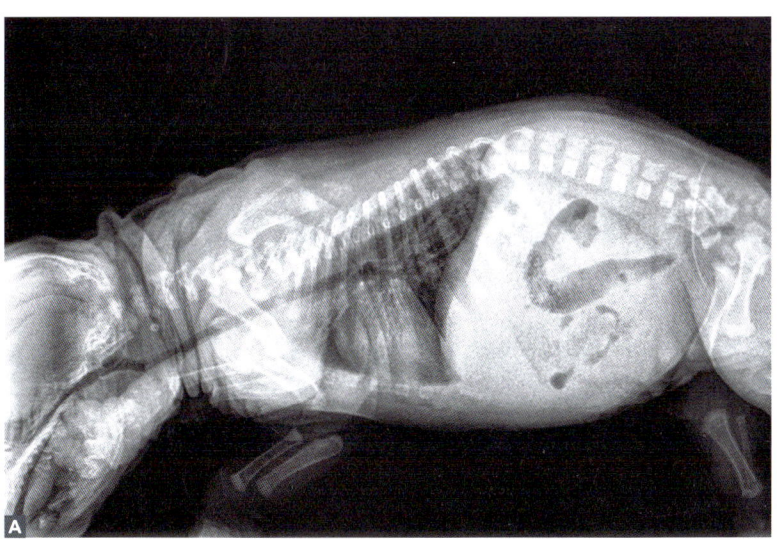

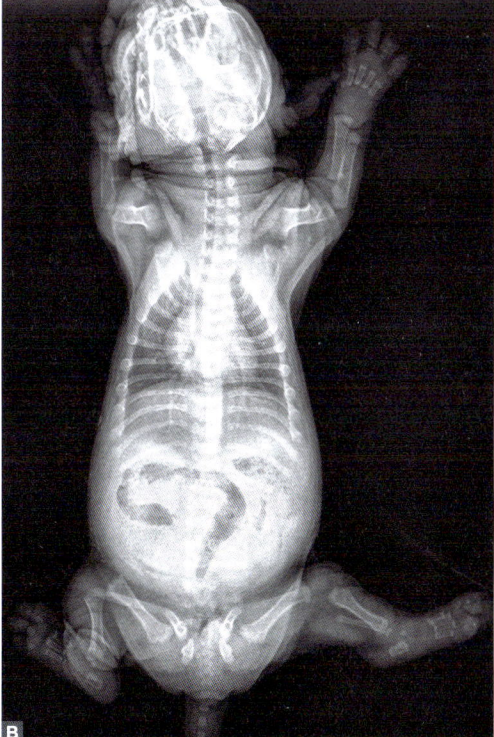

111

Rickets or hypovitaminosis D

Rickets is a rare disease of juvenile dogs and cats caused by inadequate vitamin D intake or heritable disorder affecting vitamin D metabolism or utilization.

Clinical signs are shifting lameness, difficulties walking and generalized pain.

The radiographic features are a generalized decreased bone opacity, with thinning of the cortices and reduced trabecular pattern leading to bowing and pathological fractures of the bone shafts (**fig. 11.10**). Growth plate changes are characteristic and more evident at the distal radius and ulna with widening of the physes and flaring of the metaphyses assuming a mushroom appearance. The vertebrae appear misshapen with wavy appearance of the physes or foreshortened.[1]

Osteochondral dysplasias

Osteochondral dysplasias are a group of diseases characterized by abnormal endochondral or intramembranous ossification (**table 11.1**).

Chondrodysplasia and osteochondral dysplasia result in disproportionate dwarfism.

Radiographic signs are more evident at the physes, which are wider, and at the metaphyseal regions, that appear flared. A triangular metaphyseal radiolucency can be detected, which is consistent with a retained cartilage core (**fig. 11.11**). The disease can also result in angular limb deformity.[10]

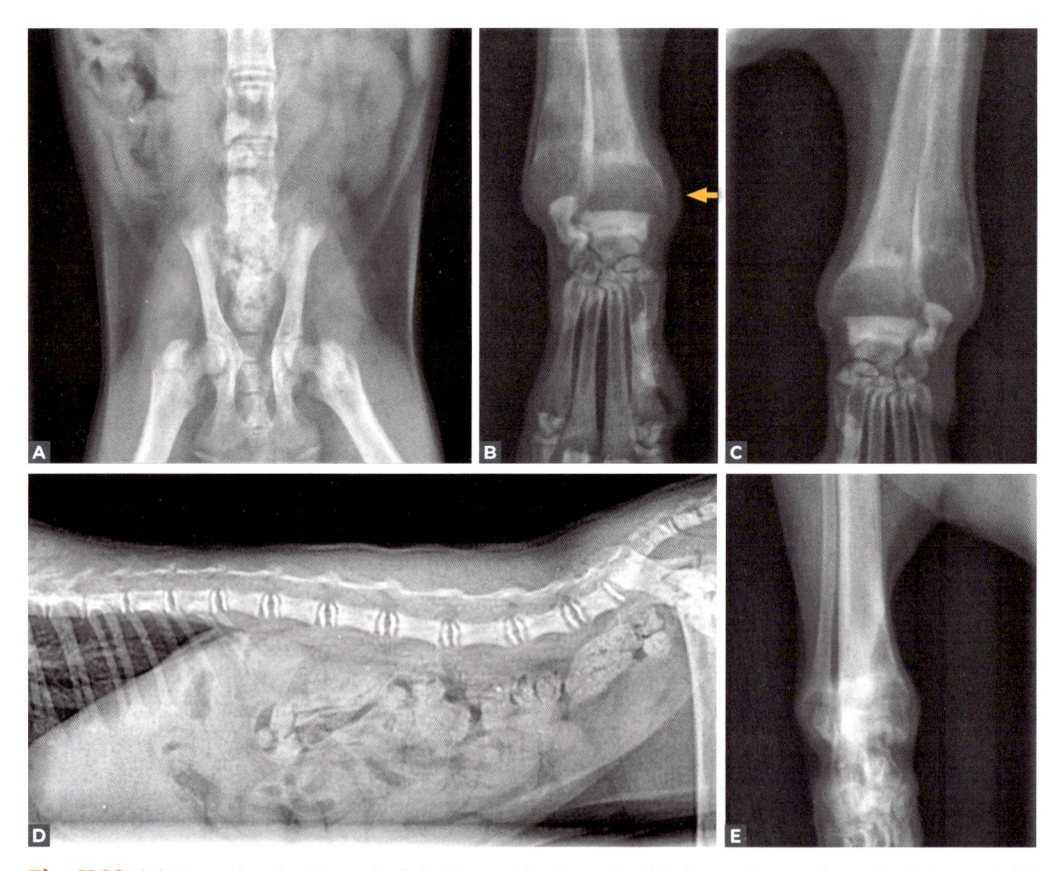

Fig. 11.10 (**A**) Ventrodorsal radiograph of the hips and lumbar spine, (**B**) dorsopalmar radiographs of the carpi, (**C**) laterolateral radiograph of the thoracolumbar spine, and (**D**) dorsoplantar radiographs of the tarsus of a four-month-old kitten presenting with bowing of the antebrachium of both legs and lordosis of the lumbar spine. There is generalized decrease radiodensity of bones, especially in the epiphyses and metaphysis. The distal growth plates of the radii, ulnae and femurs are severely widened resulting in a mushroom appearance (arrow). The physes are present and the vertebrae have a normal shape. The presumptive diagnosis is rickets or hypovitaminosis D. Courtesy of Dr. Stefanie Veraa, PhD, Dip. ECVDI.

CHAPTER 11 Metabolic bone diseases

Table 11.1 Summary of osteochondrodysplasia types in dogs and cats.

Osteochondral dysplasias	Breed	Clinical and radiographic signs
Multiple epiphyseal dysplasia	Beagle, Miniature Poodle	Epiphyseal dysplasia, short limbs, enlarged joints
Dysplasia epiphysealis hemimelica (DEH)	Boxer	Epiphyseal dysplasia and hypertrophy with delayed mineralization, mainly affecting the femurs
Osteochondrodysplasia	Bull Terrier	Epiphyseal dysplasia mainly of the femoral physes, long bone distortion, femoral neck fractures
	Scottish Fold	Irregular shape and size of the bones of the tarsus, carpus, metatarsus, metacarpus, phalanges and caudal vertebrae, progressive new bone formation around joints of advanced stages
	Scottish Deerhound	Diffuse epiphyseal dysplasia with short limbs and vertebrae
Chondrodysplasia	English Pointer (enchondrodystrophy) Alaskan Malamute Domestic shorthair and Domestic longhair cats Miniature Poodle Norwegian Elkhound Pyrenean Mountain Dog	Disproportionate dwarfism, wider physes and flared metaphyses, sclerosis of the metaphyseal side of the growth plates
Oculoskeletal dysplasia Disproportionate dwarfism, cataract and retinal detachment	Labrador Retriever	Delayed growth of the anconeal and coronoid processes of the ulna and medial epicondyle of the humerus. Retained endochondral cartilage cores may be present in costochondral junctions. Epiphyses and cuboidal bones are large and misshapen. Hip dysplasia is a common sequel
	Samoyed	Disproportionate dwarfism, cataract and retinal detachment
Hypochondroplasia	Irish setter	Mildly shorter limbs compared to littermate, variable radius and ulna bowing and carpal valgus. Epiphyses and metaphyses radiologically normal

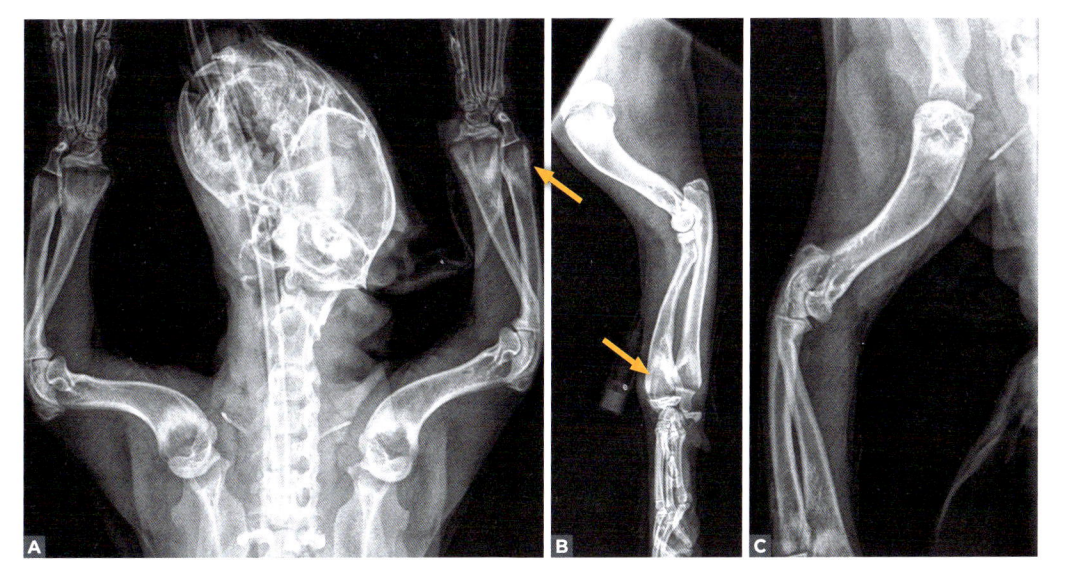

Fig. 11.11 Dorsoventral radiographs of the skull and brachia (**A**) and mediolateral (**B**) and craniocaudal (**C**) radiographs of the right brachium of a ten-month-old Domestic shorthair cat presented for intermittent lameness, bowing of the antebrachia and carpal valgus. There is severe widening of the humeral, ulnar and radial physes, flaring of the metaphysis and the presence of a triangular radiolucency of the metaphysis consistent with retained cartilage core. The long bones are short, but the skull is normal in size. The suspected diagnosis is chondrodysplasia of the Domestic shorthair cat. Courtesy of Dr Yulia Gerne, MRCVS.

References

1. Malik R. Rickets in a litter of racing greyhounds. *J Small Anim Pract* 38:109-114, 1997.
2. Stillion JR, Ritt MG. Renal secondary hyperparathyroidism in dogs. *Compend Contin Educ Vet* 31:1-19, 2009.
3. Vanbrugghe B, Blond L, Carioto L, Carmel EN, Nadeau ME. Clinical and computed tomography features of secondary renal hyperparathyroidism. *Can Vet J* 52:184-188, 2011.
4. Barczak E, O'Connell E, Mortier JR. Clinical, CT and ultrasonographic features of renal secondary hyperparathyroidism in a juvenile dog. *Vet Rec Case Reports* 8:1-6, 2020.
5. Bennett D. Nutrition and bone disease in the dog and cat. *Vet Rec* 98:313-21, 1976.
6. Tomsa K, Glaus T, Hauser B, Flückiger M, Arnold P, Wess G, et al. Nutritional secondary hyperparathyroidism in six cats. *J Small Anim Pract* 40:533-539, 1999.
7. Kawaguchi K, Braga IS, Takahashi A, Ochiai K, Itakura C. Nutritional secondary hyperparathyroidism occurring in a strain of German shepherd puppies. *Jpn J Vet Res* 41:89-96, 1993.
8. Wang P, Sorenson J, Strickland S, Mingus C, Haskins ME, Giger U. Mucopolysaccharidosis VII in a cat caused by 2 adjacent missense mutations in the GUSB gene. *J Vet Intern Med* 29:1022-1028, 2015.
9. Bojanić K, Acke E, Jones BR. Congenital hypothyroidism of dogs and cats: A review. *N Z Vet J* 59:115-122, 2011.
10. BSAVA Manual of Canine and Feline Musculoskeletal Imaging. Kirberger R, McEvoy F, editors. BSAVA British Small Animal Veterinary Association, 2016, p 92.

CHAPTER 12

Soft tissues

Barbara Posch, Antonella Puggioni and Massimo Vignoli

> **KEY POINTS**
>
> - Large dog breeds are predisposed to shoulder tendinopathies and cruciate ligament disease.
> - Tendinopathies are generally caused by strenuous repetitive exercise and often associated with dystrophic mineralization of the tendon fibers.
> - Calcaneal tendinopathy/rupture is more often caused by blunt trauma.
> - Radiography and high-frequency ultrasonography remain the initial, most accessible and cost-effective imaging tools for conditions of tendons and ligaments.
> - A combination of complementary imaging techniques, however, provides the most comprehensive assessment of tendons and ligaments, including CT for evaluating osseous structures of the shoulder and stifle and MRI, providing exquisite detail for soft tissues of shoulder, stifle and peripheral nerves.

Biceps brachii tendon

Bicipital tenosynovitis is a common cause of forelimb lameness in middle-aged, medium to large-breed dogs. Inflammation plays a role in most cases of primary bicipital tenosynovitis, presumably as a result of overuse or chronic repetitive trauma-type injury. Biceps tendinopathy may be also secondary to acute shoulder trauma, shoulder joint instability or joint mouse migration from an OCD lesion of the humeral head.[1]

Radiographs may be normal with biceps tendinopathy, especially in the acute phase. Ill-defined sclerosis and new bone formation along the bicipital groove can be a radiographic indicator of bicipital tenosynovitis (**fig. 12.1**).[1]

Skyline views (flexed cranioproximal-craniodistal oblique view) may help to identify new bone formation along the bicipital groove.[2] Other radiological signs include remodeling of the supraglenoid tubercle, dystrophic mineralization of the tendon, avulsion fractures of the attachment of the tendon and mineralized fragments within the tendon sheath (**fig. 12.2**).

Positive-contrast arthrography is a useful additional imaging tool to plain radiographs, which may demonstrate reduced or irregular filling of the biceps tendon sheath.[1]

High-frequency ultrasonography is a very useful tool for diagnosing biceps tendinopathy. The shoulder is rotated outwards and abducted to obtain a perpendicular scan plane of the biceps tendon.[3] On a transverse plane, the tendon appears as an oval, uniformly hyperechoic structure, surrounded by a scant amount of fluid within the tendon sheath. In the longitudinal plane, the tendon is composed of multiple, parallel and hyperechoic lines (fibrillar pattern) (**fig. 12.3**).[4]

SECTION II APPENDICULAR SKELETON

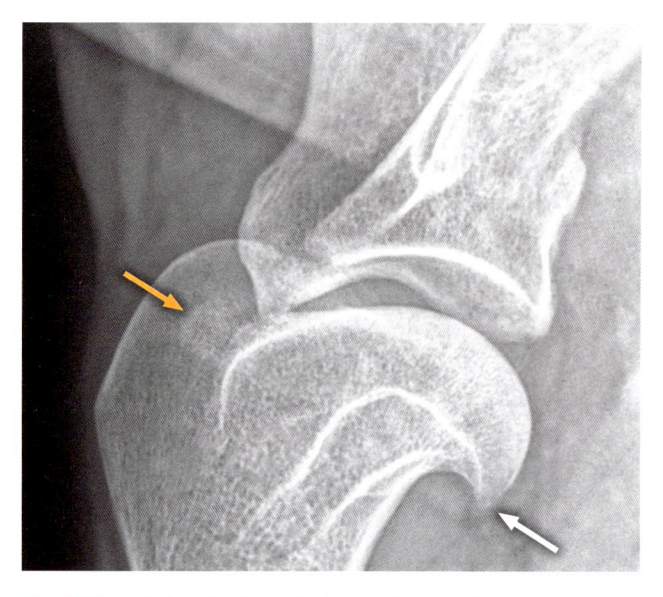

Fig. 12.1 Mediolateral radiograph of a shoulder joint of a two-year-old Small Münsterländer. Focal sclerosis is visible at the level of the bicipital groove (orange arrow) and osteophyte formation at the caudal aspect of the humeral head (white arrow).

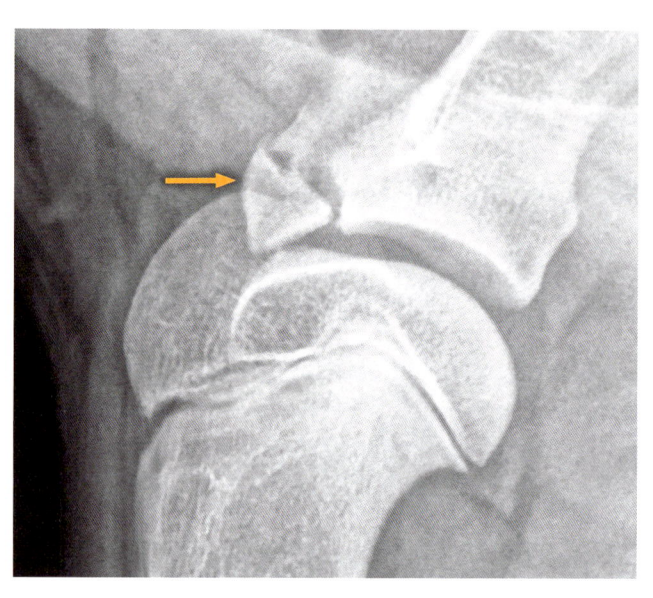

Fig. 12.2 Mediolateral radiograph of a shoulder joint of a skeletally immature six-month-old Rottweiler. An avulsion fracture of the supraglenoid tubercle is visible (arrow).

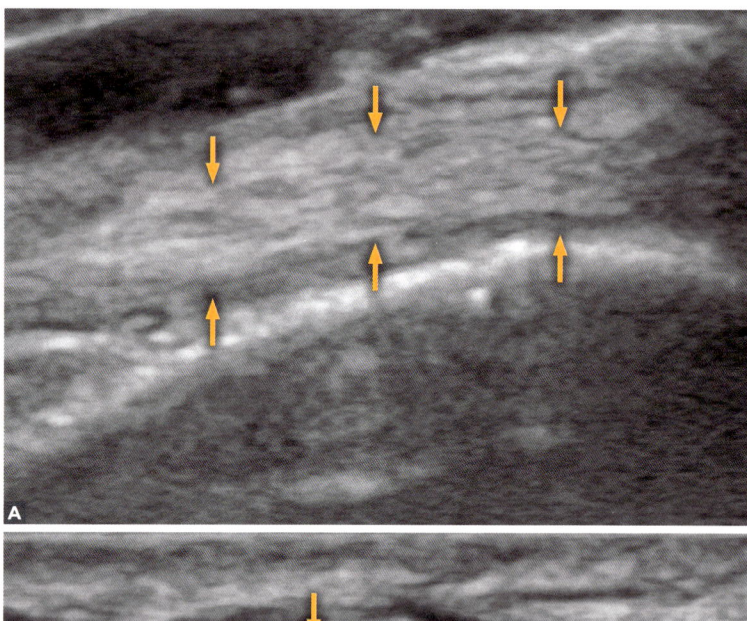

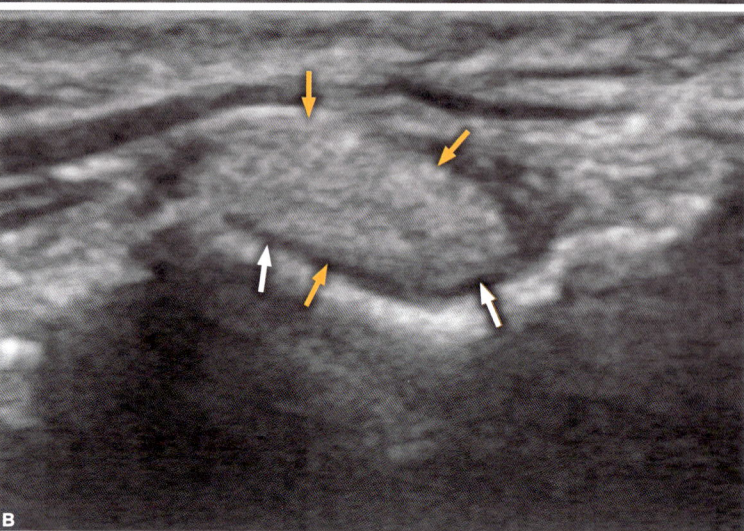

Fig. 12.3 Ultrasonographic images of a normal biceps tendon in a two-year-old Labrador Retriever. Note the normal hyperechoic echotexture with parallel tendon fiber alignment (orange arrows) in the longitudinal plane (**A**). In the transverse plane (**B**), the biceps tendon appears as a uniformly hyperechoic oval structure (orange arrows), surrounded by a thin hypoechoic rim representing normal fluid within the tendon sheath (white arrows).

Comparison with the unaffected contralateral side can be useful due to size variation of the tendon in various breeds.[2] Ultrasonographic signs of bicipital tenosynovitis include mild to severe tendon sheath effusion and irregular synovial thickening. The bicipital tendon appears mildly to severely thickened, with possibly fibrillar pattern disruption and hypoechoic areas (core lesion) caused by partial tears and/or hemorrhage (**fig. 12.4**).

With complete rupture, the fibrillar structure of the tendon is disrupted, associated with tendon sheath effusion as a result of hemorrhage.[2,3,4] In case of fracture of the supraglenoid tubercle, a bone fragment can be seen moving with the tendon during dynamic flexion and extension of the shoulder (**fig. 12.5**).[3,4]

CT is frequently used in the diagnosis of shoulder lameness. CT signs of biceps tendinopathy are tendon sheath effusion, thickened bicipital tendon, osteophytes within the bicipital groove and biceps mineralization (**fig. 12.6**).

CT has a greater sensitivity for detection of soft tissue mineralization compared to radiographs.[5] Computed tomographic arthrography (CTA) provides a superior diagnostic efficacy relative to survey CT for the assessment of the biceps tendon and tendon sheath.[6]

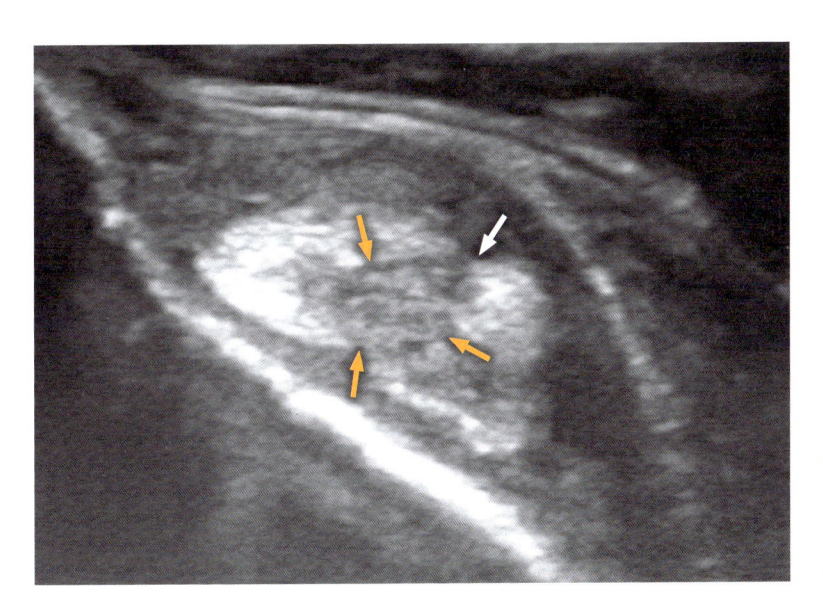

Fig. 12.4 Transverse sonographic images of a biceps tendon in a two-year-old German Shepherd with partial tear of the biceps tendon. A hypoechoic core lesion can be found in the center of the tendon, consistent with fibrillar disruption and hematoma (orange arrows). A cleft can also be noted (white arrow).

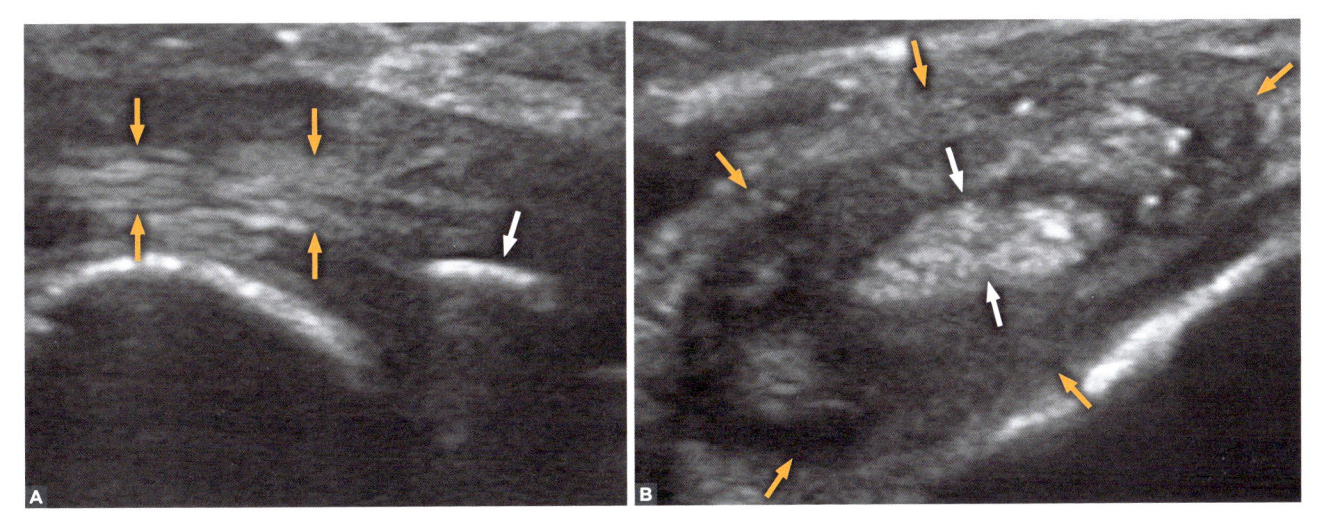

Fig. 12.5 Same dog as in fig. 12.2 with avulsion fracture of the supraglenoid tubercle. (**A**) The avulsion fragment (white arrow) is visible as a hyperechoic structure at the proximal extend of the biceps tendon (orange arrows). (**B**) Severe tendon sheath effusion is present (orange arrows) as the result of hemorrhage around the biceps tendon (white arrows).

MRI is an excellent imaging modality for the shoulder joint due to its exquisite soft tissue resolution, multiplanar imaging capabilities and large field of view.[7] The biceps tendon is best appreciated in the sagittal and transverse planes. The normal tendon is uniformly hypointense on T1W and T2W images. In the T2W image, a fine hyperintense rim of synovial fluid surrounds the biceps tendon.[8] MRI characteristics of biceps tendinopathy includes thickening of the tendon with a heterogenous and increased signal intensity in T2W and STIR images (**fig. 12.7**).[9] Progressive tendon fraying causes thinning of the tendon, which can lead to spontaneous rupture. Synovitis is seen as thickened and possibly irregular synovial lining, with strong enhancement in T1W post-contrast images.[7,9]

MRI arthrography causes distension of the tendon sheath, which may improve outlining of synovial proliferation and adhesions.[9]

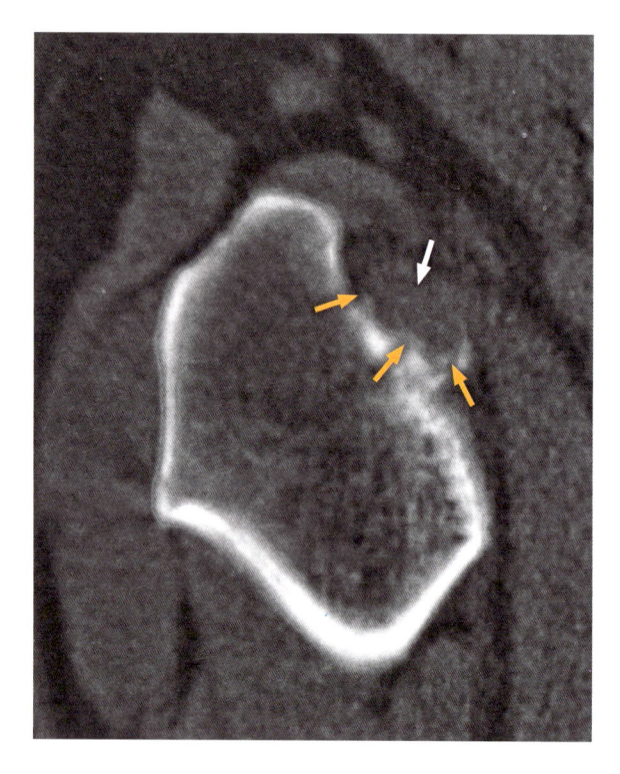

Fig. 12.6 Same dog as in fig. 12.1. Transverse CT image obtained at the level of the bicipital groove, where new bone formation is visible (orange arrows), partially encircling the biceps tendon (white arrow).

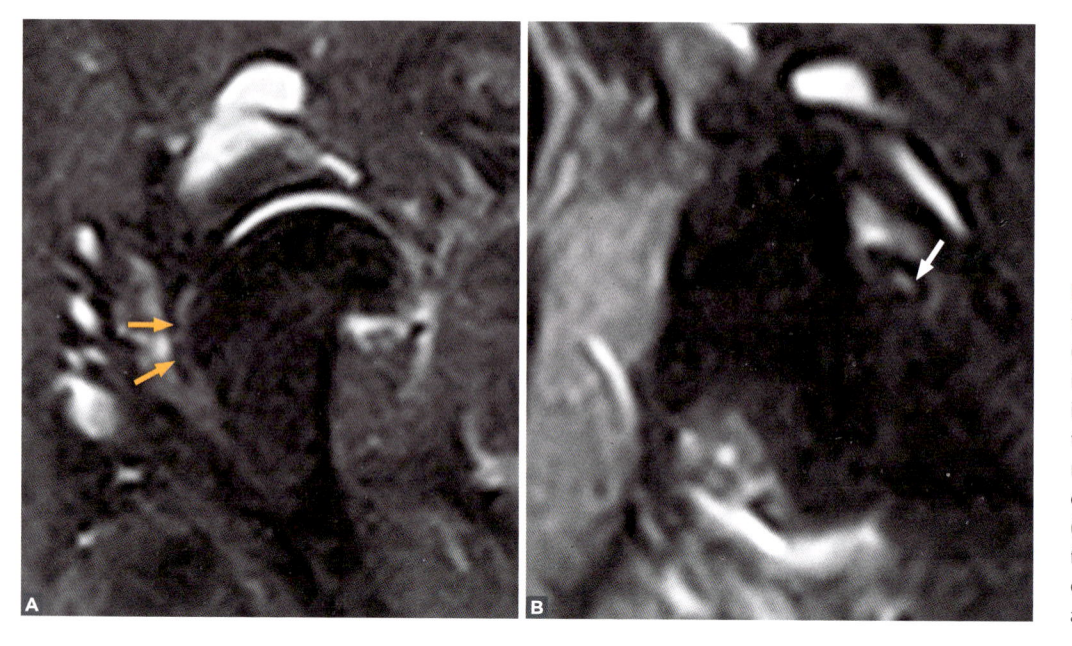

Fig. 12.7 Same dog as in figs. 12.1 and 12.6. Sagittal (**A**) and transverse (**B**) STIR images of the shoulder joint in a dog with chronic biceps tendinopathy. The proximal part of the biceps tendon is irregular and thinned (orange arrows). Note the focal hyperintensity in the center of the tendon (white arrow).

Supraspinatus tendinopathy

The supraspinatus tendon is an extraarticular active stabilizer of the shoulder and forms part, with the infraspinatus, teres minor and subscapularis, of a structure loosely analogue to the human rotator cuff, which provides stability and support to this joint. The supraspinatus in particular is responsible for shoulder extension and advancement of the limb.[10]

Damage to the rotator cuff and supraspinatus tendon can be linked to repetitive strain and strenuous activity leading to tendinosis. Clinical presentation includes mild weight bearing lameness with pain on direct palpation of the area and flexion of the shoulder. Calcifying tendinopathy can represent the chronic presentation of the condition in form of calcification at the insertion site at the greater tubercle; however, areas of mineralization in the body of the tendon are commonly reported, even bilaterally, as incidental finding in non-lame dogs. Large breed dogs and in particular Labrador Retrievers and Rottweilers are overrepresented in this particular condition. It has been postulated that mineralization, not necessarily initiated by trauma, is secondary to hypoxia causing fibrocartilaginous transformation of the tendon collagen fibers, which then undergo calcification. Mineralization has been reported to reform after surgical excision.[11] Thickening of the supraspinatus tendon can cause compression and impingement on the bicipital tendon and have a role in the development of bicipital tenosynovitis.

Mediolateral radiographic views of the shoulder can be unremarkable or show a variably sized, faint flap or a well-defined area of mineral opacity superimposed on the tendon region cranial to the scapulohumeral joint (**figs. 12.8** and **12.9**). Caudocranial or "swimmer" views might provide further information about the location and size of the fragment. It has been suggested to radiograph both legs even in the absence of contralateral lameness.[12]

When performing an ultrasonographic exam of the supraspinatus tendon it should be remembered that, as recently described,[13] the normal tendon, at its insertion on the greater tubercle, presents a thicker heterogeneously hypoechoic area, consistent with a histological region of less dense collagen. Common ultrasonographic findings of supraspinatus tendinopathy include irregular fiber pattern,

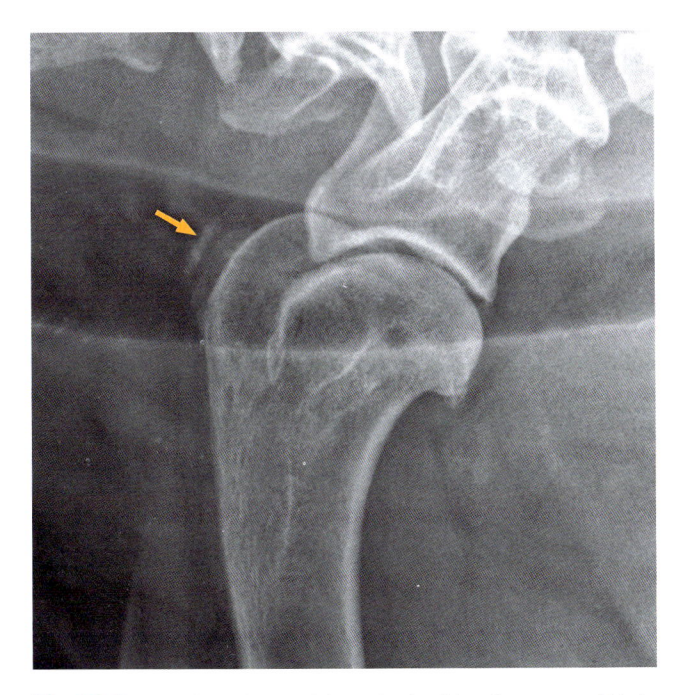

Fig. 12.8 Mediolateral view of the right shoulder of a 12-year-old Labrador Retriever presented for lameness. An elongated mineral flap is seen cranial to the proximal humerus in the region of the supraspinatus tendon. The dog had concurrent mild shoulder osteoarthritis.

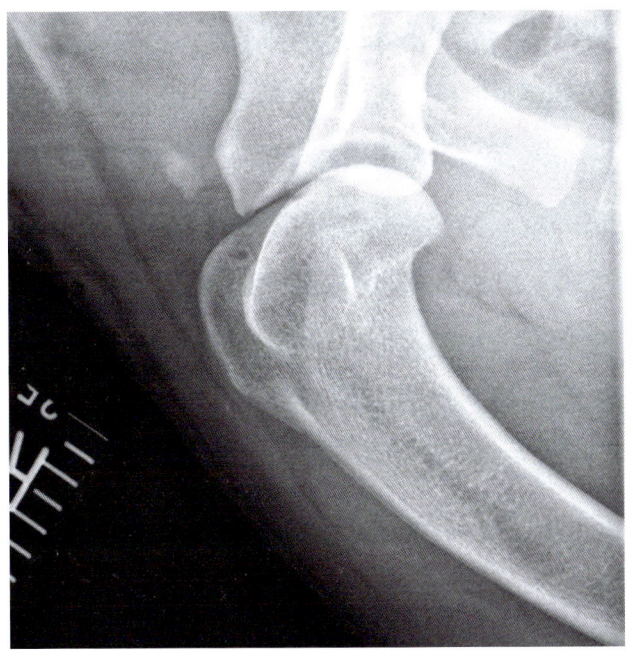

Fig. 12.9 Mediolateral view of the right shoulder of a three-year-old Pit Bull Terrier presented with a history of chronic lameness. An irregularly shaped, but clearly defined mineral fragment is seen cranial to the glenoid, in a position more proximal in the tendon compared to fig.12.8.

thickened diameter, and heterogeneous echogenicity.[14] In calcifying tendinopathy the most common finding is a hyperechoic area with acoustic shadowing; mineralizations can vary in size from 2 to 20 mm and size was not considered related to clinical severity. Focal hypoechoic areas can surround the calcifications, suggesting focal edema/hemorrhage of the tendon fibers and, therefore, an inflammatory process (**fig. 12.10**).

Computed tomography findings depend on the severity and chronicity of the condition; they vary from small mineral speckles throughout the body of the tendon, to presence of a single, large mineral fragment, to entheseophytosis of the greater tubercle (**fig. 12.11**). These findings are often incidentally detected during CT studies of the thorax of animals presented for other complaints.

The fluid rich central histological composition of the supraspinatus also affects its normal magnetic resonance features, characterized by a trilaminar appearance with central increased intensity on fluid sensitive pulse sequences. MRI features described for the tendon in normal dogs overlap with those described in dogs with suspected shoulder pathology (**figs. 12.12** and **12.13**). Increased size and central hyperintensity with compression of the biceps into the groove are possible features.[15]

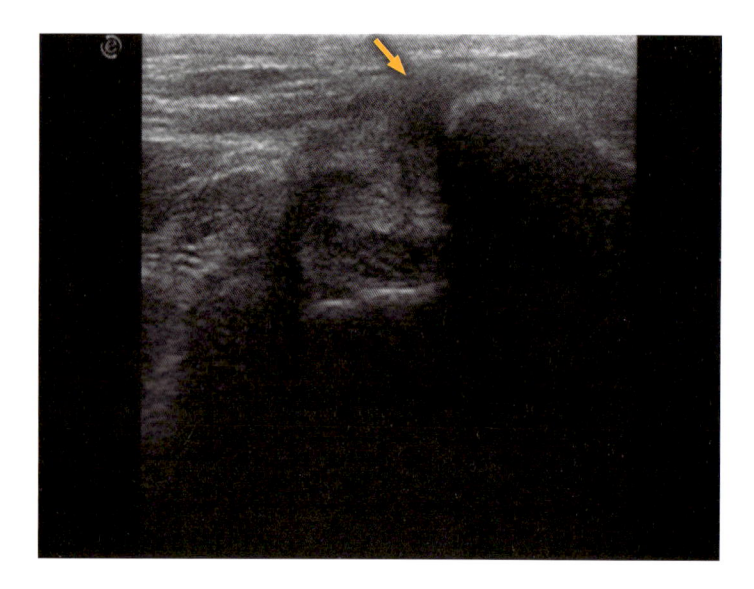

Fig. 12.10 Longitudinal sonographic image of the shoulder of an eight-year-old Labrador Retriever. Proximal is on the left; the arrow points to the hypoechoic insertion of the swollen supraspinatus tendon on the greater tubercle.

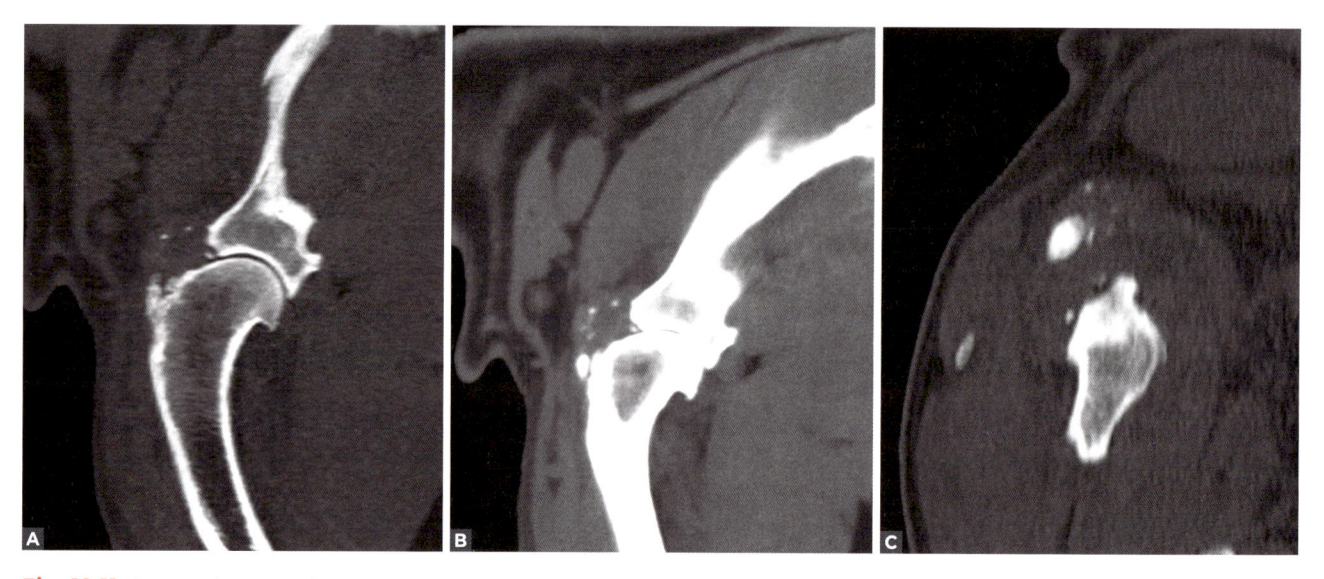

Fig. 12.11 Computed tomography images of the shoulder of a 13-year-old Labrador Retriever presented for lymphoma investigation. (**A**) Sagittal reconstruction bone algorithm; (**B**) sagittal reconstruction soft tissue algorithm; (**C**) dorsal reconstruction bone algorithm. Entheseophytosis at the tendon insertion, remodeling of the greater tubercle and multiple mineralized speckles within the body of the tendon are seen. The tendon body is increased in diameter. This was an incidental finding.

CHAPTER **12** Soft tissues

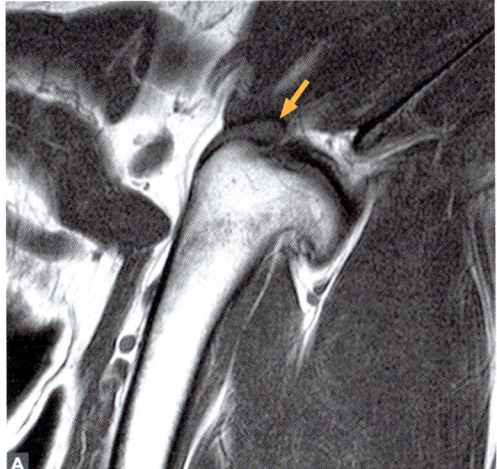

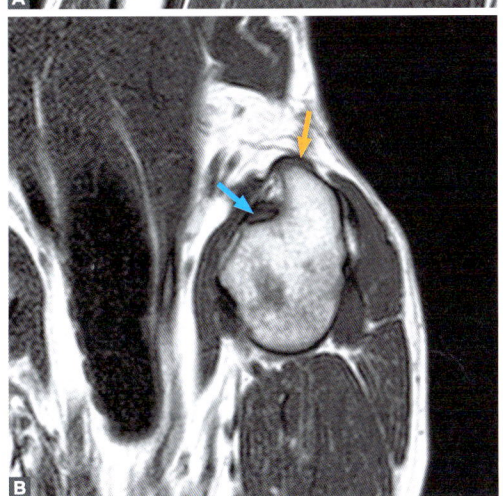

Fig. 12.12 T2W sagittal and transverse MRI images of a normal shoulder. (**B**) The orange arrow points to the supraspinatus tendon, the blue to the bicipital tendon. Is at the level of the tendon's insertion on the greater tubercle.

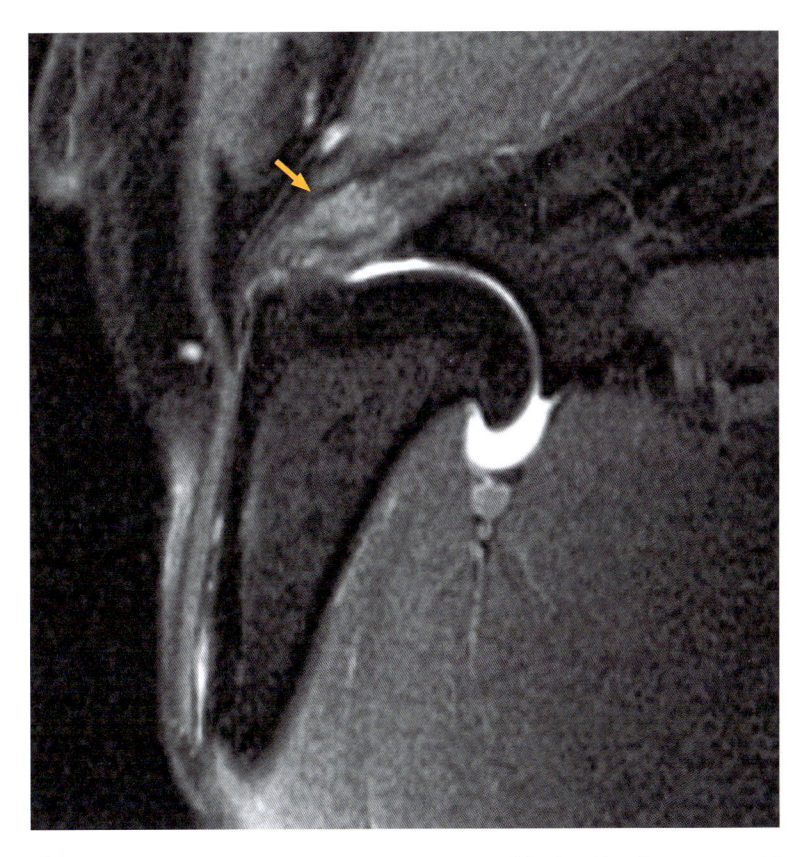

Fig. 12.13 Sagittal proton density fat saturation image of the shoulder of a seven-year-old Labrador Retriever. The arrow points to the supraspinatus tendon, which appears thickened and irregularly hyperintense.

Infraspinatus muscle contracture

Located on a lateral position, the infraspinatus muscle and tendon provide dynamic stability to the shoulder joint, its main functions being abduction and rotation of the humerus and to a lesser extent extension and flexion of the shoulder.

Injury to the tendon is reported more often in large breeds, working or hunting dogs and is considered secondary to strenuous, repetitive exercise rather than acute trauma. In some cases, the damage can lead to a muscular fibrotic contracture due to myofiber degeneration that presents four to six weeks later. While the initial damage can cause swelling and pain in the area associated with lameness; the secondary contracture is painless, but it causes a characteristic stand with abduction of the proximal humerus and a circumducted gait with reduced range of motion of the shoulder. Atrophy of the shoulder musculature can be present. Tenotomy at the insertion of the tendon is considered curative. Ossification of the infraspinatus with concurrent osteochondromatosis of the bursa has been described.[16]

Radiographs are unremarkable unless ossification is present, but are useful to rule out other shoulder conditions. If ossification is present, it shows a more caudal location compared to mineralization of biceps or supraspinatus tendons.

121

A recent study[17] followed the computed tomography evolution of an infraspinatus myopathy over the course of eight months. In the acute phase the muscle appeared enlarged, with a hypoattenuating center compared to the adjacent supraspinatus surrounded by a poorly contrast enhancing area; as the condition became chronic, the muscle appeared progressively atrophic, fibrotic and a hyperattenuating linear structure appeared in the center.

Magnetic resonance features of the acutely contracted tendon include thickening, heterogeneous signal intensity of the muscle and partially of the tendon; in chronic cases the size and the signal intensity of the muscle are decreased.[18]

Cruciate ligament disease

Cranial cruciate ligament disease (CrCLD) is the most common cause of pelvic limb lameness in dogs, frequently occurring bilaterally. CrCLD is commonly a result of chronic degeneration rather than of acute trauma. CrCLD is a relatively uncommon condition in cats and might be associated with damage to collateral ligaments and menisci. Isolated rupture of the caudal cruciate ligament (CaCL) is uncommon but can occur in conjunction with CrCLD and medial collateral ligament tears.[19]

Standard orthogonal views of the stifles remain the most important initial diagnostic step in case of CrCLD. Certain surgical procedures require special views to allow measurement of the tibial plateau angle.[19] Normal stifle radiographs do not exclude partial cranial cruciate ligament (CCL) rupture.[20] Radiographic evidence of CrCLD includes joint effusion of various degrees, resulting in compression of the infrapatellar fat pad. Signs of secondary osteoarthrosis include osteophyte formation on the trochlear ridges, both poles of the patella, fabellae, femoral epicondyles and tibia plateau (**fig. 12.14**). Subchondral cysts and sclerosis can be present in the region of the intercondylar fossa of the femur and intercondylar eminences of the tibia. Distal displacement of the popliteal sesamoid bone is associated with CrCLD. Purely traumatic rupture of the cranial cruciate ligament is uncommon but reported in young dogs, maybe accompanied by an avulsion fragment.[19,21]

High frequency ultrasonography is a useful diagnostic tool, such as for establishing the presence of joint effusion, even with no radiographic signs of osteoarthrosis.[22] However, the sensitivity to detect

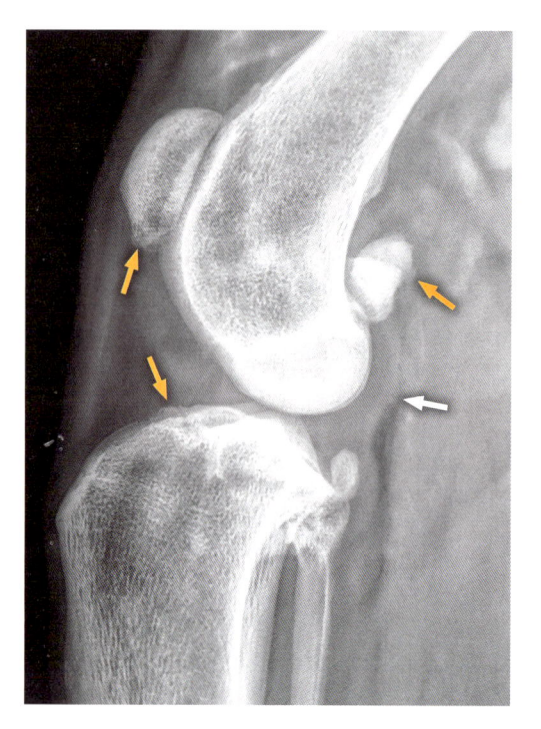

Fig. 12.14 Mediolateral radiograph of a stifle joint of a five-year-old Bobtail with CrCLD. Moderate joint effusion is present, with reduced size of the infrapatellar fat pad and caudal displacement of the caudal fascial plane (white arrow). Osteophyte formation is present at the distal pole of the patella, fabellae and tibial plateau (orange arrows).

Fig. 12.15 Sagittal PDW image of the stifle in a normal five-year-old Border Collie. The cranial (orange arrow) and caudal cruciate (white arrow) ligaments are intact, forming homogeneous hypointense bands.

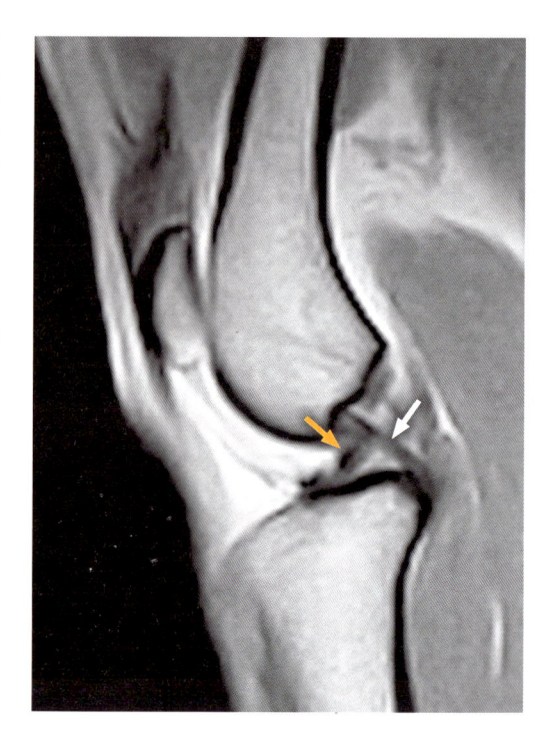

cranial cruciate ligament rupture is limited.[4,22] The CCL is best seen with the stifle fully flexed, using an infrapatellar probe position and lateral rotation of the transducer by 10-20° in the sagittal plane. The normal CCL is seen as a hypoechoic band.[4] In a recent study, a hyperechoic fibrillar pattern could be visualized in the distal third of the CCL.[20] A ruptured ligament is difficult to recognize, especially in the acute phase, but commonly associated with joint effusion and irregular osteophyte formation. With chronic cruciate ligament rupture, a small, hyperechoic and irregular ligament stump might be identified. Chronic ruptures are commonly associated with intra-articular fibrous tissue proliferation due to chronic synovitis, seen as a variably sized, hyperechoic and irregular areas.[4,22]

CT is a useful technique for evaluating osseous structures and all major soft tissue structures of the stifle joint can be clearly outlined. The ability to perform multiplanar and 3D image reconstructions is helpful for complete evaluation and surgical planning. The normal CCL is visible as a tubular structure of intermediate density, with an improved outline of its margins on the post contrast series.[21] CT features of CrCLD include joint effusion, joint capsule thickening, periarticular degenerative osseous changes and maybe small intra-articular osseous bodies.[23] CTA has shown to detect cruciate ligament tears with good accuracy.[24] The CCL is located extrasynovially, being covered by a thin synovial sheath, which normally prevents contrast from penetrating into the ligament.[20] With partial cruciate ligament tear dissection of contrast medium within the ligament occurs. Inability to trace the ligament continuously indicates complete ligament rupture.[23]

The superior soft tissue contrast of MRI is the main advantage compared to CT, which improves evaluation of cruciate ligaments and menisci, and is therefore the preferred imaging modality in people.[21] The CCL and CaCL are best appreciated on sagittal images, seen as homogeneous hypointense bands, with the CCL being slightly smaller than the CaCL.[8]

Proton density-weighted (PDW) images (**fig. 12.15**) in the sagittal plane provided the best agreement with surgical findings in the identification of CrCLD in a study.[25] Increased signal intensity on PDW and T2W images and irregular margination are associated with a partial tear. Subchondral cyst-like and bone marrow lesions at the origin and insertion of the ligament may be present. Joint effusion and osteoarthrosis are commonly observed (**fig. 12.16**).

Incompleteness or non-visualization of the ligament indicates complete rupture.[7,9,21,25] MRI arthrography is reported to improve visualization and evaluation of the CCL and CaCL.[8,21]

Fig. 12.16 Same dog as in fig. 12.14. Sagittal PDW (**A**) and dorsal GE T2* (**B**) images of the stifle in a dog with CrCLD. The cranial cruciate ligament is not clearly visible. There is distension of the joint capsule (orange arrows). Note the heterogeneous hyperintense signal in the CCL (white arrow).

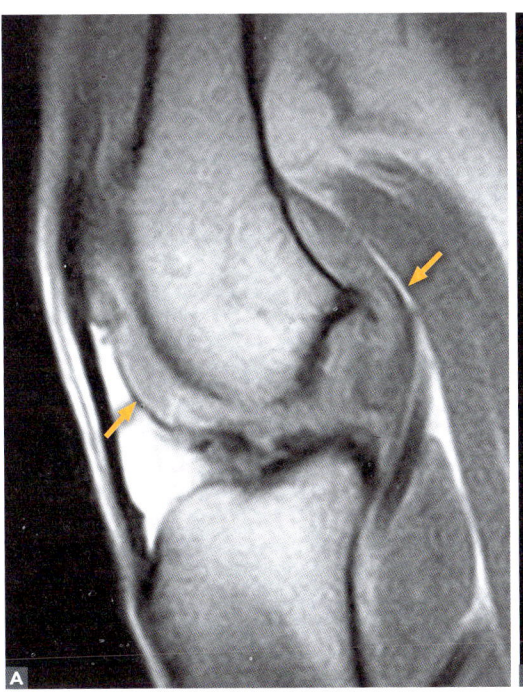

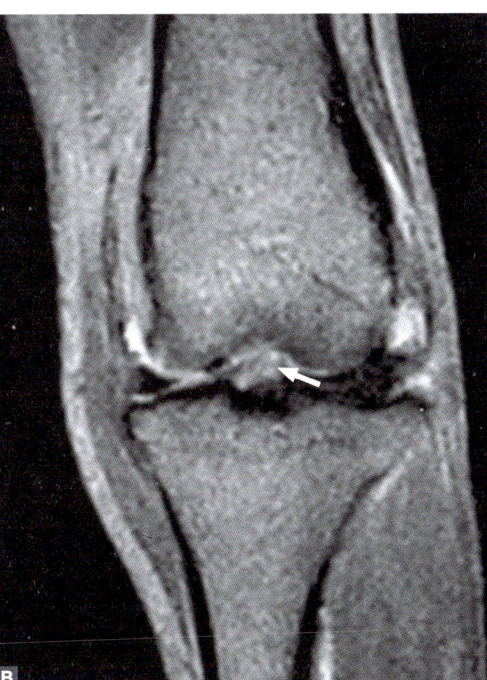

Achilles tendon tendinopathy

The Achilles tendon is a composite structure (common calcaneal tendon [CCT]) formed by three tendons contained within a sheath of connective tissue; two are separate structures, the gastrocnemius tendon (GT) and superficial digital flexor, and three are converging tendons that join to create the common tendon (CT) (gracilis, semitendinosus and biceps femoris). The three main components insert in various sites of the calcaneal tuberosity: the GT proximolaterally, the CT medially and the SDFT, which extends distally to insert on the phalanges, at the level of the tarsus broadens creating a "cap" that inserts on the calcaneus medially and laterally through retinacula. The common calcaneal tendon ensures extension of the tarsus (mostly GT and partially CT) and of the phalanges (SDFT). Injuries to the Achilles tendon can affect the whole structure or a combination of the separate components; damage to the fibers ranges from mild disruption with focal edema and hemorrhage to complete rupture of the body of the tendon to avulsion at the insertion on the calcaneal tuberosity. The etiology is most commonly traumatic (acute blunt trauma, overstretching) but can include iatrogenic and systemic causes.[26,27] A chronic, degenerative process of the tendon fibers can also lead to acute rupture. Medium to large size dogs and Dobermanns in particular are most commonly reported. Marked non-weight bearing lameness, focal swelling at the insertion on the proximal calcaneus, thickening of the tendon body, "dropped" tarsus, "crab claw stance" with flexion of the phalanges and plantigrade stand with complete flexion of the tarsus and extension of the stifle are all possible clinical presentations depending on the degree of damage of the tendon or its components and on chronicity of the lesion.[27] Some reports suggest that a plantigrade stance does not necessarily relate to a complete rupture of the tendon and it is not predictive of which of the tendon components is affected, but rather indicates that the injury involves the musculo-tendineous junction. The clawing stance is indicative of rupture of the CCT with an intact SDFT. Less commonly reported are pain or discomfort on palpation, local wounds and lacerations.

Neutral mediolateral radiographic views of the affected tarsus show one or more of the following typical radiographic features: swelling along the distal tendon and particularly severe at the insertion on the calcaneus; mineralized speckles along the body of the calcaneus; variable degree of remodeling of the calcaneal tuberosity secondary to osteophytosis/entheseophytosis; in cases of avulsion of the insertion presence of a separate, more defined mineral flap (**figs. 12.17**, **12.19** and **12.21**).

A stressed mediolateral view will exacerbate the flexion and confirm damage/rupture.

Plantarodorsal views in neutral and stressed positions (forcing a varus and valgus position of the pes) can be used to rule out concurrent damage to the tarsal collateral ligaments.

Ultrasonography is considered highly sensitive in identifying injuries to the calcaneal tendon and essential to complement the clinical exam (**figs. 12.18**, **12.20** and **12.22**); there can be inconsistency between the severity of the clinical signs and the ultrasonographic findings. Fiber disruption/degeneration can be detected in non-affected legs and a plantigrade stance doesn't always correspond to a complete rupture.

The exam is usually performed with the tarsus flexed to ensure tension of the tendon and better probe contact. As always, it is essential to image both tendons even if clinical signs are unilateral.

Ultrasonographic findings can include changes to only one or all of the components of the common calcaneal tendon such as: disruption of the fibers, hypoechoic areas, complete rupture of the fibers, mineralized speckles scattered through the fibers, large avulsed hyperechoic fragments with acoustic shadow, irregular outline of the calcaneal tuberosity.[28]

Computed tomography is not the technique of choice to diagnose rupture/damage of the CCT. When performed, typical findings include a swelling of soft tissue/fluid attenuation and heterogeneous contrast enhancement in the distal aspect of the tendon, areas of mineral attenuation scattered through the distal tendon, one large fragment of mineral attenuation in cases of avulsion at the insertion site and variable degrees of remodeling of the calcaneal tuberosity in chronic cases (**figs. 12.23** and **12.24**).

Fig. 12.17 Mediolateral views of the right and left tarsal regions of a six-year-old Boxer cross dog with a chronic history of left hindlimb lameness. There is mild to moderate swelling of the left calcaneal tendon region and encircling the calcaneal tuberosity, which shows an irregular outline with a focal region of lucency. There is also osteophytosis of the distal intertarsal joint. Milder soft tissue swelling and remodeling of the calcaneal tuberosity are also visible on the right tarsus.

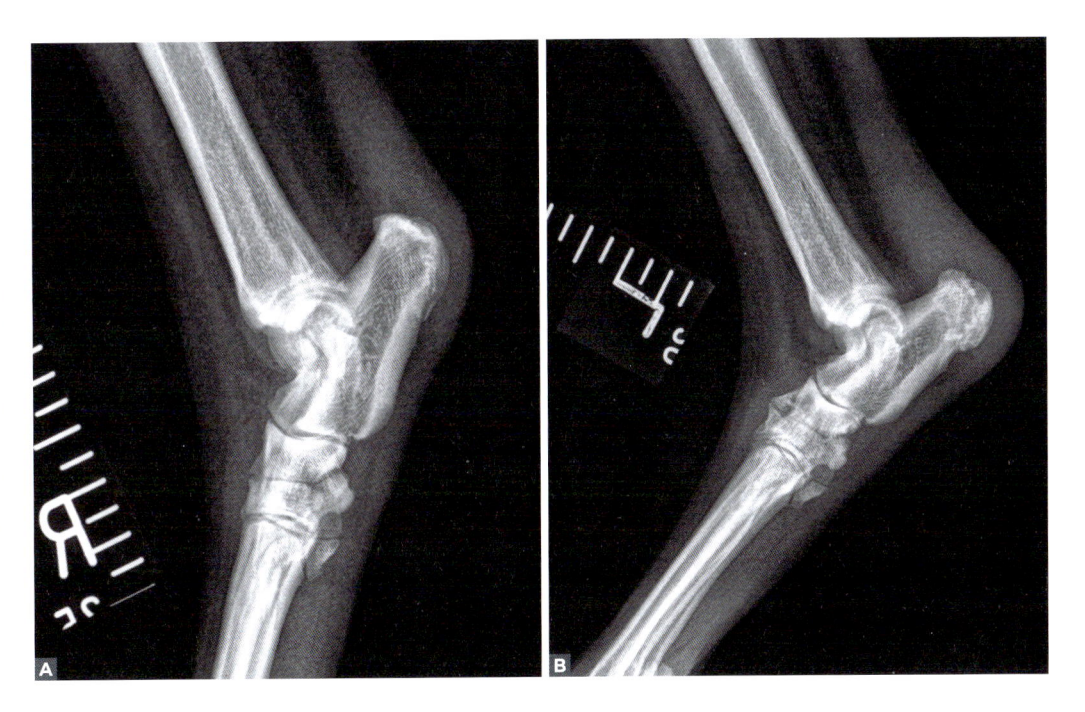

Fig. 12.18 Ultrasonographic images of the calcaneal tendon of the same dog as in fig. 12.17. (**A**) Longitudinal plane: the calcaneal tuberosity on the left leg is markedly irregular, the distal aspect of the tendon at the insertion is hypoechoic suggesting disruption of the fibers/edema. (**B**) Transverse plane at the level of the mid body of the CCT. The diameter of the left tendon is markedly increased compared to the right; the separate components cannot be seen clearly.

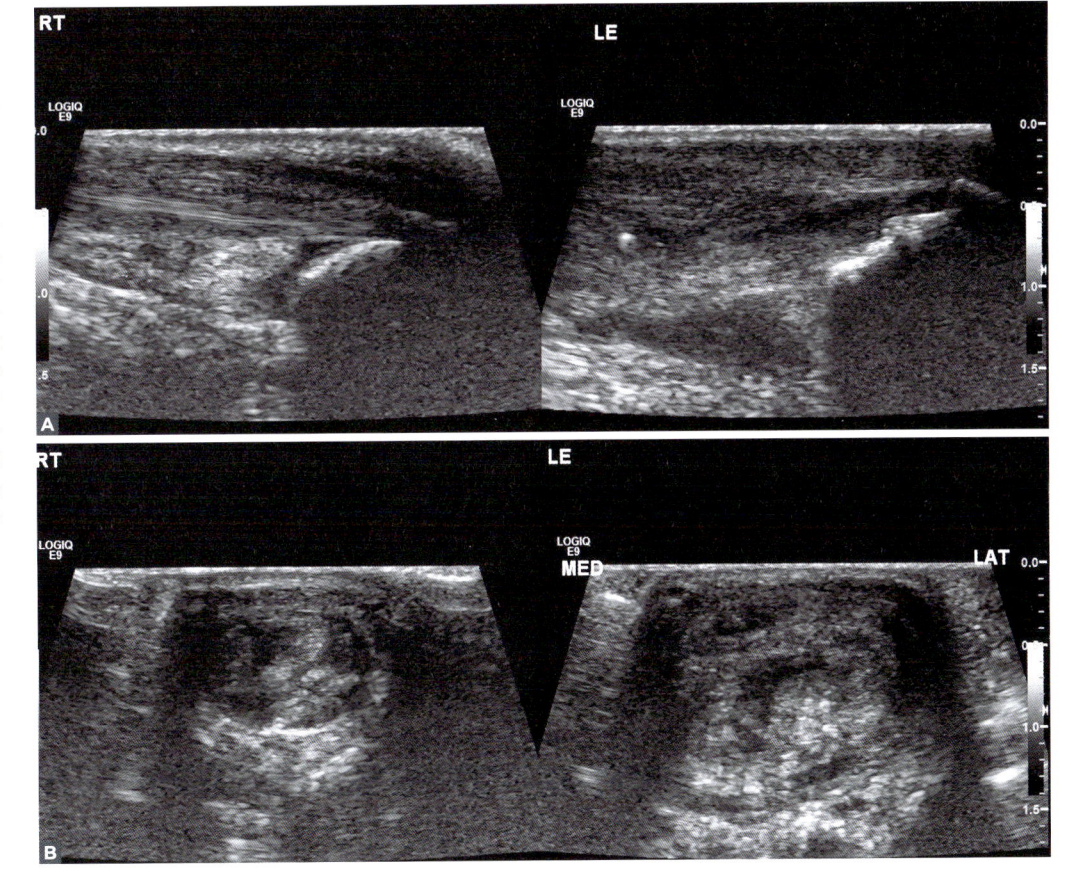

Magnetic resonance is complementary to the ultrasound exam, since the excellent contrast resolution of MRI facilitates the recognition of the single components of the CCT and, therefore, the diagnosis of specific injuries. Reported findings include T2W hyperintensity and T1W hypointensity around the tendons suggestive of edema; thickening (if swollen) or thinning (if disrupted) of the tendon; heterogeneity of signal of the tendon with strong contrast enhancement.[26]

SECTION II APPENDICULAR SKELETON

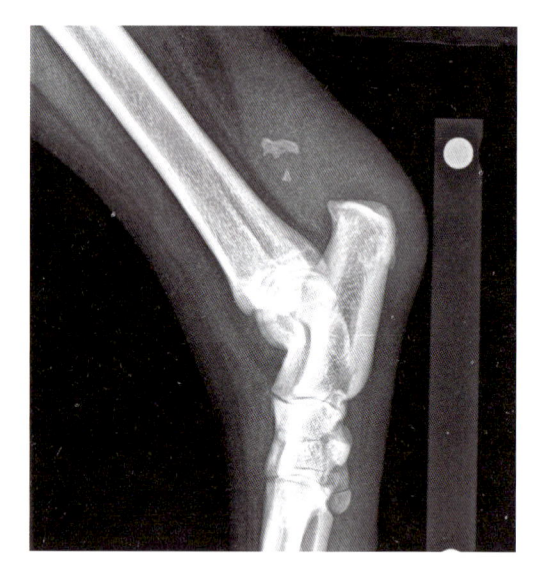

Fig. 12.19 Mediolateral view of the tarsal region of a seven-year-old Labrador Retriever presented for acute right hind lameness. There is marked swelling in the caudal tibial region immediately proximal to the calcaneus. One large mineral fragment and a smaller triangular one are seen superimposed on the swelling. The calcaneal tuberosity is irregular in shape due to a defect corresponding to the fragment. Avulsion of the insertion of the CCT.

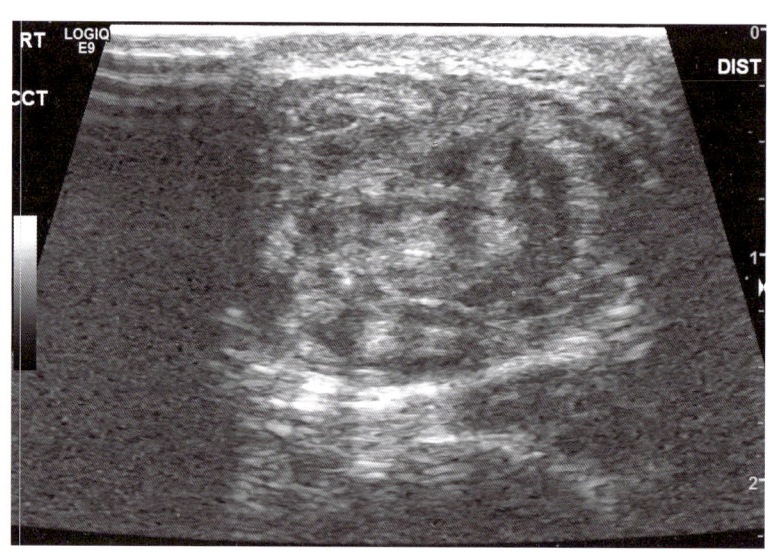

Fig. 12.20 Transverse ultrasonographic image of the same leg as in picture 12.19 at the level of maximal swelling: the diameter of the CCT is increased, the echogenicity is heterogeneous with poor distinction of the components of the tendon.

Fig. 12.21 Mediolateral views of the left tarsal region of an 11.5-year-old cat presented with a plantigrade stand and ulcerated hocks. (**A**) The radiograph was obtained in July; there is an irregular defect of the soft tissues proximal to the calcaneal tuberosity, which shows jagged outline due to new bone formation. The distal tendon is mildly thickened and a mineral fragment is seen superimposed on to it tendon. (**B**) The radiograph was obtained in January of the following year. The calcaneus has completely lost its original shape and appears bent, osteopenic, the calcaneal tuberosity has been almost completely resorbed and has an elongated, triangular shape. The CCT is no longer recognizable as a soft tissue structure separated from the tibia by subcutaneous fat. The tarsus and pes are mildly osteopenic.

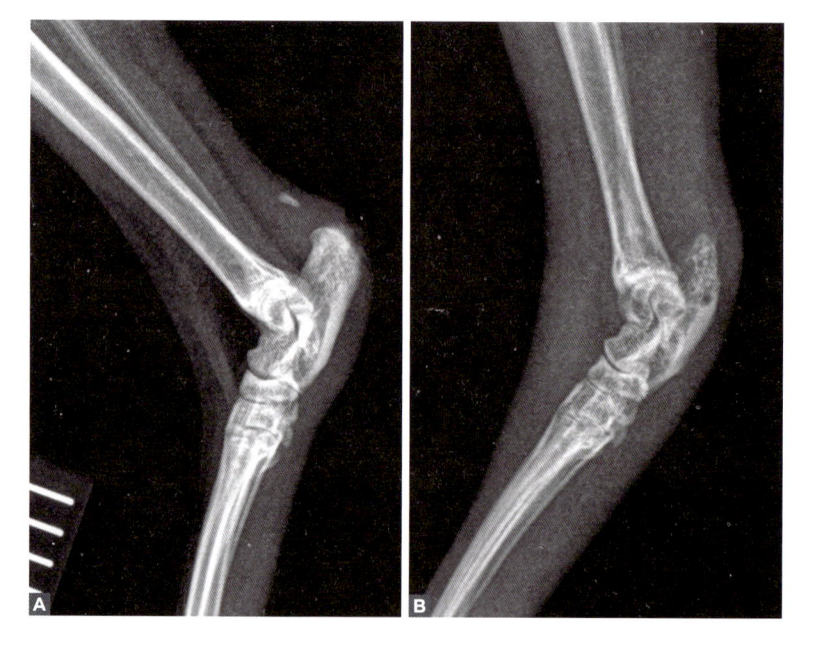

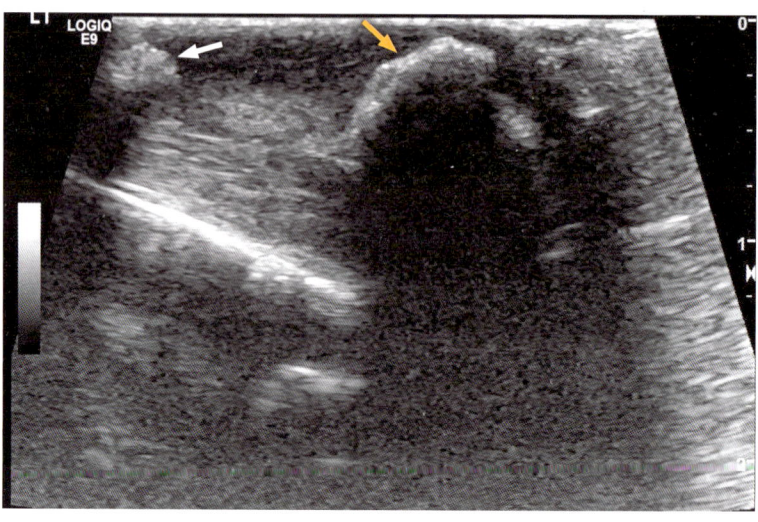

Fig. 12.22 Longitudinal ultrasonographic image of the CCT of the cat in fig. 12.21A. On the left of the image note the mineral avulsion fragment embedded in the tendon (white arrow). The calcaneal tuberosity is markedly irregular in outline (orange arrow).

Fig. 12.23 Transverse CT image of the tarsii (right is to the left) of a seven-year-old Brittany Spaniel presented for chronic lameness after running into a window. On palpation the calcaneal apparatus was intact, but a fragment could be palpated. There is irregular outline of the calcaneal tuberosity on the right tarsus.

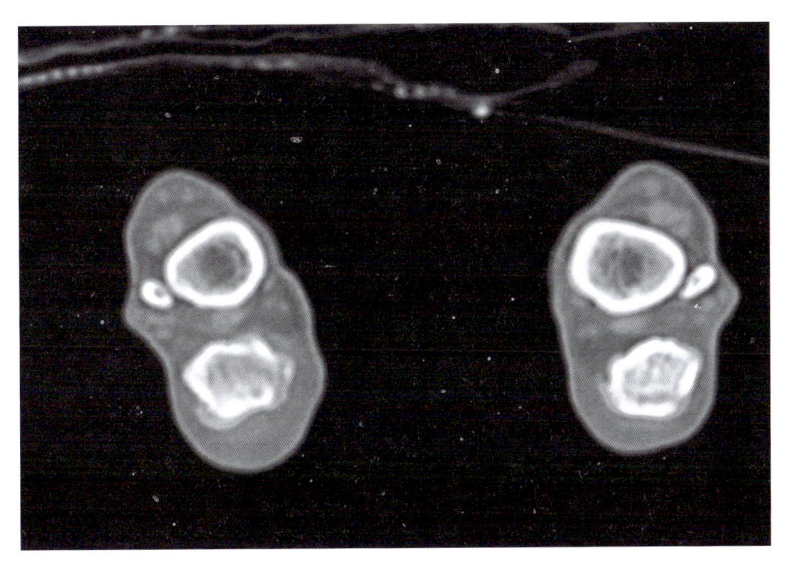

Fig. 12.24 CT sagittal reconstruction (**A**), CT transverse (**B**) and longitudinal ultrasonographic image (**C**) of the same dog as fig. 12.23. The orange arrows point to the mineralized fragment in all three images. The blue arrow on the CT image points to the calcaneus, incompletely visible due to slice thickness.

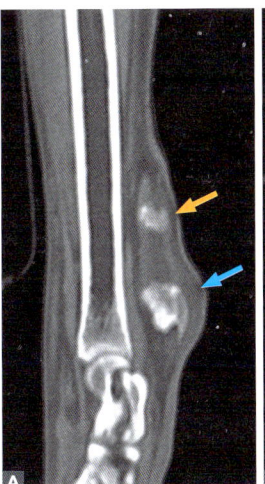

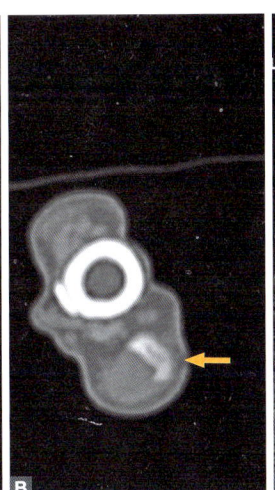

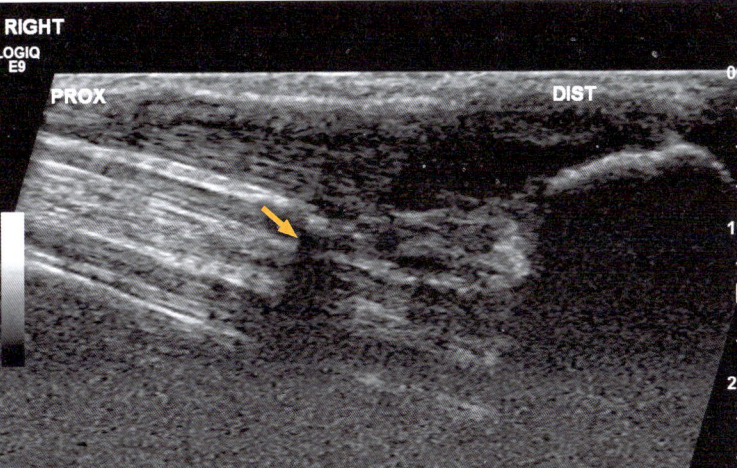

Peripheral nerves (brachial and lumbosacral plexus)

The limbs are supplied by nerves arising from either the brachial or lumbosacral plexus, which consists of a complex network of interconnected nerves formed by the ventral branches of the spinal nerves (C6-T2 and L4-S2 respectively). The most common conditions of the brachial and lumbosacral plexus include neoplasia, traumatic injuries and less commonly inflammatory disorders.[29]

Survey radiographs are often unremarkable. Slow-growing peripheral nerve sheath tumors (PNST) may occasionally cause enlargement of the intervertebral foramen and lysis of the vertebral body. Myelography increases the sensitivity for the identification of PNST but will only be of value if the tumor involves the vertebral canal.[30]

High-frequency linear transducers are preferably used to scan peripheral nerves. They appear as linear hypoechoic structures surrounded by a hyperechoic rim in the longitudinal plane. In transverse plane, nerves are circular or oval hypoechoic structures (**fig. 12.25**).[31,32,33]

Color flow Doppler is useful to differentiate adjacent vessels from a nerve.[31] The scanning technique and ultrasonographic anatomy of the brachial plexus and sciatic nerve have been described in both dogs and cats.[32,33,34,35] PNSTs of the brachial plexus have been reported in dogs as a fusiform mass of mixed echogenicity or tubular hypoechoic masses that lacks blood flow.[30,36] Ultrasonography can be

SECTION II APPENDICULAR SKELETON

Fig. 12.25 Ultrasonographic images of a normal sciatic nerve in the longitudinal plane near the greater trochanter in a two-year-old Labrador Retriever, which appears as a linear hypoechoic structure surrounded by a hyperechoic rim (arrows).

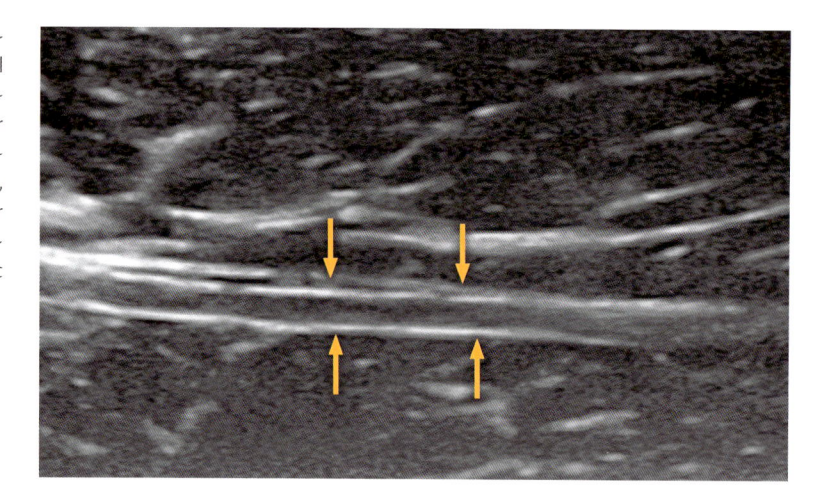

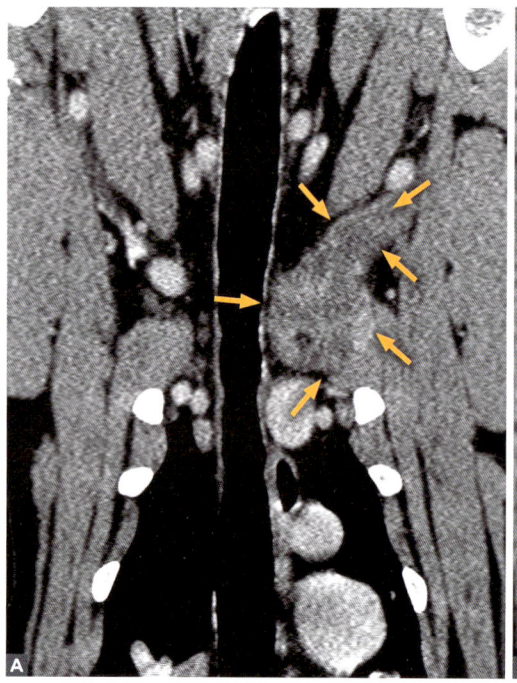

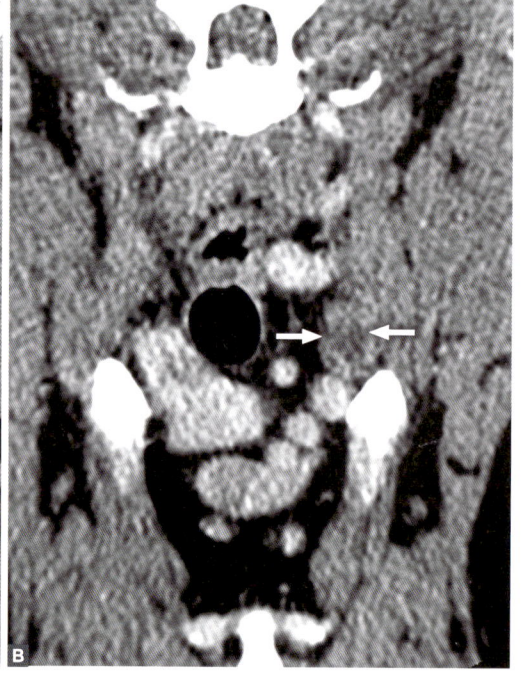

Fig. 12.26 Dorsal reconstructed (**A**) and transverse (**B**) CT images obtained at the cervicothoracic junction of a ten-year-old Labrador Retriever. A large, well-defined and heterogeneously contrast enhancing mass is identifiable in the left axilla (orange arrows), with invasion into the thoracic cavity (white arrows). The histologic diagnosis was a high grade malignant peripheral nerve sheath tumor.

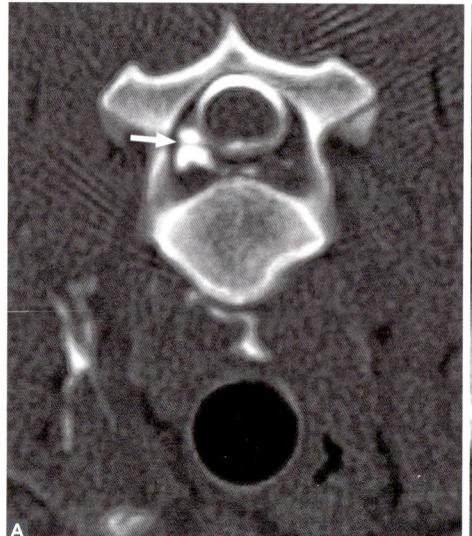

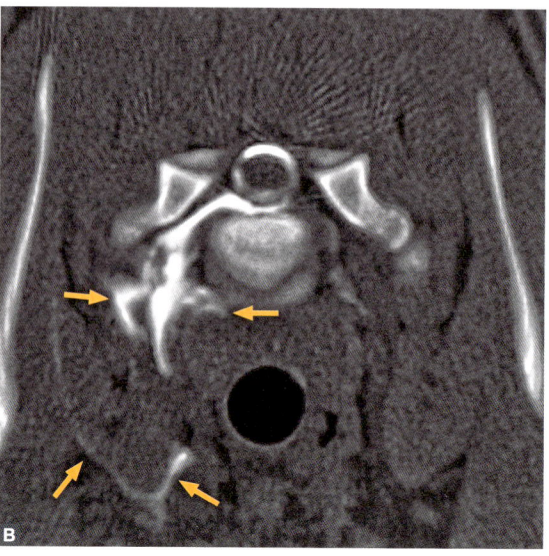

Fig. 12.27 Transverse CT images at the level of C7-T1 in a five-year-old Irish Terrier that was hit by a car, with monoplegia of the right thoracic limb. (**A**) Both ventral and dorsal nerve roots are missing and associated pseudocysts are present (white arrow). (**B**) Leakage of intrathecal contrast medium tracking from the intervertebral foramen towards the ventral paravertebral muscles can be identified (orange arrows), consistent with cerebrospinal fluid leak due to brachial plexus avulsion.

used to guide fine-needle aspirates or biopsies of the lesions. Loss of visualization of the distal segments are strongly suggestive of traumatic rupture of peripheral nerves, associated with hematoma formation in the axillary region in the acute phase.[31]

CT is a useful diagnostic tool to identify and to fully assess the extent of masses of the brachial and lumbosacral plexus, including the normal contralateral side for comparison. However, small or diffuse tumors might be difficult to detect, depending on noticeable soft tissue asymmetry and contrast enhancement.[37] CT features of brachial plexus neoplasm in dogs include a well-defined axillary mass, contrast enhancement of most masses frequently with rim enhancement, periscapular muscle atrophy and in some cases invasion into the thoracic cavity or dorsally into the vertebral canal (**fig. 12.26**).[38] CT myelography can be used to identify nerve root avulsions, based on absence of radiating linear fillings defects of the nerve roots in the contrast-enhanced subarachnoid space (**fig. 12.27**).[39]

MRI is the imaging technique of choice to investigate conditions of the peripheral nerves due to its excellent soft tissue contrast and is more sensitive for detecting masses of the brachial or lumbosacral plexus than CT (**fig. 12.28**). Straight body positioning with symmetrically positioned forelimbs is

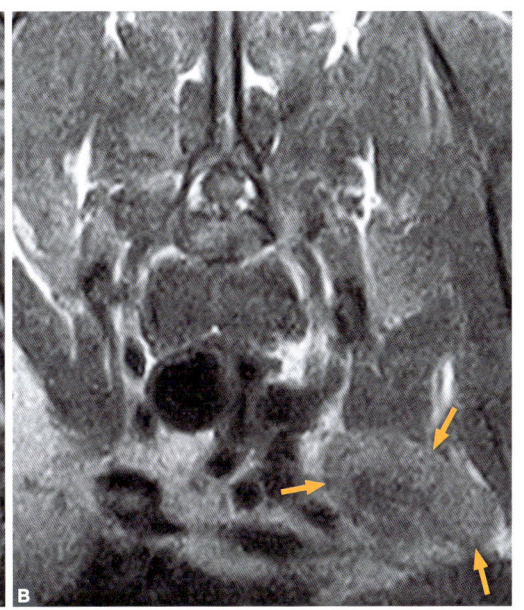

Fig. 12.28 Same dog as in fig. 12.26. Transverse STIR (**A**) and T1W (**B**) images acquired at the level of the axilla. Thickening of the left eighth cervical spinal nerve (white arrow) and a hyperintense mass (orange arrows) in the left axilla are identified on STIR image. Heterogeneous contrast enhancement of the discrete axillary mass can be noted (orange arrows).

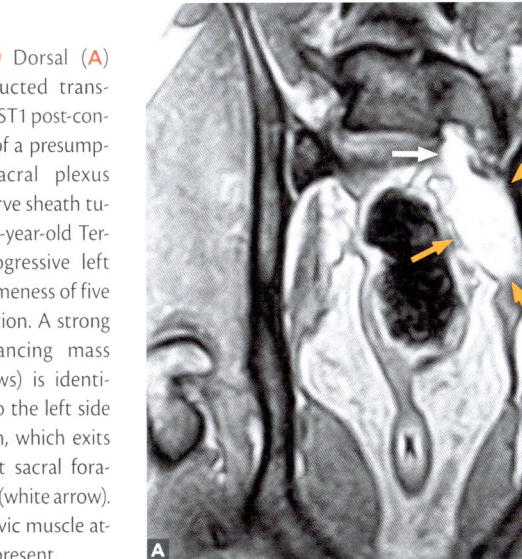

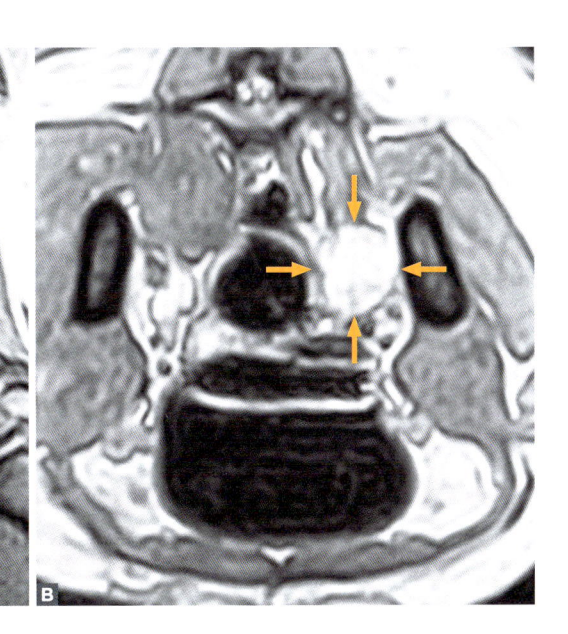

Fig. 12.29 Dorsal (**A**) and reconstructed transverse (**B**) 3D SST1 post-contrast images of a presumptive lumbosacral plexus peripheral nerve sheath tumor in a nine-year-old Terrier with progressive left pelvic limb lameness of five months duration. A strong contrast-enhancing mass (orange arrows) is identified ventral to the left side of the sacrum, which exits from the first sacral foramen cranially (white arrow). Left-sided pelvic muscle atrophy is also present.

Fig. 12.30 Same dog as in fig.12.27. Transverse STIR image at the level of C7-T1 in a dog with brachial plexus avulsion. Ill-defined hyperintensity is seen in the region of the eighth cervical spinal nerve and axillary region (arrows).

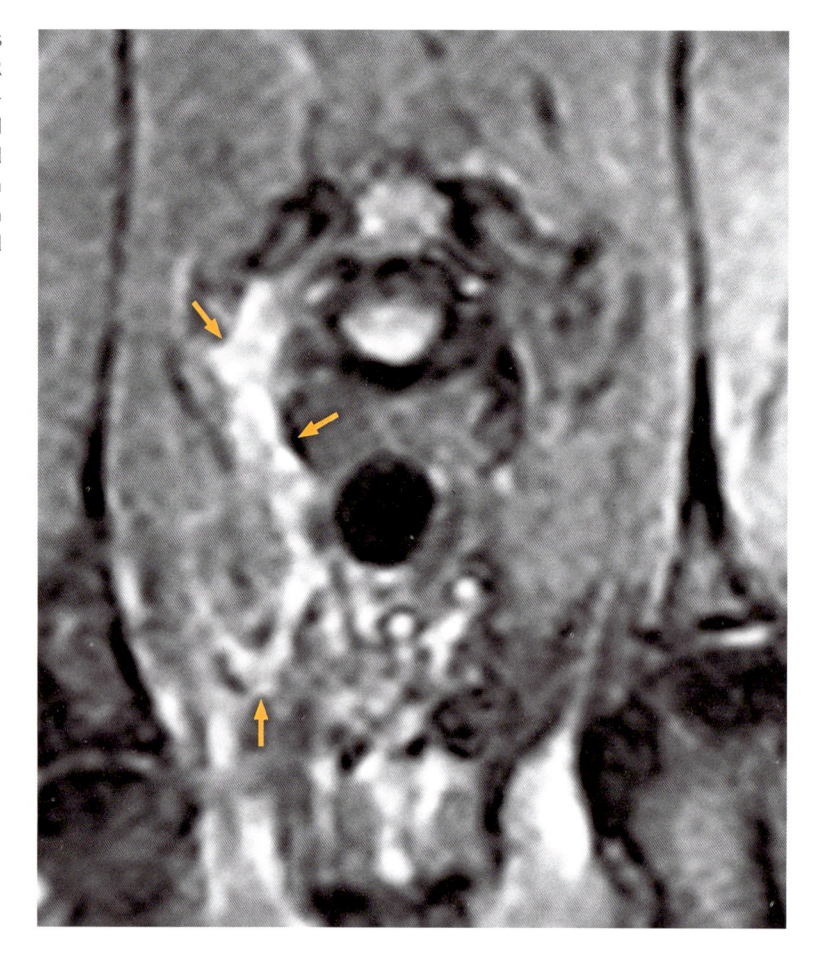

useful for comparison between the affected and healthy side, especially when a lesion is subtle. An initial large-field-of-view STIR sequence in the dorsal plane is useful for screening lesions.[29,37] MRI features of brachial plexus tumors include diffuse brachial plexus nerve thickening or discrete axillary mass, usually hyperintense on T2W images, and variable and commonly heterogeneous contrast enhancement. Ipsilateral muscle atrophy and signal intensity changes are often present.[37]

MRI features of lumbosacral plexus PNST are similar to those of brachial plexus tumors (**fig. 12.29**). Inflammatory changes of the brachial or lumbosacral nerves are rare, with both sites typically affected.[29] MRI findings in case of brachial plexus avulsion include irregular hyperintense signal in the areas of the plexus and close to the foramina on T2W and STIR images, associated with focal inflammation or edema secondary to soft tissue trauma (**fig. 12.30**).[29] Intrathecal injection of contrast medium has been used in a dog for diagnosis of traumatic dural tear.[40]

References

1. Gielen I, Van Caelenberg A, Van Bree H. The shoulder joint and scapula. In Kirberger R, McEvoy F, editors. BSAVA Manual of canine and feline musculoskeletal imaging 2nd edition, Gloucester, 2016, BSAVA publications, pp 171-188.
2. Long C, Nyland T. Ultrasonographic evaluation of the canine shoulder. *Vet Radiol Ultrasound* 40:372- 379, 1999.
3. Kramer M, Gerwing M, Sheppard C, Schimke E. Ultrasonography for the diagnosis of diseases of the tendon and tendon sheath of the biceps brachii muscle. *Vet Surg* 30:64-71, 2001.
4. D'Anjou M, Blond L. Musculoskeletal system. In Penninck D, D'Anjou M, editors. Atlas of Small animal Ultrasonography 2nd edition. Ames, Wiley Blackwell, 2015, pp 495-544.
5. Maddox T, May C, Keeley B, McConnell F. Comparison between shoulder computed tomography and clinical finding in 89 dogs presented for thoracic limb lameness. *Vet Radiol Ultrasound* 54: 358-364, 2013.
6. Eivers C, Corzo-Menéndez N, Austwick S, Thomson D, Gibson S, Handel I, Schwarz T. Computed tomographic arthrography is a useful adjunct to survey computed tomography and arthroscopic evaluation of the canine shoulder joint. *Vet Radiol Ultrasound* 59: 535-544, 2018.
7. Sage J, Gavin P. Musculoskeletal MRI. *Vet Clin North Am Small Anim Pract* 46:421-451, 2016.
8. Zalcman A, Cook C, Mai W. General features and optimized techniques for the musculoskeletal system. In Mai W, editor. Diagnostic MRI in dogs and cats. Boca Raton, FL, CRC Press, 2018, pp 130- 152.
9. Zalcman A, Cook C, Mai W. MRI of musculoskeletal diseases. In Mai W, editor. Diagnostic MRI in dogs and cats. Boca Raton, FL, CRC Press, 2018, pp 643-684.
10. Canapp SO, Canapp DA, Carr BJ, Cox C, Barrett JG. Supraspinatus tendinopathy in 327 dogs: a retrospective study. *Veterinary Evidence* 1, 2016.
11. Laitinen OM, Flo GL. Mineralization of the supraspinatus tendon in dogs: a long-term follow-up. *J Am Anim Hosp Assoc* 36:262-267, 2000.
12. Muir P, Johnson K. Supraspinatus and biceps brachii tendinopathy in dogs. *J Small Anim Pract* 35:239-243, 1994.
13. Lassaigne CC, Boyer C, Sautier L, Taeymans O. Ultrasound of the normal canine supraspinatus tendon: comparison with gross anatomy and histology. *Vet Rec* 186:e14-e14, 2020.
14. Mistieri MLA, Wigger A, Canola JC, Filho JG, Kramer M. Ultrasonographic evaluation of canine supraspinatus calcifying tendinosis. *J Am Anim Hosp Assoc* 48:405-410, 2012.
15. Pownder SL, Caserto BG, Hayashi K, Norman ML, Potter HG, Koff MF. Magnetic resonance imaging and histologic features of the supraspinatus tendon in nonlame dogs. *Am J Vet Res* 79:836-844, 2018.
16. McKee W.M, Macias C. Scurell E.J. Ossification of the infraspinatus tendon-bursa in 13 dogs. *Vet Rec* 161:846-852, 2007.
17. Mikkelsen MA, Ottesen N. CT findings in a dog with subacute myopathy and later fibrotic contracture of the infraspinatus muscle. *Vet Radiol Ultrasound* 62:E11-E15, 2021.
18. Orellana-James N, Ginja M, Regueiro M, Oliveira P, Gama A, Rodriguez-Altonaga J, et al. Sub-acute and chronic MRI findings in bilateral canine fibrotic contracture of the infraspinatus muscle. *J Small Anim Pract* 54:428-431, 2013.
19. Comerford E. The stifle joint. In Kirberger R, McEvoy F, editors. BSAVA Manual of canine and feline musculoskeletal imaging 2nd edition. Gloucester, BSAVA publications, 2016, pp 171-188.
20. Van der Vekens E, De Bakker E, Bogaerts E, Broeckx B, Ducatelle R, Kromhout K, Saunders J. High-frequency ultrasound, computed tomography and computed tomography arthrography of the cranial cruciate ligament, menisci and cranial meniscotibial ligaments in 10 radiographically normal canine cadaver stifles. *BMC Vet Res* 2019 15:146.
21. Marino D, Loughin C. Diagnostic imaging of the canine stifle: A review. *Vet Surg* 39:284-295, 2010.
22. Gnudi G, Bertonia G. Echographic examination of the stifle joint affected by cranial cruciate ligament rupture in the dog. *Vet Radiol Ultrasound* 42:266-270, 2001.
23. Samii V. Joints. In Schwarz T, Saunders J, editors. Veterinary Computed Tomography. Ames, IA, Wiley-Blackwell, 2011, pp 414-417.
24. Samii V, Dyce J, Pozzi A, Drost T, Mattoon J, Green E, Kowaleski M, Lehman A. Computed tomographic arthrography of the stifle for detection of cranial and caudal cruciate ligament and meniscal tears in dogs. *Vet Radiol Ultrasound* 50:144-150, 2009.
25. Barrett E, Barr F, Owen M, Bradley K. A retrospective study of the MRI findings in 18 dogs with stifle injuries. *J Small Anim Pract* 50:448-455, 2009.
26. Lin M, Glass EN, Kent M. Utility of MRI for evaluation of a common calcaneal tendon rupture in a dog: case report. *Front Vet Sci* 7:602, 2020.
27. Corr S, Draffan D, Kulendra E, Carmichael S, Brodbelt D. Retrospective study of Achilles mechanism disruption in 45 dogs. *Vet Rec* 167:407-411, 2010.
28. Gamble LJ, Canapp DA, Canapp SO. Evaluation of Achilles tendon injuries with findings from diagnostic musculoskeletal ultrasound in canines–43 cases. *Veterinary Evidence* 2, 2017.
29. Mai W. MRI of the brachial and lumbosacral plexus. In Mai W, editor. Diagnostic MRI in dogs and cats. Boca Raton, FL, CRC Press, 2018, pp 603-617.
30. Platt S, Graham J, Chrisman C, Collins K, Chandra S, Sirninger J, Newell S. Magnetic resonance imaging and ultrasonography in the diagnosis of a malignant peripheral nerves sheath tumor in a dog. *Vet Radiol Ultrasound* 40:367-371, 1999.
31. Hudson J, D'Anjou M., Spine and peripheral nerves. In Penninck D, D'Anjou M, editors. Atlas of Small animal Ultrasonography 2nd edition, Ames, IA, Wiley Blackwell, 2015, pp 545-562.
32. Guilherme S, Benigni L. Ultrasonographic anatomy of the brachial plexus and major nerves of the canine thoracic limb. *Vet Radiol Ultrasound* 49:577-583, 2008.
33. Anson A, Gil F, Laredo F, Soler M, Belda M, Ayala M, Agut A. Correlative ultrasound anatomy of the feline brachial plexus and major nerves of the thoracic limb. *Vet Radiol Ultrasound* 54:185-193, 2013.
34. Benigni L, Corr A, Lamb C. Ultrasonographic assessment of the canine sciatic nerve. *Vet Radiol Ultrasound* 48:428-433, 2006.
35. Haro P, Gil F, Laredo F, Ayala M, Belda E, Soler M, Agut A. Ultrasonographic study of the feline sciatic nerve. *J Feline Med Surg* 13:259-265, 2011.
36. Rose S, Long C, Knipe M, Hornof B. Ultrasonographic evaluation of brachial plexus tumors in five dogs. *Vet Radiol Ultrasound* 46:514-517, 2005.
37. Kraft S, Ehrhart E, Gall D, Klopp L, Gavin P, Tucker R, Bagley R, Kippenes H, DeHaan C, Pedroia V, Partington B, Olby N. Magnetic resonance imaging characteristics of peripheral nerve sheath tumors of the canine brachial plexus in 18 dogs. *Vet Radiol Ultrasound* 48:1-7, 2007.
38. Rudich S, Feeney D, Anderson K, Walter P. Computed tomography of masses of the brachial plexus and contributing nerve roots in dogs. *Vet Radiol Ultrasound* 45:46-50, 2004.
39. Forterre F, Gutmannsbauer B, Schmahl W, Matis U. CT myelography for diagnosis of brachial plexus avulsion small animals. *Tierarztl Prax Ausg Kleintiere Heimtiere* 26:322-329, 1998.
40. Munoz A, Mateo I, Lorenzo V, Martinez J. Imaging diagnosis: traumatic dural tear diagnosed using intrathecal gadopentate dimeglumine. *Vet Radiol Ultrasound* 50:502-505, 2009.

SECTION III

AXIAL SKELETON

CHAPTER 13

Diseases of the skull

Federico R. Vilaplana Grosso and Robson F. Giglio

> **KEY POINTS**
>
> - Radiography is good for the general examination of the head, especially bony and aerated structures such as the nose, sinuses, and tympanic bullae.
> - CT is superior to radiographs for examination of bony structures and quite sensitive for assessment of soft tissues with intravenous contrast.
> - MRI is the imaging modality of choice for examining the central nervous system and is the best modality for assessing soft tissues.
> - Head trauma can be assessed with radiography and CT, although MRI may be needed to assess intracranial lesions.

Radiography has traditionally been the first-line diagnostic imaging technique in veterinary medicine to examine the skull. Its availability, low cost, and rapidity in image acquisition recommend it for general examination of the head, especially bony and aerated structures such as the nose, sinuses, and tympanic bullae. However, the head is a complex anatomical region and radiographic examination is technically difficult and must be tailored to the specific area of interest.

Computed tomography (CT) and magnetic resonance imaging (MRI) are preferred if available. CT is excellent for examination of bony structures, and it does not have the problem of overlapping structures present in radiography. CT is also superior for examining aerated head structures and is quite useful for examining soft tissues. Finally, CT is the preferred modality for surgical and radiation planning, particularly with three-dimensional (3D) and multiplanar reconstructions.

For the examination of the central nervous system, MRI is the modality of choice as it has superior contrast resolution of soft tissues while lacking the superposition of structures. With both modalities, intravenous contrast can be used to help the assessment of soft tissue lesions and vascularization of tissues.

Other imaging techniques that may be used for the examination of the head are ultrasound and scintigraphy, although these modalities are much less frequently used. Some of the structures of the head that may be evaluated with ultrasound are the eyes, retro-orbital space, salivary glands, lymph nodes, tongue, retropharyngeal structures, soft tissue swellings, and less frequently the temporomandibular joints (TMJ) and ears. Scintigraphy is rarely used to study skull diseases.

Indications

- Head trauma.
- Congenital head abnormalities.
- Pain in the head region.
- Deformities or swelling of the head.
- Epistaxis and nasal discharge.
- Signs referring to nasal or nasopharyngeal disease.
- Exophthalmos and retrobulbar disease.
- Ear disease.
- Oral dysphagia.
- Temporomandibular disease.
- Dental disease.
- Metabolic disease that affects the head.
- Cranial nerve deficits and neurolocalization to the neurocranium.
- Post-surgical examination.

Disorders

Periodontitis

Periodontitis is part of periodontal disease, having a more severe presentation that involves inflammation of the periodontal ligament and alveolar bone. Radiographically, the lamina dura is a thin mineral opaque line which forms the wall of the alveolar socket and is parallel to the tooth root. The periodontal ligament appears as a thin lucent band between the lamina dura and tooth root and attaches the tooth and lamina dura.

For assessment of periodontitis, radiography and CT are the diagnostic imaging modalities of choice. Dental radiography is highly recommended to assess periodontal disease. It provides excellent image quality and resolution, although special equipment and good knowledge of the technique are required. Standard radiography can also be used to assess periodontitis utilizing open-mouth oblique lateral views of the maxilla and the mandible (i.e., left 20- to 30-degree dorsal right ventral or right 20- to 30-degree ventral left dorsal). Also, intraoral views of the rostral upper and lower dental arcade can be obtained.

Bone loss associated with periodontitis is presented in two patterns: vertical and horizontal. Vertical bone loss is presented as a widening of the periodontal ligament space that progresses parallel to the tooth root. Horizontal bone loss happens parallel to the alveolar margin and is the most common pattern encountered in dogs and cats.[1]

Radiographically, periodontitis is seen as a widening of the radiolucent periodontal ligament space with a vertical and/or horizontal pattern and associated thinning to loss of the lamina dura (**fig. 13.1**). The margins of the radiolucent region surrounding the tooth root may be well- or ill-defined, suggesting a less active or more active lesion, respectively. The surrounding alveolar bone may become sclerotic in chronic cases. The tooth root may become irregular with regions of lysis. With advanced disease, a larger periapical lucency may be present surrounding the tip of the affected tooth root, representing periapical abscessation (**fig. 13.2**). The maxillary fourth premolar teeth are most commonly affected by periapical abscessation. In cases of severe periodontitis or periapical abscessation, an irregular and ill-defined periosteal reaction can be seen indicating adjacent osteomyelitis.

In cats, feline odontoclastic resorptive lesions (FORL) are the most common dental disease.[2] These lesions initially start in the periodontal ligament and cementum below the gingival margin (**fig. 13.3**). Tooth fracture with loss of the tooth crown and retention of roots is a frequent sequela of FORL. CT is superior to radiography as the cross-sectional images eliminate superimposition, but the spatial resolution of radiographs is greater (**fig. 13.4**). A recent study comparing intraoral radiography and CT for detecting radiographic signs of periodontitis and endodontic disease in dogs showed that there is a high level of agreement between techniques and between observers.[3] Cone-beam CT can also be utilized to diagnose dental diseases in dogs and cats.

CHAPTER 13 Diseases of the skull

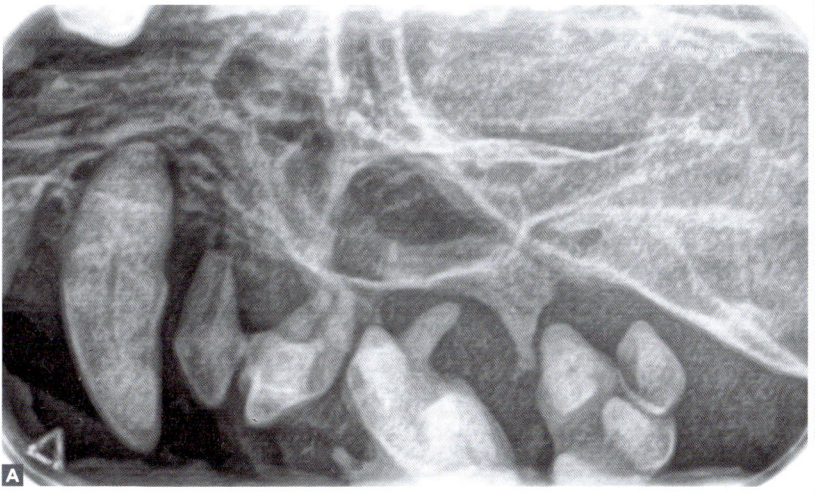

Fig. 13.1 Lateral oblique (A) and dorsoventral (B) intraoral dental radiographs of a ten-year-old spayed female Yorkshire Terrier with severe periodontitis. (A) There is marked radiolucent widening of the periodontal ligament space with loss of the lamina dura of all maxillary premolar teeth. (B) There is moderate and irregular widening of the periodontal ligament space with loss of the lamina dura of the right maxillary canine, premolar teeth, and the remaining left incisor tooth. Multiple incisor teeth are missing. The images are courtesy of Dr. Amy Stone, University of Florida, College of Veterinary Medicine.

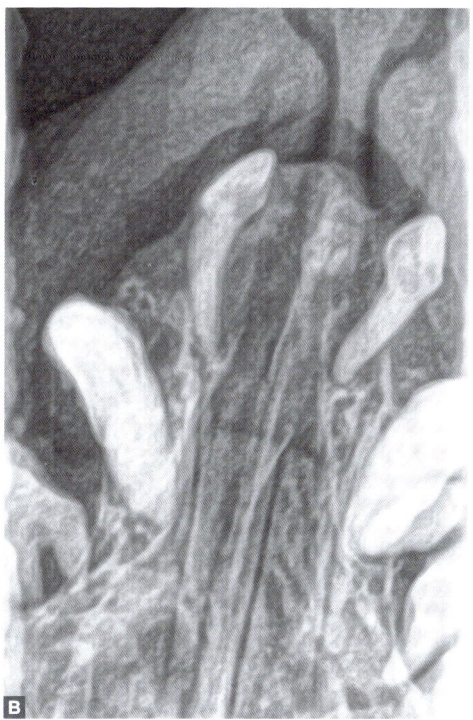

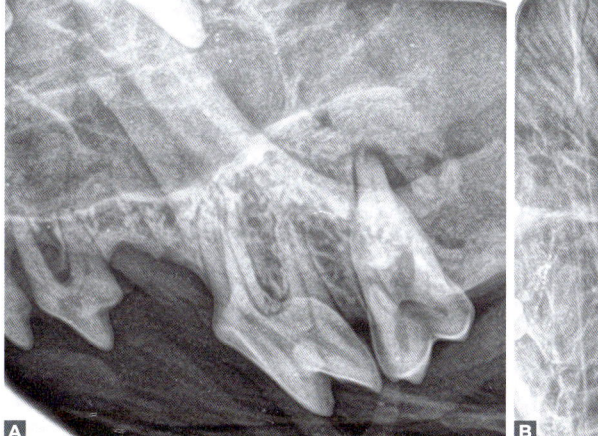

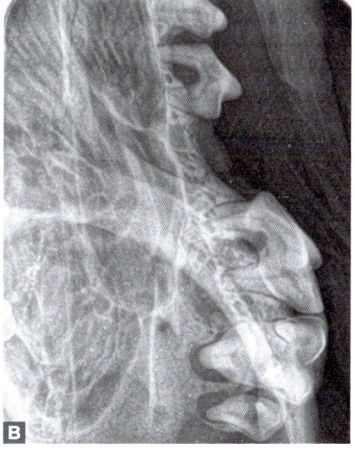

Fig. 13.2 Lateral oblique (A) and dorsoventral (B) intraoral dental radiographs of a seven-year-old neutered male Yorkshire Terrier with periapical tooth root abscessation of the first and second left maxillary molars. A large periapical lucency is seen surrounding the roots of the first and second maxillary molars. The third maxillary premolar is missing. The images are courtesy of Dr. Amy Stone, University of Florida, College of Veterinary Medicine.

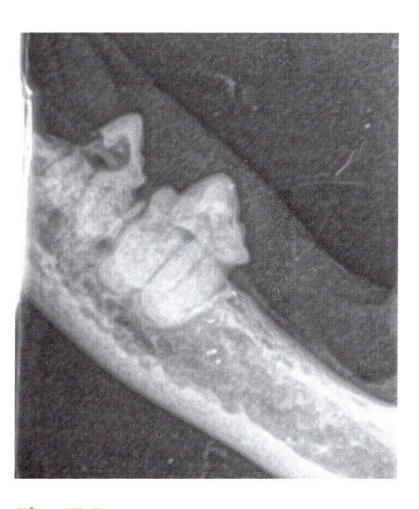

Fig. 13.3 Lateral intraoral dental radiograph of an 18-year-old spayed female Domestic shorthair cat with FORL. There is a large region of tooth crown resorption of the second mandibular premolar. The image is courtesy of Dr. Amy Stone, University of Florida, College of Veterinary Medicine.A

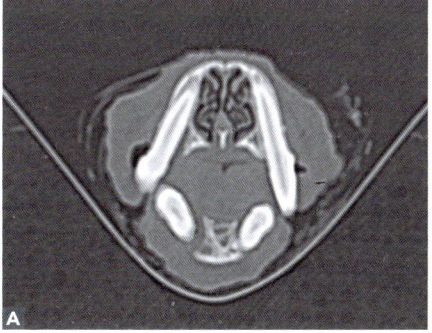

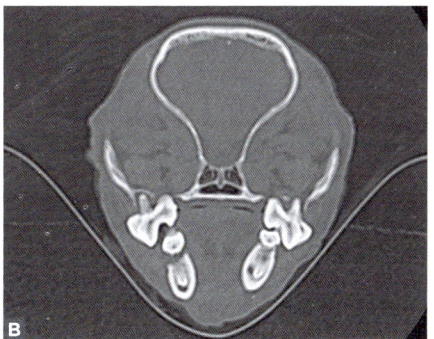

Fig. 13.4 Pre-contrast transverse CT images with a bone algorithm of a ten-year-old neutered male small mixed breed dog with severe periodontitis. (A) There is moderate to marked alveolar bone lysis surrounding the root of the right mandibular canine. (B) There is marked alveolar bone lysis surrounding the roots of both first maxillary molars, with complete lysis of the maxillary bones, and between the tooth roots of the first right mandibular molar. A large amount of tartar is also seen surrounding the buccal aspect of both first maxillary molars.

135

Oral neoplasia

Oral neoplasms account for approximately 6% of canine and 3% of feline cancers. The most common types of canine oral malignant neoplasms are fibrosarcoma, squamous cell carcinoma (SSC), and malignant melanoma. Oral fibrosarcoma in dogs affects most commonly large breeds (especially Golden Retrievers), and can affect both the mandible or the maxilla with a predilection for the palate. Oral SCC has more predilection for the rostral mandible in the dog. Radiographically, bone involvement has been noted in approximately 82% of oral SCC and 70% of oral fibrosarcomas[4] (**fig. 13.5**). Canine oral SCC rarely presents regional or distant metastasis. However, oral malignant melanomas can occur in large and small breed dogs and commonly metastasize to the regional lymph nodes and lungs. Oral SCC and malignant melanoma in dogs are commonly presented radiographically as expansile lytic lesions. Oral fibrosarcoma is mostly presented radiographically as a lytic lesion but can have components of osseous proliferation. In cats, the most common type of neoplasia is SCC,[5] which originates from the gingiva and mucosa of the maxilla, mandible, tongue, lip, sublingual area, soft palate, or tonsillar region. Oral SCC

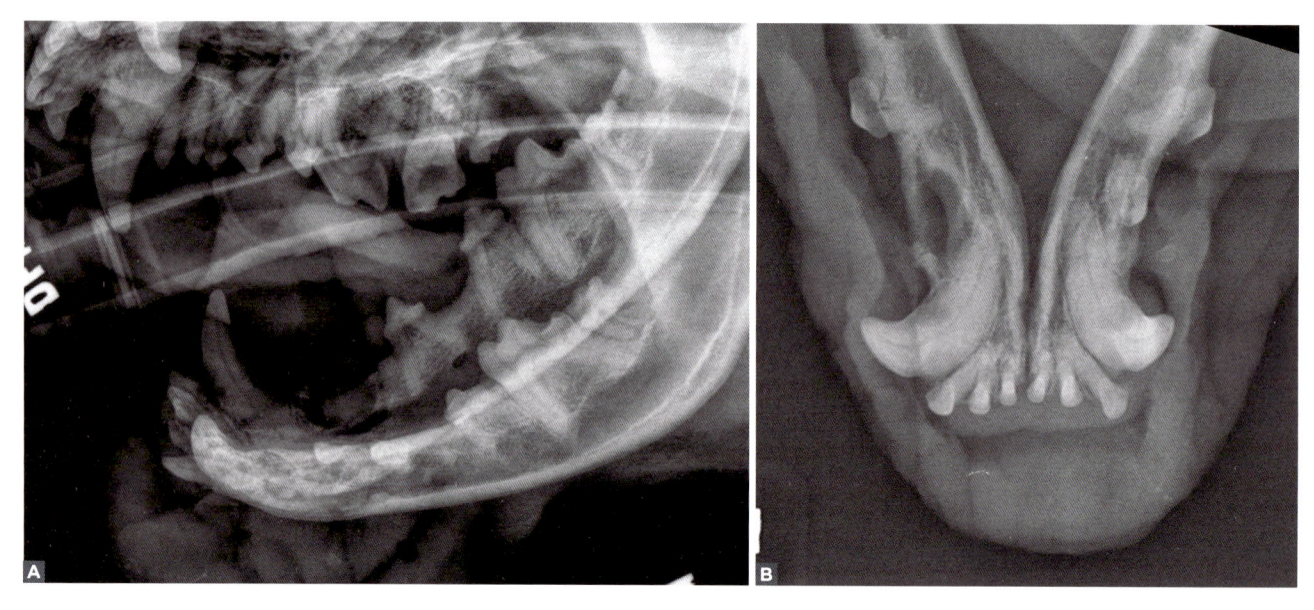

Fig. 13.5 Left 20- to 30-degree dorsal right ventral oblique (**A**) and intraoral mandibular ventrodorsal (**B**) radiographs of a 12-year-old intact male Boxer with a mandibular squamous cell carcinoma. There is a well-defined, smoothly marginated area of geographic osteolysis at the level of the right first mandibular premolar tooth, which is absent.

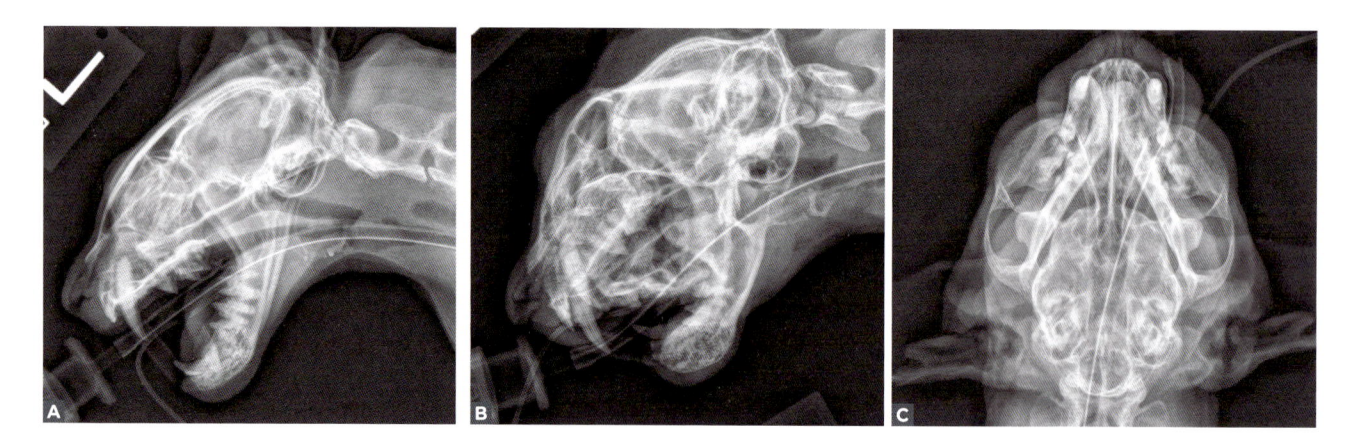

Fig. 13.6 Lateral (**A**), left 20- to 30-degree dorsal right ventral oblique (**B**), and dorsoventral (**C**) radiographs of a nine-year-old neutered male Domestic shorthair cat with a left mandibular SCC. Surrounding the left rostral mandible there is an expansile heterogenous, smoothly marginated, mixed osteolytic and osteoproliferative mass. The rostral mandibular cortex at this location is thinned and ill-defined. The left mandibular second and third incisor and canine teeth are absent. There is soft tissue thickening surrounding the bony lesion.

accounts for approximately 60-70% of feline malignant oral neoplasms. In contrast to dogs, cats with oral SCC have a poorer prognosis and are less responsive to radiotherapy. Feline SCC is primary lytic in appearance and causes expansion (**fig. 13.6**). Other less common feline oral neoplasms are fibrosarcomas. In cats, common CT features of oral SCC include sublingual and maxillary locations, marked heterogeneous contrast enhancement, and osteolysis[6] (**fig. 13.7**).

Radiographic signs associated with oral malignant neoplasms generally have an aggressive appearance with osteolytic and/or osteoproliferative expansile lesions, involvement of the cortical and medullary bone, presence of mass effect, increase in soft tissue opacity, tooth root erosion, and displacement or loss of teeth.

Radiography is poor for determining the gross tumor extent. For this purpose, CT and MRI are preferred since they provide more accurate evaluation of the tumor extent and help to discern the soft tissue and bone components of the tumor (**fig. 13.8**). For oral neoplasms with minimal bony changes, MRI may be preferred since it allows evaluation of the bone marrow and is better for assessing the soft tissues.

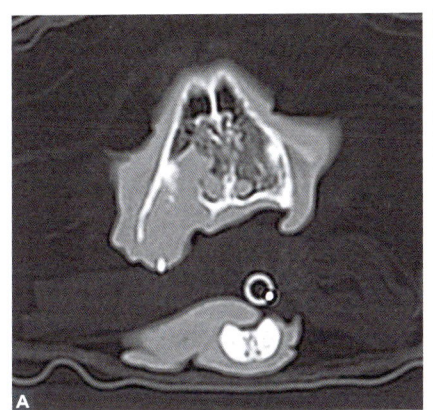

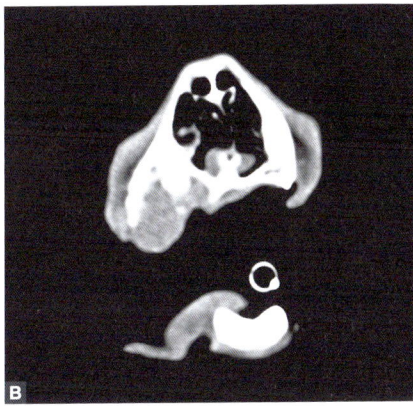

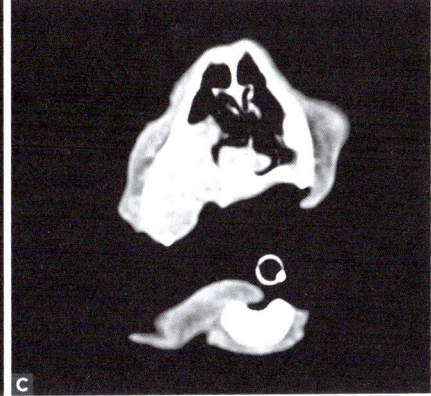

Fig. 13.7 CT transverse images with a bone (**A**) and a soft tissue algorithm, (**B**) pre-contrast, and (**C**) post-contrast, of a 21-year-old neutered male Domestic medium hair cat with a right maxillary SCC. At the level of the right maxillary canine there is an expansile, homogeneously soft tissue attenuating, heterogeneously contrast-enhancing mass causing extensive regional lysis, and expansion of the maxillary bone. There is focal lysis of the maxilla, with invasion of right ventral nasal meatus. Focal thickening of the oral soft tissues overlying the hard palate is seen.

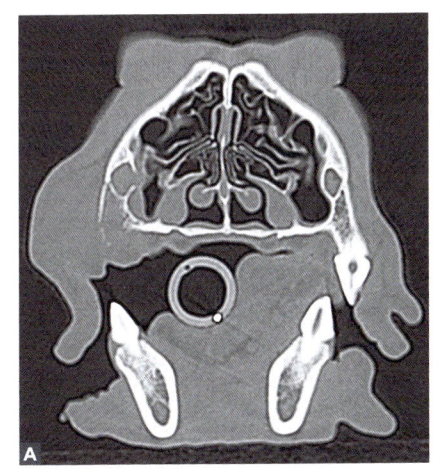

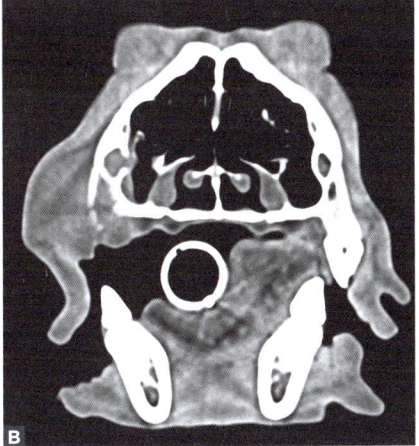

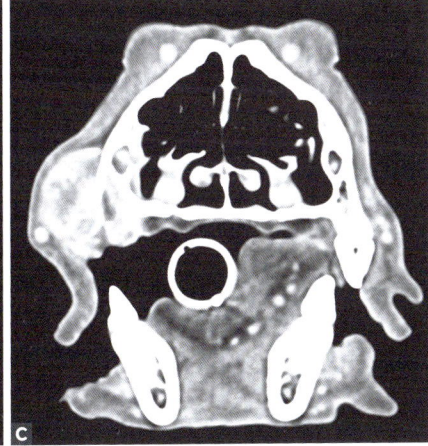

Fig. 13.8 CT transverse images with a bone (**A**) and a soft tissue algorithm, (**B**) pre-contrast, and (**C**) post-contrast, of a one-year-old neutered male mixed breed Labrador Retriever with a maxillary rhabdomyosarcoma. Centered over the caudal aspect of the right maxillary bone, at the level of the fourth maxillary premolar, there is a well-defined, rounded, and laterally smoothly marginated mass. The mass is homogeneously soft tissue attenuating and markedly contrast-enhancing. At the level of the mass, there is extensive regional lysis of the maxillary bone and absence of the fourth maxillary premolar. The mass also extends into the infraorbital canal and causes widening and mild focal lysis of the lateral aspect of the infraorbital canal, resulting in communication with the nasal cavity. Additionally, a small portion of this mass extends into the right ventral periphery of the right maxillary recess.

Primary nasal neoplasia

Tumors of the nasal cavity in dogs and cats account for approximately 1% to 2% of all neoplasms. The most common types of canine nasal neoplasms are epithelial, such as adenocarcinoma, undifferentiated carcinoma, and SCC; or mesenchymal, such as chondrosarcoma and osteosarcoma. Neuroendocrine tumors (e.g., esthesioneuroblastoma) arising from the nasal cavity typically originate from or next to the cribriform plate, extending into the nasal cavity and the cranial cavity. In dogs, epithelial neoplasms account for approximately ⅔, and mesenchymal neoplasms for about ⅓ of the nasal tumors. Canine nasal neoplasia is frequent in older, medium to large, mesaticephalic and dolichocephalic dogs. In cats, lymphoma and epithelial neoplasms, such as adenocarcinoma and SCC, are the most common tumor types. Most nasal tumors are unilateral, usually arise from the middle or caudal third of the nasal cavity, and cause local invasion with possible regional metastasis, but uncommonly distant metastasis. Feline nasal lymphoma can be bilateral and is often centered on the ventral nasal meatus and the nasopharynx.

The most valuable radiographic projections for assessing nasal disease are the intraoral DV and the open-mouth VD projections. They allow a detailed evaluation of the nasal cavity without superimposition of the mandible. Radiographic signs associated with nasal neoplasms are turbinate destruction, increased soft tissue opacity within the nasal cavity (representing tumor tissue and/or accumulated secretions or hemorrhage), a discrete soft tissue mass, erosion or destruction of the vomer, lysis affecting the facial bones adjacent to the nasal cavity, and an increase in soft tissue opacity within the frontal sinuses (e.g., secondary to obstruction of drainage or tumor extension) (**fig. 13.9**). Some of these radiographic signs are also seen with rhinitis; however, complete opacification of the nasal cavity (unilateral > bilateral), turbinate destruction, destruction of the vomer and/or facial bones and mass effect, are more suggestive of nasal neoplasia.[7] In cats, nasal lymphoma may be presented radiographically as a soft tissue mass or increased soft tissue opacity involving both nasal cavities.

CT and MRI are excellent imaging modalities for diagnosing nasal neoplasia. CT can detect subtle osteolytic and osteoproliferative changes, assess the integrity of the cribriform plate, and is used for radiation therapy planning. Compared to CT, MRI is more sensitive to determine intracranial extension of a nasal neoplasm (**fig. 13.10**).

In dogs, CT features that have been correlated with nasal neoplasia include destruction of ethmoid bones, destruction of bones surrounding the nasal cavities, abnormal soft tissue in the retrobulbar space, hyperostosis of the lateral maxilla, and areas of increased attenuation within abnormal soft tissues[8] (**fig. 13.11**).

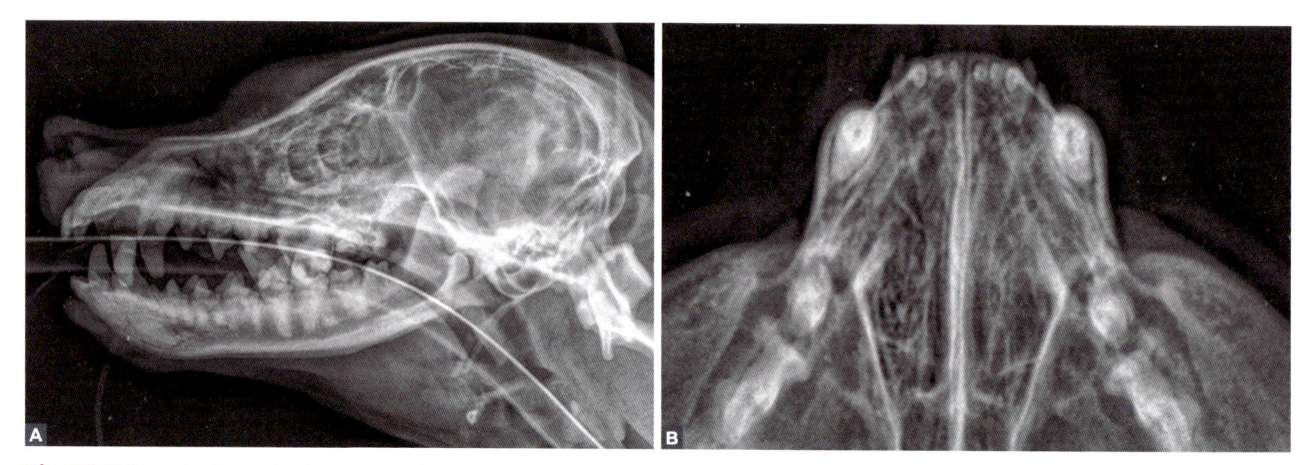

Fig. 13.9 Lateral radiograph of an 11-year-old neutered male Jack Russel terrier with a unilateral nasal carcinoma (**A**) and collimated open-mouth ventrodorsal radiograph of a 15-year-old Domestic shorthair cat with a unilateral nasal carcinoma (**B**). (**A**) There is a focal soft tissue swelling dorsal to the caudal aspect of the nasal cavity with associated irregular, ill-defined and discontinuous periosteal proliferation. (**B**) There is a focal increase in soft tissue opacity in the rostral two-thirds of the left nasal cavity with mild turbinate destruction.

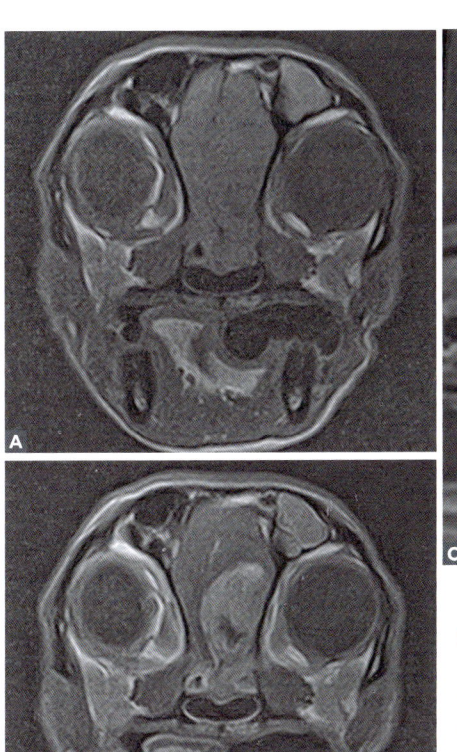

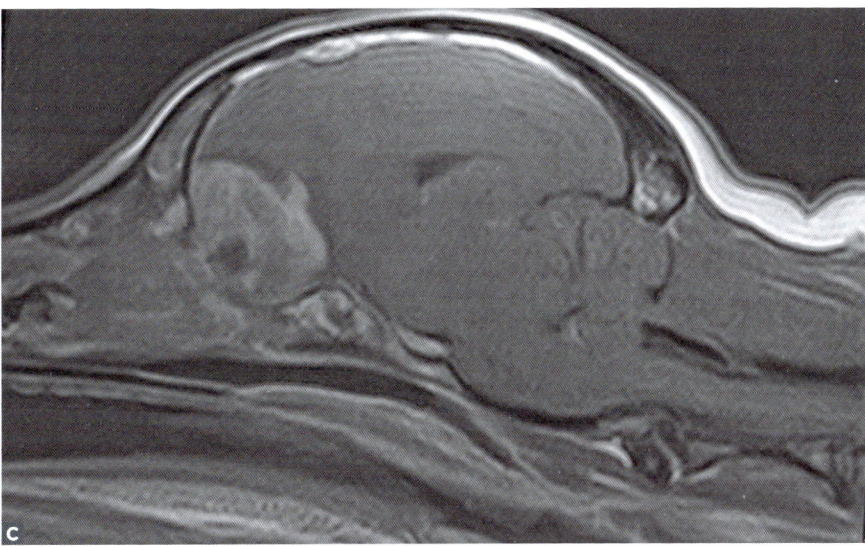

Fig. 13.10 MRI transverse pre- (**A**) and post-contrast (**B**) T1-weighted and sagittal post-contrast T1-weighted (**C**) images of a ten-year-old spayed female Miniature Schnauzer with a nasal undifferentiated carcinoma with intracranial extension. Centered on the caudal nasal cavity, mostly to the left of midline, there is a large, well-defined, mildly lobulated and heterogeneously T1 iso- to mildly hypointense mass with marked heterogeneous contrast enhancement. The mass extends into the cranial fossa, obliterating the left olfactory bulb and causing marked compression of the left frontal lobe, as well as a mild rightward midline shift of the falx cerebri rostrally. The left frontal sinus contains a large amount of T1 hyperintense material, and the mucosa is moderately contrast enhancing, compatible with obstructive sinusitis.

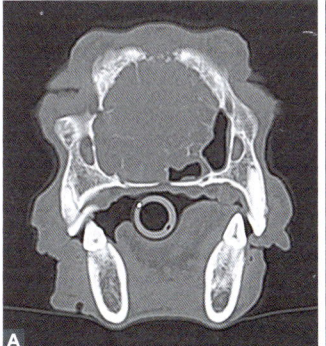

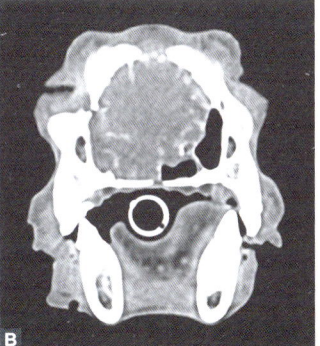

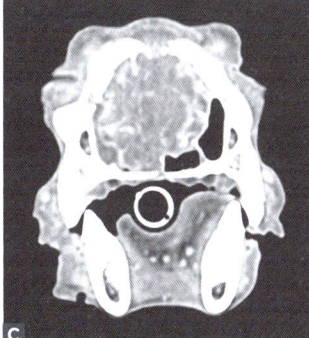

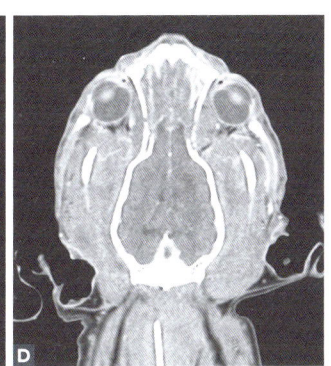

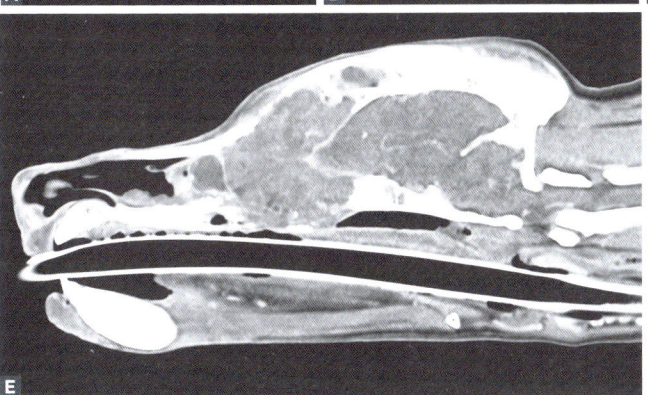

Fig. 13.11 CT transverse images with a bone (**A**) and a soft tissue algorithm, (**B**) pre-contrast, and (**C**) post-contrast, and post-contrast dorsal (**D**) and sagittal (**E**) multiplanar reconstructions with a soft tissue algorithm of a ten-year-old neutered male mixed breed dog with a nasal carcinoma. Along the right nasal cavity and extending into the caudal portion of the left nasal cavity and into the right and left frontal sinuses there is a lobulated, heterogeneously soft tissue attenuating, and heterogeneously contrast enhancing mass. There is severe osteolysis of the nasal turbinates and ethmoturbinates, cribriform plate, ventral portion of the left and right frontal bones, maxillary bone, palatine bone and right maxillary recess. There is intracranial extension of the nasal neoplasm, which is better assessed on the dorsal and sagittal multiplanar reconstructions.

Fungal rhinitis and sinusitis

Fungal infections of the nasal cavity are relatively uncommon in dogs and cats, although more common in dogs than in cats. The most frequent etiology in dogs is *Aspergillus* spp., particularly *Aspergillus fumigatus*, and *Cryptococcus neoformans* in cats. Fungal rhinitis is not always a primary disease and could be secondary to immunosuppression or foreign bodies.

▎ **Aspergillus infection** Nasal aspergillosis is a type of destructive rhinitis that typically involves the frontal sinuses. Mesocephalic and dolichocephalic, young to middle-aged dogs (<8 years) are most commonly affected. Aspergillosis can occur in cats but is much less common than in dogs. In cats, two forms are described: sino-nasal and sino-orbital. The infection starts in the nasal cavity and sinuses and may progress to the orbit, causing the sino-orbital form of this disease, which has a poor prognosis. Some of the imaging features of feline aspergillosis may include bilateral involvement, variable turbinate destruction, and a large amount of fluid and soft tissue within the nasal cavity. Multifocal bone erosion, hyperostosis, and presence of fluid and/or soft tissue within the frontal sinuses may be seen.

Radiographic examination in cases of nasal aspergillosis should include orthogonal projections of the skull, intraoral projections of the nasal cavity and maxilla, as well as a rostro-caudal projection of the frontal sinuses. Aspergillus rhinitis has been described as "destructive rhinitis" and the characteristic features are nasal turbinate lysis and hyperlucency of the nasal chamber.

Radiographic findings may also include punctate lucencies in the maxillary and nasal bone, multifocal increase in soft tissue opacity in the nasal chambers from accumulated secretion and granulomas and increased soft tissue opacity within frontal sinuses. Chronic cases may show hyperostosis and punctate lucencies within the frontal bones. It is not possible to distinguish radiographically between nasal aspergillosis and neoplasia.

CT is superior compared to radiography with a sensitivity of 88 to 92% compared to 72 to 84% on radiographs.[9] CT features of canine nasal aspergillosis include moderate to severe cavitary destruction of the nasal turbinates with the presence of a variable amount of abnormal soft tissue in the nasal passages, mucosal thickening, hyperostosis, turbinate destruction, and frontal sinus fluid/soft tissue, hyperostosis, and osteolysis (**fig. 13.12**). In earlier phases of canine nasal aspergillosis, unilateral nasal mucosal thickening and secretions are noted; however, in more chronic phases, marked turbinate destruction will result in destruction of internal structures of the affected nasal cavity. Soft tissue mass-like structures may be present within the caudal nasal cavity or frontal sinuses.

▎ **Cryptococcus infection** *Cryptococcus* spp. (*Cryptococcus neoformans* and *Cryptococcus gatti*) is the most common type of sinonasal fungal infection seen in cats. Cryptococcosis is a systemic fungal disease that can be presented in a nasal form, central nervous system form, or cutaneous form. The nasal form is the most common, and the central nervous system form is likely due to nasal infection crossing the cribriform plate into the cranial cavity. Nasal cryptococcosis is commonly presented as a chronic rhinitis that affects the nasal passages and generally causes a non-destructive hyperplastic rhinitis.

Radiographic features of nasal cryptococcosis include unilateral or, more commonly, bilateral soft tissue opacification of the nasal cavity and frontal sinuses, with variable nasal turbinate destruction which depends on the severity and the chronicity. More frequently, turbinate destruction is mild. When fungal granulomas are present, a mass-like structure may be seen with possible erosion of the adjacent bones.

CT features of feline fungal rhinitis include destruction of nasal turbinates, lysis of nasal cavity bones, uni- or bilateral masses with variable enhancement, involvement of the frontal sinuses, involvement of the nasopharynx, and extension into the orbital or facial soft tissues (**fig. 13.13**). Cryptococcal granuloma formation can happen in the nasopharynx seen as a well-defined mass.

CHAPTER **13** Diseases of the skull

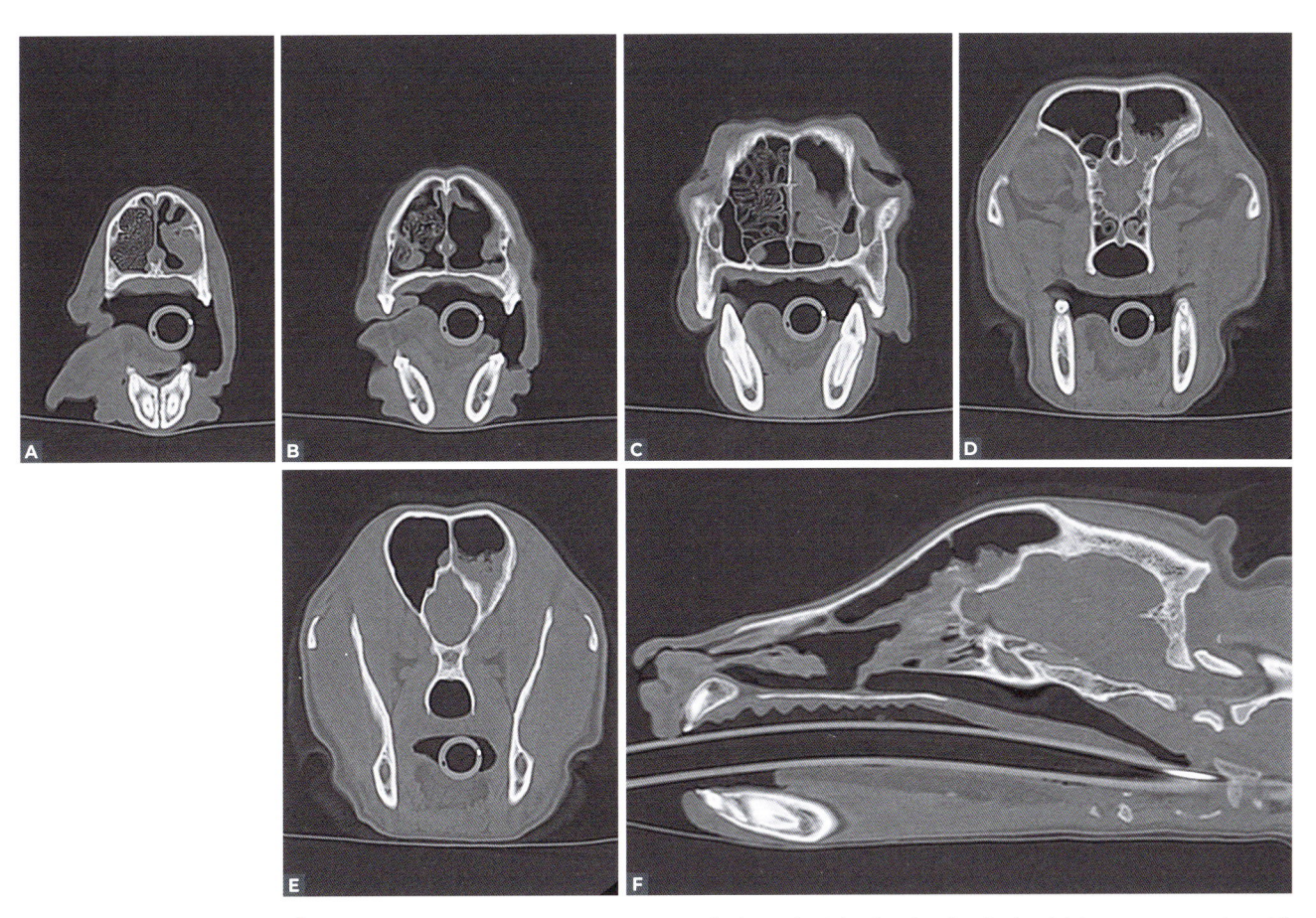

Fig. 13.12 Pre-contrast transverse CT images with a bone algorithm (**A-E**) and sagittal multiplanar reconstruction with a bone algorithm (**F**) of the head of a nine-year-old spayed female Labrador Retriever with nasal aspergillosis. Throughout the left nasal cavity there is marked turbinate and ethmoturbinate destruction. Conforming to the remainder of the nasal turbinates within the ventral aspect of the rostral and caudal nasal cavity, and within the left maxillary recess and left frontal sinus there is a moderate amount of soft tissue attenuating material. In addition, there is lysis seen on the left dorsal aspect of the cribriform plate. The left frontal and maxillary bones are also multifocally irregularly thickened, compatible with hyperostosis.

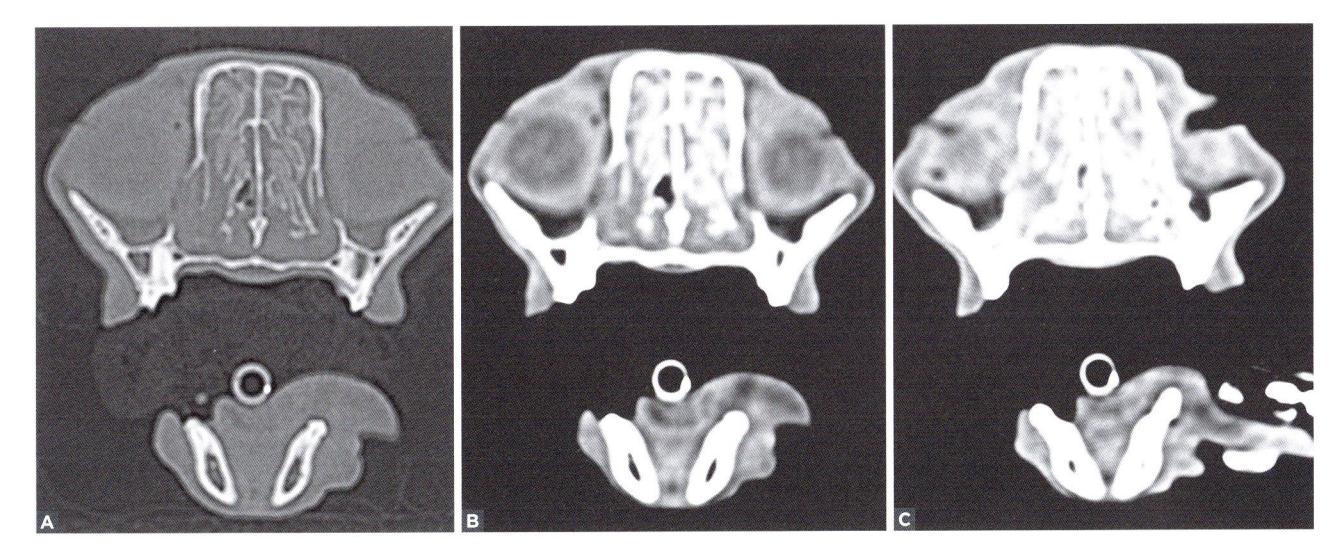

Fig. 13.13 CT transverse images with a bone (**A**) and a soft tissue algorithm, (**B**) pre-contrast, and (**C**) post-contrast of a four-year-old neutered male Domestic shorthair cat with nasal cryptococcosis. Throughout the left and right sides of the nasal cavity and maxillary recesses, there is a large amount of mixed fluid and soft tissue attenuating, heterogeneously contrast enhancing material with associated marked mucosal enhancement. There is moderate, bilateral osteolysis of the ventral aspect of the nasal turbinates. There is also osteolysis of the left and right aspects of the maxilla at the level of the orbit with mild extension of the heterogenous soft tissue attenuating material into the right orbit.

Nasopharyngeal polyp

Nasopharyngeal polyps generally occur in young cats and can extend into the external ear canal. Nasopharyngeal polyps can present with chronic rhinosinusitis, stridor from nasopharyngeal obstruction and middle and/or inner ear disease.

Radiographically, a nasopharyngeal polyp may be seen as an oval or rounded, soft tissue opaque structure within the nasopharynx. The rostral margin of the polyp is not commonly seen, but the caudal margin is generally well-defined since it is surrounded by air (**fig. 13.14**). Nasopharyngeal polyps can cause ventral displacement of the soft palate. It is common to observe radiographic evidence of middle ear disease, which, if present, indicates the tympanic bulla at the origin of the polyp. In

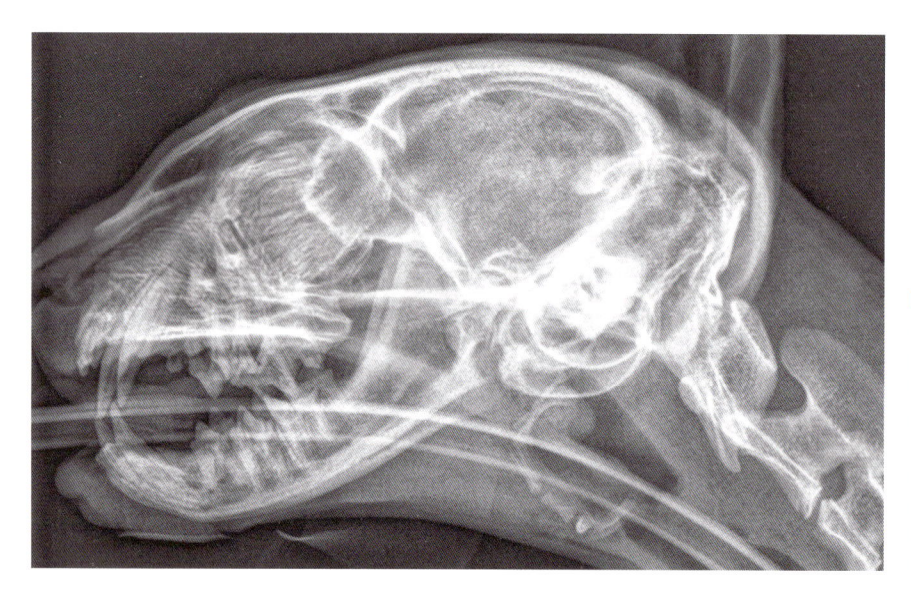

Fig. 13.14 Lateral radiograph of a one-year-old neutered male Maine Coon with a nasopharyngeal polyp and chronic otitis media. Within the nasopharynx dorsal to the soft palate there is an ovoid, caudally well-defined soft tissue opaque structure. Within the most ventrally located tympanic bulla (laterality undetermined), there is a diffuse increase in soft tissue opacity with thickening and irregularity of the tympanic bulla wall.

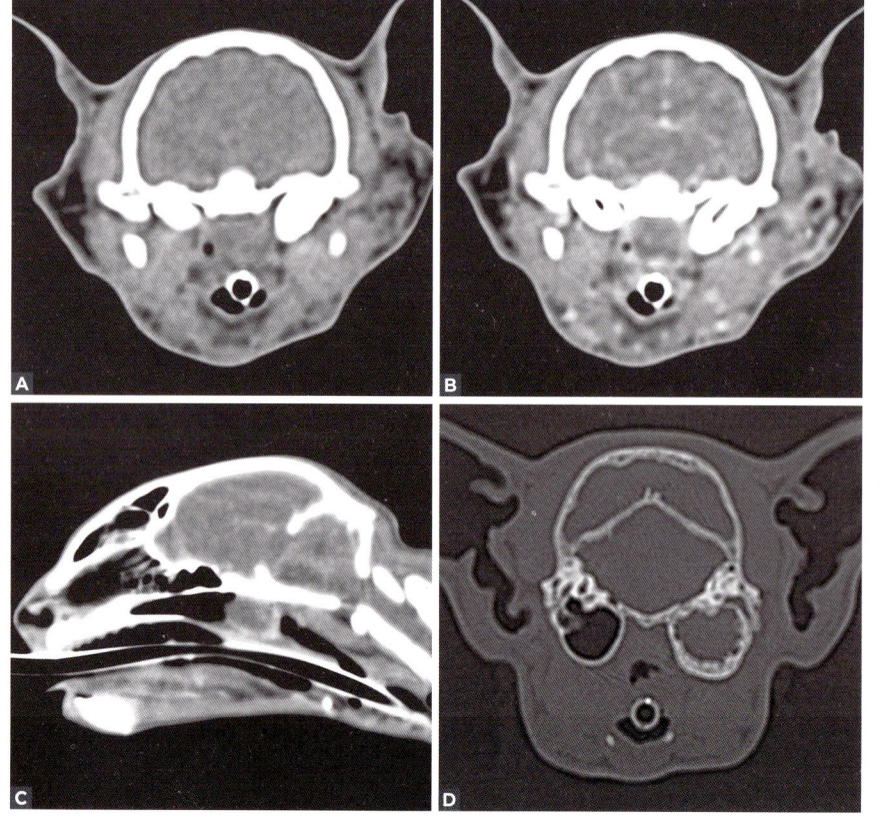

Fig. 13.15 CT transverse images with a soft tissue algorithm (**A**) pre-contrast, and (**B**) post-contrast, sagittal multiplanar reconstruction with a soft tissue algorithm (**C**), and transverse image with a bone algorithm (**D**) of a five-month-old intact female Domestic shorthair cat with a nasopharyngeal polyp and chronic left-sided otitis media. (**A-C**) There is a well-defined, oval, soft tissue attenuating mass with strong rim enhancement visible within the rostral aspect of the nasopharynx, just rostral to the level of the tympanic bullae. This mass causes complete occlusion of the lumen of the nasopharynx. (**D**) The left tympanic bulla is moderately enlarged when compared with the right and has a diffusely thickened and irregular wall. Fluid to soft tissue attenuating material is completely filling the left tympanic bulla.

cases of tympanic bulla involvement, an increase in soft tissue opacity, thickening of the bulla wall, and bulla expansion may be present.

CT and MRI are excellent modalities for detecting nasopharyngeal polyps, as well as tympanic bulla changes, and differentiating them from other nasopharyngeal diseases.

CT features of feline nasopharyngeal polyps include a well-defined pedunculated mass with strong rim enhancement, a mass-associated stalk-like structure, and an asymmetric tympanic bulla wall thickening with expansion of the tympanic bulla[10] (fig. 13.15).

MRI features of feline nasopharyngeal polyps include a well-defined mass with strong rim enhancement, mass-associated stalk-like structure, and asymmetric tympanic bulla lesions. The polyps appear hyperintense on T2-weighted images, and hypo- to isointense on T1-weighted images.

Middle and inner ear diseases

Otitis media

In dogs, otitis media is most commonly associated with an extension of otitis externa through the tympanic membrane. However, in cats, otitis media is more commonly secondary to viral or bacterial upper airway infections with secondary extension through the auditory tube. For examination of otitis media, radiography may be useful and indicated in cases of chronic otitis externa where the tympanic membrane cannot be clearly visualized or when there is clinical suspicion of otitis media even with a tympanic membrane that appears to be intact. The most useful radiographic projections include open-mouth rostrocaudal, DV or VD, and oblique laterals (i.e., left 30-degree dorsal right ventral or right 30-degree ventral left dorsal).

Radiography is not sensitive for middle ear disease in dogs and may result in false-negative diagnosis in approximately 25-40% of cases. In chronic cases, the most common radiographic findings are increased soft tissue opacity within the tympanic bulla, thickening and sclerosis of the tympanic bulla wall, new bone formation surrounding the tympanic bulla, lysis of the tympanic bulla wall and petrous temporal bone, para-aural soft tissue swelling and, less frequently, expansion of the affected tympanic bulla or presence of a nasopharyngeal mass (i.e., cats with a nasopharyngeal polyp) (fig. 13.16).

For a better examination of otitis media, CT and MRI are highly recommended. CT features of otitis media in earlier phases include the presence of soft tissue and/or fluid within the tympanic bulla and irregular thickening and enhancement of the tympanic bulla lining. In later stages, the tympanic bulla wall may become thickened and irregular, the bulla may expand, and there may lysis/erosion of the bulla wall (fig. 13.17).

MRI findings associated with otitis media in acute cases include the presence of fluid, which is hypo- to isointense on T1-weighted images and hyperintense on T2-weighted images, and irregular thickening and contrast enhancement of the mucosal lining of the bulla (fig. 13.18). In chronic cases, the fluid within the lumen becomes more proteinaceous, and there may be more tissue proliferation within the tympanic bulla. There may be expansion of the bulla, non-uniform and irregular thickening of the tympanic bulla wall, and lysis/erosions.

Otitis interna

Otitis interna is usually a consequence of extension of otitis media into the inner ear. The infection may progress by direct extension through osteolysis of the petrous temporal bone or through the internal acoustic meatus. Otitis interna cannot be diagnosed radiographically, and CT and/or MRI are necessary to evaluate the inner ear. CT can be used to assess the petrous temporal bone, including the region of the inner ear (i.e., cochlea, vestibule, and semicircular labyrinths), searching for lysis and may show evidence of brainstem involvement in post-contrast images (fig. 13.19).

SECTION III AXIAL SKELETON

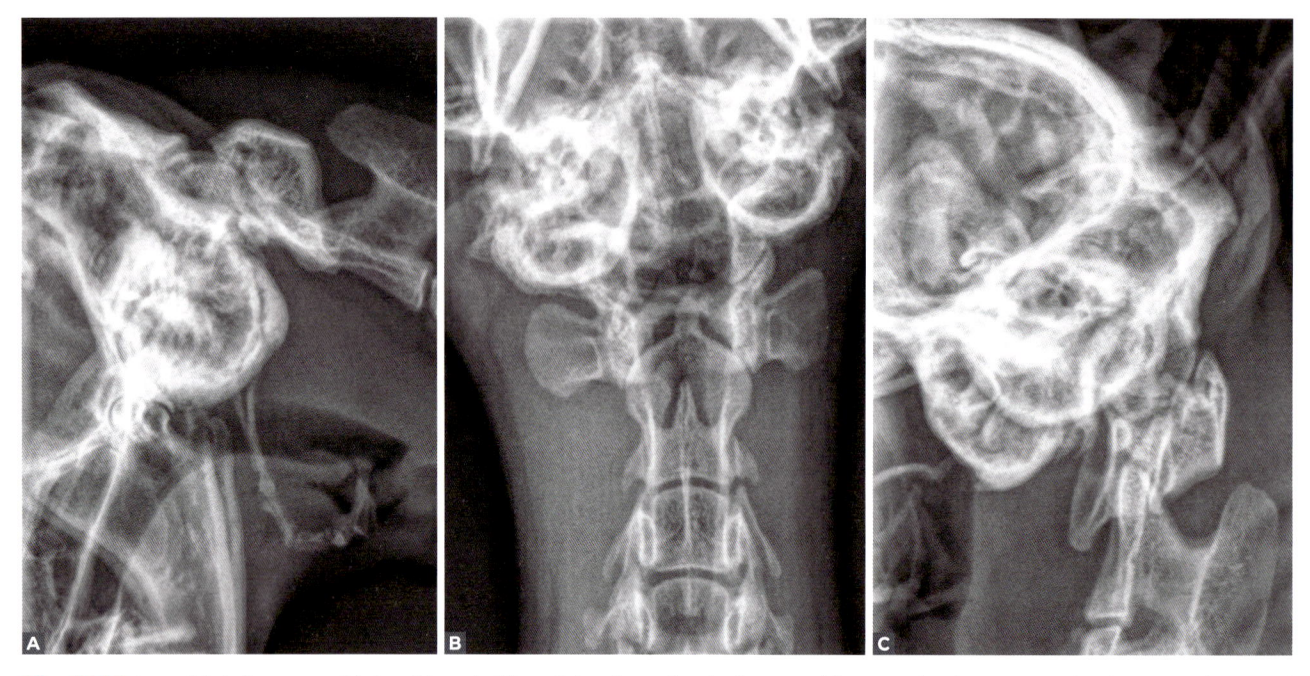

Fig. 13.16 Lateral (A), dorsoventral (B) and lateral oblique (C) radiographs of a five-year-old neutered male Domestic shorthair cat with bilateral chronic otitis media. There is marked sclerosis and nonuniform, but well-defined thickening of the wall of both tympanic bullae (R>L). The tympanic bullae are increased in soft tissue opacity.

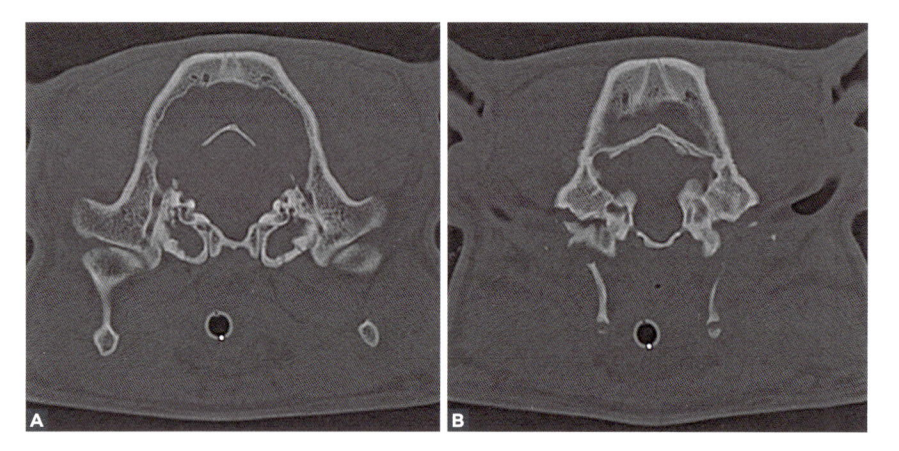

Fig. 13.17 Pre-contrast transverse CT images with a bone algorithm of a five-year-old neutered male French Bulldog with bilateral chronic otitis externa and media. (A) Both tympanic bullae are completely filled with soft tissue attenuating material, and the walls are thickened with mildly irregular internal margins. Multiple tympanic bulla wall erosions are seen as thin hypoattenuating lines. (B) There is a moderate amount of fluid to soft tissue attenuating material partially filling the lumen of the horizontal portion of the external ear canals. The walls of both external ear canals are partially mineralized.

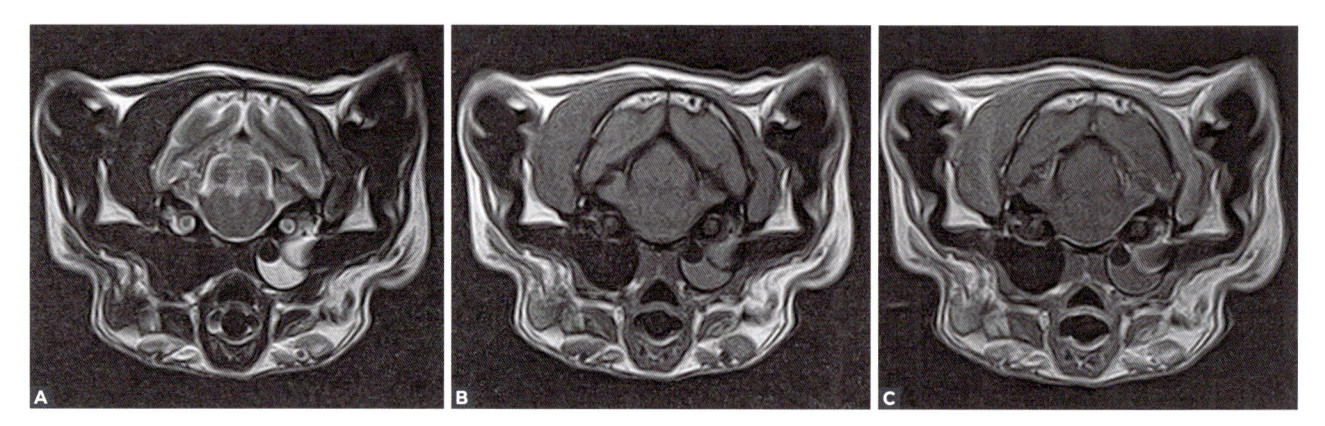

Fig. 13.18 Transverse T2-weighted (A), pre- (B) and post-contrast (C) T1-weighted images of an eight-year-old neutered male Domestic shorthair cat with left-sided otitis media and meningitis. Both compartments of the left tympanic bulla are almost completely filled with T2 hyperintense and T1 hypointense non-contrast enhancing fluid material. The mucosal lining of the left tympanic bulla is diffusely enhancing. In addition, there is mild diffuse thickening and enhancement of the meninges especially along the ventral and left ventral aspects of the neurocranium.

Fig. 13.19 Pre-contrast transverse CT image with a bone algorithm of a 12-year-old spayed female Chinese Crested with chronic otitis media and otitis interna. The right tympanic bulla is filled with homogeneous soft tissue attenuating material. The wall of the tympanic bulla is thickened and smoothly marginated. A lytic lesion is seen in the right petrous temporal bone involving the vestibule and semicircular labyrinth.

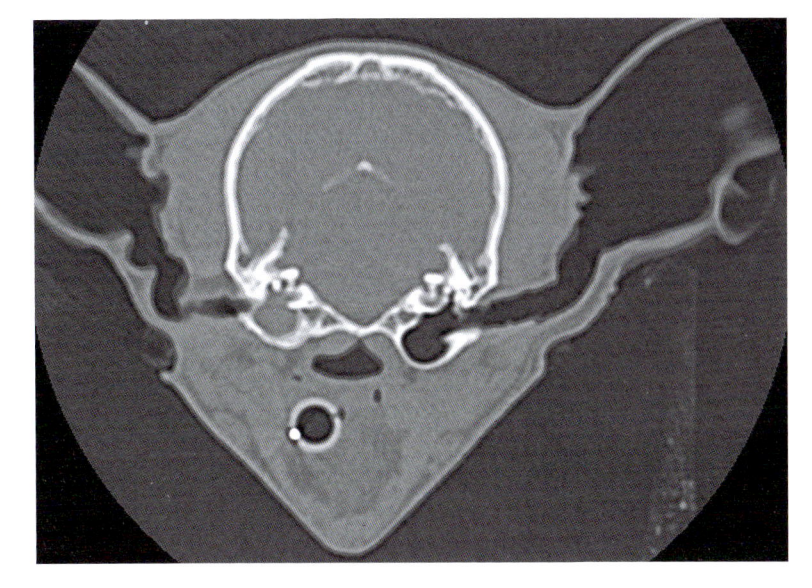

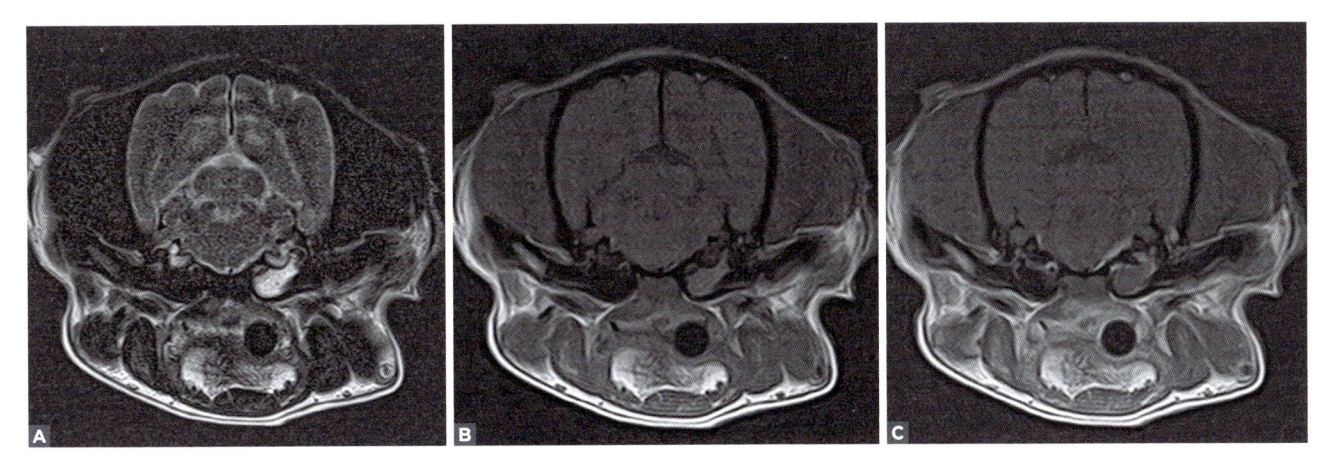

Fig. 13.20 Transverse T2-weighted (**A**), pre- (**B**) and post-contrast (**C**) T1-weighted images of a nine-year-old spayed female Yorkshire Terrier with left-sided otitis media and interna. The left tympanic bulla is filled with T2 hyperintense, T1 iso- to mildly hyperintense, non-contrast enhancing material. The mucosal lining of the tympanic bulla is contrast enhancing. Contrast enhancement is seen within the left inner ear, and there is contrast enhancement of the adjacent meninges.

MRI is superior for evaluating the soft tissue structures of the inner ear including the endolymph and perilymph, and the cranial nerves VII (facial) and VIII (vestibulocochlear). MRI findings associated with acute otitis interna include contrast enhancement of the labyrinth on post-contrast T1-weighted images with normal signal intensity in T2-weighted images (**fig. 13.20**). In chronic cases, a decrease of the normal T2-weighted hyperintense signal of the vestibule and cochlea may be noticed, with minimal to none post-contrast enhancement on T1-weighted images. Meningeal and/or cranial nerve (VII and VIII) thickening and enhancement may be seen.

Bulla effusion

Unilateral or bilateral sterile bulla effusion may occur secondary to obstruction of the auditory tube or auditory tube dysfunction secondary to a disease affecting the nerve of the tensor veli palatini muscle, a small branch of the mandibular nerve, part of the trigeminal nerve. Tympanic bulla effusion has been observed ipsilaterally in dogs with trigeminal nerve disease in approximately 30% of the cases.[11] Bulla effusion must be differentiated from otitis media, although this can be challenging. On CT, bulla effusion will appear as non-contrast enhancing fluid attenuation within the tympanic bulla

SECTION III AXIAL SKELETON

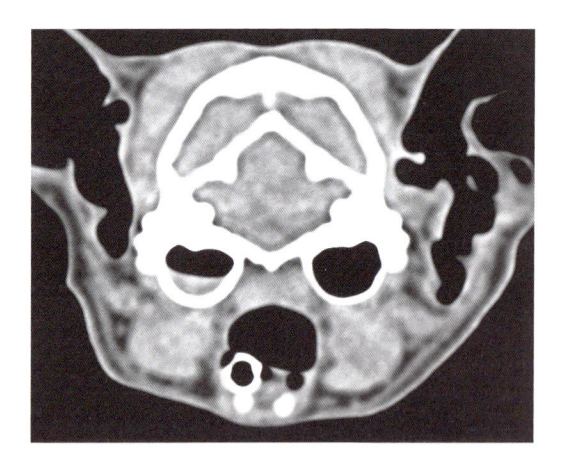

Fig. 13.21 Pre-contrast transverse CT image with a bone algorithm of a ten-year-old neutered male Domestic shorthair cat with a nasopharyngeal mass and secondary bulla effusion. Within the right tympanic bulla there is a moderate amount of fluid attenuating material with a fluid level. No contrast enhancement of the mucosa lining was noted on post-contrast images.

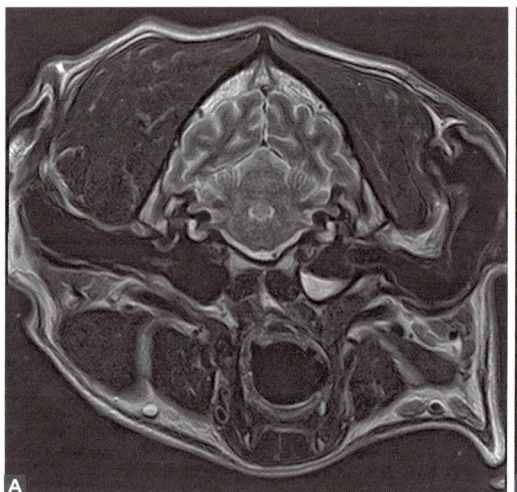

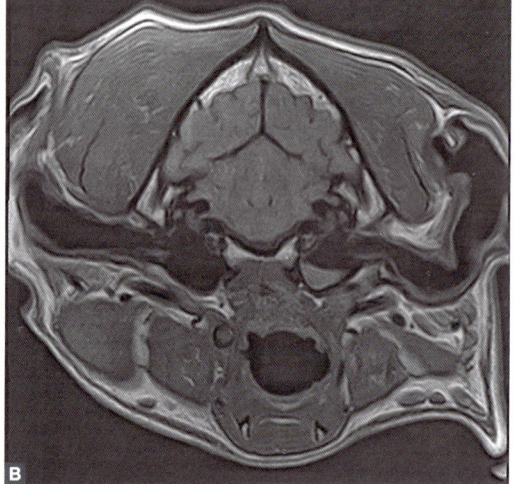

Fig. 13.22 Transverse T2-weighted (**A**), pre-contrast (**B**) T1-weighted images of a nine-year-old neutered male mixed breed dog with a left-sided trigeminal nerve sheath tumor and secondary bulla effusion. Within the dependent aspect of the left tympanic bulla there is a moderate amount of homogeneously T2 hyperintense and T1 hypointense fluid material with a fluid level. No contrast enhancement of the mucosa lining was noted on post-contrast images.

without other CT findings (**fig. 13.21**). On MRI, it will appear hyperintense on T2-weighted images and hypo- to hyperintense on T1-weighted images (**fig. 13.22**). With MRI, otitis media may be differentiated from bulla effusion since with otitis media, there will be contrast enhancement of the mucosal lining of the tympanic bulla.

Neoplasia

Neoplasms of the auricular structures are relatively uncommon in dogs and cats. Most of the auricular neoplasms originate from the external ear canal. Neoplasia within the middle and internal ear is much less common and is typically the result of direct extension of a neoplasm from a more lateral compartment. In dogs, approximately 60% of ear tumors are malignant. About 85% of auricular tumors are malignant in cats, and the most common type are ceruminous gland carcinoma, SCC, or undifferentiated carcinoma.

Radiographic findings of auricular neoplasia include swelling of the para-aural soft tissues, obliteration of the ear canal, displacement of the fascial planes, increased soft tissue opacity within the tympanic bulla, lysis and expansion of the bulla, lysis of the adjacent bony structures, and irregular and ill-defined new bone formation surrounding the bulla (**fig. 13.23**).

CT and MRI are much more sensitive modalities for the identification and assessment of auricular neoplasms. CT and MRI findings associated with malignant ear tumors include mass effect to the soft tissues with potential obliteration of the external ear canal, lysis of the adjacent bones, lysis of the bulla and the petrous and squamous part of the temporal bone, marked heterogeneous contrast enhancement and irregular and ill-defined new bone formation (**fig. 13.24**).

CHAPTER **13** Diseases of the skull

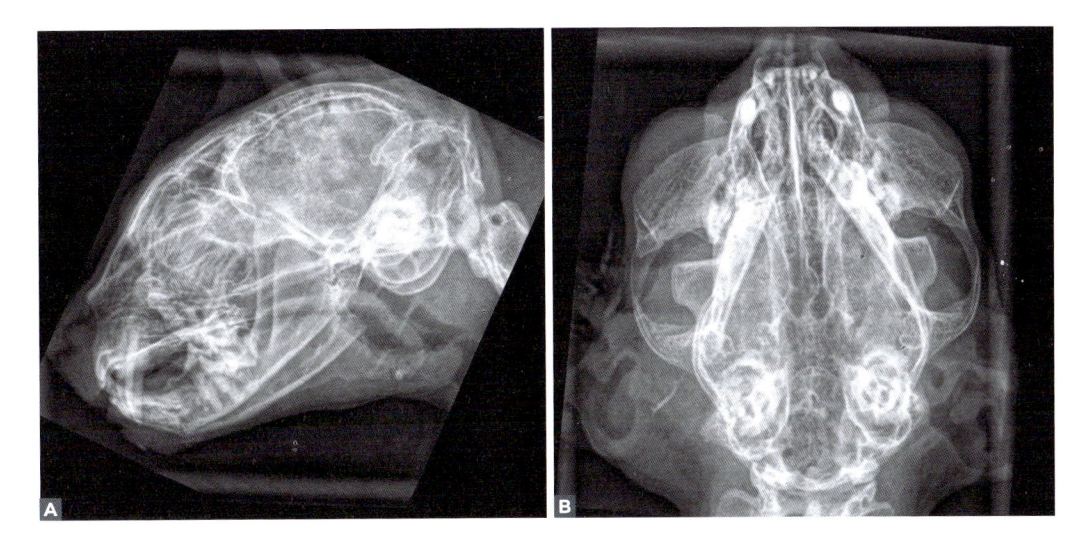

Fig. 13.23 Lateral (**A**) and dorsoventral (**B**) radiographs of a 12-year-old neutered male Domestic shorthair cat with a right-sided ceruminous gland adenocarcinoma. (**A**) There is a retropharyngeal soft tissue swelling ventrally to the atlantooccipital joint with narrowing of the nasopharynx and laryngopharynx. (**B**) A severe soft tissue swelling is noted on the right caudal aspect of the skull, centered at the external ear canal. The lumen of the right ear auricular canal is obliterated. A linear mineralization is also noted within the swelling. The lateral margin of the petrous part of the right temporal bone is irregular and ill-defined.

Fig. 13.24 CT transverse images with a bone (**A**) and a soft tissue algorithm (**B**) pre-contrast, and (**C**) post-contrast, and post-contrast dorsal (**D**) multiplanar reconstruction with a soft tissue algorithm of a 12-year-old spayed female mixed breed dog with a right-sided ceruminous gland adenocarcinoma. Centered on the right external ear canal and tympanic bulla there is an ill-defined, heterogeneously attenuating and contrast enhancing, lobular, locally expansive mass with osteolysis of the caudal and lateral aspects of the tympanic bulla, and petrous temporal bone.

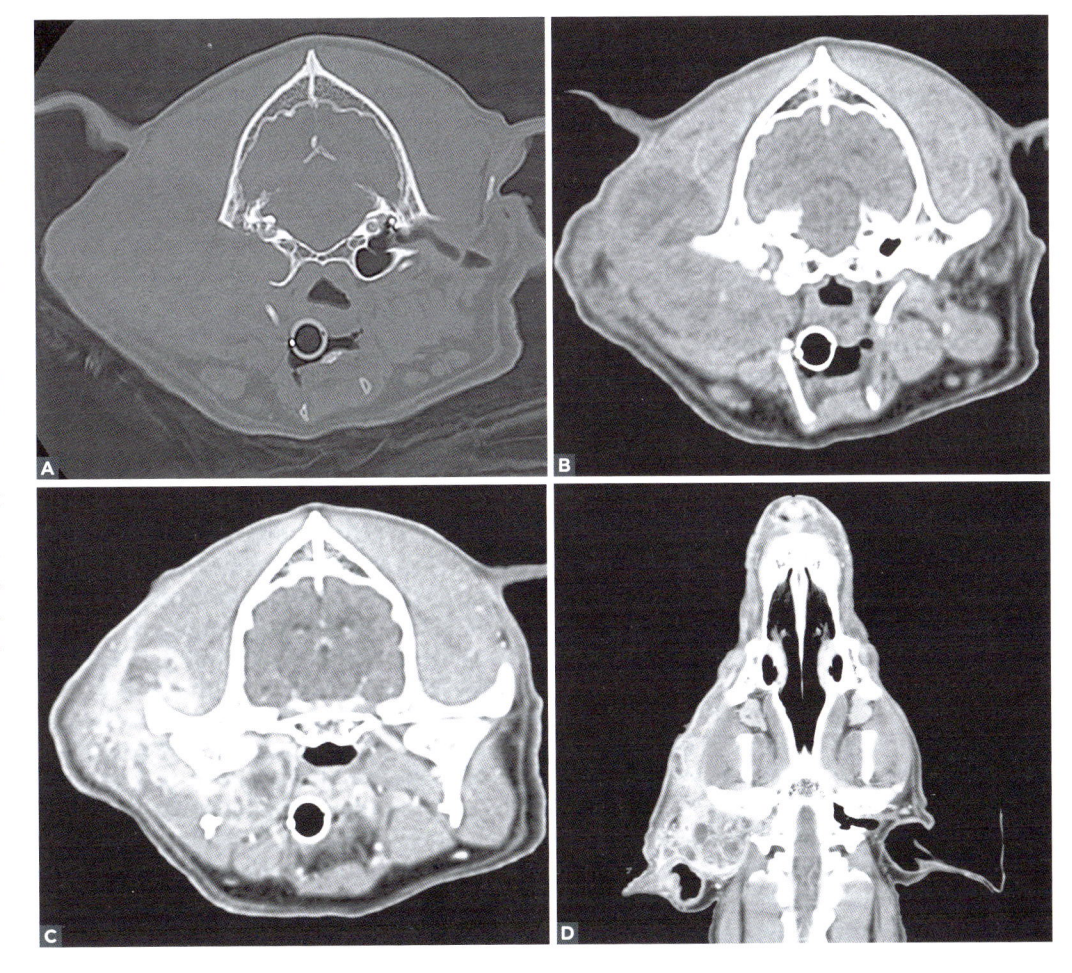

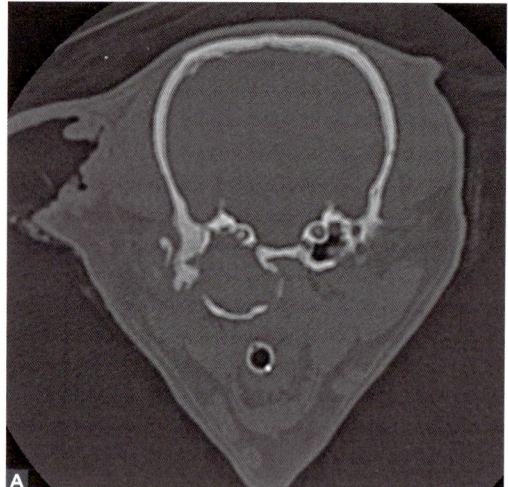

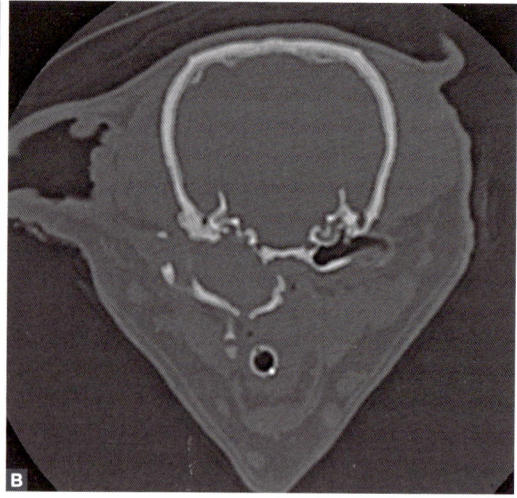

Fig. 13.25 Pre-contrast transverse CT images with a bone algorithm (A-B) of an 11-year-old spayed female Chihuahua with a right-sided cholesteatoma. The right tympanic cavity is severely expanded and filled by a soft tissue attenuating, non-contrast enhancing material causing multifocal osteolysis of the tympanic bulla wall. There is osteolysis of the ipsilateral tympanic and petrous parts of the temporal bone. There is obliteration of the right auditory ossicles and ventrolateral aspect of the inner ear, vestibule, and cochlea. The right temporal bone is increased in thickness and is sclerotic.

Aural cholesteatomas

Aural cholesteatomas are acquired epidermoid cysts originating from the tympanic bulla. They are non-neoplastic, slowly growing, cystic structures composed of a central cavity of keratin debris surrounded by keratinizing, stratified squamous epithelium. Aural cholesteatomas are mostly seen in dogs, although they have been described in cats.

Radiography can be used for the evaluation of cholesteatomas; however, MRI and especially CT are particularly useful in making the diagnosis. Radiographically cholesteatomas result in increased soft tissue opacity within the tympanic bulla, expansion of the tympanic bulla, thinning and irregularity of the tympanic bulla wall, bulla wall lysis, and surrounding ill-defined new bone formation.

CT appearance of cholesteatomas has been reported, being characterized by an expansile, tympanic cavity mass of soft tissue attenuation with non-contrast enhancing contents, variable peripheral ring enhancement, tympanic bulla wall lysis, proliferation and osteosclerosis, and sclerosis or osteoproliferation of the ipsilateral TMJ and paracondylar process[12] (fig. 13.25). Cholesteatomas can cause lysis of the petrosal part of the temporal bone.

With MRI, heterogeneous and non-contrast enhancing material may be noted within the lumen of the tympanic bulla with expansion. Secondary meningitis may also be diagnosed with MRI.

Multilobular osteochondrosarcoma

Multilobular osteochondroma (MLO), also known as multilobular tumor of bone, multilobular osteosarcoma, or chondroma rodens, is a rare malignant tumor that arise from the skull. This tumor is far more common in dogs than in cats. It has a predilection for the temporal and occipital bones, but can affect the orbit, zygomatic arch, maxilla, mandible, and hard palate. This tumor grows slowly and is locally invasive. Recurrence after attempted surgical excision is common.

MLO has typical radiographic characteristics appearing as a well-defined mass with nodular or stippled mineralized opacity, giving a "popcorn" appearance, and variable lysis of underlying bone with extension or expansion within the cranium (fig. 13.26).

CT and/or MRI are necessary to determine the degree of internal extension and potential compression of the intracranial structures. CT shows better the bony components of the mass; however, MRI is more sensitive to determine the overall extent of the mass and the intracranial changes, such as brain edema. Both imaging modalities are useful for surgical planning.

CHAPTER **13** Diseases of the skull

Fig. 13.26 Lateral (**A**), rostro-caudal (**B**) and lateral oblique (**C**) radiographs of a nine-year-old spayed female Soft-Coated Wheaten terrier with calvarial multilobular osteosarcoma. In the soft tissues adjacent to the left parietal bone there is a large, oval, ill-defined soft tissue mass, with multifocal areas of mineralization having a "popcorn" appearance. Well-defined lysis of the parietal bone is present, which is bordered by sharply marginated, well-defined osseous proliferation. The left maxillary fourth premolar is absent.

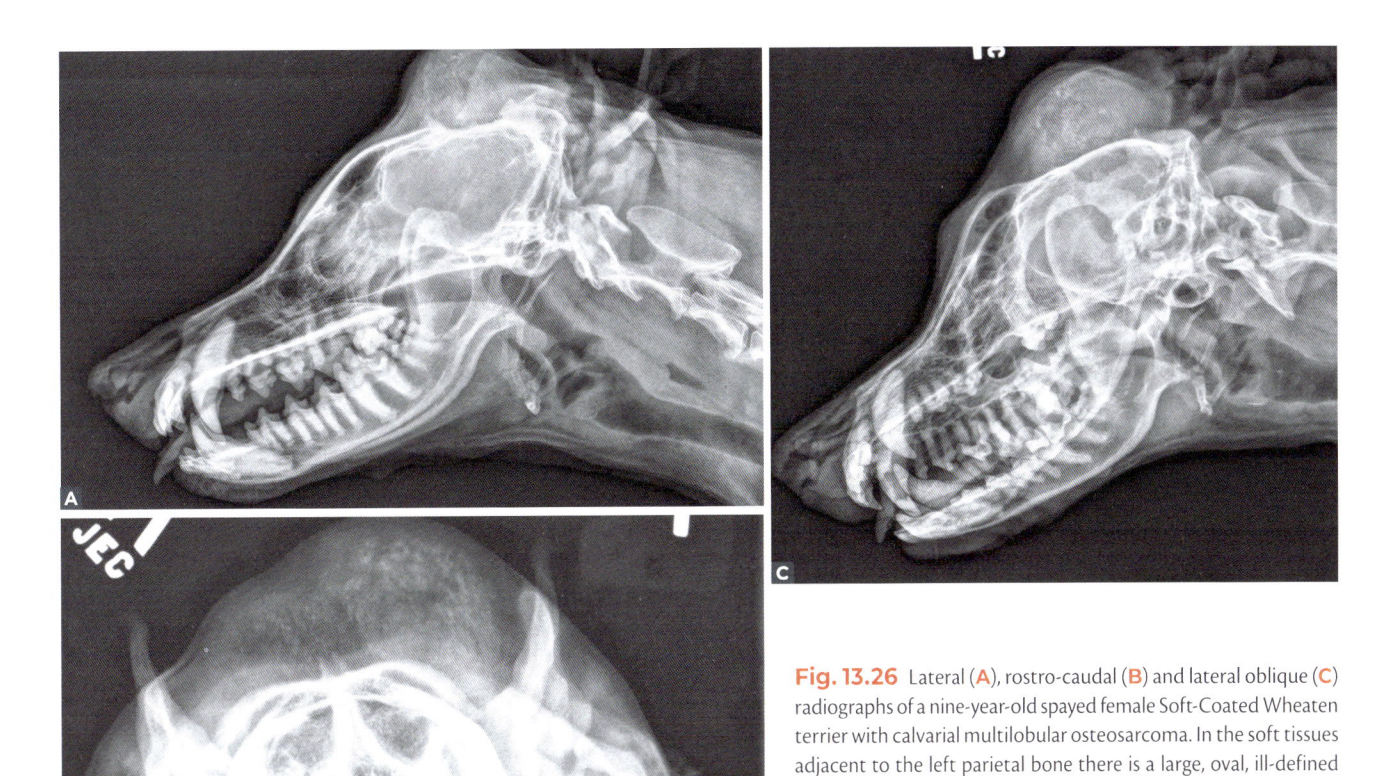

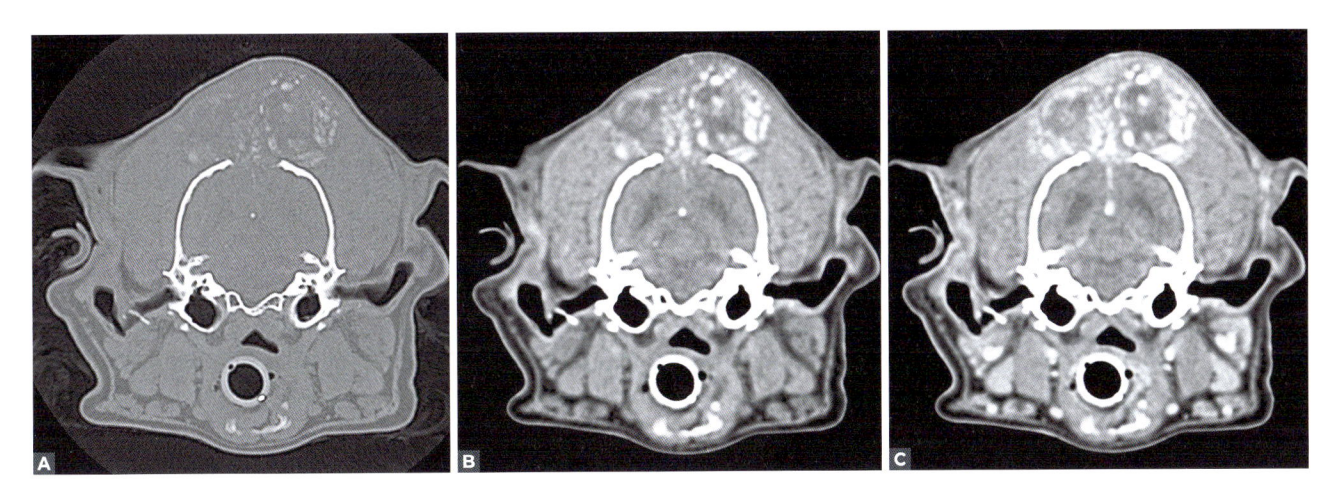

Fig. 13.27 CT transverse images with a bone (**A**) and a soft tissue algorithm (**B**) pre-contrast, and (**C**) post-contrast of the same dog as in fig. 13.26. There is an oval, lobulated, soft tissue mass with multiple punctate mineral attenuating structures within having a mineral stippled appearance, located adjacent to the central portion of the parietal bone. Mild peripheral contrast enhancement is noted. Well-marginated lysis of the parietal bone is present. This mass does not have an intracalvarial mass effect.

CT features of MLO include a round, well-defined, irregularly marginated mass with coarse and heterogeneous granular mineral attenuation, a mineral stippled appearance, and mild contrast enhancement (**fig. 13.27**). They frequently expand into the calvarium or the orbit, causing a marked mass effect. The MRI features of MLO include a mixed-signal intensity in T1-weighted, T2-weighted, and proton-weighted images with fairly large areas of post-contrast enhancement on T1-weighted images. These tumors are mostly T1- and T2-weighted hypointense.

Traumatic injury

Cranial fractures

Cranial fractures are the main type of injury related to head trauma, usually secondary to vehicle accidents, falls, bite wounds, gunshots, or other blunt trauma. Maxillary and mandibular fractures are more common than calvarial fractures. Radiographic examination is indicated for evaluating fractures, especially those affecting the mandibles.

Radiographic signs associated with calvarial fractures may include soft tissue swelling at the fracture site, subcutaneous emphysema, and visible fracture lines (**fig. 13.28**). Fractures may be simple or comminuted and depressed. Fracture lines may only be visible if the fracture line is oriented parallel to the X-ray beam. Overlapping fractures and fracture fragments may result in increased mineral opacity. Depressed fractures of the frontal sinuses are commonly associated with extensive subcutaneous emphysema. Depression fractures of the calvarium are generally associated with a worse prognosis due to the injury to the underlying brain. It is important to distinguish normal skull sutures and vascular channels from nondisplaced calvarial fractures. Fracture lines will be asymmetrical while suture lines are symmetrical (**fig. 13.29**). Fracture lines can also show tapering or widening at one end of the radiolucent line, in contrast to suture lines. Oblique and skyline radiographic projections may be necessary to show depression fractures.

CT and MRI are necessary for the examination of intracranial injuries such as brain contusions, hemorrhage, and epidural, subdural, or subarachnoid hematomas (**fig. 13.30**). CT has been shown to identify more traumatic injuries of the skull than radiography in dogs and cats (**fig. 13.31**). There is general agreement that CT is the modality of choice to evaluate the patient with acute head trauma. CT will provide a better assessment of the bone, traumatic brain injury, brain swelling, and brain herniation, and allows the creation of 3D reconstructions that are very useful for fracture assessment and surgical planning (**fig. 13.32**). Acute hemorrhage is readily identified on CT. MRI is superior for complete assessment of brain trauma. Regions of brain edema would be seen as hyperintense on T2-weighted and FLAIR images. For evaluation of hemorrhage, the T2* gradient echo sequence is the most sensitive since it will show areas of susceptibility where blood degradation products are present. With MRI, negative prognostic indicators in dogs with head trauma include the degree of

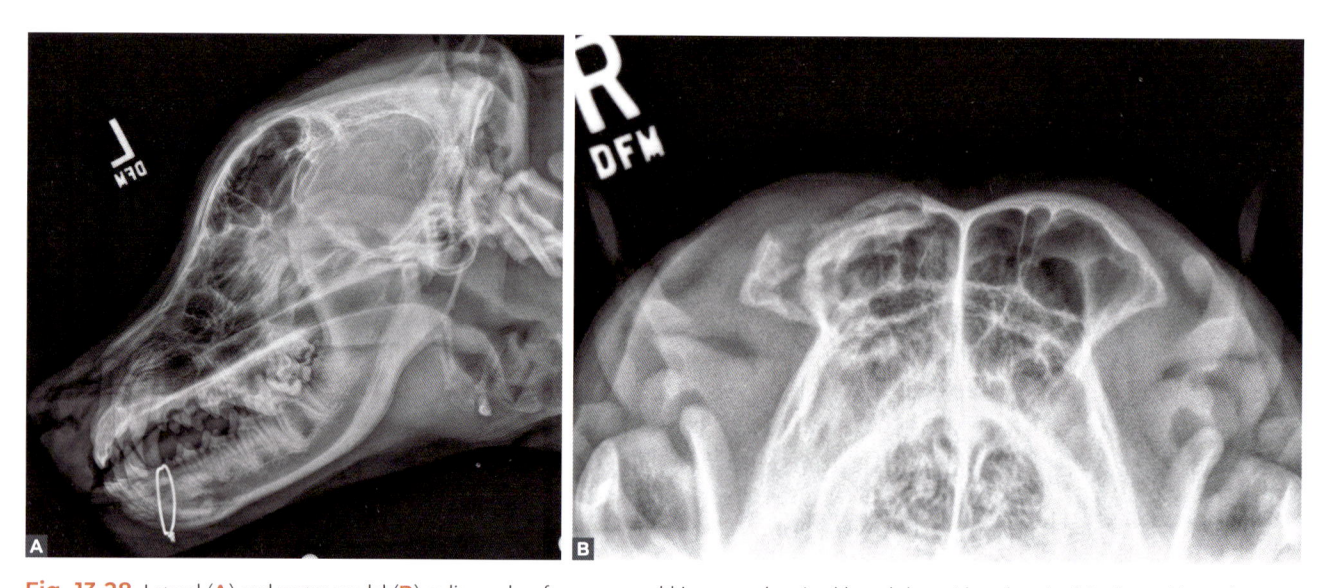

Fig. 13.28 Lateral (**A**) and rostrocaudal (**B**) radiographs of a one-year-old intact male mixed breed dog with a chronic right frontal bone fracture. Associated with the right frontal bone at the level of the frontal sinus there is a comminuted fracture with mildly ill-defined margins, and a mild amount of ill-defined new bone formation. There is moderate soft tissue thickening overlying the right frontal sinus at the fracture site. A cerclage wire is present at the rostral mandible.

CHAPTER **13** Diseases of the skull

Fig. 13.29 Lateral oblique (**A**) and lateral (**B**) radiographs of a five-year-old intact male Jack Russel Terrier that was hit by a car. (**A**) A depression fracture of the left parietal bone is noted. (**B**) Multiple fracture lines can be seen extending ventrally. Soft tissue swelling overlies the fracture site.

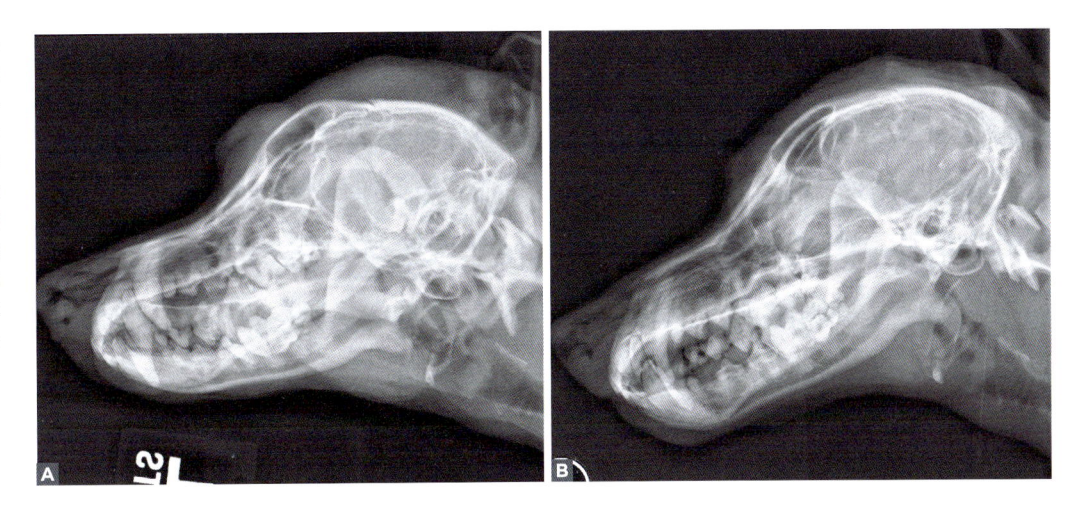

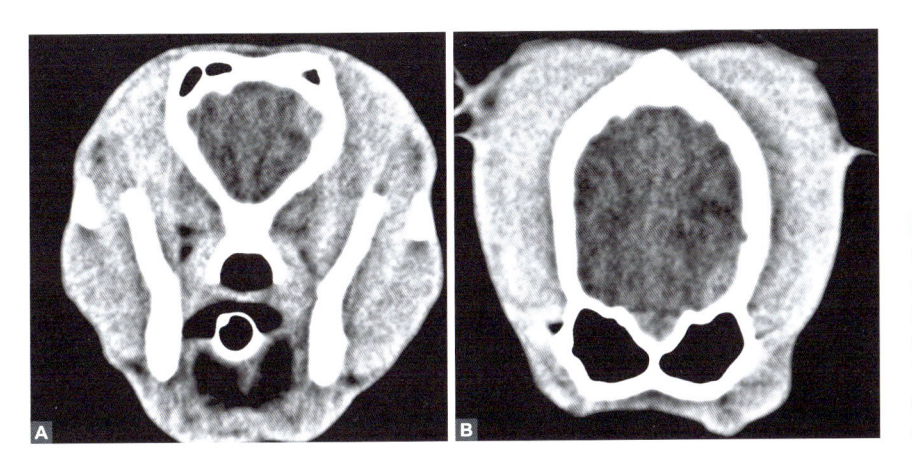

Fig. 13.30 Pre-contrast CT transverse image with a brain algorithm (**A**) and pre-contrast dorsal (**B**) multiplanar reconstruction with a brain algorithm of the same dog as in fig. 13.29 showing a large, acute, subdural hematoma. There is a broad base extra-axial hyperattenuating lesion identified on the left dorsolateral aspect of the frontal bone.

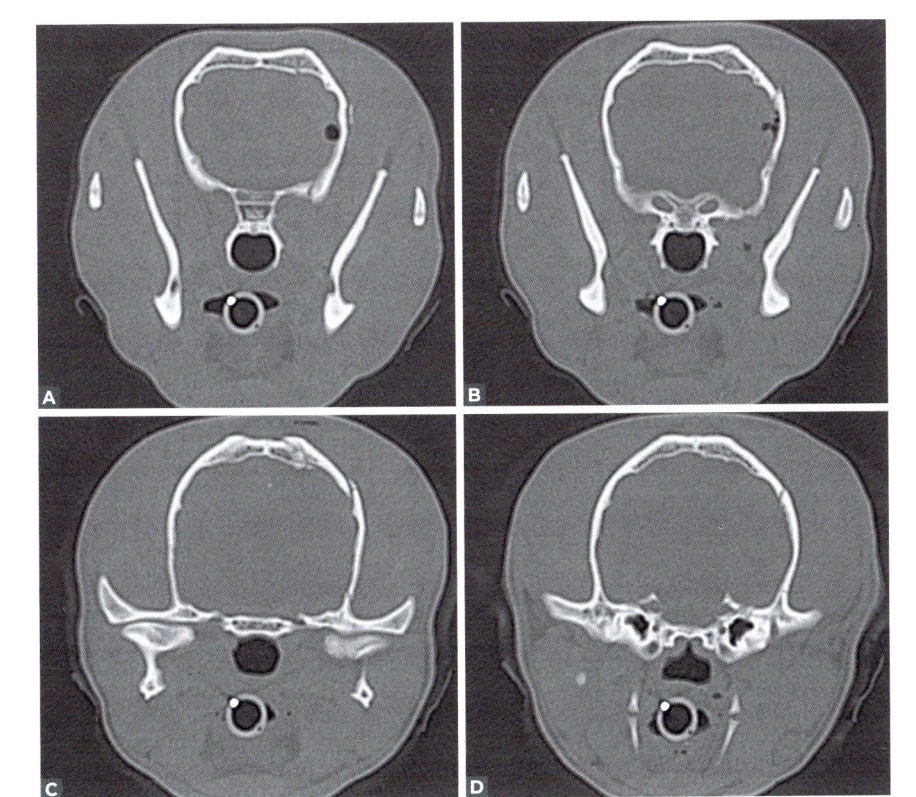

Fig. 13.31 Pre-contrast transverse CT images with a bone algorithm (**A-D**) of the same dog as in fig. 13.29. Multiple skull fractures are identified in the left side of the skull. The main fracture line involves the left temporal and left parietal bones. There is minimal depression of the fracture at the level of the parietal bone with slight overlapping of the fracture fragments. Multiple gas bubbles are identified immediately adjacent to these skull fractures within the calvarium (i.e., pneumocephalus).

151

SECTION III AXIAL SKELETON

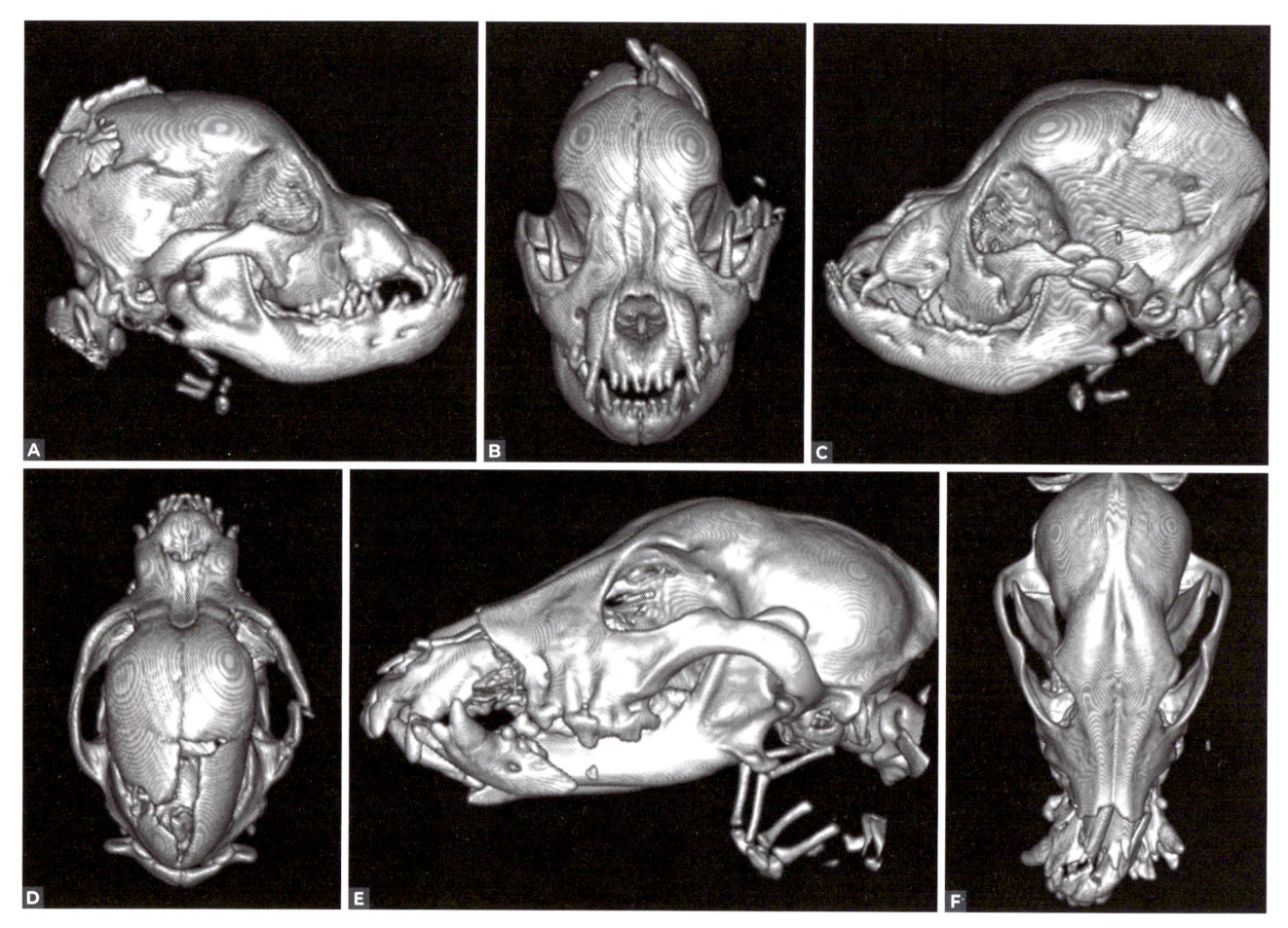

Fig. 13.32 3D reconstructions of a two-month-old female Boxer (**A-D**) attacked by another dog, and of a seven-year-old intact male Dachshund that got into a fight with a larger dog (**E-F**). (**A-D**) There are multiple calvarial fractures affecting the parietal and the occipital bones with variable degrees of comminution. Some of the fractures are depressed with displacement of multiple fragments into the cranial vault. (**E-F**) There are multiple comminuted fractures of the rostral mandible and maxilla.

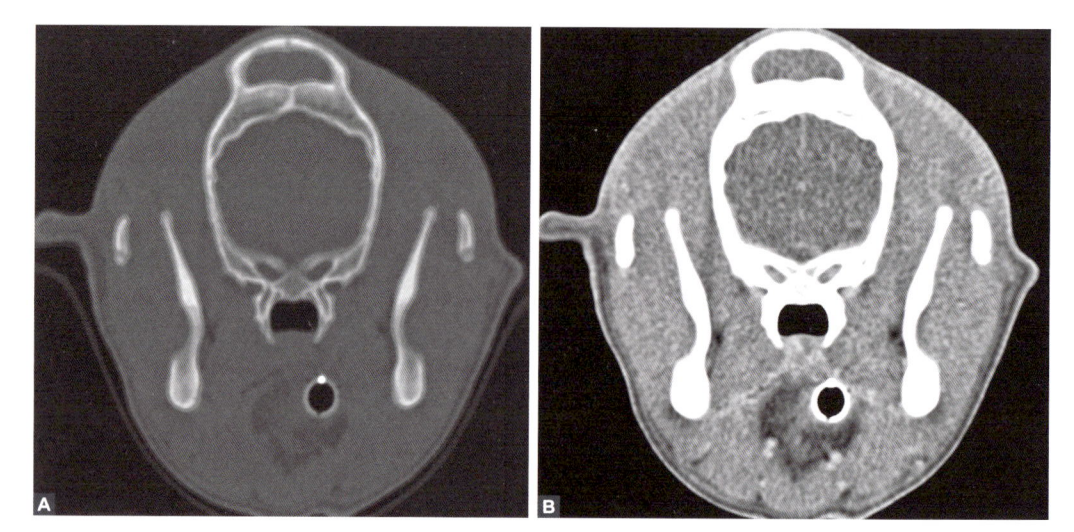

Fig. 13.33 CT transverse images with a soft tissue algorithm displayed in a bone window (**A**) and soft tissue window (**B**), post-contrast, of a five-month-old intact male mixed breed dog with a chronic hard swelling on the calvarium after unknown trauma, compatible with a subperiosteal hematoma. There is a fluid to soft tissue attenuating, non-contrast enhancing mass-like lesion with a thick, smoothly marginated peripheral mineralization dorsal to the frontal and parietal bones.

midline shift, the extent of the intraparenchymal edema and hemorrhage, the presence of brain herniation, and the presence of skull fractures, and injuries affecting the caudal fossa or both the rostral and caudal fossae. Gas may be present in the calvarium due to open trauma to the skull (i.e., pneumocephalus).

Calvarial subperiosteal hematoma

Subperiosteal hematomas may occur secondary to single or repetitive trauma to the calvarium. Calvarial subperiosteal hematomas are collections of extravasated blood between the periosteum and bone causing elevation of the periosteum. The formation of a subperiosteal hematoma can occur days to weeks after the traumatic incident. Radiographically these lesions are seen as a soft tissue swelling, which will later show periosteal reaction with a shell-like appearance. The most common location is dorsal to the frontal sinus and calvarium. CT findings include a fluid to soft tissue attenuating mass-like lesion with a thick, smoothly marginated peripheral mineralization[13] (**fig. 13.33**).

Craniomandibular osteopathy

Cranial mandibular osteopathy (CMO) is a self-limiting, non-neoplastic, proliferative bone disease that affects the skull and occasionally the long bones in young dogs between 3-8 months old. CMO affects mostly small breed dogs such as West Highland White Terrier, Scottish Terrier, and Cairn Terrier, and rarely large breed dogs. The etiology of this disease is unknown; however, it has been found that the condition in West Highland White Terriers has an autosomal recessive inheritance.[14] Radiography is an excellent imaging modality for the assessment of this disease. Radiographically, there is irregular and ill-defined periosteal new bone formation with a palisading appearance, along the mandibles (mandibular body, ramus and articular part of the mandible), the tympanic bullae and the petrous temporal bone (**fig. 13.34**). The amount and the extent of the new bone formation varies greatly between patients and is usually bilateral, but less often asymmetric or unilateral. Sometimes the calvarium and frontal bones may be affected with evidence of hyperostosis. Rarely, lesions similar to those seen in cases of metaphyseal osteopathy/hypertrophic osteodystrophy may be present in the limbs.

Fig. 13.34 Lateral radiograph of a seven-month-old intact female mixed breed shepherd dog with craniomandibular osteopathy. There is an irregular and ill-defined periosteal reaction with a palisading appearance along the mandibles, as well as thickening of the mandibular cortices. Mild soft tissue swelling is noted ventral to the region of periosteal reaction. There is no bone proliferation noted at the tympanic bullae.

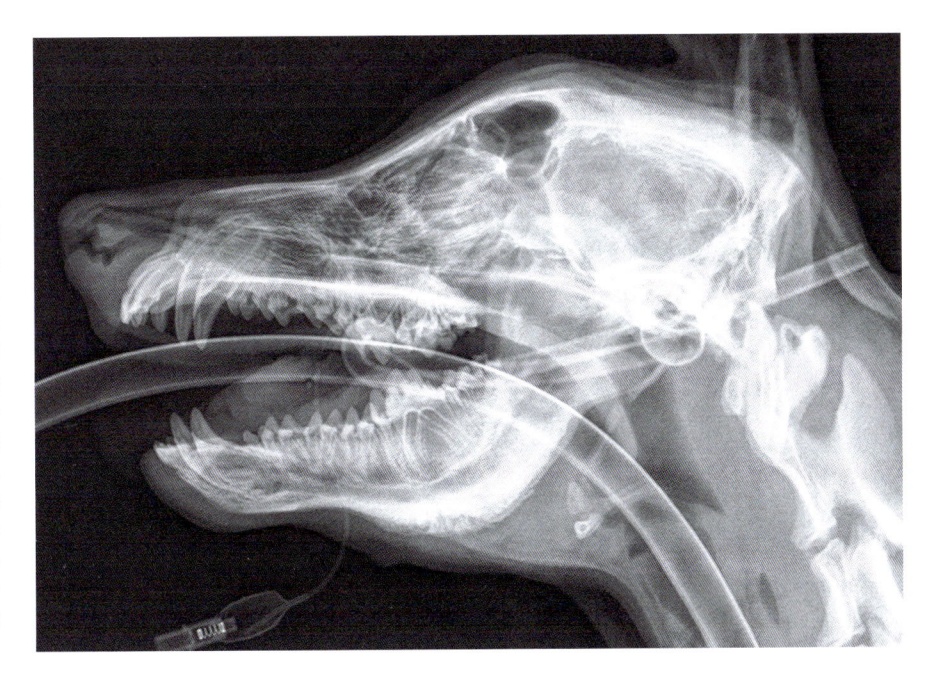

CT findings associated with CMO are similar to those described with radiography and include smooth and well-defined thickening of the mandible, tympanic bulla, petrous temporal bone and calvarium; irregular and ill-defined periosteal proliferation, possible extension of the new bone formation within the TMJs, and mild soft tissue swelling (**fig. 13.35**). Occasionally the new bone formation impinges on the TMJs, limiting jaw motion or even causing ankylosis. In such cases, assessment with CT is indicated to assess the extent of the TMJ involvement and for surgical planning (**fig. 13.36**).

Calvarial hyperostosis

Calvarial hyperostosis is a disease of juvenile large and giant breed dogs, characterized by bone proliferation similar to CMO, but mostly affecting the frontal and parietal bones. Calvarial hyperostosis has been mostly described in young (approximately 5-10 months old) Bullmastiffs of either sex, and

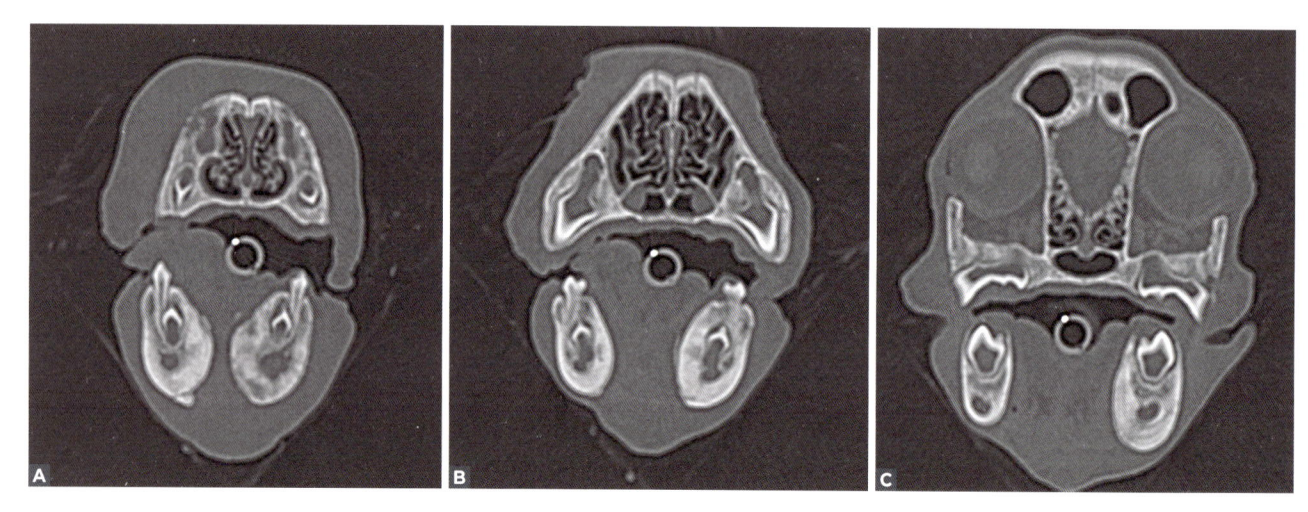

Fig. 13.35 Pre-contrast transverse CT images with a bone algorithm (**A-C**) of a four-month-old intact male West Highland White Terrier with craniomandibular osteopathy. There is asymmetric (L>R) smooth and well-defined thickening of the mandibular cortices, and a mild amount of smooth and ill-defined periosteal proliferation ventrally. The soft tissues overlying the rostral mandibles and maxilla (R>L) are moderately thickened.

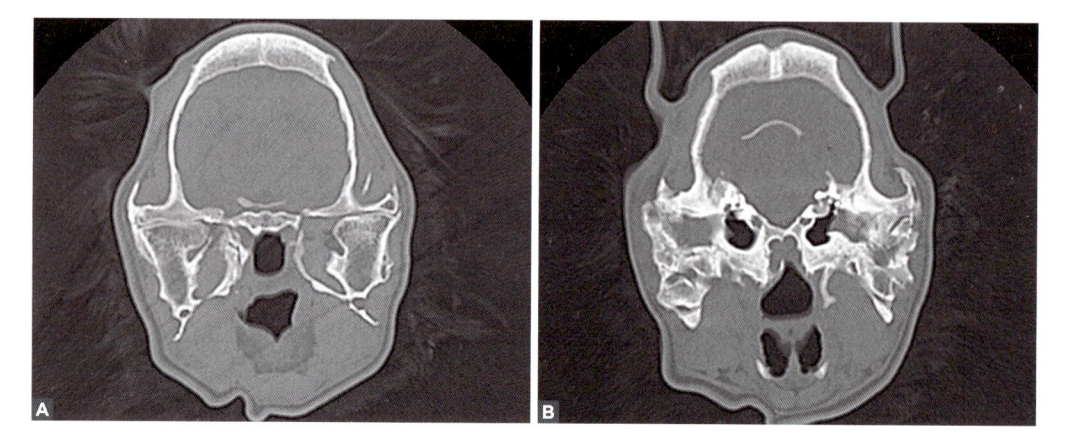

Fig. 13.36 Pre-contrast transverse CT images with a bone algorithm (**A-B**) of a two-year-old spayed female West Highland White Terrier with chronic craniomandibular osteopathy and difficulty opening the mouth. A severe amount of irregular but well-defined new bone formation is noted surrounding the temporomandibular joints, petrous part of the temporal bones, and tympanic bullae causing ankylosis of the temporomandibular joints. There is moderate to severe diffuse thickening of the dorsal aspect of the calvarium, compatible with calvarial hyperostosis. In addition, marked atrophy of the temporal and masseter muscles is also noted.

CHAPTER **13** Diseases of the skull

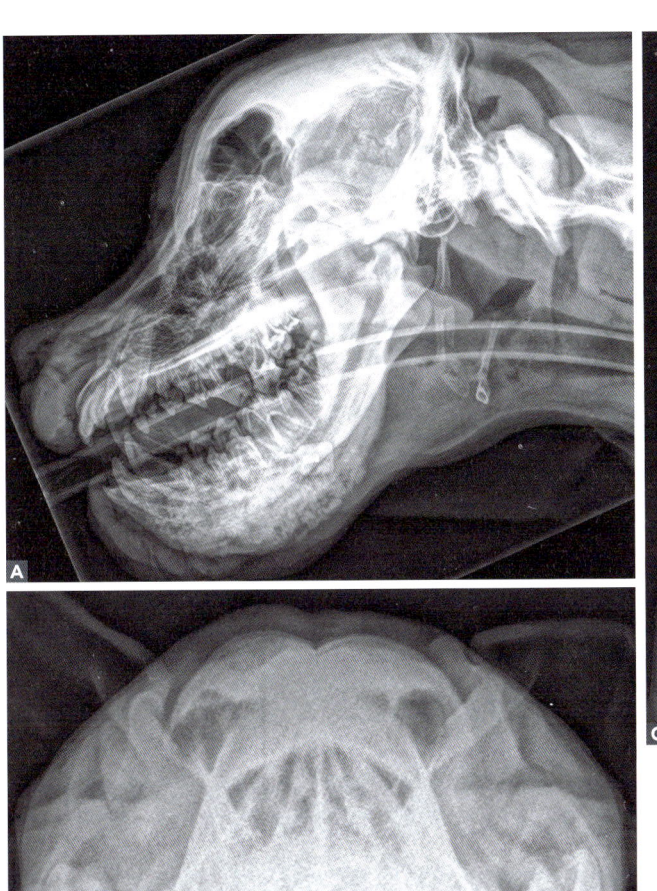

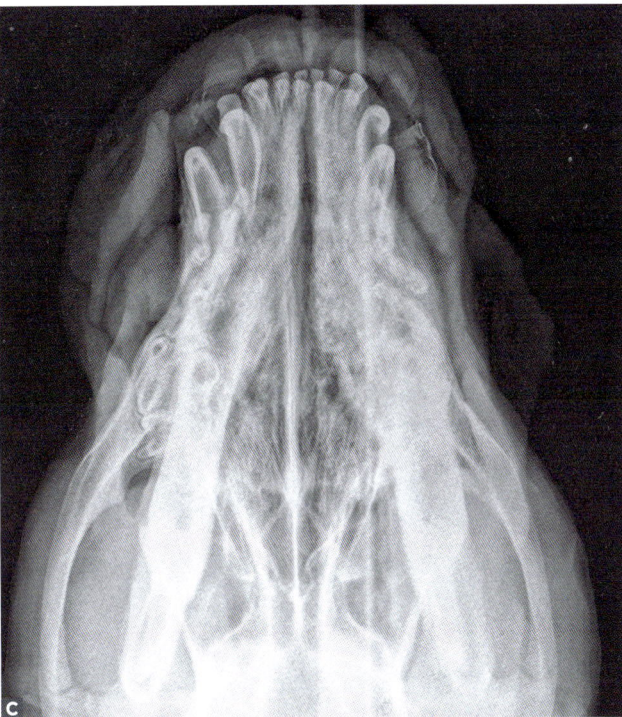

Fig. 13.37 Lateral (**A**), dorsoventral (**B**) and rostrocaudal (**C**) radiographs of a five-month-old intact male Bullmastiff with calvarial hyperostosis and craniomandibular osteopathy. There is marked and asymmetric thickening of the calvarial bones, more pronounced on the right side and better assessed on the rostrocaudal projection. Mild soft tissue swelling is also noted dorsal to the calvarium. In addition, there is an extensive and marked, asymmetric (L>R), irregular and ill-defined periosteal reaction with a palisading appearance along the ventral aspect of the mandibles.

the etiology is unknown. Clinical signs associated with this disease commonly regress with skeletal maturity and the bony lesions may disappear or persist.

Rostrocaudal and lateral radiographs are excellent for diagnosis and show exuberant bone proliferation with marked thickened and increased opacity of the calvarial bones, especially the frontal and parietal bones. Changes can be symmetrical or more often asymmetrical (**fig. 13.37**). As in CMO, lesions similar to those seen in cases of metaphyseal osteopathy/hypertrophic osteodystrophy may be seen.

CT and MRI can be used for further assessment, especially if neurological signs are present. Both modalities show thickening and sclerosis of the calvarial bones. The new bone formation can extend externally but also internally.

Temporomandibular joint subluxation, luxation and fracture

The TMJs are susceptible to dislocations and fractures, especially in cats. Dislocations may occur secondary to trauma and TMJ dysplasia. TMJ dislocation can be either complete luxation or subluxation. Malocclusion with lateral displacement of the mandible and inability to close the mouth are highly suggestive of unilateral or bilateral TMJ trauma. For the identification of temporomandibular dislocations, VD or DV and 20-degree lateral oblique radiographs are very useful. With these projections the relationship between the mandibular condyle and the mandibular fossa can be compared on both sides. Radiographically a TMJ luxation is seen as a rostro-dorsal displacement of the mandibular condyle with an empty mandibular fossa. The mandible will be displaced towards the opposite side (**fig. 13.38**). Oblique radiographic projections can be used to assess fractures of the mandibular condyle, mandibular fossa, and retroarticular process, but are technically quite challenging and must be adapted to the skull conformation of the patient.

In cases where the radiography does not confirm the presence of dislocations or fractures, CT is indicated. CT findings associated with TMJ luxation include an empty mandibular fossa, rostro-dorsal displacement of the mandibular condyle, and dental malocclusion with mandibular shift (**fig. 13.39**). With TMJ subluxation, an asymmetric joint space may be seen. Chronic cases may show TMJ degenerative joint disease. For assessment of subluxations, sagittal and dorsal plane reconstructions are helpful.

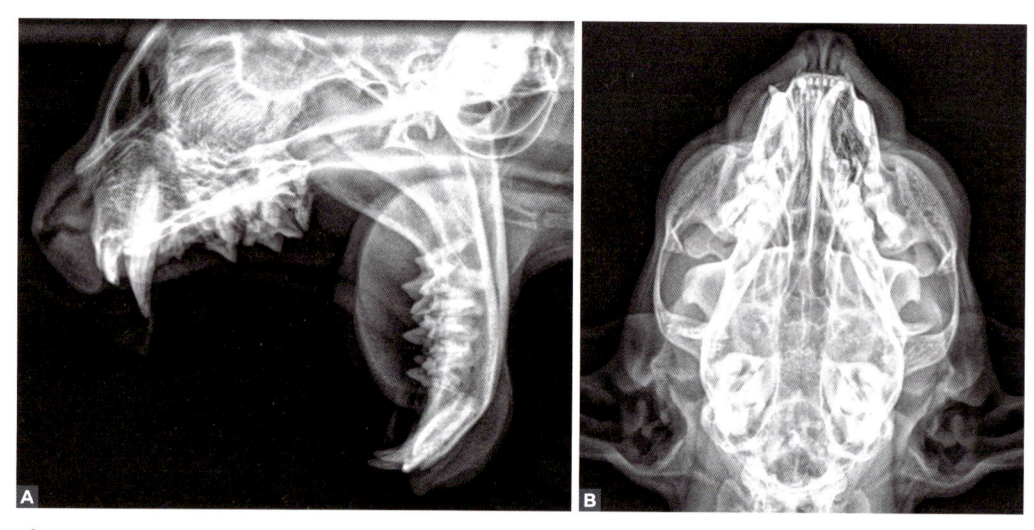

Fig. 13.38 Lateral (**A**) and dorsoventral (**B**) radiographs of a five-year-old neutered male Domestic shorthair cat with unknown trauma and a left-sided rostro-dorsal temporomandibular joint luxation. (**A**) One of the mandibular fossae is empty and the condylar process is luxated rostro-dorsally. (**B**) The left condylar process is luxated rostrally as compared with the right. In addition, there is dental malocclusion with the mandibles angled towards the right side.

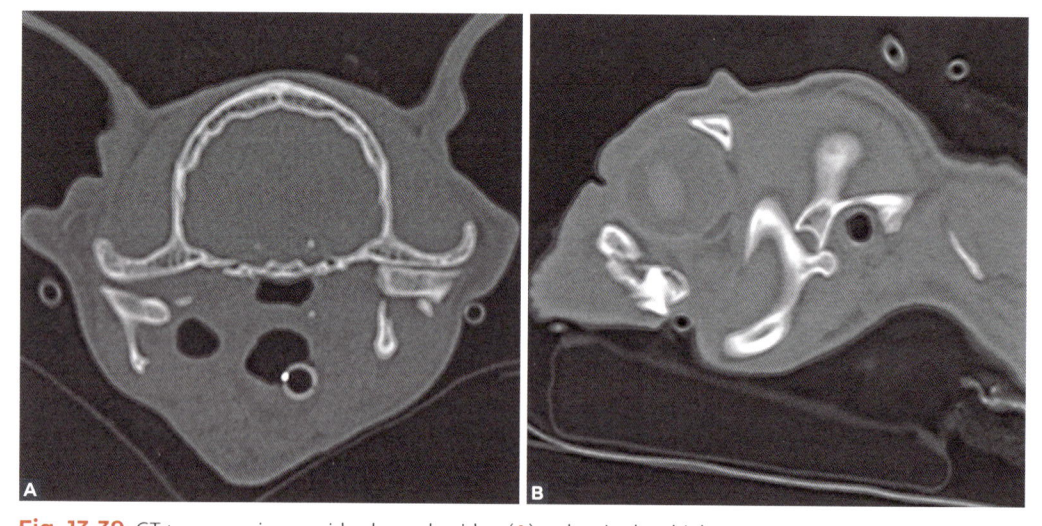

Fig. 13.39 CT transverse image with a bone algorithm (**A**) and sagittal multiplanar reconstruction with a bone algorithm (**B**) of a 13-year-old spayed female Domestic shorthair cat with a right-sided caudoventral temporomandibular joint luxation and a left-sided mandibular comminuted fracture of the left mandibular ramus immediately ventral to the condylar process. (**A**) The right temporomandibular joint space is severely widened with ventral displacement of the condylar process. Several fracture fragments and soft tissue swelling are noted ventrally to the left temporomandibular joint. (**B**) The right mandibular fossa is empty, and the condylar process is located caudoventrally.

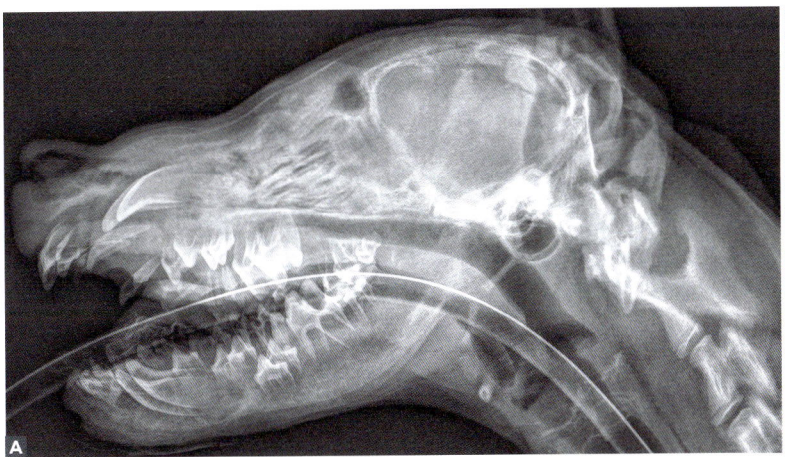

Fig. 13.40 Lateral (**A**) and dorsoventral (**B**) radiographs of a five-month-old intact male Siberian Husky with renal secondary hyperparathyroidism due to congenital renal dysplasia. There is marked osteopenia of the skull bones, more pronounced at the maxilla and mandibles, with complete loss of the lamina dura of the alveolar sockets, and the impression of "floating teeth". The visible nasal turbinates and ethmoturbinates are increased in soft tissue opacity and thickened. Mild soft tissue swelling is noted surrounding the maxilla.

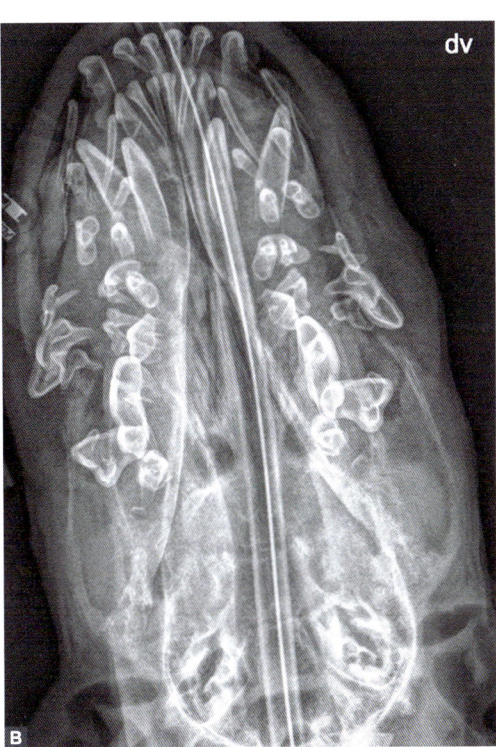

Renal secondary hyperparathyroidism: "rubber jaw"

Secondary hyperparathyroidism is usually due to dietary calcium deficiency or hypocalcemia resulting from renal disease. Renal secondary hyperthyroidism causes diffuse osteopenia affecting the skull more severely, and results in the clinical condition colloquially known as "rubber jaw" from loss of structural rigidity in the mandibles and maxilla, that become soft and pliable. In this disease the bone is absorbed and replaced by fibrous tissue and poorly organized woven bone. Renal secondary hyperparathyroidism is rare and can occur in young dogs with congenital renal dysplasia or hypoplasia, and in older dogs and cats with severe chronic kidney disease.

Radiographically, renal secondary hyperparathyroidism is seen as marked osteopenia of the skull with coarser trabeculation of the bone, more pronounced in the mandibles and maxilla, loss of the lamina dura of the alveolar bone, and increased lucency surrounding the tooth roots. The teeth retain normal opacity giving impression of "floating teeth". There is soft tissue swelling of the face from fibrous hyperplasia (**fig. 13.40**).

Brachycephalic obstructive airway syndrome

Brachycephalic breeds, such as English Bulldogs, French Bulldogs and Pugs, have anatomical abnormalities of the upper respiratory tract that may lead to increased negative pressure on inspiration and upper airway obstruction, known as brachycephalic airway syndrome. Primary components of the syndrome are stenotic nares, elongated soft palate, and possibly tracheal hypoplasia.

Radiography can be used to assess the soft palate and trachea in brachycephalic dogs with lateral radiographs of the neck and thorax. The soft palate can be assessed for thickness and elongation. The caudal aspect of the soft palate should not extend beyond the epiglottis (**fig. 13.41**).

SECTION III AXIAL SKELETON

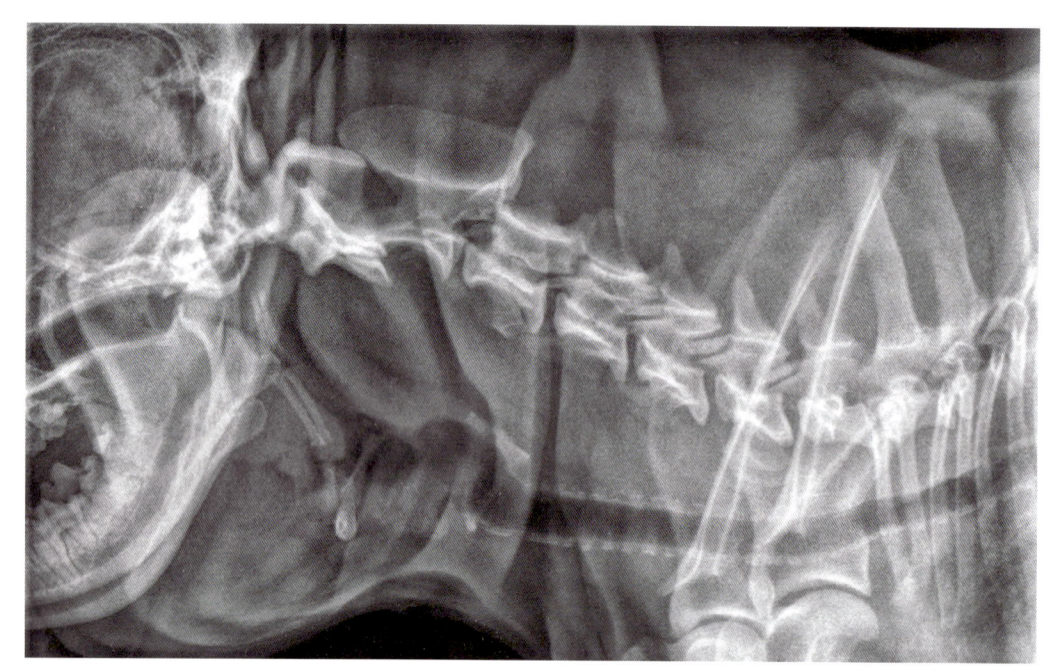

Fig. 13.41 Lateral radiograph of a one-year-old neutered male French Bulldog with brachycephalic obstructive airway syndrome. The soft palate is severely thickened and mildly elongated, extending caudally to the epiglottis. The nasopharynx and oropharynx are almost completely collapsed, with minimal gas seen within them.

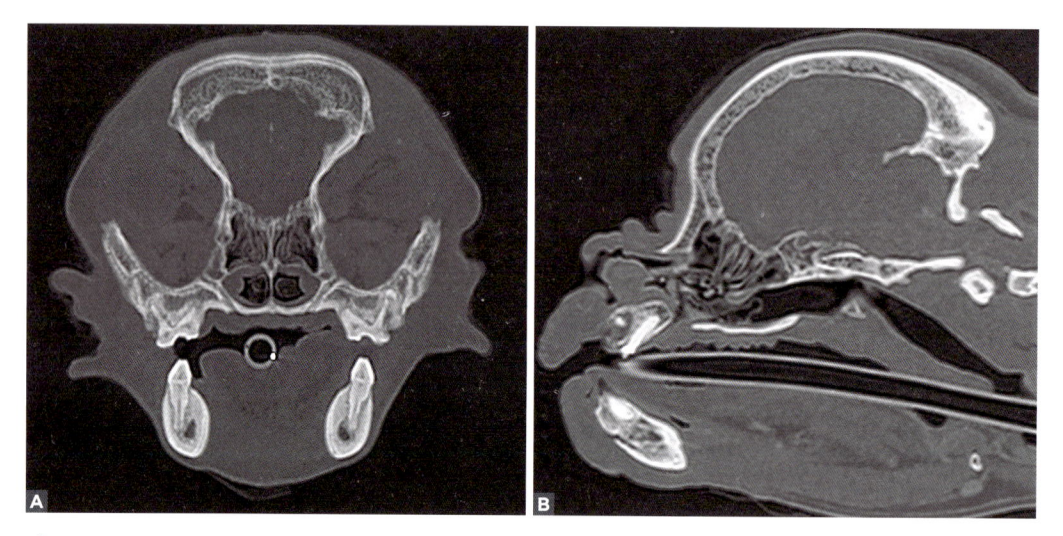

Fig. 13.42 CT transverse image with a bone algorithm (A) and sagittal multiplanar reconstruction with a bone algorithm (B) of a ten-year-old neutered male French Bulldog with brachycephalic obstructive airway syndrome. Caudal aberrant nasal turbinates are noted extending into the nasopharyngeal meatus and nasopharynx.

Another newly recognized component of the brachycephalic obstructive airway syndrome is the presence of aberrant nasal turbinates. Aberrant turbinates are structural deformities of the nasal turbinates leading to extension beyond their normal anatomic limits. CT studies have shown the presence of aberrant turbinates extending even into the nasopharynx and are thought to contribute to the upper airway obstruction[15] (fig. 13.42). CT is the preferred imaging modality for global evaluation of the airway in patients with brachycephalic airway syndrome since it allows the evaluation of the nares, nasal cavity, nasopharynx, oropharynx, retropharyngeal tissues, larynx, and trachea.

Retropharyngeal swelling and mass effect

Retropharyngeal swelling may result from inflammation, edema, hemorrhage, tumors, abscesses, hematomas, or lymphadenopathy. Lymphadenopathy may be from multicentric neoplasia such as lymphoma or metastasis from a primary malignant lesion in the oral cavity or pharynx such as SCC. Retropharyngeal foreign bodies are a common reason for retropharyngeal cellulitis and abscess formation, more frequently seen in dogs playing with sticks that penetrate the pharynx. Cats may suffer from penetration by sewing needles.

Radiography is a good imaging modality for assessing retropharyngeal swelling and mass effect, although it will usually not determine the cause. Radiography may detect presence of gas in cases of penetrating trauma or abscessation with gas-forming bacteria and may detect radiopaque foreign bodies. Ultrasonography can be used to demonstrate cavitated lesions, masses, and radiolucent retropharyngeal foreign bodies. CT is superior to radiography in assessing retropharyngeal swelling and retropharyngeal masses. MRI is also an excellent modality for evaluation of the soft tissues involving the retropharyngeal area.

Radiographic findings associated with retropharyngeal swelling and mass effect include an increase in soft tissue opacity at the level of the retropharyngeal tissues with associated narrowing of the nasopharynx, and ventral displacement and narrowing of the larynx and trachea (**fig. 13.43**). A rough rule of thumb is that the thickness of the retropharyngeal tissues should not exceed the length of the body of the axis. In case of acute penetrating trauma, gas and radiopaque foreign material may be seen in the retropharyngeal region. Soft tissue opaque foreign bodies are detected with radiography, and diagnosis requires ultrasound or CT (**fig. 13.44**).

Salivary mucocele

Salivary mucoceles or sialoceles are characterized as a collection of saliva that has leaked from a damaged salivary gland or salivary duct and has accumulated in tissues. Salivary mucoceles are often

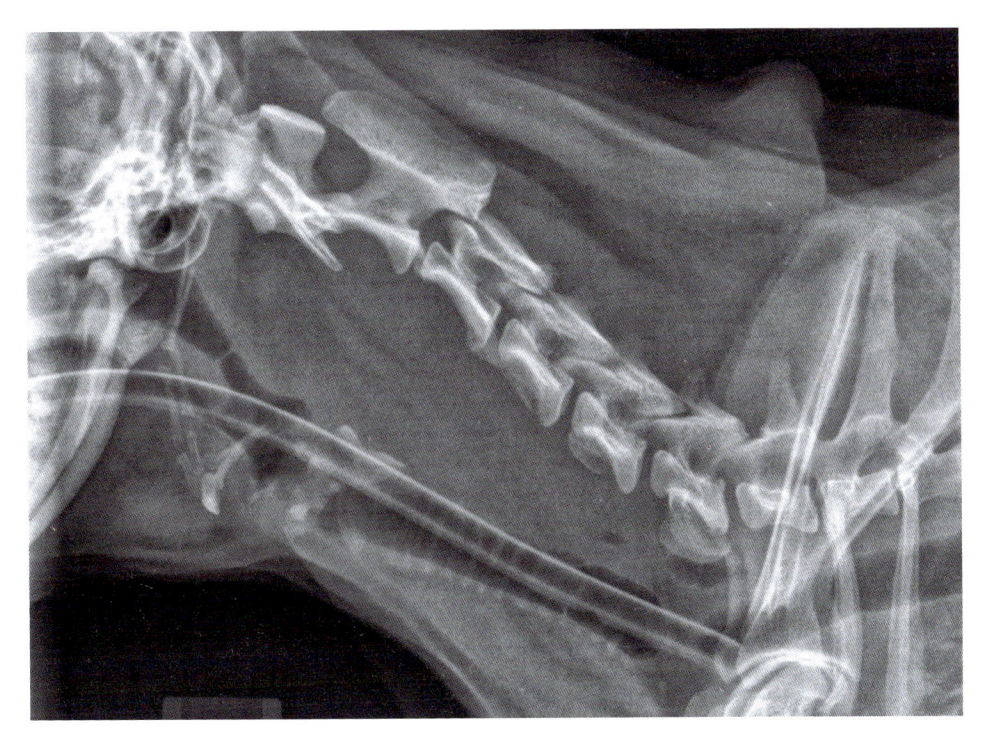

Fig. 13.43 Lateral radiograph of a nine-year-old, spayed female Dachshund with abscessation of the medial retropharyngeal lymph nodes of unknown cause with secondary retropharyngeal cellulitis. There is a severe soft tissue swelling in the retropharyngeal region extending caudally to C5 that creates a mass effect with ventral displacement of the nasopharynx, larynx and trachea.

SECTION III AXIAL SKELETON

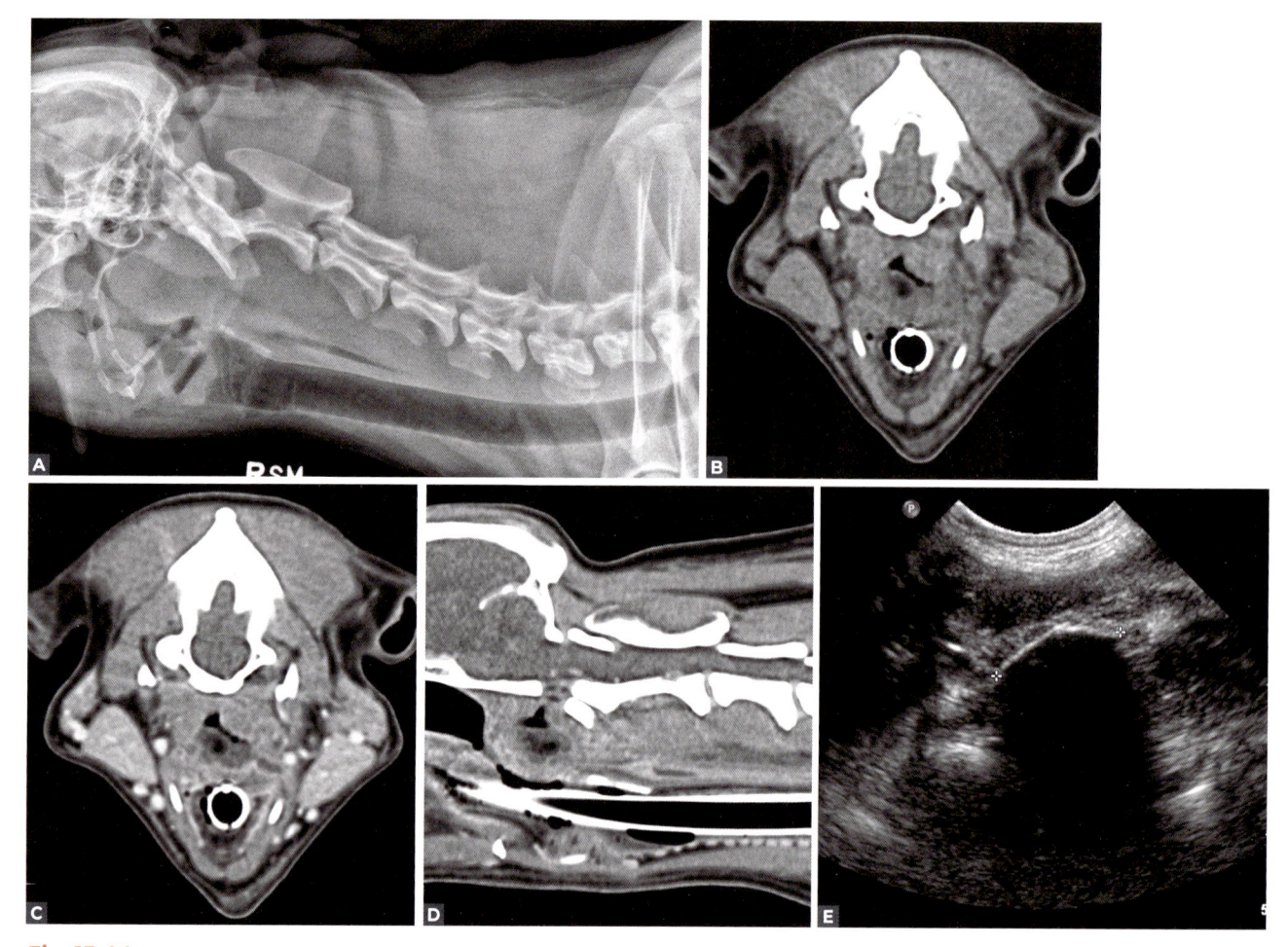

Fig. 13.44 Lateral radiograph (**A**), CT transverse images with a soft tissue algorithm (**B**, pre-contrast and **C**, post-contrast), CT post-contrast sagittal reconstruction with a soft tissue algorithm (**D**), and longitudinal ultrasound image (**E**) of a three-year-old spayed female mixed breed dog with a chronic stick impalement injury in the retropharyngeal area. (**A**) There is a moderate focal soft tissue swelling in the retropharyngeal tissues, ventral to the tympanic bullae, occipital condyles and atlas. The dorsal pharyngeal wall protrudes and has a convex contour. A small pocket of gas is noted within the swelling immediately ventral of the tympanic bullae. (**B-D**) The focal swelling is further characterized by a region of mixed fluid and soft tissue attenuation with a gas pocket dorsally and an angular hypoattenuating structure within the center of the swelling. This structure represents a wooden foreign body. (**E**) The foreign body is seen as an angular hyperechoic structure displaying clean distal acoustic shadowing. A small piece of a wooden stick was retrieved surgically.

clinically presented as a fluctuant, painless swelling of the neck or within the oral cavity. Salivary mucoceles are classified as cervical, sublingual, pharyngeal, and zygomatic, depending on the region of accumulation of saliva. Cervical mucoceles are the most common. The sublingual salivary glands are most commonly associated with salivary mucoceles.

Radiography is not sensitive for the diagnosis of salivary mucoceles, and the most common radiographic finding is soft tissue swelling ventral to the caudal part of the mandibles and around the base of the ear. Mineral opaque structures compatible with sialoliths may be detected radiographically. Administration of iodinated contrast media through the salivary ducts, also known as sialography, can be used to demonstrate a communication between a soft tissue swelling and the salivary gland, and to determine salivary duct rupture or obstruction. However, this is technically challenging, and studies are frequently non diagnostic. Ultrasonography can be used to confirm that the mass is fluid-filled. CT and MRI are superior to radiography and ultrasonography and are recommended for presurgical assessment (**fig. 13.45**). Even with CT and MRI, the communication between the salivary mucocele and salivary gland of origin may be difficult to visualize.

Fig. 13.45 Post-contrast CT transverse images with a soft tissue algorithm (**A-D**) of a two-year-old intact male Pharaoh Hound with a bilateral sublingual salivary mucocele. In both submandibular regions (L>R) there are two well-defined, regionally extensive, tubular to oval, fluid-filled structures with a thick and smooth contrast-enhancing capsule. (**B-C**) There are two small well-defined, round, smoothly marginated, mineral attenuating foci compatible with sialoliths.

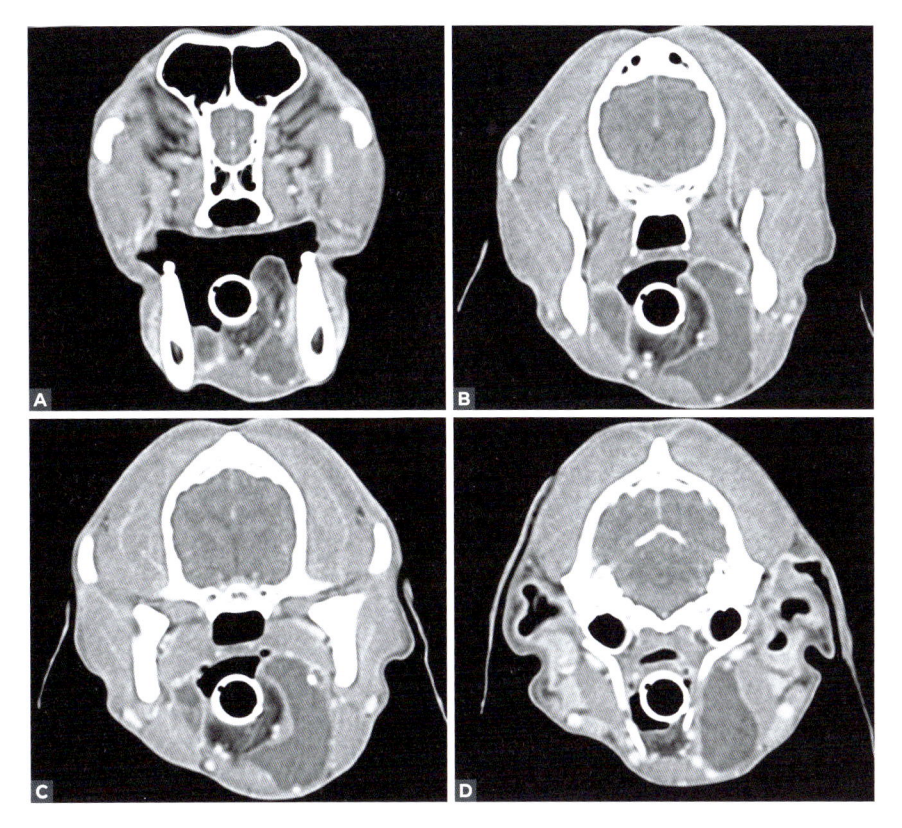

Diseases of the neurocranium

Neurological disease of the brain is rarely investigated with radiography since it lacks sensitivity, and it is almost never useful. However, it can occasionally confirm mineralized meningiomas or calvarial hyperostosis secondary to meningioma, and osseous masses affecting the calvarium. For most other intracranial diseases, MRI is the diagnostic imaging modality of choice. CT can also be used for the assessment of brain diseases but is less sensitive than MRI.

Hydrocephalus

When congenital hydrocephalus is moderate or severe, it may cause radiographic changes such as an enlarged, dome-shaped calvarium, thinned bones, smooth appearance of the inner surface of the calvarium, and open cranial fontanelles and sutures. For a confirmation of hydrocephalus, an ultrasound may be performed via open fontanelles to assess ventricular dilation and cerebral atrophy. If the calvarial bones are very thin but there is no open fontanelle, ultrasound imaging can often be performed by maximizing power and gain settings or using low frequency transducers. Ideally, a CT or better, MRI, will assess the severity of ventricular dilation.

Caudal occipital malformation syndrome/occipital dysplasia

This syndrome mostly affects small and toy breeds and especially Cavalier King Charles Spaniels. Radiographically, sometimes an enlarged foramen magnum may be seen, which will have a keyhole shape. This malformation has been infrequently associated with the presence of clinical signs. In other cases, signs of atlanto-occipital overlap and/or atlanto-axial instability may be identified, which tend to have more clinical relevance. For the examination of this syndrome, MRI is the modality of choice since it allows the cerebral parenchyma and spinal cord to be assessed. The most frequent MRI findings of this syndrome are cerebellar hernia, syringohydromyelia, and, on lesser occasions, obstructive hydrocephalus. When surgical treatment is considered, CT is an excellent modality to be used.

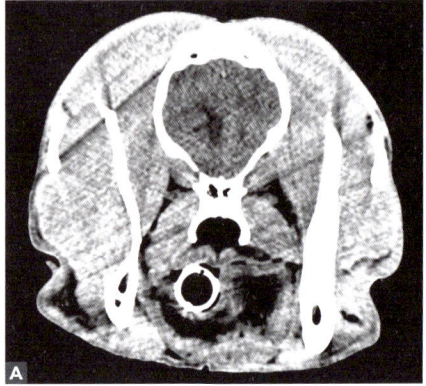

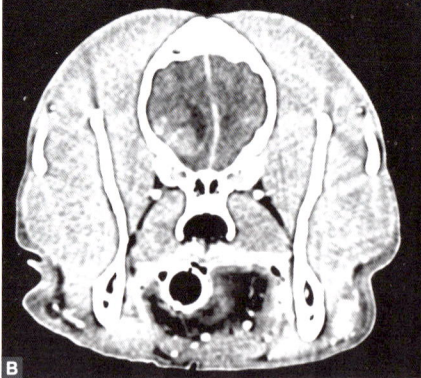

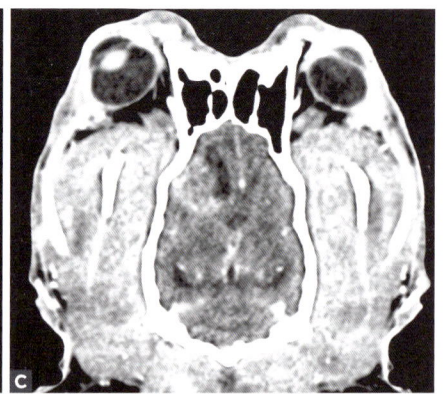

Fig. 13.46 Pre- (**A**) and post-contrast (**B**) CT transverse images, and dorsal (**C**), sagittal (**D**) post-contrast CT images with a brain window of a seven-year-old Boxer with seizures and a confirmed diagnosis of glioma. (**A-B**) Within the right ventral aspect of the right frontal lobe there is an ill-defined and rounded mass that is primarily isoattenuating to the surrounding brain parenchyma with a large fluid attenuating region medially. After administration of contrast, the mass enhances heterogeneously and shows a periperhal contrast enhancing rim surrounding the fluid filled region. The mass results in a mild leftward midline with clear deviation of the falx cerebri on post-contrast images (**B-C**).

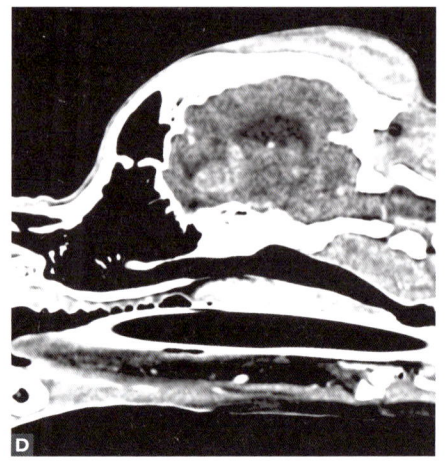

Other brain disorders

For the assessment of other diseases of the brain (inflammatory, infectious, vascular, metabolic, toxic, and degenerative), it is necessary to perform a CT or, in most cases, an MRI, which is much more sensitive (**fig. 13.46**).

References

1. Bannon KM. Clinical canine dental radiography. *Vet Clin North Am Small Anim Pract* 43:507-32, 2013.
2. Reiter AM, Mendoza KA. Feline odontoclastic resorptive lesions. An unsolved enigma in veterinary dentistry. *Vet Clin North Am Small Anim Pract* 32:791-837, 2002.
3. Campbell RD, Peralta S, Fiani N, Scrivani PV. Comparing intraoral radiography and computed tomography for detecting radiographic signs of periodontitis and endodontic disease in dogs: an agreement study. *Front Vet Sci* 3:68, 2016.
4. Gardner H, Fidel J, Haldorson G, et al. Canine oral fibrosarcomas: a retrospective analysis of 65 cases (1988-2010). *Vet Comp Oncol* 29:40-47, 2015.
5. Bilgic O, Sanchez MD, Lewis JR. Feline oral squamous cell carcinoma: clinical manifestations and literature review. *J Vet Dent* 32:30-40, 2015.
6. Gendler A, Lewis JR, Reetz JA, et al. Computed tomographic features of oral squamous cell carcinoma in cats: 18 cases (2002-2008). *J Am Vet Med Assoc* 236:319-325, 2010.
7. Russo M, Lamb CR, Jakovljevic S. Distinguishing rhinitis and nasal neoplasia by radiography. *Vet Radiol Ultrasound* 41:118-24, 2000.
8. Thrall DE, Robertson ID, McLoad DA, et al. A comparison of radiographic and computed tomographic findings in 31 dogs with malignant nasal cavity tumours. *Vet Radiol* 30:59-66, 1989.
9. Saunders JH, van Bree H. Comparison of radiography and computed tomography for the diagnosis of canine nasal aspergillosis. *Vet Radiol Ultrasound* 44:414-9, 2003.
10. Oliveira CR, O'Brien RT, Matheson JS, Carrera I. Computed tomographic features of feline nasopharyngeal polyps. *Vet Radiol Ultrasound* 53:406-11, 2012.
11. Kent M, Glass EN, de Lahunta A, Platt SR, Haley A. Prevalence of effusion in the tympanic cavity in dogs with dysfunction of the trigeminal nerve: 18 cases (2004-2013). *J Vet Intern Med* 27:1153-8, 2013.
12. Travetti O, Giudice C, Greci V, et al. Computed tomography features of middle ear cholesteatoma in dogs. *Vet Radiol Ultrasound* 51:374-379, 2010.
13. Nowak A, King R, Anson A. Canine calvarial subperiosteal hematomas are fluid to soft tissue attenuating mass-like lesions with smoothly marginated peripheral mineralization on CT. *Vet Radiol Ultrasound* 62:44-53, 2021.
14. Padgett GA, Mostosky UV. The mode of inheritance of craniomandibular osteopathy in West Highland White terrier dogs. *Am J Med Genet* 25:9-13, 1986.
15. Ginn JA, Kumar MS, McKiernan BC, Powers BE. Nasopharyngeal turbinates in brachycephalic dogs and cats. *J Am Anim Hosp Assoc* 44:243-249, 2008.

CHAPTER 14

Brachycephalic obstructive airway syndrome

Susanne AEB Boroffka and Gert ter Haar

> **KEY POINTS**
>
> - Brachycephalic airway syndrome (BAS) is characterized by upper airway obstruction and narrow dimensions of the nasal cavity and pharynx.
> - Elongated thickened soft palate, stenotic nares, soft tissue thickening in the nasopharynx, aberrant conchae, and enlargement of the tongue base are common abnormalities in BAS.
> - Skull conformation anomalies in brachycephalic breeds lead to compression of nasal passages.
> - Computed tomography is the modality of choice for imaging brachycephalic airway syndrome as it will clearly depict all the skull structures.

Brachycephalic airway syndrome (BAS) is characterized by increased upper airway resistance and obstruction caused by multiple anatomic abnormalities of the nasal cavity, nasopharynx, pharynx, larynx, and trachea.[1-6] BAS is commonly found in brachycephalic dog breeds, such as the English and French Bulldog, Pug, Boston Terriers, Pekingese, Shih Tzu, Pomeranian, Chihuahua, etc. There are also feline breeds, such as the Persian, affected by similar brachycephalic changes. All brachycephalic breeds have a short and wide skull,[1-5] leading to narrow luminal airway dimensions and reduced air passage[8] with significantly altered nasal and pharyngeal anatomy.[1-5] The anatomical abnormalities affect brachycephalic dogs in the entire respiratory tract, including the middle ears.[7,8]

Ultrasonographic and conventional radiographic evaluation of the airway structures in the head (**fig. 14.1**), neck, and thoracic cavity can occasionally be sufficient for the treatment of patients that present with acute respiratory distress (e.g., aspiration pneumonia) or evaluation of the tracheal di-

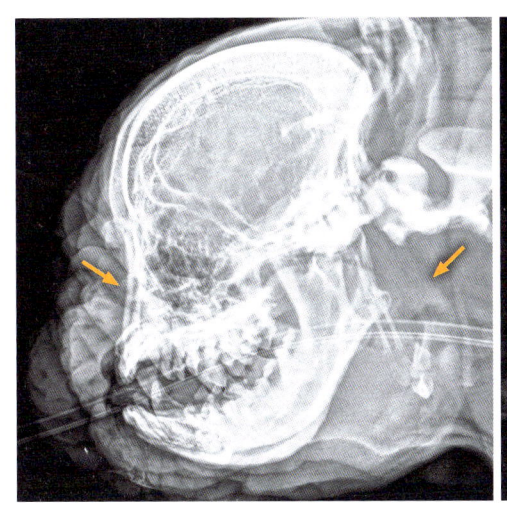

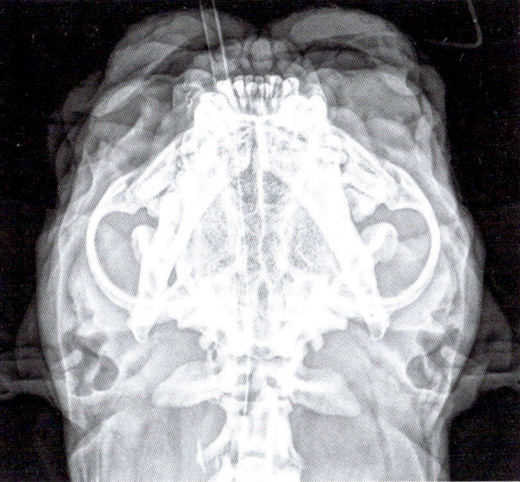

Fig. 14.1 Lateral and dorsoventral radiographs of the head of a French Bulldog showing an extremely short nose, no frontal sinuses, and a thickened soft palate.

ameter. However, for a complete and detailed evaluation of the congenital anatomical and secondary acquired abnormalities, a high-resolution computed tomographic (CT) evaluation is recommended. It allows for assessment of the degree of brachycephaly of the skull and, more specifically, for objective evaluation of the nares and ventral alae, nasal cavity and sinuses, nasopharyngeal dimension, the presence of aberrant conchae, degree of turbinate protrusion, the thickness and length of the soft palate, tympanic bulla anatomy and middle ear effusion and cricoid and tracheal dimensions.[1-9] As abnormalities of the upper airways will affect the structures in the lower airways and vice versa, CT evaluation of the entire respiratory tract should be performed to allow proper evaluation of the prognosis and treatment planning in the brachycephalic patient and this will therefore be described in this chapter. In patients with suspected dynamic airway collapse, such as nasopharyngeal and/or tracheal collapse, videofluoroscopic evaluation may be recommended.[7-15]

Nares

Stenotic nares are a common congenital condition of brachycephalic breeds in both dogs and cats. The dorsolateral nasal cartilages are medially displaced, impinging on the external nasal opening and dramatically decreasing the available lumen to a vertical slit with nearly complete obstruction (**fig. 14.2**).[15]

Nasopharyngeal cranial and caudal turbinates

Nasopharyngeal turbinates are common findings in brachycephalic dogs.[7] Some authors found a prevalence of caudal aberrant turbinates of 100% in clinically healthy English Bulldogs, which varied from a minimal grade (17,5%), a mild grade (70%), to a moderate grade (12,5%).[8] Pugs are reported to have even more frequently higher grades of nasopharyngeal turbinate protrusion.[7] The clinical significance and specific contribution to increased airway resistance are not known (**figs. 14.3-14.6**).

Some authors demonstrated that CT may aid in obtaining data on nasal mucosal contact, caudal aberrant nasal turbinates, and septal deviations. In their study, nasal mucosal contact and caudal aberrant nasal turbinates were significantly more prevalent in brachycephalic dogs than in normocephalic dogs, whereas no significant difference was seen in prevalence or the angle of septal deviation.[14]

Increased mucosal contact points are described by one study, showing that there is basically more contact between the turbinates and less air, partly the result of the aberrant rostral turbinates.[15]

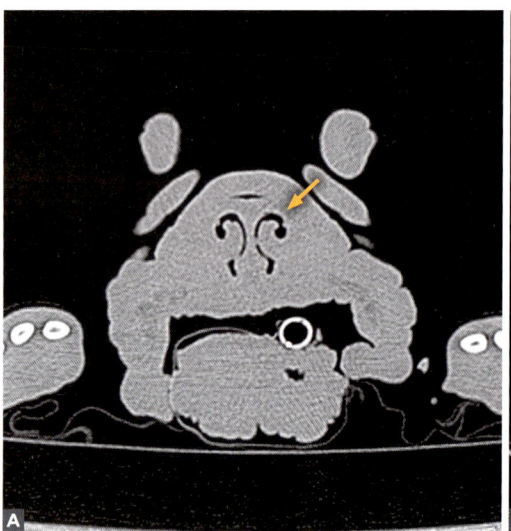

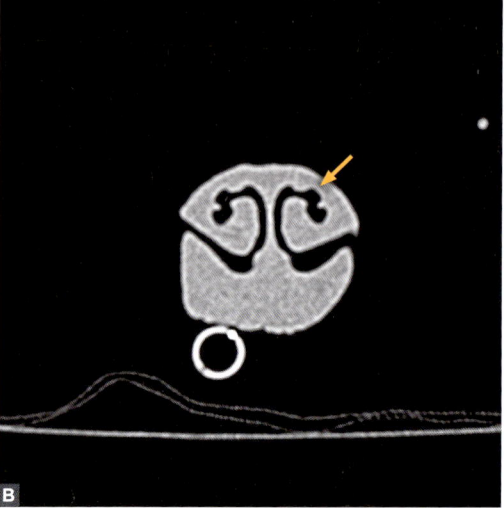

Fig. 14.2 Transverse computed tomography images in bone window of a French Bulldog and a Dachshund illustrating the stenotic nasal alae with a narrowed nasal vestibule caused by thickened ventral alae in comparison with the normal anatomy of the Dachshund.

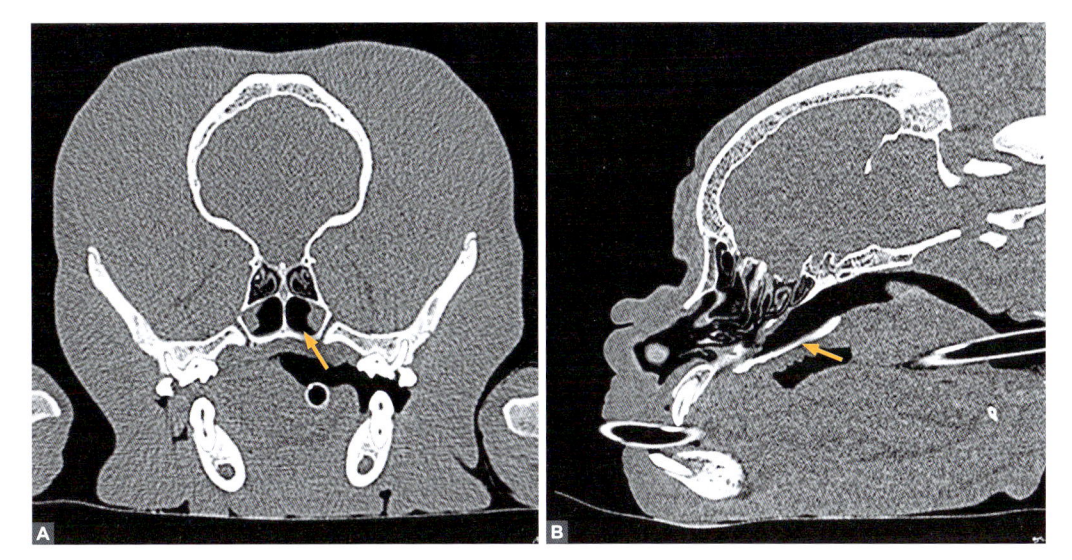

CHAPTER **14** Brachycephalic obstructive airway syndrome

Fig. 14.3 Transverse CT image and sagittal MPR in bone window of a French Bulldog without caudal aberrant turbinates at the level of the nasopharyngeal meatuses.

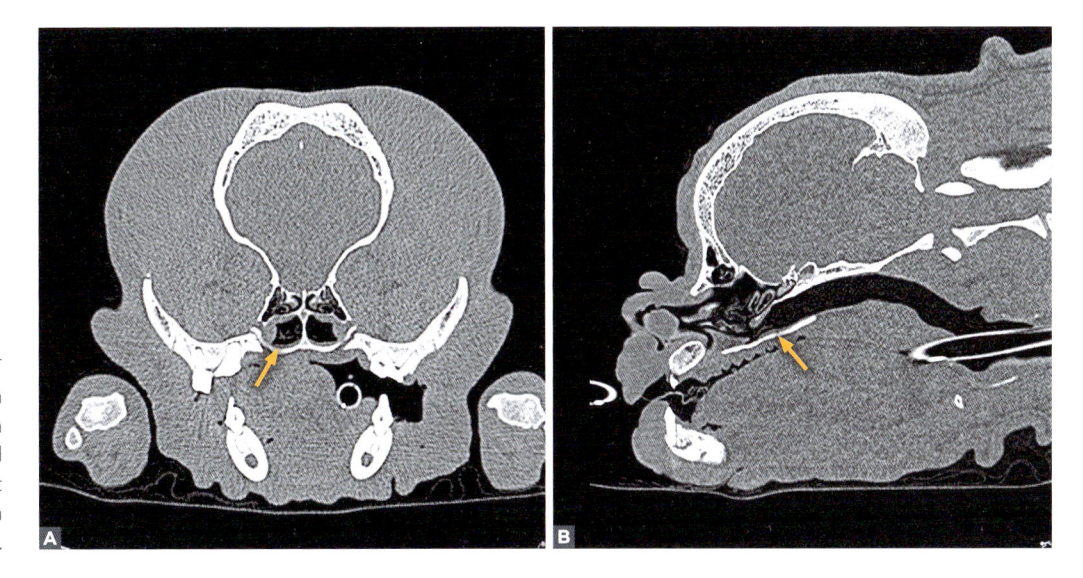

Fig. 14.4 Transverse CT image and sagittal MPR in bone window of a French Bulldog with unilateral grade 3 caudal aberrant turbinates visible within the ventral nasal meatuses.

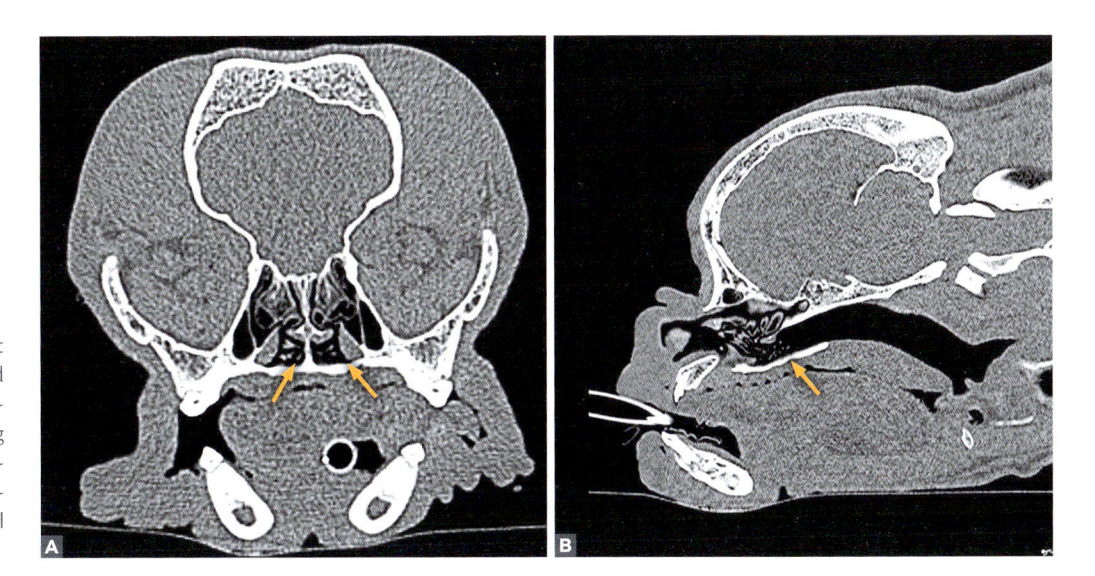

Fig. 14.5 Non-contrast transverse CT image and sagittal MPR in bone window of a French Bulldog with bilateral grade 3 caudal aberrant turbinates visible within the ventral nasal meatuses.

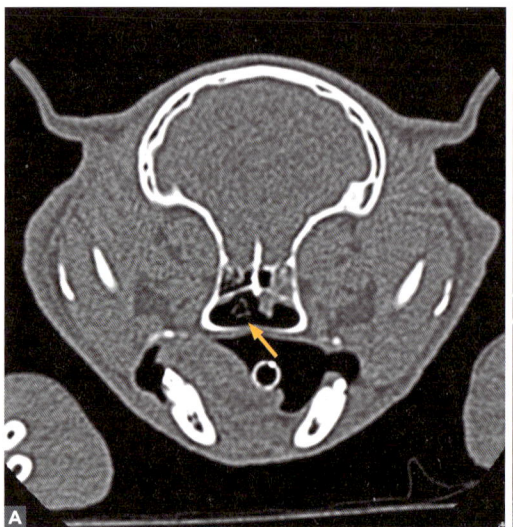

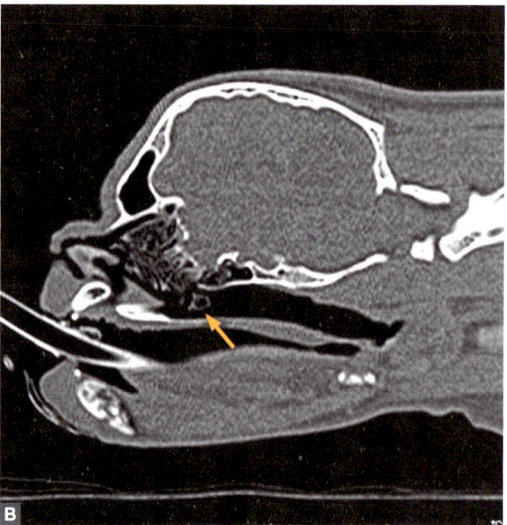

Fig. 14.6 Transverse CT image and sagittal MPR in bone window of an Exotic cat with bilateral grade 3 caudal aberrant turbinates visible within the ventral nasal meatuses.

Frontal sinus

In the brachycephalic breeds, the frontal sinuses are either underdeveloped or absent.

Nasopharyngeal dimensions

In brachycephalic breeds, the ventral meatus, choanae, and cranial nasopharyngeal dimensions may be very narrow.
A study demonstrated with CT that the upper airway morphology showed that the smallest nasopharyngeal cross-sectional areas were located dorsal to the caudal end of the soft palate in Pugs and French Bulldogs.[12] Pugs had a smaller nasopharyngeal cross-sectional area despite smaller soft palate dimensions than French Bulldogs.
In Pugs, a dorsal rotation of the maxillary bone, rudimentary or absent frontal sinuses, and ventral orientation of the olfactory bulb result in an even shorter craniofacial measurement than in English or French Bulldogs (**fig. 14.7**).

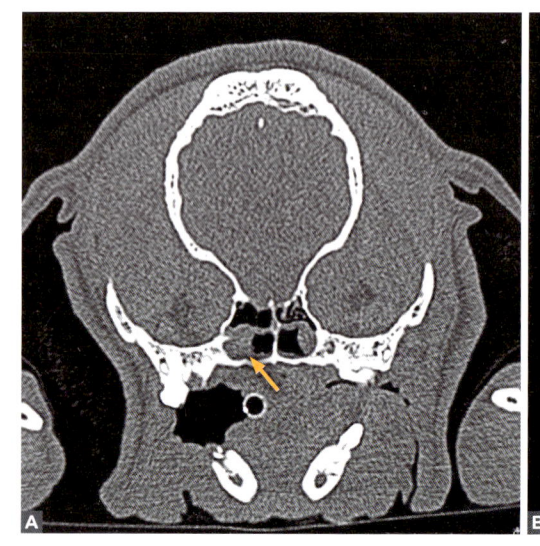

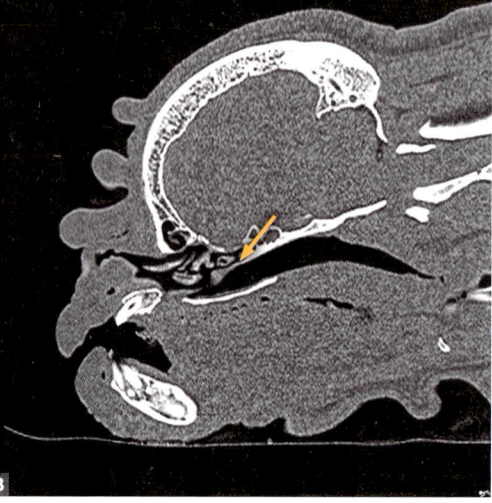

Fig. 14.7 Transverse CT image and sagittal MPR in bone window of a Pug illustrating the dorsal rotation of the maxillary bone, rudimentary or absent frontal sinuses, and ventral orientation of the olfactory bulb resulting in an even shorter craniofacial measurement. Furthermore, the thickened mucosa in the nasal meatus is visible.

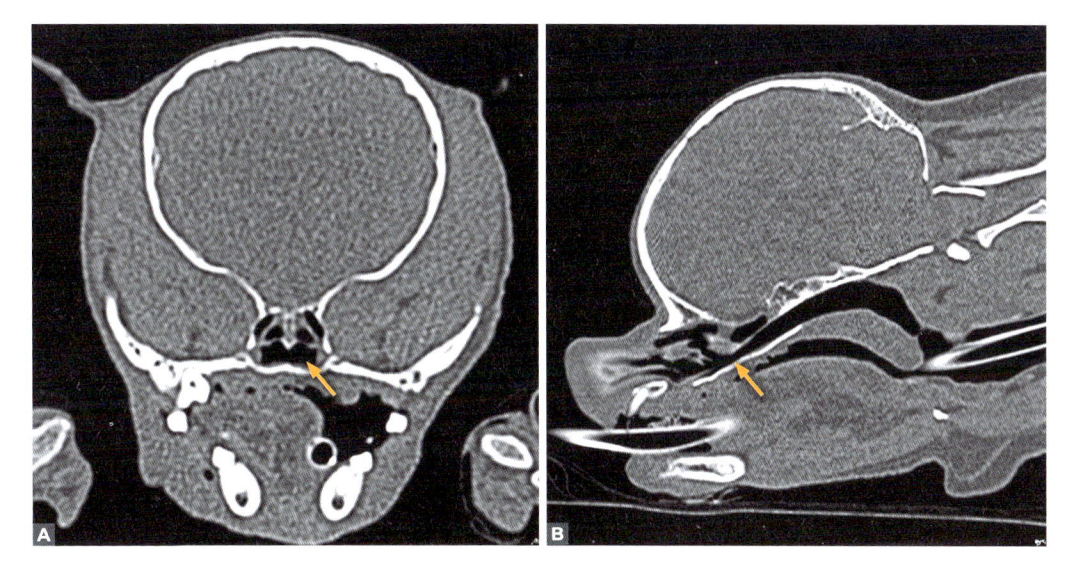

Fig. 14.8 Transverse CT image and sagittal MPR in bone window of a Chihuahua illustrating the narrow nasopharynx with the smallest dimensions located at the rostral part of the nasopharynx.

There are differences in brachycephalic breeds as to the precise anatomical configuration of the nasopharynx, cricoid, and trachea. Wijsman et al. have demonstrated that the nasopharynx is remarkably narrow in Chihuahuas and Pomeranians, with the smallest dimensions located at the rostral part of the nasopharynx (**fig. 14.8**).

Pharynx and soft palate

Relative macroglossia has been described in brachycephalic compared to mesaticephalic dogs. The overly long and thick tongue in brachycephalic breeds is thought to contribute to a dorsal displacement of the soft palate, causing narrowing of the nasopharynx. An increased normalized total tongue volume in brachycephalic breeds was demonstrated when compared to mesaticephalic breeds. A decrease in total outlined air area indexed to the total soft tissue area at certain levels in the oropharynx and nasopharynx in brachycephalic dogs was described (**fig. 14.9**).[6]

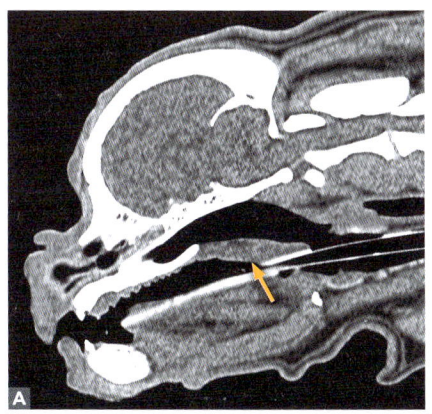

Fig. 14.9 (**A-C**) Sagittal MPR in soft tissue window of different French Bulldogs and (**D**) a Landseer, illustrating different degrees of elongated and thickened and the normal soft palates, respectively. In the Landseer, the normal nasopharynx is also visible compared to the French Bulldogs and the Chihuahua in fig. 14.8B.

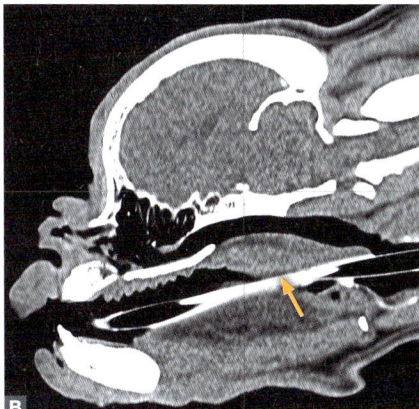

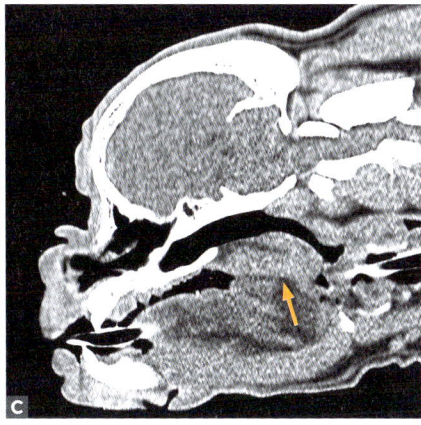

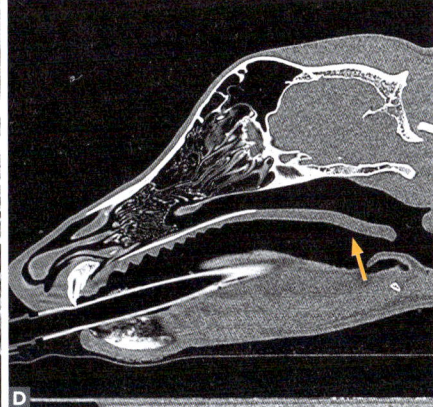

SECTION III AXIAL SKELETON

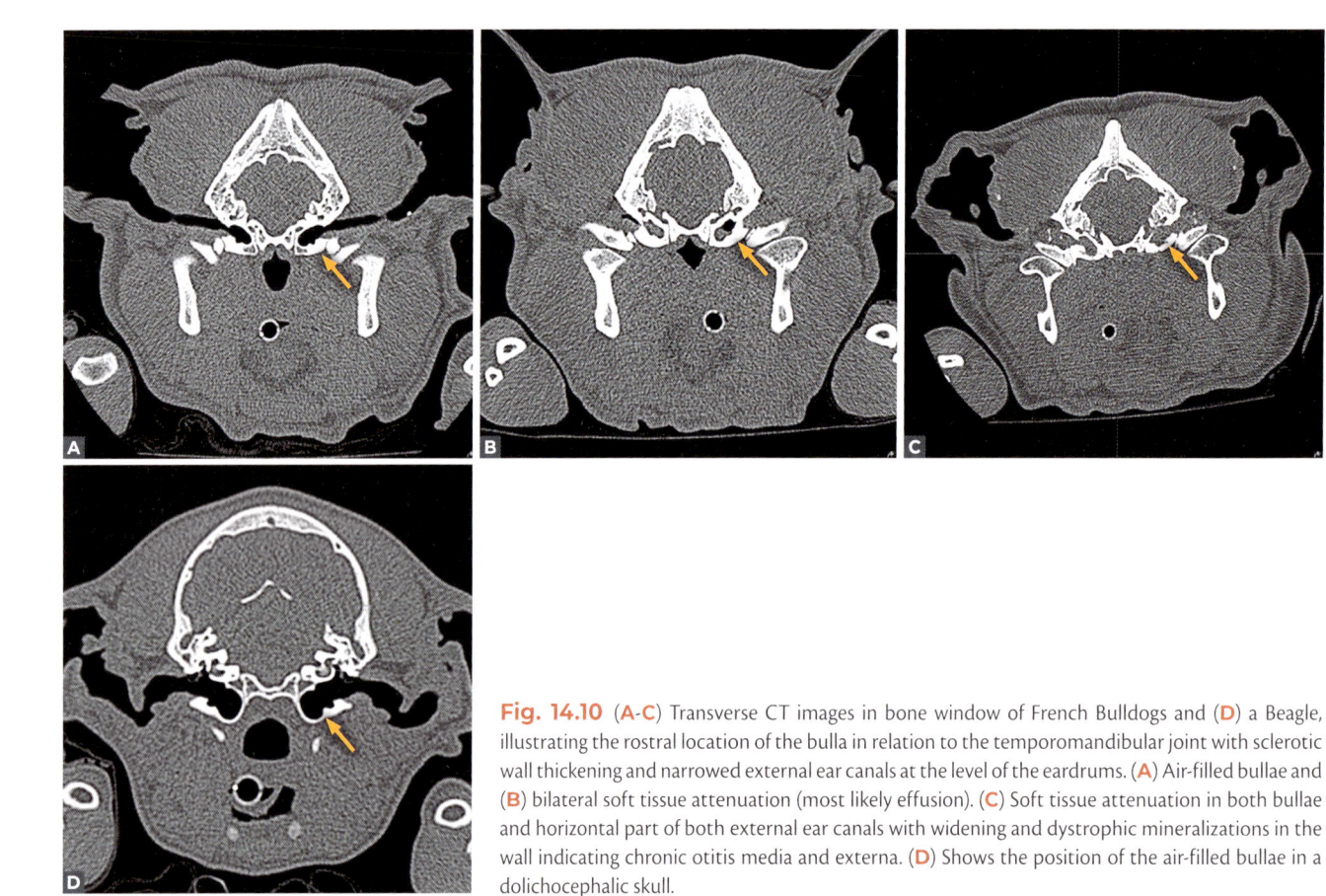

Fig. 14.10 (A-C) Transverse CT images in bone window of French Bulldogs and (D) a Beagle, illustrating the rostral location of the bulla in relation to the temporomandibular joint with sclerotic wall thickening and narrowed external ear canals at the level of the eardrums. (A) Air-filled bullae and (B) bilateral soft tissue attenuation (most likely effusion). (C) Soft tissue attenuation in both bullae and horizontal part of both external ear canals with widening and dystrophic mineralizations in the wall indicating chronic otitis media and externa. (D) Shows the position of the air-filled bullae in a dolichocephalic skull.

Bullae

Brachycephalic dogs and cats are predisposed to bulla effusion because of their skull conformation with a more rostral location of the bulla in relation to the temporomandibular joint, bulla wall thickening, and auditory tube dysfunction leading to middle ear effusion, which needs to be differentiated from otitis media (**fig. 14.10**).

Larynx

The cross-sectional area of the cricoid was found to be significantly smaller in dogs of brachycephalic breeds (Pugs, French Bulldogs, English Bulldogs, and Boston Terriers) compared to mesaticephalic breeds (Jack Russell Terriers and Labradors). In addition, the shape of the cricoid cartilage was more vertically oval (and not the normal circular form) in Pugs and French Bulldogs when compared to mesaticephalic breeds and English Bulldogs (**fig. 14.11**).[13] A significant correlation between the severity of laryngeal collapse with bronchial collapse has been described, especially in Pugs.

Trachea

To evaluate the tracheal diameter (TD), traditionally, the tracheal diameter on radiographs is compared to the thoracic inlet (TI). The normal TD:TI ratio in nonbrachycephalic dogs is up to 0.2 and in brachycephalic dogs up to 0.16, even though in the English Bulldog, 0.12 is used. Tracheal hypoplasia is defined when the TD:TI ratio is less and has been described in a study to occur in approximately 13% of brachycephalic dogs. In the English Bulldog, it has been reported that a ratio of 9% was found without showing clinical signs.[11] However, radiographic evaluation of the tracheal dimensions is not very accurate; CT evaluation and comparison with endoscopic assessment are recommended. The left main bronchus often shows dorsoventral flattening (**figs. 14.12-14.14**).[13]

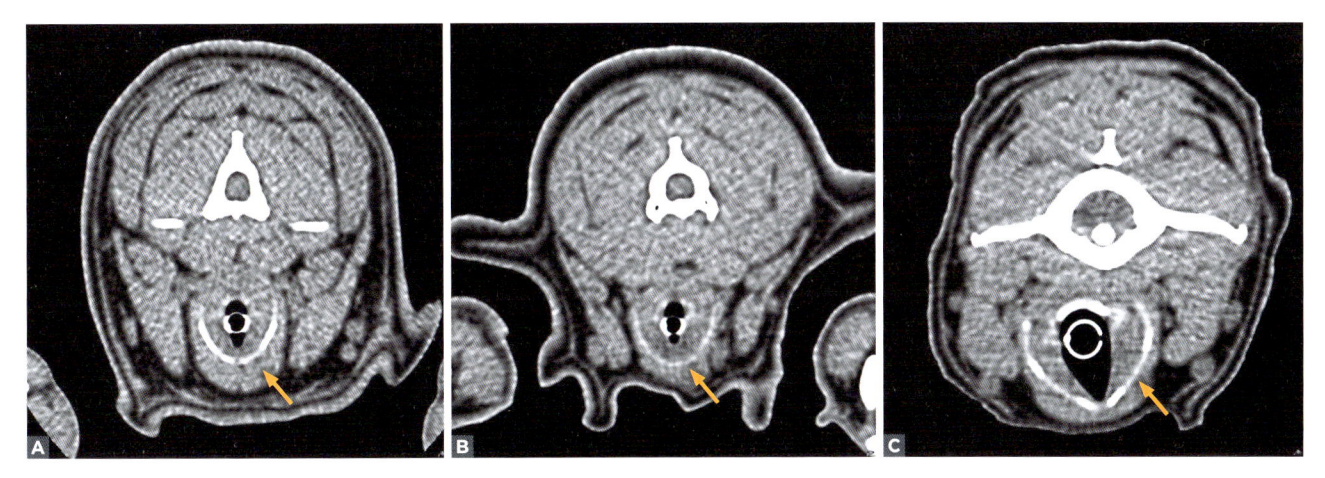

Fig. 14.11 Transverse CT images in bone window of a French Bulldog, a Pug, and a Shepherd dog, illustrating the smaller cross-sectional area of the larynx in the French Bulldog and Pug as compared to the Shepherd dog.

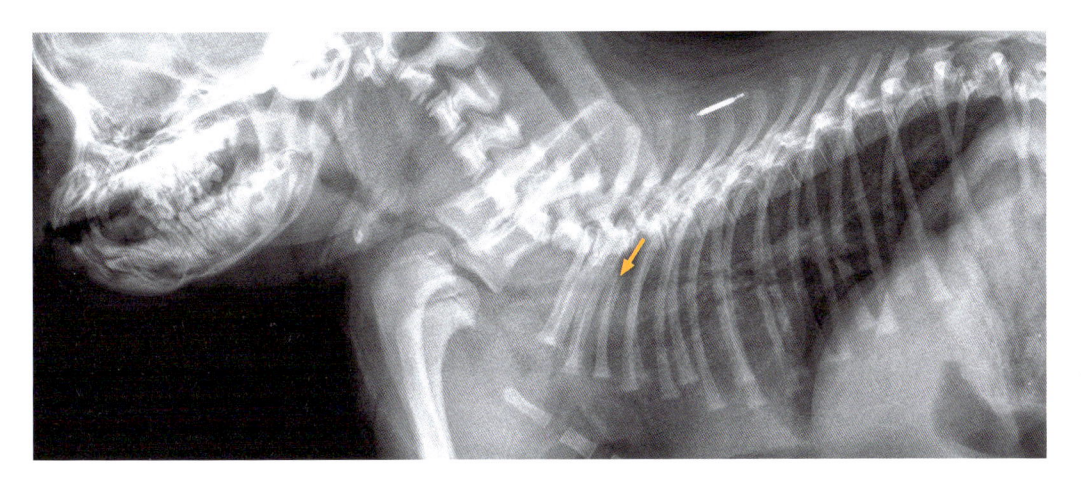

Fig. 14.12 Lateral radiograph of a four-month-old Pug with severe narrowing of the dorsoventral diameter of the trachea.

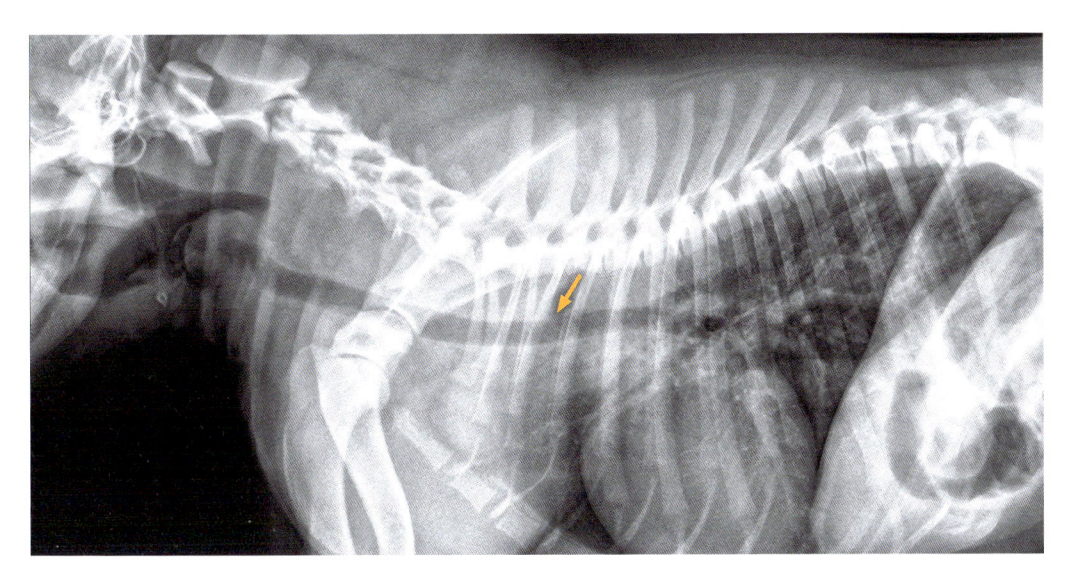

Fig. 14.13 Lateral radiograph of an adult French Bulldog with mild narrowing of the dorsoventral diameter of the trachea.

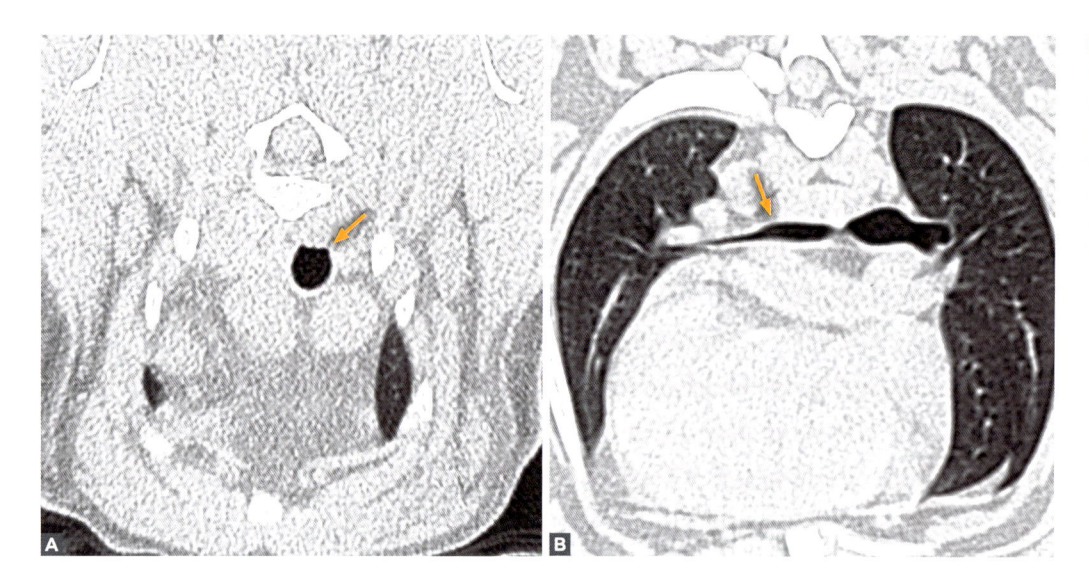

Fig. 14.14 Transverse CT images in lung window of a French Bulldog at the level of the thoracic inlet (A) and carina (B) illustrating the narrow tracheal diameter and dorsoventral flattening of the left main bronchus.

References

1. Dupre G, Heidenreich D. Brachycephalic syndrome. *Vet Clin North Am Small Anim Pract* 46:691-707, 2016.
2. Ter Haar G, Oechtering GU. Brachycephalic airway disease. In Brockman DJ, Holt DE, Haar G (editors). BSAVA Manual of Canine and Feline Head, Neck and Thoracic Surgery 2nd edition. Cheltenham, BSAVA, 2018, pp 82-87.
3. Brown D, Gregory S. Brachycephalic airway disease. In Brockman DJ, Holt DE, Haar G (editors). BSAVA Manual of Canine and Feline Head, Neck and Thoracic Surgery. Cheltenham, BSAVA, 2005, pp 84.
4. Ter Haar G, Sanchez R. Brachycephaly-related diseases. *Veterinary Focus* 27, 2017.
5. Grand JG, Bureau S. Structural characteristics of the soft palate and meatus nasopharyngeus in brachycephalic and non-brachycephalic dogs analysed by CT. *J Small Anim Pract* 52: 232-239, 2011.
6. Siedenburg JS, Dupré G. Tongue and upper airway dimensions: a comparative study between three popular brachycephalic breeds. *Animals* 11: 662, 2021.
7. Vilaplana Grosso F, Ter Haar G, Boroffka SAEB. Gender, weight, and age effects on prevalence of caudal aberrant nasal turbinates in clinically healthy English bulldogs: a computed tomography study and classification. *Vet Radiol Ultrasound* 56:486-493, 2015.
8. Mielke B, Lam R, Haar GT. Computed tomographic morphometry of tympanic bulla shape and position in brachycephalic and mesaticephalic dog breeds. *Vet Radiol Ultrasound* 58:552-558, 2017.
9. Salguero R, Herrtage M, Holmes M, Mannion P, Ladlow J. Comparison between computed tomographic characteristics of the middle ear in nonbrachycephalic and brachycephalic dogs with obstructive airway syndrome. *Vet Radiol Ultrasound* 57:137-143, 2016.
10. Kaye BM, Boroffka SAEB, Haagsman AN, Ter Haar G. Computed tomographic, radiographic, and endoscopic tracheal dimensions in English bulldogs with grade 1 clinical signs of brachycephalic airway syndrome. *Vet Radiol Ultrasound* 56:609-616, 2015.
11. Regier PJ, Vilaplana Grosso F, Stone H, van Santen E. Radiographic tracheal dimensions in brachycephalic breeds before and after surgical treatment for brachycephalic airway syndrome. *Can Vet J* 61:971-976, 2020.
12. Heidenreich D, Gradner, Kneissl S, Dupre G. Nasopharyngeal dimensions from computed tomography of Pugs and French bulldogs with brachycephalic airway syndrome. *Vet Surg* 45:83-90, 2016.
13. Rutherford L, Beever L, Bruce M, ter Haar G. Assessment of computed tomography derived cricoid cartilage and tracheal dimensions to evaluate degree of cricoid narrowing in brachycephalic dogs. *Vet Radiol Ultrasound* 58:634-646, 2017.
14. Auger M, Alexander K, Beauchamp G, Dunn M. Use of CT to evaluate and compare intranasal features in brachycephalic and normocephalic dogs. *J Small Anim Pract* 57:529-536, 2016.
15. Oechtering GU, Pohl S, Schlueter C, Lippert JP, Alef M, Kiefer I, Ludewig E, Schuenemann. A novel approach to brachycephalic syndrome. 1. Evaluation of anatomical intranasal airway obstruction. *Vet Surg* 45:165-172, 2016.

CHAPTER 15

Eye and orbit

Susanne Boroffka and Rick F. Sánchez

KEY POINTS

- Ultrasound (US) is the modality of choice for imaging the eye and is to perform in the awake animal under topical anesthesia.
- Ocular ultrasonography enables imaging of the ocular structures in patients with opaque ocular media or if the eye is not directly visible.
- Computed tomography (CT) and magnetic resonance imaging (MRI) are the modalities of choice for the detection and definition of orbital disease.
- CT is superior for the examination of patients with suspected orbital disease involving the bony structures.
- MRI enables high-resolution imaging of orbital soft tissues and brain, including the intracranial optic nerve, optic chiasm, and visual cortex.

Diagnosis, prognosis, and clinical management of ocular and orbital disease depend on an accurate description of the anatomic detail in patients with opaque ocular media, and/or orbital disease. The skull is a complex anatomical structure with superimposing shadows of bone, soft tissue, and air-filled spaces.[1-5] Modern imaging techniques allow for the precise description of the location, extent, size, character, and structures of ocular and orbital pathology. This facilitates the planning of biopsies and treatments, and it increases the prognostic value.[1-7]

Anatomy of the eye and orbit

Ultrasonography is the technique of choice for evaluation of the eye though it may be used to assess elements of the orbital contents. Computed tomography is used to evaluate the bony orbit and to search for metastatic disease, while MRI may be used for targeted assessment of soft tissues.[1-6] High-frequency transducers (7.5 to 50 MHZ) are recommended for US examination of the eye and orbit, as they offer the best resolution possible.[3-6]

Ocular US is performed preferably without sedation to avoid ventromedial rotation and retraction of the eye. The transducer is positioned over the cornea (i.e., cornea contact method), at the corneoscleral limbus or sclera (i.e., transscleral or conjunctival contact method), or over the eyelid (i.e., transpalpebral method), the latter of which reduces image quality (**fig. 15.1A**). The examiner applies one drop of an ocular topical anesthetic 2 minutes prior to the exam, followed by a lubricant tear to protect the eye from the potentially irritating ultrasound gel, and then ultrasound gel between the transducer and the cornea to prevent direct corneal contact and inadvertent epithelial trauma. Horizontal and vertical images are acquired. Oblique planes may offer additional information.

SECTION III AXIAL SKELETON

The "cornea contact method" and a dorsal approach via the temporal muscle (**fig. 15.2A**) are advised for examination of the orbit.[3] After the exam the gel is gently wiped from the eyelids and the remaining gel is flushed with sterile saline from the ocular surface.

The healthy globe is a well-delineated structure with an anechoic interior except for the echogenic interfaces of the cornea, iris, ciliary body, anterior and posterior lens capsule, and scleroretinal rim. (**figs. 15.1B** and **15.1C**). The cornea forms two parallel hyperechoic curvilinear lines with the anechoic stroma in between. The sclera lacks an anechoic middle layer. The lens capsule forms a convex and a concave hyperechoic curvilinear interface that lies between the echogenic ciliary body mounds and tapers off at the lens equator. The iris forms two elongated echogenic leaflets with the pupil gap in the center. The anterior and posterior chambers, lens nucleus and cortex, and the vitreous are anechoic in the absence of disease or degenerative changes. The echogenic choroid, retina, and sclera cannot be identified separately, forming the scleroretinal rim. The optic disc is visible in the ventrolateral, internal aspect of the posterior wall of the globe, as a slightly recessed or elevated, hyperechoic area. The anterior portion of the optic nerve is hypoechoic, undulating, approximately 2 mm in diameter, and extends into the orbit.[1-3, 7]

The extraocular rectus muscles and retractor bulbi are thin hypoechoic bands dorsal, ventral, lateral, and medial to the optic nerve, whereas the oblique muscles have not been identified with US

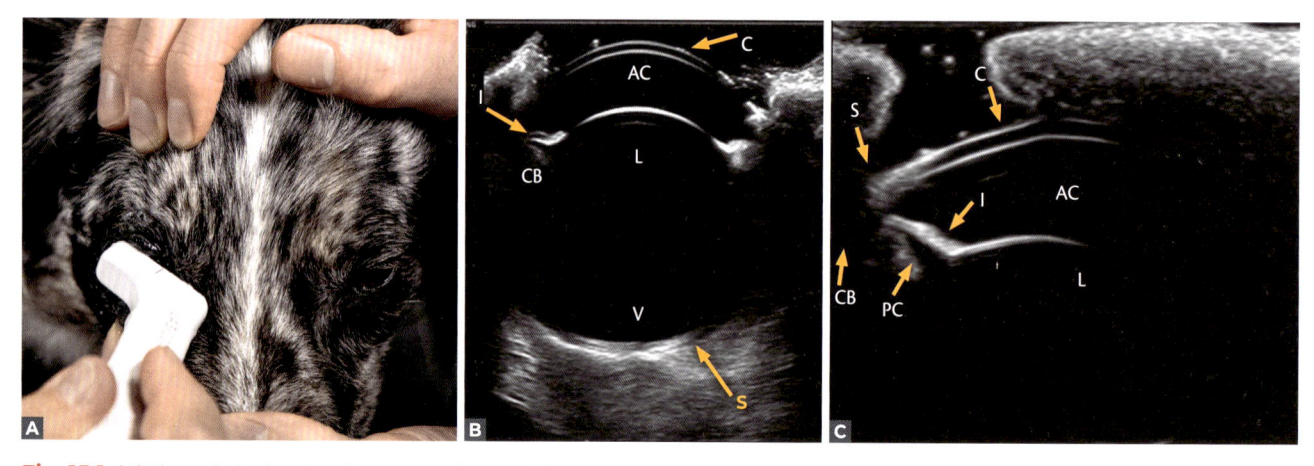

Fig. 15.1 (**A**) The probe is placed on the cornea and oriented horizontally to the globe using a high-frequency transducer (18 MHz). (**B**) Horizontal ultrasound image of a normal eye. The globe is surrounded by the three-layered scleroretinal rim (S). The anterior and posterior chambers and the vitreous body (V) are anechoic. (C, cornea; L, lens; CB, ciliary body; AC, anterior chamber; I, iris). (**C**) Horizontal ultrasound image of a normal anterior segment of the eye. The anterior and posterior chambers are anechoic. (C, cornea; L, lens; CB, ciliary body; AC, anterior chamber; I, iris; PC, posterior chamber; S, scleroretinal rim).

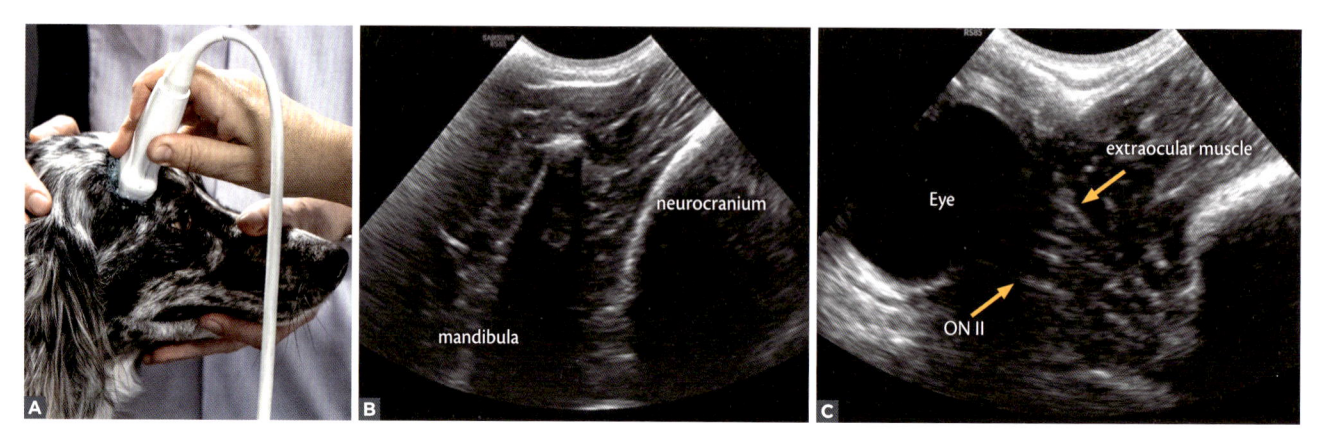

Fig. 15.2 (**A**) The probe is placed on the temporal muscle caudal to the orbital ligament using the dorsal approach and oriented horizontally to the head using a curved array transducer (8 MHz). (**B**) Transverse ultrasound image of the normal orbital space showing the mandibula and bony margin of the neurocranium. The normal temporal muscle is located between the bony structures. (**C**) Longitudinal ultrasound image of the normal orbital space showing the normal hypoechoic optic nerve (ON II) and extraocular muscle.

(**figs. 15.2B** and **15.2C**). There is hyperechoic orbital fat between the extraocular muscles and the optic nerve and surrounding the periorbita. The bony orbit is a hyperechoic line with distal acoustic shadowing.[3] It is not always possible to differentiate every individual structure.

Pre- and post-contrast CT of the eye and orbit is performed in sternal recumbency in bone and soft tissue algorithm with thin slices. The scan should include the head and retropharyngeal lymph nodes. Computed tomography is valuable for evaluating the bony structures, though a high-quality CT may be sufficient to determine if there is inflammation or neoplastic disease of the soft tissues.[1-5] The scleroretinal rim shows well-defined enhancement after intravenous contrast injection. The lens is hyperattenuating but poorly delineated, and the anterior chamber and vitreous are hypoattenuating. The iris is thinly visible, and the ciliary body and posterior chamber are not visible. The optic disc has a small hyperattenuating rim with a hypoattenuating core. The low attenuation of the orbital fat facilitates the identification of orbital structures (**fig. 15.3**).

Magnetic resonance imaging should include transverse pre- and post-contrast T1- and T2-weighted, FLAIR and proton density, and fat suppression sequences with the thinnest slice thickness possible.[1-3,8,9] T1-weighted images of the orbit are characterized by the high signal intensity of the orbital fat, whereas the lens has low signal intensity and the extraocular muscles, optic nerve, ciliary body, and iris have intermediate signal intensity. The signal intensity of the vitreous lies between that of the

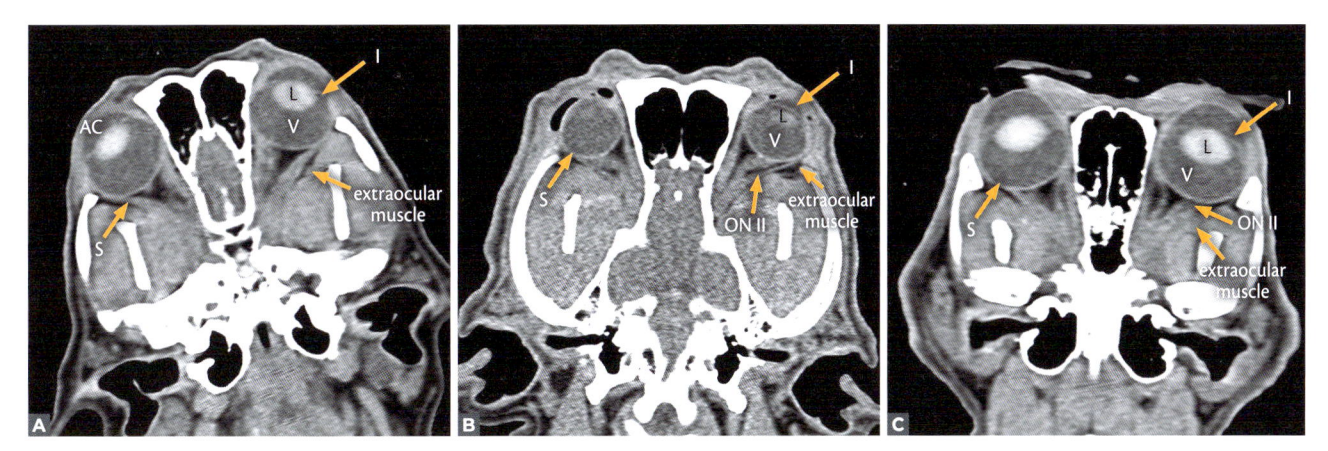

Fig. 15.3 (**A**) Dorsal plane reconstruction in soft tissue window of a Dachshund that shows the normal ocular and orbital structures. L, lens; AC, anterior chamber; I, iris; S, scleroretinal rim. (**B**) Dorsal plane reconstruction in soft tissue window of a Dachshund that shows the normal ocular and orbital structures. L, lens; AC, anterior chamber; I, iris; S, scleroretinal rim; ON II, optic nerve.

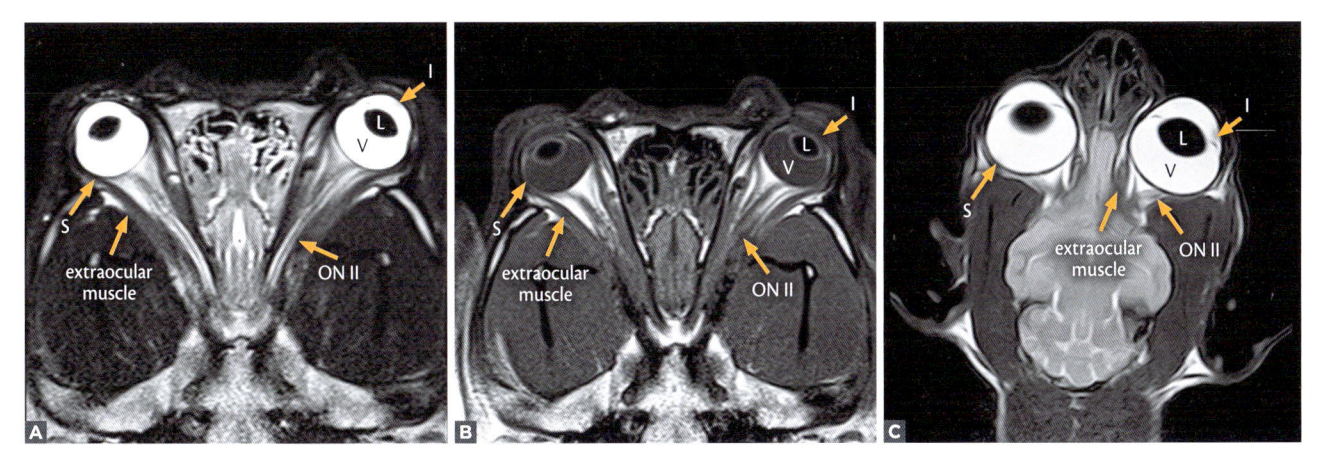

Fig. 15.4 (**A**) Dorsal T2W MRI image of a Bernese Mountain dog showing the normal ocular and orbital structures. L, lens; AC, anterior chamber; I, iris; S, scleroretinal rim; ON II, optic nerve. (**B**) Post-contrast dorsal T1W MRI image of a Bernese Mountain dog showing the normal ocular and orbital structures. L, lens; AC, anterior chamber; I, iris; S, scleroretinal rim; ON II, optic nerve. (**C**) Dorsal TW MRI image of a Domestic shorthair cat showing the normal ocular and orbital structures. L, lens; AC, anterior chamber; I, iris; S, scleroretinal rim; ON II, optic nerve.

lens and extraocular muscles and the signal intensity of the lens capsule lies between that of the orbital fat and extraocular muscles.

T2-weighted images show high signal intensity of fluid with a signal intensity order from high to low being: vitreous and aqueous, brain, extraocular muscles, optic nerve and iris, eyelids and skin, fat, and lens and air (**fig. 15.4**).

Malformations

True anophthalmia occurs rarely. Microphthalmia may present with or without other congenital abnormalities, such as persistent hyperplastic tunica vasculosa lentis/persistent hyperplastic primary vitreous (PHTVL/PHPV), with or without a persistent hyaloid artery seen as a linear structure between the posterior lens and optic disc, lenticonus, cataract, and/or retinal detachment (**fig. 15.5**). Doppler examination might help determine if blood flow is present within a persistent hyaloid artery. However, ocular movement often disturbs the color blood flow signal obscuring microvasculature flow, while microbubble contrast use has been shown to help in those cases.[10]

Ocular degenerative disorders

Cataracts

Various types of cataractous changes might affect the lens. Ultrasound examination is used for pre-cataract screening to measure the size of the lens for choosing the adequate intraocular lens implant and to evaluate the health status of the posterior lens capsule, vitreous, and retina. Increased lens echoes of varying severity may be visible within the lens nucleus, cortices, and even the capsule (**fig. 15.6**).[7, 11, 12] Ultrasound may be used to assess the position of the lens in cases with primary or secondary lens (sub-)luxation. The lens may dislocate into the anterior chamber (anterior luxation) or into the degenerative (i.e., liquified) vitreous (i.e., posterior luxation) (**fig. 15.7**).

Cataracts and other lens changes may be seen on CT and MRI images, though these modalities are not normally used clinically for this purpose.

Vitreous

Vitreous degeneration may be visible on ultrasound as single or multiple echogenic, mobile foci, or hyperechoic lines (i.e., vitreal membranes, protein aggregates). Asteroid hyalosis appears as multiple strong, pinpoint foci that do not move with ocular movement if the vitreous gel is intact. Otherwise, the asteroid hyalosis will swirl in a liquified vitreous (i.e., vitreous syneresis) during ocular movement (**fig. 15.6C**).[11,12]

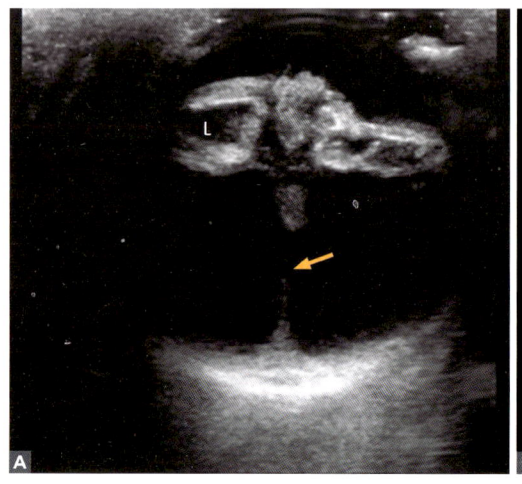

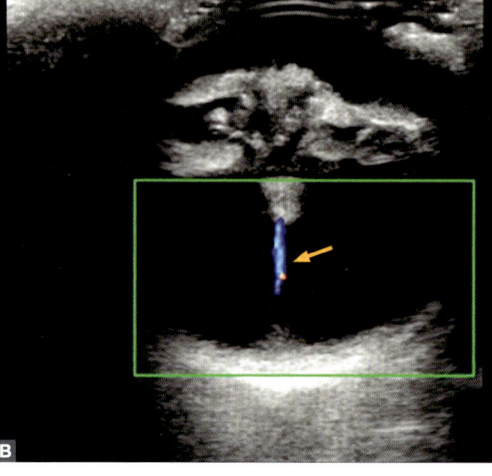

Fig. 15.5 (**A**) Horizontal ultrasound image of a nine-month-old Rhodesian Ridgeback showing the hyperechoic lens (cataract) with an abnormal heterogeneous and flattened shape (L). There is a persistent hyaloid artery (arrow) visible expanding from the posterior lens (L) to the optic nerve area. (**B**) Color Doppler horizontal image illustrates the blood flow within the persistent hyaloid artery suggesting patency.

CHAPTER **15** Eye and orbit

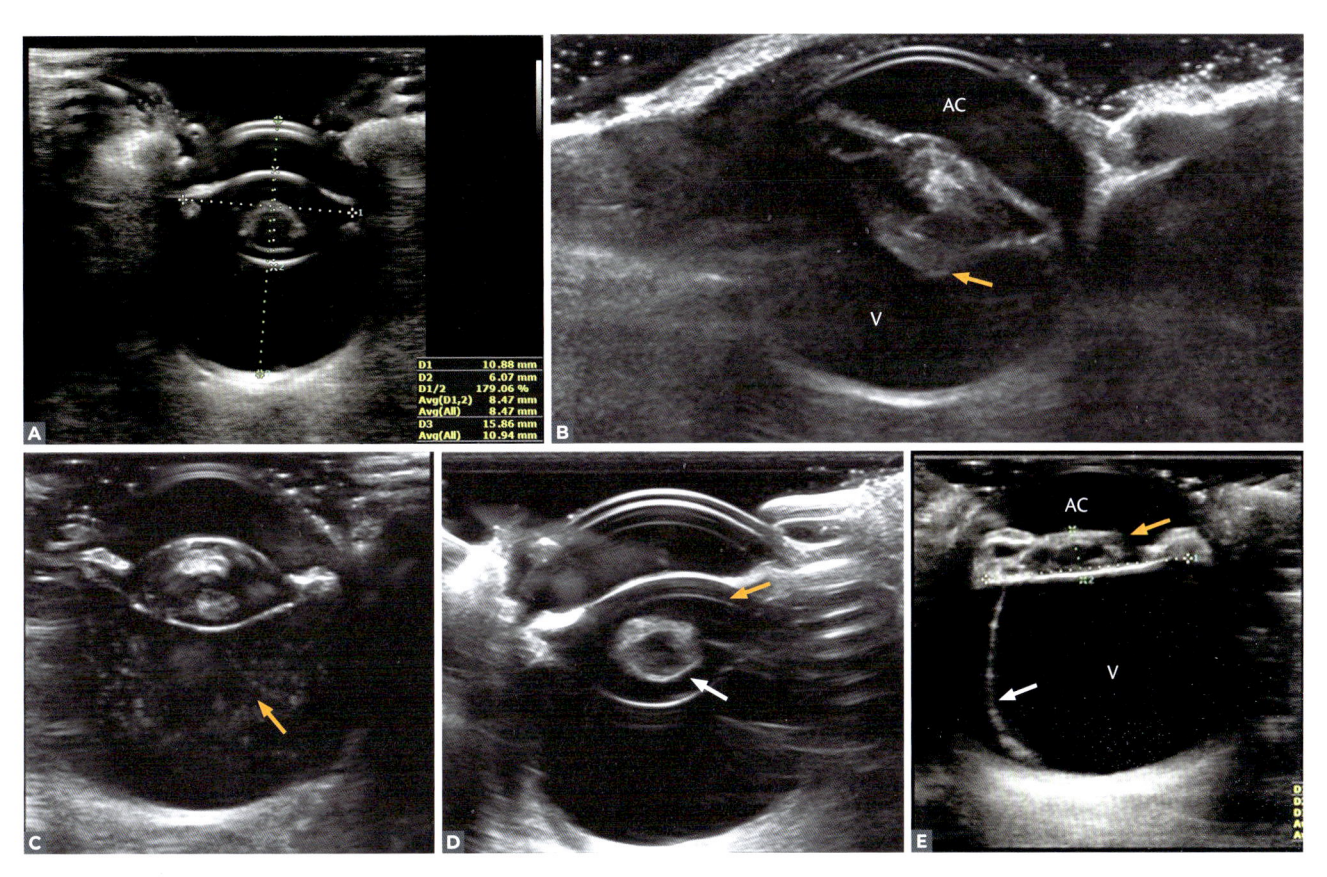

Fig. 15.6 (**A**) Horizontal ultrasound image of a one-year-old Shiba Inu showing the hyperechoic lens (cataract) with smooth anterior and posterior lens capsule. The measurement for presurgical cataract evaluation is illustrated, showing there is microphthalmos present. (**B**) Horizontal ultrasound image of a two-year-old Abyssinian cat showing the hyperechoic lens (cataract) with posterior lenticular plaque (arrow). V, vitreous; AC, anterior chamber. (**C**) Vertical ultrasound image of a nine-year-old mixed breed dog showing the hyperechoic lens with smooth anterior and posterior lens capsule. There are echogenic foci visible in the vitreous (arrow). (**D**) Horizontal ultrasound image of a one-year-old Cavalier King Charles Spaniel showing the hyperechoic nucleus of the lens (cortical cataract) with smooth anterior and posterior lens capsule (orange arrow). There is also nucleus sclerosis visible (white arrow). (**E**) Horizontal ultrasound image of a ten-year-old mixed breed dog showing the hyperechoic flattened lens with smooth anterior and posterior lens capsule (hypermature cataract) (orange arrow). There is lateral retinal detachment visible (white arrow). The measurement for presurgical cataract evaluation is illustrated.

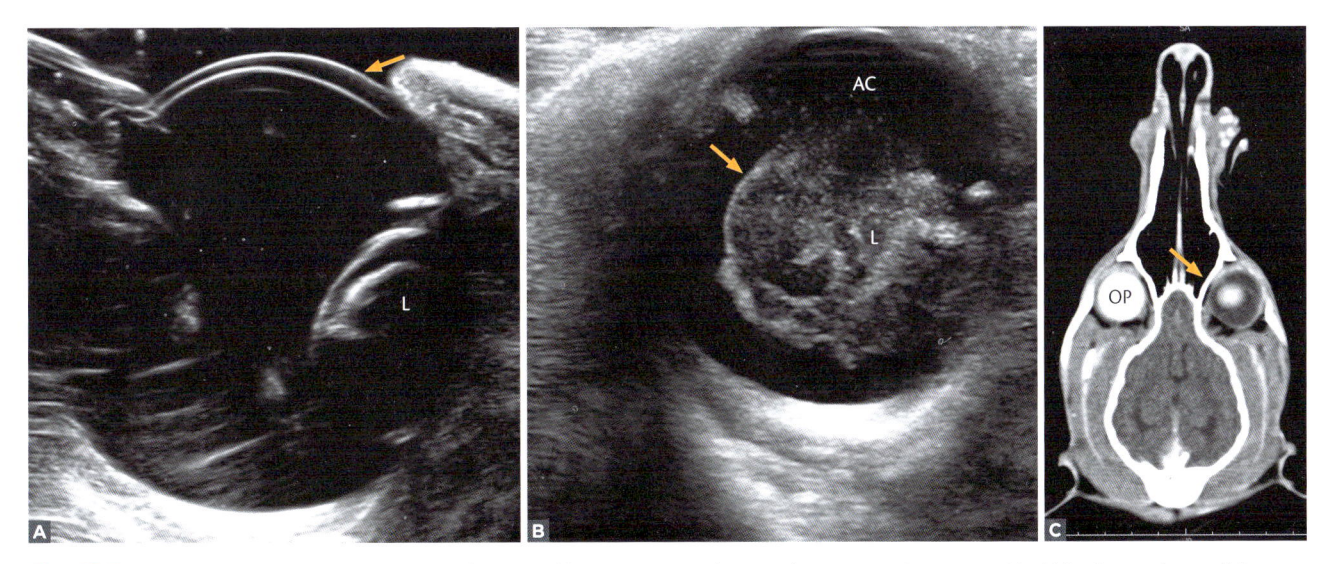

Fig. 15.7 (**A**) Horizontal ultrasound image of a five-year-old Boston Terrier showing the asymmetric cornea with thickening at the medial aspect (arrow). The anechoic lens is dislocated medially (L) illustrating the lens luxation. (**B**) Vertical ultrasound image of a 12-year-old Yorkshire Terrier showing echogenic lens (cataract) dislocated ventrally (L) illustrating the chronic lens luxation. (**C**) Dorsal MPR CT-image in soft tissue window shows the ocular prosthesis of the left eye (OP) and the lens luxation in the right eye (arrow).

Retina

A focal or complete retinal detachment may be diagnosed with ultrasound as a thin echogenic line between the ora ciliaris retinae (i.e., ora serrata) and the optic nerve, with an underlying anechoic or echogenic space. Total retinal detachment gives rise to two concave lines the apex of which meet at the optic nerve and are often referred to as having a "seagull" appearance.[17, 20] Retinal detachment is seldomly diagnosed through CT or MRI. On T1W and T2W MRI images subretinal fluid (edema and/or blood) appears hyperintense to the vitreous (**fig. 15.6E**).[11]

Ocular and orbital inflammatory disease and infections

Obstruction of the nasolacrimal apparatus

The third eyelid, eyelids, and nasolacrimal apparatus (NSA) that drains tears to the nose are also visible with CT. The NSA is composed of two openings (i.e., upper punctum and lower punctum) found in the medial edge of the conjunctival side of the eyelids, each of which leads to a short subconjunctival canaliculus that empties into the nasolacrimal sac, which sits on the lacrimal bone and continues as a fine intraosseous passage (i.e., the nasolacrimal duct) that ends in the nasopharyngeal area or the nasal vestibule. Foreign bodies, tumors or inflammation can obstruct the lacrimal sac or the interosseous duct. The NSA is best investigated with CT pre- and post-contrast. The latter requires injecting ≤1ml of contrast with a lacrimal cannula through the upper punctum while observing for a small drop of contrast to appear through the lower punctum, which is then closed with gentle finger pressure before injecting <0.5ml more. Patients with unilateral signs should also have contrast injected in the unaffected side, as it may be used for comparison.

Endophthalmitis, panophthalmitis, and orbital cellulitis

Endophthalmitis affects the anterior and posterior ocular cavities, while panophthamitis also affects the tunics of the globe (i.e., corneosclera and uvea), and may be caused by infectious agents (i.e., septic endophthalmitis/panophthalmitis) including a variety of bacteria, fungi, and feline infectious peritonitis, although it may also be aseptic (i.e., immune-mediated), degenerative, neoplastic,

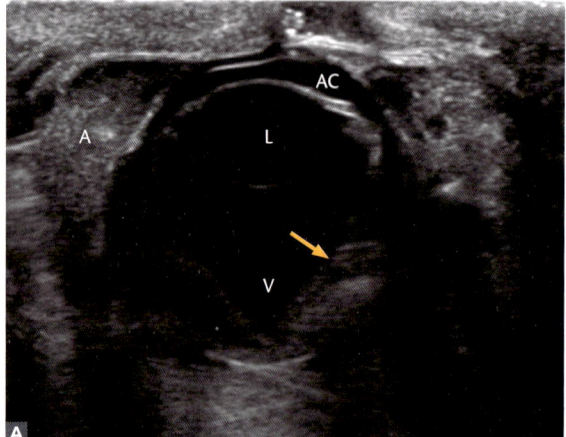

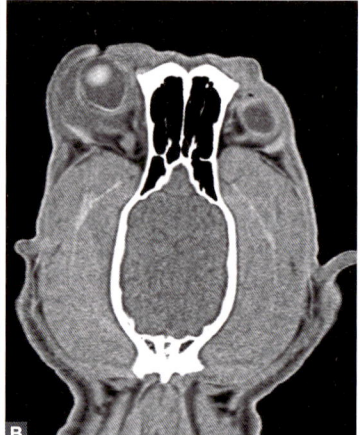

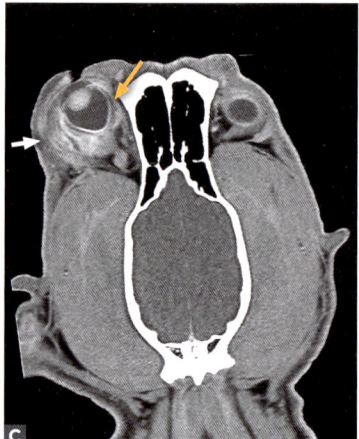

Fig. 15.8 (**A**) Horizontal ultrasound image of a six-month-old Bernese Mountain dog showing the severely thickened scleral wall and deformation of the vitreal cavity with suspicion of retinal detachment (arrow). At the lateral aspect of the globe there is the suspicion of an abscess caused by severe diffuse scleritis. A, abscess; L, lens; AC, anterior chamber; V, vitreous. (**B**) Pre- and post-contrast dorsal MPR CT image of a six-month-old Bernese Mountain dog showing the severely thickened scleral wall and deformation of the globe with suspicion of retinal detachment (orange arrow). At the lateral aspect of the globe there is the suspicion of an abscess (white arrow) caused by severe diffuse scleritis.

CHAPTER 15 Eye and orbit

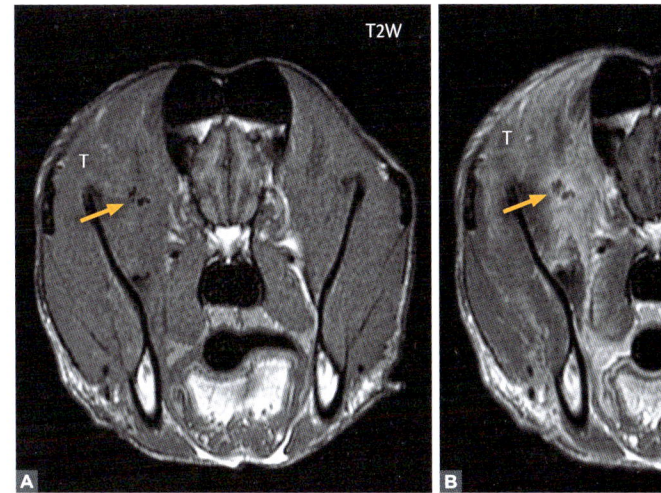

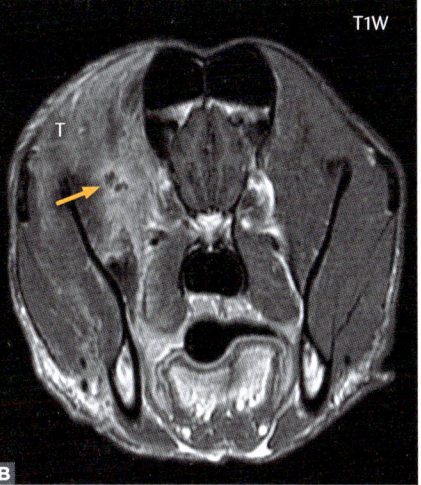

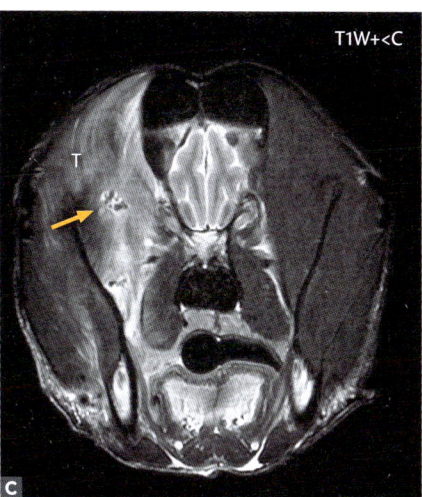

Fig. 15.9 (A-C) Transverse T2W and pre- and post-contrast T1W MRI images of a five-year-old hunting dog show the abnormal T2W hyperintense and T1W isointense signal of the temporal muscle (T) with severe heterogenous contrast enhancement (temporal myositis). In the mid region, there is low signal intensity linear structure (arrow), suspicious for a foreign body. (D) Ultrasound image of the same patient using the dorsal approach. There is a small hyperechoic linear structure with acoustic shadowing visible, demonstrating the foreign body (arrow).

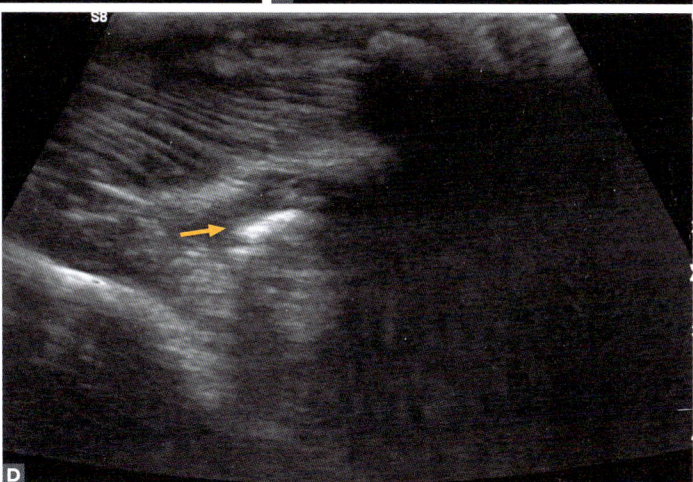

or traumatic in nature, including trauma caused by migrating foreign bodies. Imaging may show thickening of intraocular structures and the scleroretinal rim with strong post-contrast enhancement on CT and MRI images, possible retinal detachment, possible deformation of the globe, and orbital fat that is often ill-defined (**fig. 15.8**).[1-3]

Orbital cellulitis may be caused by penetrating foreign bodies (i.e., often via the oral cavity or conjunctival sac) (**fig. 15.9**), bite wounds, dental disease, or hematogenous spread of infectious organisms. On US it takes the appearance of a diffuse increased echogenicity with blurring of the margins of the orbital structures with or without a discrete cavitary lesion (i.e., abscess). Imaging with CT and MRI enables the visualization of the extension of an inflammatory process within the orbit and possible intracranial extension, and of for the evaluation of dental disease, such the presence of periapical abscesses.[13-17]

Extraocular polymyositis

This is a rare, unilateral or bilateral, idiopathic disease with a predisposition in young Golden Retrievers, that is believed to be immune-mediated and affects single or multiple extraocular muscles. The acute presentation is associated with exophthalmos. Ultrasonography may show enlarged, hypoechoic muscles.[1-3, 18, 19] An increase in volume and loss of definition of the extraocular muscles is visible on CT and MRI, with strong enhancement and increased T2W signal intensity, respectively. Atrophy and fibrosis of the extraocular muscles are associated with the chronic stage of untreated or severe cases, or cases with a delayed diagnosis (**fig. 15.10**).

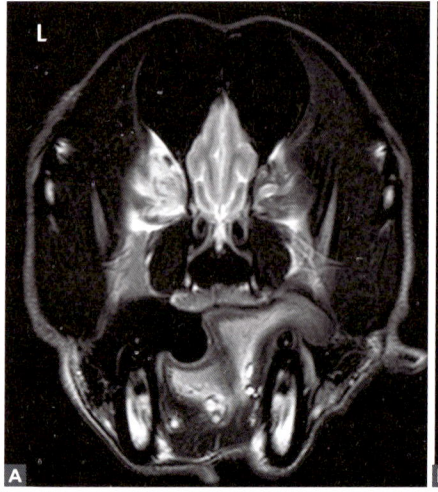

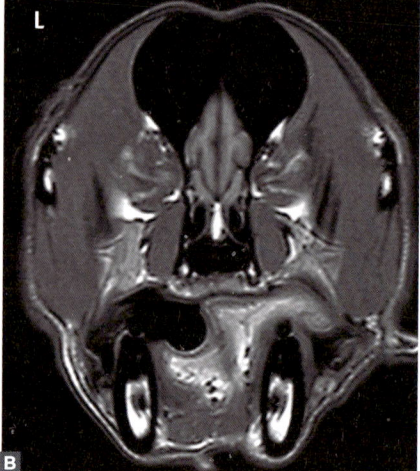

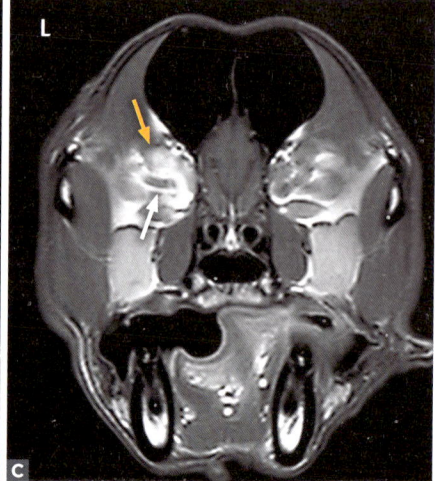

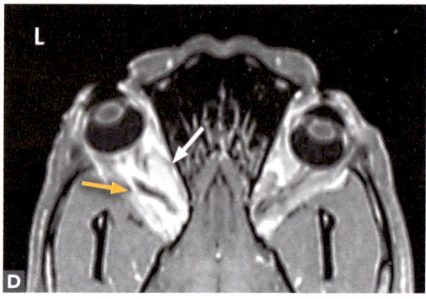

Fig. 15.10 (**A-C**) Transverse T2W and pre- and post-contrast T1W MRI images of a three-year-old Labrador Retriever showing the left-sided abnormal T2W hyperintense and T1W isointense signal of the mildly thickened extraocular muscles (orange arrow) with severe heterogenous contrast enhancement (extraocular polymyositis). The left optic nerve is also thickened with contrast enhancement of the nerve sheath of the optic nerve (white arrow). (**D**) Dorsal post-contrast T1W MRI images of a three-year-old Labrador Retriever showing the left-sided mildly thickened extraocular muscles (orange arrow) with severe heterogenous contrast enhancement (extraocular polymyositis). The left optic nerve is also thickened with contrast enhancement of the nerve sheath of the optic nerve (white arrow).

Optic neuritis

This presents as a uni- or bilateral inflammation of the optic nerve caused by a localized form of meningitis of unknown origin (i.e., previously referred to as granulomatous meningoencephalitis), or infectious, neoplastic, or idiopathic immune-mediated diseases. The optic nerve and accompanying meninges may appear normal or thickened. The optic nerve might appear hypoechoic on US, while CT and MRI images usually show a strong enhancement of the optic nerve sheath. Depending on what part of the optic nerve is affected, intraocular changes at the level of the papilla (i.e., papillary swelling, peripapillary hemorrhage and/or bullous retinal detachment) might also be visible on US evaluation of the posterior pole (**figs. 15.10D** and **15.11**).[1-3, 13-17]

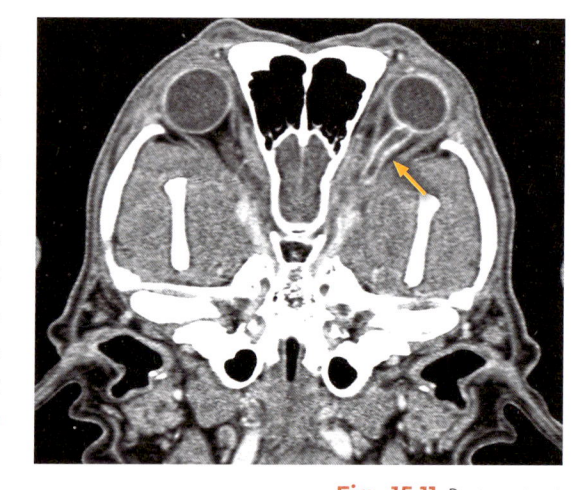

Fig. 15.11 Post-contrast dorsal MPR CT image in soft tissue window of a four-year-old Labrador Retriever showing the contrast enhancement of the nerve sheath of the right optic nerve suggestive of optic nerve neuritis (arrow).

Trauma

Blunt or penetrating trauma may result in anterior displacement of the eye (i.e., globe proptosis), bleeding (i.e., hyphema if hemorrhage in the anterior chamber, intravitreal or retrobulbar), retinal detachment, globe rupture, and fractures of the orbital bones with associated disruption of the normal orbital anatomy. Brachycephalic breeds are predisposed to globe proptosis.

Scleral rupture on US is often seen as an ill-defined scleroretinal rim in an eye with echogenic material in the ocular cavities and possible retinal detachment,[20] while CT and/or MRI images show an irregular contour of the globe with decreased volume (**fig. 15.12**). Leakage of T2W hyperintense and T1W hypointense vitreous through the scleroretinal rim may also be visible on MRI.

Orbital fractures are best visualized on CT images and 3D reconstructions may enable insight into the dislocation of bone fragments with alteration of the orbit. Acute fractures are usually sharply marginated, whereas chronic fractures may show ill-defined margins with callus formation. Orbital soft tissue damage may show as a mass effect due to hemorrhage and edema, while orbital emphysema will show as air artifacts on CT and signal void on MRI images (**fig. 15.15**).

Intraocular and orbital foreign bodies

Often, foreign bodies cannot be visualized. Their appearance varies depending on their nature, size, shape, and location. Ocular and orbital foreign bodies may appear on US as a hyperechoic structure with shadowing (plant-like material) or a comet tail artifact (metal) and surrounded by hypoechoic tissue. Foreign bodies on CT may appear as hyperattenuating structures occasionally surrounded by hypoattenuating tissue, while on MRI they may be recognized as a signal void that does not correspond to an anatomic structure (**figs. 15.9** and **15.13**).[1-3, 13, 14]

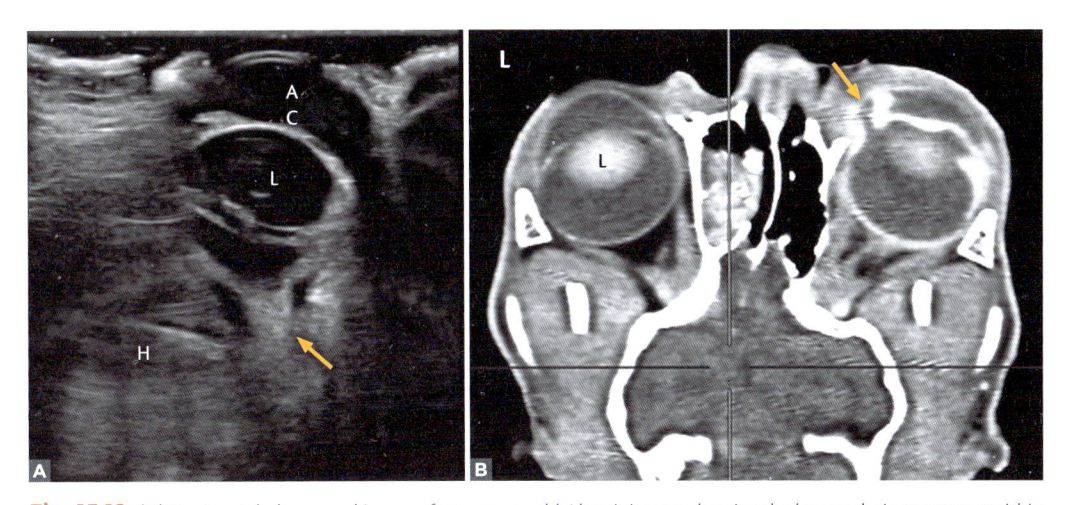

Fig. 15.12 (**A**) Horizontal ultrasound image of a two-year-old Abyssinian cat showing the hyperechoic structures within the vitreous (V), which appears decreased in size. The anterior chamber (AC) and lens (L) are unremarkable. A hyperechoic linear structure interrupting the posterior wall was suspected to correspond to a globe rupture (arrow). In the retrobulbar space, the normal anatomical structures are no longer visible and replaced by amorphous echogenic structures most likely representing hemorrhage (H). (**B**) Post-contrast dorsal MPR CT image in soft tissue window of a two-year-old Domestic shorthair cat with a history of being hit by a car. There is an abnormal conformation of the medial aspect of the right globe with suspicion of rupture of the globe (arrow) at the corneoscleral transition. The iris is mildly thickened. The anterior chamber and vitreous are unremarkable.

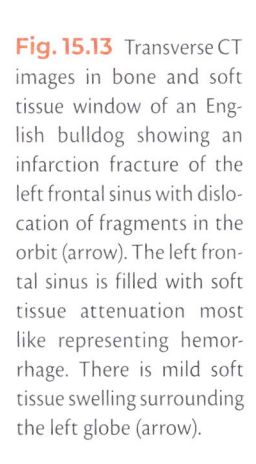

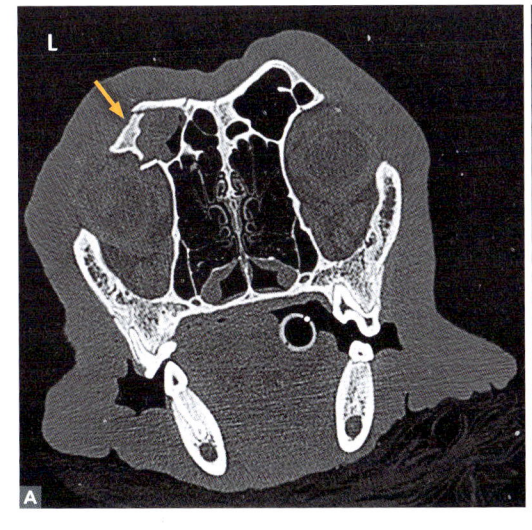

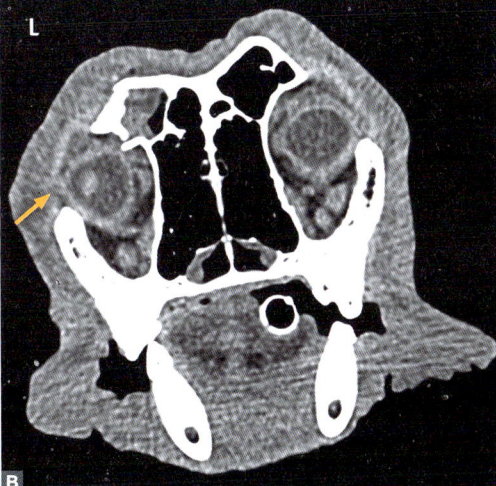

Fig. 15.13 Transverse CT images in bone and soft tissue window of an English bulldog showing an infarction fracture of the left frontal sinus with dislocation of fragments in the orbit (arrow). The left frontal sinus is filled with soft tissue attenuation most like representing hemorrhage. There is mild soft tissue swelling surrounding the left globe (arrow).

Ocular and orbital tumors

Ocular tumors are imaged as a soft tissue mass associated with the iris and/or ciliary body. Melanocytoma/melanoma and adenoma/carcinoma are the most common primary tumors of the uvea, and lymphoma is one of the commonest secondary tumors. Post-traumatic sarcoma is rare, but it has been reported in cats. Uveal tumors may cause inflammatory-like disease (i.e., uveitis-masquerade syndrome), hyphema, and/or glaucoma. Tumors arising from the posterior segment include medulloepitheliomas. Masses of the optic papilla or nerve include astrocytoma and meningiomas. Ultrasound can easily depict intraocular tumors, but CT and MRI may detect more detailed orbital invasion. MRI may diagnose melanoma with a hyperintense signal on T1W and hypointense on T2W images due to the paramagnetic properties of melanin in the mass (**figs. 15.15-15.18**).[1-3, 14-17, 21] Orbital tumors including primary neoplasia and local extension from neoplasia of the adjacent structures are mostly malignant and include carcinomas, sarcomas (such as myxosarcomas and feline restrictive orbital myofibroblastic sarcoma), round-cell tumors, and meningioma. Imaging findings are altered orbital anatomy caused either by diffuse increase or a mass lesion with heterogenous or homogenous, mild to strong contrast enhancement with or without local bone

Fig. 15.14 Horizontal ultrasound image of a seven-year-old German Pointer showing several linear hyperechoic structures in the anterior chamber of the left eye. There was the suspicion of a foreign body, most likely a grass awn (orange arrow). The cornea (C) is mildly thickened, and the stroma is echogenic. In the vitreous (V) there are several echoes visible. The scleroretinal rim is also mildly thickened with a hypoechoic structure (white arrow).

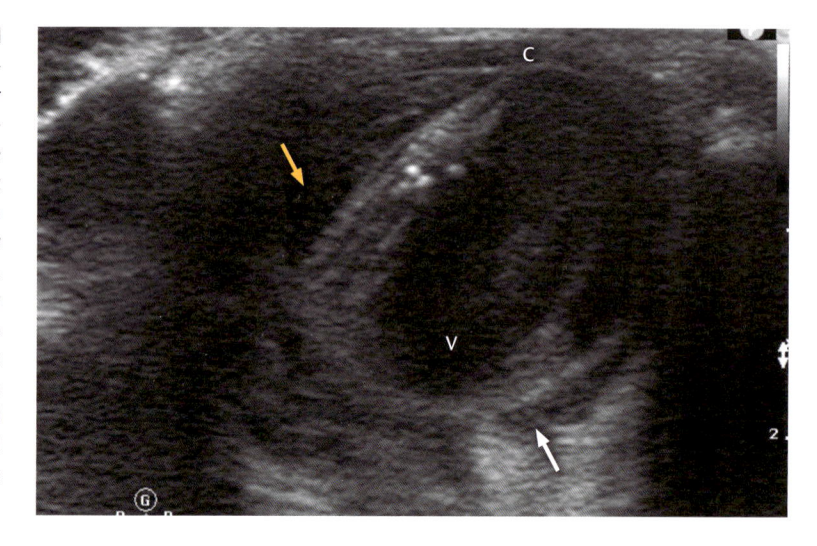

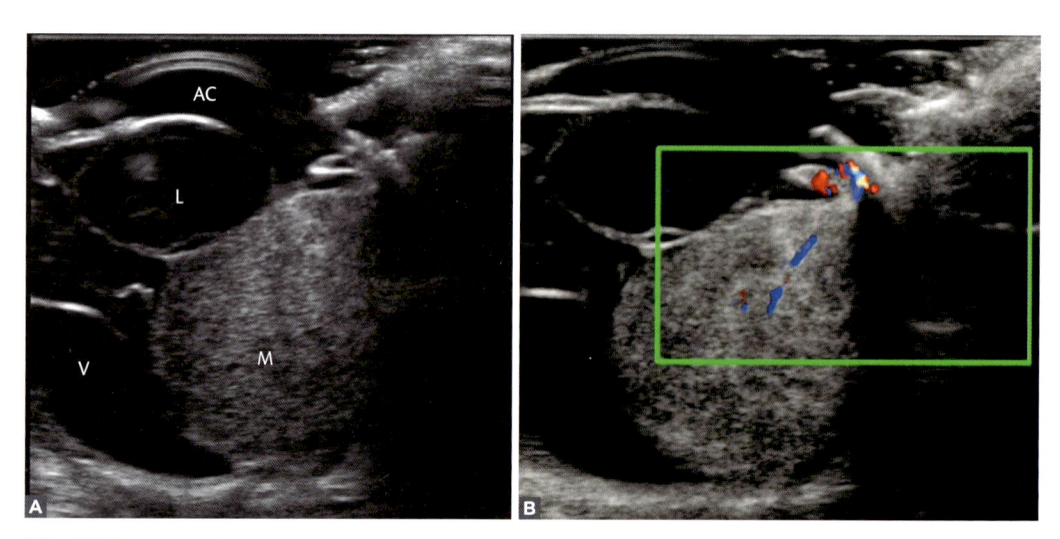

Fig. 15.15 Horizontal ultrasound image of a nine-year-old Flatcoated Retriever showing a large mass tumor originating from the medial ciliary body invading the vitreous (V) and mildly dislocating the lens (L). The structure is homogenous and echogenic. The anterior chamber is unremarkable (AC). The color Doppler image illustrates blood flow within the mass.

CHAPTER 15 Eye and orbit

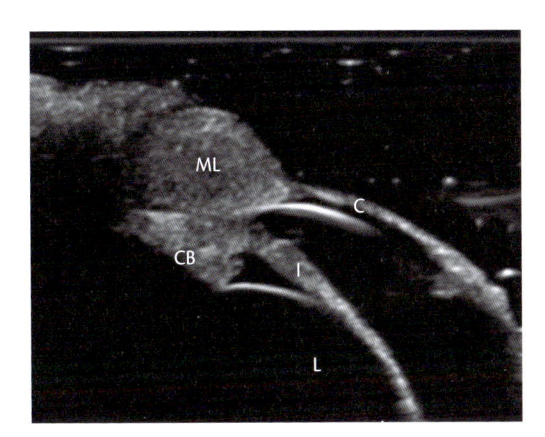

Fig. 15.16 Vertical ultrasound image of the anterior segment of a White Shepherd dog showing the small mass lesion (M) at the transition zone from the cornea (C) to the sclera. There is no invasion in the ciliary body (CB) and iris (I) visible. Histopathology confirmed the suspected diagnosis of a melanocytoma.

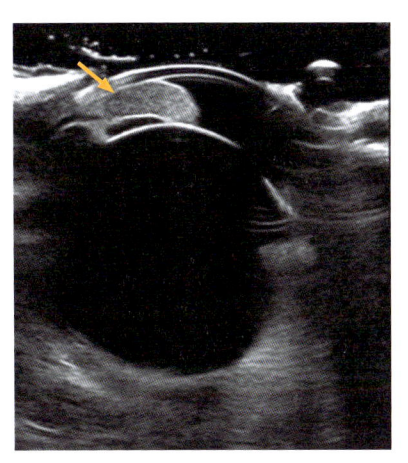

Fig. 15.17 Horizontal ultrasound image of a 12-year-old Domestic shorthair cat showing the severely thickened lateral iris with a homogenous echogenic structure (arrow). Histopathology confirmed the suspected diagnosis of melanoma.

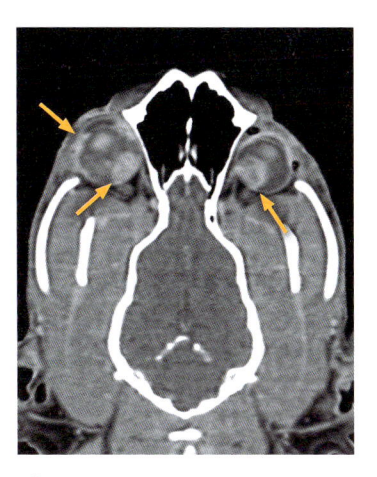

Fig. 15.18 Post-contrast dorsal MPR CT image of a seven-year-old Labrador Retriever showing contrast-enhancing masses in both eyes suspicious of metastatic disease (arrows). The ciliary body of the left eye appears prominent.

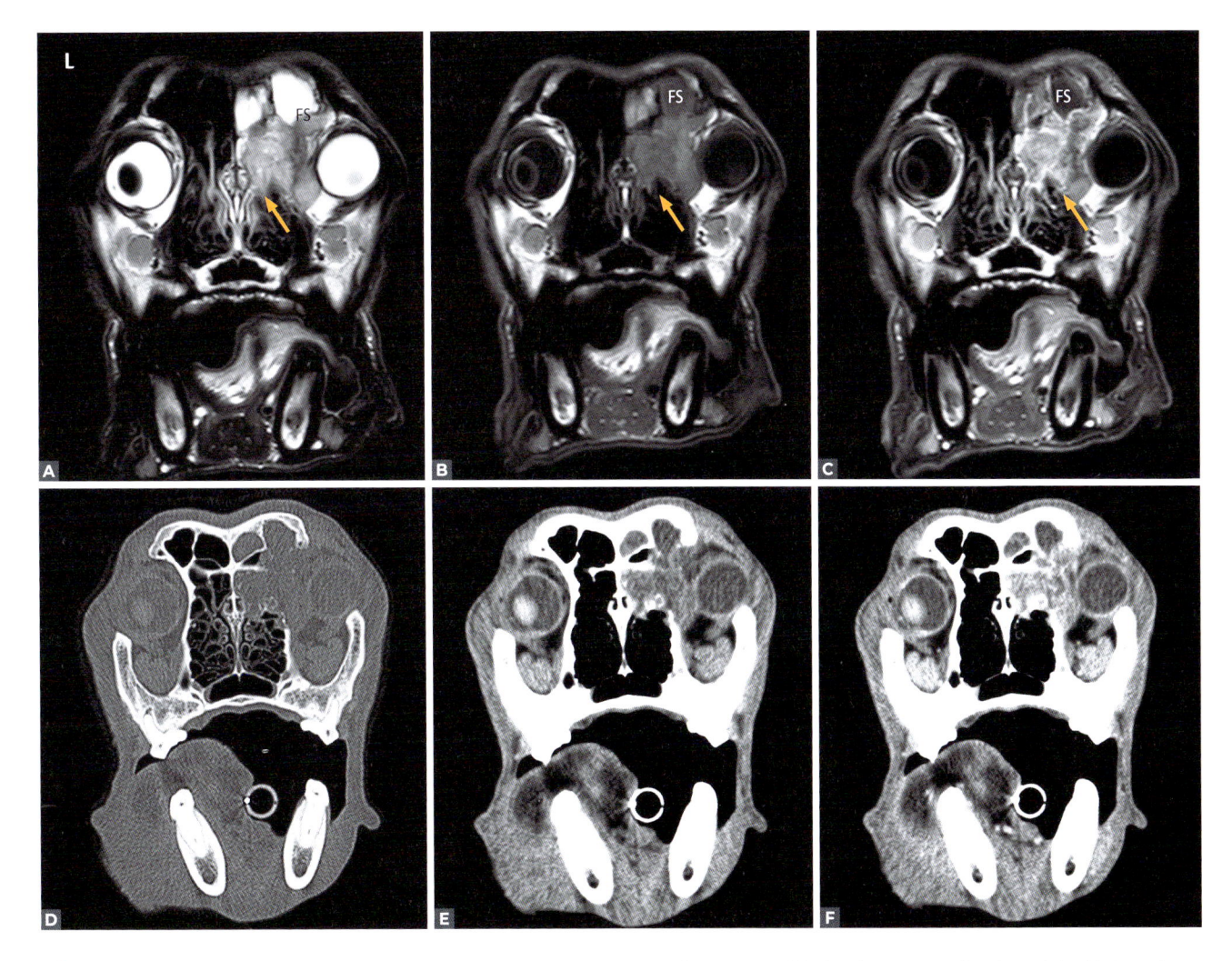

Fig. 15.19 (**A-C**) Transverse T2W and pre- and post-contrast T1W MRI images of a nine-year-old Labrador Retriever showing a right-sided nasal neoplasm tumor invading the right orbit. The mass shows a heterogenous signal with severe heterogenous contrast enhancement and mild displacement of the right eye (arrow). The right frontal sinus is filled with fluid signal (FS). (**D-F**) Pre- and post-contrast transverse CT-image in bone and soft tissue window of the same nine-year-old Labrador Retriever showing the aggressive tumor originating in the caudal right nasal cavity and invading the right orbit.

Fig. 15.20 Pre- and post-contrast T1W MRI images of a Bouvier with acute blindness showing a broad-based and well-defined homogeneous contrast-enhancing mass lesion at the level of the optic chiasma.

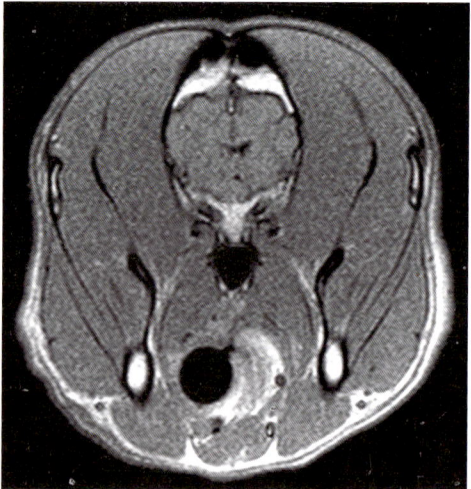

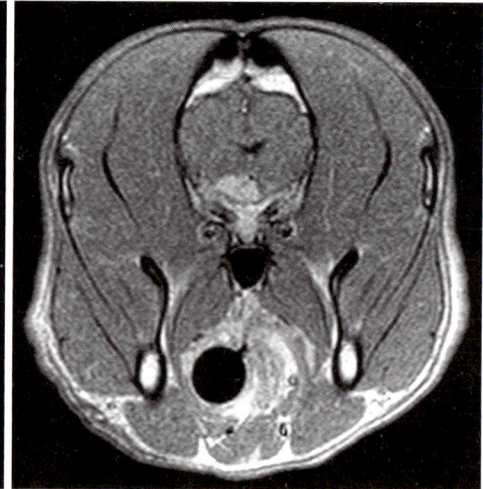

destruction or new bone formation. Neoplastic orbital mass lesions show on US, CT, and MRI images more often with well-defined margins as compared to inflammatory disease. Bony destruction of the medial bony wall will appear in the US as heterogenous with defects. CT and MRI enable detailed evaluation of the involvement of the surrounding bones, nasal cavity, optic nerve, and cranium (**figs. 15.19** and **15.20**).

References

1. Dennis R, Johnson PJ, McLellan GJ. Diagnostic imaging of the eye and orbit. In Gould D, McLellan GJ (editors). BSAVA Manual of Canine and Feline Ophthalmology 3rd edition. Wiley Blackwell, 2014, pp 24-50.
2. Penninck D, Daniel GB, Brawer R, Tidwell AS. Cross-sectional imaging techniques in veterinary ophthalmology. *Clin Tech Small Anim Pract* 16:22-39, 2001.
3. Pizzirani MS, Penninck D, Spaulding K. Eye and orbit. In Penninck D, d'Anjou MA (editors). Atlas of Small Animal Ultrasonography 2nd edition. Wiley Blackwell, 2015, pp 19-54.
4. Boroffka SAEB, Voorhout G. Direct and reconstructed multiplanar computed tomography of the orbits of healthy dogs. *Am J Vet Res* 60:1500-1507, 1999.
5. Salguera R, Johnson V, Williams D, et al. CT dimensions, volumes and densities of normal canine eyes. *Vet Rec* 176:386, 2015.
6. Manchip KEL, Sansom PG, Donaldson D, Warren-Smith C. Magnetic resonance imaging of the normal canine eye using a T1-weighted volumetric acquisition. *Vet Rec* 189:e505, 2021.
7. Boroffka SAEB, Voorhout G, Verbruggen AM, Teske E. Intraobserver and interobserver repeatability of ocular biometric measurements obtained by means of B-mode ultrasonography in dogs. *Am J Vet Res* 67:1743-1749, 2006.
8. Boroffka SAEB, Görig C, Auriemma E, et al. Magnetic resonance imaging of the canine optic nerve. *Vet Radiol Ultrasound* 49:540-544, 2008.
9. Dennis R. Use of magnetic resonance imaging for the investigation of orbital disease in small animals. *J Small Anim Pract* 41:145-155, 2000.
10. Boroffka SAEB, Verbruggen AM, Boeve MH, Stades FC. Ultrasonographic diagnosis of persistent hyperplastic tunica vasculosa lentis/persistent hyperplastic primary vitreous in two dogs. *Vet Radiol Ultrasound* 39:440-444, 1998.
11. van der Woerdt A, Wilkie DA, Myer CW. Ultrasonographic abnormalities in the eyes of dogs with cataracts: 147 cases (1986-1992). *J Am Vet Med Assoc* 203:838-841, 1993.
12. Wilkie DA, Gemensky, Metzler AJ, Colitz CM, et al. Canine cataracts, diabetes mellitus and spontaneous lens capsule rupture: a retrospective study of 18 dogs. *Vet Ophthalmol* 9:328-334, 2006.
13. Hoyt L, Greenberg M, MacPhail C, Eichelberger B, Marolf A, Kraft S. Imaging diagnosis – magnetic resonance imaging of an organizing abscess secondary to a retrobulbar grass awn. *Vet Radiol Ultrasound* 50:646-648, 2009.
14. Boroffka SAEB, Verbruggen AM, Grinwis GCM, Voorhout G, Barthez PY. Assessment of ultrasonography and computed tomography for the evaluation of unilateral orbital disease in dogs. *J Am Vet Med Assoc* 230:671-680, 2007.
15. Armour MD, Broome M, Dell'Anna G, Blades NJ, Esson DW. A review of orbital and intracranial magnetic resonance imaging in 79 canine and 13 feline patients (2004-2010). *Vet Ophthalmol* 14:215-226, 2011.
16. Dennis R. Use of magnetic resonance imaging for the investigation of orbital disease in small animals. *J Small Anim Pract* 41:145-155, 2000.
17. Morgan RV, Ring RD, Ward DA, Adams WH. Magnetic resonance imaging of ocular and orbital disease in 5 dogs and a cat. *Vet Radiol Ultrasound* 37:185-192, 1996.
18. Allgoewer I, Blair M, Basher T, et al. Extraocular muscle myositis and restrictive strabismus in 10 dogs. *Vet Ophthalmol* 3:21-26, 2000.
19. Joslyn S, Richards S, Boroffka S, et al. Magnetic resonance imaging contrast enhancement of extra-ocular muscles in dogs with no clinical evidence of orbital disease. *Vet Radiol Ultrasound* 55:63-67, 2014.
20. Rampazzo A, Eule C, Speier S, Grest P, Spiess B. Scleral rupture in dogs, cats, and horses. *Vet Ophthalmol* 9:149-155, 2006.
21. Bell CM, Schwarz T, Dubielzig RR. Diagnostic features of feline restrictive orbital myofibroblastic sarcoma. *Vet Pathol* 48:742-750, 2011.

CHAPTER 16

Vertebral column

Ruth Dennis

KEY POINTS

- Survey radiography is a useful initial imaging modality for investigation of diseases of the vertebral column, and will show lesions involving bone, some disc space changes and larger paraspinal soft tissue masses.
- High quality images with careful patient positioning and including orthogonal views are usually required.
- Demonstration of spinal cord compression, deviation or swelling requires myelography, although this is not without a degree of risk to the patient.
- A thorough appreciation of spinal anatomy and variants, such as transitional vertebrae, is important.
- MRI is the modality of choice for spinal imaging as it will depict all the spinal structures clearly.
- CT is excellent for bone and some disc lesions but demonstration of spinal cord compression or swelling often requires CT myelography.

Imaging techniques for the spine

Survey radiography

Survey radiography is a valuable tool for investigation of spinal disease, especially for lesions involving bone.[1] Signs of disc disease may also be evident (see later), although some disc lesions may not be currently clinically relevant and myelography, MRI or CT are needed to confirm the site and degree of any resulting spinal cord compression. It is important to include the whole area of potential pathology; for example, neurological deficits in the pelvic limbs may result from lesions as far cranially as the T3 spinal cord segment. If neoplasia is suspected, thoracic radiographs should also be obtained to look for lung metastases and in patients with suspected trauma, thoracic radiography and abdominal radiography or ultrasonography should be performed for detection of associated pathology such as diaphragmatic hernia, pneumothorax or ruptured bladder.

Appropriate restraint for radiography is important as radiographs obtained in conscious patients are likely to be suboptimally positioned and only large lesions will be evident. Sedation or general anesthesia is generally required for diagnostic images; the more subtle the radiographic changes the better the images must be. Trauma patients must be handled with great care, and this is described in the section on trauma.

Positioning aids such as radiolucent foam wedges of different sizes are required to pad the patient so that the spine lies in a straight line parallel to the table top for lateral radiographs (**fig. 16.1**). Sandbags should not be included in the primary beam as they generate scattered radiation.

SECTION III AXIAL SKELETON

In most patients, multiple radiographs with different centering points are required for accurate depiction of the spine, especially of the disc spaces, due to the geometry of the diverging X-ray beam. Orthogonal views (i.e., lateral and VD) are usually required; oblique projections are occasionally helpful. Stressed views can be obtained in certain circumstances but care must be taken if such positioning might increase the risk to the spinal cord, for example the flexed lateral radiograph for detection of atlantoaxial subluxation. In the caudal neck and at the lumbosacral junction flexed and hyperextended positioning can be employed to demonstrate instability, and a flexed VD projection of the lumbosacral junction with the pelvic limbs pulled cranially is a useful way of seeing the lumbosacral disc space clearly.[2]

Myelography

Myelography involves the injection of a low-osmolarity, iodine-based contrast medium into the subarachnoid space, thus surrounding the spinal cord and demonstrating areas of spinal cord swelling (intramedullary lesions, **figs. 16.2A** and **16.2B**) or compression (intradural-extramedullary lesions, **figs. 16.2C** and **16.D**; extradural lesions, **figs. 16.2E** and **16.2F**).[3]

Fig. 16.1 (**A**) Schematic view of a dog in lateral recumbency showing how the spine can sag towards the table top, resulting in poor positioning for radiography and inaccurate depiction of vertebrae and disc spaces. (**B**) Radiolucent foam pads placed under the mid neck and mid lumbar areas in order to align the spine straight, level and parallel to the table top.

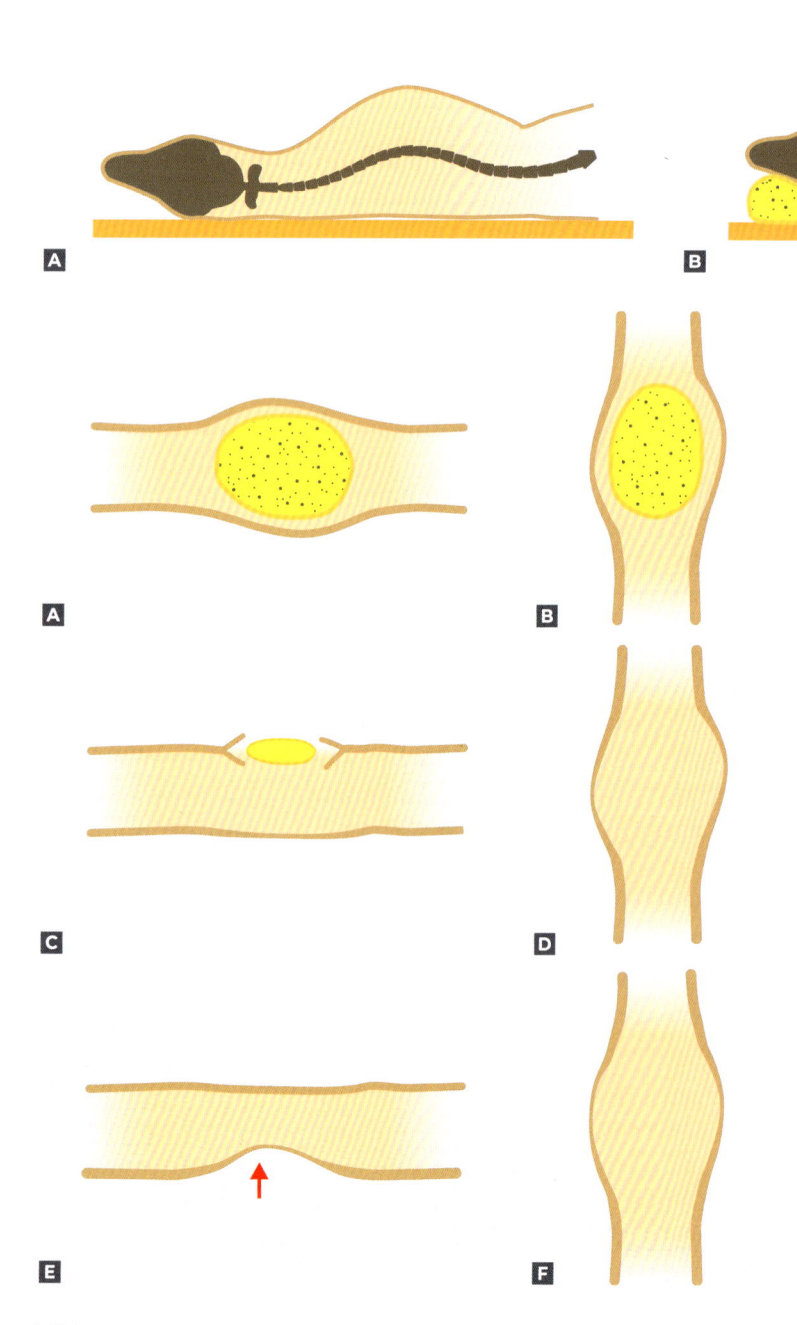

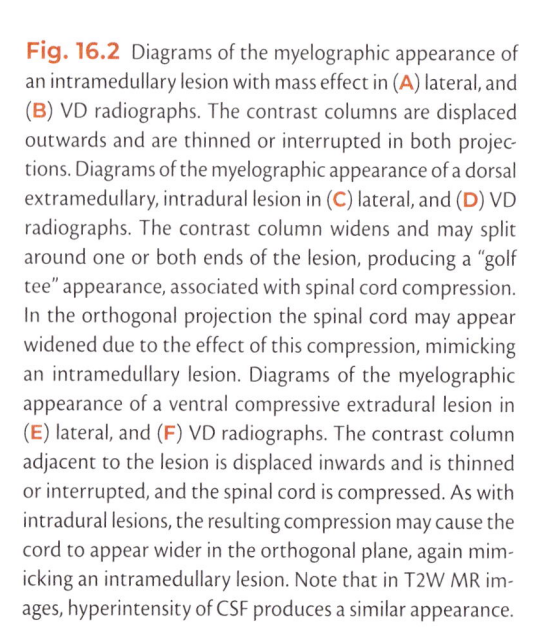

Fig. 16.2 Diagrams of the myelographic appearance of an intramedullary lesion with mass effect in (**A**) lateral, and (**B**) VD radiographs. The contrast columns are displaced outwards and are thinned or interrupted in both projections. Diagrams of the myelographic appearance of a dorsal extramedullary, intradural lesion in (**C**) lateral, and (**D**) VD radiographs. The contrast column widens and may split around one or both ends of the lesion, producing a "golf tee" appearance, associated with spinal cord compression. In the orthogonal projection the spinal cord may appear widened due to the effect of this compression, mimicking an intramedullary lesion. Diagrams of the myelographic appearance of a ventral compressive extradural lesion in (**E**) lateral, and (**F**) VD radiographs. The contrast column adjacent to the lesion is displaced inwards and is thinned or interrupted, and the spinal cord is compressed. As with intradural lesions, the resulting compression may cause the cord to appear wider in the orthogonal plane, again mimicking an intramedullary lesion. Note that in T2W MR images, hyperintensity of CSF produces a similar appearance.

Myelography is especially helpful in cases in which survey radiographs are normal, and to demonstrate the significant site of disc disease. Prior to injection, CSF may be collected for analysis if required; contrast medium is then injected with care either into the *cisterna magna* between the skull and C1 (cisternal myelography) or into the ventral lumbar subarachnoid space at L5-L6 (dogs) or L6-L7 (cats). The technique is not without risk to the patient and untoward sequelae include seizures, temporary or permanent worsening of neurological signs, cardiorespiratory arrest and needlestick injuries of the brainstem. Following injection of the contrast medium, lateral and VD radiographs should be acquired routinely but oblique projections can also be helpful, especially for demonstrating the exact location of compressive extradural lesions such as disc extrusions.[4] A DV projection is preferred to a VD for the cervicothoracic junction, as contrast medium will pool dependently under gravity. Although many patients now undergo investigation with MRI or CT, which are safer, radiographic myelography is still occasionally used and CT myelography using smaller amounts of contrast medium can be performed.

Magnetic resonance imaging

For most purposes, magnetic resonance imaging (MRI) is the preferred technique for spinal imaging due to its excellent soft tissue and acceptable bone detail; however, when fine bone detail is essential computed tomography (CT) is preferred. MRI scanning may be performed in ventral, dorsal or lateral recumbency depending on the size of the patient and the shape of the radiofrequency coil used. Whichever recumbency is used, the spine should be as straight as possible to facilitate acquisition of diagnostic sagittal images. For most purposes T2-weighted (T2W) images yield the most information due to the high contrast between spinal cord, CSF and epidural fat, discs, vertebrae and surrounding soft tissues (**fig. 16.3A**). However, other sequences which may be of value depending on the pathology under investigation include pre- and post-contrast T1W (the latter ideally with fat suppression in high field units) (**fig. 16.3B**), STIR and T2* gradient echo. Sagittal and transverse image planes are used routinely but the dorsal plane is also very useful and is often overlooked; oblique planes are also occasionally employed.

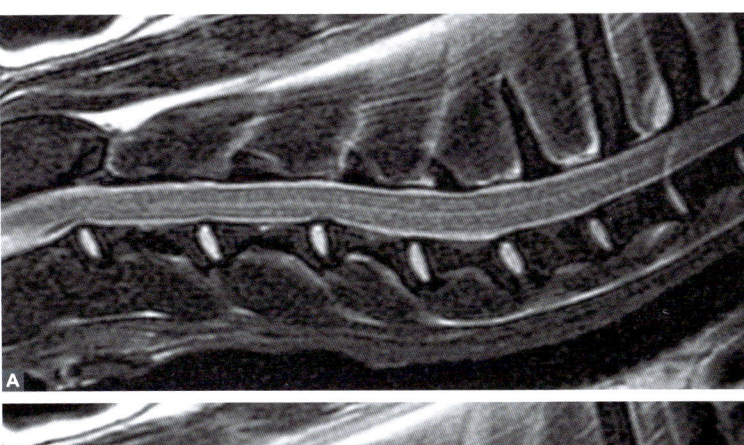

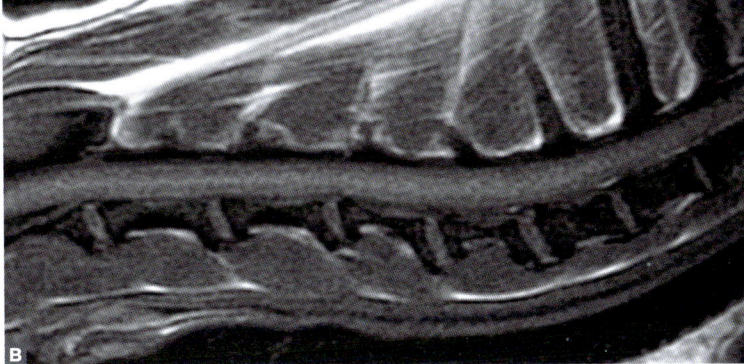

Fig. 16.3 (**A**) Normal sagittal T2W MRI image of the cervical spine of a Border Collie. CSF in the subarachnoid space and central canal of the spinal cord and hydrated disc material are hyperintense. (**B**) Normal sagittal T1W MRI image of the cervical spine in the same dog. CSF and hydrated disc material are hypointense and contrast between the subarachnoid space and the spinal cord is much poorer than with T2W.

When scanning the thoracolumbar spine, it can be hard to identify individual vertebrae unless the lumbosacral junction is included in the field of view. A useful tip is to identify the location of the celiac and cranial mesenteric arteries in a sagittal image which includes the lumbosacral junction and to note this for subsequent scans obtained more cranially. They usually lie close to L1, but their precise position varies between individuals.

Flexion/extension scans and traction studies are possible but a detailed description of spinal MRI technique is beyond the scope of this chapter.[5]

Computed tomography

For spinal CT, dorsal recumbency is best as it reduces the effect of respiratory motion. However, if the thorax and/or abdomen are also to be scanned ventral recumbency may be preferred, and if patient manipulation should be minimized lateral recumbency may be safest. If CT myelography is to be performed, lateral or ventral recumbency may be more practical. As with MRI, the spine should be as straight as possible to facilitate reconstruction of the primary transverse images into the sagittal plane. Depending on the area scanned, the thoracic or pelvic limbs should be restrained cranially or caudally away from the scanning field of view to reduce artefact. For the lumbosacral junction, scanning with the area in both flexion and extension may be useful.

Tube voltage should be 100-120 kVp and tube current 200 mA with a slice width of 1-2 mm.[6] Low and high frequency reconstruction algorithms should be used to provide soft tissue and bone windows respectively. For soft tissue the images should be displayed using a window level (WL) of 100 HU and window width (WW) of 300 HU and for bone WL 500 HU and WW 3000. The soft tissue study may be repeated following intravenous injection of iodinated contrast medium, using 600-800 mg L/kg body weight (**fig. 16.4**). Non-ionic contrast media have a lower osmotic pressure than ionic media, resulting in fewer side-effects. CT myelography can also be performed as described radiographically using non-ionic media but with a smaller dose of contrast medium to avoid blooming artifact (e.g., 60 mg L/kg body weight).

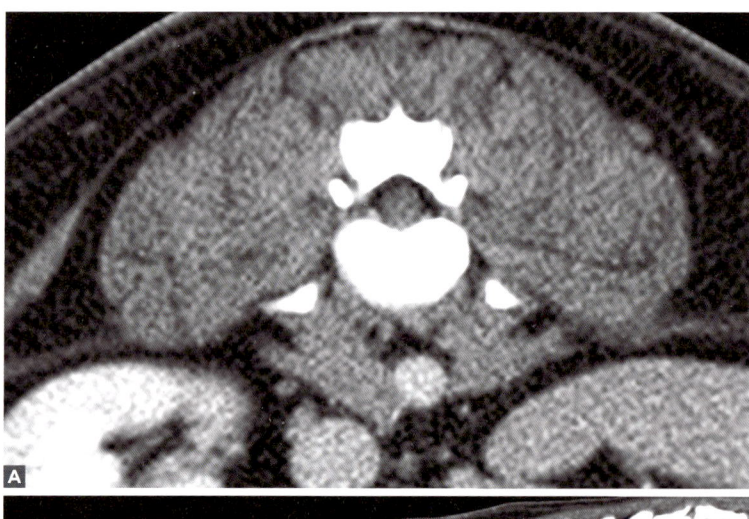

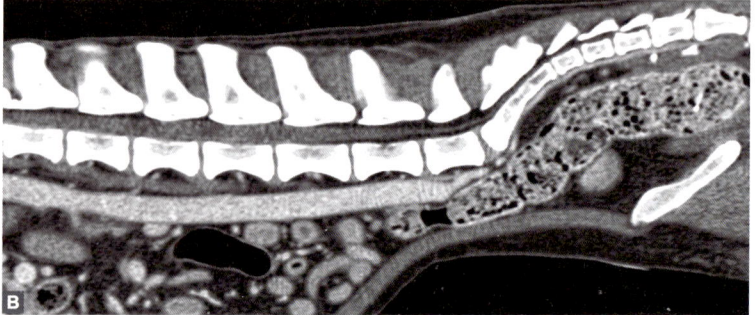

Fig. 16.4 (**A**) Transverse, contrast-enhanced CT image of the spine at L1-L2 in an English Mastiff using a soft tissue window. The spinal cord is of soft tissue opacity and is surrounded by hypoattenuating epidural fat. Enhancing blood in the venous sinuses is seen bilaterally, ventrolateral to the cord. In a bone window, much finer definition of the vertebrae would be shown. (**B**) Sagittal CT reconstruction (post-contrast soft tissue window) of a normal lumbosacral spine in a Hungarian Vizsla. Hypoattenuating fat outlines the cauda equina.

CHAPTER 16 Vertebral column

Normal radiographic spinal anatomy

A typical vertebra consists of a body or centrum, lateral pedicles, a dorsal lamina and various processes (cranial and caudal articular processes, transverse processes ± spinous, accessory and mamillary processes). Most vertebrae have three centers of ossification at birth (body and each side of arch) with epiphyses or endplates appearing at three to four weeks. The main centers fuse at two to four months and the endplate physes fuse at seven to nine months (can be delayed in neutered cats). Vertebral bodies are roughly rectangular and are longer in the cat than the dog.

Cervical vertebrae (fig. 16.5)

▌ **C1 (atlas)** Large lateral wings for muscle attachment; concave cranial facets articulate with occipital condyles allowing mainly up-and-down movement. Three centers of ossification at birth – one each for lateral part and one for the ventral arch, which replaces a vertebral body. No endplates.

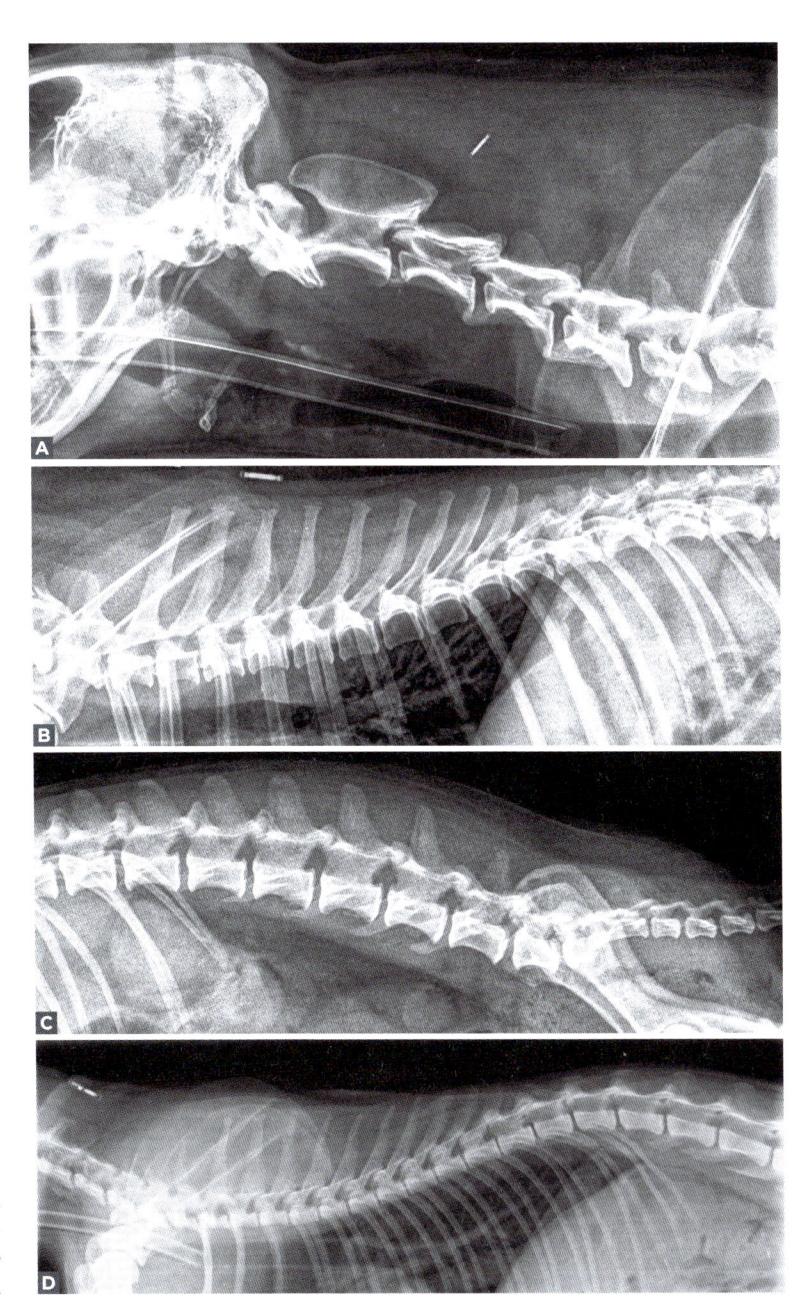

Fig. 16.5 Lateral radiographs of the (**A**) cervical spine in a Labrador Retriever; the (**B**) thoracic spine and (**C**) lumbosacral spine in a Terrier cross; and (**D**) the mid part of the spine (C3 to L4) in a Domestic shorthair cat. See text for description.

▌ **C2 (axis)** The dens or odontoid peg represents the original body of C1. The apical ligament of the dens extends cranially in three parts, the central part to the ventral margin of the *foramen magnum* and lateral alar ligaments to sites just medial to the occipital condyles. The transverse atlantal ligament holds the dens against the floor of the atlas. There is a large dorsal spinous process and small, caudally-directed transverse processes. Four centers of ossification are present at birth; dens, body and lateral parts of arch, and shortly afterwards centers of ossification for cranial and caudal endplates appear (there is occasionally also a center at the cranial tip of the dens). Atlantoaxial articulation allows rotation of the neck.

▌ **C3, C4 and C5** Progressively taller dorsal spinous processes.

▌ **C6** Characteristic large transverse process projecting ventrally.

▌ **C7** First pair of ribs articulate with its transverse processes.

Thoracic vertebrae

The total number of thoracic and lumbar vertebrae is quite constant at 20 (usually 13 and 7 respectively although variations are common – see Transitional vertebrae). Thoracic vertebral bodies are relatively short. Their dorsal spinous processes are tall cranially but reduce in size from T7 or 8; they are angled caudally as far as the anticlinal vertebra T11, which is vertical, and those behind are angled cranially. Articular processes lie in the dorsal plane to T1-T10 and then in the sagittal plane. The disc space T10-T11 is often narrower than its neighbors in both dogs and cats and this should not be mistaken for disc disease.

Lumbar vertebrae

The ventral margins of vertebral bodies L3 and L4 are ill-defined in large dogs due to the diaphragmatic crural attachments. The dorsal spinous processes are short and broad, and that of L7 may be absent. Transverse processes are directed cranioventrally: care must be taken not to confuse transverse processes superimposed over disc spaces in lateral radiographs with mineralized disc material. In chondrodystrophic breeds of dog premature bony fusion leads to the presence of shorter pedicles, a small dorsoventral vertebral canal diameter and relative reduction in the size of the subarachnoid space, hence they are more likely to suffer spinal cord compression due to disc disease.

Sacrum

A four-sided wedge-shaped structure consisting of three fused components of which S1 is much the largest. The ventral surface is concave. Two pairs of dorsal sacral foramina for nerves and vessels represent intervertebral foramina. Dorsally, the median sacral crest is composed of the fused dorsal spinous processes. The wings of the sacrum are enlarged, roughened lateral parts which articulate with the iliac wings.

Caudal (coccygeal) vertebrae

Six to 23 in number. V- or Y-shaped hemal arches articulate ventrally with Cd4-Cd6 to protect the median coccygeal artery. Vertebrae near the tail base have a recognizable structure but those further back are simple rods.

Anatomy textbooks should be consulted for further details of spinal anatomy (discs, ligaments, muscles, spinal cord, spinal nerves, meninges, subarachnoid and epidural spaces, vascular structures).

Congenital and developmental spinal diseases

Alterations in number of vertebrae
Real, e.g., six or eight lumbar vertebrae, four sacral (however, the total number of vertebrae is usually constant, apart from the tail). Apparently, due to the presence of transitional vertebrae.

Transitional vertebrae
Vertebrae with anatomical features of two adjacent groups, bilaterally or unilaterally. Usually not clinically significant unless (a) used as surgical landmarks; or (b) unilateral transitional vertebra at the lumbosacral junction cause secondary changes.
Examples of transitional vertebrae include:

- Occipitoatlantoaxial malformations (see below).
- C7 with vestigial ribs.
- T13 lacking one or both ribs; L1 with one or two ribs; elongated transverse processes or vestigial structures at the thoracolumbar junction instead of ribs (**fig. 16.6A**).
- Sacralization of L7 or lumbarization of S1 (**fig. 16.6B**) – last lumbar segment fused to ilium or first sacral segment with vestigial transverse process(es). This may predispose to cauda equina syndrome and, if symmetrical, to pelvic tilting and secondary hip dysplasia-like changes on the "up" side.

Hemivertebrae
Mostly in screw-tailed breeds (Pug, English and French Bulldog, Boston Terrier) because of selection for deformed vertebrae in the tail. Mainly seen the thoracic spine, often leading to kyphosis, lordosis

Fig. 16.6 (A) VD radiograph of an asymmetrical transitional vertebra at the thoracolumbar junction, in this case an abnormal T13. On one side a thickened and elongated transverse process mimics a rib and on the other side the rib is vestigial and arises from a transverse process. (B) VD radiograph of an asymmetrical transitional vertebra at the lumbosacral junction in a German Shepherd dog. The first sacral segment is fused to the ilial wing on one side but shows a lumbar transverse process on the other side. This has resulted in tilting of the pelvis creating a hip dysplasia-like defect on the side with the sacroiliac fusion, which lies more dorsally when the dog is upright.

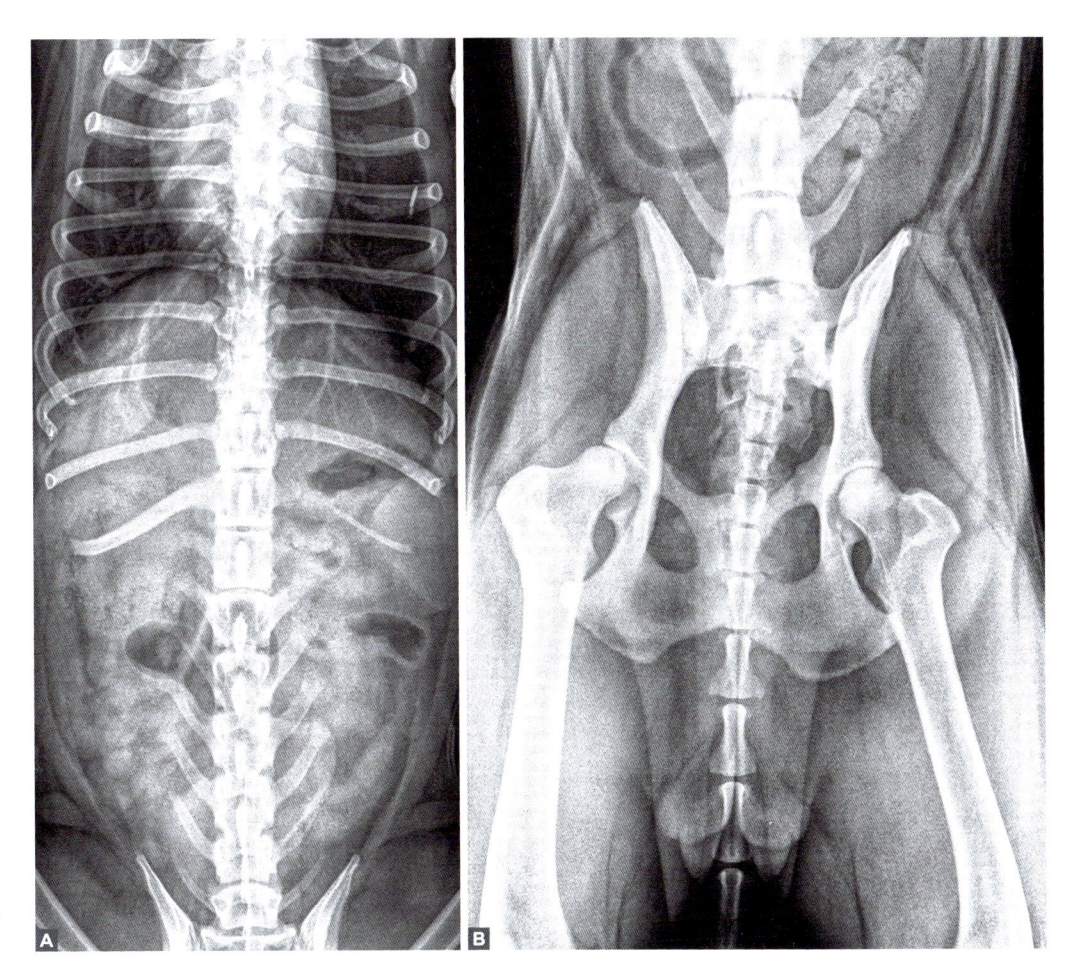

and scoliosis, although this is not usually physically apparent (**fig. 16.7A**). The vertebral bodies are incompletely formed, being short and wedge- or trapezoid-shaped, resulting in crowding of ribs and remodeling of adjacent vertebrae. "Butterfly vertebrae" have a central sagittal cleft so that on the VD radiograph they appear as two triangles with the apices touching.

Hemivertebrae are often clinically silent but sometimes cause significant vertebral canal stenosis and spinal cord compression, clinical signs usually occurring before skeletal maturity and most often in Pugs. Radiographic or CT myelography, or MRI (**fig. 16.7B**) are required to demonstrate spinal cord compression.

In Manx cats, which are bred to have very reduced or absent tails, sacrocaudal dysgenesis is usually present, comprising multiple malformed vertebrae. In severe cases, there are associated neurological deficits. Spina bifida and meningocele may be present.

Fused or block vertebrae

Vertebrae may show minor fusion via articular or spinous processes, or more obvious vertebral body fusion with reduction or loss of the disc space (**fig. 16.8**). Complex anomalies can result in spinal deviation. The resultant rigidity of a portion of the spine predisposes to disc extrusion on either side of the fused segment.

Atlantoaxial subluxation

A number of congenital spinal malformations affect the craniocervical junction, the most common of which is atlantoaxial subluxation.[7] This affects mainly toy dog breeds although it is also reported

Fig. 16.7 (**A**) Lateral thoracic radiograph of a seven-month-old Pug with paraparesis secondary to the presence of a mid-thoracic hemivertebra. The body of T7 is hypoplastic ventrally and is therefore wedge-shaped, causing focal kyphosis and vertebral canal stenosis. The caudal end of the T6 vertebral body is correspondingly remodeled. (Note that C7 is a transitional vertebra, bearing a pair of ribs). (**B**) Sagittal T2W MRI image of the same dog showing severe spinal cord compression above the T6-T7 disc space; no disc nucleus is evident.

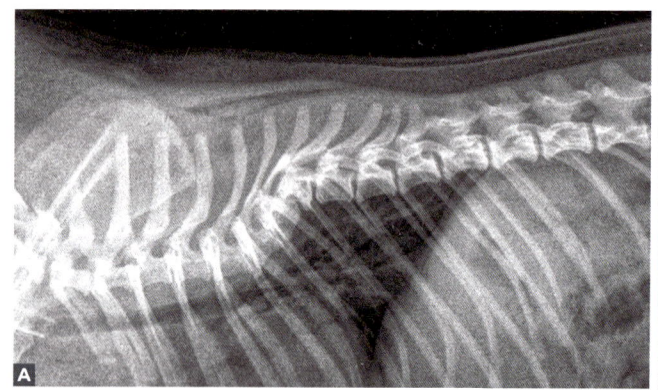

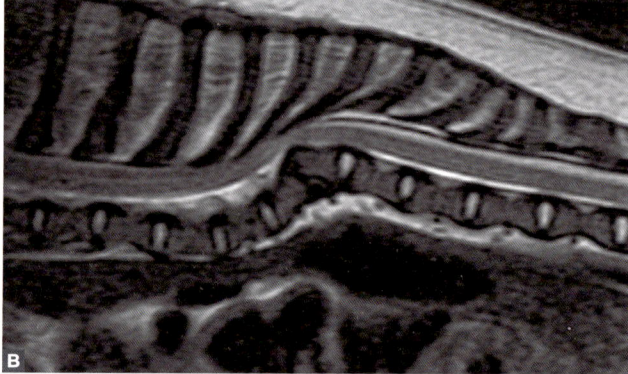

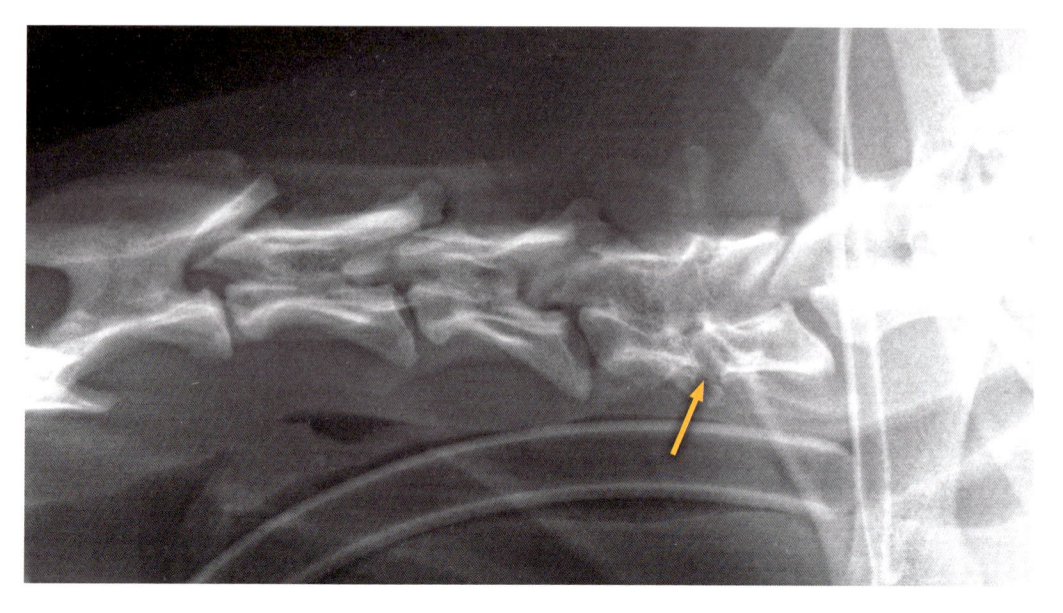

Fig. 16.8 Radiograph of a C5-C6 block vertebra in a ten-month-old Pointer. The two vertebrae are largely fused together but a vestigial space between them is still just visible (arrow). This was an incidental finding, but the dog is at risk of disc prolapse at the disc spaces on either side in the future, due to rigidity of this section of the spine.

sporadically in larger dogs and cats. Clinical signs due to atlantoaxial instability and spinal cord compression can arise at any age, often induced by minor trauma. Causative deformities include aplasia or hypoplasia of the dens, separation or non-fusion of the center of ossification of the dens and stretching or rupture of the transverse ligament of the atlas. The dens may also be misshapen and/or angled dorsally. Atlantoaxial subluxation can also result from C1 or C2 fractures and incomplete ossification of the atlas.

Atlantoaxial subluxation leads to instability between the atlas and axis, allowing abnormal flexion at this joint. This causes ventral cord compression by the dens if it is intact or by the cranial end of the body of C2. Radiographically, the normal comma-shaped intervertebral foramen between the two vertebrae widens on gentle flexion of the neck, although this manoeuvre must be undertaken with care (**figs. 16.9A** and **16.B**). Overlap of the spinous process of C2 and the neural arch of C1 is greatly reduced or absent. The dens itself is best assessed in a VD or lateral oblique radiograph if cross-sectional imaging is not available. Atlantoaxial subluxation is often accompanied by an ab-

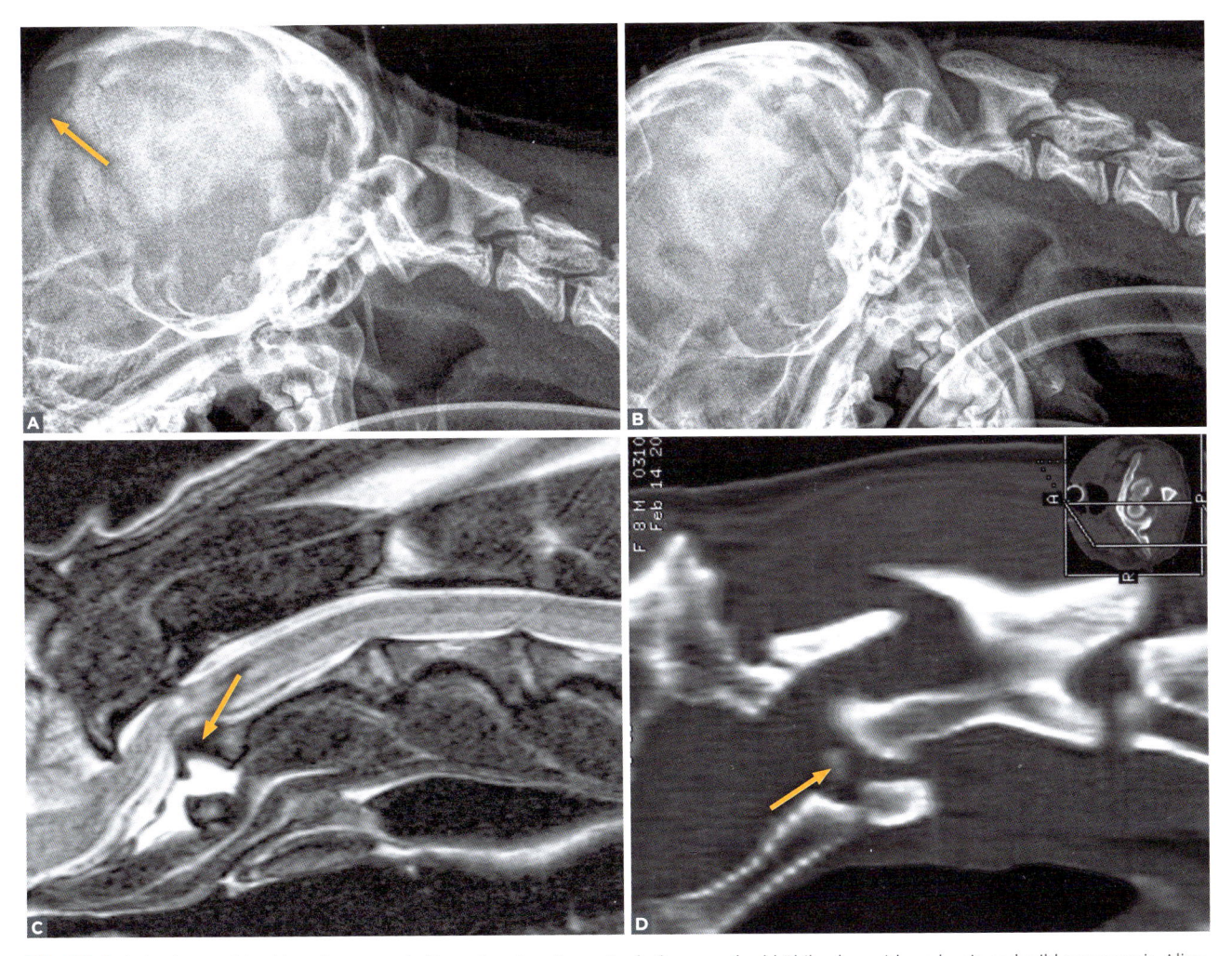

Fig. 16.9 (**A**) Atlantoaxial subluxation: extended lateral neck radiograph of a five-month-old Chihuahua with neck pain and mild tetraparesis. Alignment of C1 and C2 appears normal; the region of the dens is obscured by the wings of the atlas. A large open fontanelle is also visible in this projection (arrow). (**B**) The same dog with the atlanto-occipital area in a gently-flexed position, showing widening of the C1-C2 intervertebral foramen and reduced overlap of the spinous process of C2 on the neural arch of C1. (**C**) Sagittal T2W MRI image of the cranial cervical spine of an 11-month-old Cocker Spaniel with tetraparesis due to atlantoaxial subluxation. The dens is intact but is displaced dorsally from the body of C1 (arrow), indicating that the transverse ligament is incompetent. The spinal cord at this level is severely compressed and shows areas of both hyperintense and hypointense signal suggestive of hemorrhagic contusion. (**D**) Sagittal CT reconstruction (bone window) of a six-month-old German Shepherd dog with atlantoaxial subluxation secondary to an occipitoatlantoaxial malformation (OAAM). There is cranial and dorsal displacement of C2 relative to an abnormal C1, causing severe vertebral canal stenosis. A small, separate dens fragment is visible cranially (arrow). A complete understanding of the nature of this complex anomaly required careful examination of all three imaging planes together with 3D reconstructions.

normally-short C1 neural arch and sometimes by other cranial cervical malformations. Atlantoaxial instability can be seen with MRI (**fig. 16.9C**) and in sagittal CT reconstructions (**fig. 16.9D**), and MRI will also demonstrate secondary spinal cord contusion or atrophy. Both techniques are helpful for assessing the dens and MRI will also depict the transverse ligament.

Occipitoatlantoaxial malformations

Occipitoatlantoaxial malformations (OAAM) comprise a variety of abnormal morphologies involving fusion and/or abnormal shape of the occipital bone, C1 and/or C2. The effective sites of motion in the cranial cervical spine are altered and instability such as atlantoaxial subluxation may also be present. Neural compression frequently results and is best demonstrated using MRI, although CT is useful for demonstration of the bony defects (**fig. 16.9D**).

Incomplete ossification of C1

The atlas normally forms from three centers of ossification, two lateral portions and a midline ventral arch. Occasionally, defects in ossification or fusion lead to incompetence of its ring-like anatomy and resulting atlantoaxial instability. The ossification defects may be visible radiographically but CT or MRI are preferred diagnostic tools: in particular, MRI will demonstrate secondary spinal cord injury better.

Syringohydromyelia secondary to Chiari-like malformation

Most of the clinical signs arising from Chiari-like malformation of the skull (caudal occipital malformation) are due to secondary syringomyelia, which forms as a result of altered CSF flow at the foramen magnum ensuing from impaction of the cerebellar vermis or vermian herniation. The changes usually progress from birth to middle age and mainly affect the cervical area, although in some dogs the whole spinal cord can be affected. The condition typically affects small breeds of dogs, in particular the Cavalier King Charles Spaniel, and screening schemes exist based on assessment of MRI images, this being the best tool for detection of syringomyelia. Survey radiographs will be normal in most cases although on myelography the spinal cord may diffusely swollen and the subarachnoid space markedly narrowed (**fig. 16.10A**); however, cisternal injection of contrast medium can be hazardous in affected dogs due to cord swelling and attenuation of the subarachnoid space. MRI demonstrates widening

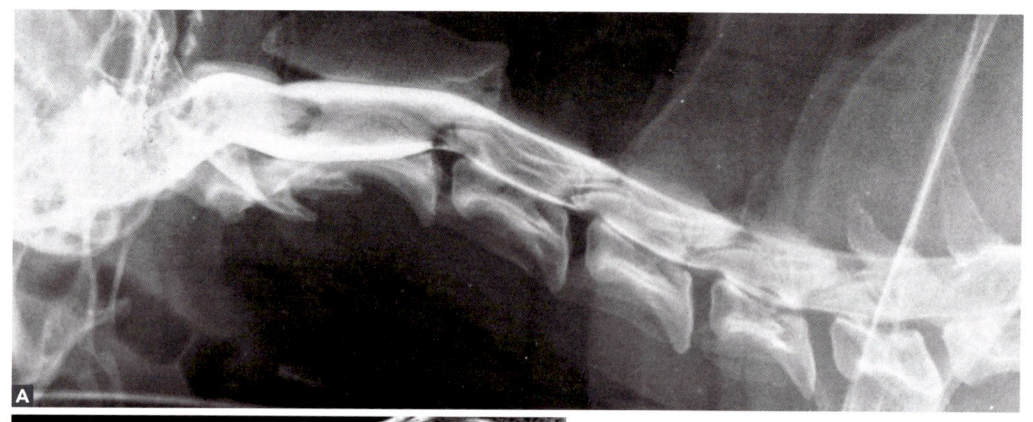

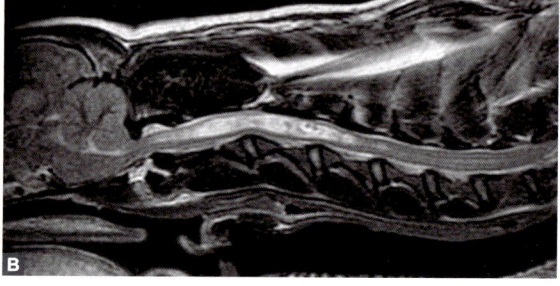

Fig. 16.10 (**A**) Myelogram of an 18-month-old Cavalier King Charles Spaniel with syringomyelia. Subjectively the spinal cord is mildly swollen caudal to C2 and the subarachnoid space is attenuated, but MRI was needed for confirmation. However, the myelogram ruled out disc disease as a cause of neck pain. (**B**) Sagittal T2W image of the caudal fossa and neck of an eight-year-old Cavalier King Charles Spaniel with Chiari-like malformation and severe syringomyelia from C2 to C4. Hyperintense signal with the cord shows accumulation of CSF, causing compression of parenchyma and spinal cord swelling. Variations of signal intensity within the syrinx are due to flow artefact.

of the central canal of the spinal cord or more overt fluid accumulation centrally, which may appear sacculated (**fig. 16.10B**). In some dogs, syrinxes are seen as slits in the cord parenchyma and ill-defined cord edema may also be evident. CT will show more severe cases of syringomyelia.

Articular process dysplasia

Dysplasia (aplasia or hypoplasia) of caudal vertebral articular processes is commonly seen in screw-tailed breeds of dogs, especially in Pugs. The deformity is usually in the caudal thoracic spine and may be unilateral, bilateral or asymmetrical. Resulting microinstability can lead to fibrosis and a constrictive myelopathy with resultant neurological deficits;[8] affected dogs are usually middle-aged. Secondary disc extrusions or arachnoid diverticula can also ensue.

Radiographically, the deformed processes may be visible in both lateral and VD radiographs, although they are easily overlooked. In lateral radiographs there is reduction in size of the processes and loss of dorsal margination of the intervertebral foramen; in VD radiographs the characteristic W-shape of the caudal articular processes is absent or reduced. The changes are also visible in high-quality MRI images although CT is more sensitive for the bony deformity. Secondary spinal cord compression is well demonstrated in MRI and may be seen in CT, but radiographically requires myelography.

Cranial thoracic stenosis

Bony stenosis of the cranial thoracic spine is occasionally seen in large dogs, especially of mastiff-type breeds. Most cases are in males and neurological signs, when present, manifest before skeletal maturity. Vertebral stenosis is the result of over-large and malpositioned articular processes, which can cause dorsolateral spinal cord compression. The most severely affected sites are usually T2-T3 and T3-T4. Diagnosis requires MRI, CT or radiographic myelography.

Spina bifida

An embryonic neural tube fusion defect results in a midline cleft in the dorsal spinous process or vertebral arch of varying sizes, or in complete absence of the arch, affecting one or more vertebrae. Duplication of the spinous process of affected vertebrae may be visible radiographically.

Spina bifida occulta comprises bony changes only without involvement of neural tissue and is an incidental finding. However, in other cases, mainly in brachycephalic dogs and in Manx cats in the lumbosacral area, a meningocele or myelomeningocele is also present in which the meninges and sometimes the terminal spinal cord exit the spine to attach to the skin, causing tethering of the spinal cord and a dorsal, subcutaneous skin dimple. The skin connection may remain closed (spina bifida cystica) or can open to the exterior (spina bifida aperta), discharging CSF and being open to infection. The bony defects may be hard to spot radiographically but CT or MRI will show them well, and radiographic or CT myelography will depict associated dural sac involvement (**fig. 16.11A**). However, MRI is required to demonstrate the extent of the deformity and to show whether there is a meningocele or a myelomeningocele (**fig. 16.11B**). There may also be tethering of the spinal cord and/or lipoma formation.

Dermoid sinuses

Spinal dermoid sinuses are also caused by a failure of neural tube closure and lack of differentiation between spine and skin so that a sinus tract exists between the two areas, containing elements such as hair follicles and sebaceous glands. Dermoid sinus tracts are classified depending on their length, the most serious being grade IV, in which the tract extends from the vertebral canal to the skin surface giving rise to a risk of septic meningomyeltitis. Dermoid sinuses are usually seen in the cranial thoracic or cervical areas and the Rhodesian Ridgeback is predisposed.

Contrast sinography can be performed radiographically or with CT to investigate the depth of the track, but MRI will yield the best soft tissue information.

Sacral osteochondrosis

Osteochondrosis has been reported to affect the lumbosacral joint, usually the dorsal margin of the cranial sacral endplate and less often the caudal L7 endplate.[9] Clinical signs of cauda equina syndrome may ensue, although this is usually due to secondary degenerative disc disease. The German Shepherd dog is most frequently affected, with a strong male preponderance, although the condition has been seen in other large breeds.

Radiographically, the dorsal margin of the affected endplate margin is blunted, remodeled and sclerotic, and occasionally mineralized fragments are visible (**fig. 16.12**). In the VD projection the subchondral defect is usually lateralized. As the affected area is also the site of attachment for fibers of the dorsal annulus fibrosis, secondary disc herniation is common. Both CT and MRI will demonstrate mineralized osteochondral fragments, subchondral sclerosis and remodeling.

Cartilaginous exostoses and angiomatosis

Please see Neoplasia section.

Arachnoid diverticula

Please see Miscellaneous section.

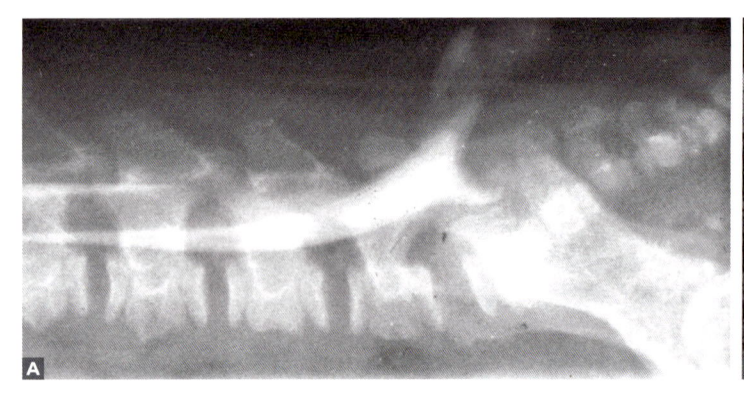

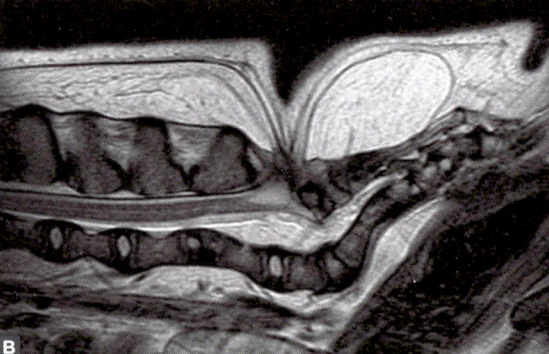

Fig. 16.11 (**A**) Lumbosacral myelographic radiograph of a six-week-old English Bulldog puppy with paraparesis. The dural sac exits the vertebral canal between the neural arches of L7 and S1, extending into an area of dorsal soft tissue swelling. The diagnosis is spina bifida with meningocele. (**B**) Sagittal T2W MRI image of a five-month-old English Bulldog with paraparesis and incontinence. A meningocele, possibly also with neural content, exits the vertebral canal between the neural arches of L6 and L7 and extends into overlying subcutaneous fat, tethered to the skin. A large depression is seen in the soft tissues dorsally, which developed as the dog grew. A lipoma lies above the sacrum.

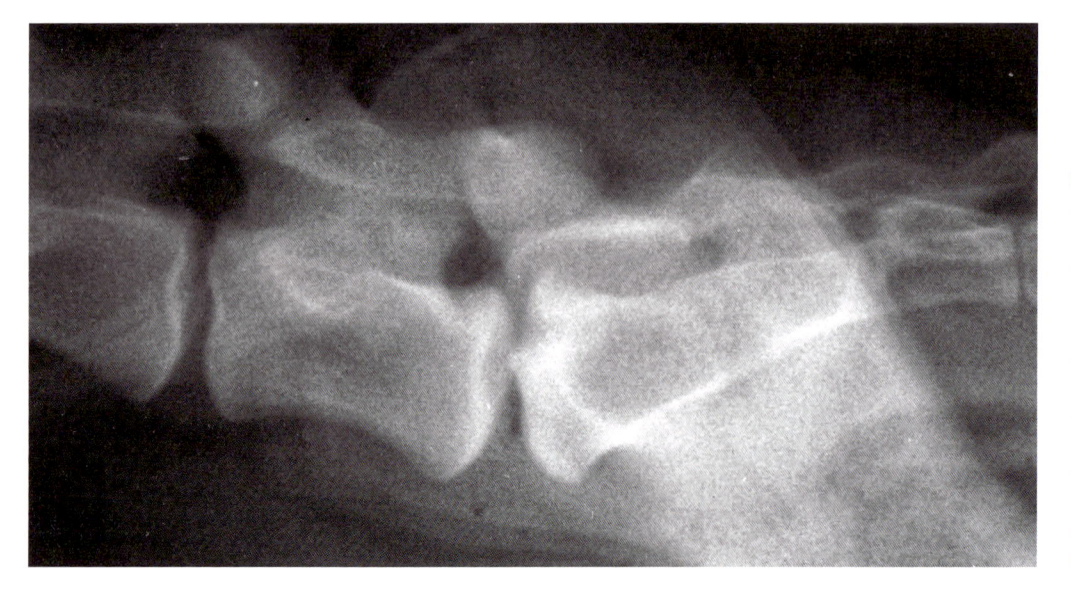

Fig. 16.12 Lateral radiograph of the lumbosacral junction in a one-year-old German Shepherd dog with lumbosacral pain. The craniodorsal margin of the sacrum is sclerotic and markedly remodeled, projecting dorsally into the vertebral canal. A radiolucent streak in the disc space may be due to vacuum phenomenon caused by disc degeneration.

Degenerative spinal diseases

Spondylosis deformans

Spondylosis is common in older dogs and cats and usually arises without apparent cause although it is predisposed to by sites of instability or chronic disc prolapse, especially at the lumbosacral junction and in the caudal neck. The spondyles are spurs of new bone which arise from the ventral aspect of the vertebral endplates and enlarge in a curved manner cranially or caudally towards the adjacent vertebra: they may also extend laterally and be visible in VD radiographs. At some sites ankylosis may occur. Sometimes a crescentic mass of new bone may be seen ventral to a disc space, especially at the lumbosacral junction, which seems to represent a similar process beginning in soft tissue. The new bone is smoothly-marginated and well-trabeculated and is easily differentiated in location and contour from reactive new bone secondary to infection (**fig. 16.13**).

Even when severe and dramatic, spondylosis is rarely of clinical significance, although occasionally osteophytes dorsolateral to the vertebral endplate may impinge on a spinal nerve as it exits the intervertebral foramen causing spinal pain or lameness. Fusion of adjacent vertebrae resulting in reduced mobility of that segment can predispose to adjacent disc extrusion.[10]

Elderly cats frequently show multiple sites of thoracic disc space collapse and mild spondylosis: this is an incidental finding and is not associated with clinical signs (**fig. 16.14**).

Spondylitis, with bone proliferation extending the length of the vertebral bodies, may be seen at T8-T11 in dogs with *Spirocerca lupi* infection together with an adjacent esophageal mass.

Fig. 16.13 Lumbosacral spinal radiograph of an eight-year-old Boxer with severe spondylosis and osteoarthrosis of the synovial joints. Large ventral spondyles have fused in places, bridging several vertebrae. Dorsolateral spondylosis on the cranial endplate of L3 is superimposed over the vertebral canal, and new bone has also arisen between spinous processes of L2, L3 and L4 (so-called "kissing spines"). Despite the severity of the changes these findings were detected incidentally during abdominal radiography, although the dog's mobility is likely to have been reduced.

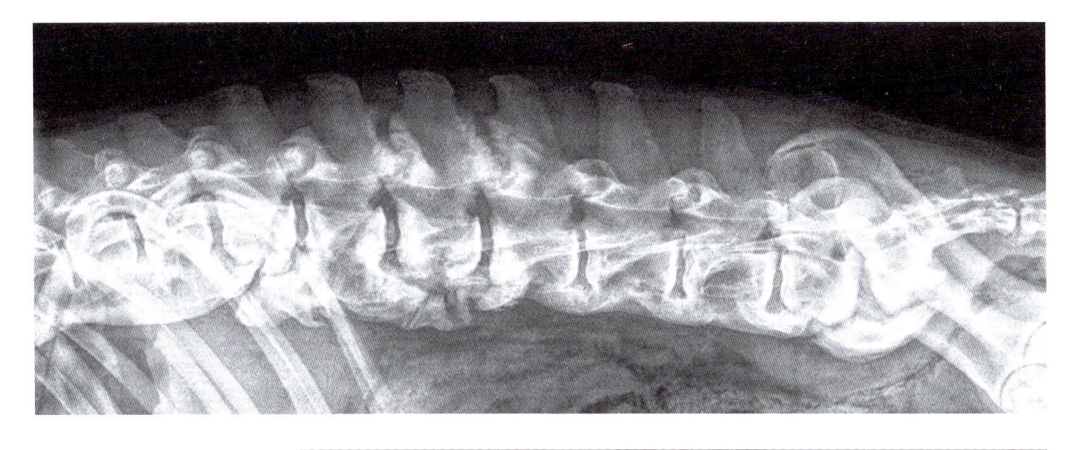

Fig. 16.14 Lateral thoracic radiograph of a twelve-year-old Domestic shorthair cat. Narrowing of multiple thoracic disc spaces together with the presence of small spondyles is a common finding in older cats. Ageing changes are also seen in the costal cartilages.

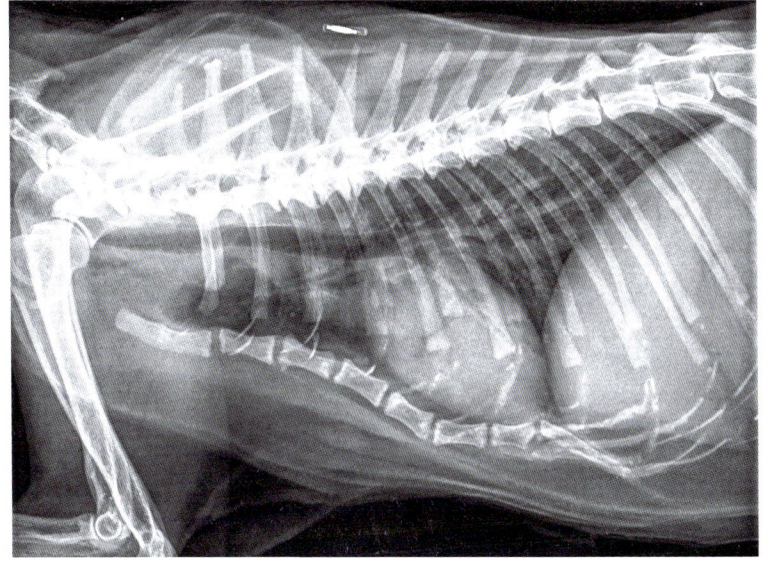

Spinal osteoarthrosis

The vertebral dorsal articular processes form synovial joints and can therefore develop osteoarthritis as an aging change. Spinal osteoarthritis can also occur secondary to discospondylitis, trauma and instability, and cervical osteoarthritis may arise in young dogs of large breeds (notably the Great Dane) leading to "Wobbler" syndrome. Radiologically, spinal osteoarthritis appears as enlargement, irregularity and sclerosis of the processes with narrowing of the joint space (**fig. 16.13**). Severe spinal osteoarthritis can cause dorsolateral spinal cord compression, demonstrated using MRI or CT.

Disseminated idiopathic skeletal hyperostosis

Disseminated idiopathic skeletal hyperostosis (DISH) or Forestier's disease in man has also been described in dogs: the cause is unknown. The main feature is spinal new bone described as "flowing" spondylosis, which extends further along the ventral aspect of the vertebral body than does normal spondylosis and which often fuses; spinal synovial joint osteoarthritis and pseudoarthrosis between dorsal spinous processes may also occur. Periarticular new bone in some limb joints, prominence of trochanters and tuberosities and enthesiopathies have also been described. In man, several criteria for diagnosis of disseminated idiopathic skeletal hyperostosis are required, including flowing anterolateral ossification of at least four adjacent vertebrae, relative absence of degenerative disc changes and lack of other signs of spinal degeneration such as osteoarthritis. In the veterinary literature there are only sporadic case reports and there is no consensus for diagnosis. As with spondylosis, fusion of adjacent vertebral segments causes rigidity which predisposes to disc disease on either side.[10]

Dural ossification (ossifying pachymeningitis)

Round or elliptical bone plaques may form on the inner surface of the dura mater and may coalesce to form a tube around the spinal cord, mainly in older, large breed dogs. Dural ossification is clinically insignificant unless a plaque lies at the site of intended CSF tap or myelographic injection. Small plaques <2 mm diameter are not seen radiographically but larger areas produce a very fine, mineral opacity line best seen ventral to the lumbar spinal cord crossing disc spaces. In cases of disc prolapse or other extradural lesion the dural ossification may be deviated creating an "automyelogram". The plaques are easily seen in CT images and may also be recognized in MRI as discrete dural areas of signal void.

Differential diagnosis: mineralized, herniated disc material; mineralized dorsal longitudinal ligament; small dorsolateral spondyles.

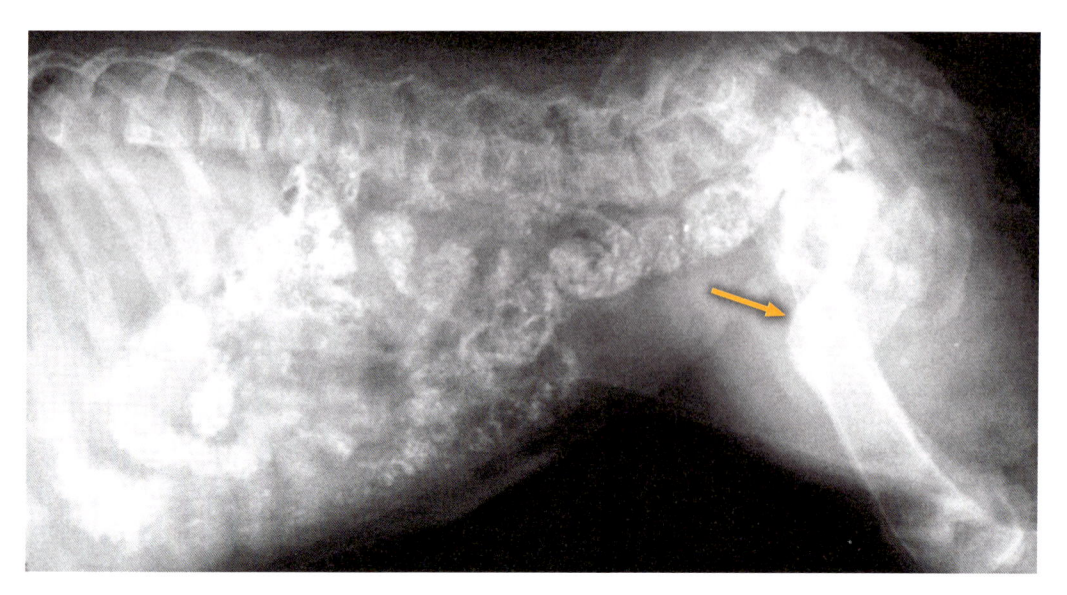

Fig. 16.15 Lateral abdominal and spinal radiograph of a 13-week-old Afghan Hound puppy with nutritional secondary hyperparathyroidism. Compared with the soft tissues the skeletal structures show reduced radiopacity, and the cortices are thinned. There is lumbosacral lordosis and a folding fracture in one femur (arrow). The puppy had been on an all-meat diet but had recently been fed a diet with mineral content, hence the increased radiopacity of the intestinal contents.

Metabolic spinal diseases

Nutritional secondary hyperparathyroidism (juvenile osteoporosis)
This metabolic condition is seen in puppies and kittens on all-meat diets, which are low in calcium. The growing skeleton is poorly mineralized and prone to folding fractures, which in the spine can result in deformity such as lordosis and in neurological deficits. Radiographically the bones show cortical thinning and reduced radiopacity compared with soft tissues; folding fractures are seen as ill-defined bands of sclerosis resulting in vertebral shortening and angulation of long bones (**fig. 16.15**). Differential diagnosis is osteogenesis imperfecta, a rare, inherited and congenital collagen defect which causes generalized osteopenia with multiple folding fractures occurring due to the brittle state of the bones.

The following diseases may have combined congenital/developmental and metabolic causes.

Congenital hypothyroidism
A rare, developmental metabolic disease which causes retardation of endochondral ossification and disproportionate dwarfism, mainly in Boxer dogs. There is delayed closure of physes and epiphyseal dysplasia throughout the skeleton including vertebral end plates, which are characteristically pointed. The spine may be kyphotic and the vertebrae are abnormally short. Affected dogs also have short, broad heads, protuberant tongues and mental dullness; osteoarthritis is a sequel to the epiphyseal dysplasia. Differential diagnosis: inherited chondrodysplasia.

Pituitary dwarfism
Pituitary dwarfism is due to a lack of growth hormone, and in small animals mainly affects German Shepherd dogs causing delayed physeal closure, proportionate dwarfism and a poor hair coat. Some cases also have skeletal changes similar to those with hypothyroidism, and osteopenia may be present.

Mucopolysaccharidosis and hypervitaminosis A
Mucopolysaccharidoses are a group of inherited lysosomal storage diseases which mainly affect cats of Siamese ancestry, although they can also occur in dogs. Like congenital hypothyroidism, mucopolysaccharidosis causes epiphyseal dysplasia, resulting in short vertebral bodies and wide disc spaces. Exuberant periosteal new bone forms, especially in the cervical spine, where the vertebrae may be massively remodeled with proliferative new bone causing ankylosis. Dens hypoplasia may also be present and epiphyseal dysplasia in the limb joints leads to severe osteoarthritis. Changes are usually evident radiographically by six months and are progressive. Affected cats have characteristic short, broad faces and may also suffer from hip dysplasia and *pectus excavatum*.
Differential diagnosis: hypervitaminosis A, seen in young adult cats fed on raw liver diets: it can coexist with nutritional secondary hyperparathyroidism resulting in osteopenia. Similar proliferative bony spinal changes to mucopolysaccharidosis are seen and the elbow, hip and stifle may also be affected. Both diseases are rare.

Inflammatory and infectious spinal diseases

Spondylitis and discospondylitis
Spondylitis and discospondylitis most often arise in larger and older male dogs and are rare in cats. They are usually secondary to bacterial infection elsewhere in the body (e.g., urinary tract, endocarditis) and in young animals can be associated with portosystemic shunts. Infection may also be caused by tracking foreign bodies, especially in the lumbar area. However, if diagnosed at one site the whole spine should be radiographed since multiple disc spaces may be involved, especially with fungal infections. Clinical signs include pyrexia, lethargy, spinal pain, paraspinal swellings and dis-

charging sinuses, and in some cases, there are neurological deficits. Diagnosis is based on the typical radiographic appearance but can sometimes be confirmed by blood or urine culture. MRI and CT are more sensitive for detection of early or mild changes.

Spondylitis There may be a mottled, sclerotic trabecular pattern to the affected vertebral body with poorly defined periosteal new bone along its ventral margin, with an appearance atypical for simple spondylosis (**fig. 16.16A**). Often two or more adjacent vertebrae may be affected. Inhaled grass awns may track along the diaphragmatic crura to the ventral margins of L3 and L4 causing spondylitis of these vertebrae, but note that the normal diaphragmatic crural attachments at these sites can also produce slight convexity of the ventral cortex in larger dogs. Localized soft tissue swelling may be evident. MRI and CT also show heterogeneous architecture suggestive of inflammation with contrast enhancement of the affected vertebral body, periosteal new bone and changes in adjacent soft tissues (**fig. 16.16B**). Differential diagnosis: vertebral neoplasia.

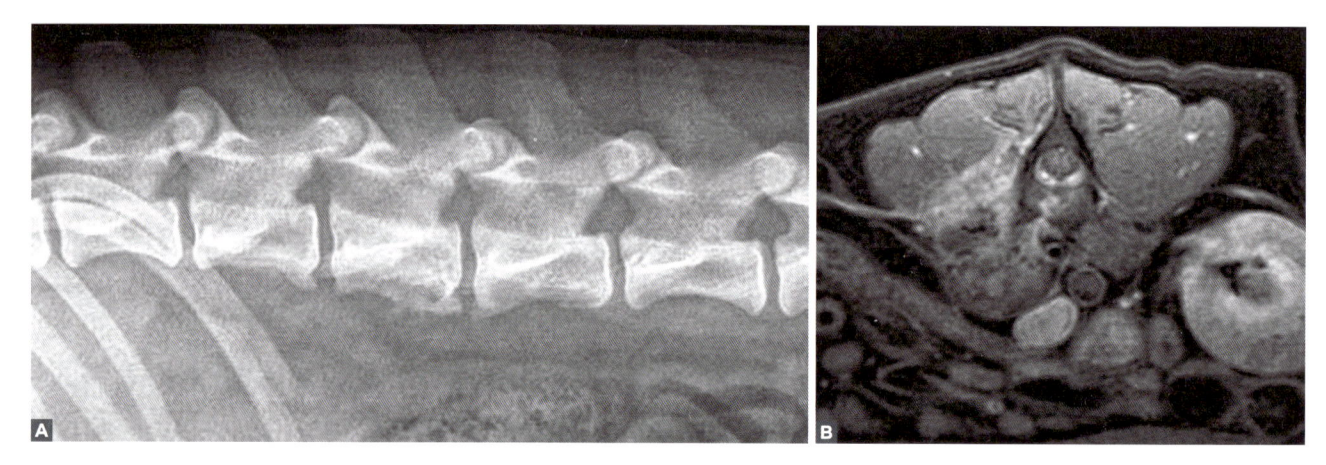

Fig. 16.16 (A) Lateral lumbar radiograph of a two-year-old English Springer Spaniel with lumbar pain and unilateral soft tissue swelling. The radiograph shows subtle heterogeneity in the trabecular pattern of the vertebral body of L3 and solid but irregular periosteal new bone along the ventral margins of L2 and L3. However, there is no evidence of endplate osteolysis which would suggest discospondylitis. (B) A transverse, post-contrast T1W MRI image with fat suppression at the level of mid L3 in the same dog shows marked, unilateral swelling and inflammation of paralumbar muscle and a track of inflammation extending into the vertebral body. Other MRI images suggested the presence of a foreign body, and a grass awn was retrieved under ultrasonographic guidance.

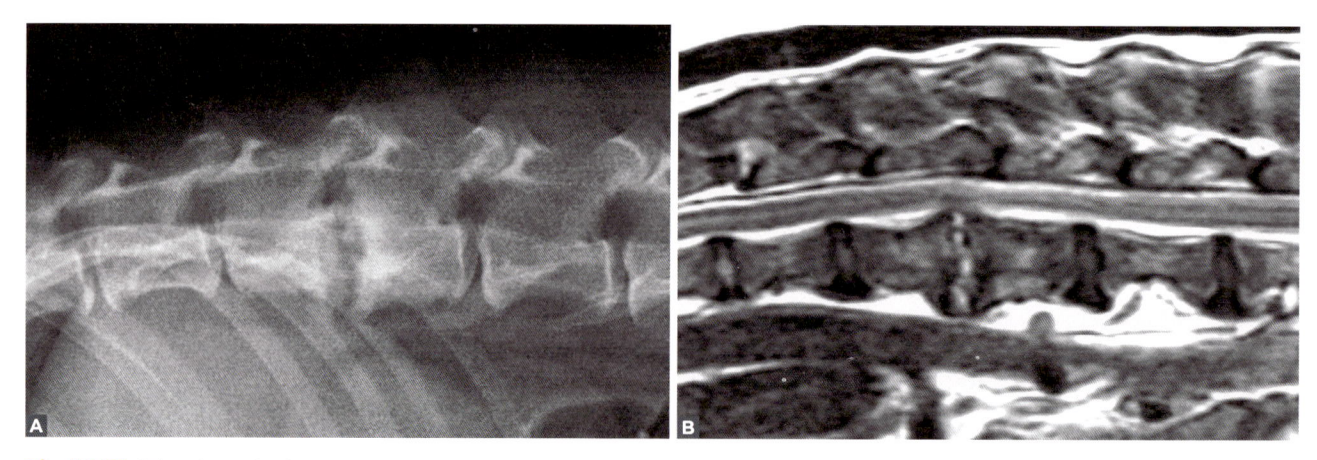

Fig. 16.17 (A) Radiograph of chronic discospondylitis at L1-L2 in a seven-year-old English Springer Spaniel. The margins of the disc space are irregular due to osteolysis of the adjacent vertebral endplates making the vertebrae shorter than normal. The ends of the vertebral bodies show increased opacity, probably due to a combination of true sclerosis and superimposition of new bone. Ventrally there is both spondylosis and more diffuse periosteal new bone, and dorsally the intervertebral foramen is reduced in size with proliferative changes affecting the articular processes. (B) Sagittal T2W MRI image of the same dog one week later. The L1-L2 disc space is narrowed and contains an uneven streak of very hyperintense (therefore hydrated) material. The vertebral endplates are irregular and show mildly increased signal intensity. New bone is present along the ventral margins of both vertebrae. The overlying spinal cord is slightly unclear and hyperintense but is not seen to be compressed. A contrast study showed marked enhancement of the affected vertebrae and surrounding soft tissues indicating inflammation. Note that the remaining discs in the field of view show incidental age-related dehydration.

▌**Discospondylitis** The affected disc space is irregularly marginated due to osteolysis of the vertebral endplates, and in the early stages may be narrowed and/or show slight subluxation. Sclerosis of the adjacent parts of the vertebral bodies is often evident, and proliferative changes may also be seen in the dorsal synovial joints. Chronic infection results in shortening of vertebral bodies due to more extensive osteolysis, vertebral body sclerosis, widening of the disc space and surrounding remodeling spondylosis (**fig. 16.17A**). The lumbosacral junction is a predisposed site.

Differential diagnosis: degenerative lumbosacral disease (at the lumbosacral junction superimposition of the iliac wings means that the disc space may be hard to assess); disc disease with indentation of endplates due to Schmorl's nodes.

MRI is a sensitive modality for detection of discospondylitis, showing changes earlier than with radiography. A number of features are characteristic.[11] There is a streak of abnormally-high signal intensity in the affected disc space on T2W scans due to increased water content with hyperintense signal in STIR images in the adjacent parts of the vertebrae on either side of the affected disc space (**fig. 16.17B**). Endplate irregularity is usually best detected in T1W and T2*GE images, although CT is more sensitive for early bone changes. In both MRI and CT, contrast enhancement of material within and surrounding the disc space may be intense, especially in more chronic cases. Surrounding soft tissue pathology can also be seen.

Associated neurological deficits may arise when proliferating inflammatory tissue extends into the vertebral canal or subluxation occurs, causing spinal cord compression, and these require MRI or radiographic/CT myelography for detection.

Vertebral physitis

Physitis results from infection arising in the region of vertebral growth plates. Affected animals are usually less than two years old and therefore the physes are either open or have recently closed. Bacteria are deposited at the physis probably because of slow-flowing arterial blood, and the resulting osteomyelitis creates a wide, ill-defined band of lucency between the endplate and the vertebral body. Progression to vertebral collapse and kyphosis has been reported.

Differential diagnosis: healing Salter-Harris fracture, although these are usually displaced.

Meningomyelitis

Meningomyelitis may be non-infectious (e.g., part of a meningoencephalitis syndrome) or infectious (e.g., secondary to discospondylitis). In most cases MRI is required for diagnosis and shows focal or diffuse areas of spinal cord swelling, T2W hyperintensity and modest contrast enhancement, which may be nodular. Meningitis may also be present (**fig. 16.18**). Radiographic or CT myelography may demonstrate spinal cord swelling in severe cases. Myelography is best avoided as it will cause significant worsening of clinical signs.

Spinal epidural empyema

Purulent material within the epidural space is known as empyema, and is uncommon. It may arise without obvious cause (idiopathic) or be secondary to discospondylitis, tracking foreign body or paraspinal abscessation. Clinical signs include pyrexia, spinal pain and a rapidly-progressing myelopathy. Diagnosis is best made using MRI, which shows unstructured epidural mass lesions with peripheral, diffuse or heterogeneous contrast enhancement causing spinal cord compression and T2W hyperintensity. Radiographic or CT myelography will show only spinal cord compression due to epidural mass effect, and is non-specific. However, causative discospondylitis may be identified.

Spinal foreign bodies

A variety of foreign bodies have been reported within the spinal epidural or subarachnoid spaces, including aberrant *Dirofilaria immitis* parasites, fragments of wood (e.g., from a pharyngeal stick injury),

SECTION III AXIAL SKELETON

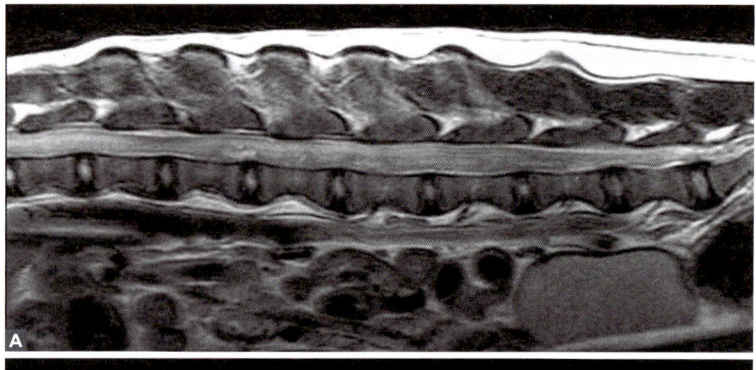

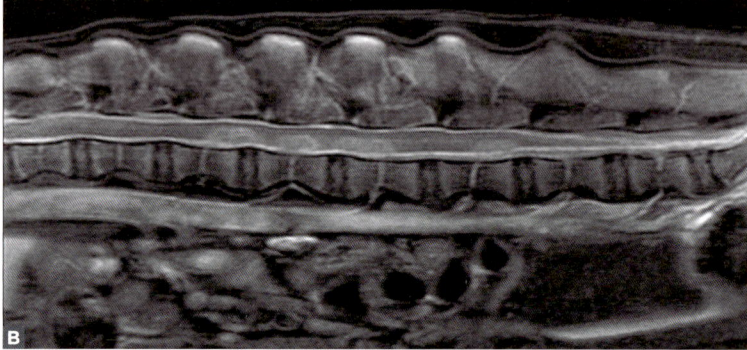

Fig. 16.18 (A) Sagittal T2W MRI image of the lumbar spine of a seven-month-old Spaniel cross with pyrexia and back pain. The spinal cord and cauda equina are diffusely swollen, compressing the subarachnoid space, and show patchy, ill-defined hyperintensity. (B) Post-contrast T1W MRI image with fat suppression of the same area shows several semi-defined areas of contrast enhancement within the cord and marked meningeal inflammation. Enhancement of the tips of the spinous processes is a normal finding in a young dog. Lumbar CSF analysis showed a mixed pleocytosis and the final diagnosis was meningomyelitis of unknown origin.

grass awns and porcupine quills. Extramedullary mass lesions and signal changes are seen as for empyema, but the foreign material itself may not be identifiable.

Paraspinal abscessation

Extensive soft tissue swelling surrounding abscess cavities and sinus tracts are usually the result of migrating vegetal foreign bodies and is mainly seen in dogs. MRI is the diagnostic tool of choice for its ability to depict soft tissue changes, its superior spinal images and the spatial information it gives prior to surgery. The iliopsoas muscles are most often affected, although changes can extend epaxially as well. Large foreign bodies such as intact grass seeds may be seen as areas of signal void surrounded by an area of inflammation (contrast enhancement), but most foreign material will have macerated by the time clinical signs are evident. CT will show larger areas of cavitation and inflammation but radiography is unlikely to be helpful except for depicting secondary spondylitis. In some patients, grass awns may be identified and retrieved using ultrasonography.

Idiopathic sterile inflammation of epidural fat

Inflammation of epidural fat may occur without known cause or by extension from paraspinal or retroperitoneal inflammation: resulting mass effect causes neurological deficits and requires surgical decompression. MRI is the diagnostic technique of choice but radiographic or CT myelography will show spinal cord compression. The imaging features may be similar to epidural empyema.

Spinal neoplasia

Spinal tumors have a variable clinical course and can present surprisingly acutely, mimicking other disease processes, especially if tumors involving bone cause pathological fracture. Spinal masses can be classified according to their location as intramedullary (35%), intradural-extramedullary (15%) and extradural (50%); pain is generally greatest with extradural tumors. Although most patients are older, young animals can be affected by benign osteochondromata, developmental angiomatosis and neural tumors.

Bony radiographic changes may or may not occur and radiographic or CT myelography or MRI is usually needed for diagnosis or assessment of severity.

Intramedullary (spinal cord) tumors

Various neural tumors may arise in the spinal cord and peripheral nerve sheath tumors may invade the cord: predilection sites are the brachial and lumbar intumescences. Most canine intramedullary tumors are gliomas: spinal lymphoma occurs in both dogs and cats either as a solitary focus or as part of more widespread disease, and is the commonest spinal tumor in cats in which it may arise at any location. Survey radiographs are usually normal, although occasionally subtle widening of the vertebral canal is evident due to pressure remodeling. Radiographic myelography may demonstrate localized spinal cord swelling as subarachnoid space thinning and displacement in both lateral and VD projections (**fig. 16.19A**).

CT can show spinal cord swelling even without myelography, as surrounding epidural fat will be attenuated. Most cord tumors will enhance after intravenous injection of contrast medium. MRI will demonstrate cord swelling and focal signal change, especially in T2W images, but surrounding edema is also likely to be present and, therefore, the underlying tumor itself may be better delineated in post-contrast T1W images (**fig. 16.19B**).

Extramedullary-intradural tumors

These masses arise in the subarachnoid space although they may also infiltrate the spinal cord and/or extend extradurally, and the origin of large masses is often impossible to define. The commonest intradural tumors in dogs are meningiomas, especially in the cervical area; lymphoma is also prevalent in cats. Peripheral nerve sheath tumors often have an intradural component although may involve all three locations. The developmental tumor nephroblastoma typically arises in young dogs in an intradural location between T9 and L3; German Shepherd dogs are predisposed.

Survey radiographs are usually unremarkable although subtle enlargement of the affected intervertebral foramen is occasionally seen with peripheral nerve sheath tumors that also have an extradural component. Radiographic and reformatted sagittal and dorsal CT myelographic images should be examined carefully for the typical appearance of subarachnoid widening outlining a filling defect ("golf tee sign", **fig. 16.20A**) and associated cord compression in one plane, with corresponding cord widening in the

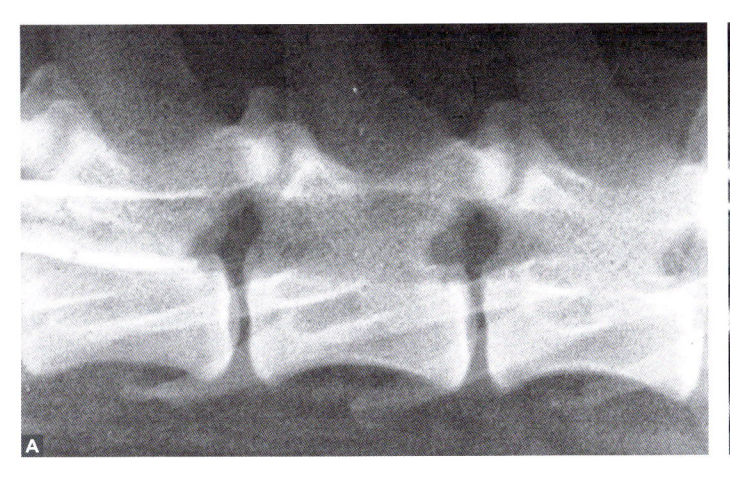

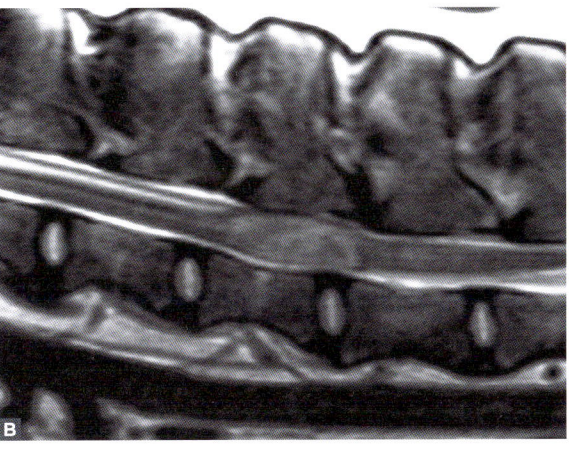

Fig. 16.19 (**A**) Myelogram in the mid-lumbar area of a seven-year-old Golden Retriever with paraparesis. The dorsal and ventral contrast columns diverge, thin and halt rather abruptly suggesting spinal cord swelling. The vertebral canal through the next vertebra is widened due to smooth remodeling of the neural arch; this suggests pressure atrophy due to slow expansion of the spinal cord. The presumptive diagnosis was an intramedullary mass, likely to be neoplastic, but further imaging and histopathology were not performed. (**B**) Sagittal T2W MRI image of the mid-lumbar spine in a three-year-old Boxer with paraparesis. The spinal cord is markedly swollen by the presence of a well-defined, hyperintense, intramedullary mass and the surrounding subarachnoid space is occluded. The central canal of the spinal cord is slightly widened cranial to the mass, due to its obstructive effect, and caudally a small area of less well-defined hyperintensity is seen. The final diagnosis was lymphoma.

SECTION III AXIAL SKELETON

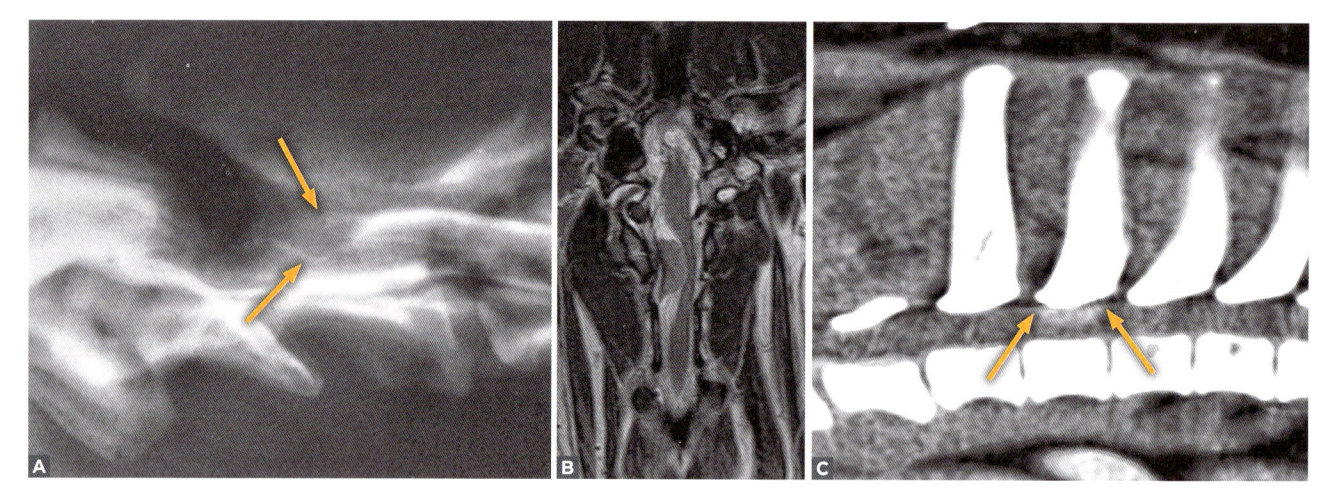

Fig. 16.20 (A) Myelogram of the cranial cervical spine in a nine-year-old Boxer with slowly-progressive tetraparesis and neck pain. The dorsal contrast column is interrupted and caudal to this area is seen to widen and split around an intradural filling defect (arrow). The ventral column is depressed and thinned. On post mortem examination a meningioma was found. (B) Dorsal plane T2W MRI image of the cranial cervical spine of a nine-year-old German Shepherd dog with tetraparesis, showing a well-defined, slug-shaped, intradural mass lateral to the spinal cord causing severe cord compression. The subarachnoid space containing hyperintense CSF is widened cranial and caudal to the mass. Post-contrast T1W images showed marked, homogeneous enhancement of the mass. A meningioma was removed surgically. The cranial cervical spine is a predilection site for meningiomas. (C) Sagittal CT reconstruction (post-contrast soft tissue window) of a five-year-old Flat-coated Retriever with a three-month history of slowly-progressive, generalized stiffness and occasional vocalization, responding to pain killers. A well-defined, extramedullary mass is seen causing spinal cord compression. Apparent dural tails cranially and caudally (arrows) and external fat opacity suggest that the mass is most likely to be intradural-extramedullary. A histological diagnosis was not made but it was thought likely to be a meningioma.

orthogonal plane. If the tumor has also invaded the spinal cord, general cord swelling may be seen. With MRI, T2W and STIR sequences, in which CSF is hyperintense, will give the same appearance of subarachnoid widening delineating a filling defect (**fig. 16.20B**). Intradural tumors are likely to show contrast enhancement, and dural tails are commonly seen with meningiomas (**fig. 16.20C**).

Extradural tumors

▍ **Spinal tumors not involving bone** Small soft tissue tumors within and confined to the vertebral canal produce no radiographic changes in survey radiographs, although many extradural tumors involve bone to some extent and changes are visible when sufficiently severe. Myelography will show the extent of resulting cord compression. MRI is the technique of choice for diagnosis although contrast-enhanced CT may also be useful (**fig. 16.21**).

▍ **Spinal tumors involving bone** Primary malignant bone tumors in the spine are less common than in the appendicular skeleton. The commonest type in the dog is osteosarcoma and in the cat is fibrosarcoma, but the imaging features are non-specific for tumor type. Primary vertebral tumors are usually solitary (monostotic), affecting any part of the vertebra with sparing of the endplates and disc spaces. They predominantly show aggressive features of osteolysis with varying degrees of periosteal reaction and/or tumor bone (**fig. 16.22A**). Adjacent soft tissue swelling may be evident and pathological collapse of weakened bone can occur.

MRI and CT, as expected, show loss of normal bone architecture, primarily through osteolysis of cortices and trabecular bone. In MRI images normal bone marrow fat signal is replaced by varying degrees of hyperintensity in T2W and STIR images and hypointensity in T1W (**fig. 16.22B**). T2*GE images are sensitive for areas of mineral loss. With both CT and MRI, uneven contrast enhancement of the tumor will occur and both techniques will show the extent of surrounding soft tissue changes and spinal cord compression (**fig. 16.22C**).

Differential diagnosis: osteomyelitis, especially fungal, for more proliferative tumors.

CHAPTER **16** Vertebral column

Fig. 16.21 Sagittal T2W MRI image of the mid-lumbar spine in an eight-year-old Bullmastiff with progressive ambulatory paraparesis. A well-defined soft tissue mass compresses the spinal cord from the dorsal aspect. It is surrounded by hyperintense epidural fat and the dura (the dark line) is displaced ventrally. There is no visible bone involvement.

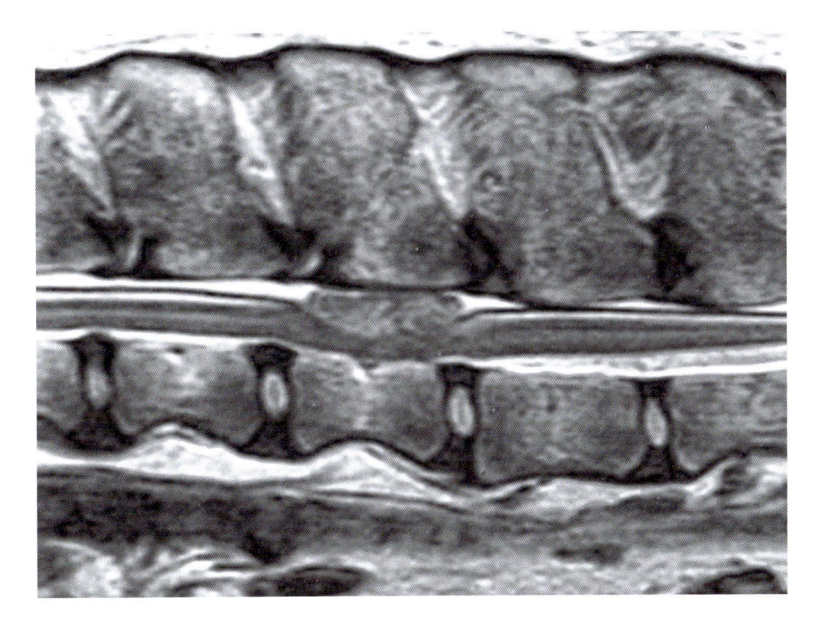

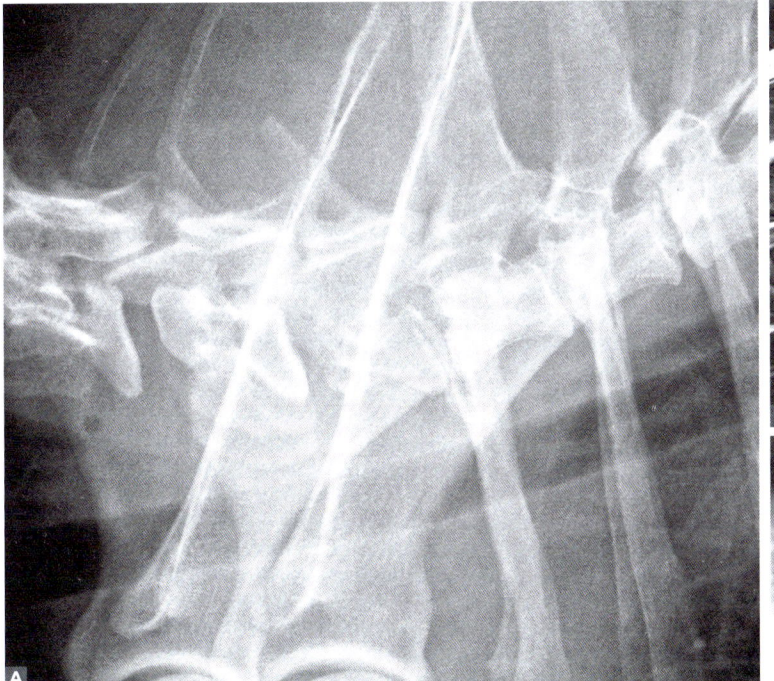

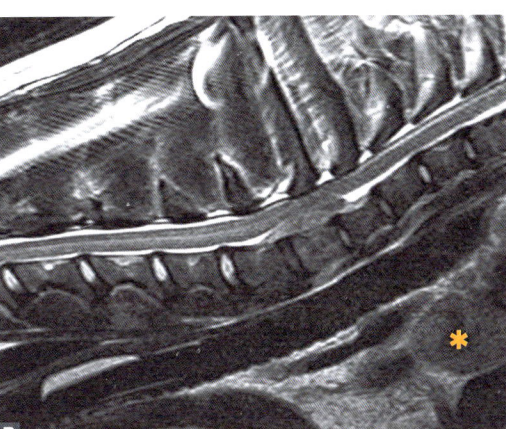

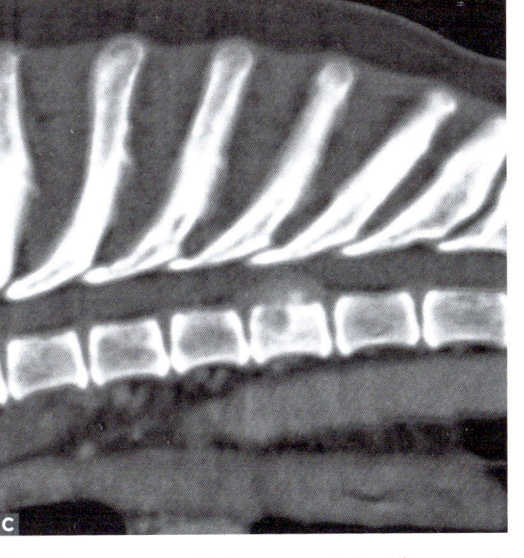

Fig. 16.22 (**A**) Lateral radiograph of the cervicothoracic spine in a ten-year-old Labrador Retriever with severe neck pain and thoracic limb lameness. There is reduced radiopacity of the vertebral body of C7 with loss of clarity of its cranial and dorsal margins indicating diffuse osteolysis, and narrowing of the C6-C7 disc space. MRI confirmed the presence of a vertebral mass causing spinal cord compression, but the dog was euthanized and a histopathological diagnosis was not made. Malignant neoplasia was assumed. (**B**) Sagittal T2W image of the cervicothoracic spine in a four-year-old English Bull Terrier with a one-month history of worsening neck pain and tetraparesis localized to the C6-T2 neural segments. Abnormal tissue which is mildly hyperintense to the spinal cord infiltrates the body of T1 and extends into the vertebral canal causing spinal cord elevation and compression. The study also showed mediastinal lymphadenopathy (asterisk) and lung metastases. Malignant neoplasia with metastasis was diagnosed but the dog was euthanized and a histological diagnosis was not made. (**C**) Sagittal CT reconstruction (post-contrast soft tissue window) of the thoracic spine of an eight-year-old Labrador Retriever with acute onset of reluctance to walk four days previously and diffuse spinal pain. There is focal osteolysis with surrounding sclerosis in the vertebral body of T8 with an overlying, partly-mineralized soft tissue mass in the vertebral canal causing severe spinal cord compression. The dog was taken home for palliative care: a histological diagnosis was not made but osteosarcoma or other primary tumor was suspected as no other lesions were detected.

203

▌ **Metastatic vertebral tumors** These are likely to be multiple, and arise especially from carcinomas: skeletal metastases are uncommon but the spine is a predilection site. Osteolysis predominates but differentiation between primary and secondary vertebral tumors cannot be made radiographically, although polyostotic disease is suggestive of metastasis. Metastases are less likely to invade the vertebral canal and cause spinal cord compression than are primary tumors. Ill-defined periosteal new bone on the ventral margins of the lumbosacral vertebrae and on the iliac wings is highly suggestive of prostatic carcinoma in male dogs.

▌ **Plasma cell myeloma (multiple myeloma)** Plasma cell myeloma (multiple myeloma) is a tumor of bone marrow stem cells which produces secondary bone lesions. These are characteristically osteolytic with a discrete, "punched out" appearance and may be solitary or multiple; in the latter case confluence of multiple lesions often produces a moth-eaten bone appearance and pathological fractures may occur. The spine and pelvis are typical sites although the long bones, ribs and sternebrae can also be affected (**fig. 16.23A**). Extension into the vertebral canal and spinal cord compression is uncommon. Radiography and CT show areas of osteolysis: in MRI the soft tissue in the lytic areas appears homogeneous and contrast-enhancing; they are usually mildly expansile without breaching the vertebral cortices (**fig. 16.23B**). Both CT and MRI are superior to radiography for detection of smaller lesions: MRI STIR sequences are highly sensitive due suppression of the normal fat signal in surrounding bone marrow, the lesions then being obvious as focal hyperintensities. Multifocal lesions with these imaging characteristics are highly suggestive of multiple myeloma.[12]

▌ **Osteochondroma** Osteochondroma is a form of skeletal dysplasia due to aberrant endochondral ossification, and is considered to be a benign developmental tumor. When multiple,

Fig. 16.23 (**A**) Lateral lumbar radiograph of a six-year-old Golden Retriever with multiple myeloma. Numerous well-defined areas of osteolysis of varying size affect all vertebrae, producing a marbled appearance to the bone. Other parts of the skeletal system were also affected, including the pelvis, ribs and sternum. (**B**) Sagittal T2W MRI image of the thoracolumbar spine (T7-L3) of an eight-year-old Golden Retriever with multiple myeloma. Several areas of homogeneous, hyperintense bone infiltrate are seen, showing mild mass effect in places without causing aggressive osteolysis. Affected areas include the vertebral bodies of T9, T10, T11 and L3, the spinous processes of T8 and T9 and the neural arch of T10. Other areas of hyperintense bone signal may represent smaller lesions or uneven distribution of bone marrow fat; further sequences were needed to clarify this.

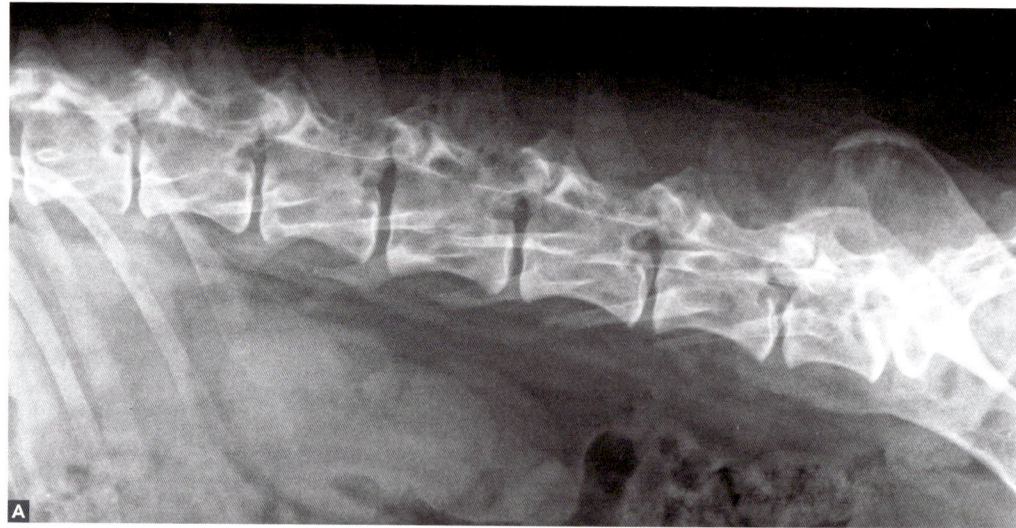

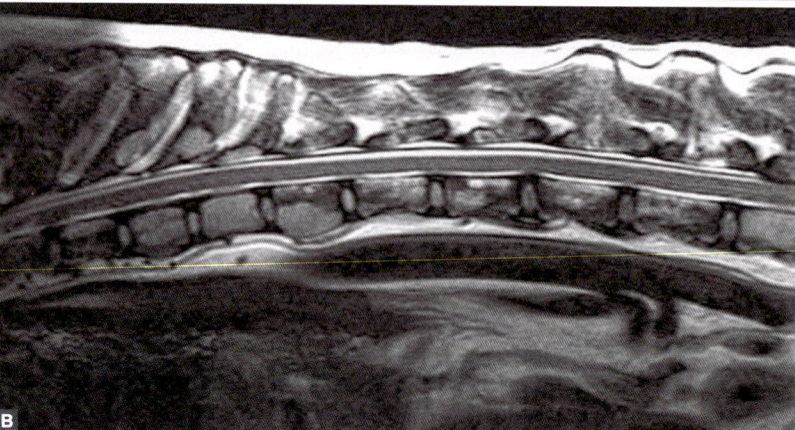

Fig. 16.24 (A) Cranial thoracic spinal radiograph of an 11-year-old Labrador Retriever with cranial thoracic pain and neurological deficits localizing to the C6-T2 spinal cord segments. There is complete lysis of the spinous process and neural arch of T2, partial lysis with pathological fracture of the spinous process of T1 and sclerosis with loss of normal trabecular pattern of the spinous process of T3. Aggressive osteolysis of several adjacent bones suggests malignant soft tissue neoplasia and biopsy revealed fibrosarcoma. (B) Sagittal post-contrast T1W MRI image of the lumbosacral area of a 13-year-old Domestic shorthair cat with pelvic limb paresis and incontinence. The site of previous removal of a superficial soft tissue mass (fibrosarcoma) is indicated by an oil capsule, which is hyperintense in MRI images. An extensive, enhancing soft tissue mass extends into the vertebral canal causing severe compression of the cauda equina.

osteochondromata are referred to as "multiple cartilaginous exostoses". They arise in skeletally immature animals at cartilaginous sites, forming masses which reduce in size or resolve with skeletal maturity, and they can arise at a variety of locations including vertebrae, causing clinical signs due to spinal cord compression. Radiographically, they are seen as smoothly-bordered, expansile, cauliflower-like outgrowths from cartilaginous areas such as growth plates, costochondral junctions, iliac wing crests and vertebral spinous and articular processes. Occasionally malignant transformation to osteosarcoma occurs.

Imaging shows spinal lesions as small, expansile areas of bone usually arising from the neural arch or articular processes: the cortex and medullary cavity merge with underlying bone with no osteolysis or periosteal reaction. Radiographically, myelography is required for demonstration of cord compression. The general appearance is of a non-aggressive lesion and the diagnosis is usually obvious given the typical young age of the patient.

In cats, osteochondromata can also occur in older animals, and there is a possible association with FeLV. Although uncommon, the spine may be a predilection site. Lesions here may be smaller and more sclerotic than the typical canine lesion.

▍ **Angiomatosis** Angiomatosis is a non-neoplastic, developmental vertebral condition seen in young cats, in which a vascular malformation arises due to proliferation of well-defined blood vessels. The lesions are expansile and have a mottled, sclerotic appearance containing multiple, punctate foci of radiolucency. The vertebral pedicles are most commonly affected, and this can cause spinal cord compression. Irregular contrast enhancement occurs with MRI and CT, due to the vascular nature of the lesions.

Differential diagnosis, considering the signalment of the patient, is osteochondroma, but angiomata tend to have a more aggressive appearance.

▍ **Paraspinal tumors** Soft tissue malignancies arising in a paraspinal location may invade adjacent vertebrae, usually affecting more than one bone. Mesenchymal tumors such as fibrosarcoma are commonest in dogs, and lymphoma in cats. Osteolysis tends to predominate with little or no evidence of new bone and in the thoracic area rib heads may also be destroyed (**fig. 16.24**). However, some extradural soft tissue tumors enter or exit the vertebral canal via intervertebral foramina without causing osteolysis. In the thoracic area, paraspinal tumors may be seen highlighted against air in the lungs; elsewhere they may be hard to appreciate unless there is a large mass or fascial plane displacement. Extradural lymphoma is the commonest spinal tumor in cats, which are usually FeLV positive.

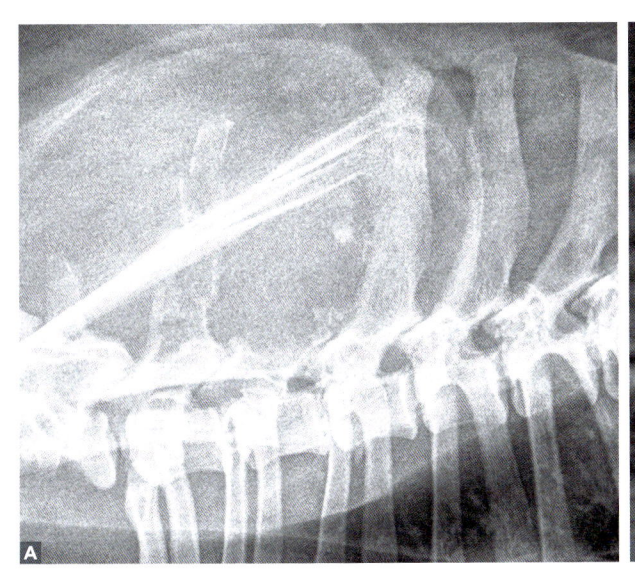

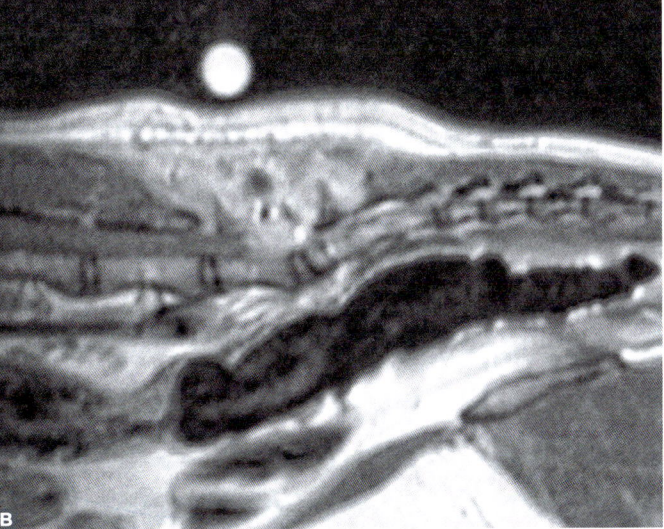

Spinal trauma

Dogs and cats with spinal trauma must be handled carefully in case instability of the spine leads to further cord damage. General anesthesia should be avoided in the first instance since this will abolish protective muscle spasm. The affected area should be splinted if possible or the patient placed on a back board, and lateral radiographs obtained first. Use of a cassette tray or a radiolucent board raised slightly off the table top will allow cassettes to be positioned without moving the animal. The orthogonal (VD) view is essential in order to detect lateral displacement; this can be obtained using a horizontal X ray beam. However, displacement at the time of radiography may be much less than that at the time of impact as it may be reduced by protective muscle spasm, so spinal cord damage is likely to be underestimated.

Fractures and subluxations

About two thirds of spinal trauma cases are due to impacts with motor vehicles; other causes include fights, falls from heights and head-on injuries. Combinations of fracture and subluxation are common. Subluxations often occur at the junctions between movable and rigid sections of spine, e.g., at either end of the rib cage and at the lumbosacral junction, whereas those within the thoracic area are usually minor because of the stabilizing effect of the rib cage. Fractures and subluxations of the sacrum or tail in cats ("tail pull injuries") may cause avulsion of cauda equina nerves leading to subsequent problems with urination and defecation. In the cranial neck, dislocation at the occipitoatlantal junction may occur without fracture, and C1 or C2 fractures often cause atlantoaxial subluxation. Delayed spinal cord compression following trauma can develop months later due to subsequent callus formation, and the owners should be warned of this possibility.

Initial imaging assessment may be with radiography but one study showed that radiography cannot be used to rule out potentially unstable vertebral lesions reliably.[13] Additional information can be supplied by CT and/or MRI in many cases, and this is recommended if surgical stabilization of complex fractures is contemplated. CT is ideal for more subtle bone lesions whereas MRI is more sensitive for spinal cord and paraspinal soft tissue damage.[14,15] With CT, multiplanar reformatting and 3D surface rendering are useful tools. The main goal of imaging is to determine whether or not the spine is unstable and this can be assessed using the three compartment model adapted from medical imaging in which the spine is divided into three compartments, dorsal (laminae, pedicles, articular processes, spinal processes and supporting soft tissues), middle (dorsal longitudinal ligament, dorsal part of vertebral body and dorsal annulus fibrosus) and ventral (the rest of the vertebral body, ventral annulus fibrosus and the ventral longitudinal ligament). If two of the three compartments are damaged the spine is likely to be unstable. Following spinal trauma, the patient should also be checked for other injuries such as ruptured diaphragm, pneumothorax, fractured ribs and damaged abdominal viscera using imaging techniques as appropriate.

▌ Fractures Major fractures of vertebral bodies are usually obvious radiographically, since displacement of fragments is common (**fig. 16.25A**). Careful assessment should be made for fragments which could be within the vertebral canal. Salter I fractures of the vertebral physes with slipping of the endplate can occur in skeletally immature animals. Compression fractures of vertebrae can occur due to trauma (especially in cats) (**fig. 16.25B**) or to pathological weakening of the vertebral body due to neoplasia, osteopenia, infection or bone cysts (**fig. 16.25C**). Compression fractures are subtle and are easily overlooked: the VD is often the more helpful projection. Signs to look for are loss of the rectangular shape of the vertebral body, a band of ill-defined increase in opacity, angulation of the spine and loss of parallelity of the adjacent disc spaces. Fractures of articular processes are also subtle and may be best seen on the VD view where the two sides are seen separately. Fractures of transverse and spinous processes are less important. MRI and CT will give more precise information about the nature of fractures and their effect on the spinal cord (**fig. 16.26**).

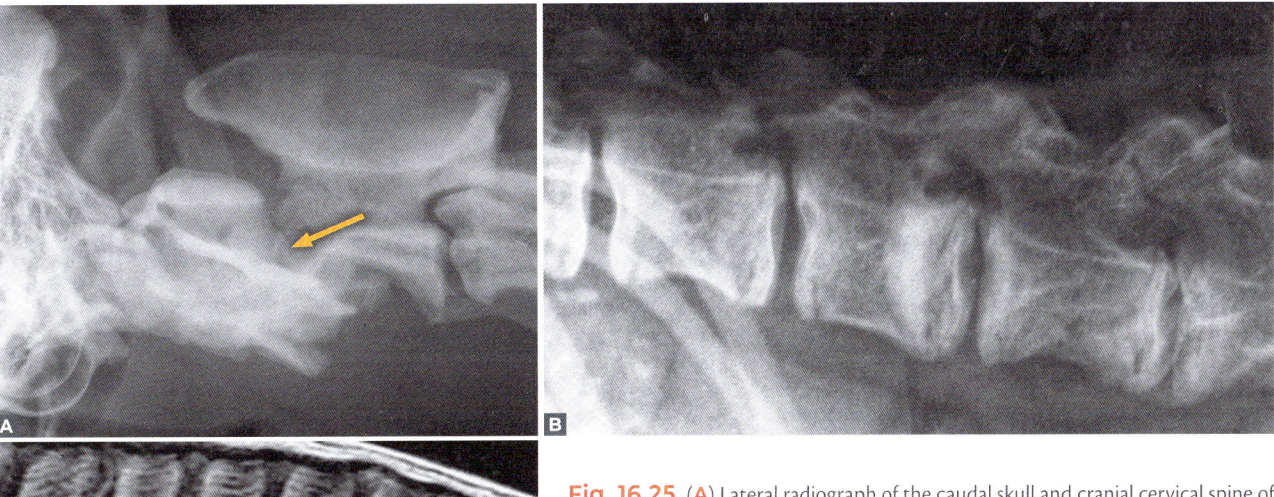

CHAPTER 16 Vertebral column

Fig. 16.25 (A) Lateral radiograph of the caudal skull and cranial cervical spine of a five-year-old German Shepherd dog which was tetraplegic after being hit by a car. There is atlantoaxial subluxation with overriding of C2 on C1 due to a comminuted C2 fracture but even with multiple radiographic projections its exact nature was unclear, preventing surgical planning (one fracture line is arrowed). CT was not available and so MRI was performed. (B) Radiographic appearance of a compression fracture of the vertebral body of L2 in a five-month-old crossbred dog which had been hit by a car. The bone is shortened but alignment remains normal. An ill-defined sclerotic band is seen where the bone has been compacted. (C) Sagittal T2W MRI image of the thoracic spine of a nine-year-old crossbred dog with acute paraparesis. The vertebral body of T5 is markedly shortened and misshapen due to a pathological compression fracture. Abnormal, hyperintense tissue is seen in the bone protruding dorsally and causing spinal cord compression. No external soft tissue mass is visible and primary bone neoplasia was considered likely.

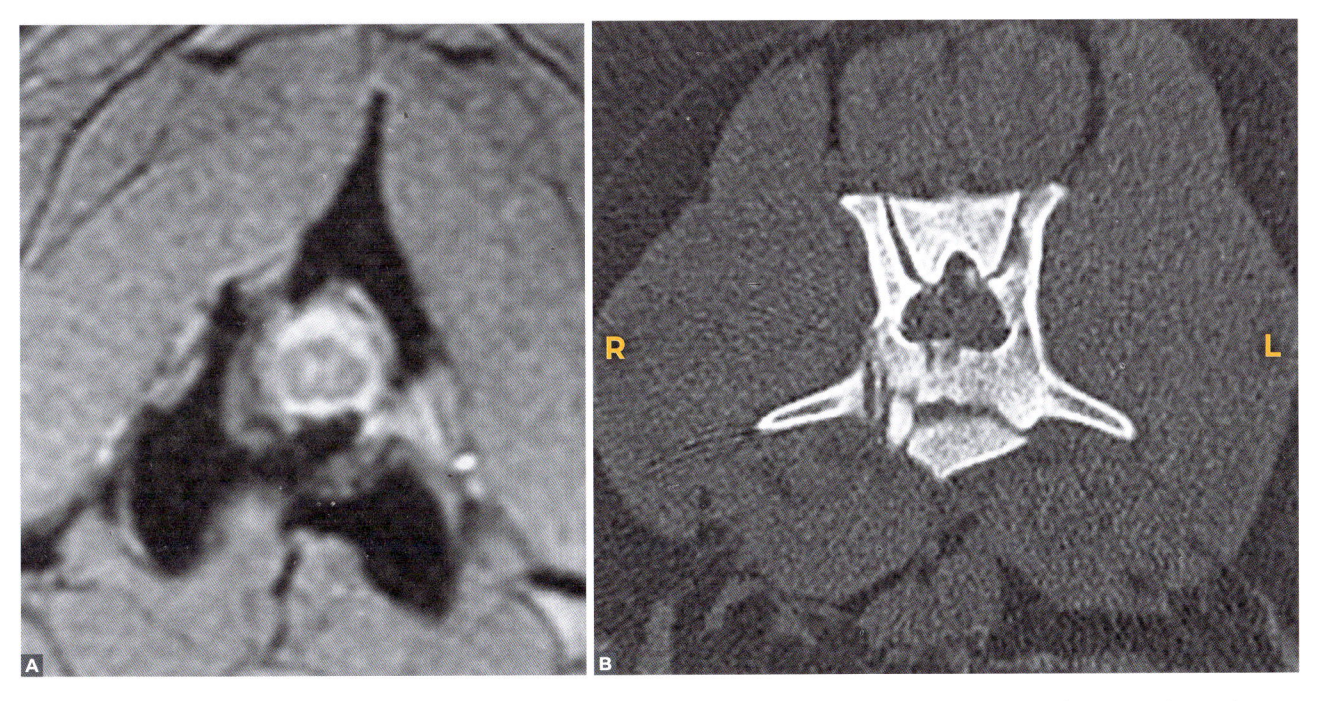

Fig. 16.26 (A) Transverse T2*GE MRI image of the dog in fig. 16.25A at the level of mid C2, clearly depicting the conformation of major fracture lines and showing that the spinal cord was not compressed despite fragment displacement. The dog made a full recovery after surgical stabilization. CT would also have demonstrated any non-displaced fissures and surface rendered CT images would also have been useful in giving 3D information; however, information about the state of the spinal cord would have been inferior. (B) Transverse CT bone window image of a comminuted fracture of L4 in an 18-week-old Airedale Terrier puppy which had been hit by a car. In this image comminuted fractures of the vertebral body are seen together with fractures of both pedicles, the base of the right transverse process and the left cranial articular process. This level of bony detail would not be evident with either radiography or MRI.

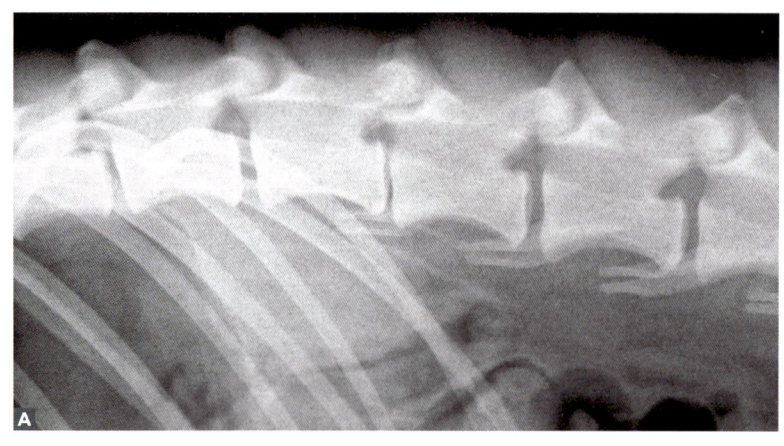

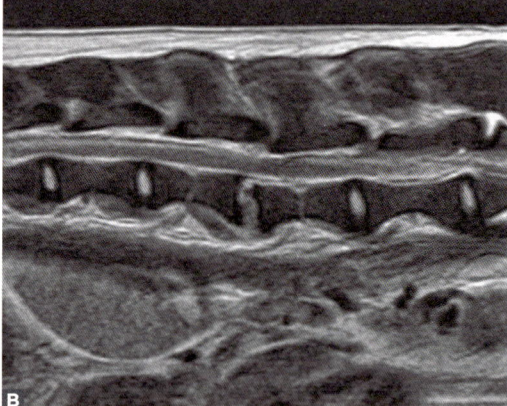

Fig. 16.27 (**A**) Radiograph of the thoracolumbar spine of a four-year-old Irish Red Setter suffering spinal pain and mild paraparesis after being hit by a car. The L1-L2 disc space and intervertebral foramen are narrowed and there is slight ventral displacement of L2 relative to L1. This displacement is mild but may have been more severe at the time of impact, hence the integrity of the spinal cord is not known. (**B**) Sagittal T2W MRI image of the same dog showing widening of the affected disc space and more obvious vertebral subluxation, indicating that the site is unstable. The disc annulus is disrupted both dorsally and ventrally and the subluxation suggests that all three spinal compartments are damaged. However, despite some loss of clarity of the epidural space and dorsal dura at the site, the spinal cord appears to be neither compressed nor obviously contused.

▌**Subluxations** Subluxations at a disc space usually result in narrowing or wedging of the disc space and intervertebral foramen with changes in width of the dorsal articular joint space (for traumatic disc extrusion, see the section on disc disease). Slight stepping of the dorsal or ventral margins of the vertebral body is likely and small chip fractures are common due to ligament avulsion (**fig. 16.27**). Rotational subluxation usually occurs in the cervical spine and is best seen on the VD radiograph as malalignment of dorsal spinous processes.

▌**Gunshot wounds** Gunshot wounds can involve the spine, and although the spinal cord is relatively protected. Ballistic fractures are usually comminuted and most have extensive associated soft tissue injury. Radiographs are useful for assessment and artefacts caused by the metallic fragments will degrade both CT and MRI images.

Spinal cord and dural injury

Milder blunt trauma can cause spinal cord contusion in the absence of bony changes; injuries causing fracture and/or subluxation will inevitably result in more severe cord damage including compression, stretching and transection. An important goal of cross-sectional imaging is to assess the likely degree of cord damage in order to provide a prognosis. Cord contusion is best seen in MRI as T2W hyperintensity (edema) and signal void with susceptibility artefact in T2*GE images (hemorrhage). In CT images, these changes may be hypodense and hyperdense respectively, when severe. With both modalities, contrast enhancement is likely to be minimal but contrast medium uptake by cord parenchyma indicates grave damage. Compressive epidural hemorrhage may be detected.

Traumatic dural laceration has been reported in association with blunt trauma and explosive disc extrusion, and may occur spontaneously in athletic dogs. Myelography shows extravasation of contrast medium into surrounding soft tissues.

Disc disease

Disc prolapse usually occurs in a dorsal direction because the normal annulus fibrosus is thinnest dorsally. Hansen types I and II disc prolapse are commonest but other types of disc prolapse have been recognized since the use of MRI in veterinary patients.

Whilst survey radiographs can be suggestive, confident radiographic diagnosis usually requires myelography, and is essential if surgery is to be performed. For suspected thoracolumbar disc extrusions lumbar puncture should be carried out as secondary cord swelling may prevent contrast medium from a cervical puncture from outlining the affected site adequately. VD and oblique radiographs should be obtained as well as laterals as these will show the distribution of extruded disc material relative to the cord, especially when it is circumferential.[16] Difficulties with diagnosis may arise from both technical and pathoanatomical problems, and have been usefully reviewed in a well-illustrated paper.[17]

Although MRI is usually the technique for choice for imaging disc disease, CT is also valuable. The relative merits of MRI, CT and radiographic myelography have been reviewed.[18]

Hansen type I disc extrusion

Type I intervertebral disc extrusions occur mainly in chondrodystrophic dogs in which the nucleus pulposus can undergo chondroid degeneration and mineralization from a very young age. Subsequent acute rupture of the overlying annulus fibrosis and dorsal longitudinal ligament may occur, with extrusion of mineralized material into the vertebral canal causing spinal cord concussion and compression and acute or subacute clinical signs. In the cervical area, these disc extrusions usually occur at the more cranial disc spaces; in the thoracolumbar area most extrusions are in the caudal thoracic or cranial lumbar areas due to the greater mechanical load at this site; disc extrusion cranial to T11 is unusual due to the intercapital ligaments and greater stability of the area. However, similar clinical signs can arise from any disease T3-L3 and so the whole area should be radiographed. Interestingly large dogs, especially German Shepherd dogs, may suffer from extrusions in the cranial thoracic spine (T2-T5). Cats are occasionally affected by disc extrusions, usually in the mid lumbar area. Occasionally, a small lateralized extrusion may occur at a site of chronic type II change, resulting in acute clinical signs.

Survey radiographs may give both false-positives and false-negatives, but the following features may be seen (**fig. 16.28A**):

- Disc space and intervertebral foraminal narrowing – compare with those on either side, but beware of artefactual narrowing due to positioning and the geometry of the diverging X-ray beam. The narrowing should be consistent in all images of the area, including the VD. Note that the anticlinal disc space (usually T10-T11) is often slightly narrowed.
- Mineralized disc material with a dorsal spur extending towards or into the vertebral canal. Beware of overlying rib heads and accessory or transverse processes, and obliquely-projected endplates, which mimic mineralized disc material. Note that mineralized disc material which remains within the disc space and is rounded dorsally is unlikely to be significant, and many chondrodystrophic dogs will have multiple, incidental, mineralized discs.
- Opacification of the intervertebral foramen.
- Gas within a disc space under stress ("vacuum phenomenon") is a non-specific sign of disc degeneration.
- Endplate sclerosis and spondylosis – these suggest a chronic lesion, which may not be the current problem.

Myelographic images must be assessed for evidence of extradural spinal cord compression; cord swelling may also be seen adjacent to the site of compression. Although usually ventral or ventrolateral over a disc space, extruded material may lie anywhere since it can migrate along the vertebral canal or even dorsal to the cord: oblique radiographs should be acquired as well as conventional lateral and VD, in order to detect ventrolateral or dorsolateral cord compression (**fig. 16.28B**). Extensive extradural compression suggests secondary hemorrhage due to laceration of the vertebral venous sinuses. Opacification of the central canal or cord itself at the site of pathology is a grave prognostic sign since it indicates myelomalacia, with leakage of contrast medium into the cord.

Extrusion of a discrete nodule of mineralized or non-mineralized disc material laterally into an intervertebral foramen can occur (foraminal extrusion). These cause severe pain by compressing

SECTION III AXIAL SKELETON

spinal nerve roots, without neurological deficits. Mineralized foraminal extrusions may be seen radiographically whereas those which are non-mineralized require MRI for diagnosis. Radiographic and CT myelography are generally unhelpful.

MRI and CT are frequently used for diagnosis of disc disease. Overall, MRI is superior for detection of disc changes since even very early disc degeneration will result in loss of signal of the nucleus in T2W scans; heavily mineralized disc material appears as a signal void in all sequences. In addition, MRI depicts changes within the cord itself. Following extrusion, disc material is seen in the epidural space and since epidural fat and CSF are of different signal intensity to the spinal cord, compression is readily appreciated (**fig. 16.28C**). Annular tears may sometimes be seen in high-quality transverse and sagittal images. Associated epidural hemorrhage resulting from rupture of venous sinuses appears as dispersed signal void in T2*GE images which is heterogeneous in other sequences. Associated

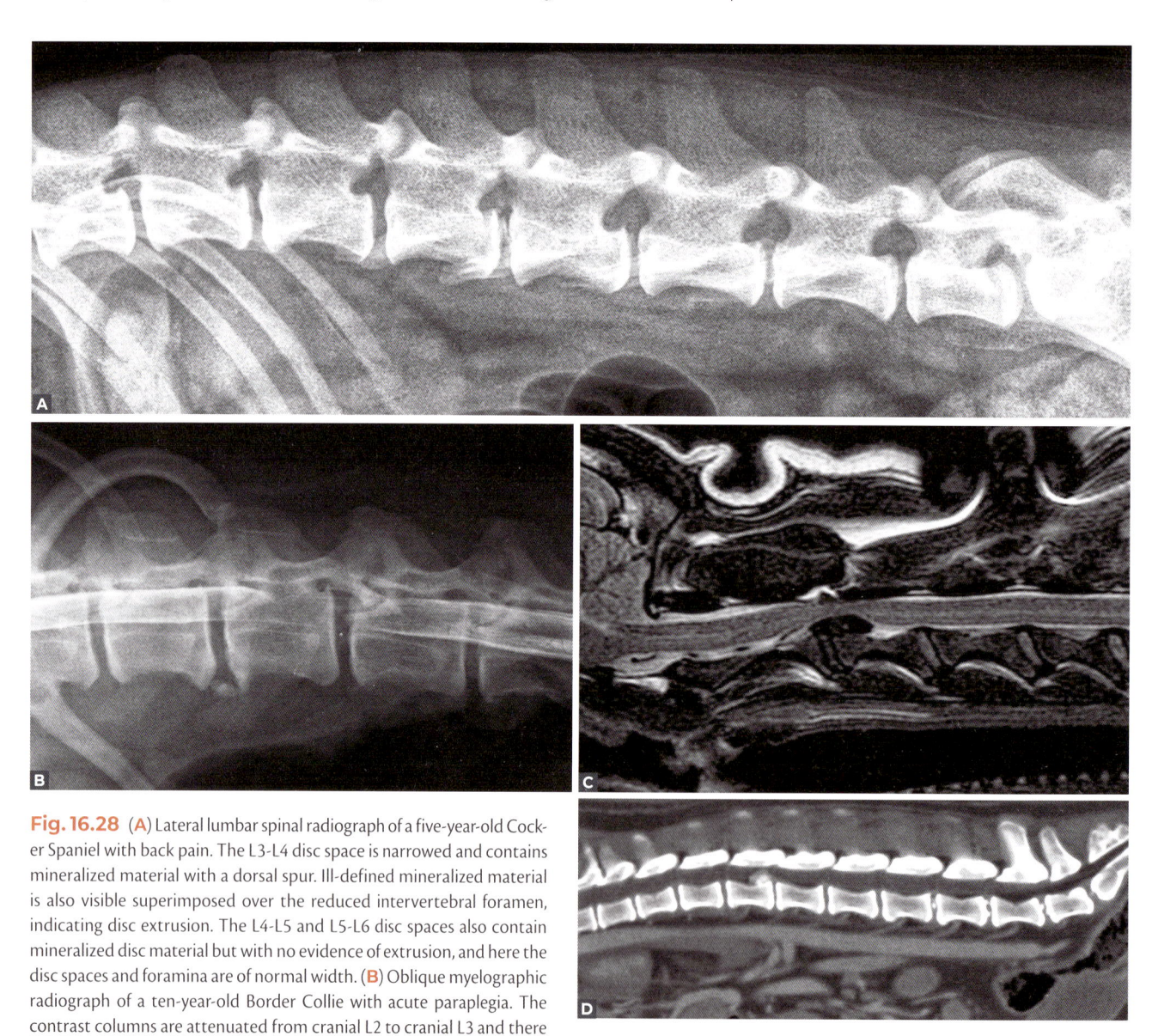

Fig. 16.28 (**A**) Lateral lumbar spinal radiograph of a five-year-old Cocker Spaniel with back pain. The L3-L4 disc space is narrowed and contains mineralized material with a dorsal spur. Ill-defined mineralized material is also visible superimposed over the reduced intervertebral foramen, indicating disc extrusion. The L4-L5 and L5-L6 disc spaces also contain mineralized disc material but with no evidence of extrusion, and here the disc spaces and foramina are of normal width. (**B**) Oblique myelographic radiograph of a ten-year-old Border Collie with acute paraplegia. The contrast columns are attenuated from cranial L2 to cranial L3 and there is inward displacement of the dorsolateral column suggesting the presence of extruded disc material ± hemorrhage in this location, causing spinal cord compression. The extrusion originated from the L2-L3 disc space. (**C**) Large disc extrusion at C2-C3 in a five-year-old Cocker Spaniel with severe neck pain shown in a sagittal T2W MRI image. The extruded material is of signal void, suggesting that it is largely mineralized. The C2-C3 disc space is slightly narrowed and residual disc material is more hypointense than those more caudally. The spinal cord is elevated and severely compressed but is of normal signal intensity. (**D**) Sagittal CT reconstruction image (post-contrast soft tissue window) of the lumbar spine of a three-year-old French Bulldog with acute back pain and paraplegia. Narrowing of the L1-L2 disc space due to extrusion of a large volume of mineralized disc material is seen. Mineralized disc material is also visible in disc spaces T11-T12, L4-L5, L5-L6, L6-L7 and L7-S1.

Fig. 16.29 (**A**) Sagittal T2W MRI image of the cranial thoracic spine of a ten-year-old English Setter with ataxia and paraparesis. All visible discs are degenerate and T2-T3 shows moderate dorsal protrusion causing slight elevation and compression of the spinal cord. There is also evidence of dorsal bony stenosis at T3, T4 and T5 (confirmed in transverse images). The central canal of the spinal cord is mildly dilated cranially to the obstructive effect. (**B**) Sagittal CT reconstruction (post-contrast soft tissue window) of the lumbosacral spine of an 11-year-old Labrador Retriever undergoing abdominal CT. A moderate disc protrusion is visible at the lumbosacral junction, causing elevation of the cauda equina (arrow). However, neural compression is not evident with the dog lying in this position, as hypoattenuating epidural fat is still visible dorsally. Ventral spondylosis suggests chronicity. This was an incidental finding.

spinal cord damage, both acute and chronic, is well demonstrated in T2W images in which cord edema appears as diffuse hyperintensity and cord swelling. Ascending myelomalacia appears similar, but usually covers a much larger length of cord cranial to the extrusion. In about one third of cases, paraspinal muscle signal changes are seen, although their cause is not yet fully understood.

In CT, mineralized disc material appears hyperattenuating and therefore extruded mineralized disc material within the vertebral canal is readily appreciated (fig. 16.28D). Non-mineralized extruded material is of similar attenuation to spinal cord but may be outlined by adjacent epidural fat; epidural hemorrhage may appear mildly hyperdense. CT myelography is required to show the extent of cord compression ± reactive swelling, and delineates non-mineralized extruded material more clearly. CT images should always be reformatted in the sagittal and dorsal planes as these show any narrowed disc spaces, and location, lateralization and the length of compressed areas better. Entry of contrast medium into the cord itself suggests myelomalacia but otherwise cord changes such as edema and hemorrhage are not visible.

Hansen type II disc protrusion

Type II intervertebral disc protrusion usually occurs in non-chondrodystrophic dogs and consists of fibroid degeneration of the nucleus pulposus with hypertrophy and/or bulging of the overlying annulus fibrosus and dorsal longitudinal ligament into the vertebral canal, resulting in chronic signs. Partial annular tears may also be present but nuclear material remains confined. Disc protrusions often occur at sites of instability such as the caudal neck and at the lumbosacral junction; protrusions in the cranial thoracic area are sometimes seen in large dogs, especially German Shepherd dogs.

Survey radiographs of disc protrusions are often normal but, in some cases, the affected disc space is narrowed or wedge-shaped. Mineralization of disc material is not usually seen. Since the condition is chronic, endplate sclerosis and spondylosis are also often present. Disc protrusions are often a component of caudal cervical spondylomyelopathy ("Wobbler" syndrome) and cauda equina syndrome. Myelography is required for diagnosis and shows extradural cord compression from the midline ventral aspect. Since the condition is chronic, cord swelling is not seen and the cord may even have atrophied. Disc protrusions in the caudal neck and at the lumbosacral junction may have a dynamic component and the degree of compression will reduce when traction or flexion respectively is applied; in the case of cord atrophy in the neck, the cord remains narrow and instead the subarachnoid space fills with contrast medium in the dynamic image.

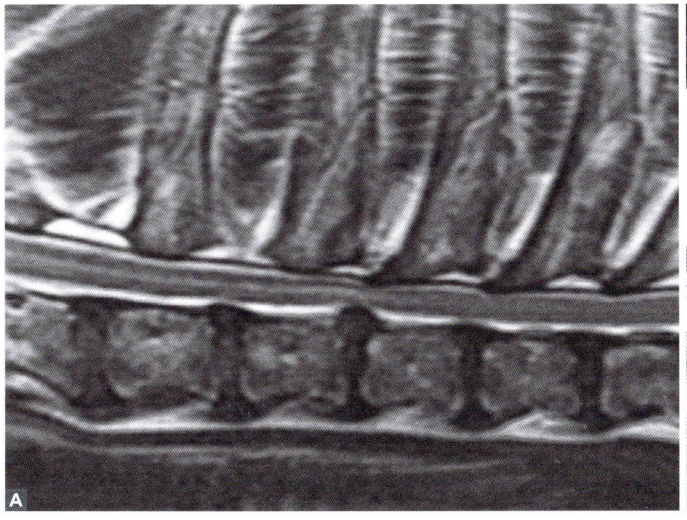

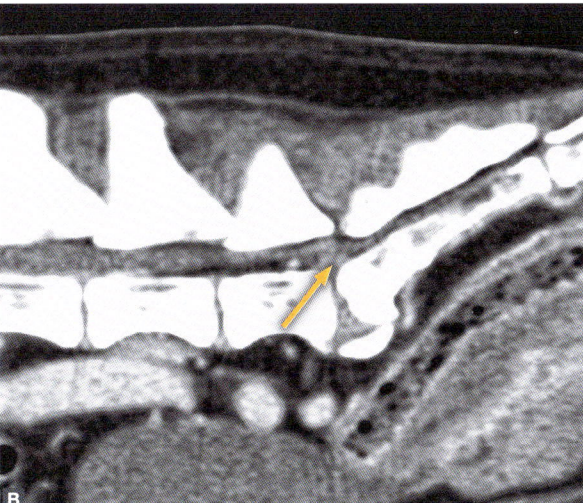

In MR images, signs of disc protrusions include disc degeneration, disc space narrowing and/or wedging, and thickening and dorsal bulging of the signal void structure which represents the combined annulus and dorsal longitudinal ligament (fig. 16.29A). If the overlying cord has atrophied, CSF is still visible around an attenuated section. In such cases, a small area of central cord T2W hyperintensity is often seen, likely to represent gliosis. Following traction, partial flattening of the protruded tissue may be seen in some cases, which assists surgical planning.

In CT images, disc space narrowing may again be seen in reformatted sagittal images with the protruding disc evident as a well-defined dome of mildly hyperattenuating soft tissue extending into the vertebral canal (**fig. 16.29B**). CT myelography shows the severity of cord displacement and compression but changes within the cord parenchyma are not visible. However, it may be impossible to differentiate type I from type II disc lesions using CT.

Traumatic disc extrusions (acute hydrated nucleus pulposus extrusion)

Non-degenerate discs may extrude acutely following internal trauma caused by a sudden athletic movement of the spine (e.g., jumping, running). In these cases, hydrated nucleus pulposus is forcefully extruded through a tear in the dorsal annulus but, being soft, will spread out within the vertebral canal. This type of disc extrusion was first recognized in MRI, and most often occurs in the mid neck in smaller breeds of dogs; it has not been described in cats.

Survey radiographs inconsistently show disc space narrowing; radiographic and CT myelography demonstrates shallow, ventral, extradural cord compression centered above a disc space. These extrusions are clearly seen in MRI. In T2W images, subtle disc space narrowing and reduction in nuclear volume is evident. Overlying the disc space and extending cranially and caudally is a shallow mound of hyperintense signal which is isointense to epidural fat and CSF in T2W, therefore is not clearly seen; however, in T1W images the extruded material, isointense to hydrated disc but hypointense to fat, is clearly outlined. In transverse T2W images the compressed cord adopts a characteristic "seagull" shape in cross section. Since the extruded material is soft, cord edema is not usually seen. Two other types of acute disc extrusion are recognized in MRI only, and as such are beyond the scope of this chapter: these are high-velocity, low-volume disc extrusions, also known as acute, non-compressive nucleus pulposus extrusions (ANCNPE) and intramedullary extrusions. The reader is directed to relevant references for further information.

Schmorl's nodes (intravertebral disc herniation)

Schmorl's nodes are well described in humans and are recognized but unusual in small animals. They are more common in humans because of vertical stance and the cartilaginous rather than bony nature of the end plate. Weakening of the vertebral end plate predisposes to herniation of disc material into the bone, potentially causing pain but often clinically silent. Radiographic signs include disc space narrowing, vacuum phenomenon, discrete end plate indentation and vertebral body lucencies with varying degrees of surrounding sclerosis. The lumbosacral disc space may be predisposed.

Differential diagnosis: discospondylitis.

Spinal infarcts (fibrocartilaginous emboli)

These are a clinical differential diagnosis for acute disc extrusions, often occurring during strenuous exercise and causing peracute, non-progressive paresis or plegia, usually in non-chondrodystrophic breeds. Fibrocartilaginous material from the nucleus pulposus enters the spinal cord vasculature (the exact mechanism is unclear) producing an ischemic myelopathy due to infarction. Spinal cord infarction can also arise due to other causes of emboli such as endocarditis. Survey radiographs are normal; radiographic and CT myelography show focal, mild spinal cord swelling in some cases but may also be normal: in these cases, the diagnosis is made by excluding disc extrusion.

MRI is the technique of choice for diagnosis; in peracute cases no changes are seen but disc extrusion is excluded. After several hours the lesion appears as a semi-defined area of T2W cord hyperinten-

Fig. 16.30 (**A**) Sagittal T2W MRI image of the cervicothoracic spine of an eight-year-old Staffordshire Bull Terrier with peracute tetraparesis, worse on the right side, and right Horner's syndrome, localized to the C6-T2 spinal cord segments. The spinal cord is swollen at the level of C6 and shows pronounced, ill-defined T2W hyperintense signal. The disc nucleus at C6-C7 is hydrated but is slightly reduced in volume and was considered possibly to be the source of a fibrocartilaginous embolus (arrow). No extramedullary material was identified to suggest extrusion into the vertebral canal. (**B**) Dorsal T2W MRI image at the same level, showing the predominantly right-sided nature of the changes.

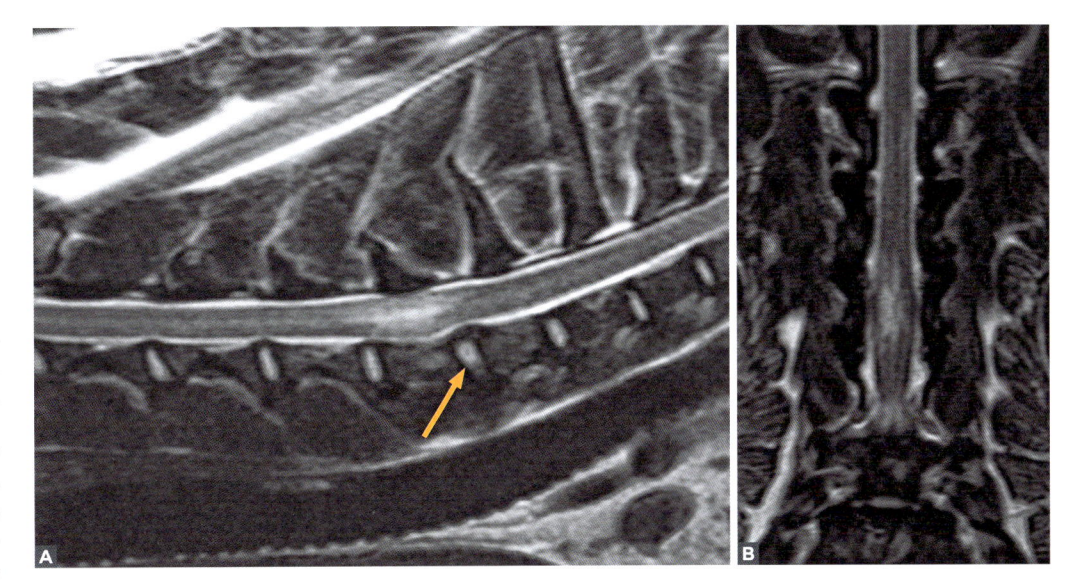

sity with or without mild cord swelling: the lesions are usually not above disc space and are often lateralized, corresponding to neurological deficits (**figs. 16.30**). In cases of longer clinical duration, mild contrast enhancement may be seen.

Miscellaneous – mixed etiology

Cauda equina syndrome

Cauda equina syndrome is a complex of clinical signs produced either by primary disease of the cauda equina such as myelitis or neoplasia or, more commonly, by changes in the surrounding tissues which cause cauda equina compression. Due to the anatomy in this area, clinical signs of cauda equina syndrome can arise because of pathology anywhere from L5 caudally, but the lumbosacral disc space is the most commonly-affected site. The condition has similarities to "Wobbler" syndrome in that vertebral canal stenosis and neural compression can result from a combination of bony and soft tissue changes. The purposes of imaging are (a) to identify the site(s) of compression, and (b) to determine the etiology, as this may affect treatment.

Causes include congenital, developmental, degenerative, inflammatory, traumatic, neoplastic and vascular etiologies affecting bone, discs, spinal cord, nerve roots or meninges and are listed in **box 16.1**. Bony changes are often seen in survey radiographs (**fig. 16.31A**), but false-positives and negatives are common since (a) many of the radiographic changes associated with cauda equina syndrome are seen in dogs without clinical signs; and (b) some dogs have lesions confined to soft tissues. A flexed VD projection may be helpful as it gives a much clearer view of disc space pathology and endplate changes.[2] Contrast studies can be used for further investigation especially if stressed views are important, although in most cases MRI will give more information. CT can also be helpful although yields less information than MRI (**fig. 16.29B**).

Radiography should also be used to examine the caudal abdomen and pelvic limbs for primary or secondary lesions of the colon, bladder and prostate gland which might mimic the clinical signs of cauda equina syndrome and thoracic radiography should be performed if neoplasia is suspected. CT and ultrasonography may also be used for these purposes.

The most appropriate radiographic contrast study is myelography, which allows examination of the lumbosacral junction in a high percentage of cases as well as demonstrating lesions further cranially. However, in some dogs the dural sac does not extend far enough caudally for myelography to be diagnostic. Discography and epidurography may also be used at the lumbosacral junction but both

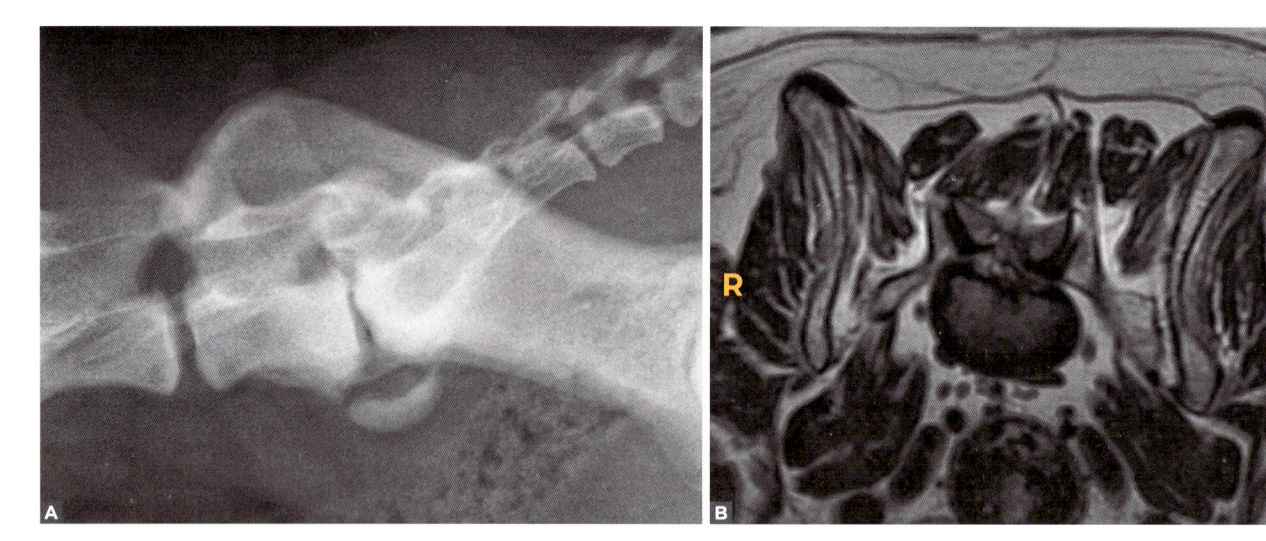

Fig. 16.31 (**A**) Lateral lumbosacral radiograph of an eight-year-old Labrador Retriever with pelvic limb stiffness, reluctance to climb stairs and lumbosacral discomfort on manipulation. Several radiographic features indicate degenerative disc disease at this site although myelography or cross-sectional imaging is needed to demonstrate the nature and degree of any cauda equina compression. The disc space is collapsed and contains a small accumulation of gas indicating a vacuum phenomenon. There is ventral and probably lateral spondylosis; increased radiopacity of the vertebral endplates may be due to a combination of sclerosis and superimposed lateral spondylosis. There is subtle ventral subluxation of S1 relative to L7. (**B**) Transverse T2W MRI image at the level of the lumbosacral junction in a four-year-old German Shepherd dog with clinical signs of cauda equina syndrome. The dog has an asymmetrical transitional vertebra forming the first sacral segment, with a reduced sacral wing articulating with the ilium on the left side (right of image) and a transverse process on the right (left of image), resulting in subtle rotatory misalignment. There is stenosis of the vertebral canal and intervertebral foramina due to a combination of anatomical and degenerative changes, which included a lumbosacral disc protrusion.

BOX 16.1 CAUSES OF CAUDA EQUINA SYNDROME

Degenerative lumbosacral stenosis (DLSS) is the commonest cause in large breeds, notably the German Shepherd dog. The syndrome includes type II disc protrusion, hypertrophy of the *ligamentum flavum* and dorsal articular joint degeneration, and is thought to be an attempt by the soft tissues to stabilize an unstable joint.

- Primary vertebral canal stenosis is due to short pedicles and/or large dorsal articular processes; mainly small and medium dog breeds.
- Asymmetrical transitional vertebrae (mainly German Shepherd dogs) may predispose to lumbosacral disc disease by breaking the spine/pelvis axis, although transitional vertebrae occasionally cause stenosis in their own right.
- Osteochondrosis of the sacral end plate is seen mainly in male German Shepherd dogs. Stenosis is usually due to secondary changes including disc disease, rather than to primary osteochondrosis. Such dogs may present at a younger age than many other dogs with cauda equina syndrome.
- Fractures and luxations may produce immediate clinical signs or delayed signs due to instability or callus formation. Oblique fractures of L7 are the commonest finding.
- Subluxation may occur between L7 and S1.
- Instability may lead to dynamic compression and predisposes to disc degeneration.
- Disc disease type II >> type I at the lumbosacral junction is common and may be predisposed to by instability and sacral osteochondrosis.
- Spondylosis – lateral spondyles may contribute to foraminal stenosis and spinal nerve compression.
- Infection – discospondylitis, spondylitis and extension from adjacent abscesses may occur at the lumbosacral junction. This is a predilection site for discospondylitis, possibly because its mobility predisposes it to microfractures within which infection settles.
- Neoplasia of soft tissue or bony structures.
- Cauda equina neuritis.
- Cauda equina infarcts (fibrocartilaginous emboli).
- Spina bifida ± myelomeningocele.
- Scarring post-surgery.
- Neurogenic intermittent claudication – vascular dilation in the presence of a stenosis causes further neurological compression and ischemia.

Clinical differential diagnoses for cauda equina syndrome include hip dysplasia, stifle disease, degenerative myelopathy and iliac thrombosis.

of these studies can be difficult to interpret. Compression of the cauda equina occurs ventrally with disc disease, sacral osteochondrosis and other ventral soft tissue masses, whereas dorsal and/or lateral compression occurs with hypertrophy of the *ligamentum flavum* and lateral some bony deformities. Flexion/extension myelography is the technique of choice for radiographic diagnosis of lumbosacral spondylopathy in large breeds since it may be a dynamic problem. In normal dogs, the length, diameter and shape of the terminal dural sac change minimally between flexion and extension. In some affected dogs, cauda equina compression can be shown myelographically with the spine in a neutral position and with alleviation on flexion; hyperextension will demonstrate worsening of the compression. In less severely affected dogs, compression is only visible on extension.

MRI has become the technique of choice for investigation of cauda equina syndrome, where available, as it is non-invasive and gives excellent contrast between all of the bony and soft tissues. Stressed views may be possible with some scanners, depending on the shape of the radiofrequency coil. Disc protrusion causes elevation of the dural sac and loss of epidural fat signal around the cauda equina. Nerve root compression due to foraminal stenosis may be evident on parasagittal and transverse views, a diagnosis that cannot be made radiographically (**fig. 16.31B**). However, caution should be exercised in diagnosis when the MRI features are not dramatic since many middle-aged dogs of larger breeds have clinically silent disc protrusions at the lumbosacral junction, potentially giving rise to false-positives diagnoses. Studies have shown that there is poor correlation between the clinical signs of cauda equina compression and the degree of apparent stenosis on MRI. CT can also be helpful for investigation of cauda equina syndrome, especially following intravenous contrast administration and/or myelography.

Caudal cervical spondylo(myelo)pathy; "Wobbler" syndrome

Synonym: cervical vertebral malformation/malarticulation syndrome.

This condition has similarities to CES, with characteristic clinical signs due to an extradural compressive cervical myelopathy arising from a number of different bony and soft tissue causes, often in combination. Developmental vertebral canal stenosis due to bony malformation gives rise to a juvenile form, but the clinical condition is more often seen in middle-aged dogs due to secondary degenerative disease. Large and giant dogs are principally affected, especially the Doberman and Great Dane, with a male preponderance. Other large breeds and Basset Hounds are occasionally affected. If there is also a dynamic component, spinal cord compression is worsened in certain positions, usually hyperextension. Causes of cervical spondylomyelopathy are listed in **box 16.2**.

Survey radiographs show only bony lesions (**figs. 16.32A** and **16.33A**); they are often indicative of pathology but are not conclusive since they may suggest the wrong lesion site, and the nature and severity of spinal cord compression cannot be assessed. Features visible include the following:

- Deformity and upward tilting of vertebral bodies, becoming trapezoid to triangular in shape ("ploughshare appearance").
- Wedging and/or narrowing of the disc space cranially.
- Ventral spondylosis.
- Ventral angulation of the cranial end of the neural arch.
- Enlargement, sclerosis and loss of definition of articular processes.
- Stepping between vertebral bodies on flexion: interpret with caution since a degree of vertebral stepping is present in the normal dog on flexion of the neck.

Myelography is essential for accurate diagnosis of the site, nature and severity of spinal cord compression, by demonstrating the effects of soft tissue as well as bone pathology, by outlining disc protrusions and by allowing dynamic studies (**fig. 16.32B**). However, many dogs show temporary clinical deterioration after myelography, especially if stressed views have been performed, and the owners should be warned of this. The DV rather than the VD position should be used for the caudal neck to encourage contrast pooling under gravity at the site of interest. Traction radiographs using

SECTION III AXIAL SKELETON

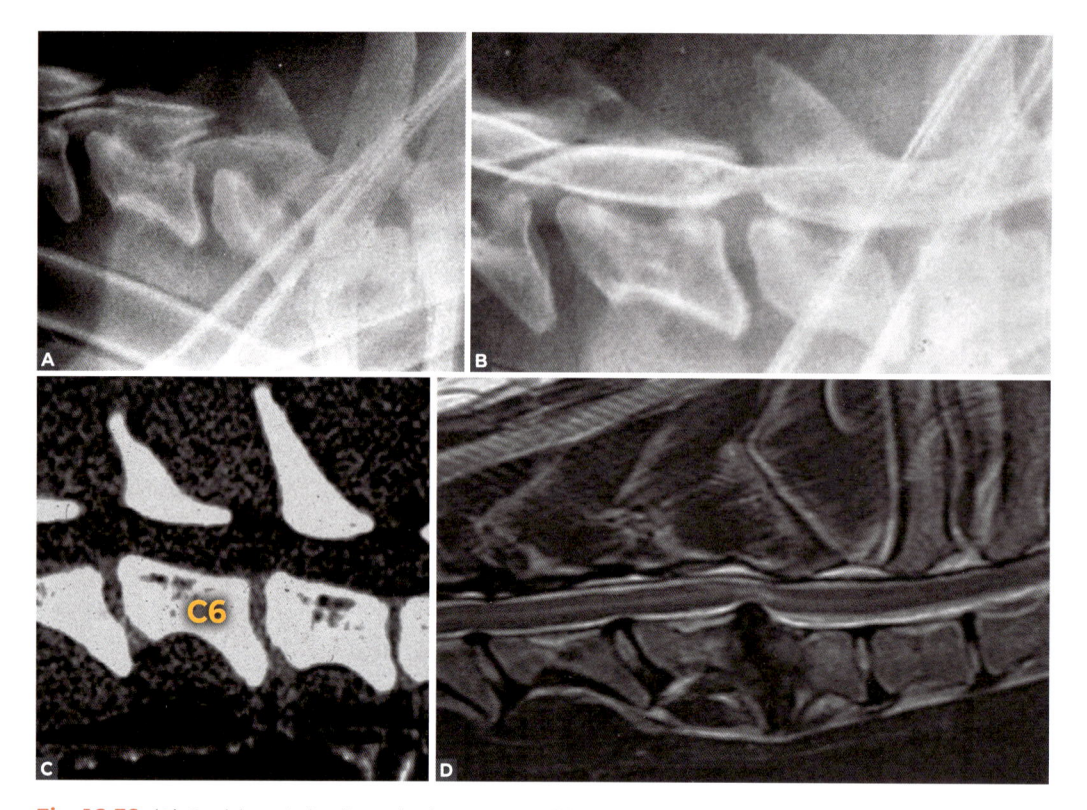

Fig. 16.32 (A) Caudal cervical radiograph of a seven-year-old Dobermann with ataxia. The centrum of C7 is abnormal in shape with upward tilting of its cranial end causing dorsoventral vertebral canal stenosis and wedging of the C6-C7 disc space. (B) Myelographic image of the same dog with mild traction applied. The ventral contrast column is markedly elevated above the disc space indicating disc protrusion. The spinal cord is reduced in depth but the dorsal subarachnoid space is still visible, hence the cord must be atrophied. The disc space is slightly wider than in (A) due to the effect of traction. (C) Sagittal CT reconstruction (post-contrast soft tissue window) of the caudal cervical spine of a six-year-old Dobermann Pinscher with ataxia, pelvic limb paresis and thoracic limb hypermetria. The cranial end of the vertebral body of C6 is tilted slightly dorsally, resulting in stepping between C5 and C6, wedging of the disc space and mild vertebral canal stenosis. (D) Sagittal T2W MRI image of a six-year-old Dobermann with a similar deformity. The body of C7 is misshapen and in addition there is ventral C6-C7 spondylosis. The disc space is narrowed and disc space within is dehydrated and protruding (type II disc protrusion). The overlying spinal cord is reduced in depth and shows a central streak of hyperintense signal (gliosis), but the dorsal subarachnoid space remains patent, indicating that the cord is atrophied.

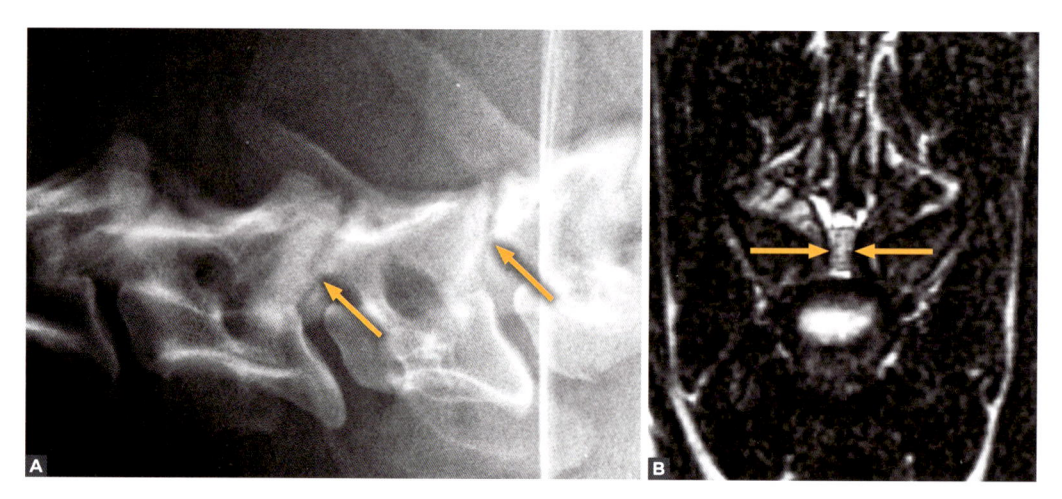

Fig. 16.33 (A) Caudal cervical radiograph of 17-month-old male Great Dane with clinical signs of cervical spondylopathy. Enlarged, irregular and sclerotic articular processes are seen at C5-C6 and C6-C7 (arrows) whereas those at C4-C5 appear normal. This is likely to have resulted in lateral or dorsolateral vertebral canal stenosis and spinal cord compression. (B) Transverse T2W MRI image of the spine at the level of C6-C7 in a two-year-old male Great Dane with clinical signs of cervical spondylopathy. There is very severe lateral vertebral canal stenosis and spinal cord compression due to vertebral malformation (arrows). MRI of dogs of this size and conformation can be technically challenging.

a weight of 20-25% body weight will show alleviation of ventral extradural compression if bulging and redundancy of the soft tissues has occurred, and will differentiate this from hypertrophy and "static" tissue. Traction is a safe procedure as it does not worsen any cord compression present. If hyperflexion is performed it should involve the whole neck and care should be taken not to occlude the endotracheal tube. Hyperextension is the riskiest maneuver since it often exacerbates both dorsal and ventral cord compression. Chronic cord compression may result in cord atrophy, i.e., a reduced cord diameter which does not increase with traction radiography.

CT will show bony lesions (**fig. 16.32C**), and is the best technique for depicting purely bony changes of articular processes. However, CT myelography is required to confirm the site and severity of resulting spinal cord compression, which is the main purpose of imaging. As with radiographic myelography, traction can be applied. However, the superior soft tissue detail of MRI makes this the optimum technique: one study showed that MRI appeared to be more accurate in predicting the site, severity and nature of spinal cord compression than myelography[19] (**figs. 16.32D** and **16.33B**). Chronic cord compression often results in focal central cord hyperintensity in T2W images, due to gliosis, edema and/or central canal dilation as a result of atrophy: this has a bearing on prognosis. Traction studies can be performed, and will distinguish between cord compression and cord atrophy as well as indicating which patients may benefit from distraction surgery.

Arachnoid diverticula (subarachnoid "cysts")

Spinal arachnoid diverticula (SAD) are focal, fluid-filled dilations of the subarachnoid space which can cause a progressive, compressive myelopathy.[20] The etiology of these pseudocysts is not known and may be congenital and/or secondary to inflammation, microtrauma or altered CSF dynamics, but their presence often in dogs less than one year of age and in littermates suggests a developmental factor in many cases. Most affected dogs are of small breeds with a lesion in the caudal thoracic or cervical spine, but the Rottweiler is predisposed to cervical arachnoid diverticula. They may be associated with caudal articular process aplasia or dysplasia around the thoracolumbar junction, especially in Pugs, or with hemivertebrae or disc disease. Patients with clinical signs usually respond to decompressive surgery. Survey radiographs are usually normal, although in some cases the articular process changes may be evident. Myelography demonstrates a characteristic bulbous, dorsal dilation of the subarachnoid space which forms a teardrop-shaped pouch which has a blunted caudal margin, but which is occasionally reversed (**figs. 16.34A** and **16.34B**). The caudal margin of the distension may be partly or completely sealed by coarse subarachnoid trabeculae hindering the passage of contrast medium.

BOX 16.2   CAUSES OF CERVICAL SPONDYLOMYELOPATHY

Bone lesions
- Vertebral body malformations – upward tilting of the cranial end of the vertebral body results in dorsoventral stenosis of the vertebral canal and wedging of the disc space and occurs especially in the caudal neck (C7, C6) in the Dobermann. Subsequent type II disc protrusion is common.
- Enlarged dorsal articular processes cause dorsolateral spinal cord compression, especially in the caudal neck in large, male Great Danes. They may present at a young age, or later due to secondary degenerative change.
- Vertebral canal stenosis due to shortening of vertebral pedicles and lowering of the neural arch at the cranial end of the affected vertebra occurs especially in the cranial neck and in Basset Hounds, often involving multiple sites.

Soft tissue lesions
- Type II disc protrusion with hypertrophy of the annulus fibrosus and dorsal longitudinal ligament is seen mainly in the caudal neck in middle-aged Dobermanns and Dalmatians.
- Hypertrophy of the ligament flavum dorsally and the joint capsules dorsolaterally contributes to stenosis, which may therefore be circumferential.

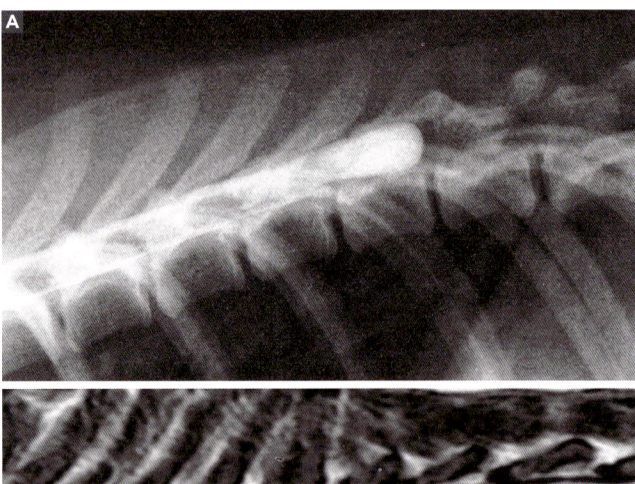

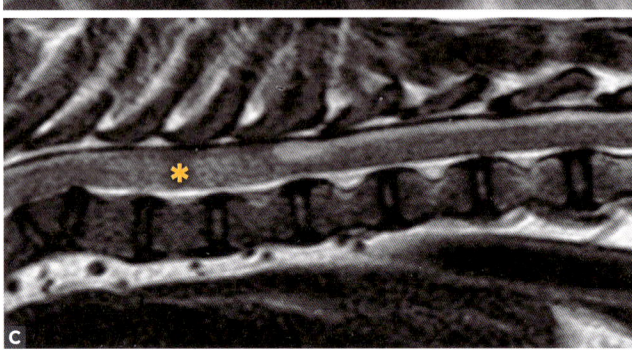

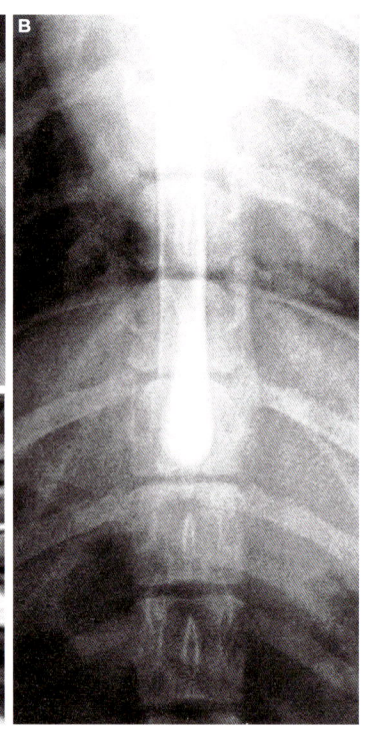

Fig. 16.34 (**A**) Lateral myelographic study centered on the caudal thoracic spine in an eight-month-old Tibetan Spaniel with paraparesis. The contrast medium terminates abruptly at the level of caudal T10, with distension of the subarachnoid space and a convex caudal contour. No contrast medium passes beyond. (**B**) Ventrodorsal radiograph showing left lateralization of the diverticulum and resulting spinal cord compression. (**C**) Sagittal T2W MRI image of the caudal thoracic spine of a four-year-old French Bulldog with a cranially-directed arachnoid diverticulum. The dorsal subarachnoid space widens progressively in a cranial direction before terminating abruptly with a teardrop-shaped conformation. There is corresponding spinal cord compression but cranial to this area the cord is mildly swollen and shows diffuse hyperintensity (asterisk). No potentially causative vertebral anomaly is evident.

Myelography also shows cord narrowing at the site of the lesion. In MRI images spinal cord swelling and T2W hyperintense signal are usually seen adjacent to the blunt end of the diverticulum (**fig. 16.34C**) whereas CT is preferred to look for any associated osseous changes.

References

1. Dennis R. Radiographic examination of the canine spine. *Vet Rec* 121:31-35, 1987.
2. McKee WM, Dennis R. Radiology Corner: lumbosacral radiography. *Vet Radiol Ultrasound* 44:655-656, 2003.
3. Llabres Diaz F. Practical contrast radiography 4. Myelography. *In Practice* 27:502-510, 2005.
4. Gibbons SE, Macias M, De Stefani A, Pinchbeck GL, McKee WM. The value of oblique versus ventrodorsal myelographic view for lesions lateralization in canine thoracolumbar disc disease. *J Small Anim Pract* 47:658-662, 2006.
5. Dennis R. Optimal magnetic resonance imaging of the spine. *Vet Radiol Ultrasound neuroimaging supplement* 52:S72-S80, 2011.
6. Drees R, Dennison SE, Keuler NS, Schwarz T. Computed tomographic imaging protocol for the canine cervical and lumbar spine. *Vet Radiol Ultrasound* 50:74-79, 2009.
7. Cerda-Gonzalez S, Dewey CW. Congenital diseases of the craniocervical junction in the dog. *Vet Clin North Am Small Anim Pract* 40:121-141, 2010.
8. Lourinho F, Holdsworth, McConnell JF, Gonçalves R, Gutierrez-Quintana R, Morales C, Lowrie M, Trevail R, Carrera I. Clinical features and MRI characteristics of presumptive constrictive myelopathy in 27 pugs. *Vet Radiol Ultrasound* 61:545-554, 2020.
9. Hanna FY. Lumbosacral osteochondrosis: radiological features and surgical management in 34 dogs. *J Small Anim Pract* 42:272-278, 2001.
10. Ortega M, Gonçalves R, Haley A, Wessmann A, Penderis J. Spondylosis deformans and diffuse idiopathic skeletal hyperostosis (DISH) resulting in adjacent segment disease. *Vet Radiol Ultrasound* 53:128-134, 2012.
11. Carrera I, Sulllivan M, McConnell F, Gonçalves R. Magnetic resonance imaging features of discospondylitis in dogs. *Vet Radiol Ultrasound* 52:125-131, 2011.
12. Wyatt S, De Risio L, Driver C, José-López R, Pivetta M, Beltran E. Neurological signs and MRI findings in 12 dogs with multiple myeloma. *Vet Radiol Ultrasound* 60: 409-415, 2019.
13. Kinns J, Mai W, Seiler G, Zwingenberger A, Johnson V, Cáceres A, Valdés-Martinez A, Schwarz T. Radiographic sensitivity and negative predictive value for acute canine spinal trauma. *Vet Radiol Ultrasound* 47:563-570, 2006.
14. Gallastegui A, Davies E, Zwingenberger AL, Nykamp S, Rishniw M, Johnson PJ. MRI has limited agreement with CT in the evaluation of vertebral fractures of the canine trauma patient. *Vet Radiol Ultrasound* 60:533-542, 2019.
15. Johnson P, Beltran E, Dennis R, Taeymans O. Magnetic resonance imaging features of suspected vertebral instability associated with fracture or subluxation in eleven dogs. *Vet Radiol Ultrasound* 53:552-559, 2012.
16. Squires A, Brisson BA, Holmberg DL, Nykamp SG. Use of the ventrodorsal myelographic view to predict lateralization of disc material in small-breed dogs with thoracolumbar intervertebral disc extrusion: 104 cases (2004-2005). *J Am Vet Med Assoc* 230:1860-1865, 2007.
17. Lamb CR. Common difficulties with myelographic diagnosis of acute intervertebral disc prolapse in the dog. *J Small Anim Pract* 35:549-558, 1994.
18. Robertson I, Thrall DE. Imaging dogs with suspected disc herniation: pros and cons of myelography, computed tomography and magnetic resonance. *Vet Radiol Ultrasound neuroimaging supplement* 52:S81-S84, 2011.
19. Da Costa RC, Parent J, Dobson H, Holmberg D, Partlow G. Comparison of magnetic resonance imaging and myelography in 18 Doberman Pinscher dogs with cervical spondylopathy. *Vet Radiol Ultrasound* 47:523-531, 2006.
20. Da Costa RC, Cook LB. Cystic abnormalities of the spinal cord and vertebral column. *Vet Clin North Am Small Anim Pract* 46:277-293, 2016.

SECTION **IV**

THORAX

CHAPTER **17**

Thoracic wall, diaphragm, and pleura

Chee Kin Lim and Hock Gan Heng

> **KEY POINTS**
>
> ▌ Good knowledge of thoracic anatomy and pathology is required to understand the imaging features of diseases of the thoracic wall, the diaphragm, and the pleura.
> ▌ The combined use of different imaging modalities may help to increase sensitivity and specificity of diagnosing diseases of the thoracic wall, the diaphragm, and the pleura.
> ▌ Specific radiographic positions/views may help to delineate lesion(s) that may not be detected on a standard position/view.
> ▌ Some diseases may be dynamic (e.g., sliding hiatal hernia) and fluoroscopic evaluation may be required for diagnosis.
> ▌ There may be multiple abnormalities such as pleural effusion and pleural mass that contribute to a similar presenting sign.

Thoracic wall anatomy

The thoracic wall surrounds the thoracic cavity and is comprised of the skin, subcutaneous fat, muscles, ribs, costal cartilages, parietal pleura, vessels, and nerves. The thoracic cavity is bordered dorsally by the thoracic spine, ventrally by the sternum, cranially by the thoracic inlet, and caudally by the diaphragm (**fig. 17.1**).

Dogs and cats normally have 13 thoracic vertebrae, 13 pairs of ribs, and eight sternebrae. The first nine ribs have costal cartilages that articulate with the sternebrae. The costal cartilages of the 10th to 12th ribs unite with the costal cartilage of the ninth rib to form the costal arch on each side. The last pair of ribs (the 13th ribs) are known as the floating ribs because the cartilages are not attached and end in the musculature.[1] The thoracic spinal nerves give rise to the intercostal nerves, which together with the intercostal arteries and veins run along the caudal margin of each rib.

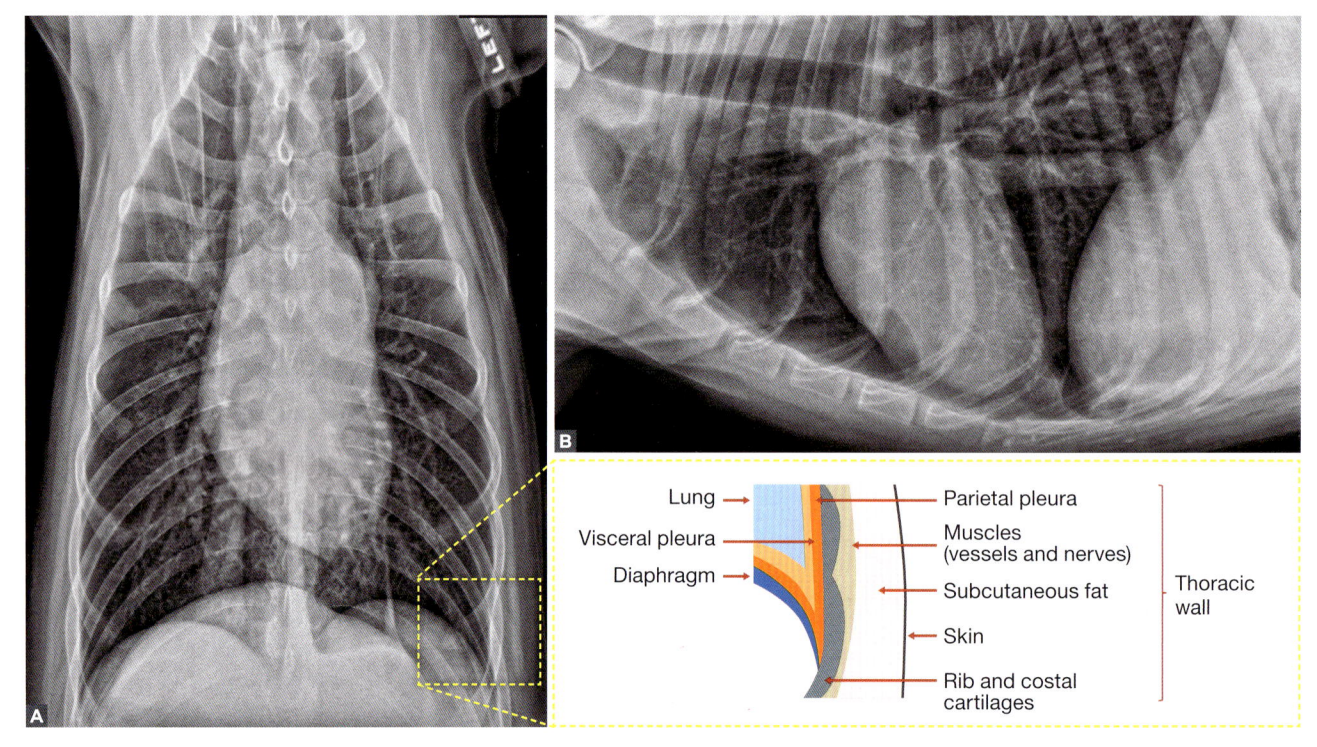

Fig. 17.1 (**A**) Ventrodorsal and (**B**) right lateral view of the thorax of a dog with a schematic representation of the components of the thoracic wall in (**A**).

Barrel chest in lower airway disease

Barrel chest refers to a maximally expanded thoracic cavity with the ribs oriented perpendicular or almost perpendicular to the spine rather than being angled caudally on the dorsoventral or ventrodorsal view (**fig. 17.2**). On the lateral view, the dorsoventral height of the thoracic cavity may be increased with cranial bowing of the ribs and outward bowing of the sternebrae on lateral view.[2] Barrel chest occurs secondary to increased intrathoracic volume such as a large volume of pleural effusion, tension pneumothorax, large mediastinal or pulmonary tumors, pulmonary emphysema, or obstructive lower airway disease causing air trapping (i.e., obstructive tracheobronchitis or chronic obstructive pulmonary disease).[2,3]
A barrel chest is a normal breed-specific appearance in some dog breeds such as the Bulldogs and Boston Terriers.[2]

Thoracic wall trauma

Common thoracic wall trauma that may be detected with imaging include soft tissue swelling/edema, subcutaneous or soft tissue emphysema, rib fracture, malpositioned ribs/widened intercostal space due to intercostal muscle tear, vertebral or sternal fracture/subluxation/luxation. These pathologies may be detected using radiography (**fig. 17.3**) or computed tomography (CT) and, to some extent, thoracic ultrasonography. Careful evaluation for symmetry and homogenous opacity of the thoracic wall is important. Rib fracture with displacement is easily identified on radiographs. However, non-displacing rib fractures may be difficult to detect. Thus, thoracic radiography of three or four views is crucial in a traumatic patient. Computed tomography is probably the most reliable imaging modality to detect most of these pathologies; however, direct access to CT may be limited to referral veterinary institutions.

CHAPTER 17 Thoracic wall, diaphragm, and pleura

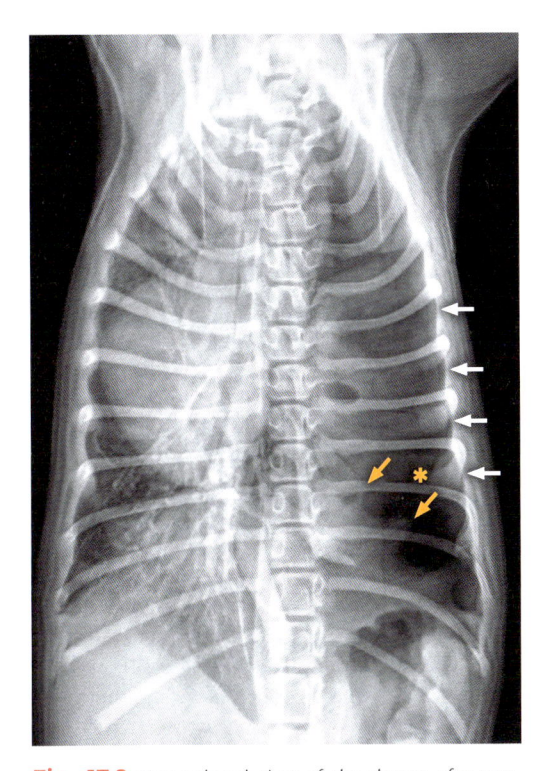

Fig. 17.2 Ventrodorsal view of the thorax of a two-month-old Pomeranian with barrel chest due to left-sided tension pneumothorax (asterisk). The thoracic cavity is markedly expanded with widened intercostal spaces, outward bulging of the pleural margin (white arrows), and "tenting" of the diaphragm (orange arrows). The cardiac silhouette is displaced towards the right hemithorax. Courtesy of Dr. Amy Zalcman, DACVR.

Fig. 17.3 (**A**) Dorsoventral and (**B**) right lateral view of the thorax of a six-year-old Chihuahua bitten by another dog. There is diffuse thoracic wall soft tissue thickening and emphysema (white arrows) with acute traumatic fractures of the left fifth and sixth ribs (orange arrows). There is also widening of the left sixth intercostal space (orange asterisk) and caudal displacement of the left seventh rib due to intercostal muscle tear. There is concurrent moderate increased soft tissue opacification of the caudal subsegment of the left cranial lung lobe and left caudal lung lobe due to contusion/hemorrhage and a few small gas bubbles within the pleural space, consistent with mild pneumothorax (white asterisk). Courtesy of Dr. Elisabet Dominguez, DECVDI.

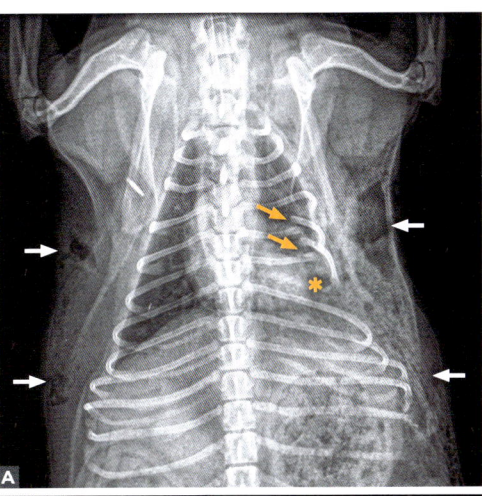

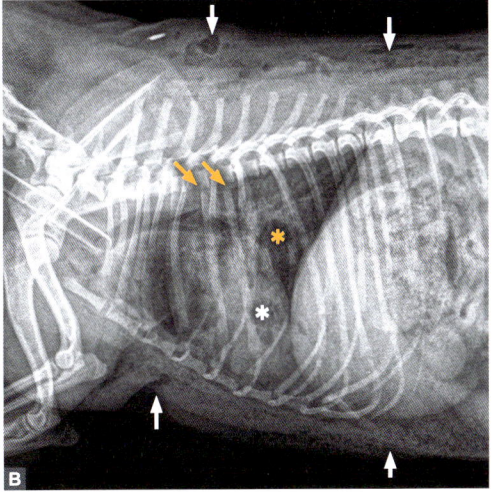

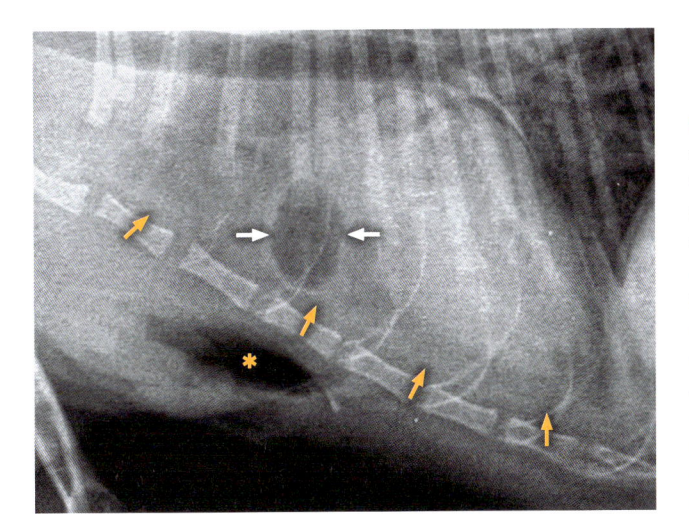

Fig. 17.4 Right lateral view of the thorax of a four-year-old Domestic shorthair cat with ventral thoracic wall soft tissue thickening and emphysema (asterisk) due to a dog bite wound. There is concurrent mild increased soft tissue opacification (fluid) within the pleural space with mild retraction of the ventral lung margins, consistent with secondary pleural effusion (orange arrows). An ovoid-shaped gas opacity is noted within the mid-ventral thoracic cavity, consistent with pneumothorax (white arrows). Courtesy of Prof. Robert M. Kirberger, DECVDI.

Thoracic wall injuries usually have associated injuries to the pleurae and lungs. For example, rib fractures or penetrating thoracic wall injury may cause concurrent pneumothorax or pleural effusion (**fig. 17.4** and **fig. 17.5**). "Flail chest" refers to a segment of the thoracic wall that can move paradoxically due to segmental fractures of consecutive ribs from trauma.[4] This results in respiratory compromise with direct trauma to the lungs and decreased ventilation. Concurrent pneumothorax and pulmonary contusions are noted in more than 50% of the dogs with flail

221

SECTION IV THORAX

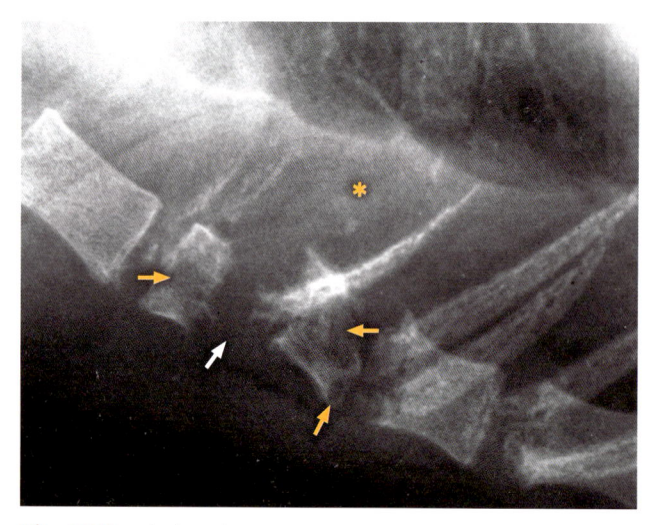

Fig. 17.5 Right lateral view of a ten-year-old Boerboel with sternebral osteomyelitis characterized with mixed moth-eaten to permeative lysis of the fourth and fifth sternebrae (orange arrows) and pathological fracture of the fourth sternebra (white arrow). There is also concurrent moderate retraction of the ventral margins of the lung lobes with the pleural space filled with homogeneous soft tissue opacity/pleural effusion (asterisk). Courtesy of Prof. Robert M. Kirberger, DECVDI.

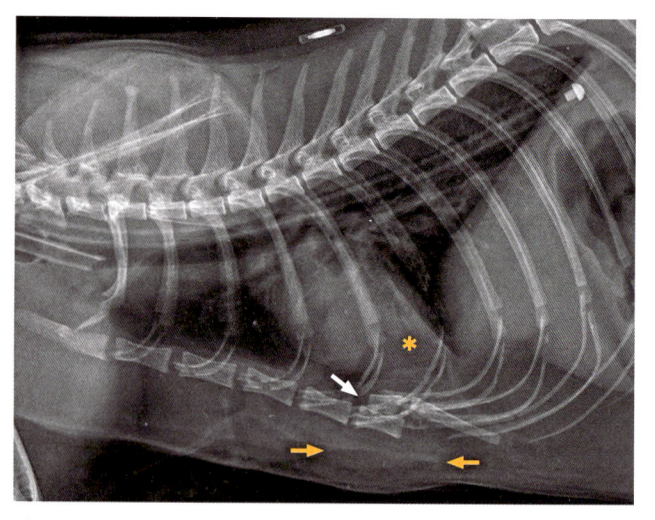

Fig. 17.6 Right lateral view of the thorax of a six-year-old American Domestic shorthair with acute traumatic sternal luxation characterized by overriding of the sixth and seventh sternebrae (white arrow). There is a moderate amount of associated ventral thoracic wall soft tissue thickening (orange arrows), most likely due to hemorrhage or edema. There is also moderate soft tissue opacification of the caudal subsegment of the left cranial lung lobe with faint air bronchograms and lobar signs, most likely due to pulmonary contusion/hemorrhage given the concurrent acute traumatic event in this region (asterisk).

thorax due to bite wounds on thoracic radiographs.[5] Changing the orientation or/and inverting the grayscale of thoracic radiographs may make it easier for some novices to examine the rib and detect rib fractures.[6]

Acute traumatic sternal luxation is typically accompanied by concurrent thoracic wall soft tissue injury (i.e., thickening and emphysema) and intrathoracic changes (i.e, pleural effusion, pneumothorax, or pulmonary/contusion/hemorrhage) (**fig. 17.6**). Chronic sternal subluxation may be seen as incidental findings on thoracic radiography with no other secondary changes or obvious clinical significance.

Pectus excavatum and pectus carinatum

Pectus excavatum is an abnormal sternal conformation characterized by dorsal (inward) deviation of the sternebrae and dorsoventral narrowing of the thoracic cavity. Most pectus excavatum is congenital in cats and dogs, with a possible familial cause suggested in Bengal kittens, and is a common skeletal manifestation of heritable mucopolysaccharidosis VI in Siamese cats.[7] Severe congenital pectus excavatum may lead to compression of the heart (**fig. 17.7**), and surgical correction may be required. Acquired pectus excavatum has been reported in a dog and a cat with the presence of a dynamic component in the cat, secondary to chronic obstructive upper airway disease (**fig. 17.8**).[8,9] In the case of dynamic pectus excavatum caused by upper airway obstruction, the sternum may be intermittently deviated dorsally rather than being static in location.

Pectus carinatum refers to an abnormal sternal conformation characterized by ventral (outward) deviation of the sternebrae and dorsoventral widening of the thoracic cavity (**fig. 17.9**). Pectus carinatum is less common compared to pectus excavatum and is usually an incidental finding with lesser few reported secondary complications and clinical signs.

CHAPTER **17** Thoracic wall, diaphragm, and pleura

Fig. 17.7 Right lateral view of the thorax of a four-month-old Domestic shorthair cat with congenital pectus excavatum characterized by static, marked dorsal deviation of the caudal sternebrae (arrow).

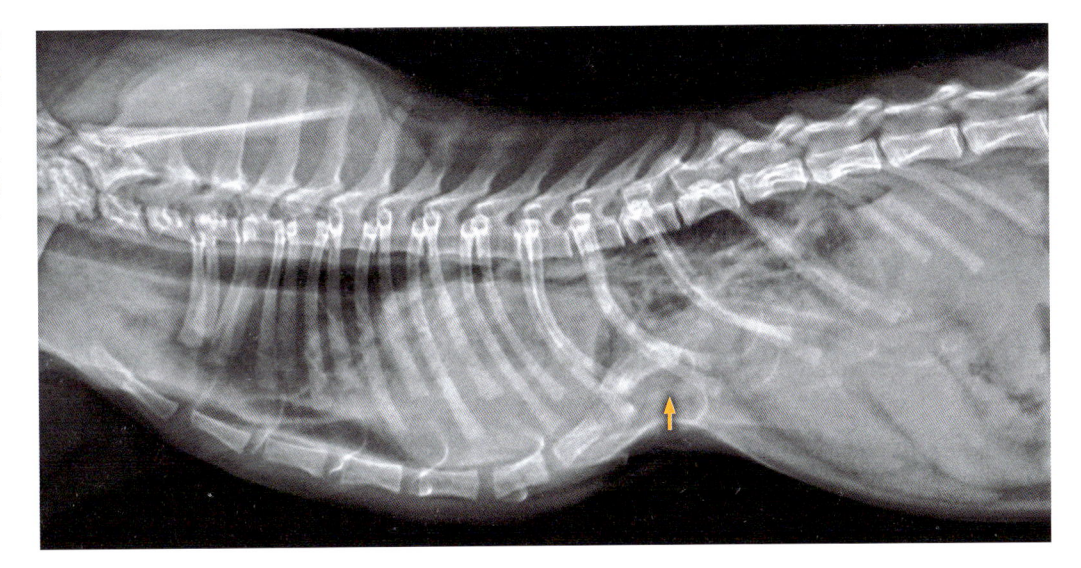

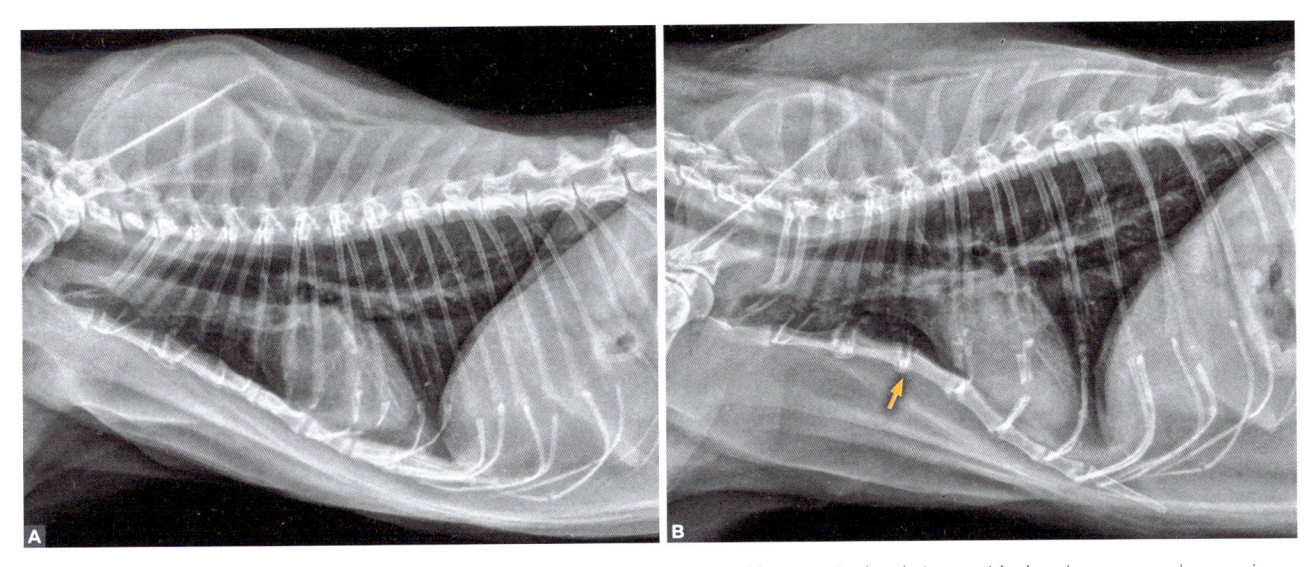

Fig. 17.8 (**A**) Left lateral and (**B**) right lateral views of the thorax of an 11-year-old Domestic shorthair cat with chronic upper respiratory airway disease, taken two minutes apart. The sternum is in a normal anatomic location on the left lateral view, but there is a moderate dorsal deviation of the mid sternebrae noted on the right lateral view consistent with acquired dynamic pectus excavatum (arrow). © Canadian Veterinary Medical Association - Can Vet J. 2021 Jul;62(7):751-754.

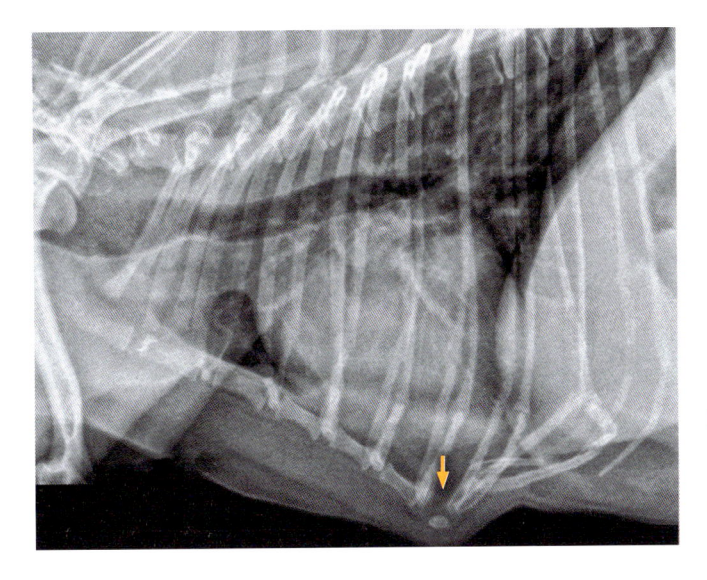

Fig. 17.9 Left lateral view of the thorax of a five-year-old English Bulldog with pectus carinatum (arrow), characterized by marked ventral deviation of the mid to caudal sternebrae.

223

Thoracic wall neoplasia

Primary neoplasia may develop from any of the structures of the thoracic wall but malignant lesions most commonly derive from the ribs. Adipose masses such as lipoma and infiltrative lipoma are commonly seen within the fascial planes of the thoracic wall.[10] Malignant liposarcomas are rare. Lipomas are typically well marginated, round to oval-shaped, and with homogeneous fat opacity (on radiography) or attenuation (on CT). Occasionally, there may be small regions of increased soft tissue opacity or attenuation within the lipoma due to necrosis (**fig. 17.10**), hemorrhage, or fibrosis. Infiltrative lipomas tend to be more irregular in shape, more hyperattenuating than the surrounding fat, and have internal linear striations (i.e., residual muscular bands). Other invasive soft tissue sarcomas or carcinomas of soft tissue origin are also seen occasionally. Primary rib neoplasms are usually sarcomas with osteosarcoma and chondrosarcoma being more common, but metastatic carcinoma to the rib has also been reported (**fig. 17.11**).[11-13] The radiographic appearance of primary rib neoplasia is similar to other bone neoplasia such as cortical lysis with or without associated soft tissue swelling.

Thoracic wall neoplasia can be detected and evaluated using radiography, CT, or ultrasound. CT is the preferred modality to evaluate the extent and margins of the thoracic wall neoplasia for surgical treatment planning. Larger thoracic wall masses including both rib neoplasia and soft tissue neoplasia may bulge into the parietal pleural, resulting in an "extrapleural sign", which is typically seen as a well-demarcated broad-based convex mass with tapered peripheral margins (**fig. 17.12**).[2] The "extrapleural sign" is a useful key finding to differentiate a thoracic wall mass from a pulmonary mass, and they usually do not move along with the lungs during respiratory motion when observed in fluoroscopy or ultrasonography, given its non-pulmonary origin. Any thoracic wall masses regardless of etiology may cause an "extrapleural sign"; however, common non-neoplastic causes include osteomyelitis, abscess, foreign body reaction, and granuloma involving the thoracic wall structures. Sternal lymphadenopathy may also produce an "extrapleural sign".[2] In the authors' personal experience, ultrasound-guided sampling of the extrapleural soft tissue is usually feasible and may aid in obtaining a definitive diagnosis (**fig. 17.13**, **video 17.1**).

> **VIDEO 17.1**
> Videoclip of focal transcutaneous thoracic ultrasonography revealing a large hypoechoic mass surrounding the lytic right fifth rib. Biopsy of the mass confirmed osteosarcoma.

Diaphragm anatomy

The diaphragm is a dome-shaped musculotendinous structure that forms the caudal boundary of the thoracic cavity, separating the thoracic and abdominal cavities.[14] The diaphragm consists of a V-shaped central tendon and a peripheral muscular portion that is subdivided into lumbar, costal, and sternal parts. The intact normal diaphragm is an important muscle of respiration. In general, the diaphragm contracts during inspiration (the diaphragmatic silhouette will flatten) and relaxes during expiration (the diaphragmatic silhouette will be displaced cranially) rhythmically during respiration. The actual diaphragm is normally not visible as it is thin, and silhouettes with the liver and abuts the cranial margins of the liver to form the so-called "diaphragmatic silhouette", which is seen as the central cupula, the left crus and the right crus.[15]

The normal diaphragm also has three openings for major structures to pass between the thoracic and abdominal cavities:

- Aortic hiatus: located dorsally (for aorta, azygous vein, and thoracic duct).
- Esophageal hiatus: located centrally (for esophagus and vagal nerves).
- Caval foramen: located at the right crus (for caudal vena cava).

CHAPTER 17 Thoracic wall, diaphragm, and pleura

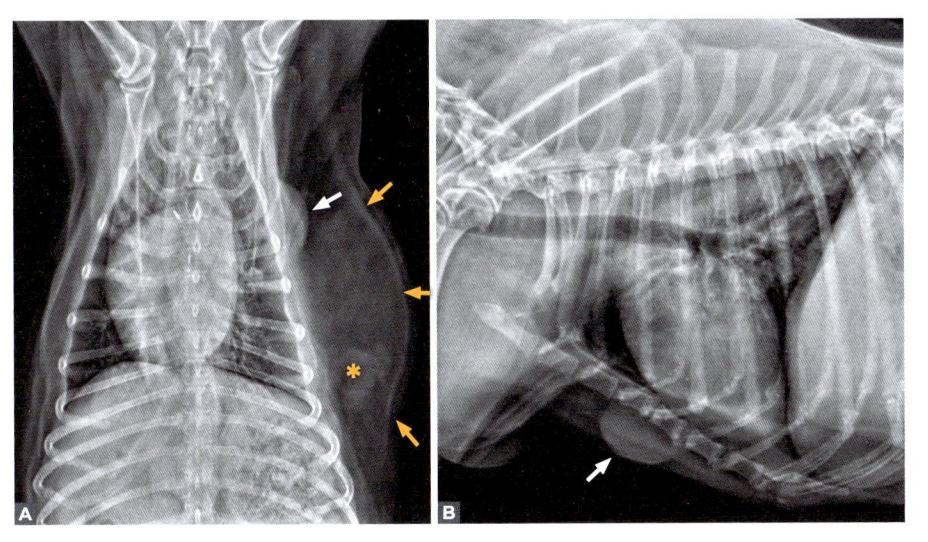

Fig. 17.10 (A) Ventrodorsal view and (B) right lateral view of the thorax of a 15-year-old mixed breed dog with a large and broad-based fat opaque thoracic wall subcutaneous lipoma (orange arrows) with a focal region of necrosis (asterisk) characterized by lobulated soft tissue opacity within the caudal aspect. Another smaller subcutaneous lipoma is also noted at the left cranioventral aspect of the thoracic wall (white arrow).

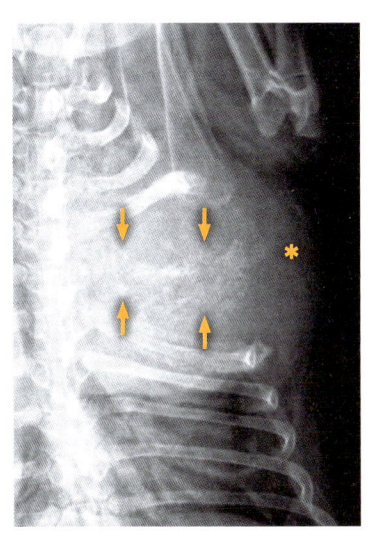

Fig. 17.11 Dorsoventral view of the thorax of a 13-year-old mixed breed dog with osteosarcoma of the left fifth rib. There is severe lysis of the fifth rib (arrows) with marked mass effect centered at the rib displacing the adjacent ribs towards cranially and caudally and causing a broad-based thoracic wall soft tissue swelling (asterisk). There is diffuse increased soft tissue opacification of the entire left cranial lung lobe.

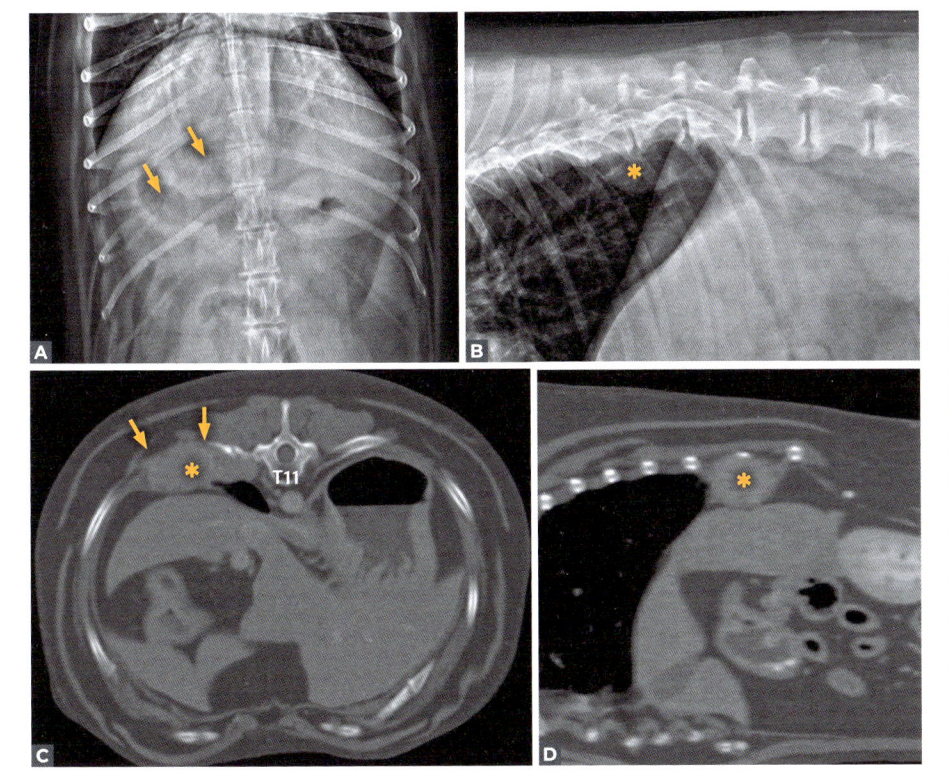

Fig. 17.12 (A) Ventrodorsal and (B) left lateral radiographic views, corresponding transverse CT (C) and sagittal multiplanar reconstructed plane (D) images of an eight-year-old Labrador Retriever with solitary plasma cell tumor of the right 11th rib. There is severe lysis of the right 11th rib (orange arrows) with moderate a local soft tissue thickening mass, causing an "extrapleural sign" (asterisk). The right and left 13th ribs are hypoplastic.

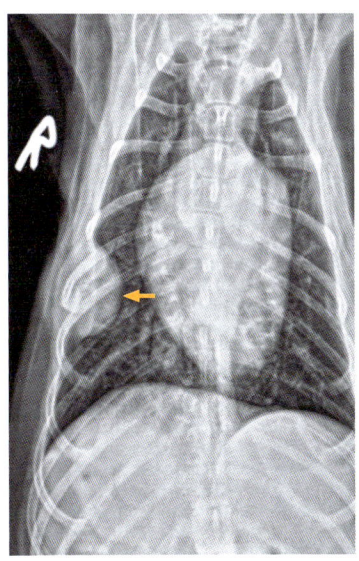

Fig. 17.13 Ventrodorsal view of the thorax of a ten-year-old Beagle with a broad-based soft tissue mass bulging into the parietal pleura at the level of the right 5th rib causing an "extrapleural sign" (orange arrow).

225

SECTION IV THORAX

On lateral views, the dorsal margin of the diaphragmatic crura attached to the ventral aspect of either the L4 or L5 vertebral body and forms the lumbodiaphragmatic recess. The cranioventral margin of the diaphragmatic silhouette usually ends at the xiphoid process.[15]

On the right lateral view, the crura appear parallel and the right crus is displaced more cranially than the left crus by the abdominal organs. The caudal vena cava can be seen merging with the more cranial crus at the caval foramen (**fig. 17.14A**). On the left lateral view, the crura appear to cross or are "Y-shaped", and the left crus is displaced more cranially than the right crus. The caudal vena cava can be seen merging with the more caudal crus (**fig. 17.14B**).[15]

The diaphragm typically appears as a single dome-shaped structure on the dorsoventral view (**fig. 17.15A**), and two or three separate dome-shaped structures on the ventrodorsal view (**fig. 17.15B**). However, the position and shape of the diaphragm can vary substantially depending on beam centering and respiratory phase.[15]

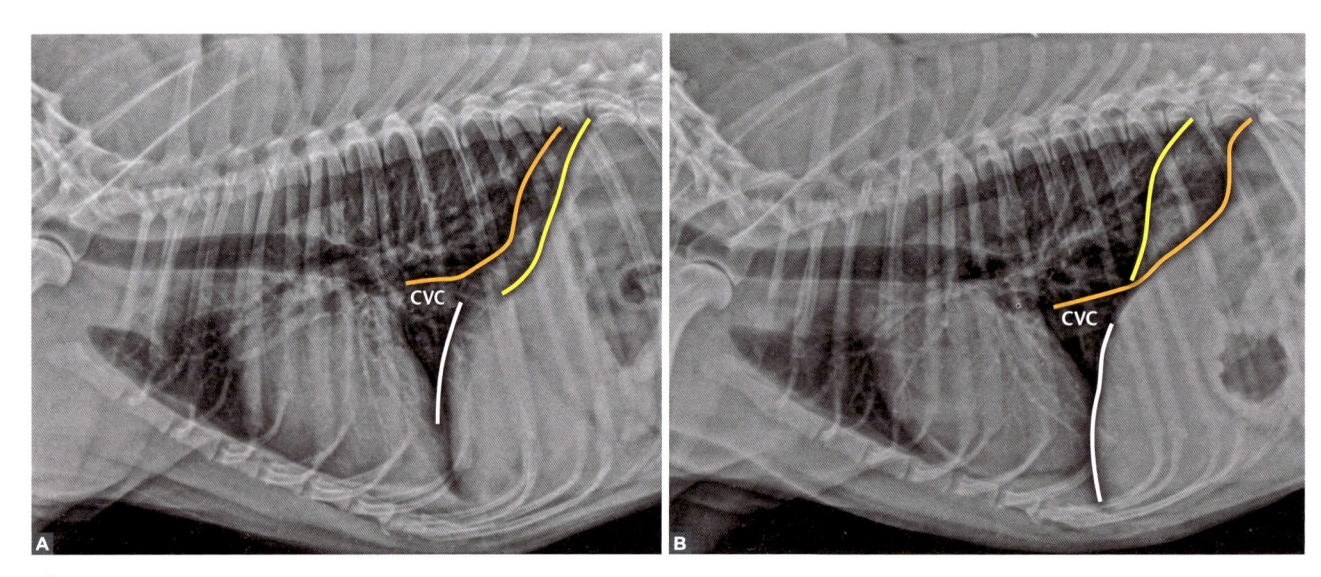

Fig. 17.14 (**A**) Right lateral and (**B**) left lateral thoracic views of the thorax of a six-year-old Labrador Retriever. The orange line represents the right diaphragmatic crus (usually continuous with the caudal vena cava); the yellow line corresponds to the left diaphragmatic crus; the white line outlines the diaphragmatic cupula. CVC, caudal vena cava.

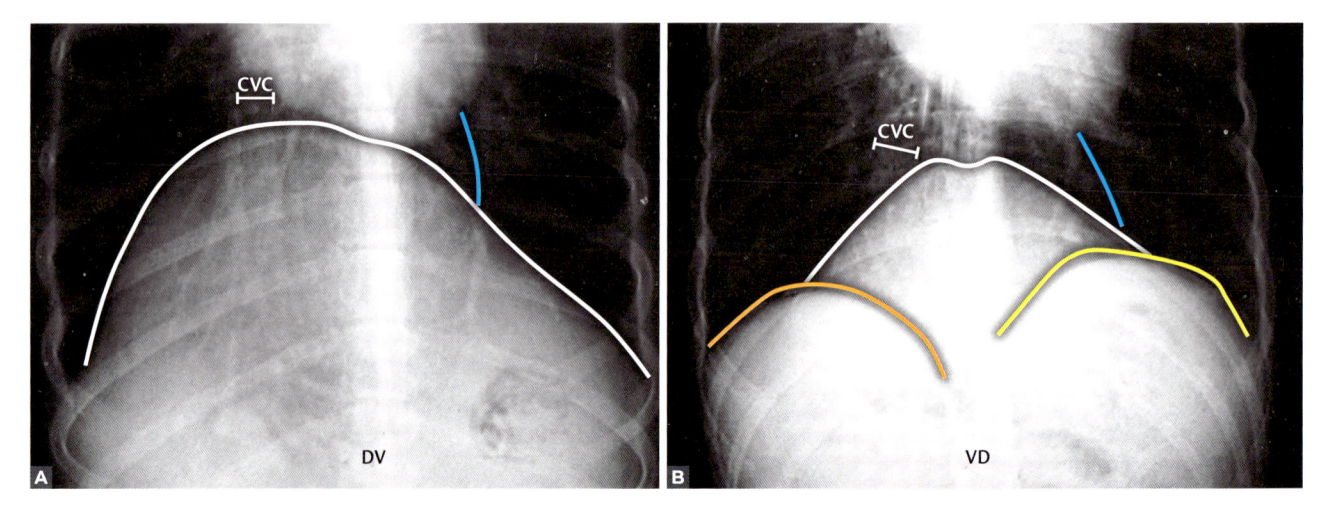

Fig. 17.15 (**A**) Dorsoventral and (**B**) ventrodorsal views of the thorax of a six-year-old Labrador Retriever. The orange line represents the right diaphragmatic crus; the yellow line corresponds to the left diaphragmatic crus; the white line outlines the diaphragmatic cupula; the blue line points to the caudoventral mediastinal reflection. CVC, caudal vena cava. Courtesy of Prof. Robert M. Kirberger, DECVDI.

Diseases of the diaphragm

Diaphragmatic hernia is the most common disease of the diaphragm. Diaphragmatic hernia is characterized by displacement of abdominal viscera into the thorax through a defect in the diaphragm. Diaphragmatic hernias can be categorized into traumatic (i.e., diaphragmatic rupture) or congenital (i.e., peritoneopericardial diaphragmatic hernia, hiatal hernia, and peritoneopleural hernias) in origin.[16]

Diaphragmatic rupture

Diaphragmatic rupture or traumatic diaphragmatic hernia is almost exclusively due to blunt trauma to the abdomen, with up to 85% of cases documented in one study due to motor vehicle accidents.[17] Diaphragmatic rupture usually involves the muscular portion of the diaphragm and can affect either side.[18] This will result in cranial herniation of abdominal viscera into the thoracic cavity.

Radiography is the most commonly used imaging technique to diagnose diaphragmatic rupture. The most consistent radiographic findings of diaphragmatic rupture are the presence of abdominal viscera within the thoracic cavity with partial or complete loss of the diaphragmatic border (**fig. 17.16**). Pleural effusion may also be noted, particularly in cases of chronic liver herniation.[17]

The most commonly herniated abdominal viscus is the liver. The stomach, small intestines, and spleen are often herniated in left-sided diaphragmatic rupture, while the small intestines and pancreas may also be herniated in right-sided diaphragmatic rupture.[19] Common radiographic features of diaphragmatic rupture are the presence of gas-filled gastrointestinal tract in the thorax, presence of soft tissue opacity in the pleural cavity (liver, spleen, or pleural effusion), and reduced volume of liver, stomach, and/or small intestine and spleen in the abdomen. Other thoracic structures such as the heart, the mediastinum, and the lungs may be obscured or displaced depending on the amount and location of the herniated abdominal viscera within the thoracic cavity.

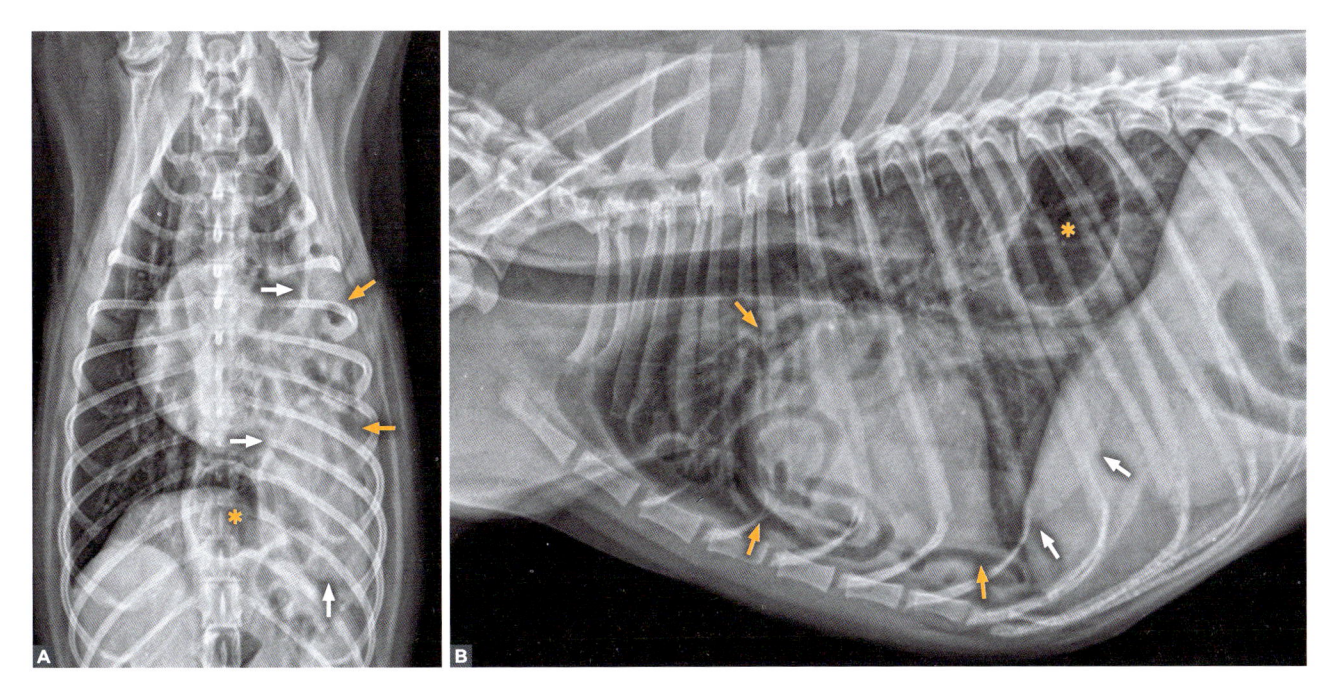

Fig. 17.16 (**A**) Ventrodorsal and (**B**) left lateral views of the thorax of a Whippet with a diaphragmatic rupture from a motor vehicle accident. The stomach (asterisk), small intestines (orange arrows), and the spleen (white arrows) are herniated into the left hemithorax.

Congenital diaphragmatic hernia

Approximately 15% of diaphragmatic hernias are congenital. These are often clinically silent and may be diagnosed in patients of any age. This includes peritoneopericardial diaphragmatic hernia, hiatal hernia, and pleuroperitoneal hernia.[20]

Peritoneopericardial diaphragmatic hernia

Peritoneopericardial diaphragmatic hernia (PPDH) is characterized by defective midline closure in the embryo resulting in a persistent communication between the pericardial sac and peritoneum. There is variable herniation of the abdominal viscera into the pericardial sac. Peritoneopericardial diaphragmatic hernia may or may not cause clinical signs and many are incidental findings.

The most consistent radiographic finding with peritoneopericardial diaphragmatic hernia is moderate or severe enlargement of the cardiac silhouette. This may be rounded but often has a bizarre irregular shape. Unlike patients with cardiomegaly or pericardial effusion, the cardiac silhouette may have a non-uniform opacity from the presence of omentum and mesentery (**fig. 17.17**). The gas-filled stomach or intestine may be visible within the pericardium. Reduced liver volume or absent abdominal viscera are important secondary signs supporting the diagnosis. The ventral diaphragmatic and caudal cardiac borders are usually contiguous. In cats, the identification of a distinct curvilinear soft tissue opacity between the heart and diaphragm known as the dorsal peritoneopericardial mesothelial remnant is a consistent finding for peritoneopericardial hernia (**fig. 17.18**).[21] Ultrasonography or a limited gastrointestinal contrast study may also aid in confirming a diagnosis of peritoneopericardial diaphragmatic hernia.

The liver and gallbladder are most commonly herniated abdominal viscera, followed by omentum, intestines, spleen, pancreas, and falciform fat.

Hiatal hernia

Hiatal hernia refers to the protrusion of abdominal viscera through the esophageal hiatus into the mediastinum. Hiatal hernias can occur in both dogs and cats. There are four types of hiatal hernia:

- Type I (sliding hiatal hernia) is the most common, with the abdominal esophagus and part of the stomach (including the caudal esophageal sphincter) displaced cranially into the esophageal hiatus (**fig. 17.19**).[22] English Bulldogs, Chinese Shar Peis, and other brachycephalic dogs such as French Bulldogs, and Boston Terriers are overrepresented.

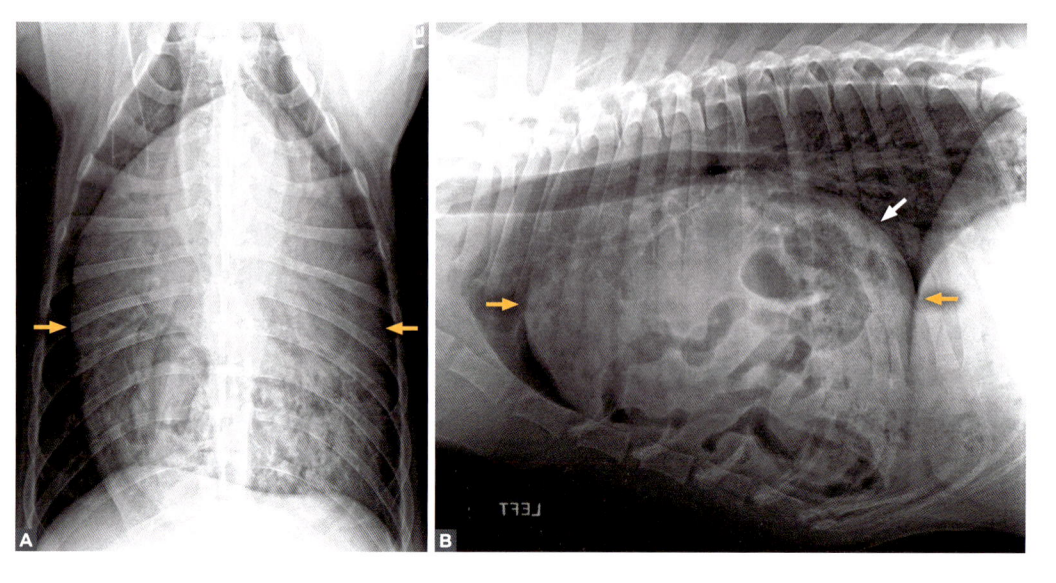

Fig. 17.17 (**A**) Ventrodorsal and (**B**) left lateral views of the thorax of a Labrador Retriever with peritoneopericardial diaphragmatic hernia. The cardiac silhouette is markedly enlarged with smooth margins (orange arrows) and the caudal cardiac border is convex in shape (white arrow). Gas-filled intestinal segments are noted within the enlarged cardiac silhouette.

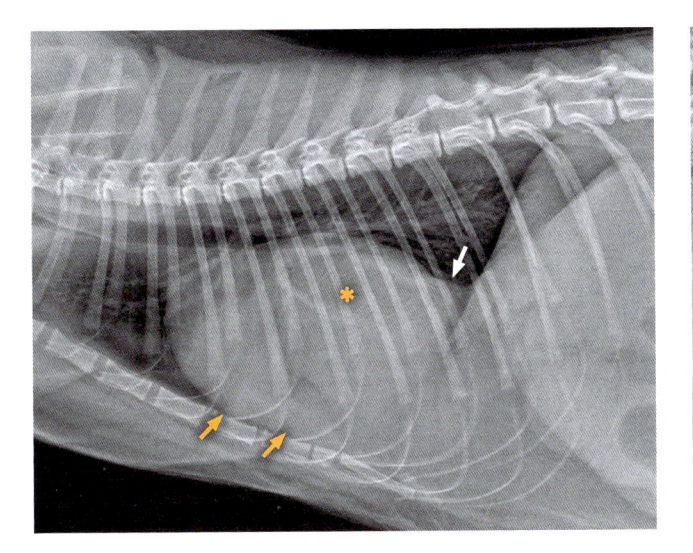

Fig. 17.18 Left lateral view of the thorax of a two-year-old American Domestic shorthair cat with peritoneopericardial diaphragmatic hernia. The cardiac silhouette is markedly enlarged, has non-uniform soft tissue opacity, and is contiguous with the diaphragmatic cupula. A dorsal peritoneopericardial mesothelial remnant is present (white arrow). The liver is herniated into the pericardiac sac (orange arrows), and the heart is displaced caudodorsally (asterisk).

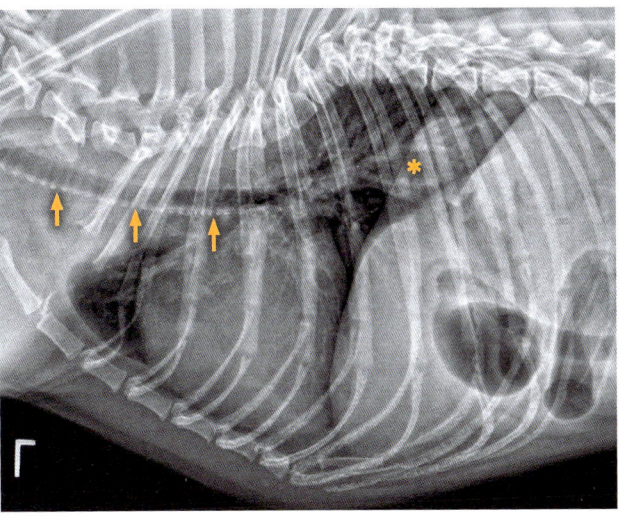

Fig. 17.19 Left lateral view of a two-year-old English Bulldog diagnosed with brachycephalic obstructive airway syndrome and sliding hiatal hernia (asterisk) characterized by an ill-defined and smoothly marginated soft tissue opaque structure at the caudodorsal mediastinum. There is also concurrent mild tracheal hypoplasia characterized by relatively smaller tracheal diameter (orange arrows).

- Type II (paraesophageal hernia) is characterized by herniation of part of the stomach into the mediastinum adjacent to the esophagus, but the caudal esophagus into remains in place at the hiatus.[22, 23]
- Type III and IV hiatal hernias are considered uncommon and rarely reported.

There is current lack of information regarding the relative sensitivities and specificities of each diagnostic modality for diagnosing hiatal hernia in the veterinary literature. Videofluoroscopic evaluation is more useful than radiography in diagnosing sliding hiatal hernia (**video 17.2**) and also aids in diagnosing gastroesophageal reflux, hypomotility, or esophageal redundancy).[22, 24] Computed tomography is also useful to classify the type of hiatal hernia and to better identify the herniated organs for presurgical planning.[24]

Pleuroperitoneal diaphragmatic hernia

Pleuroperitoneal hernia or true diaphragmatic is a rare congenital subtotal diaphragmatic defect that enables the abdominal viscera to enter the thoracic cavity. However, the peritoneal membrane of the diaphragm remains intact, thereby preventing direct communication between the pleural and peritoneal cavities.[25]

The radiographic findings of pleuroperitoneal diaphragmatic hernia are rather similar to those seen in diaphragmatic rupture, except that the peritoneal membrane of the diaphragm is still intact.[26]

There are only several to a few cases of pleuroperitoneal diaphragmatic hernia reported.[25-29] In dogs, the liver or stomach is often displaced cranially while in cats falciform fat is displaced cranially into the thoracic cavity. Pleuroperitoneal diaphragmatic hernia can occasionally be misdiagnosed as a pulmonary mass (**fig. 17.20**).[26] This is because the herniated liver or summation of herniated falciform fat often has a soft tissue opacity and has well-defined margins due to containment by the peritoneal membrane. Positive contrast peritoneography, ultrasonography, or CT angiography in particular are useful in distinguishing pleuroperitoneal diaphragmatic hernia from a pulmonary mass.[26, 30] With CT angiography, the vasculature may be traceable into the herniated structure and

VIDEO 17.2

Videofluoroscopy of sliding hiatal hernia with barium meal in a seven-year-old Bischon Frisé. There is sliding hiatal hernia and concurrent esophageal dysmotility. Courtesy of Dr. Federico Vilaplana-Grosso, DECVDI, DACVR.

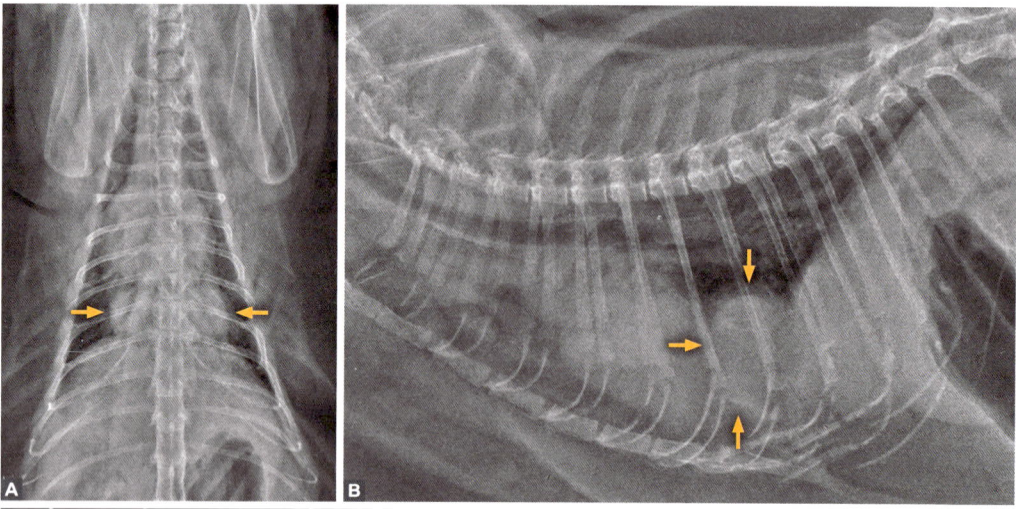

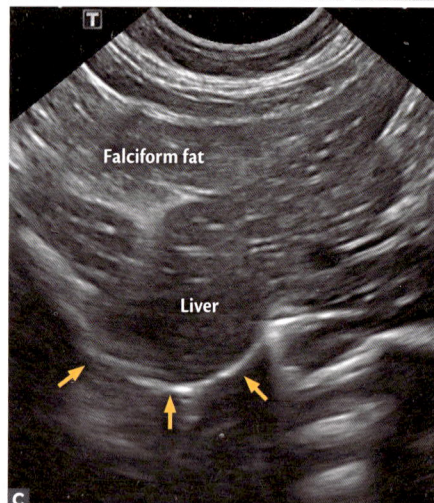

Fig. 17.20 (**A**) Ventrodorsal and (**B**) left lateral views of the thorax, and (**C**) transhepatic abdominal ultrasonography of a nine-year-old Ragdoll cat with pleuroperitoneal diaphragmatic hernia confirmed on surgery. The liver, which appears as a rounded soft tissue mass (arrows), is noted between the cardiac silhouette and the diaphragmatic silhouette, causing partial effacement of the caudal cardiac border, as well as the mid and ventral portions of the diaphragmatic silhouette. On ultrasonography, the cranioventral portion of the liver parenchyma is herniated into the thoracic cavity but is confined by the peritoneal membrane of the diaphragm (arrows).

VIDEO 17.3

Fluoroscopy of bilateral diaphragmatic paralysis in an 11-year-old Pomeranian. Note that both diaphragmatic crura and cupula are cranially displaced with lack of diaphragmatic excursion. The movement of the diaphragm is due to compensatory abdominal muscle contraction from respiration. Courtesy of Dr. Federico Vilaplana-Grosso, DECVDI, DACVR.

the Hounsfield unit of fat tissue can easily be determined. Tension gastrothorax, which is an acute life-threatening condition has been reported in five Cavalier King Charles spaniel dogs with congenital pleuroperitoneal diaphragmatic hernia when the stomach is herniated into the thoracic cavity through the defect of the left crus of the diaphragm.[29]

Unilateral and bilateral diaphragmatic paralysis

Diaphragmatic paralysis may be caused by pneumonia, trauma, phrenic neuropathy, diaphragmatic myopathy, or idiopathic causes.[31] It may be presented as unilateral or bilateral, temporary, or permanent.

Fluoroscopy and ultrasonography (B-mode and M-mode) are considered the mainstay for diagnosing diaphragmatic paralysis in veterinary medicine.[31, 32] On the ventrodorsal/dorsoventral radiographs, the crura are asymmetrical with the paralyzed crus being cranially located. Both imaging modalities have the advantage of detecting the paralyzed diaphragm in real-time, usually characterized by diminished diaphragmatic excursion. Nevertheless, bilateral diaphragmatic paralysis may be more challenging to diagnose, particularly if the patient is tachypneic (**video 17.3**).

Pleura

The pleura lining consists of a single layer of mesothelial cells overlying a thin layer of vasculature and lymphatics. The parietal pleura lines the inner surface of the thoracic wall (costal parietal pleura), the diaphragm (diaphragmatic parietal pleura), and the mediastinum (mediastinal parietal pleura), while the pulmonary pleura or visceral pleura lines the surface of the lungs. The pleural cavity is the space between the visceral and parietal pleura, and it surrounds all the lung lobes (**fig. 17.21**).[33] Under normal physiologic conditions, a scant amount of pleural fluid is present and is not normally detectable on radiography, CT, or ultrasonography.

Occasionally, very thin pleural fissure lines or interlobar fissures (**fig. 17.22** and **fig. 17.23**) may be visible due to the X-ray beam being oriented perpendicular parallel to the plane of the pleural division or due to incidental pleural thickening in older patients.

In dogs, the right and left pleural cavities can communicate via the fenestrated caudoventral mediastinal pleura.[34] Therefore, bilateral pleural disease is not uncommon.

In cats, the mediastinal pleura is often intact or non-fenestrated, therefore unilateral pleural disease is more common.[35]

Pleural effusion

Presence of pleural effusion is typically characterized by widening of interlobar fissures and retraction of lungs from the thoracic wall with soft tissue opacity (fluid) within the pleural cavity on radiography (**fig. 17.24**) and CT. On radiography, pleural effusion will cause partial to complete effacement of the cardiac silhouette and diaphragmatic silhouette. The interlobar fissure is wider at the peripheral margin of the thorax and narrower at the perihilar region. The psoas minor muscle in cats extends more cranially than in dogs, therefore one should not confuse the more cranial attachment of the psoas minor muscle at the T12-T13 vertebra in cats with pleural effusion on the lateral radiographic views (**fig. 17.25**).

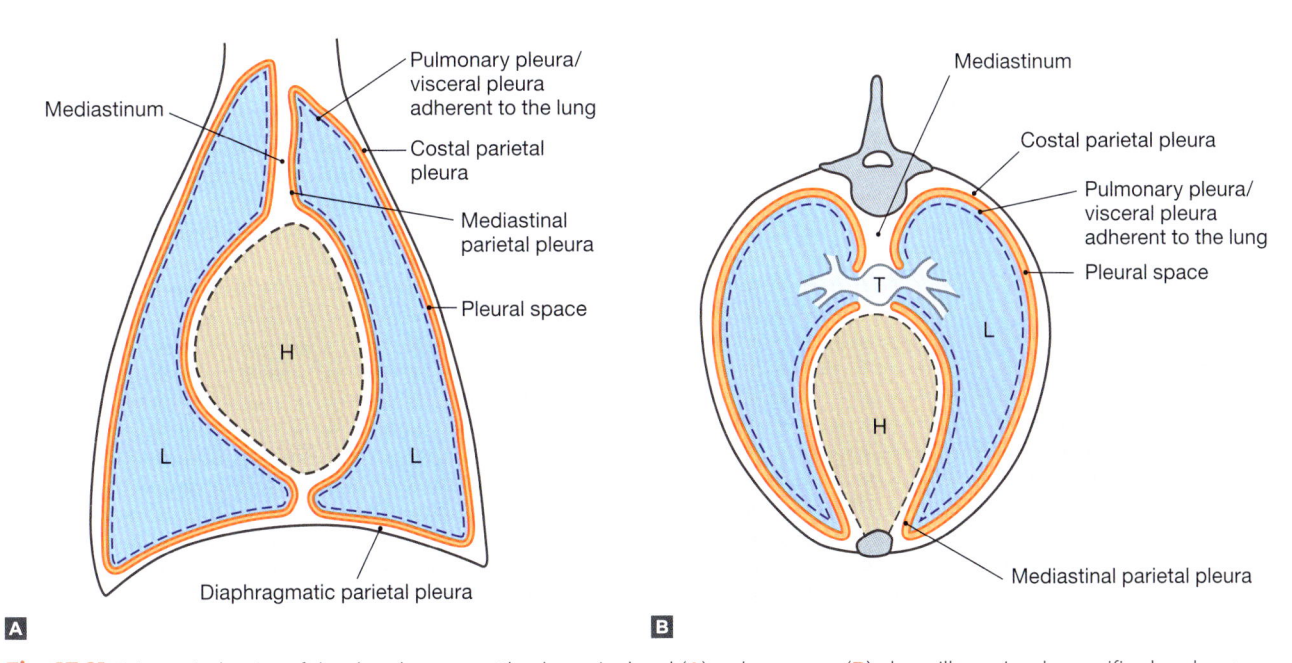

Fig. 17.21 Schematic drawing of the pleural anatomy. The thorax in dorsal (**A**) and transverse (**B**) planes illustrating the specific pleural anatomy. (**A**) Note the continuity of the costal, mediastinal, and diaphragmatic parts of the parietal pleura and the pulmonary/visceral pleura that intimately lines the surface of the lungs. (**B**) Note how the mediastinal pleura is reflected onto the lung to become pulmonary/visceral pleura. The lung is depicted by navy blue dotted line and the heart is depicted black dotted line. H, heart; L, lung; T, trachea.

SECTION IV THORAX

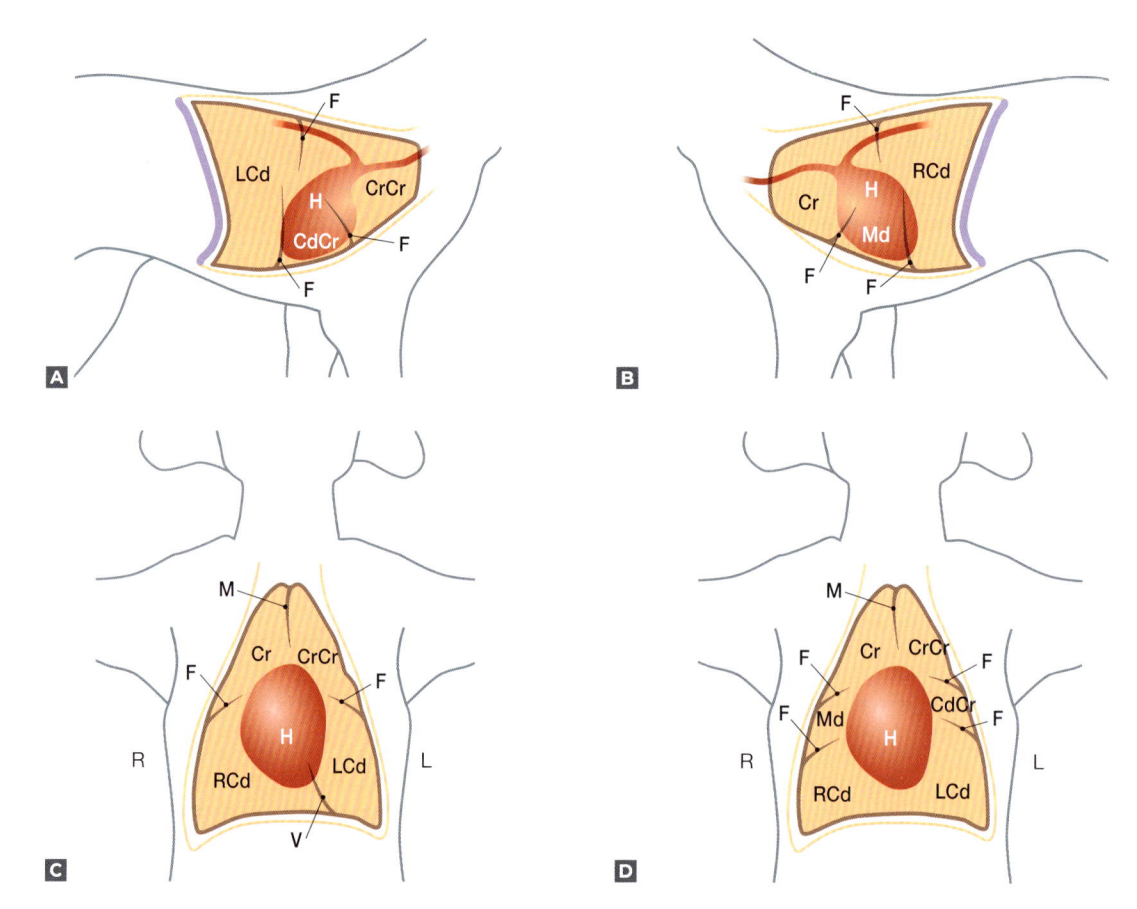

Fig. 17.22 Schematic drawing of the location of the interlobar fissures with different positionings. (A) In left lateral recumbency, interlobar fissures of the left lungs are more likely to be visible. (B) In right lateral recumbency, interlobar fissures of the right lungs are more likely to be visible. (C) In dorsal recumbency, interlobar fissures on the dorsal aspect of the lungs are more likely to be visible. (D) In sternal recumbency, interlobar fissures on the ventral aspect of the lungs are more likely to be visible. Ac, Accessory lung lobe; CdCr, caudal subsegment of left cranial lung lobe; Cr, right cranial lung lobe; CrCr, cranial subsegment of left cranial lobe; F, interlobar fissure; H, heart; LCd, left caudal lung lobe; M, mediastinal reflection; Md, right middle lung lobe; RCd, right caudal lung lobe; V, caudoventral mediastinal reflection.

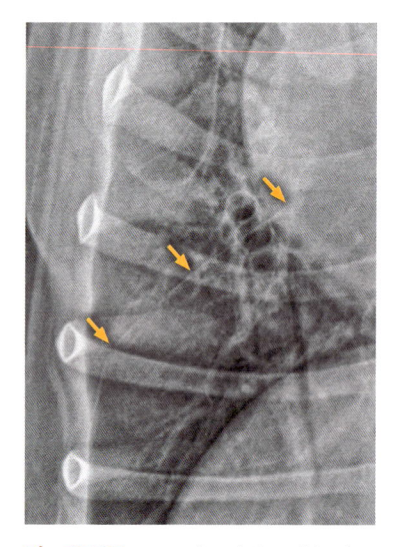

Fig. 17.23 Ventrodorsal view of the thorax of a seven-year-old Dachshund with a very thin pleural fissure line (arrows) between the right middle and right caudal lung lobes.

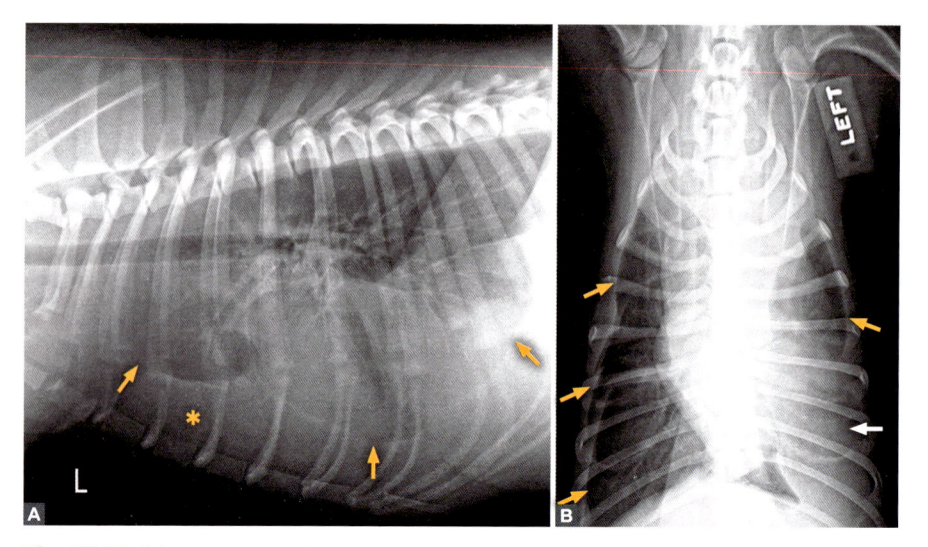

Fig. 17.24 (A) Left lateral and (B) ventrodorsal views of the thorax of a three-year-old Border Collie with pleural effusion (asterisk), retracted margins of the lungs with widened interlobar fissure (orange arrows), and consolidation of the left caudal lung lobe (white arrow).

232

CHAPTER **17** Thoracic wall, diaphragm, and pleura

It is important to understand the difference in the distribution of the pleural effusion between the dorsoventral and ventrodorsal views, particularly when trying to detect small volumes of pleural effusion (**fig. 17.26**).

On dorsoventral view, the fluid accumulates in the ventral aspect of the thorax, causing varying degree (depending on the amount of the pleural effusion) of moderate border effacement of the cardiac silhouette and the diaphragm. Mild retraction of the lung margins and a widening of the interlobar fissures may be visible.

Fig. 17.25 (**A**) Lateral thoracic view of a cat and (**B**) lateral thoracic view of a dog. The psoas minor muscle in the cat is seen as a triangular soft tissue opacity between the caudodorsal margins of the caudal lung lobes and the T12 and T13 vertebrae (arrow). This should not be confused with pleural effusion. The psoas minor muscle is not normally identifiable in the dog (**B**).

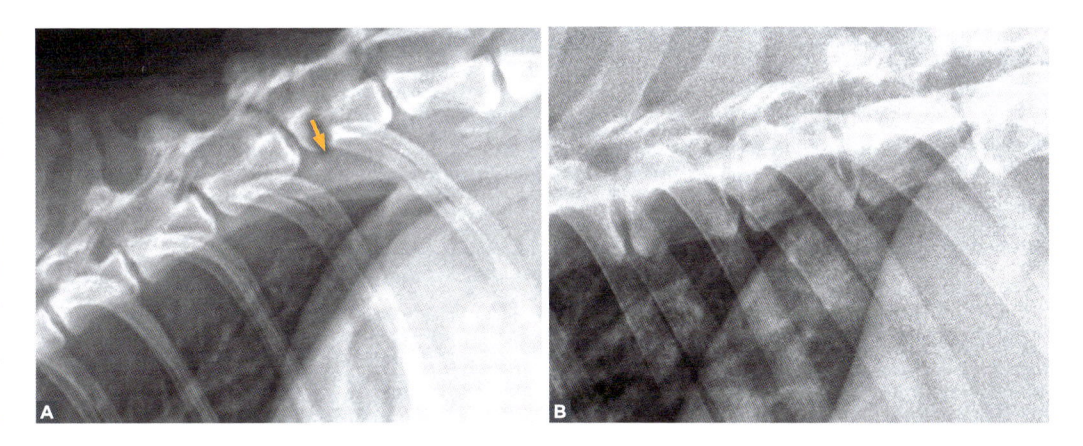

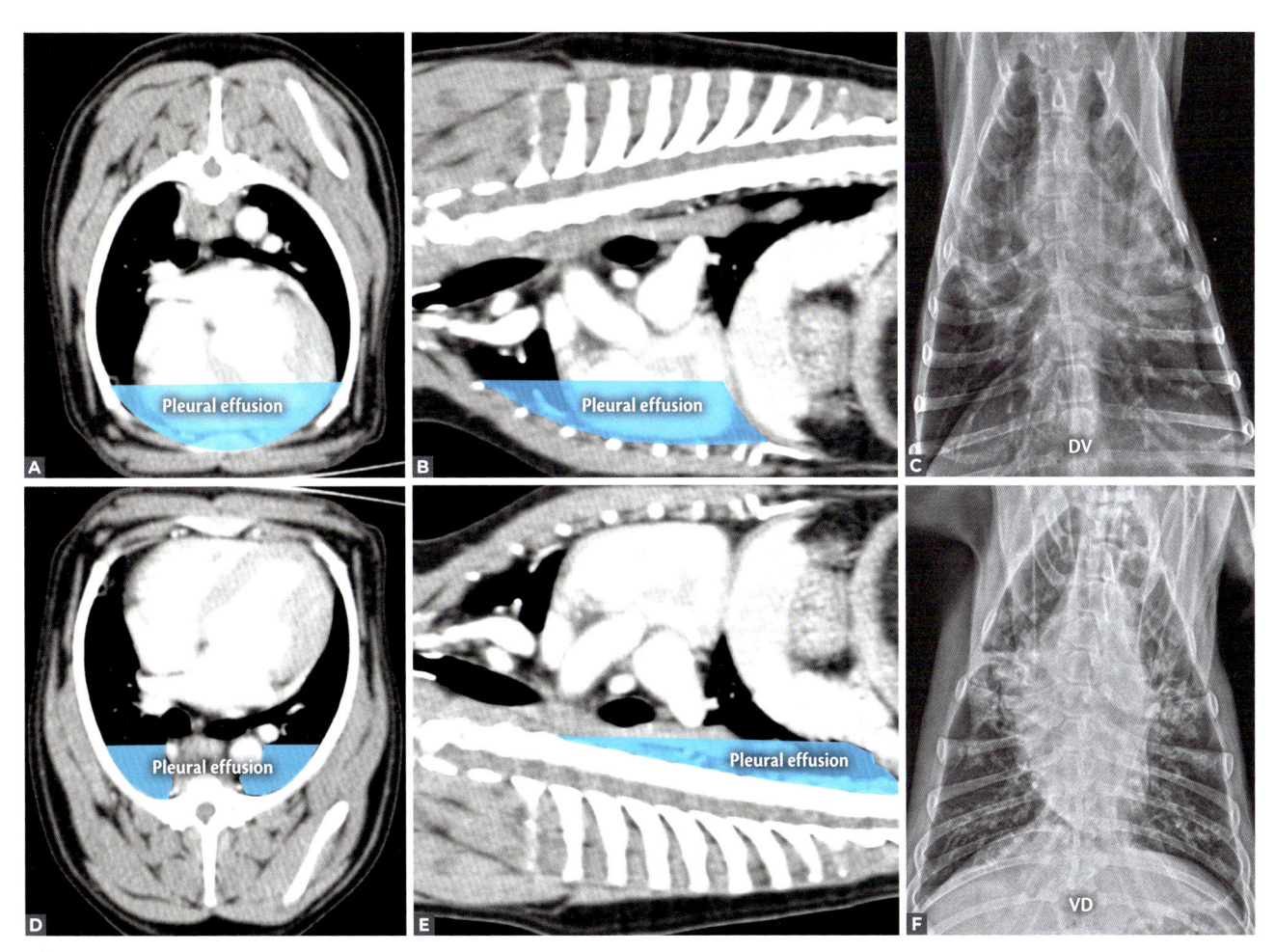

Fig. 17.26 (**A**, **B**) With the patient in sternal recumbency, the pleural effusion will gravitate at the ventral aspect of the thoracic cavity. (**C**) Therefore, on dorsoventral view, the pleural effusion will cause border effacement of the cardiac silhouette. (**D**, **E**) With the patient in dorsal recumbency, the pleural effusion will gravitate at the dorsal aspect of the thoracic cavity, within the paraspinal gutter instead of surrounding the heart. (**F**) Therefore, on ventrodorsal view, the small amount of pleural effusion does not cause border effacement of the cardiac silhouette and can be overlooked.

233

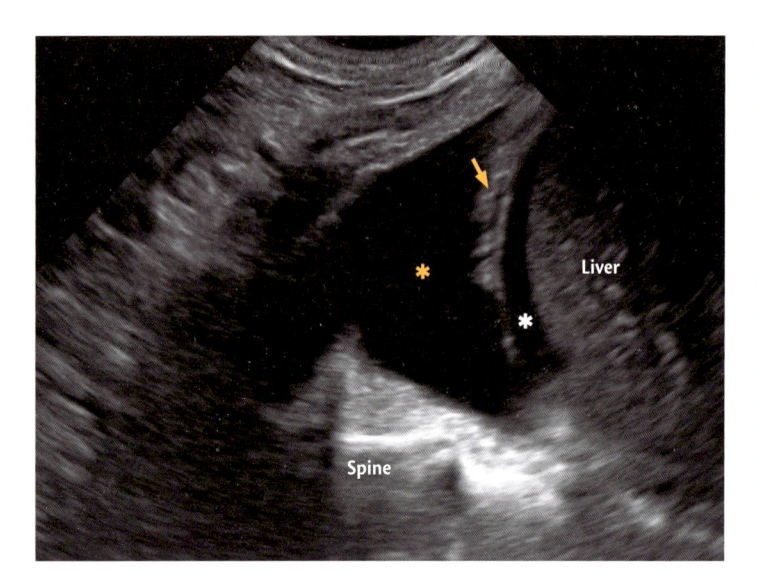

Fig. 17.27 Transthoracic ultrasonography of an eight-year old mixed breed dog with a large amount of anechoic pleural effusion (orange asterisk) through the mild left 11th intercostal space. A small amount of peritoneal effusion is also noted (white asterisk) between the diaphragm (orange arrow) and the liver. The bicavitary anechoic effusion is most likely due to hypoalbuminemia from the underlying protein-losing enteropathy. Courtesy of Dr. Federico Vilaplana-Grosso, DECVDI, DACVR.

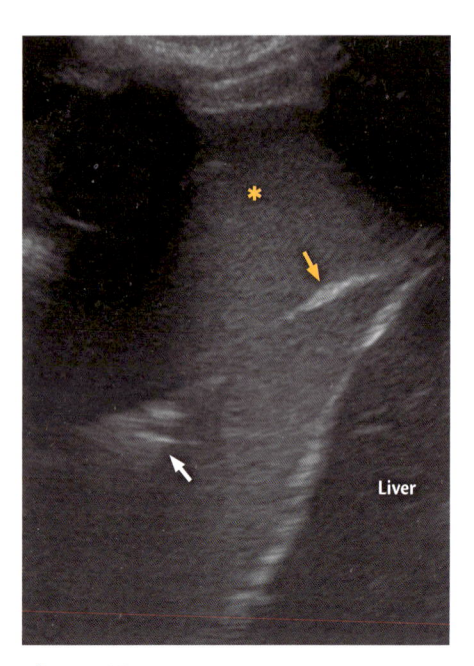

Fig. 17.28 Transthoracic ultrasonography of a three-year-old Springer Spaniel dog with pyothorax through the left dorsal 11th intercostal space window. A large amount of echogenic pleural effusion (asterisk) with a hyperechoic fibrinous tag (orange arrow) are noted. The left caudal lung lobe is atelectatic (white arrow). Courtesy of Dr. Carlo Anselmi, DECVDI.

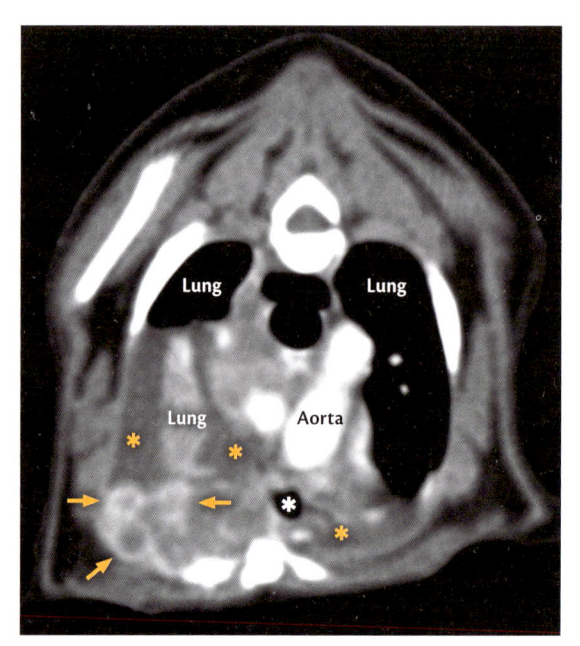

Fig. 17.29 Transverse CT image of the thorax of a nine-year-old Domestic shorthair cat with pleural effusion (orange asterisks) and contrast-enhancing nodules (orange arrows) due to pleural carcinomatosis. Note that the ventral portion of the right cranial lung lobe is atelectatic. There is also a small, iatrogenic gas bubble (white asterisk) in the mid-ventral aspect of the thoracic cavity due to prior thoracocentesis.

On ventrodorsal view, the fluid accumulates in the dorsal aspect of the thorax. The lung margins may have a varying degree (depending on the amount of pleural effusion) of rounding and retraction with widening of the interlobar fissures. The cardiac silhouette is usually visible if the amount of pleural effusion is small; however, border effacement of the heart and diaphragm may eventually occur with an increasingly larger amount volume of pleural effusion.

Pleural effusion can be divided into transudates, exudates, hemorrhage, neoplastic effusion, and chyle.[36] The exact nature of the pleural effusion (i.e., blood or pus or chyle or transudate) cannot be determined based on radiographic appearance as all fluid has the same radiographic capacity.

Sampling of the pleural effusion via thoracocentesis for cytology and analysis is often needed to determine the exact type and nature of the fluid present.

The presence of pleural effusion may cause a variable degree of effacement of the normal thoracic structures and other intrathoracic pathologies. Thoracic ultrasonography is a useful imaging modality to visualize the intrathoracic structures, potential thoracic pathology, and the appearance of the pleural effusion.[37] When the pleural fluid is anechoic, it is suggestive of either transudate, modified transudate, or chylous effusion. When the fluid is echogenic (or speckled), it is suggestive of it being either cellular, fibrinous, or proteinaceous (exudates, hemorrhage, or neoplastic effusions) fluid (**fig. 17.27** and **fig. 17.28**). The sonographic appearance of fluid is not reliable, and sampling should be performed. The presence of irregular pleural thickening or pleural masses and echogenic fibrinous strands may indicate a more chronic effusion, pleuritis, or pleural neoplasia. However, thoracic ultrasonography is limited by the ribs and aerated lung and cannot provide an overview of the entire thoracic cavity.

CT can provide a global overview of the entire thoracic cavity and is more sensitive than radiography in detecting pleural masses or nodules (i.e., pleural carcinomatosis or mesothelioma) or other intrathoracic pathologies due to its ability to detect contrast-enhancing lesions. On radiography, these pathologies may be masked by the presence of pleural effusion as both have similar soft tissue opacity (**fig. 17.29**).

Pneumothorax

Pneumothorax can be classified as traumatic, spontaneous, or iatrogenic.[38] Traumatic pneumothorax can be due to blunt trauma or penetrating thoracic wall injuries. Spontaneous pneumothorax refers to pneumothorax with no known traumatic or iatrogenic causes such as spontaneous rupturing of pulmonary bulla/bleb or secondary to pre-existing lung disease. Possible causes of iatrogenic pneumothorax include thoracostomy tube placement or removal, needle thoracocentesis, dehiscence of thoracotomy incisions, celiotomy with undetected diaphragmatic hernia, bronchoscopy, tracheal rupture associated with intubation in cats, intermittent positive-pressure ventilation, or percutaneous lung fine-needle aspiration of the lung.

On radiographic images, pneumothorax is characterized by retraction of the lungs from the thoracic wall and spine with interposed gas. There will be a lack of lung markings (vasculature) extending to the periphery of the thorax. The cardiac apex may also be displaced from the sternum on lateral views. In general, lateral views are considered more sensitive for the detection of pneumothorax than dorsoventral or ventrodorsal views (**fig. 17.30**).[34] Occasionally, skin folds can mimic pleural gas. The skin fold, however, typically extends beyond the thoracic cavity and is usually oriented differently to the lung lobe margin (**fig. 17.31**).

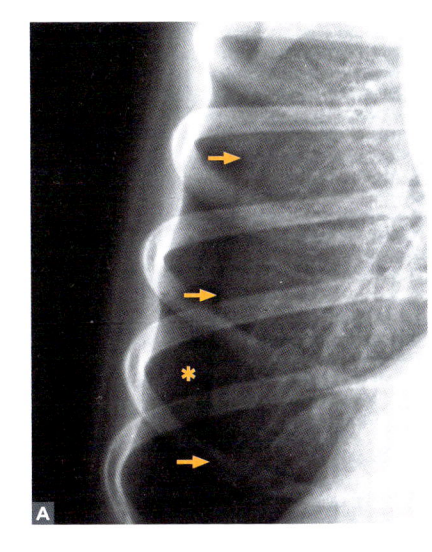

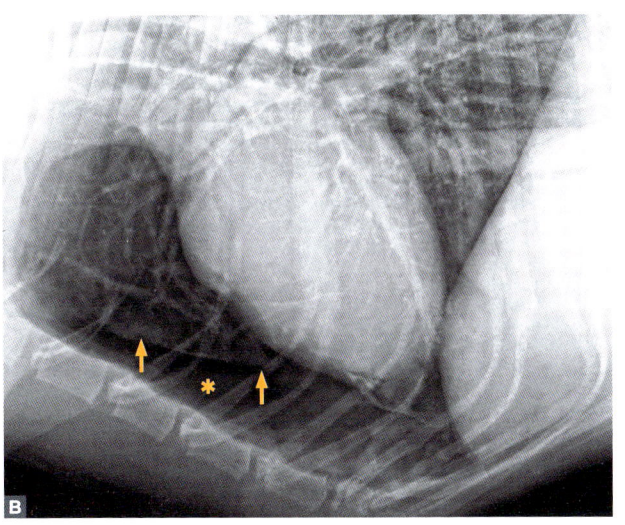

Fig. 17.30 (**A**) Ventrodorsal and (**B**) left lateral views of the thorax of a five-year-old neutered male Boxer dog with spontaneous pneumothorax. Note the retraction of the lung lobes from the thoracic margins (orange arrows) due to the presence of free gas (asterisk) within the pleural cavity.

SECTION IV THORAX

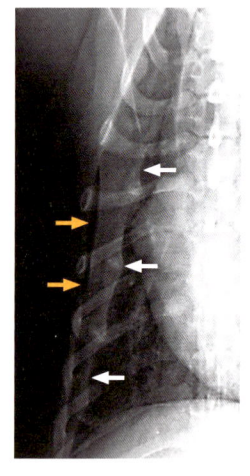

Fig. 17.31 Ventrodorsal view of the thorax of a three-year-old Bassett Hound with a skin fold artifact and "normal" bowed ribs conformation in this breed, mimicking both pneumothorax (orange arrows) and pleural effusion (white arrows).

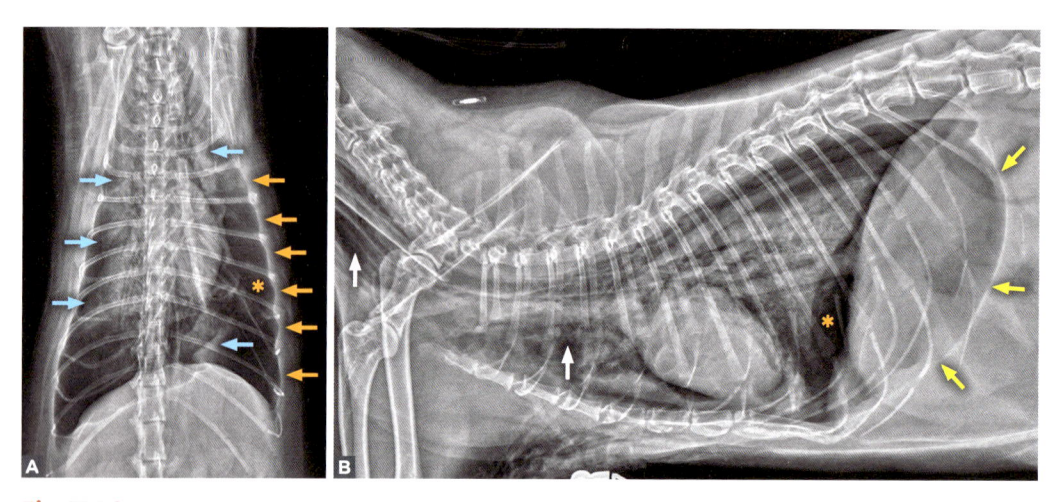

Fig. 17.32 (**A**) Ventrodorsal and (**B**) right lateral views of a ten-year-old American Domestic shorthair cat with tension pneumothorax (asterisk), and overdistension of the left hemithorax characterized by widened intercostal spaces, outward bulging of the pleural margin (orange arrows) and caudal displacement of the diaphragm (yellow arrows). There is also associated moderate multilobar pulmonary atelectasis characterized by increased soft tissue opacification of multiple lung lobes (blue arrows). There are also concurrent marked cervical fascial emphysema and pneumomediastinum, characterized by gas within the cervical fascial plane and the mediastinum (white arrows).

Fig. 17.33 (**A**) Dorsoventral radiographic view and (**B**) dorsal reconstructed CT image of the thorax of a two-year-old Chihuahua with tension pneumothorax (asterisks), right middle lung lobar emphysema (orange arrows), right cranial and right caudal lung lobes atelectasis (white arrows) and marked leftward shift of the heart. Note the barrel chest of the patient due to the tension pneumothorax and lobar emphysema. Courtesy of Dr. Federico Vilaplana-Grosso, DECVDI, DACVR.

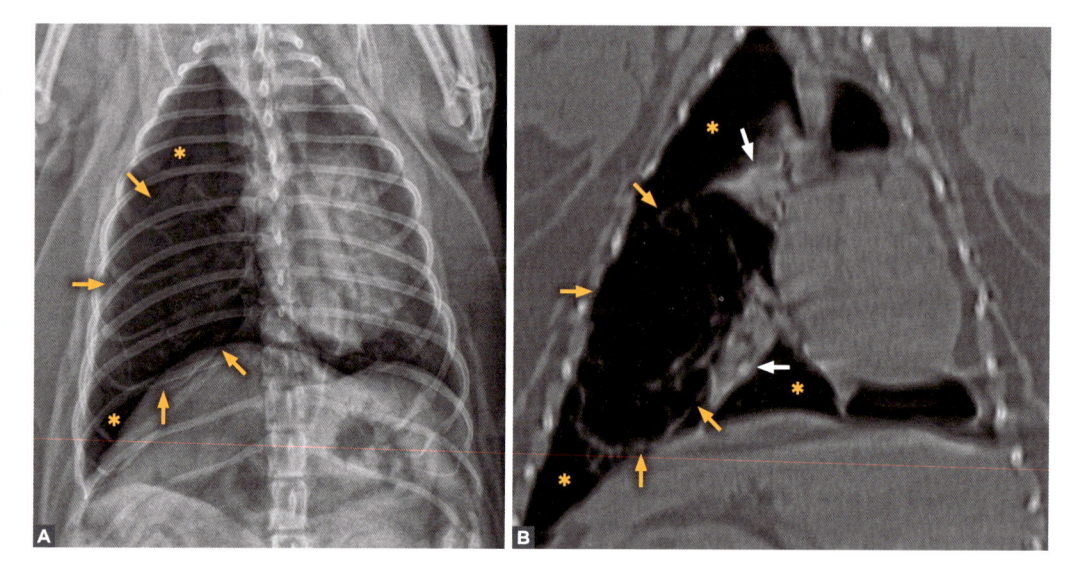

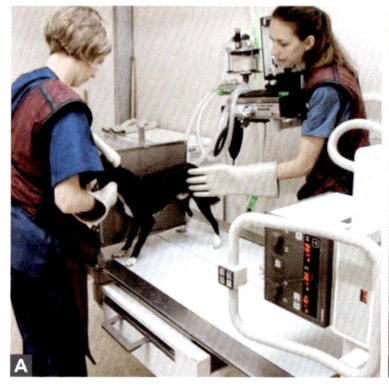

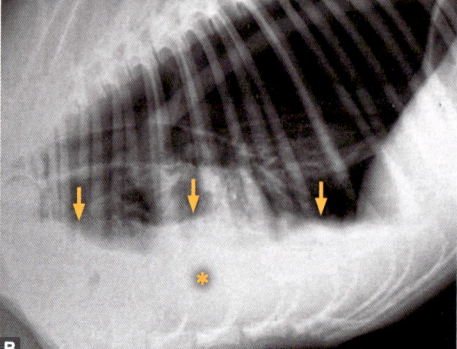

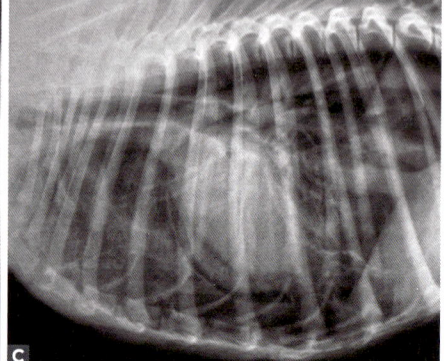

Fig. 17.34 Positioning (**A**), standing left to right laterolateral view using horizontal beam (**B**), and conventional right lateral recumbency view (**C**) of the thorax of a three-year-old mixed breed dog with hydropneumothorax. Note that the pleural effusion (asterisk) will gravitate and form a horizontal "fluid line" (arrows) while the free gas (pneumothorax) will rise to the upper part of the thorax on the standing lateral view. Courtesy of Prof. Robert M. Kirberger, DECVDI.

CHAPTER 17 Thoracic wall, diaphragm, and pleura

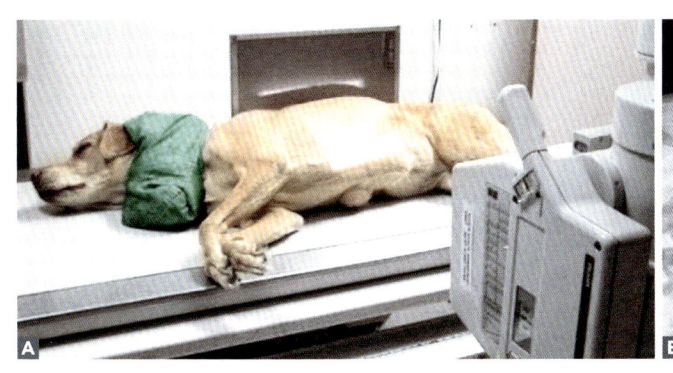

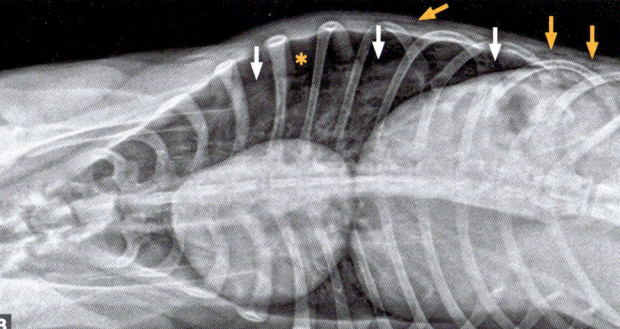

Fig. 17.35 Positioning (**A**) and ventrodorsal view (**B**) of the thorax of a four-year-old mixed breed dog on right lateral recumbency using a horizontal beam. There is mild pneumothorax characterized by accumulation of gas within the non-gravity-dependent aspect of the left pleural cavity (asterisk) and retraction of the left lung lobes from the thoracic wall (white arrows). There is also concurrent very mild subcutaneous emphysema (orange arrows).

Fig. 17.36 Transverse CT image of the thorax of an 11-year-old Labrador Retriever with spontaneous mild pneumothorax, characterized by a small amount of gas within the pleural cavity (asterisks) secondary to a small ruptured bleb (orange arrow). Courtesy of Dr. Amy Zalcman, DACVR.

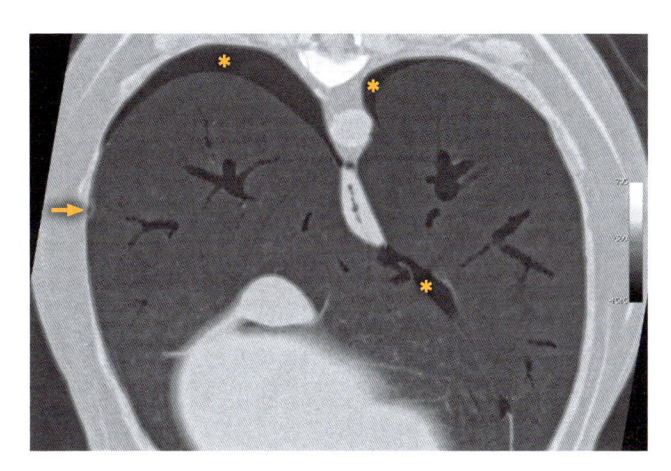

Tension pneumothorax may occur when the pleural gas pressure exceeds the atmospheric pressure. This is typically characterized by the presence of a large amount of gas within the pleural cavity, severe lung lobe atelectasis, overdistension of the thorax with a barrel-shaped appearance, and caudal displacement or flattening of the diaphragm (**fig. 17.32**). In unilateral tension pneumothorax, the cardiac silhouette is shifted towards the opposite side due to the increased pleural gas pressure (**fig. 17.33**).

Horizontal beam radiography

A standing lateral radiograph or ventrodorsal radiograph with the patient in lateral recumbency using a horizontal beam is the best method for detecting a small volume pneumothorax (**fig. 17.34** and **fig. 17.35**).[39] Free gas within the pleural cavity will typically rise to the upper part of the thorax. Radiography is usually sufficient to diagnose pneumothorax. Computed tomography is often used in patients with suspected spontaneous pneumothorax to rule out ruptured bulla or bleb (**fig. 17.36**) or other underlying lung diseases but often cannot confirm the location of the etiologic lesion and thoracotomy or thoracoscopy are often required for diagnosis.[40]

Thoracic ultrasound may also be helpful in diagnosing pneumothorax, particularly as a quick initial screening tool in severely dyspneic or stressed patients. The diagnosis of pneumothorax is made when the normal gliding movement of the visceral pleural margin is not seen, whereas air in the pleural space does not move with respiration.

Chronic restrictive pleural disease or chronic restrictive/fibrosing pulmonary disease

Fibrosis of the visceral pleura or fibrosing pleuritis may develop due to chronic inflammatory pleural effusion such as pus, chyle, or hemorrhage.[41] This may lead to thickening and contraction of the visceral pleura of the lungs and restricting and reducing lung volume. Following therapeutic centesis of the pleural fluid, the lungs remain collapsed, even with continuous drainage. As a result, lung

SECTION IV THORAX

margins appear rounded, lacking the acute lobar margins of the normal lung (**fig. 17.37**).[42] Severe fibrosing pleuritis have has been reported in dogs and cats with chronic chylothorax.[41]

Thoracic bellows

The thoracic bellows mechanism includes the rib cage and the diaphragm.[43] Chronic pulmonary or pleural disease resulting in loss of pulmonary compliance may cause thoracic bellows abnormalities. Non-traumatic stress fractures of multiple ribs may occur secondary to chronic respiratory distress. Severe inspiratory effort or coughing may result in contraction of the diaphragm and simultaneous pulling of the serratus dorsalis muscle, causing increased bending forces, shearing forces, and chronic microtrauma, leading to stress fractures at the proximal aspect of the ribs and the 8th-12th ribs are most commonly affected (**fig. 17.38**).[43] The presence of multiple rib fractures with varying degrees of healing, a history of chronic respiratory signs, and no history of trauma should alert the clinician to the diagnosis of thoracic bellows abnormalities.

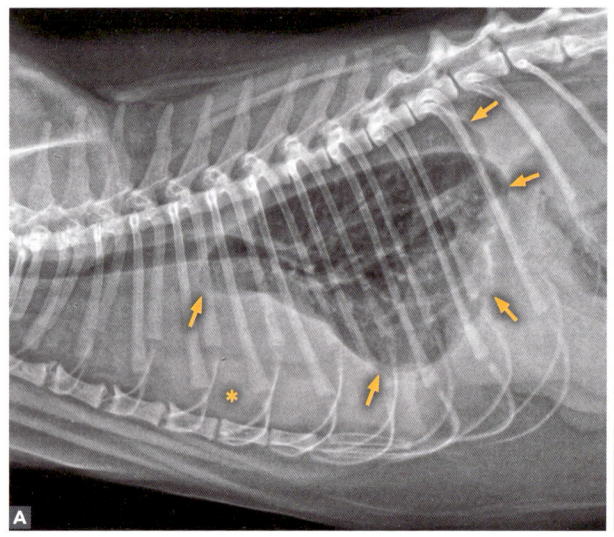

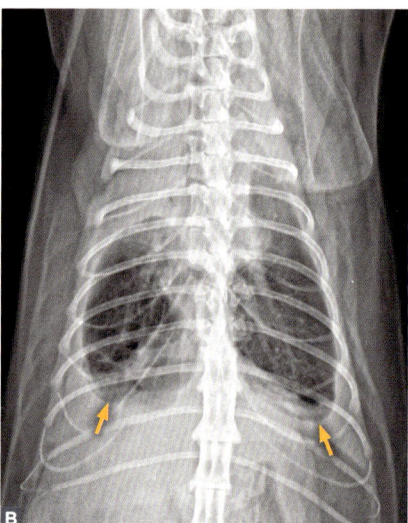

Fig. 17.37 (**A**) Right lateral and (**B**) ventrodorsal views of a 16-year-old British shorthair cat with chronic chylothorax and restrictive (fibrosing) pleuritis. There is a moderate amount of pleural effusion (asterisk) characterized by increased soft tissue opacification (fluid) within the pleural cavity, and the margins of the caudal lung lobes are rounded and retracted from the thoracic wall due to restrictive pleural fibrosis (arrows). The right cranial, right middle, and left cranial lung lobes are completely atelectatic with no visible aeration. Courtesy of Dr. Elisabet Dominguez, DECVDI.

Fig. 17.38 Ventrodorsal view of the thorax of a three-year-old Domestic shorthair cat with feline asthma. There is a diffuse bronchial lung pattern, atelectasis (increased soft tissue opacification) of the right middle lung lobe (asterisk) and pulmonary overinflation. These changes are consistent with chronic feline asthma with small airway obstruction. There are partly healed fractures of the right 9th to 13th ribs (arrows). The rib fractures are likely stress fractures secondary to the primary respiratory disease. Courtesy of Dr. Federico Vilaplana-Grosso, DECVDI, DACVR.

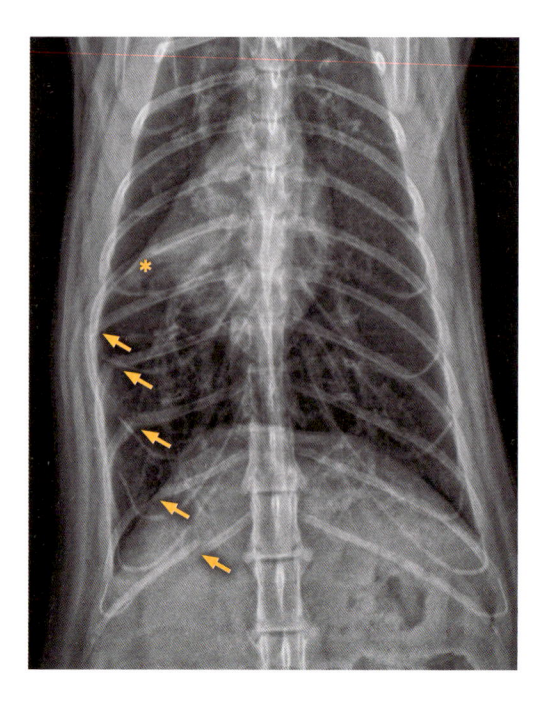

References

1. Evans HE, de Lahunta A. The skeleton. In Evans HE, de Lahunta A (editors). Miller's Anatomy of the Dog. St. Louis, Elsevier Saunders, 2013, pp 80-157.
2. Suter PF. Lesions of the thoracic wall, extrapleural diseases. In Suter PF (editor). Thoracic Radiography: A Text Atlas of Thoracic Diseases of the Dog and Cat. Wettswill, Switzerland, Peter F. Suter, 1984, pp 161-177.
3. Suter PF. Lower airway and pulmonary parenchymal diseases. In Suter PF (editor). Thoracic Radiography: A Text Atlas of Thoracic Diseases of the Dog and Cat. Wettswill, Switzerland, Peter F. Suter, 1984, pp 517-682.
4. Parry A, Lamb C. Radiology of thoracic trauma in the dog and cat. In Practice 32:238-246, 2010.
5. Scheepens ET, Peeters ME, L'eplattenier HF, Kirpensteijn J. Thoracic bite trauma in dogs: a comparison of clinical and radiological parameters with surgical results. J Small Anim Pract 47:721-726, 2006.
6. Lamb CR, Parry AT, Baines EA, Chang YM. Does changing the orientation of a thoracic radiograph aid diagnosis of rib fractures? Vet Radiol Ultrasound 52:75-78, 2011.
7. Charlesworth TM, Sturgess CP. Increased incidence of thoracic wall deformities in related Bengal kittens. J Feline Med Surg 14:365-368, 2012.
8. Kurosawa TA, Ruth JD, Steurer J, Austin B, Heng HG. Imaging diagnosis. Acquired pectus excavatum secondary to laryngeal paralysis in a dog. Vet Radiol Ultrasound 53:329-332, 2012.
9. Lim CK, Heng HG, Guptill LF. Presumed acquired dynamic pectus excavatum in a cat. Can Vet J 62:751-754, 2021.
10. Spoldi E, Schwarz T, Sabattini S, Vignoli M, Cancedda S, Rossi F. Comparisons among computed tomographic features of adipose masses in dogs and cats. Vet Radiol Ultrasound 58:29-37, 2017.
11. Feeney DA, Johnston GR, Grindem CB, Toombs JP, Caywood DD, Hanlon GF. Malignant neoplasia of canine ribs: clinical, radiographic, and pathologic findings. J Am Vet Med Assoc 180:927-933, 1982.
12. Pirkey-Ehrhart N, Withrow SJ, Straw RC, Ehrhart EJ, Page RL, Hottinger HL, Hahn KA, Morrison WB, Albrecht MR, Hedlund CS, et al. Primary rib tumors in 54 dogs. J Am Anim Hosp Assoc 31:65-69, 1995.
13. Clarke BS, Mannion PA, White RA. Rib metastases from a non-tonsillar squamous cell carcinoma in a dog. J Small Anim Pract 52:163-167, 2011.
14. Hermanson JW E. The muscular system. In Evans HE, de Lahunta A (editors). Miller's Anatomy of the Dog. St. Louis, Elsevier Saunders, 2013, pp 185-280.
15. Grandage J. The radiology of the dog's diaphragm. J Small Anim Pract 15:1-18, 1974.
16. Levine SH. Diaphragmatic hernia. Vet Clin North Am Small Anim Pract 17:411-30, 1987.
17. Wilson GP, Newton CD, Burt JK. A review of 116 diaphragmatic hernias in dogs and cats. J Am Vet Med Assoc 159:1142-1145, 1971.
18. Garson HL, Dodman NH, Baker GJ. Diaphragmatic hernia. Analysis of fifty-six cases in dogs and cats. J Small Anim Pract 21:469-481, 1980.
19. Sullivan M, Reid J. Management of 60 cases of diaphragmatic rupture. J Small Anim Pract 31:425-430, 1990.
20. Wilson GP, Hayes HM Jr. Diaphragmatic hernia in the dog and cat: a 25-year overview. Semin Vet Med Surg Small Anim 1:318-326, 1986.
21. Berry CR, Koblik PD, Ticer JW. Dorsal peritoneopericardial mesothelial remnant as an aid to the diagnosis of feline congenital peritoneopericardial diaphragmatic hernia. Vet Radiol 31:239-245, 1990.
22. Ellison GW, Lewiq DD, Phillips L, Tarvin GB. Esophageal hiatal hernia in small animals: literature review and a modified surgical technique. J Am Anim Hosp Assoc 23:391-399, 1987.
23. Miles KG, Pope ER, Jergens AE. Paraesophageal hiatal hernia and pyloric obstruction in a dog. J Am Vet Med Assoc 193:1437-1439, 1988.
24. Phillips H, Corrie J, Engel DM, Duffy DJ, Holt DE, Kendall AR, Schmiedt CW, Vetter A, Meren IL, Follette C, Schaeffer DJ, Mayhew PD, Marks SL. Clinical findings, diagnostic test results, and treatment outcome in cats with hiatal hernia: 31 cases (1995-2018). J Vet Intern Med 33:1970-1976, 2019.
25. Cariou MP, Shihab N, Kenny P, et al. Surgical management of an incidental diagnosed true pleuroperitoneal hernia in a cat. J Feline Med Surg 11:873-877, 2009.
26. Voges AK, Bertrand S, Hill RC, et al. True diaphragmatic hernia in a cat. Vet Radiol Ultrasound 38:116-119, 1997.
27. Feldman DB, Bree MM, Cohen BJ. Congenital diaphragmatic hernia in neonatal dogs. J Am Vet Med Assoc 153:942-944, 1968.
28. Valentine BA, Cooper BJ, Dietze AE, Noden DM. Canine congenital diaphragmatic hernia. J Vet Intern Med 2:109-112, 1988.
29. Rossanese M, Pivetta M, Pereira N, Burrow R. Congenital pleuroperitoneal hernia presenting as gastrothorax in five cavalier King Charles spaniel dogs. J Small Anim Pract 60: 701-704, 2019.
30. Parry A. Positive contrast peritoneography in the diagnosis of a pleuroperitoneal diaphragmatic hernia in a cat. J Feline Med Surg 12:141-143, 2010.
31. Vignoli M, Toniato M, Rossi F, Terragni R, Manzini M, Franchi A, Pozzi L. Transient post-traumatic hemidiaphragmatic paralysis in two cats. J Small Anim Pract 43:312-316, 2002.
32. Choi M, Lee N, Kim A, Keh S, Lee J, Kim H, Choi M. Evaluation of diaphragmatic motion in normal and diaphragmatic paralyzed dogs using M-mode ultrasonography. Vet Radiol Ultrasound 55:102-108, 2014.
33. Evans HE, de Lahunta A. The respiratory system. In Evans HE, de Lahunta A (editors). Miller's Anatomy of the Dog. St. Louis, Elsevier Saunders, 2013, pp 338-360.
34. Kern DA, Carrig CB, Martin RA. Radiographic evaluation of induced pneumothorax in the dog. Vet Radiol Ultrasound, 35:411-417, 1994.
35. Dennis R, Kirberger RM, Barr Frances, Wrigley RH. Other thoracic structures: pleural cavity, mediastinum, thoracic oesophagus, thoracic wall. In Dennis R, Kirberger RM, Barr F, Wrigley RH (editors). Handbook of Small Animal Radiology and Ultrasound - Techniques and Differential Diagnoses. St. Louis, Elsevier, 2010, pp 199-228.
36. Briola C, Zoia A, Rocchi P, Caldin M, Bertolini G. Computed tomography attenuation value for the characterization of pleural effusions in dogs: A cross-sectional study in 58 dogs. Res Vet Sci 124:357-365, 2019.
37. Larson MM. Ultrasound of the thorax (noncardiac). Vet Clin North Am Small Anim Pract 39:733-745, 2009.
38. Pawloski DR, Broaddus KD. Pneumothorax: a review. J Am Anim Hosp Assoc 46:385-397, 2010.
39. Lynch KC, Oliveira CR, Matheson JS, Mitchell MA, O'Brien RT. Detection of pneumothorax and pleural effusion with horizontal beam radiography. Vet Radiol Ultrasound 53:38-43, 2012.
40. Au JJ, Weisman DL, Stefanacci JD, et al. Use of computed tomography for evaluation of lung lesions associated with spontaneous pneumothorax in dogs: 12 cases (1999-2002). J Am Vet Med Assoc 228:733-737, 2006.
41. Fossum TW, Evering WN, Miller MW, Forrester SD, Palmer DR, Hodges CC. Severe bilateral fibrosing pleuritis associated with chronic chylothorax in five cats and two dogs. J Am Vet Med Assoc 201:317-324, 1992.
42. Suess RP Jr, Flanders JA, Beck KA, Earnest-Koons K. Constrictive pleuritis in cats with chylothorax: 10 cases (1983-1991). J Am Anim Hosp Assoc 30:70-77, 1994.
43. Hardie EM, Ramirez O, Clary EM, Kornegay JN, Correa MT, Feimster RA, Robertson ER. Abnormalities of the thoracic bellows: stress fractures of the ribs and hiatal hernia. J Vet Intern Med 12:279-287, 1998.

CHAPTER 18

Mediastinum

Ehren M. McLarty

KEY POINTS

- Radiography is an appropriate screening tool for mediastinal disease, although CT is often indicated for precise localization of disease.
- Adult brachycephalic dogs usually have a large volume of fat in the cranial mediastinum, which should not be mistaken for a mass.
- Mediastinal lymphadenopathy is most commonly associated with round cell neoplasia.
- Sternal lymphadenopathy can be an indicator of intra-abdominal disease.
- Thymic epithelial tumors and lymphoma are the most common cranial mediastinal masses.
- Cranial mediastinal cysts have a similar radiographic appearance to other masses but are non-contrast enhancing on CT.
- Tracheobronchial lymphadenopathy causes a mass effect dorsal to the carina, most often associated with lymphoma or fungal infection.
- Paraesophageal empyema causes a caudodorsal midline mass and is often associated with mediastinitis, pleural effusion, and bronchopneumonia.
- Mediastinal hemorrhage causes diffuse, V-shaped mediastinal widening.
- Pneumomediastinum causes increased conspicuity of mediastinal structures and may extend to or originate from the cervical fascia and retroperitoneal space.
- Contrast videofluoroscopy is necessary to identify esophageal dysmotility.
- Generalized megaesophagus may be congenital, associated with systemic disease or idiopathic, while segmental esophageal dilation is caused by vascular ring anomalies, foreign bodies, strictures, and rarely esophageal neoplasia.
- Gastroesophageal reflux and hiatal herniation are common diseases of the hiatal region, often occur together, and are best diagnosed by contrast videofluoroscopy.
- Esophageal neoplasms are rare but both carcinomas and sarcomas may occur with carcinomas more common in cats and sarcomas from *Spirocerca lupi* infection in dogs.

Normal mediastinum

The mediastinum is defined as the space between the right and left pleural sacs and contains the trachea and the carina, the esophagus, the heart and great vessels, the thoracic duct, numerous lymph nodes, and the thymus or thymic remnants (**fig. 18.1**). The mediastinum also contains a small amount (in the appropriately conditioned animal) of adipose tissue surrounding the soft tissue organs. On ventrodorsal radiographs, the width of the mediastinum is less than, or equal to, that of the spine, but may be wider in obese patients. In adult brachycephalic dogs, a large volume of fat is usually present in the cranial mediastinum, and it appears wider than in other dogs. The cranial margin of the mediastinum is defined by the thoracic inlet where it communicates with the cervical fascial planes, which enables gas or fluid in this region to extend to the mediastinum and vice versa. Caudally, the mediastinum is bounded by the diaphragm, but communicates with the retroperitoneal space through the aortic hiatus. The mediastinum can be divided into three regions for discussion, although there is certainly overlap of pathology between these regions, particularly when generalized mediastinal diseases (such as mediastinitis, pneumomediastinum, or effusion) are present. The cardiac silhouette is a convenient landmark with which to define these regions: the cranial mediastinum (cranial to the cardiac silhouette), the middle mediastinum (including the heart and region dorsal to the heart), and the caudal mediastinum (between the cardiac silhouette and the diaphragm). Additionally, the mediastinum can be divided for discussion into dorsal and ventral compartments in reference to the trachea and carina.[1,2]

Cranial Mediastinum

Thymus In the juvenile dog or cat, the thymus is a pyramidal or cone-shaped structure that is found in the ventral cranial mediastinum, just cranial to the heart. On lateral radiographic projections it may contribute to increased soft tissue opacity in the cranial mediastinum but does not have distinct margins. On dorsoventral or ventrodorsal projections, it can be seen as a triangular soft tissue structure at the left margin of the cranial mediastinum, immediately cranial to or abutting the cardiac silhouette (this is sometimes referred to as the "sail sign"). On computed tomography (CT) the thymus is iso-attenuating to muscle and mildly contrast-enhancing.

Lymph nodes Lymph nodes in the cranial mediastinum include the sternal lymph nodes, which are positioned just dorsal to the cranial sternum, and the cranial mediastinal lymph nodes which are found in the center or dorsal aspect of the cranial mediastinum. When normal, these lymph nodes are not visible on radiographic projections and are often not seen on magnetic resonance images (MRI), CT or ultrasound. In a large dog, normal lymph nodes may be visualized on ultrasound and have a similar appearance and size to other lymph nodes (moderately echogenic, ovoid to fusiform, around 5 mm in width). Normal sternal and cranial mediastinal lymph nodes are usually visualized on CT images as small, soft tissue attenuating, ovoid to elliptical structures surrounded by fat. Sternal lymph nodes are usually paired and have a visible hypoattenuating hilus while cranial mediastinal lymph nodes are often smaller and variable in number, without a distinct hilus.[3]

Great vessels The aortic root and descending aorta are normally visible on radiographs. On lateral projections, the aortic root is seen at the craniodorsal aspect of the cardiac silhouette. On ventrodorsal and dorsoventral projections the aortic root may form a slight bulge along the left cranial margin of the cardiac silhouette and the left margin of the descending aorta can often be seen just to the left of the vertebrae, coursing across the cardiac silhouette in a slightly oblique orientation and converging on midline at the diaphragmatic hiatus. Branches of the aortic root are sometimes visible in the region of the dorsocranial mediastinum on lateral projections and, when seen end-on, may give the false impression of small pulmonary nodules.

Fig. 18.1 Orthogonal thoracic projections of a normal five-year-old mixed breed dog (**A-B**) and a normal nine-month-old Domestic shorthair cat (**C-D**). Normal mediastinal structures are labeled as follows: *t*, trachea; *a*, aorta; *c*, caudal vena cava. The craniodorsal mediastinum, which includes the superimposed cranial vena cava, brachiocephalic trunk, subclavian arteries, cranial mediastinal lymph nodes, and mediastinal adventitia is indicated by the white arrows. In the dog, the caudal mediastinal reflection is indicated by the orange arrow and the cranial mediastinal reflection by the yellow arrow. The mediastinal lymph nodes, esophagus, and smaller vessels are not visible.

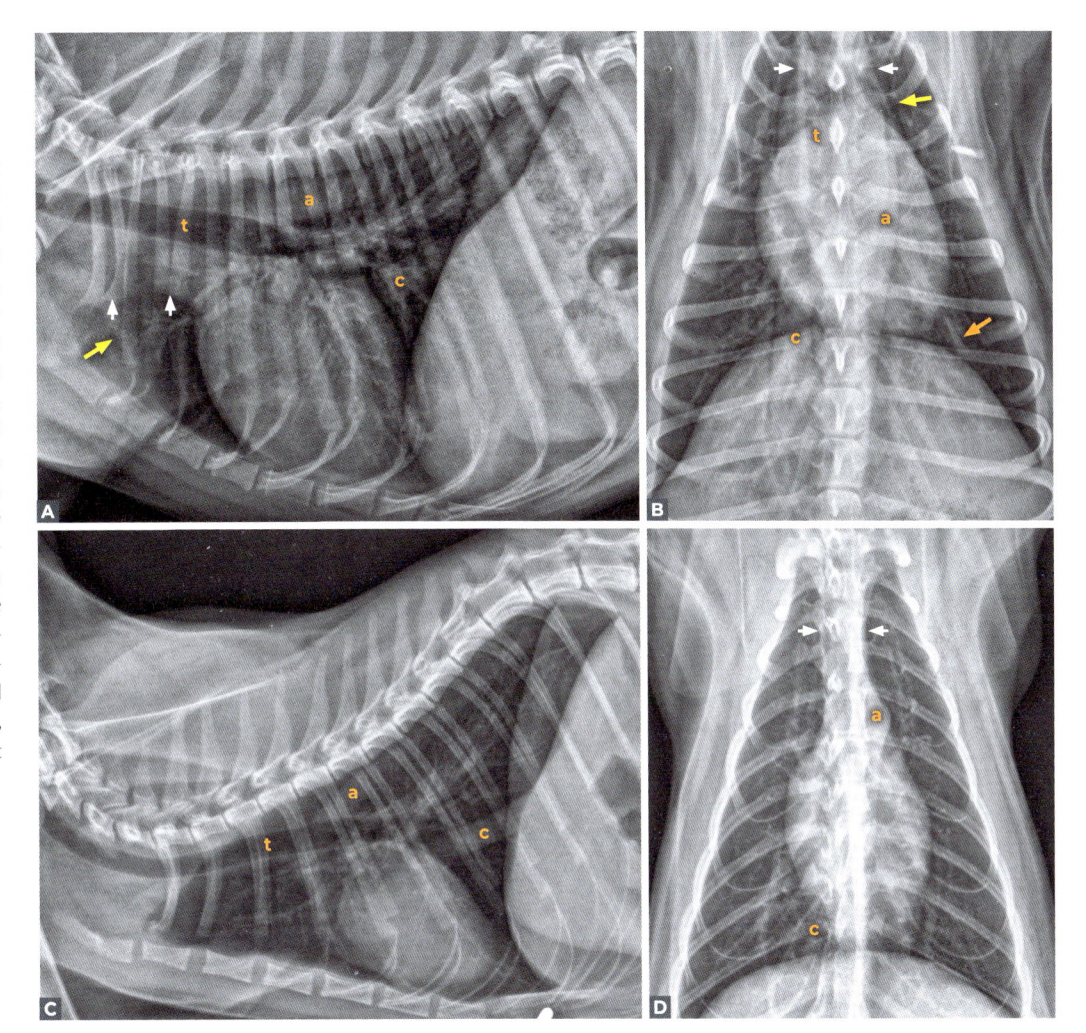

The cranial vena cava is usually not visible on radiographs but contributes to the overall soft tissue opacity in the cranial mediastinum. It can be easily visualized on CT, particularly when intravenous contrast is administered. The majority of the cranial vena cava can be visualized by a combination of ultrasonography of the cranial mediastinum and echocardiography.

▌ **Cranial mediastinal reflection** The right cranial lung lobe extends slightly to the left of midline. This causes a normal slight leftward positioning of the pleura bounding the cranial mediastinum and may be seen as an oblique soft tissue band superimposed on the right and left cranial lung lobes on lateral radiographs. On the dorsoventral or ventrodorsal projection this is seen as an oblique linear soft tissue structure slightly to the left of midline, in a similar location as the thymus.

Dorsal mediastinum

▌ **Aorta** The descending aorta continues from the aortic root in the dorsal thorax, immediately ventral to the spine. The aorta is immediately bounded by mediastinal pleura laterally, with adjacent aerated lung, making it visible on radiographs in most dogs and cats. The aorta traverses the diaphragm dorsal to the esophagus and vena cava, continuing in the retroperitoneal space.

▌ **Trachea and carina** The intrathoracic trachea and carina are contained within the cranial mediastinum, positioned in the dorsal third of the mediastinum. The carina (bifurcation of the trachea into the left and right principal bronchi) is positioned just dorsal to the heart base. Displacement of the trachea is an important indicator of mass effect within the mediastinum and helpful for determining the origin of the mass effect. The lumen of the trachea is normally clearly defined on radiography, CT, or MRI due to the gas filling it. The outer margin of the tracheal wall is typically not seen on radiographs due to the presence of adjacent soft tissue and/or opaque structures within the mediastinum (border effacement). The trachea is covered in greater detail in chapter 21.

▍ **Tracheobronchial lymph nodes** There are multiple lymph nodes in the region of the carina; most dogs have at least one cranial and one caudal to each principal bronchus (four in total). When normal, these lymph nodes are not visible on radiographs and difficult to visualize on CT or MRI.

▍ **Esophagus** The esophagus traverses the entire mediastinum at a similar level to the trachea, often overlapping with the trachea. The esophagus is typically not visible on radiographs, although the caudal thoracic esophagus is inconsistently visible in the caudal mediastinum on any projection. Fluid or gas in the esophagus may occur normally in the sedated patient, or from swallowing or eructation during imaging (**fig. 18.2**).

The esophagus is readily visualized on CT and MRI, often containing some fluid or gas due to anesthesia-induced relaxation of the esophageal muscles and sphincters. The portion of the esophagus in the middle mediastinum is typically not visible with ultrasonography due to surrounding aerated lung. The most caudal esophagus is often visible on transdiaphragmatic ultrasound, particularly in smaller patients. The lower esophageal sphincter is normally positioned in the abdomen, caudal to the diaphragm.

Caudal mediastinum

▍ **Vena cava** The caudal vena cava is normally visible on radiographs as a short tubular structure extending from the cardiac margin to the diaphragm. It is ventral to the caudal esophagus and superimposed on the accessory lung lobe. The caudal vena cava is readily visualized on CT and MRI and can usually be seen traversing the diaphragm via abdominal ultrasonography.

▍ **Caudal mediastinal reflection** The parietal pleurae bounding the mediastinum are oriented in a median sagittal plane. However, in the caudal thorax the pleurae deviate to the left to

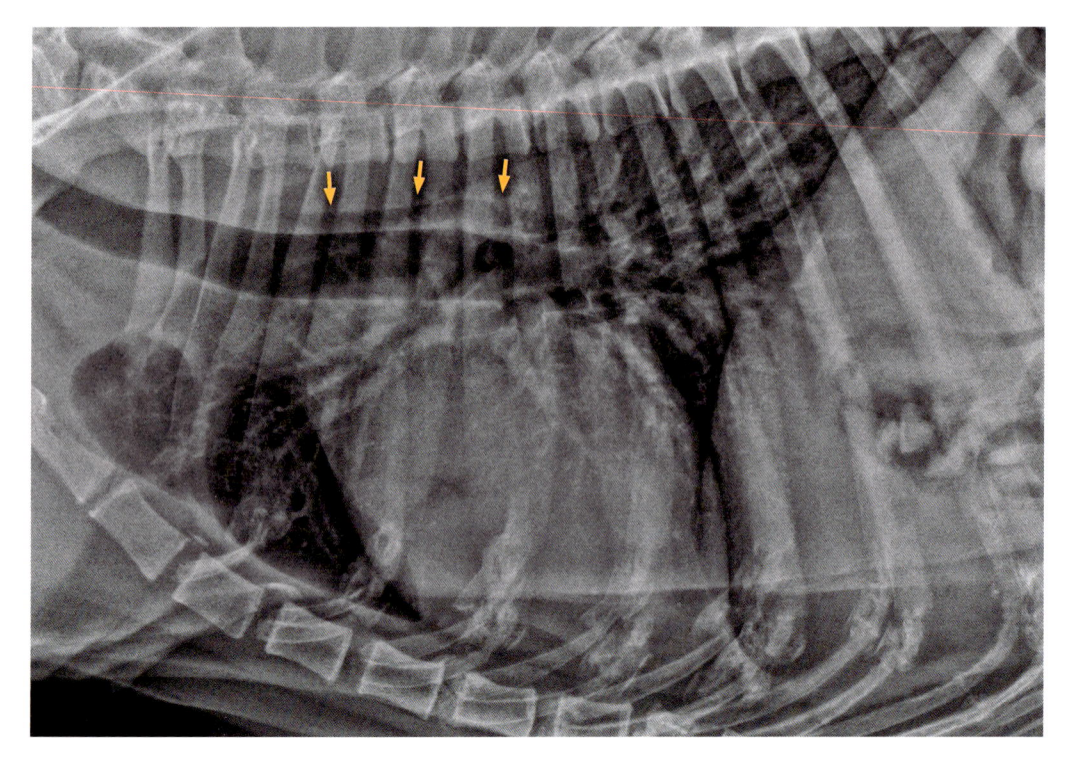

Fig. 18.2 Right lateral radiograph of the thorax of a ten-year-old Labrador Retriever showing a small amount of gas in the thoracic esophagus (arrows). This gas was seen only on one projection and is incidental, secondary to sedation or swallowing.

accommodate the accessory lung lobe and wrap around the caudal vena cava. This creates a thin, soft tissue band extending from the cardiac apex to the cupola of the diaphragm, in the left caudal thorax on dorsoventral or ventrodorsal radiographs. This normal structure may become widened with mediastinal effusions, infiltrative disease, or inflammation and in morbidly obese patients.

▌ Mediastinal serous cavity The mediastinal serous cavity is a potential space bordered by a thin serous membrane that lies to the right of the esophagus in the caudodorsal mediastinum. It is derived from the greater omentum and does not normally communicate with the rest of the mediastinum. This structure is not visible on any imaging modality in the normal patient.

Imaging modalities

Radiography

Radiography is the most common imaging modality utilized for evaluation of the mediastinum: it is accessible, reasonably priced, and relatively easy to perform while providing good anatomic detail of the major mediastinal structures. The contrast provided by the adjacent air-filled lungs aids in recognition of mediastinal pathology. Radiography, however, does have several limitations. Since most of the mediastinal structures are soft tissue opaque, natural contrast within the mediastinum is poor, often inhibiting precise localization of pathology. The mediastinum is normally a very narrow space and differentiating mediastinal from pulmonary or cardiac pathology can also be difficult due to superimposition.[4] Radiography is generally a good screening tool to identify mediastinal pathology, but more detailed information may be needed to precisely localize and characterize lesions.

Computed tomography

CT provides better differentiation of mediastinal structures by removing the problem of superimposition and improving contrast resolution. In dogs and cats CT often provides more precise localization and diagnosis of mediastinal pathology.[5] CT of the thorax, including the mediastinum, is best performed with the patient under general anesthesia using breath holds to prevent respiratory motion artifact.

Ultrasound

Ultrasound can be a useful tool for evaluating some portions of the mediastinum. The cranial mediastinum can be assessed from a thoracic inlet approach as well as from a lateral-parasternal approach (similar to echocardiography).[6] From these positions the region of the thymus, heart base, and cranial mediastinal lymph nodes can be assessed. The most caudal portion of the mediastinum can usually be assessed from a subxyphoid transdiaphragmatic approach. The caudal esophagus and lower esophageal sphincter as well as fluid, masses, diaphragmatic hernias, or other pathology in the caudal mediastinum can be visualized from this position. In very large or obese patients, mediastinal visibility with this approach may be limited by depth or fat. The remainder of the mediastinum, particularly the mid-dorsal mediastinum, cannot be assessed by ultrasound in patients with normally aerated lungs due to the gas interference.

Magnetic resonance imaging

MRI can provide high contrast images of the mediastinum, but the utility of this modality is usually limited by respiratory motion and little information regarding the use of MRI in imaging of the mediastinum has been reported in the veterinary literature. It is worth noting that portions of the mediastinum are often included in MRI imaging of the vertebral column, a relatively common procedure, and careful attention to this portion of the image may result in unexpected but clinically relevant findings (**fig. 18.3**).

SECTION IV THORAX

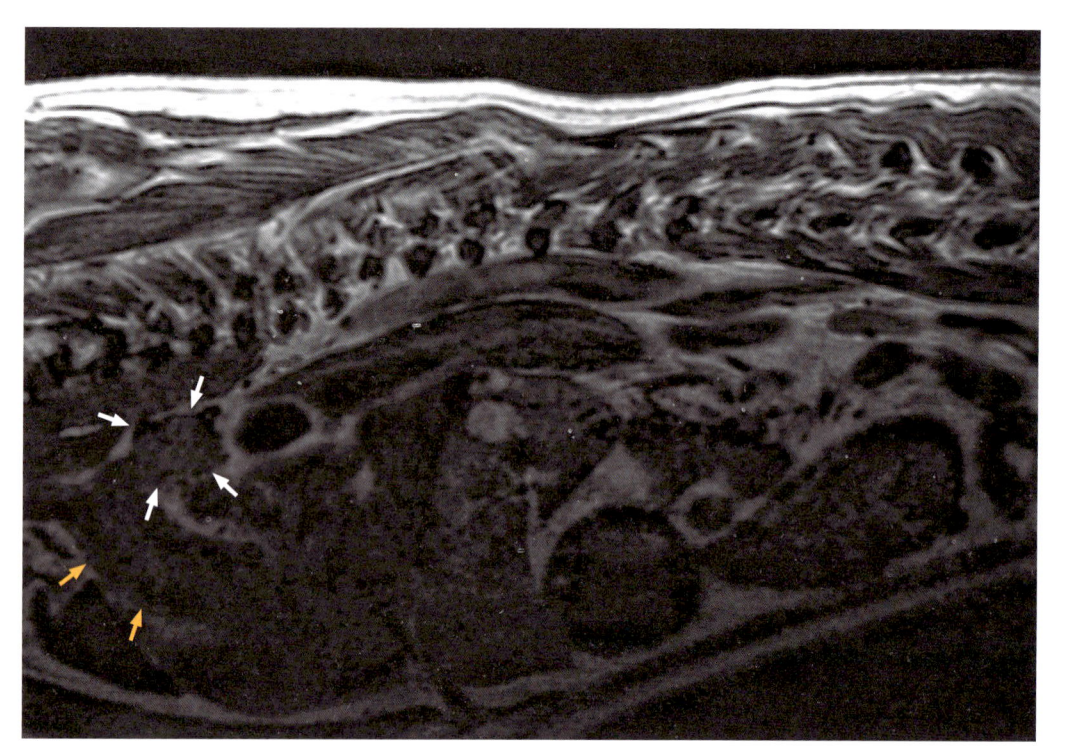

Fig. 18.3 Sagittal T1 pre-contrast MRI of a seven-year-old Bulldog showing a small heart base mass (white arrows) adjacent to the aortic root (orange arrows). A heart base mass, suspected to be a chemodectoma, was confirmed on echocardiogram. This was identified incidentally while imaging the vertebral column for suspected discospondylitis.

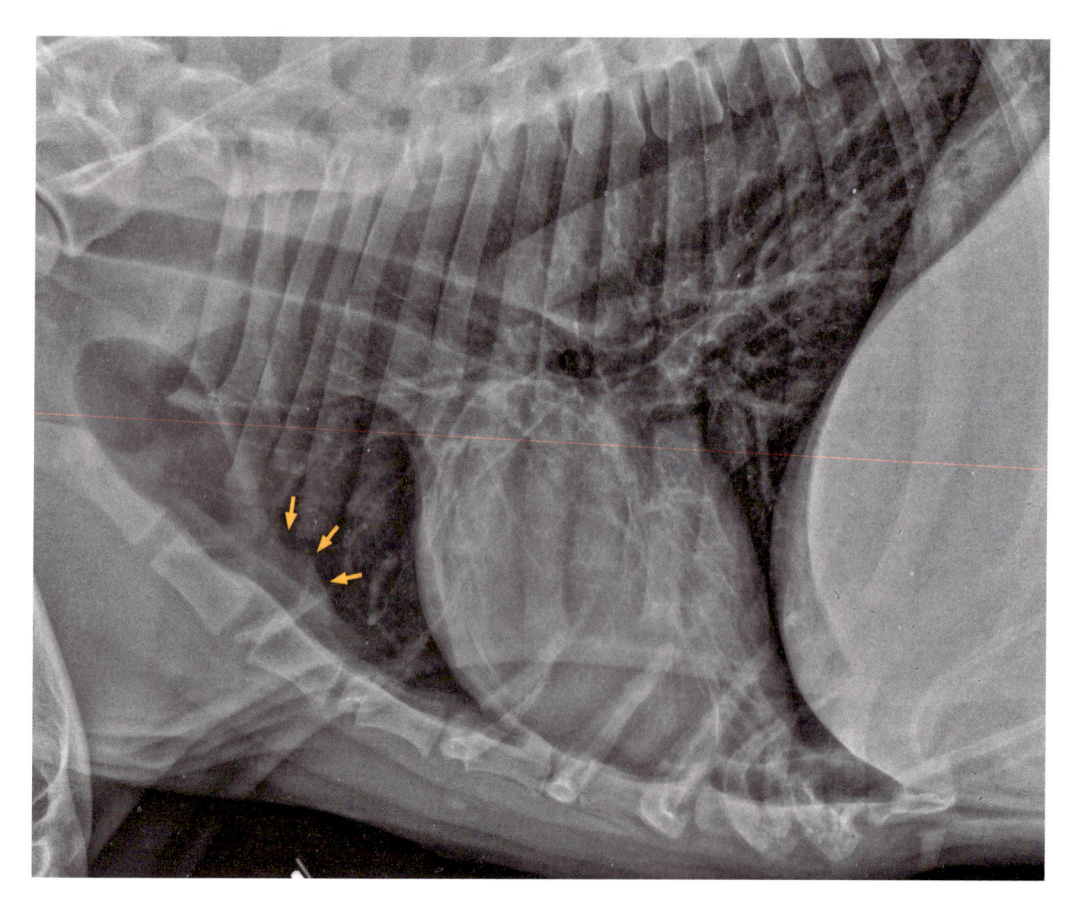

Fig. 18.4 Right lateral radiographic projection of a five-year-old Weimaraner showing an enlarged sternal lymph node (arrows). There is concurrent decreased peritoneal serosal detail and abdominal distention. The patient was diagnosed with hemoabdomen and a splenic tumor.

Contrast studies and fluoroscopy

Contrast radiography is a useful technique for evaluating the esophagus. The administration of barium or iodinated contrast material improves visualization of the course of the esophagus as well as providing information about esophageal dilation or stricture and mucosal disruptions. Fluoroscopy with contrast provides similar information, but additionally allows real-time evaluation of esophageal peristalsis and movement of fluid and food boluses. Information on the technical aspects of performing contrast studies is covered in chapter 25. Fluoroscopy is also a useful tool for real-time evaluation of the trachea, carina, and other respiratory structures.

Mediastinal masses

Cranial mediastinum

Cranial mediastinal masses commonly arise from the regional lymph nodes, thymus, or heart base. Masses from these origins will appear as an abnormal or increased soft tissue opacity in the cranioventral mediastinum on lateral radiographic projections and widening of the mediastinum on dorsoventral or ventrodorsal projections. Large masses may cause dorsal deviation of the trachea and caudal deviation of the heart. Border effacement with the cranial margin of the heart is common. The presence of pleural or mediastinal fluid can obscure cranial mediastinal masses and if the mass is large or slightly off midline, it can be difficult to distinguish between a mediastinal or pulmonary origin. Cranial mediastinal masses have a more variable appearance on CT and ultrasound, as detailed below, but the appearance of a mass effect will be similar.

▎ **Sternal and cranial mediastinal lymphadenopathy** Enlarged sternal lymph nodes (fig. 18.4) are visible on radiography as a soft tissue structure with a discrete convex dorsal margin dorsal to the second to third sternebral segments. Enlarged sternal lymph nodes are apparent in a similar location on cross-sectional imaging modalities and can often be visualized on ultrasound with a parasternal approach. The sternal lymph nodes receive lymphatic drainage from the peritoneal cavity, and thus are a common site of reactive inflammation or metastasis from abdominal disease. The sternal lymph nodes also drain the thymus, ribs, and thoracic body wall muscles.[7,8] Round cell neoplasms are the most common primary conditions in patients with sternal lymphadenopathy. Hemoabdomen from hemangiosarcoma has also been reported as a common cause of sternal lymphadenopathy in dogs. Whether this is due to metastatic disease or reactivity secondary to the hemoabdomen is unknown, but in some cases the sternal lymphadenopathy has been reported to resolve after resolution of the hemoabdomen. Cats may be more likely to have a primary inflammatory condition, with feline infectious peritonitis (FIP) being a common etiology.[8] In general, enlarged sternal lymph nodes should prompt evaluation for abdominal/peritoneal disease as well as systemic inflammatory conditions and round cell neoplasms. Mild cranial mediastinal lymph node enlargement appears as increased soft tissue opacity ventral to the trachea. Soft tissues ventral to the trachea usually have a concave outline which may become convex with lymph node enlargement. More severe cranial mediastinal lymphadenopathy has a similar appearance to other cranial mediastinal masses as described above. Enlarged cranial mediastinal lymph nodes will be readily visualized on CT ventral to the trachea and adjacent to the cranial vena cava, jugular veins, and brachiocephalic trunk. Cranial mediastinal lymph node enlargement can be visualized on ultrasound from a thoracic inlet or parasternal approach.

The cranial mediastinal lymph nodes receive lymphatic drainage from numerous structures of the mediastinum, thoracic wall and pleura, abdominal wall (but not the peritoneal cavity), and cervical region as well as from other thoracic lymph nodes.[2] Evaluation of cranial mediastinal lymph nodes is warranted in patients with round cell neoplasia, particularly those with multicentric lymphoma as cranial mediastinal involvement in these patients is a negative prognostic indicator.[9] Other considerations for enlarged cranial mediastinal lymph nodes include other metastatic neoplasia and systemic mycotic infection.

■ **Thymic epithelial tumors and lymphoma** Thymic epithelial tumors and lymphoma are the most common causes of cranial mediastinal masses in dogs and cats.[10] Thymic epithelial tumor is an umbrella term that encompasses thymomas, atypical thymomas, and thymic carcinomas. Lymphoma may arise from the thymus, remnant thymic tissue, or any of the regional lymph nodes. Thymic epithelial tumors and lymphoma are difficult to differentiate based on imaging alone; however, some features have been identified that may increase specificity for tumor type. When compared to lymphoma, thymic epithelial tumors are more likely to have two or more discrete margins on lateral radiographic projections and cause rightward shift of the cardiac silhouette on dorsoventral or ventrodorsal projections (**figs. 18.5** and **18.6**).[11] Thymic epithelial tumors are typically more heterogeneous on pre- and post-contrast CT images (**fig. 18.7**) and more commonly exhibit cystic cavitation and heterogeneity on ultrasound images, while lymphoma is more typically homogeneous on CT, lacks cavitations on ultrasound, and is more likely to encircle the vena cava.[10,12]

Myasthenia gravis, which can lead to megaesophagus, is sometimes a paraneoplastic syndrome seen in both dogs and cats with thymic epithelial tumors. Megaesophagus has been reported in up to 40% of dogs with thymic epithelial tumors. The presence of concurrent megaesophagus should increase the suspicion of thymic epithelial neoplasia in a patient with a cranial mediastinal mass. Pleural effusion is present in about half of both dogs and cats with mediastinal lymphoma (**fig. 18.8**).[13,14] Other non-imaging findings that may increase suspicion for lymphoma in patients with cranial mediastinal masses include FeLV infection in cats and hypercalcemia in dogs.

■ **Other neoplasia** Tumors that occur at the heart base are also contained within the cranial mediastinum. The most common heart base tumors are chemodectomas, arising from the aortic body (**fig. 18.9**). These tumors are most common in brachycephalic breeds and can be an incidental finding. Radiography is a specific but insensitive imaging modality for evaluating heart base tumors.[15] Unless very large, heart base masses are often difficult to delineate due to border effacement with the cardiac silhouette. Secondary radiographic signs suggestive of a heart base mass include enlargement of the cardiac silhouette, ill-defined increased soft tissue opacity and mediastinal widening at the dorsocranial margin of the heart, and focal dorsal and/or rightward deviation of the distal trachea. Cross-sectional imaging improves visualization of heart base masses by removing superimposition. Heart base tumors are typically mildly heterogeneous on pre- and post-contrast CT images and may invade adjacent vasculature (e.g., cranial vena cava) as well as displacing the trachea, esophagus, or vasculature.[16] Heart base tumors can also be identified on echocardiography.

Many other tumor types may occur in the cranial mediastinum, but all are rare. Reported cranial mediastinal neoplasms include ectopic thyroid carcinoma, neuroendocrine tumor, anaplastic carcinoma, fibroma, lipoma, and a variety of non-lymphoid sarcomas.[17]

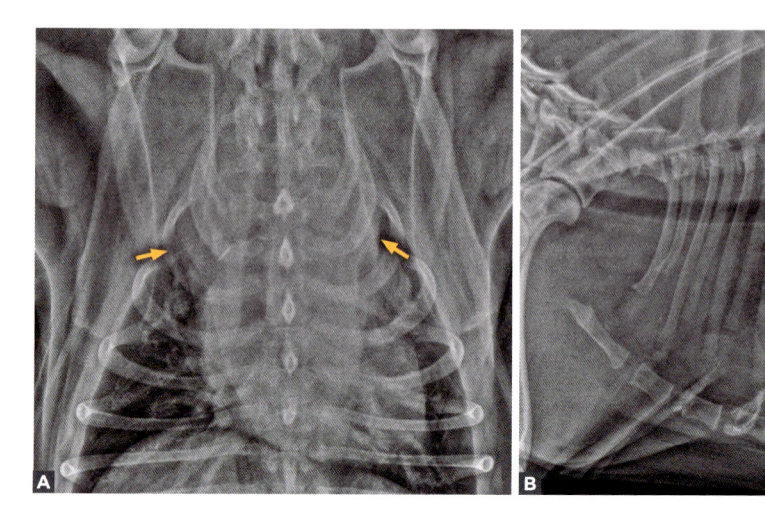

Fig. 18.5 Dorsoventral (**A**) and right lateral (**B**) thoracic projections of a seven-year-old Boxer with an ill-defined cranial mediastinal mass causing marked widening of the cranial mediastinum (arrows) and elevation of the trachea. The cranial cardiac margin is obscured by the mass. This patient was diagnosed with lymphoma.

CHAPTER 18 Mediastinum

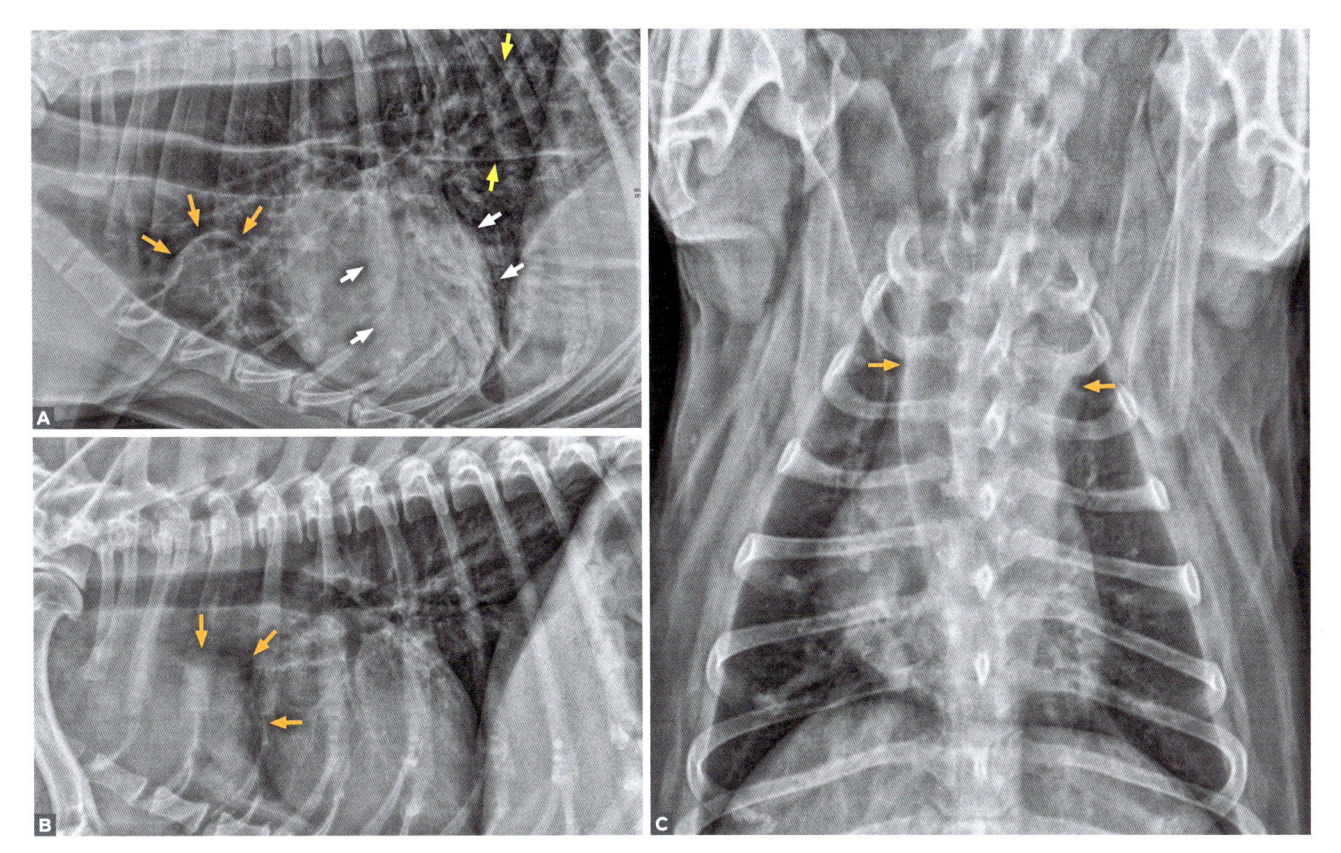

Fig. 18.6 (**A**) Left lateral projection of a nine-year-old mixed breed dog with a small thymoma (orange arrows) and concurrent megaesophagus (yellow arrows). An alveolar lung pattern is present in the right middle lung lobe indicating this patient also has aspiration pneumonia (white arrows). (**B**) Right lateral projection of a twelve-year-old mixed breed dog with a moderately large thymoma (arrows). This mass has relatively distinct dorsal and caudal margins. (**C**) Dorsoventral projection of the same patient in B showing widening of the cranial mediastinum (arrows).

Fig. 18.7 Transverse (**A**) and sagittal (**B**) plane, post-contrast CT images of the thorax of a ten-year-old Golden Retriever showing a thymoma in the cranial mediastinum (orange arrows). The mass is heterogeneously attenuating due to numerous small cystic cavitations. This thymoma is not large enough to cause deviation of the trachea or heart. Megaesophagus is not present in this patient (white arrows).

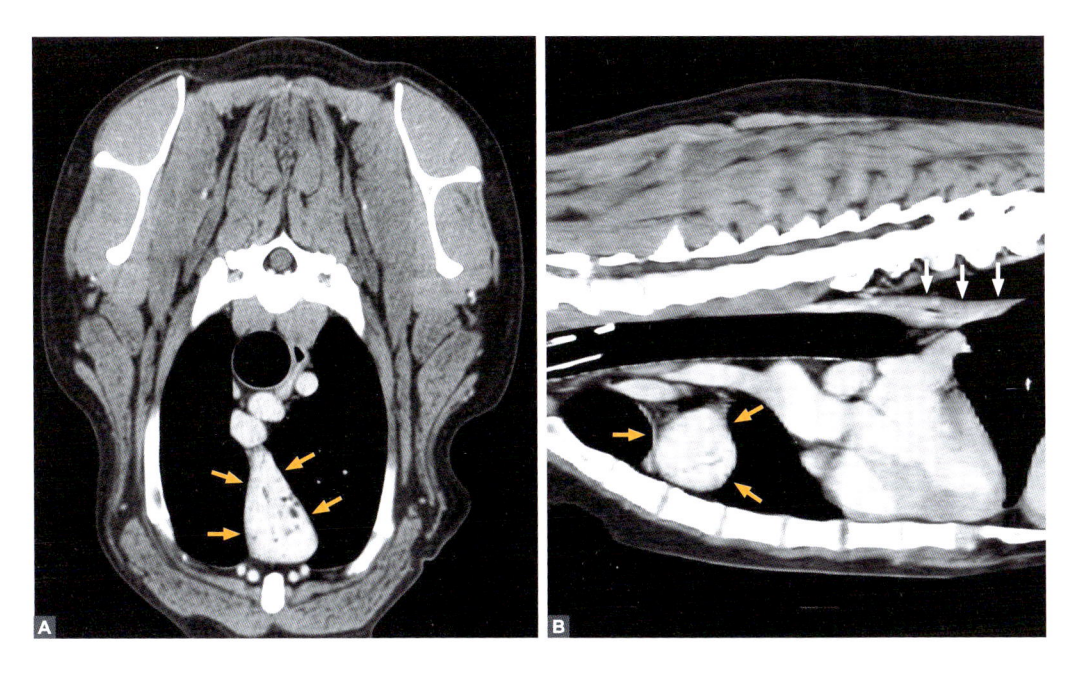

249

SECTION IV THORAX

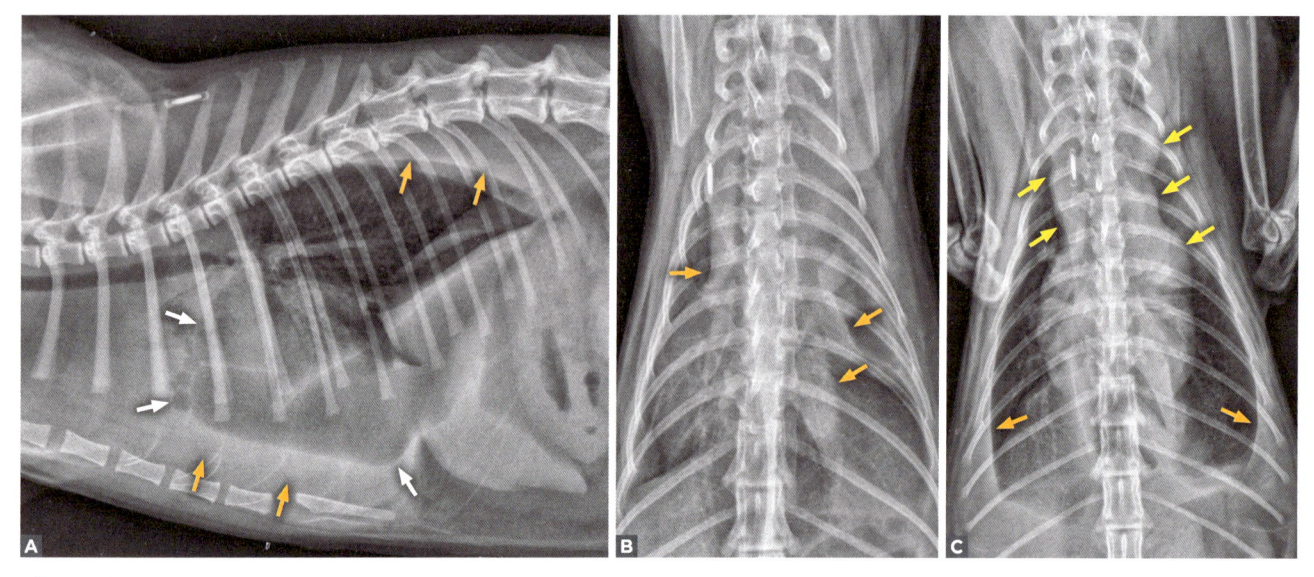

Fig. 18.8 Right lateral (A), dorsoventral (B), and ventrodorsal (C) radiographs of a 15-month-old Domestic shorthair cat. On lateral and dorsoventral projections pleural fluid (orange arrows) hampers evaluation of the cranial mediastinum; however, slight caudal displacement of the carina is suspicious for a mediastinal mass. On the ventrodorsal projection a cranial mediastinal mass with undulant borders can be seen (yellow arrows). There is also a moderate volume pneumothorax (white arrows), due to previous thoracocentesis. The patient was diagnosed with lymphoma and tested positive for feline leukemia virus.

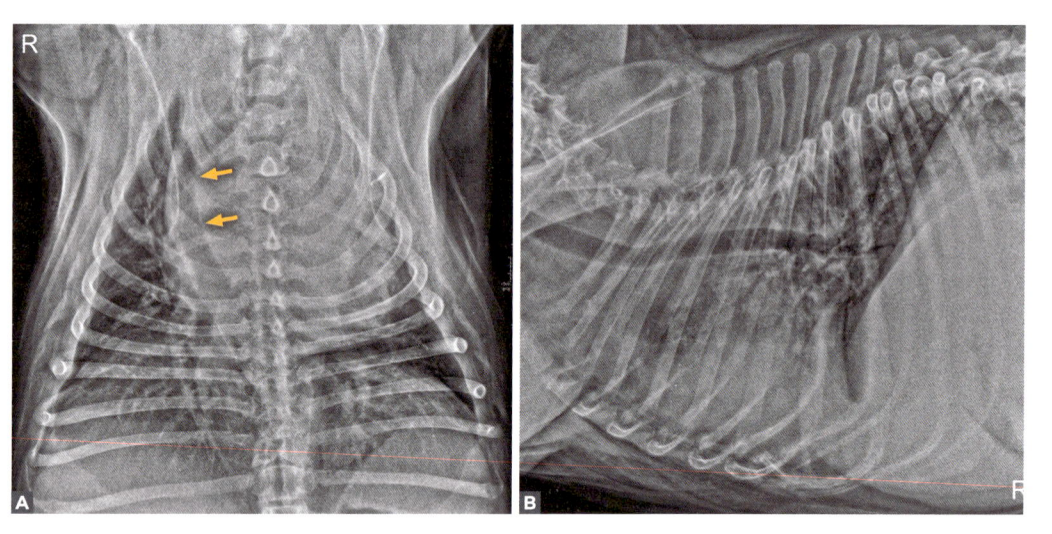

Fig. 18.9 Dorsoventral (A) and right lateral (B) thoracic projections of a ten-year-old English Bulldog with a heart base mass (suspected chemodectoma). The trachea (arrows) is markedly deviated to the right by a large soft tissue opaque mass that causes border effacement with the heart. The mass does not have well-defined margins on the lateral projection.

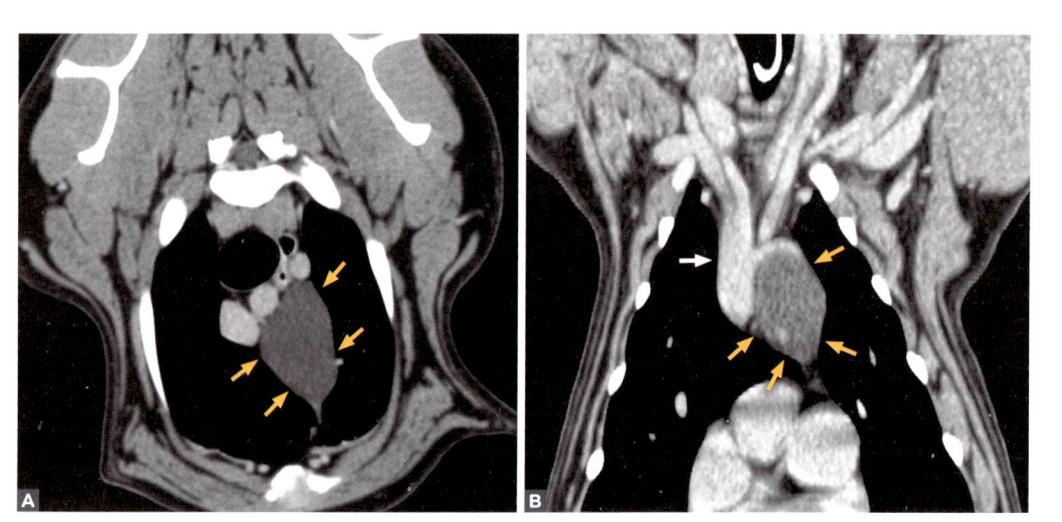

Fig. 18.10 Transverse (A) and dorsal (B) plane post-contrast CT images of an eight-year-old Australian Shepherd with a branchial cyst. The cyst (orange arrows) is non-contrast enhancing. It is positioned immediately cranial to the heart and in close association with the cranial vena cava (white arrow).

▮ **Cysts** Cranial mediastinal cysts (fluid-filled masses lined by epithelial cells) may arise from multiple tissues of origin. Most commonly, these cysts arise from remnant tissues of the middle branchial pouches, thyroglossal duct, or the duct connecting the parathyroid glands and thymic primordium. Despite the embryonic origin of these tissues, cysts are most commonly identified in older animals and are often an incidental finding, although branchial cysts have been associated with respiratory signs.[18] Cysts have also been reported arising from pleural tissue and lymph nodes can sometimes form cyst-like structures (fluid-filled cavities, but not lined by epithelium). Cranial mediastinal cysts have a similar radiographic appearance to other cranial mediastinal masses, often with well-defined borders. On CT and ultrasound these cysts are thin-walled and fluid-filled (**fig. 18.10**). The fluid will be hypoattenuating and non-contrast enhancing on CT and anechoic on ultrasound. Pleural effusion may be seen concurrently with branchial cysts.[18]

Dorsal mediastinum

Masses affecting the dorsal mediastinum typically arise from the tracheobronchial lymph nodes, esophagus, or mediastinal serous cavity. Hiatal and paraesophageal hernias, as well as gastroesophageal intussusception, will also cause a mass effect in the caudal dorsal mediastinum (esophageal pathology will be discussed later in the chapter). Neoplasms of the vertebral column, rib heads, or hypaxial musculature may also extend into the dorsal mediastinum, causing ventral displacement of the heart, trachea, and carina. Masses arising from these components of the dorsal body wall are typically broad based with no defined dorsal margin due to border effacement.

▮ **Tracheobronchial lymphadenopathy** Enlarged tracheobronchial lymph nodes are easily visualized on CT and MRI and can be seen on radiographs as one or more ovoid soft tissue structures dorsal to the carina (**fig. 18.11**). If large enough, they can cause ventral deviation of the carina and caudal lobar bronchi on lateral radiographic projections and widening of the angle between the principal bronchi on ventrodorsal or dorsoventral projections. Tracheobronchial lymphadenopathy is most commonly associated with lymphoma or fungal infections, although other round cell or metastatic neoplasms should also be considered.[19]

▮ **Mediastinal serous cavity** Pathology of the mediastinal serous cavity typically causes distention and will appear as a well-defined mass in the plane of the esophagus on radiographs, typically extending from the carina to the diaphragm (**fig. 18.12**). Due to its normal position to the right of the esophagus, mass effects originating from the mediastinal serous cavity may appear slightly more right-sided on dorsoventral or ventrodorsal projections and left dorsal displacement of the esoph-

Fig. 18.11 Dorsoventral (**A**) and right lateral (**B**) thoracic radiographs of a one-year-old Greyhound. There is a convex soft tissue margin dorsal to the carina on the lateral projection (orange arrows) and mild displacement of the principal bronchi on the dorsoventral projection (yellow arrows) representing enlarged tracheobronchial lymph nodes. A focal bronchointerstitial pulmonary pattern is present in the cranioventral lung (white arrow). The patient was diagnosed with coccidiomycosis.

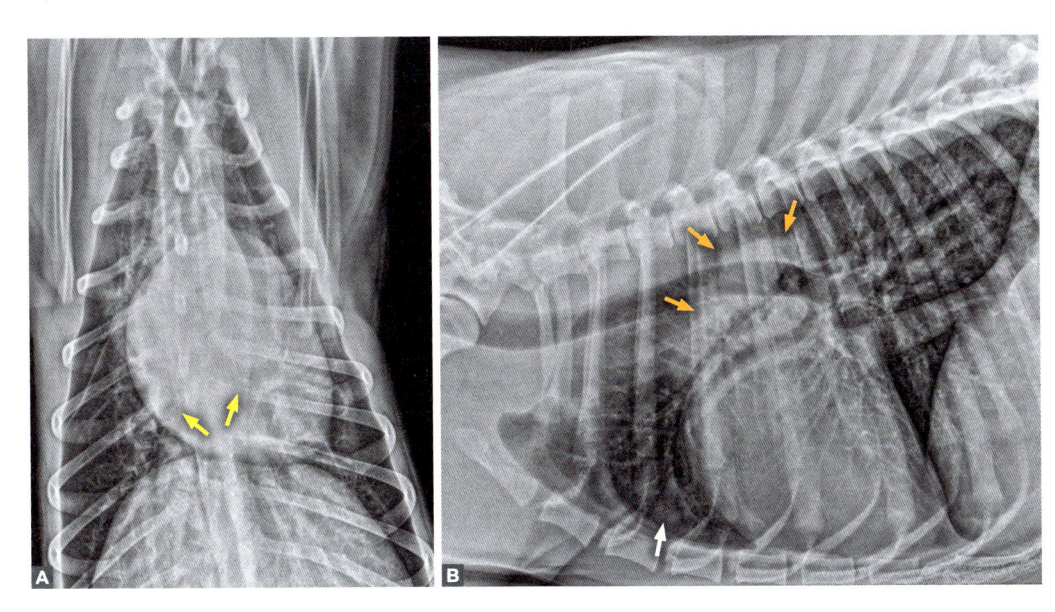

SECTION IV THORAX

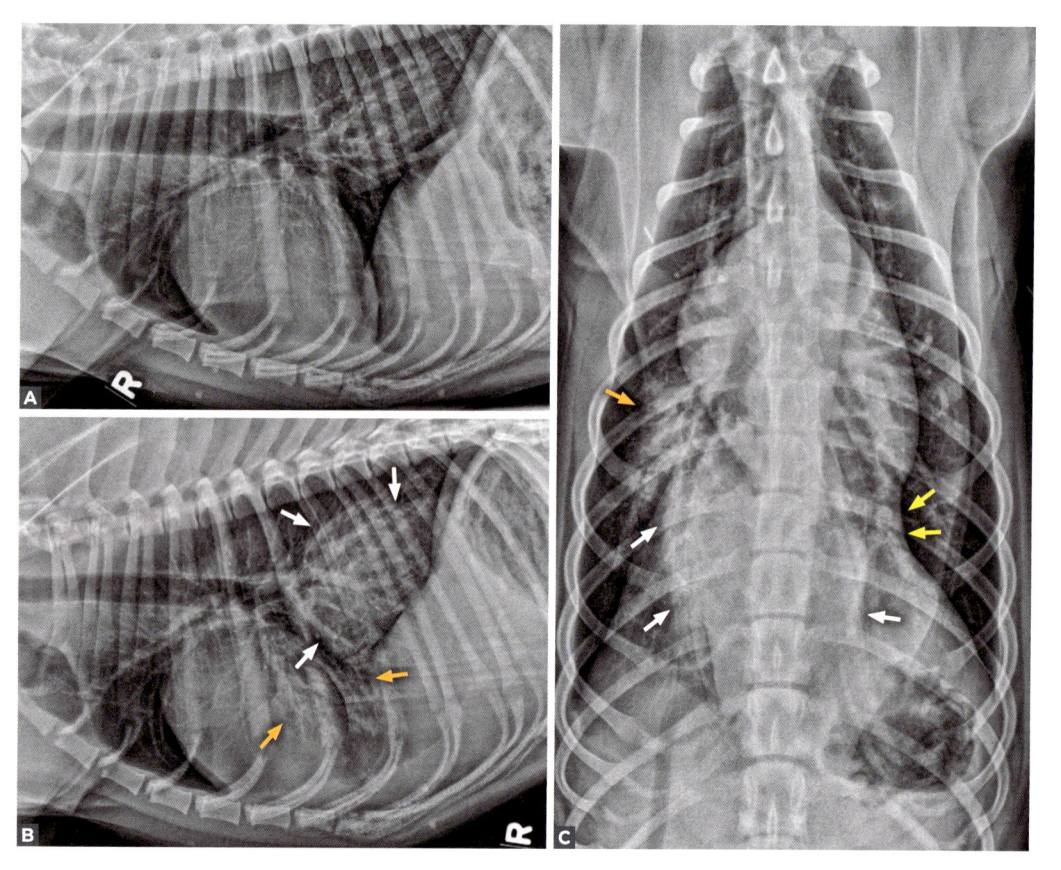

Fig. 18.12 Right lateral (**A-B**) and dorsoventral (**C**) thoracic projections of a ten-month-old Labrador Retriever. The right lateral projection in (**A**) was acquired 5 days prior to the other two projections. (**A**) There is poorly defined increased soft tissue opacity in the caudodorsal mediastinum. (**B-C**) There is a large, soft-tissue opaque mass in the caudal mediastinum (white arrows), slightly to the right of midline and extending to the caudal mediastinal reflection (yellow arrows). There is a patchy alveolar pulmonary pattern affecting the caudal subsegment of the left cranial, right middle, both caudal, and accessory lung lobes (orange arrows). The patient was diagnosed with paraesophageal empyema.

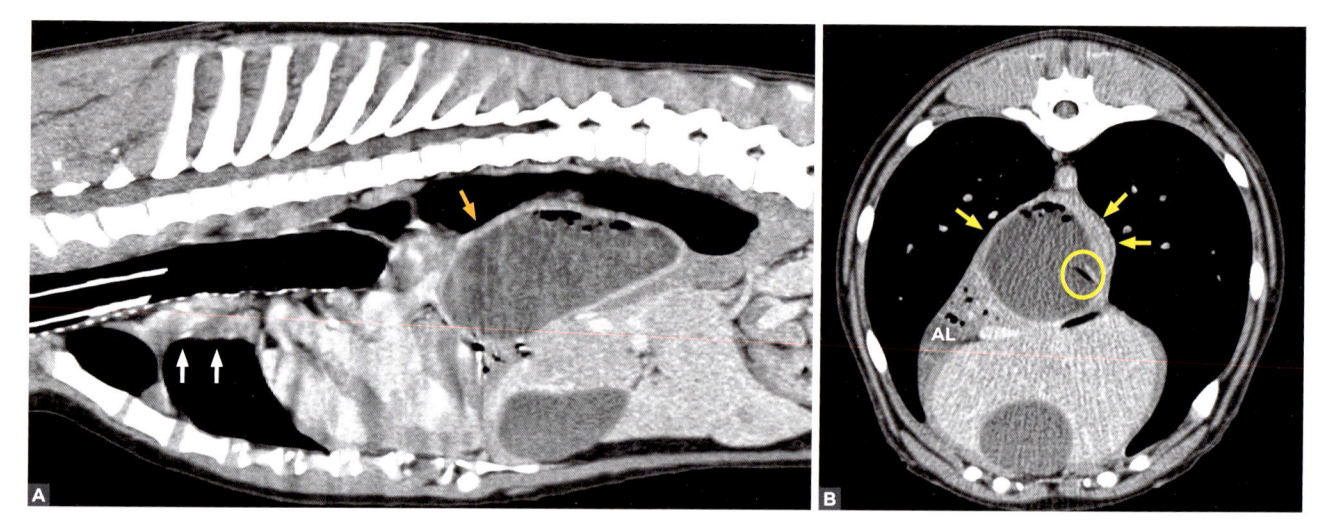

Fig. 18.13 Sagittal (**A**) and transverse (**B**) post-contrast CT images of the same patient as in Figure 18-12. There is a fluid- and gas-filled mass bounded by a contrast enhancing rim of tissue in the right caudodorsal mediastinum (orange arrows). This is consistent with empyema of the mediastinal serous cavity. A hyperattenuating object is also seen at the left ventral margin of the mass (yellow circle), which was found to be a grass awn at surgery. Concurrent broncho pneumonia, including the accessory lung lobe (AL), and thickened mediastinal adventitia consistent with mediastinitis (white arrows) are also present. The yellow arrows indicate the position off the esophagus.

agus may be appreciated if a contrast esophagram is performed. On CT, masses or effusions in the mediastinal serous cavity usually have well defined borders limited by the normal serous membrane and can be differentiated from esophageal masses.

The most common pathology affecting the mediastinal serous cavity is empyema, also known as paraesophageal abscessation. Paraesophageal abscess/empyema appears on CT as a fluid-filled structure in the caudal mediastinum, to the right of and ventral to the esophagus, and bounded by thickened, contrast-enhancing walls (fig. 18.13).[20] Paraesophageal empyema has been reported in both dogs and cats and is frequently associated with adjacent pyogranulomatous pneumonia. Pleural and/or mediastinal effusion may also be seen. Paraesophageal empyema has been associated with migrating grass awns and other plant materials and rarely with esophageal perforation.

Mesothelioma of the mediastinal serous cavity has also been reported. On CT this appears as a well-defined, fluid-filled structure in the caudal dorsal mediastinum with frond-like projections of contrast-enhancing tissue extending into the fluid from the peripheral serous membrane.[20]

Caudoventral mediastinum

Caudoventral mediastinal masses are rare in both dogs and cats. Abscesses or granulomas are most common. Metastatic neoplasia is also occasionally seen. On radiographs masses in the caudoventral mediastinum can be difficult to differentiate from pulmonary masses, especially masses of the accessory lung lobe, which crosses midline and surrounds the caudal vena cava. In fact, caudal thoracic masses, regardless of lateral or midline location, are statistically more likely to be pulmonary in origin than mediastinal.[4] Diaphragmatic masses, hernias, or eventrations may also cause a mass effect in the caudoventral mediastinum (diaphragmatic pathology is discussed in chapter 17). Caudal mediastinal masses are often visible on ultrasound by a transdiaphragmatic abdominal approach but remain difficult to differentiate from accessory lung lobe masses. Differentiation of caudal mediastinal masses from pulmonary masses is vastly improved with CT.

Abscesses and granulomas

Abscesses and granulomas can be seen in all regions of the mediastinum and may be due to a variety of etiologies, including migrating or penetrating foreign material and systemic fungal infections. Abscesses and granulomas will appear similar to other mediastinal masses on radiographs but may be accompanied by mediastinal and/or pleural effusion, leading to border effacement (fig. 18.14).

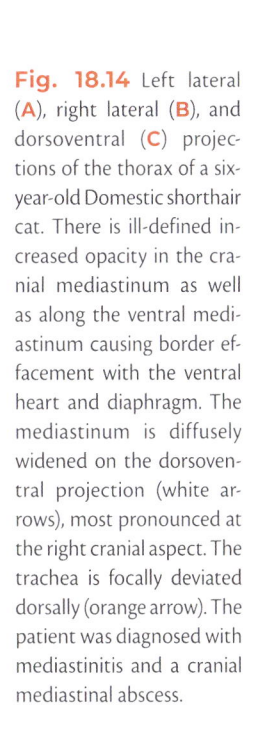

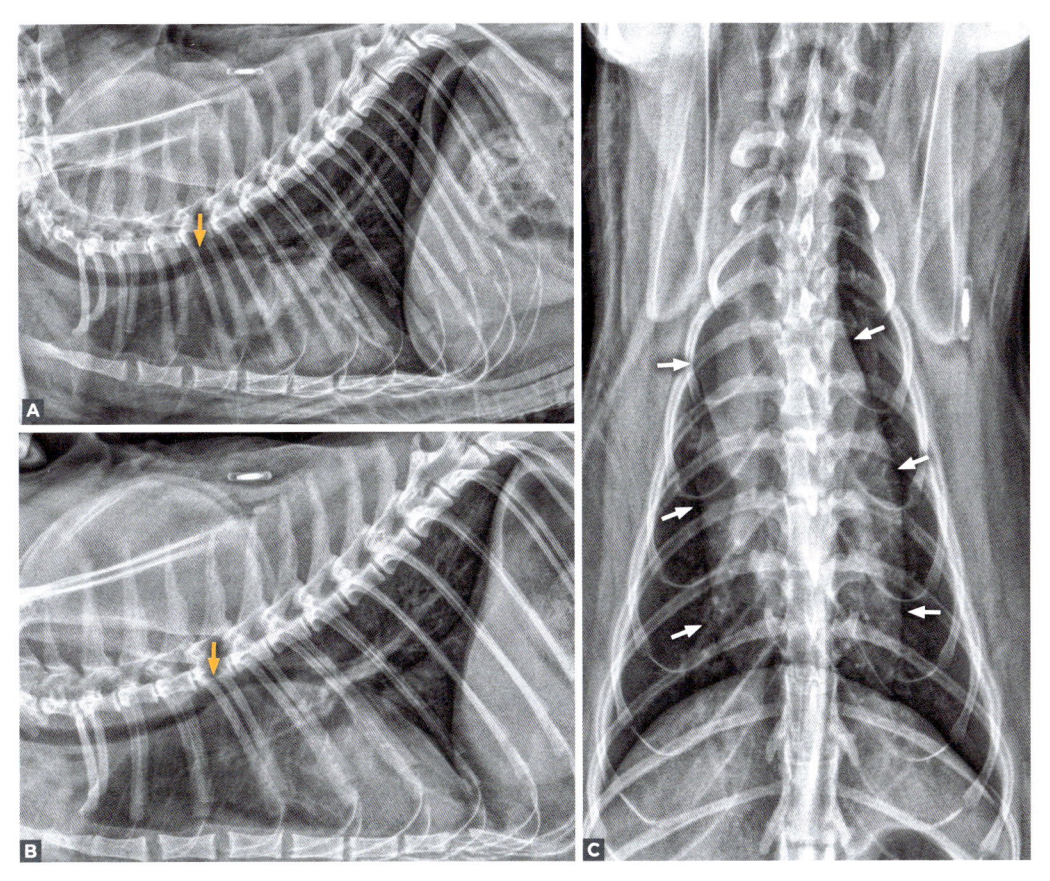

Fig. 18.14 Left lateral (A), right lateral (B), and dorsoventral (C) projections of the thorax of a six-year-old Domestic shorthair cat. There is ill-defined increased opacity in the cranial mediastinum as well as along the ventral mediastinum causing border effacement with the ventral heart and diaphragm. The mediastinum is diffusely widened on the dorsoventral projection (white arrows), most pronounced at the right cranial aspect. The trachea is focally deviated dorsally (orange arrow). The patient was diagnosed with mediastinitis and a cranial mediastinal abscess.

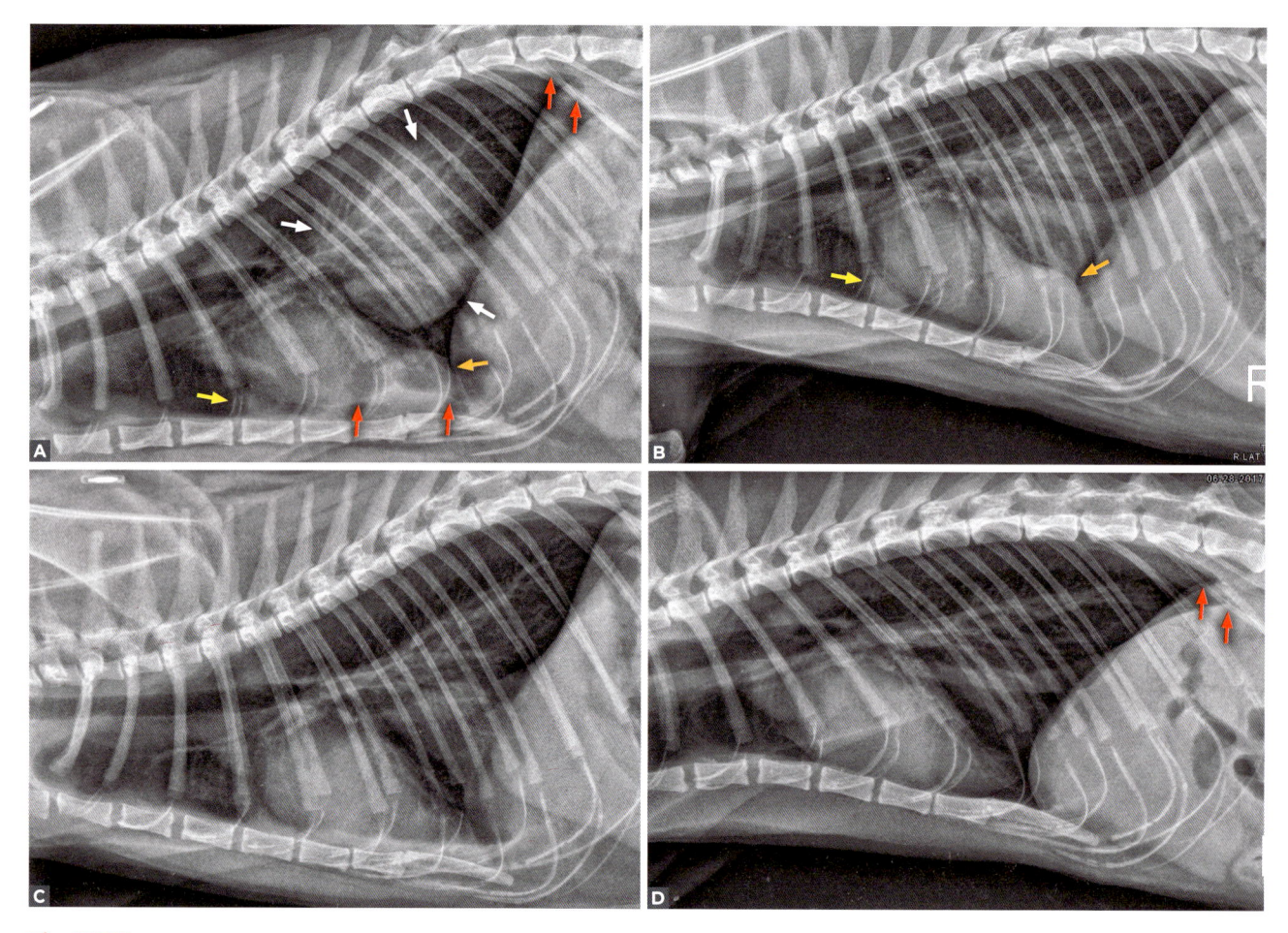

Fig. 18.15 Right lateral thoracic radiographs of a five-to-seven-year-old Domestic shorthair cat at initial diagnosis (A) and at various time points (B-D) following diagnosis with cryptococcosis. At diagnosis (A) a large soft tissue mass is seen in the caudodorsal mediastinum (white arrows), and a smaller mass is seen in the caudoventral mediastinum causing border effacement with the heart (orange arrow). A small amount of amorphous soft tissue opacity is seen at the cranioventral margin of the heart (yellow arrow). There is also mild retraction of the lung lobes indicating pleural effusion (red arrows). After two months (B) the larger mass is slightly smaller and more ill-defined while the ventral mass (orange arrow) appears larger and there is a more definitive nodule cranial to the heart (yellow arrow). At eleven months (C) all the masses have decreased in size and minimal to no pleural effusion is appreciated. At thirty months (D) there is ill-defined soft tissue opacity caudal to the heart, but discrete masses are no longer seen. There is mild persistent retraction of the caudodorsal tips of the lung (red arrows) which may indicate scant pleural fluid or fat deposition.

On ultrasound or CT abscesses will typically appear fluid-filled centrally (though the fluid may be more echogenic and attenuating than cystic fluid) with thick walls that contrast-enhance on CT. Gas may be seen within abscesses, appearing as lucent foci on radiographs, hyperechoic foci that cast a dirty shadow on ultrasound, and negatively attenuating foci on CT. Migrating foreign material, such as sticks or grass awns can occasionally be seen on CT, appearing as linear hyperattenuating structures.

Systemic fungal infections may involve the regional lymph nodes as well as causing discrete granulomatous masses, particularly in the caudal mediastinum. The most common fungal infection to present this way is cryptococcosis in cats, which often causes multiple mediastinal masses along with pleural effusion and pulmonary lesions (figs. 18.15 and 18.16).[21] Other infections that may cause primary granulomatous mediastinal masses include *Histoplasma* spp., *Blastomyces* spp., and atypical bacteria including *Actinomyces* spp. and *Nocardia* spp.[22-24]

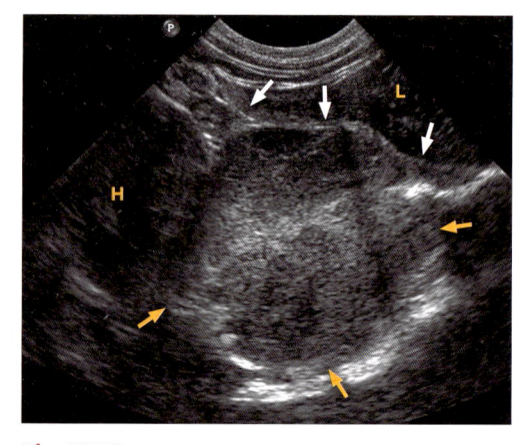

Fig. 18.16 Transdiaphragmatic ultrasound image of the largest mass (orange arrows) in the same patient as in fig. 18.15. The mass is hyperechoic to liver (L) and heart (H) and mildly heterogeneous. The mass abuts and slightly displaces the diaphragm causing an atypical undulant margin (white arrows).

Diffuse mediastinal conditions

Mediastinitis

Mediastinitis may occur with or without mediastinal abscesses and is caused by similar etiologies including penetrating trauma, esophageal perforation, migrating foreign material, and fungal infections. Mediastinitis is often associated with pyothorax and pleural effusion.[25] In addition to fluid, mediastinitis usually causes thickening of the mediastinal pleura and/or adventitia. This may appear as irregular and asymmetric mediastinal borders on radiography, with thickened, contrast enhancing tissue and wispy or dependent fluid visible on CT. Thickened, heterogeneous mediastinal tissue may also be evident on ultrasound.

Mediastinal hemorrhage

The most common cause of mediastinal hemorrhage is anticoagulant rodenticide toxicity, but other coagulopathies, trauma, or neoplasms may also cause mediastinal hemorrhage.

The radiographic signs of mediastinal hemorrhage include generalized increased opacity and widening of the mediastinum, typically most pronounced cranially. The mediastinal widening on dorsoventral and ventrodorsal projections often forms a V-shape cranially, with the most cranial aspect of the mediastinum widest, and narrowing towards the heart (**fig. 18.17**).

Mediastinal hemorrhage associated with anticoagulant rodenticide toxicity or other coagulopathies is often seen concurrently with hemorrhage in other areas, including the pleural space, pulmonary parenchyma, and dorsal tracheal membrane, all of which may be seen on thoracic radiographs.[26] Clinical signs are usually caused by these other sites of hemorrhage (e.g., hemoptysis, tachypnea, or increased respiratory effort) and not directly caused by the mediastinal hemorrhage. If the hemorrhage is severe enough, signs of hypovolemic shock (such as tachycardia and pale mucous membranes) may be seen. Because of communication with the cervical tissues and retroperitoneal space, hemorrhage in these regions may also extend to the mediastinum. Mediastinal hemorrhage caused by trauma is also typically seen with concurrent pleural and pulmonary hemorrhage as well as osseous trauma.

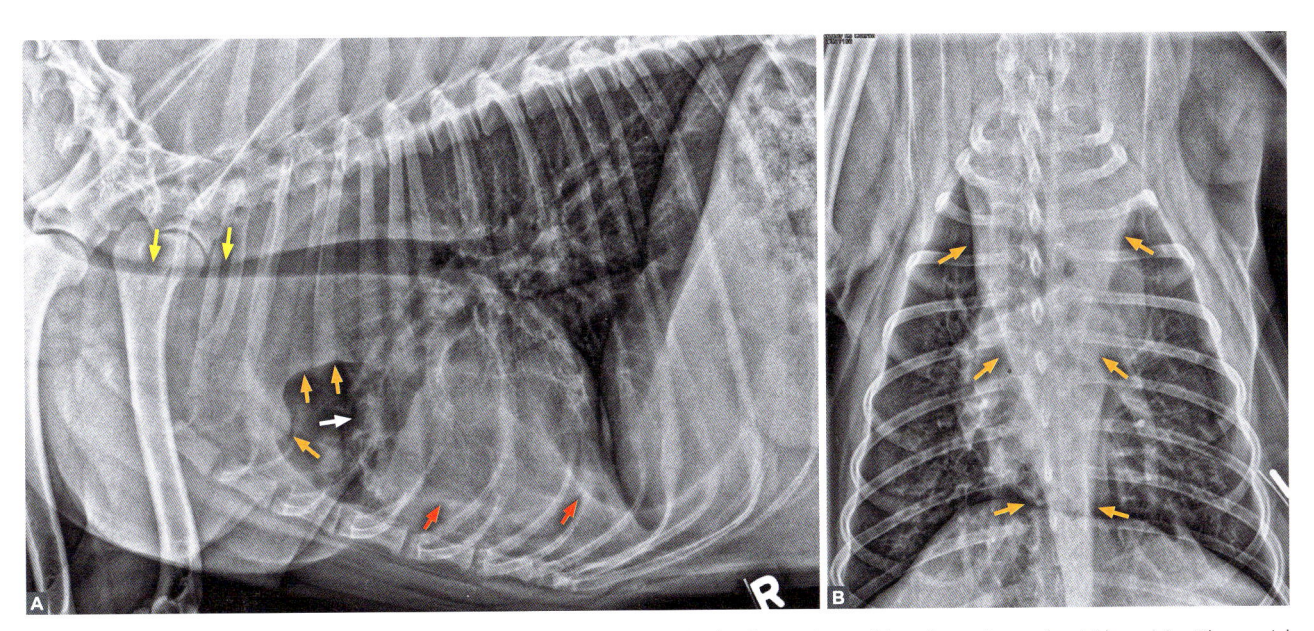

Fig. 18.17 Right lateral (**A**) and dorsoventral (**B**) projections of a six-year-old Labrador Retriever with anticoagulant rodenticide toxicity. The cranial mediastinum is diffusely widened (orange arrows), most pronounced cranially, the dorsal tracheal membrane attenuates the tracheal lumen at the level of the thoracic inlet (yellow arrows), there is slight rounding and retraction of the lung lobes ventrally (red arrows), and there is a focal interstitial pulmonary pattern cranioventrally (white arrow). These findings are consistent with mediastinal, tracheal, pleural, and pulmonary hemorrhage.

Pneumomediastinum

Pneumomediastinum refers to free gas in the mediastinum and radiographic findings are characterized by increased contrast of mediastinal structures. Radiographic signs of pneumomediastinum include increased conspicuity of the great vessels (such as the aorta and its major branches, cranial vena cava, and azygous vein), visibility of the external margins of the trachea, increased conspicuity of the caudal esophagus, and elevation of the cardiac silhouette from the sternum.[27,28] On CT, pneumomediastinum is easily identified by the presence of negatively attenuating gas within the borders and between the structures of the mediastinum.

The most common cause of pneumomediastinum in dogs is trauma, while in cats hyperbaric injury from general anesthesia with endotracheal intubation is the most common etiology.[27,28] Other causes of esophageal or tracheal disruption (including penetrating trauma, erosive neoplasia, and iatrogenic disruption) should be considered (**fig. 18.18**). Alveolar or bronchial injury may cause pneumomediastinum as air tracks along the bronchi and may occur from blunt trauma, positive pressure ventilation/hyperbaric injury, chronic cough, or severe vomiting. Gas tracking from cervical fascial emphysema, either from penetrating trauma, surgical intervention, extrathoracic tracheal injury, or jugular venipuncture (especially in a fractious patient, or when multiple attempts have been made), may also lead to pneumomediastinum. Pneumomediastinum may progress to pneumothorax but pneumomediastinum as a sequel to pneumothorax does not occur.

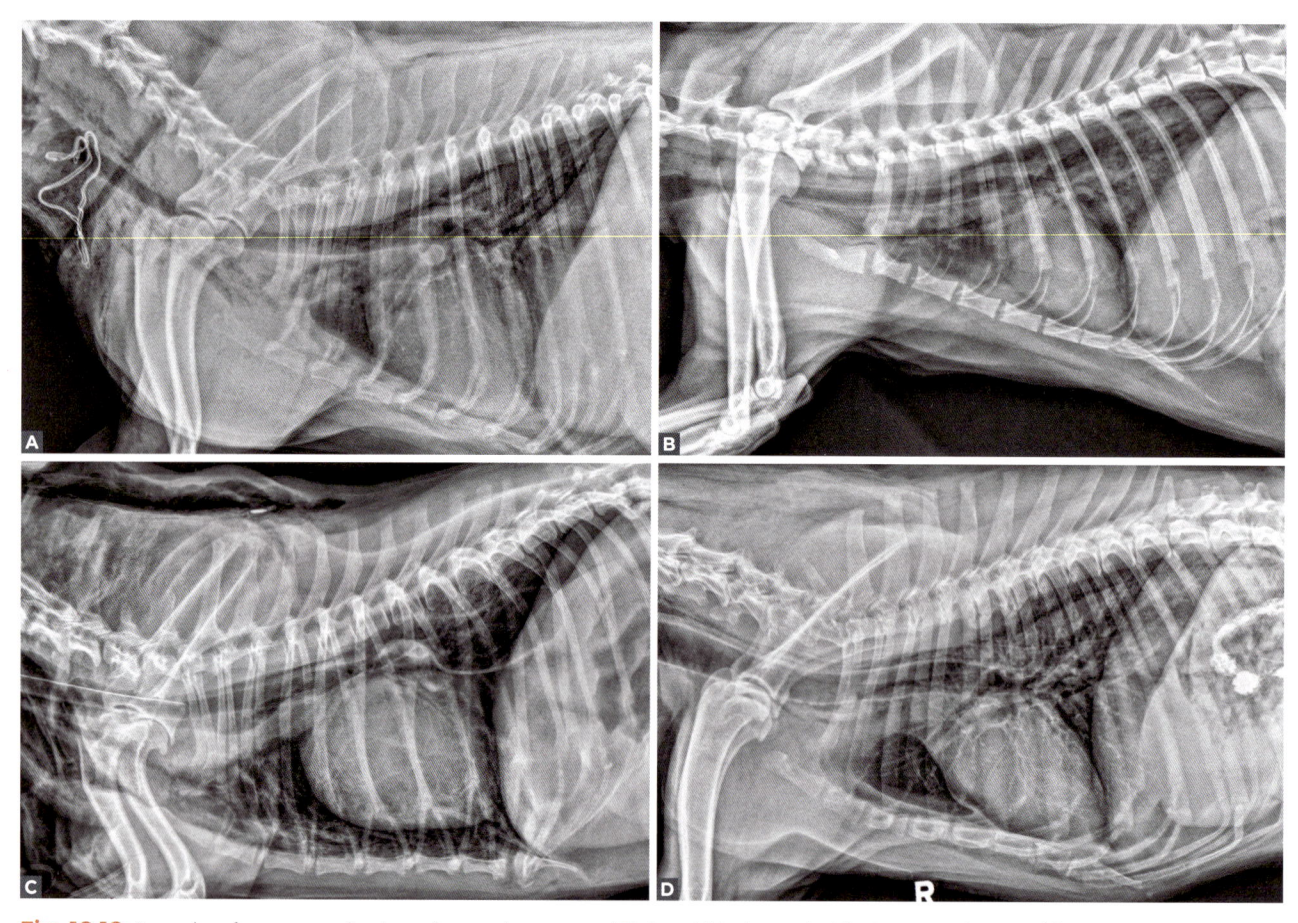

Fig. 18.18 Examples of pneumomediastinum from various causes. (**A**) Gas within the cervical fascia progressing to mild pneumomediastinum in a 15-year-old Boston Terrier with a cervical laceration. (**B**) Moderate pneumomediastinum in a three-year-old Domestic longhair cat following blunt trauma. Gas is also seen along the fascial planes of the neck and extending into the retroperitoneum, outlining the aorta. (**C**) An eleven-year-old Pekingese that developed severe pneumomediastinum and subcutaneous emphysema while under general anesthesia for a dental procedure. Iatrogenic tracheal perforation was suspected. (**D**) Mild pneumomediastinum, cervical gas, and pneumoretroperitoneum in a four-year-old Chow-Cow with a history of previous esophageal stricture treated with balloon dilation. There is also a metallic foreign body in the stomach. On endoscopy there was severe esophagitis in the region of the previous stricture. Esophageal perforation during passage of the foreign body was suspected.

Esophageal diseases

Esophageal contrast studies

Contrast radiography and fluoroscopy are particularly useful tools for evaluating the esophagus. Contrast radiography is indicated when a luminal esophageal mass, esophageal foreign body, vascular ring anomaly, acquired esophageal stricture, or esophageal perforation is suspected. Contrast radiography can be useful in differentiating esophageal masses (in which the contrast typically passes through the mass) from paraesophageal masses (in which the contrast is displaced by the mass). Fluoroscopy is similarly useful for these indications but also provides real-time functional information and is therefore most used in patients with suspected esophageal dysmotility, hiatal herniation, or esophageal stricture. Liquid barium is the preferred contrast agent in most cases; however, if esophageal perforation is suspected non-ionic iodinated contrast, diluted to be isotonic with plasma with water, should be used to avoid the severe inflammatory response that occurs with barium leakage.[29]

Redundant esophagus

The normal esophagus typically follows a relatively straight course between the thoracic inlet and diaphragm; however, in some brachycephalic dogs a U-shaped redundant ventral loop of the esophagus may be present at the thoracic inlet (fig. 18.19). This loop of the esophagus is typically not visible on radiographs, but a crescent-shaped gas pocket is sometimes visible just ventral to the trachea. The deviation of the esophagus is easily seen with contrast radiography or fluoroscopy. While food material, particularly large boluses, may be slightly delayed passing through the loop, a redundant esophageal loop is almost always an incidental finding.

Lower esophageal sphincter abnormalities

Gastroesophageal reflux is a common finding in patients with regurgitation or dysphagia. A small amount of reflux is normal but should be infrequent and rapidly cleared back into the stomach. Gastroesophageal reflux appears as mild widening and increased conspicuity of the caudal esophagus on radiographs (fig. 18.20 and video 18.1). When imaging with videofluoroscopy, liquid or food material is seen to move retrograde from the stomach into the caudal esophagus (fig. 18.21). Frequent instances, large volumes, or prolonged retention of reflux are indications of gastroesophageal reflux disease.

Chalasia of the lower esophageal sphincter is lack of contraction of the lower esophageal sphincter. This results in the sphincter remaining open continuously allowing constant reflux or to-and-fro movement across the sphincter. Radiographic findings will appear similar to gastroesophageal reflux and the open sphincter is typically visible on cross-sectional imaging. Lack of contraction and reflux are best visualized using videofluoroscopy.

VIDEO 18.1 Gastroesophageal reflux

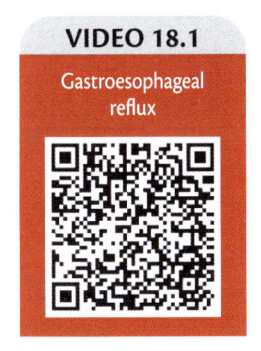

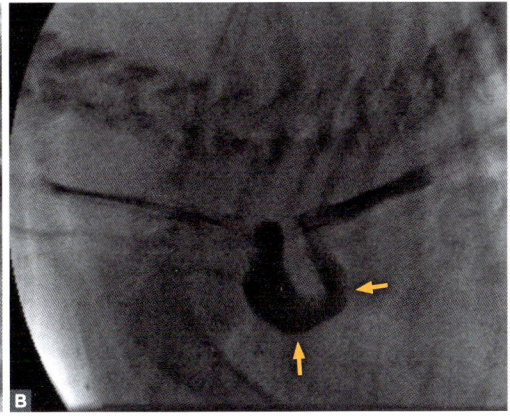

Fig. 18.19 Lateral radiograph (A) and fluoroscopic image (B) showing redundant esophagus (arrows) in a seven-month-old English Bulldog.

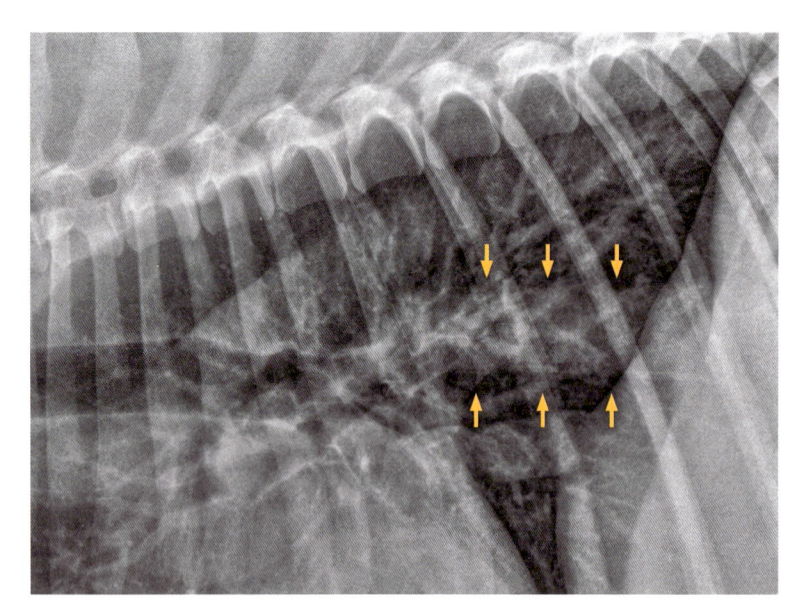

Fig. 18.20 Right lateral thoracic radiograph of a ten-year-old Labrador Retriever showing gastroesophageal reflux. Reflux of fluid into the caudal esophagus causes mild widening and increased opacity of the esophagus caudal to the cardiac base (arrows). This reflux may be secondary to sedation or underlying gastroesophageal reflux disease.

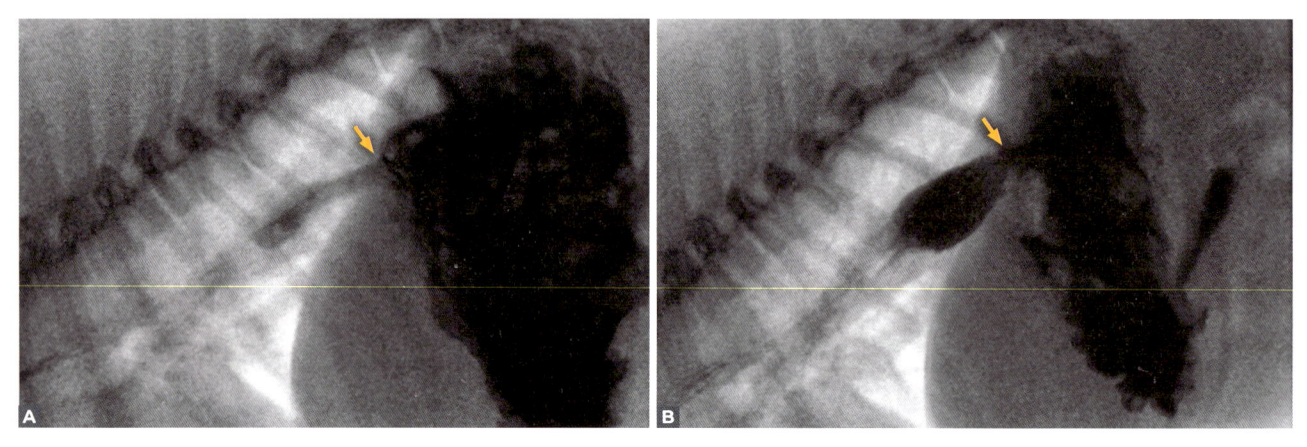

Fig. 18.21 Two fluoroscopic frames showing gastroesophageal reflux in a ten-month-old French Bulldog. Liquid containing positive contrast has moved retrograde from the stomach through the lower esophageal sphincter (arrows) back into the caudal esophagus. The amount of reflux seen in (**A**), if quickly stripped back into the stomach, could be considered normal. However, the large volume of reflux seen in (**B**) is abnormal.

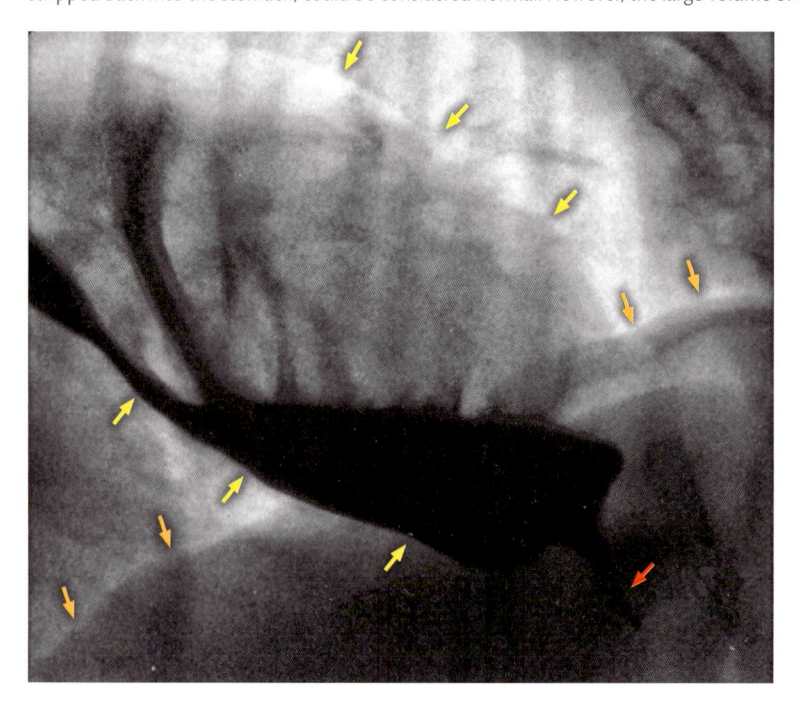

Fig. 18.22 Esophageal achalasia in a 12-year-old Belgian Malinois. The patient is upright resulting in a more vertical orientation of the esophagus. The head is toward the upper left and the diaphragm is indicated by the orange arrows. The lower esophageal sphincter remains tightly contracted despite presentation of a bolus of liquid barium. Only a thin column of liquid is able to pass through (red arrow). Marked esophageal dilation is also present (yellow arrows).

VIDEO 18.2
Chalasia of the lower esophageal sphincter

The lower esophageal sphincter may also exhibit a lack of relaxation or asynchronous relaxation, not appropriately coordinated with bolus presentation.[29] Failure of relaxation of the lower esophageal sphincter is termed achalasia, while inappropriately timed opening is termed dyssynchrony. Achalasia and dyssynchrony of the lower esophageal sphincter result in megaesophagus with retention of fluid, food, and gas, visible on radiographs, cross-sectional imaging, and videofluoroscopy (fig. 18.22 and video 18.2).

Esophageal dysmotility

▍ **Sedation** Most sedatives cause some reduction in esophageal motility leading to mild gas distention and gastroesophageal reflux. For this reason, sedation should be avoided when performing esophageal contrast studies, although small doses of acepromazine may be used with minimal effect on esophageal motility.[29] Mild gas and fluid distention of the esophagus secondary to sedation is frequently seen on thoracic radiographs. These findings are also commonly seen on CT and MRI in patients under general anesthesia.

▍ **Megaesophagus** Generalized megaesophagus is readily apparent on radiographs (fig. 18.23). Most commonly there is gas distention of the esophagus; however, distention with fluid and/or food material are also possible. Severe, gas-filled megaesophagus may cause superimposition of the dorsal esophageal wall on the spine on lateral radiographs and may be overlooked. Contrast radiography or fluoroscopy are generally not recommended in patients with megaesophagus due to the risk of aspiration pneumonia; however, fluoroscopy may be indicated if lower esophageal sphincter dysfunction is suspected to be a contributing cause. Megaesophagus may be primary (congenital or acquired idiopathic) or may be secondary to a variety of other diseases such as myasthenia gravis, hypoadrenocorticism, hypothyroidism, tetanus, and dysautonomia.[29] Secondary aspiration pneumonia is common, usually affecting the dependent lung lobes.

▍ **Dysmotility without megaesophagus** Reduced motility of the esophagus without concurrent esophageal distention may also be seen in patients with regurgitation. Esophageal dysmotility is incompletely understood but may be due to a variety of underlying etiologies. The same primary conditions that lead to secondary megaesophagus may cause non-dilated esophageal dysmotility in the early phases. Esophagitis is another common cause of esophageal dysmotility. In patients in

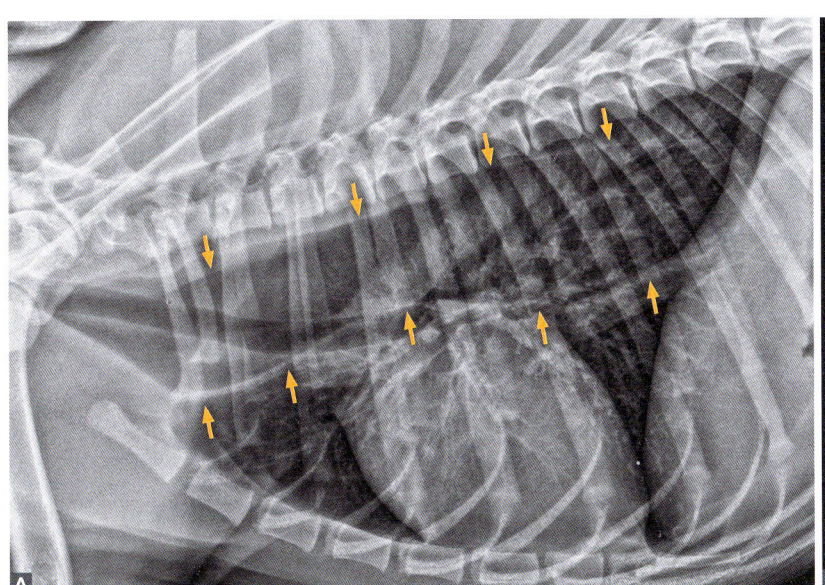

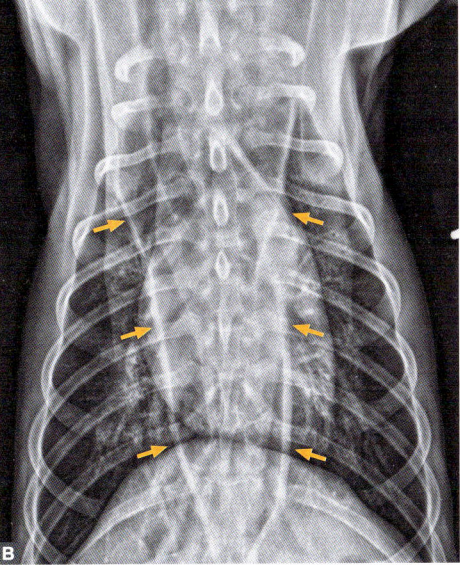

Fig. 18.23 Right lateral (**A**) and dorsoventral (**B**) thoracic radiographs of a seven-month-old Labrador Retriever. The esophagus is diffusely distended, primarily with gas, visible on both projections (arrows). The patient was diagnosed with presumptive congenital megaesophagus.

which no other underlying etiology is identified, a primary neuromuscular disorder is suspected. Esophageal dysmotility has been associated with dysautonomia in dogs and cats and occurs in higher frequency in dogs with geriatric onset laryngeal paralysis.[30,31] Contrast videofluoroscopy is required to diagnose esophageal dysmotility. Findings include abnormal primary and secondary peristaltic waves as well as overall increased transit time (**video 18.3**). Parameters that have been suggested in young dogs include <5 cm aboral movement of bolus by primary peristalsis, bolus retention after two or more secondary peristaltic waves, decreased number of peristaltic waves, and esophageal transit time >5 seconds.[32]

Esophagitis is a general term for inflammation of the esophagus and may result from gastroesophageal reflux (particularly when this occurs under general anesthesia), chronic vomiting, esophageal foreign body, hiatal hernia, ingestion of caustic materials (including tetracycline antibiotics administered without food or water), and rarely *Pythium insidiosum* infection in dogs.[33] Plain or contrast radiography may indicate secondary gas or fluid retention in the esophagus, but the primary role of radiography in patients with suspected esophagitis is to exclude concurrent anatomic abnormalities. Contrast fluoroscopy will demonstrate reduced motility, as well as gastroesophageal reflux or hiatal herniation if present. Esophagitis secondary to reflux or hiatal herniation is typically most pronounced in the caudal esophagus. Mucosal irregularity may also be appreciated with contrast radiography or fluoroscopy and may be seen on CT images. Endoscopy is the diagnostic modality of choice for confirming esophagitis.

Segmental esophageal disorders

Obstruction of the esophagus will result in segmental dilation of the esophagus proximal to the site of obstruction. Causes of esophageal obstruction include congenital vascular ring anomaly, foreign bodies, acquired strictures and rarely esophageal neoplasia.

▌ **Vascular ring anomaly** Vascular ring anomalies are developmental abnormalities of the aortic root and adjacent great vessels that result in encirclement and external constriction of the esophagus and trachea. This typically results in dilation of the esophagus cranial to the vascular ring and may also cause focal tracheal narrowing. Several vascular ring anomalies have been reported in dogs and cats.[34,35] The most common is persistent right aortic arch, in which the embryonic right (rather than left) aortic arch enlarges and becomes the ascending aorta. The left ductus arteriosus develops normally, becoming the *ligamentum arteriosum* at birth, which passes from the left-sided main pulmonary artery to the anomalous right aortic arch, resulting in a complete ring around the esophagus and trachea. Other reported anomalies that may contribute to vascular ring formation include double aortic roots, aberrant subclavian arteries, bicarotid trunk, and persistent right ligamentum arteriosum.

The primary radiographic finding in patients with vascular ring anomalies is dilation of the cranial thoracic esophagus with abrupt narrowing at the cardiac base (**fig. 18.24**). On contrast radiography or videofluoroscopy contrast and food material will be seen to lodge in this cranial dilation with minimal gas or liquid material passing through the site of constriction. The caudal esophagus typically remains empty and non-dilated. In patients with a persistent right aortic arch, the trachea will be deviated toward the left side of the cranial mediastinum. Additionally, the descending aorta will be seen on midline or slightly to the right, instead of to the left of midline. CT angiography is indicated to characterize the exact arrangement of anomalous and aberrant vessels for surgical planning. The vascular structures can usually be readily identified on post-contrast images; repeated short post-contrast series at multiple time points immediately following contrast administration may be helpful for differentiating arterial and venous structures. The *ligamentum arteriosum* is typically too small to resolve, but abrupt and focal narrowing of the esophagus can be appreciated between the aortic root and main pulmonary artery in patients with a typical persistent right aortic arch anomaly.[34]

CHAPTER **18** Mediastinum

VIDEO 18.4
Esophageal stricture

▎**Stricture** Esophageal strictures most commonly form secondary to esophagitis or mechanical esophageal damage (such as from foreign bodies). Esophageal stricture results in segmental narrowing of the esophagus with orad dilation of the esophagus (**fig. 18.25** and **video 18.4**). The esophagus caudal to a stricture is typically normal/empty but may become distended with gastroesophageal reflux or eructation. Strictures may be variably complete; the narrower the stricture the more pronounced the adjacent dilation, fluid, food, and gas accumulation, and clinical signs. The stricture itself is usually not visible on radiographs, although the abrupt cessation of gas or fluid distention is suggestive. Esophageal stricture may not be readily visualized on CT either, if minimal proximal dilation is present. Gas distention of the esophagus using a Foley catheter may help in determination of the

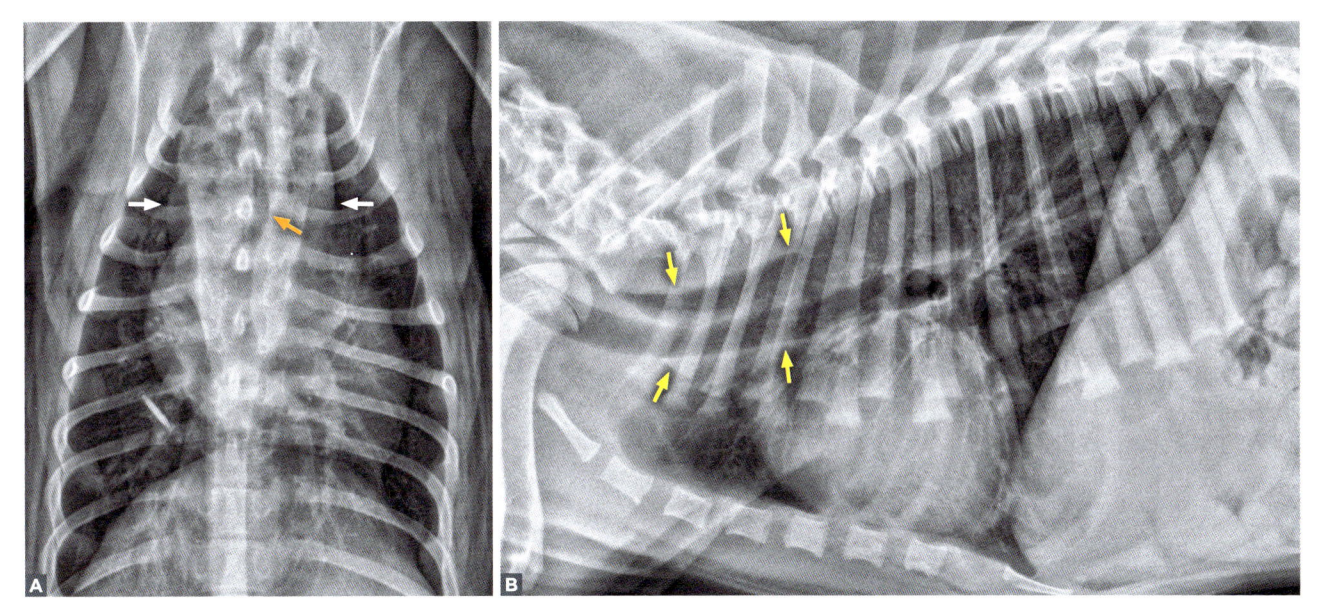

Fig. 18.24 Dorsoventral (**A**) and right lateral (**B**) thoracic radiographs of a three-month-old Labrador Retriever with persistent right aortic arch. There is focal leftward deviation of the trachea at the level of the heart base (orange arrow) and dilation of the esophagus cranial to the heart base (yellow arrows). On the dorsoventral projection the cranial mediastinum appears generally widened (white arrows) which likely represents a combination of segmental esophageal dilation, the right aortic arch, and normal thymus. A left-sided aortic arch is not visualized.

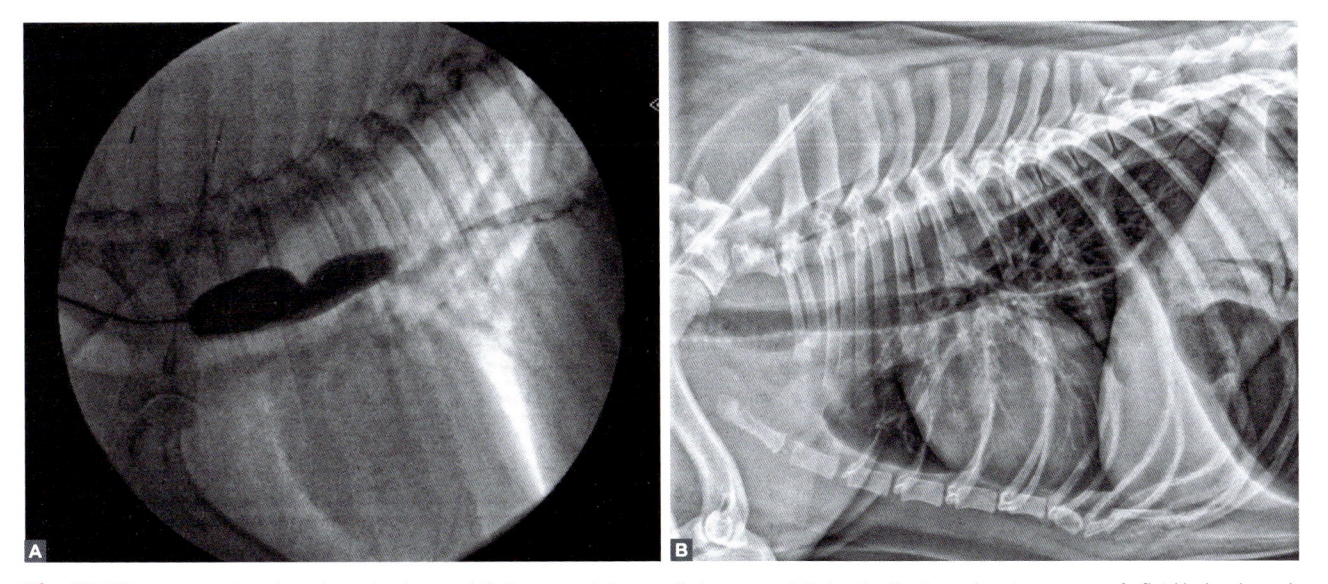

Fig. 18.25 Two examples of esophageal strictures. (**A**) Fluoroscopic image of a four-year-old Labrador Retriever showing passage of a fluid bolus through a region of focal esophageal narrowing at the level of the heart base. The esophagus orad to this narrowing is mildly dilated. (**B**) Lateral thoracic radiograph of a one-year-old French Bulldog with mild gas-dilation of the cervical esophagus, narrowing of the esophageal gas column through the cranial thorax, and moderate dilation of the caudal esophagus caudal to the heart base. The patient was diagnosed with a long cranial thoracic esophageal stricture.

SECTION IV THORAX

presence and location of an esophageal stricture. Contrast radiography and videofluoroscopy are the most useful non-invasive diagnostic procedures for identifying esophageal strictures. Administration of barium-soaked kibble is particularly helpful in identifying strictures as more liquid materials may still be able to pass through.[29] The focal narrowing and inability of the esophagus to distend during swallowing of a bolus will be readily apparent on fluoroscopic images.

▌ **Foreign bodies and esophageal perforation**   Esophageal foreign bodies may lodge anywhere in the esophagus and can usually be identified on radiographs. Radiopaque foreign bodies (such as bones, teeth, or fishhooks) are particularly apparent; soft tissue opaque foreign bodies can be difficult to delineate.[36] Focal esophageal dilation with gas accumulation proximal and/or distal to the foreign body may partly outline it, assisting diagnosis. Some foreign bodies have heterogeneous opacity with internal small pockets of air (**fig. 18.26**). Secondary esophageal perforation is uncommon but if perforation has occurred pneumomediastinum or pneumothorax may be seen as well as evidence of mediastinitis and mediastinal or paraesophageal abscessation. Positive contrast material may be administered to confirm luminal foreign material but may preclude subsequent endoscopy. If there is concern for perforation of the esophagus, nonionic iodinated contrast can be used with caution as aspiration of hypertonic contrast will induce life threatening pulmonary edema. Delayed diagnosis and treatment of an esophageal foreign body is associated with increased risk of perforation or severe esophagitis and subsequent stricture formation.

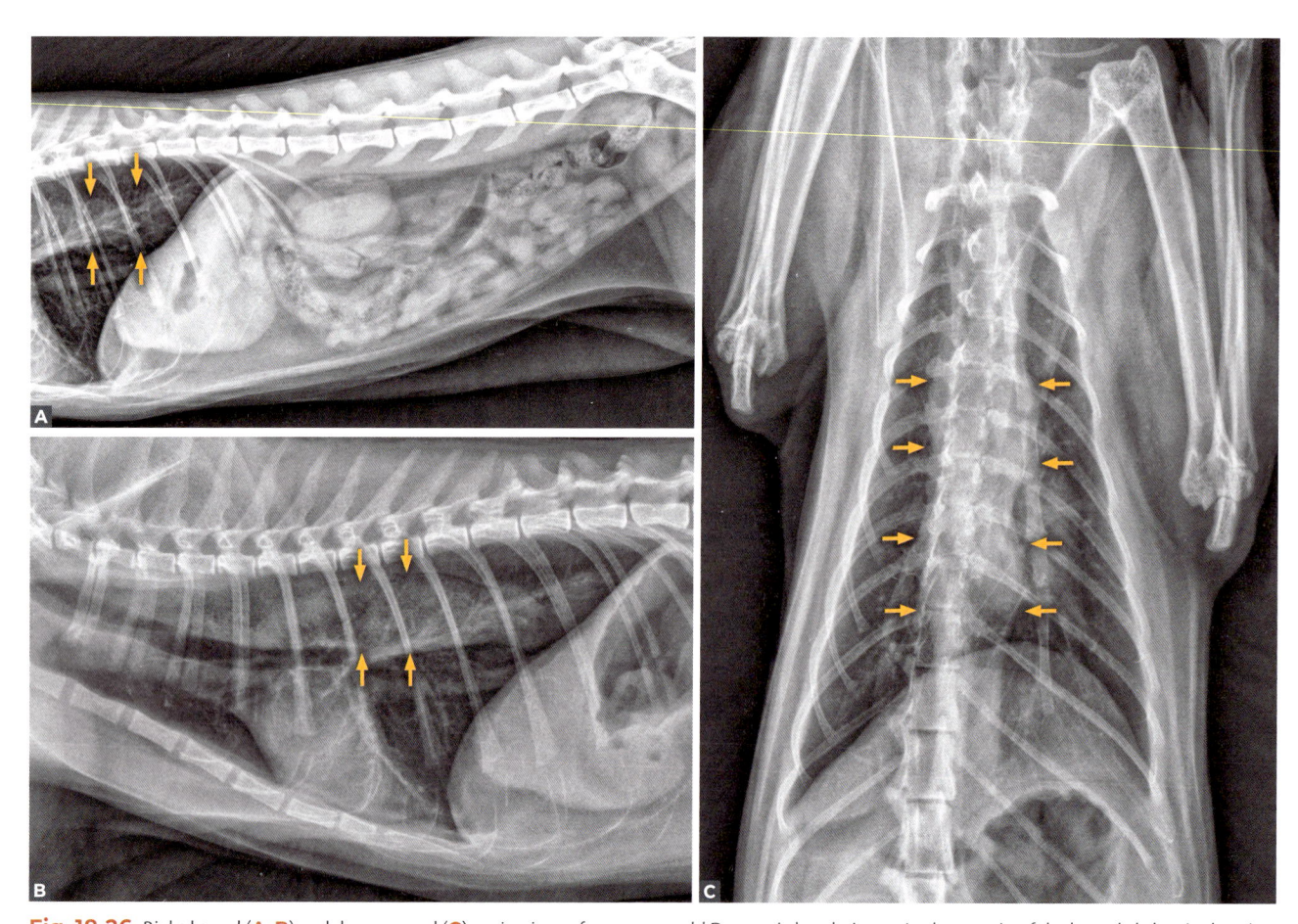

Fig. 18.26 Right lateral (**A**, **B**) and dorsoventral (**C**) projections of a two-year-old Domestic longhair cat. At the margin of the lateral abdominal projection (**A**) there is increased opacity with undulant margins in the region of the esophagus. This is further defined on dedicated thoracic radiographs. The mid to caudal esophagus is moderately distended by heterogeneous soft tissue opaque material that has undulant margins. A thin rim of gas separates luminal content from esophageal wall at the dorsal aspect. The patient was diagnosed with an esophageal trichobezoar (hairball).

Hiatal herniation

The caudal most aspect of the esophagus normally sits within the cranial abdomen where it joins the cardia of the stomach and forms the lower esophageal sphincter. Herniation of the abdominal esophagus, cardia, and part of the gastric fundus can occur at the esophageal hiatus. Hiatal herniation may be classified as type I, "sliding", in which the lower esophageal sphincter and cardia/fundus move cranial to the diaphragm; type II, "paraesophageal", in which the cardia/fundus move cranial, adjacent to the caudal esophagus, without herniation of the lower esophageal sphincter; type III, which includes both sliding and paraesophageal components; and type IV, in which additional abdominal contents (such as liver or small intestine) herniate through the esophageal hiatus.[37] Type I, or sliding, hiatal hernias are by far the most common and are most frequently diagnosed in brachycephalic breeds. This predisposition may be related to chronic upper airway obstruction due to brachycephalic obstructive airway syndrome. Sliding hiatal hernias occur uncommonly in cats.

Sliding hiatal hernias can be seen on radiographs with the primary finding being a soft tissue mass-like structure in the dorsocaudal thorax, slightly to the left of midline, that is confluent with the diaphragmatic margin. Gas from the esophageal or gastric lumen may be seen within this soft tissue mass; gastric rugal folds may be visible if a portion of the fundus is included in the hernia. Given the usually dynamic nature of hiatal hernias, it is common to see the hernia on some but not all projections, which rules out other caudodorsal mediastinal masses (**fig. 18.27** and **video 18.5**). Similarly, sliding hiatal herniation on CT or MRI may be diagnosed by the presence of the lower esophageal sphincter and/or a portion of the fundus cranial to the diaphragm. Radiography, CT, and MRI can provide definitive diagnosis of hiatal herniation; however, they rely on fortuitous timing of acquisition and are not sensitive modalities for dynamic hernias. Fluoroscopy is the preferred imaging modality for diagnosis of patients with suspected hiatal herniation, although a negative study does not definitively rule out hiatal herniation. Sliding hiatal herniation is diagnosed on fluoroscopy by demonstration of the lower esophageal sphincter and portion of the stomach cranial to the dia-

VIDEO 18.5
Hiatal herniation

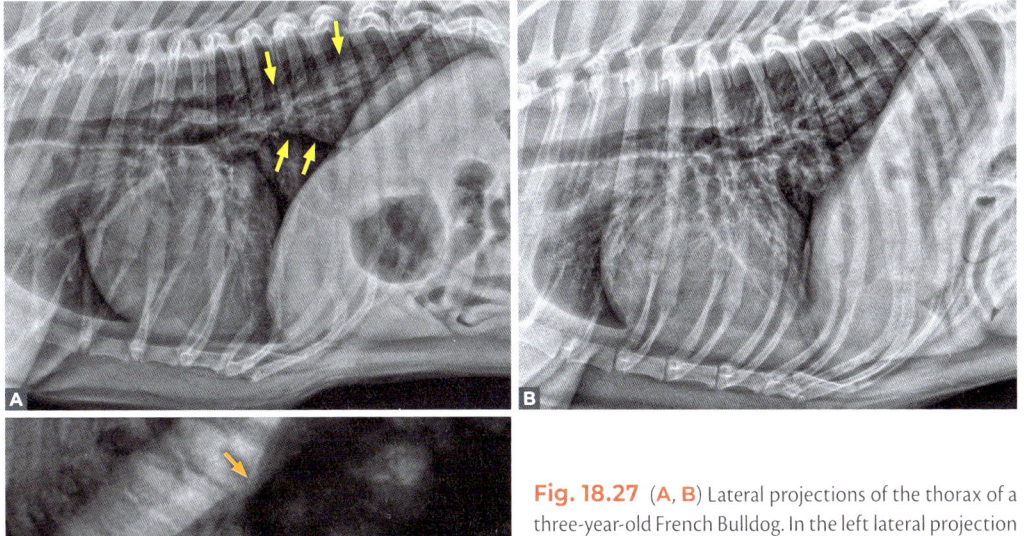

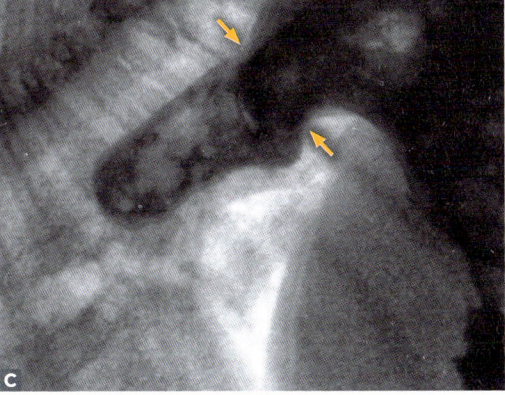

Fig. 18.27 (**A**, **B**) Lateral projections of the thorax of a three-year-old French Bulldog. In the left lateral projection (**A**) an ovoid soft tissue opacity is seen in the caudodorsal thorax that is confluent with the diaphragmatic margin (yellow arrows). This opacity is not present in the right lateral projection (**B**) and the fundus is in a normal position in the cranial abdomen. (**C**) Lateral fluoroscopic image of a hiatal hernia in another three-year-old French Bulldog. The region of the lower esophageal sphincter as well as the gastric cardia are cranially displaced into the caudodorsal thorax (orange arrows). Gastroesophageal reflux mixed with gas is also present cranial to this.

phragm. Gastroesophageal reflux usually occurs with herniation events. Mild cranial excursion of the lower esophageal sphincter without reflux may occur frequently during a study in association with respiration in dogs with hiatal hernia. Full stomach and sternal position are associated with greater likelihood of observing herniation. External pressure applied to the cranial abdomen may also encourage herniation.[29] Dynamic herniation may be observed on ultrasound while viewing the region of the esophageal hiatus.

Spirocerca lupi infection

Neoplasms of the esophagus are uncommon in cats and dogs but can arise from multiple cell types. Squamous cell carcinoma, adenocarcinoma, leiomyosarcoma, leiomyoma, plasmacytoma, and metastatic neoplasia have been reported in dogs. Squamous cell carcinoma is the most common esophageal neoplasm in cats. Granulomas from *Spirocerca lupi* infection, a nematode parasite of dogs in tropical and subtropical climates, may undergo malignant transformation to sarcomas. Esophageal neoplasms may occur anywhere along the length of the esophagus. In dogs, leiomyomas and sarcomas most commonly occur in the caudal esophagus (from heart base to cranial abdomen) with a predilection of leiomyomas and leiomyosarcomas for the lower esophageal sphincter.[38] On radiographs, caudal esophageal masses will be seen as variably sized and shaped soft tissue masses in the dorsal mediastinum (midline or just to the left of midline on dorsoventral or ventrodorsal projections). Esophageal masses often have ill-defined margins but are usually distinct from the dorsal thoracic wall unless very large (**fig. 18.28**). Gas within the esophagus and esophageal dilation may also be seen. Contrast radiography or fluoroscopy are useful to demonstrate the course of the esophageal lumen relative to the mass as well as to identify mucosal irregularities. CT is preferred for definitive localization and assessing viability of surgical resection.

Spirocerca lupi infection is reported primarily in dogs (and rarely other species) with a worldwide tropical/subtropical distribution, although most reports are from Israel, Mediterranean regions, or African countries. The primary radiographic finding is a dorsocaudal thoracic mass, consistent with an esophageal origin. Esophageal masses associated with active *S. lupi* infection represent granulo-

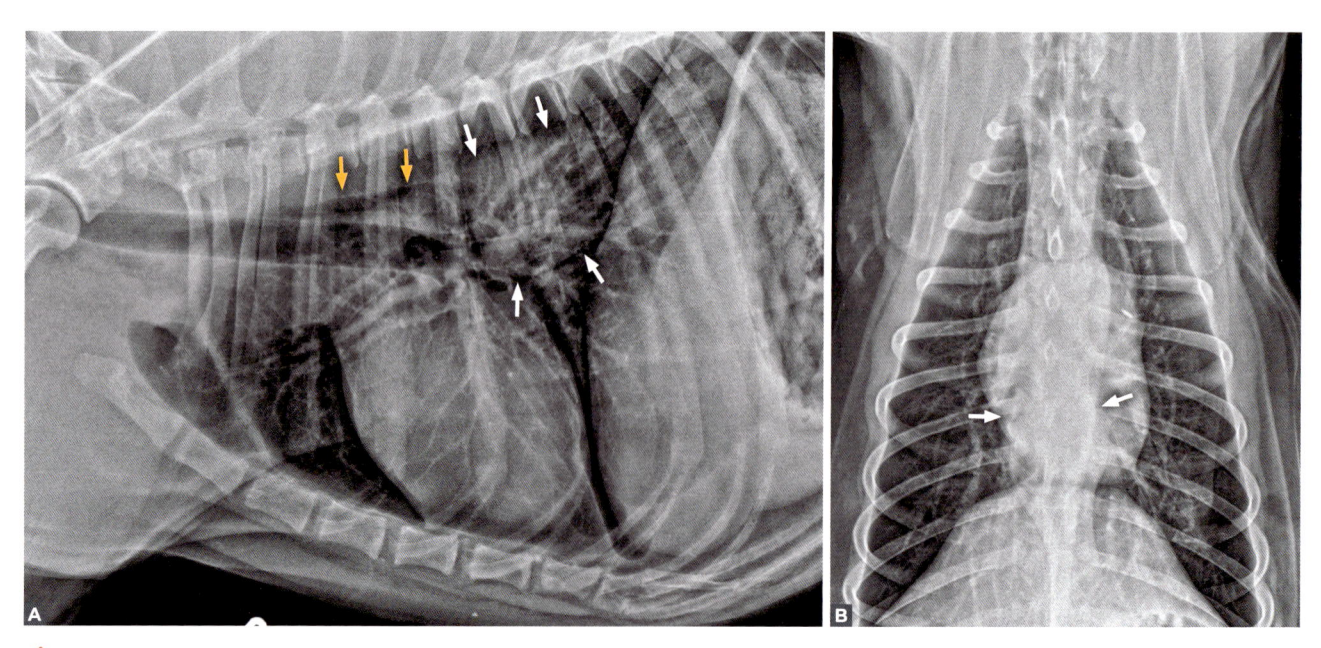

Fig. 18.28 Right lateral (**A**) and dorsoventral (**B**) thoracic projections of an eight-year-old Golden Retriever. On radiographs an ill-defined, round to ovoid soft tissue opaque mass is seen in the midline dorsal thorax (white arrows). The mass appears to be separate from the diaphragm and dorsal body wall and is in the region of the esophagus (orange arrows). CT showed an irregular, heterogeneous mass arising from the esophageal wall and extending into the esophageal lumen. Histopathology was consistent with a sarcoma.

mas and contain adult worms. These granulomas extend into the esophageal lumen and may be variable in size and number. Chronic *S. lupi* infection has been associated with esophageal osteosarcoma, fibrosarcoma, and undifferentiated sarcoma, from malignant transformation of granulomas. Mineralization of the mass may occur with malignant transformation. Other reported radiographic findings include lamellar or mildly irregular periosteal proliferation along the ventral aspect of thoracic vertebral bodies (representing spondylitis), aortic mineralization, and occasionally segmental aortic dilation which are all attributed to larval migration from the aorta to the esophagus. Contrast radiography or fluoroscopy improves sensitivity for small nodules or masses, which typically appear as luminal filling defects. CT improves delineation of esophageal masses and improves sensitivity for secondary findings, including spondylitis, aortic mineralization, and aortic aneurysm.[39]

References

1. The respiratory system. In Hermanson JW, de Lahunta A, Evans HE (eds). Miller and Evan's Anatomy of the Dog 5th edition. St. Louis, Elsevier, 2018, pp 405-407.
2. Thrall DE. Canine and feline mediastinum. In Thrall DE (editor). Textbook of Veterinary Diagnostic Radiology 7th edition. St. Louis, W.B. Saunders, 2018, pp 649-669.
3. Kayanuma H, Yamada K, Maruo T, Kanai E. Computed tomography of thoracic lymph nodes in 100 dogs with no abnormalities in the dominated area. J Vet Med Sci 82:279-285, 2020.
4. Ruby J, Secrest S, Sharma A. Radiographic differentiation of mediastinal versus pulmonary masses in dogs and cats can be challenging. Vet Radiol Ultrasound 61:385-393, 2020.
5. Prather AB, Berry CR, Thrall DE. Use of radiography in combination with computed tomography for the assessment of noncardiac thoracic disease in the dog and cat. Vet Radiol Ultrasound 46:114-121, 2005.
6. Konde LJ, Spaulding K. Sonographic evaluation of the cranial mediastinum in small animals. Vet Radiol 32:178-184, 1991.
7. Baines E. BSAVA Manual of Canine and Feline Thoracic Imaging. In Schwarz T, Johnson V (editors). BSAVA Manual of Canine and Feline Thoracic Imaging, Wiley Blackwell, 2008, pp 177-199.
8. Smith K, O'Brien R. Radiographic characterization of enlarged sternal lymph nodes in 71 Dogs and 13 Cats. J Am Anim Hosp Assoc 48:176-181, 2012.
9. Starrak GS, Berry CR, Page RL, Johnson JL, Thrall DE. Correlation between thoracic radiographic changes and remission/survival duration in 270 dogs with lymphosarcoma. Vet Radiol Ultrasound 38:411-4188, 1997.
10. Reeve EJ, Mapletoft EK, Schiborra F, Maddox TW, Lamb CR, Warren-Smith CMR. Mediastinal lymphoma in dogs is homogeneous compared to thymic epithelial neoplasia and is more likely to envelop the cranial vena cava in CT images. Vet Radiol Ultrasound 61:25-32, 2020.
11. Oura TJ, Hamel PE, Jennings SH, Bain PJ, Jennings DE, Berg J. Radiographic differentiation of cranial mediastinal lymphomas from thymic epithelial tumors in dogs and cats. J Am Anim Hosp Assoc 55:187-193, 2019.
12. Patterson MME, Marolf AJ. Sonographic characteristics of thymoma compared with mediastinal lymphoma. J Am Anim Hosp Assoc 50:409-413, 2014.
13. Fabrizio F, Calam AE, Dobson JM, Middleton SA, Murphy S, Taylor SS, Schwartz A, Stell AJ. Feline mediastinal lymphoma: a retrospective study of signalment, retroviral status, response to chemotherapy and prognostic indicators J Feline Med Surg 16:637-644, 2014.
14. Moore EL, Vernau W, Rebhun RB, Skorupski KA, Burton JH. Patient characteristics, prognostic factors and outcome of dogs with high-grade primary mediastinal lymphoma. Vet Comp Oncol 16:E45-E51, 2018.
15. Guglielmini C, Toaldo MB, Quinci M, Romito G, Luciani A, Cipone M, Drigo M, Diana A. Sensitivity, specificity, and interobserver variability of survey thoracic radiography for the detection of heart base masses in dogs. J Am Vet Med Assoc 248:1391-1398, 2016.
16. Yoon J, Feeney DA, Cronk DE, Anderson KL, Ziegler LE. Computed tomographic evaluation of canine and feline mediastinal masses in 14 patients. Vet Radiol Ultrasound 45:542-546, 2004.
17. Liptak JM, Kamstock DA, Dernell WS, Ehrhart EJ, Rizzo SA, Withrow SJ. Cranial mediastinal carcinomas in nine dogs. Vet Comp Oncol 6:19-30, 2008.
18. Liu S, Patnaik AK, Burk RL. Thymic branchial cysts in the dog and cat. J Am Vet Med Assoc 182:1095-1098, 1983.
19. Jones BG, Pollard RE. Relationship between radiographic evidence of tracheobronchial lymph node enlargement and definitive or presumptive diagnosis. Vet Radiol Ultrasound 53:486-491, 2012.
20. Gendron K, McDonough SP, Flanders JA, Tse M, Scrivani PV. The pathogenesis of paraesophageal empyema in dogs and constancy of radiographic and computed tomography signs are linked to involvement of the mediastinal serous cavity. Vet Radiol Ultrasound 59:169-179, 2018.
21. Trivedi SR, Sykes JE, Cannon MS, Wisner ER, Meyer W, Sturges BK, Dickinson PJ, Johnson LR. Clinical features and epidemiology of cryptococcosis in cats and dogs in California: 93 cases (1988-2010). J Am Vet Med Assoc 239:357-369, 2011.
22. Boyd N, Thomason J, Pohlman L, Anselmi C. Mediastinal histoplasmosis with cardiac involvement in a cat. J Vet Cardiol 31:15-22, 2020.
23. Gilor C, Graves TK, Barger AM, O'Dell-Anderson K. Clinical aspects of natural infection with *Blastomyces dermatitidis* in cats: 8 cases (1991-2005). J Am Vet Med Assoc 229:96-99, 2006.
24. Schmidt M, Wolvekamp P. Radiographic findings in ten dogs with thoracic actinomycosis. Vet Radiol 32:301-306, 1991.
25. Mellanby RJ, Villiers E, Herrtage ME. Canine pleural and mediastinal effusions: a retrospective study of 81 cases. J Small Anim Pract 43:447-451, 2002.
26. Blocker TL, Roberts BK. Acute tracheal obstruction associated with anticoagulant rodenticide intoxication in a dog. J Small Anim Pract 40:577-580, 1999.
27. Broek A van den. Pneumomediastinum in seventeen dogs: aetiology and radiographic signs. J Small Anim Pract 27:747-757, 1986.
28. Thomas EK, Syring RS. Pneumomediastinum in cats: 45 cases (2000-2010). J Vet Emerg Crit Care 23:429-435, 2013.
29. Pollard RE. Imaging evaluation of dogs and cats with dysphagia. ISRN Vet Sci 2012:1-15, 2012.
30. Levine JS, Pollard RE, Marks SL. Contrast videofluoroscopic assessment of dysphagic cats. Vet Radiol Ultrasound 55:465-471, 2014.

31. Stanley BJ, Hauptman JG, Fritz MC, Rosenstein DS, Kinns J. Esophageal dysfunction in dogs with idiopathic laryngeal paralysis: a controlled cohort study. *Vet Surg* 39:139-149, 2010.
32. Bexfield NH, Watson PJ, Herrtage ME. Esophageal dysmotility in young dogs. *J Vet Intern Med* 20:1314-1318, 2006.
33. Sellon RK, Willard MD. Esophagitis and esophageal strictures. *Vet Clin North Am Small Animal Pract* 33:945-967, 2003.
34. Morgan KRS, Bray JP. Current diagnostic tests, surgical treatments, and prognostic indicators for vascular ring anomalies in dogs. *J Am Vet Med Assoc* 254:728-733, 2019.
35. Bascuñán A, Regier PJ, Case JB, Singh A, Balsa I, Flanders J, Thieman-Mankin K, Ham KM. Vascular ring anomalies in cats: 20 cases (2000-2018). *Vet Surg* 49:265-273, 2020.
36. Thompson HC, Cortes Y, Gannon K, Bailey D, Freer S. Esophageal foreign bodies in dogs: 34 cases (2004-2009). *J Vet Emerg Crit Care* 22:253-261, 2012.
37. Reeve EJ, Sutton D, Friend EJ, Warren-Smith CMR. Documenting the prevalence of hiatal hernia and oesophageal abnormalities in brachycephalic dogs using fluoroscopy. *J Small Anim Pract* 58:703-708, 2017.
38. Willard MD. Alimentary neoplasia in geriatric dogs and cats. *Vet Clin North Am Small Anim Pract* 42:693-706, 2012.
39. Merwe LL van der, Kirberger RM, Clift S, Williams M, Keller N, Naidoo V. *Spirocerca lupi* infection in the dog: A review. *Vet J* 176:294-309, 2008.

CHAPTER 19

Congenital and acquired cardiac diseases

L. Abbigail Granger and Serena Crosara

> **KEY POINTS**
>
> ▎ Consistently correct positioning is essential when obtaining images for suspected cardiac disease to avoid shape alterations and misdiagnosis.
> ▎ Cardiac disease can be assessed with good-quality radiographs, and ultrasound images obtained in M-mode, B-mode and color Doppler to assess structural changes, function, and blood flow and to detect cardiac failure.
> ▎ Left-sided congestive cardiac failure causes pulmonary venous congestion and is usually characterized by pulmonary edema, which is best diagnosed by radiographs.
> ▎ Right-sided congestive cardiac failure causes systemic venous congestion and is usually characterized by pleural effusion, hepatomegaly and peritoneal effusion, and may be confirmed by radiographs or ultrasonography.
> ▎ A sound knowledge of the normal cardiovascular blood flow and the anatomy and physiology of congenital cardiac anomalies is essential for understanding imaging abnormalities and for formulating a diagnosis or differential diagnoses.
> ▎ The heart size can be objectively evaluated using the ratio of cardiac size to vertebral length, called vertebral heart score.
> ▎ Echocoardiography is superior to radiographs for the assessment of the cardiac valves, the myocardial function and the presence of heart defects.
> ▎ Radiography is better for confirmation of congestive cardiac failure and for assessment of treatment response.

Radiographic evaluation of the cardiopulmonary vascular system requires a quality thoracic radiographic study with attention to exposure settings, positioning, and phase of respiration during exposure to obtain images of diagnostic quality. The forelimbs must be extended to avoid cranial thoracic crowding and superimposition. A complete thoracic study requires at least one lateral view and a dorsoventral (DV) and ventrodorsal (VD) view. The appearance of the cardiovascular structures varies between radiographic views, as detailed in **table 19.1**.

The heart is a three-dimensional structure with complex internal anatomy whose radiographic interpretation is simplified to assess its shape and size. Therefore, especially when cardiac evaluation is the purpose of a thoracic study, obliquity must be eliminated as poor positioning can alter the cardiac shape (**fig. 19.1**). The beam is centered at the caudal margin of the scapula, which is the landmark for the center of the heart when the forelimbs are extended. Views centered at the diaphragm or further caudal will make the heart appear rounder and can lead to an incorrect diagnosis.

SECTION IV THORAX

The heart, pericardium, and fluid contained within the pericardium and middle mediastinum cumulatively create the radiographic cardiac silhouette. Therefore, alterations in size and shape of the cardiac silhouette may be related to abnormalities not only within the heart but also to pericardial or middle mediastinal disease. The appearance of the cardiac silhouette varies among dogs due to the broad spectrum of thoracic conformations (**fig. 19.2**). Breed-specific thoracic conformations can be categorized as deep-chested, intermediate, or barrel-chested. These variations in thoracic shape

Table 19.1 Variation in cardiac shape and vascular visibility between thoracic radiographic views.

Lateral views

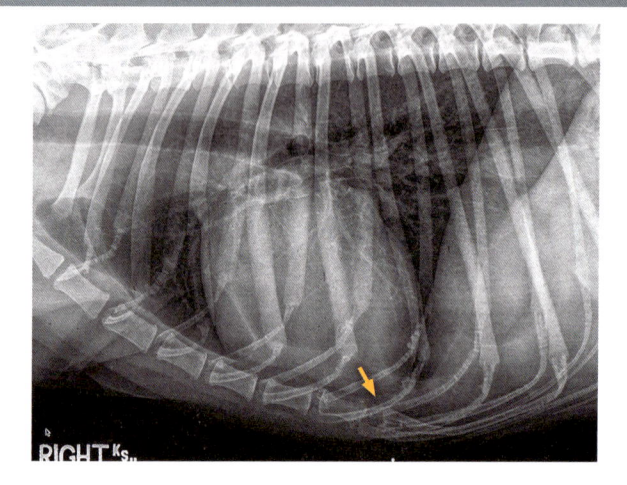

Right
- Heart elongated
- Apex contacts sternum (arrow)

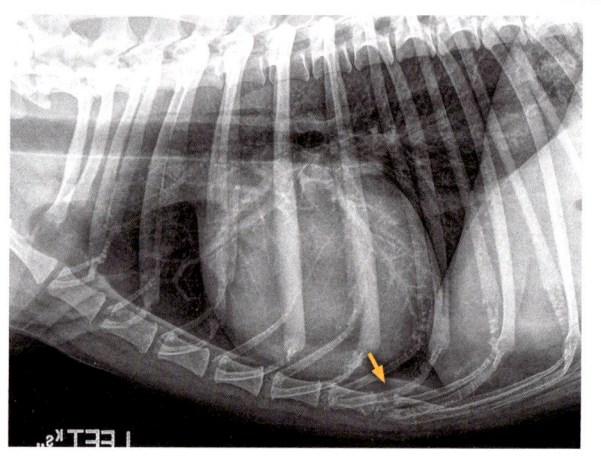

Left
- Heart rounded
- Apex appears elevated from sternum (arrow)

Orthogonal views

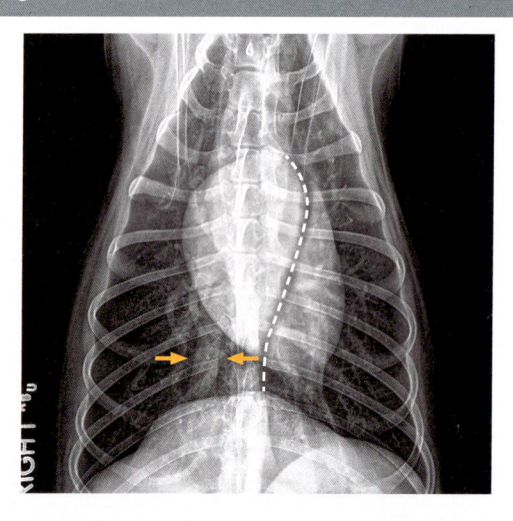

Ventrodorsal
- Heart elongated
- Increased distance between cardiac apex and diaphragm
- Apex closer to midline
- Accessory lung lobe better aerated and better assessed
- Caudal vena cava better seen (arrows)

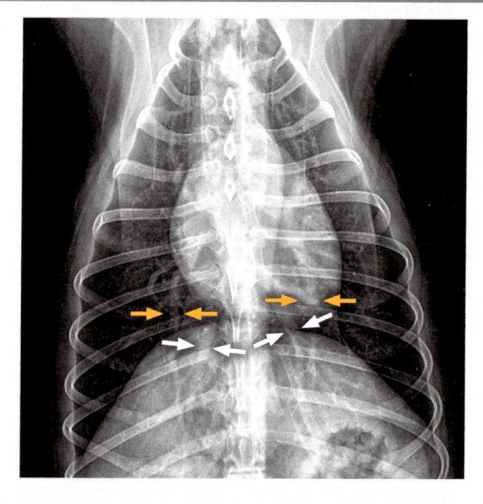

Dorsoventral
- Heart rounded
- Contact between diaphragm and cardiac apex
- Apex positioned further to the left
- Caudal lung lobes better aerated and better assessed
- Caudal lobar arteries (between orange arrows) and veins (between white arrows) better seen

Fig. 19.1 (**A**) Correctly positioned and (**B**) oblique radiographic views of the same dog obtained in the same study. (**B**) Obliquity is identified by positioning the sternum towards the right (orange arrows) and the spine, which is positioned towards the left (yellow arrows) rather than being superimposed as in (**A**). This level of obliquity creates the false impression of a bulge in the 1-2 o'clock position mimicking main pulmonary arterial dilation.

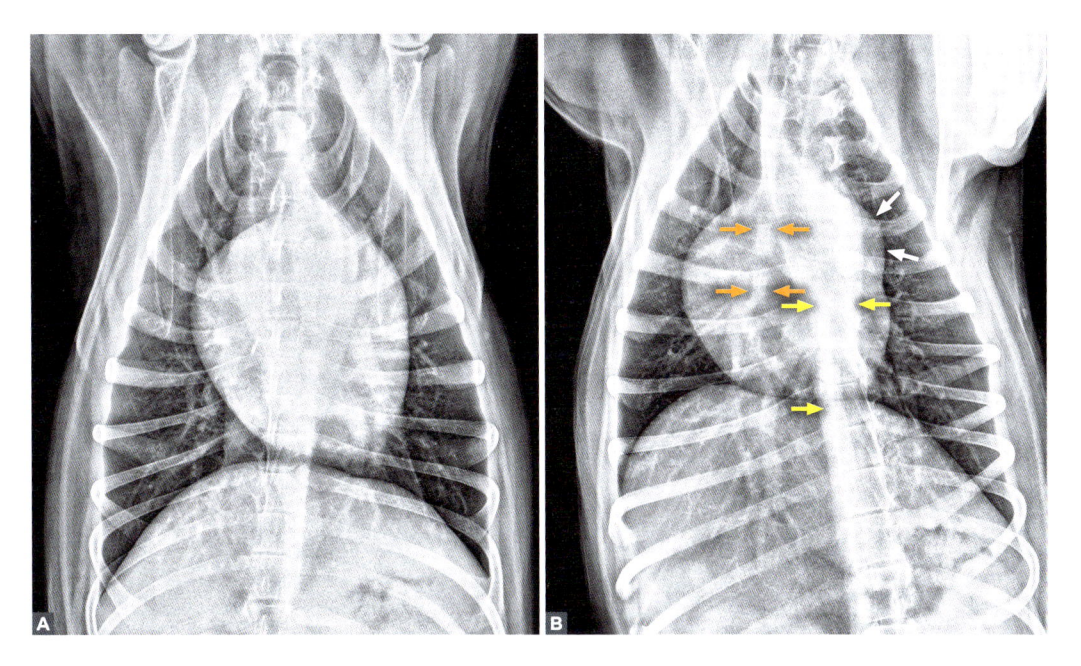

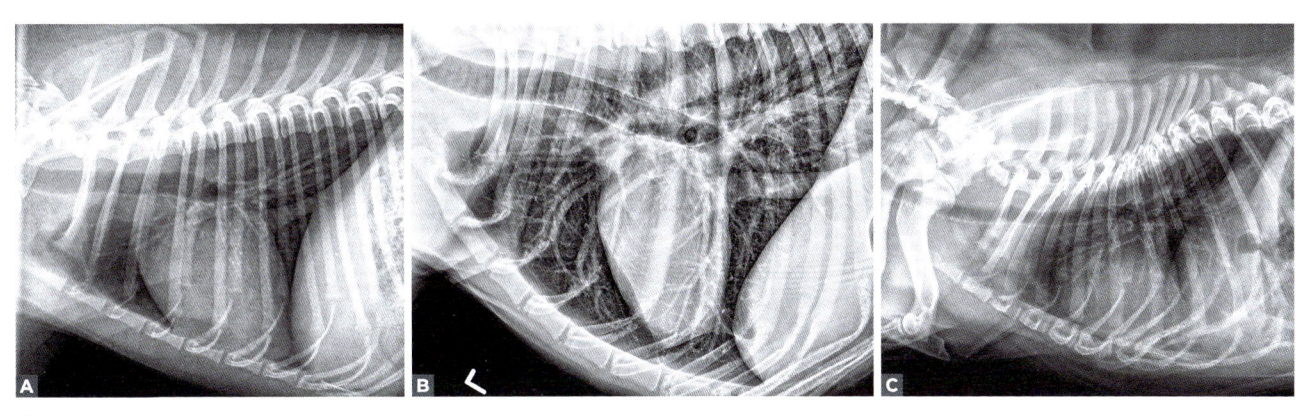

Fig. 19.2 Lateral thoracic radiographs in three dog breeds illustrating the variation that can occur with thoracic conformation. (**A**) The Yorkshire Terrier, (**B**) the Great Dane, and (**C**) the English Bulldog are all radiographically normal, but each has differing relative cardiac size and shape related to the breed's thoracic conformation.

affect the apparent size and shape of the cardiac silhouette requiring incorporation into the cardiac radiographic interpretation. Cats have little variation in conformation and appearance; however, fat deposition may influence the size and visibility of the cardiac silhouette (**fig. 19.3**).

Radiography and echocardiography are complementary methods to evaluate the heart and are often used in combination to provide a complete clinical picture of the disease. Indications for cardiac imaging are shown in **box 19.1**. Echocardiography is more sensitive to detect mild cardiomegaly and is the main modality used to assess cardiac function. Radiography is the test of choice for determining the presence of overt cardiac failure and is useful for initial diagnosis and serial monitoring of cardiomegaly. The echocardiographic exam allows the direct evaluation of cardiac function, the anatomy of the chambers and valves, the pericardium, and the extracardiac structures. The echocardiographic exam is generally performed with the patient in lateral recumbency scanning from beneath through an opening in the table because this technique reduces interference from the lung. The choice of the transducer depends on the patient's size. Low frequency probes (e.g., 5-7.5 MHz) allow more penetration but limited spatial resolution and are suitable for medium-large breed dogs. High frequency probes (e.g., 7.5-10 MHz) do not penetrate as well but have better spatial resolution and are suitable for small breed dogs and cats.

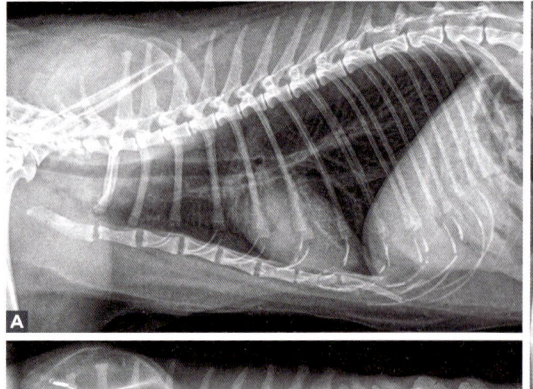

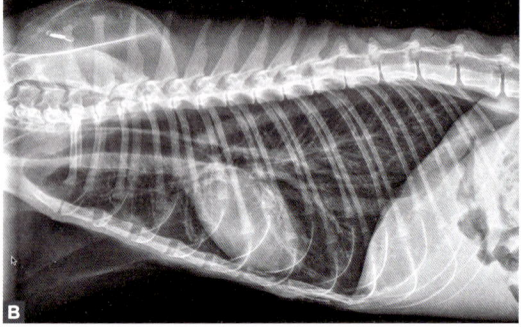

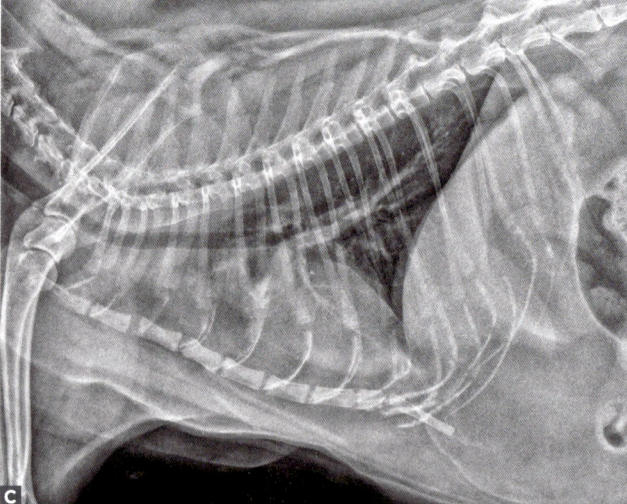

Fig. 19.3 Lateral radiographs in normal cats having various body condition scores. In cats having normal (**A**) and emaciated (**B**) body condition scores, the cardiac silhouette is well identified, and there is no significant morphological variation between cat breeds. (**C**) In obese cats, the cardiac silhouette can be partly obscured and somewhat more difficult to assess.

BOX 19.1 INDICATIONS FOR CARDIAC IMAGING.

- Audible murmur
- Exercise intolerance
- Coughing
- Dyspnea
- Increased lung sounds
- Cyanosis
- Syncope
- Abdominal distension/jugular pulses
- Heartworm infection
- Serial monitoring of previously diagnosed cardiac disease
- Screening in predisposed breeds

Considerations prior to radiographic interpretation of the heart

A thorough assessment of the cardiac silhouette, alterations of the great vessels and pulmonary vessels, and recognition of cardiac failure (right- or left-sided) can assist with creating an appropriate list of differential diagnoses and guide management. Signalment data such as species, breed, and age are useful to refine a differential diagnosis list for cardiac patients. Under many circumstances, the underlying cause of cardiomegaly should be confirmed with echocardiography. In cases where cardiac disease is suspected but the heart is radiographically normal, echocardiography should be used to confirm normal or abnormal.

Diagnosis of specific cardiac diseases requires a thorough evaluation of the cardiac and non-cardiac structures of the thorax. To arrive at an appropriate differential diagnosis list or definitive diagnosis, all of the abnormalities and normal findings must be synthesized. Thorough knowledge of normal and abnormal anatomy and physiology related to cardiac disease is the foundation of a diagnosis. Radiographic findings must be correlated with clinical signs and physical examination. The normal cardiovascular blood flow as shown in **fig. 19.4** requires frequent consideration, in addition to alterations in blood flow that occur with congenital cardiac anomalies, to predict and recognize chamber and vascular enlargements that appear with specific cardiac diseases. Understanding the physiology

Fig. 19.4 Normal flow of blood through the cardiovascular system.

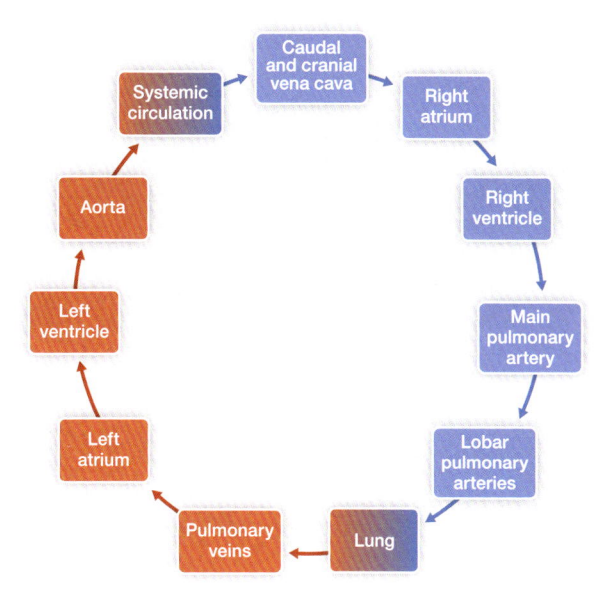

of congenital cardiac anomalies and how they affect morphology through alterations in blood flow and pressure is a more reliable approach to diagnosis than memorizing differential diagnoses for each cardiac bulge or vascular enlargement.

Cardiac radiographic anatomy

Knowledge of the normal radiographic appearance and topographic anatomy of the heart is required to recognize the abnormal. The heart size can be evaluated by subjective assessment (**box 19.2**) or objectively using a ratio of cardiac size to vertebral length, called a vertebral heart score (**fig. 19.5**). The cardiac shape is equally important in determining the presence of disease as alterations in cardiac shape may not necessarily affect cardiac size. Poorly positioned and/or centered radiographs will distort the cardiac silhouette and cause overdiagnosis or missed diagnoses. Inconsistent positioning and centering also preclude reliable serial monitoring of progression of the disease. Keeping in mind that breed

---

BOX 19.2 CARDIAC SIZE RELATIVE TO THE THORACIC CAVITY.

Canine

Lateral view
- Height of the heart is less than ⅔ the dorsoventral diameter of the thorax
- Width of the heart is 2.5-3.5 intercostal spaces
- Two-thirds of the width of the heart is cranial to the carina (right side of the heart) and ⅓ is caudal (left side of the heart)
- Trachea is nearly parallel to the sternum

Ventrodorsal view
- Left cardiac margin flatter than the right
- Width of the cardiac silhouette less than ⅔ the width of the thorax
- Cardiac apex positioned slightly left to the midline

Feline

Lateral view
- Height of the heart is less than ⅔ the dorsoventral diameter of the thorax
- Width of the heart is 2-3 intercostal spaces
- Trachea diverges from the spine and is nearly parallel to the sternum
- Increased tracheal divergence from spine with age

Ventrodorsal view
- Left cardiac margin is flat
- Width of the cardiac silhouette is less than ½ the width of the thorax
- Apex positioned moderately left to the midline

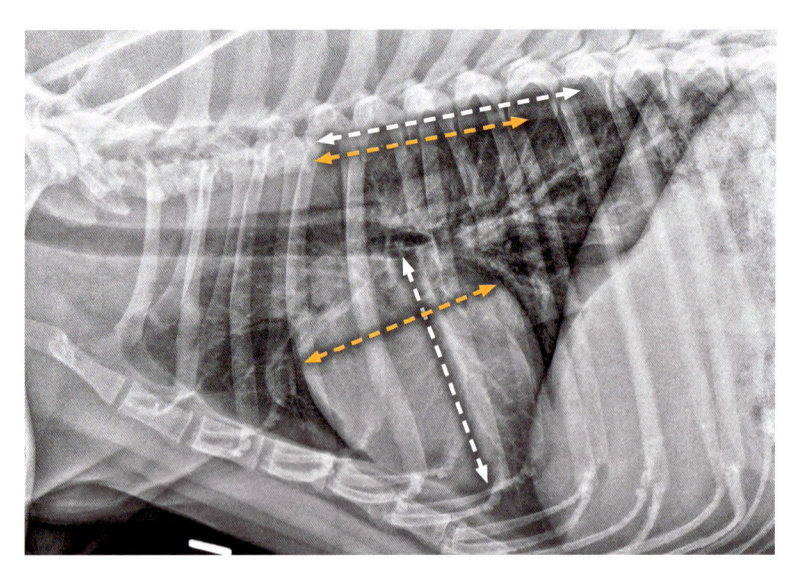

Fig. 19.5 Technique for performing the vertebral heart scale (VHS).[2] A line is drawn along the long axis of the heart from the level of the cardiac base (white) to the cardiac apex. A second line is drawn along the short axis of the heart from the level of its intersection with the dorsal caudal vena cava margin and extends to the cranial cardiac margin so that the second line is perpendicular to the original line (orange). Both lines are then transposed onto the thoracic spine from the level of the cranial endplate of T4 extending caudally. The number of vertebrae encompassed within these lines constitutes the VHS, which measures 10 in this case.

variations exist, the normal canine and feline cardiac silhouette can be assessed as shown in **box 19.2**. In an effort to provide an objective assessment of cardiac size regardless of breed conformation, a numerical index was developed to measure canine and feline cardiac size.[2-4] On the right lateral view, a line is drawn along the long axis of the heart from the cardiac base (at the tracheal bifurcation) to the cardiac apex. A second line is drawn along the short axis of the heart from the dorsal margin of the junction of the caudal vena cava to the cranial cardiac margin so that the line is perpendicular to the long axis line. Both of these measurements are then transposed onto the thoracic spine from the cranial endplate of T4 extending caudally. The number of vertebrae encompassed within these lines constitutes the vertebral heart scale (VHS) as shown in **fig. 19.5**. Most normal dogs (98%) have a VHS less than 10.6.[2,4] Some normal dogs will fall above this value. Several breed-specific VHS ranges have been published to address variation in normal values from thoracic conformation.[5-8] The reported upper limit of the VHS in cats is 8.0.[3] Accurate assessment of cardiac size is only possible with well-positioned and centered radiographs.

Changes in cardiac shape from disease can occur without increase in size (most notably in diseases characterized by concentric hypertrophy). An over-reliance on measurements in radiographic interpretation without consideration of alteration of shape can lead to misclassification of a heart as normal when it is not. The greatest value in performing a VHS is to make an objective determination of cardiac size for the relatively less experienced reader and, more importantly, to objectively measure changes in size over time. The left heart chambers are known to rapidly increase in size over the last year prior to the onset of left-sided cardiac failure in Cavalier King Charles Spaniels having mitral valvular endocardiosis.[9,10] The rate of change of increasing cardiac size increase (measured in ΔVHS/month) is predictive of imminent cardiac failure.[10] The absolute VHS measurement steadily increased from visit to visit after diagnosis of mitral endocardiosis until diagnosis of failure, but the rate of change of the VHS was consistent until the interval immediately prior to the onset of failure with a cutoff value of ≥0.08 VHS/month having a large positive effect on probability of onset of failure within a year and rates measuring ≤ 0.06 VHS/month having a low probability of imminent failure within a year.[10]

When cardiomegaly occurs, it usually affects a single chamber or side (left-sided or right-sided cardiomegaly). Sometimes, all chambers of the heart are enlarged (generalized cardiomegaly). Even in these cases, one side often predominates. To arrive at an appropriate differential list, specific chamber enlargement should be identified as indicated by alterations in size and/or shape. Therefore, bulges of the cardiac silhouette must be anatomically correlated to specific chambers and vessels. This can be accomplished by way of the clock-face analogy shown in **table 19.2**.

CHAPTER 19 Congenital and acquired cardiac diseases

Table 19.2 Times corresponding to specific cardiac chambers using the clock-face analogy.

Lateral view

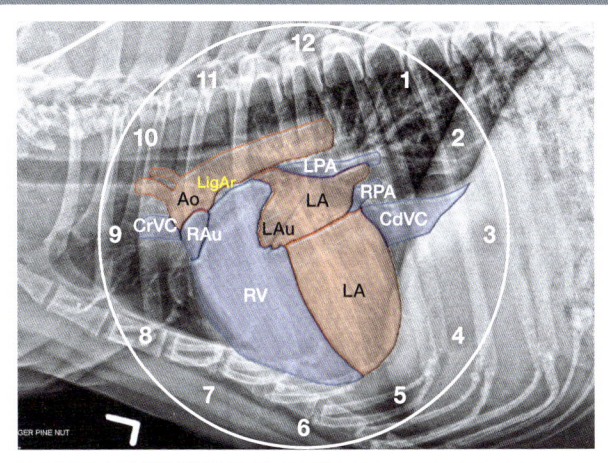

Time	Cardiac chamber(s)
12:00-3:00 (caudal cardiac base)	Left atrium (LA) and left auricle (LAu)
3:00-5:00 (caudal cardiac apex)	Left ventricle (LV)
5:00-8:00 (cranial cardiac apex)	Right ventricle (RV)
8:00-11:00 (cranial cardiac base)	Right auricle (RAu), main pulmonary artery (MPA), ascending aorta and arch (Ao)

Ventrodorsal view

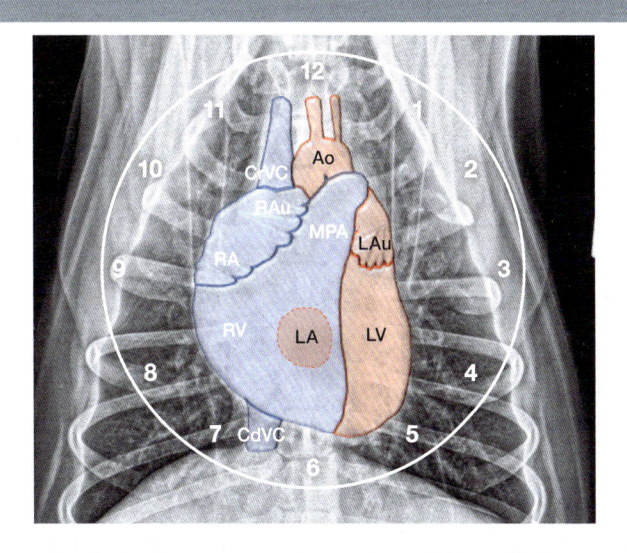

Time	Cardiac chamber(s)
11:00-1:00	Aorta (Ao)
1:00-2:00	Main pulmonary artery (MPA)
2:00-3:00	Left auricle (LAu)
3:00-5:00	Left ventricle (LV)
5:00-9:00	Right ventricle (RV)
9:00-11:00	Right atrium (RA) and right auricle (Rau)
Center dial (between mainstem bronchi)	Left atrium (LA)

SECTION IV THORAX

Chambers of the heart are located within specific segments along the clock. The clock-face analogy is similar in cats, except that the left atrium is located more to the left of the cardiac silhouette rather than dorsally at the caudal cardiac base like it is in dogs.
The echocardiographic exam includes standard views, adapted from human echocardiogra-

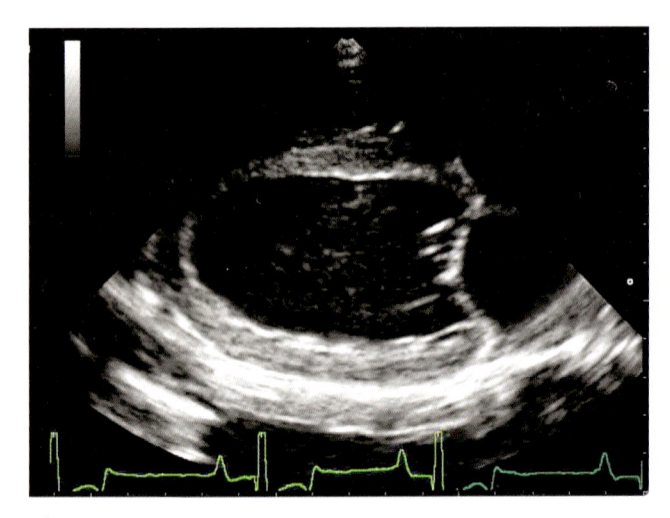

Fig. 19.6 Greyhound. Right parasternal long axis view. The probe is positioned close to the sternum, with the cursor toward the scapula, aligned with the long axis of the heart, which looks horizontal in this view. The left side is visible, and the right ventricle and atrium are mildly visible on the top of the screen. The mitral valve leaflets (anterior leaflet is dorsal, posterior leaflet is ventral) close below the insertion plane. From this view is possible to measure the ventricular and atrial volumes.

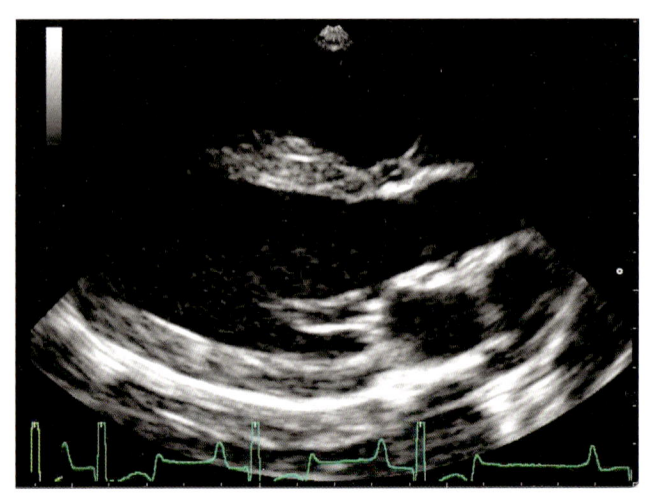

Fig. 19.7 Greyhound. Right parasternal long axis, five chambers view, systolic frame. The probe is mildly rotated counterclockwise from the right parasternal long axis to visualize the left ventricle outflow tract and the aorta. The left atrium is partially cut off. The aortic annulus and the valvular leaflets are visible. In the figure, the leaflets are open. This view is used to measure the aortic annulus and to study the LVOT and evidence the presence of a perimembranous interventricular septum defect.

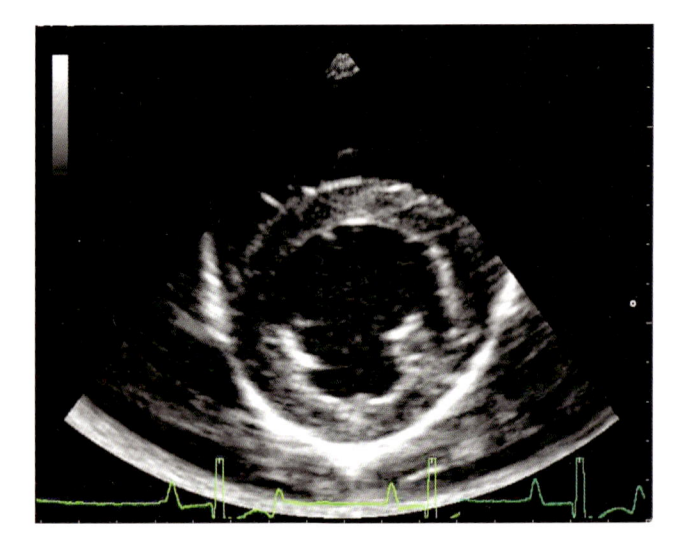

Fig. 19.8 Greyhound. Right parasternal short axis view, at the level of the papillary muscles. This view is obtained by rotating the probe 90° counterclockwise, from the right parasternal long axis view. The left ventricle is visible as a round structure in the middle of the image, with a typical "mushroom shape" for the presence of the two papillary muscles. The right ventricle ("half-moon" shape) embraces the left ventricle, and it is visible on the top of the screen. The view is correctly obtained if the mushroom is straight, and the cursor can be placed in the middle of the papillary muscles to obtain the M-mode.

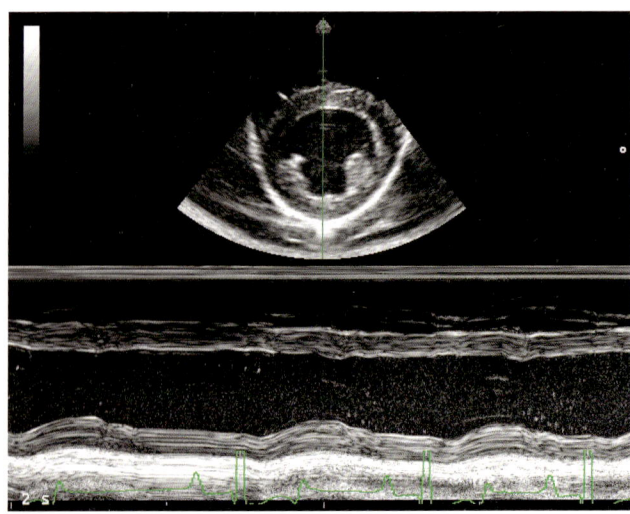

Fig. 19.9 Greyhound. M-mode obtained from the right parasternal short axis view at the level of the papillary muscles. From top to bottom, the following structures are visible: the right ventricle, the interventricular septum, the left ventricle, and the posterior wall. The M-mode technique allows the measurement of the cardiac chambers in systole and diastole by referring to the ECG. The ventricular volumes, the ejection fraction, and the shortening fraction are calculated with the Teicholz formula from the linear measurements.

phy in order to obtain uniform images. Obtaining proper images allows an immediate, subjective evaluation of cardiac morphology, myocardial function, and valvular motion. Objective measurements obtained from standard views can be compared to published normal data ranges for specific breeds and species and can be used for objective sequential assessments of disease progression (**figs. 19.6-19.14**).

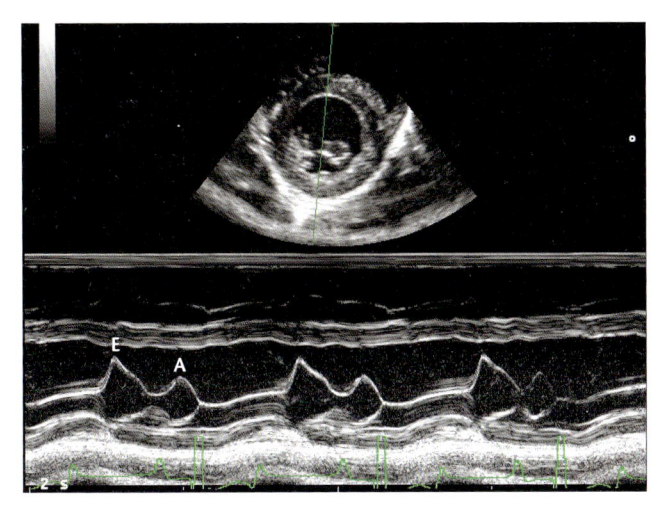

Fig. 19.10 Greyhound. M-mode obtained from the right parasternal short axis view at the level of the mitral valve. The mitral leaflets are visualized during the cardiac cycle. The typical "M-shape" is obtained because of the opening of the mitral valve during the early diastole (E) and late diastole (A). The anterior leaflet of the mitral valve is visible at the top, the posterior leaflet below. This view is used to measure the EPSS (E point septal separation), which is the distance between the E point and the interventricular septum.

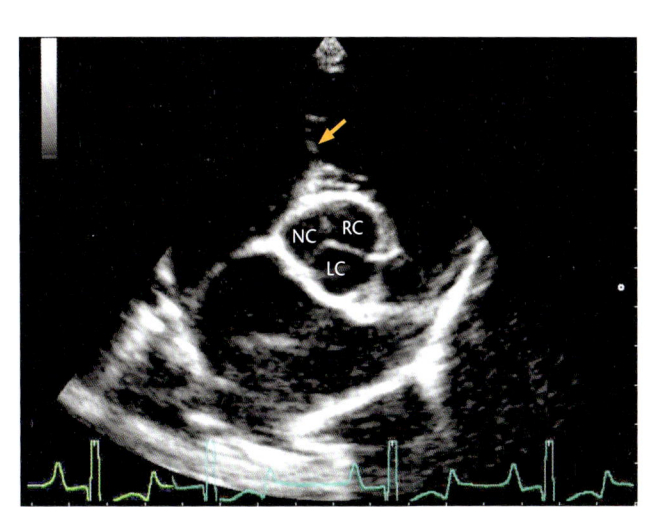

Fig. 19.11 Greyhound. Right parasternal short axis view at the level of the heart base. In the middle of the image, the aortic root and the three aortic sinuses of Valsalva are visible: the non-coronary sinus (NC), the right coronary sinus (RC), and the left coronary sinus (LC). From the bottom of the screen, clockwise, the following structures are visible: the left atrium and auricle, the right atrium, the tricuspid valve (arrow), the right ventricular outflow tract, and the pulmonary annulus. From this view is possible to measure the left atrium to aortic root ratio.

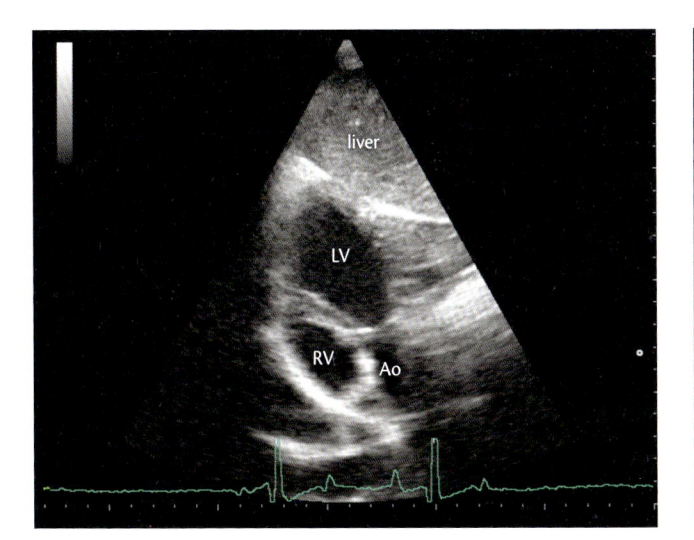

Fig. 19.12 Mongrel dog. Subcostal view. This view is obtained with the probe positioned behind the sternum and the cursor toward the spine. The ultrasound beam passes through the liver and the diaphragm. The beam is perfectly aligned with the left ventricle (LV) and the ascending aorta (Ao), thus allowing the correct measurement of the aortic flow velocity. The right ventricle (RV) is partially visible on the bottom.

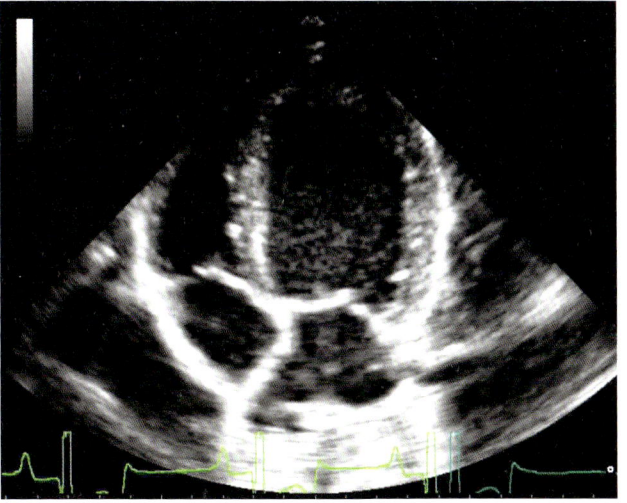

Fig. 19.13 Greyhound. Left apical view. The probe is positioned close to the sternum, at the level of the heart apex, and oriented toward the dog head with the cursor toward the spine. The beam is perfectly aligned with the long axis of the left ventricle, and it is perpendicular to the mitral plane. The correct alignment is obtained when the left ventricular apex is visible. From this view, it is possible to obtain the ventricular and atrial volumes, the diastolic transmitral flow and the tissue Doppler at the level of the mitral plane.

Fig. 19.14 Greyhound. Left apical view optimized for the right side. The left side is partially cut off, and the aorta must not be visible. From this view, the diameters and volumes of the right ventricle and right atrium can be obtained. The TAPSE (tricuspid annular plane systolic excursion) is calculated by placing the cursor on the tricuspid annulus at the level of the right ventricular free wall.

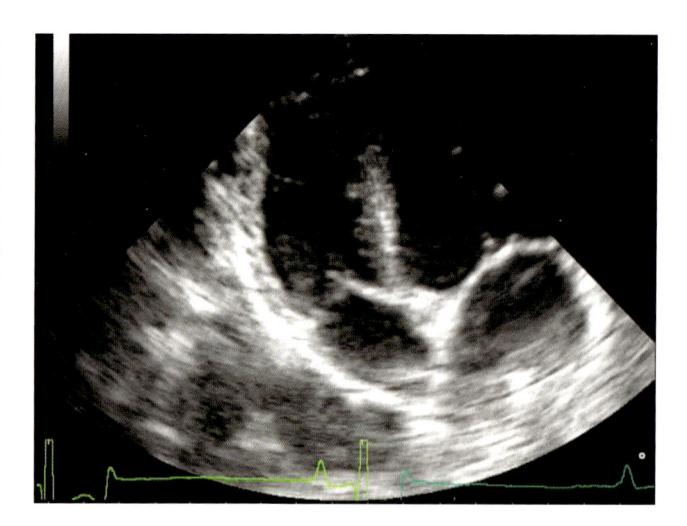

Cardiac hypertrophy

Cardiac diseases are caused by congenital or degenerative anatomical abnormalities that result in alteration of normal blood flow patterns and/or pressures or by primary myocardial disease. Alterations in flow patterns result in morphologic changes of the heart and/or vasculature, primarily due to increased blood volume and secondarily increased chamber volume over time, called eccentric hypertrophy. An increase in blood volume in the left ventricle may occur from multiple causes. Possible causes include an incompetent aortic valve, allowing the return of blood from the aorta to the left ventricle during diastole, an increase in circulating left-sided volume due to a congenital left-to-right shunt (patent ductus arteriosus, ventricular septal defect, atrial septal defect), or increased flow through the left heart due to a dysplastic or degenerative mitral valve causing continual recirculation between the left atrium and ventricle. With this increase in blood volume, the left ventricle dilates, causing eccentric hypertrophy of the myocardium and increased luminal size. In the left ventricle, an increase in pressure can occur due to stenosis of the aortic valve through which the left ventricle must transit blood forward. This increase in pressure results in thickening of the cardiac muscle and a decrease in actual luminal size called concentric hypertrophy. Concentric hypertrophy can be severe without alteration of the outer shape or size of the heart, particularly when affecting the left ventricle. As a result, concentric hypertrophy tends to be less radiographically evident when compared to eccentric hypertrophy.

Pressure overload and hypertrophic cardiomyopathy cause concentric hypertrophy, while volume overload and dilated cardiomyopathy cause eccentric hypertrophy of ventricles. The atria respond in a different manner to pressure overload than the ventricles do. When the left or right atrium undergoes a pressure overload, it will only dilate (eccentric hypertrophy) like that seen with volume overload in

Table 19.3 Eccentric versus concentric hypertrophy of the heart.

Eccentric hypertrophy	Concentric hypertrophy

- Increased chamber volume
- More radiographically evident
- Due to:
  - Volume overload
  - Myocardial dysfunction caused by dilated cardiomyopathy (DCM)
  - Coronary artery disease
	- Increased wall thickness/decreased chamber volume
	- Not seen radiographically until severe
	- Due to:
	  - Pressure overload
	  - Myocardial dysfunction caused by some cardiomyopathies (e.g., HCM)

the ventricles. For example, the right atrium may dilate due to an increased volume from a dysplastic tricuspid valve, or it may also dilate due to increased pressure from a stenotic tricuspid valve.[11]

Recognizing each type of cardiac hypertrophy is important for proper interpretation of thoracic studies and recognizing the limitations of thoracic radiology in diagnosing heart disease. Diagnoses characterized by concentric hypertrophy are less apt to be radiographically evident because the increased wall thickness may not alter the outer contour of the cardiac silhouette. The myocardium and blood are indistinguishable on a survey radiograph, and an echocardiogram or contrast angiocardiogram would be needed to confirm and quantify any hypertrophy. The main differences between eccentric and concentric hypertrophy are highlighted in **table 19.3**. A radiographically normal heart can have a clinically significant disease, and determination of cardiac normality should never be made on subjective assessment of size or VHS measurement alone. At the echocardiographic examination, eccentric hypertrophy is characterized by increased diastolic, and sometimes systolic, ventricular diameters and atrial dilation. The systolic function can be variably affected, based on the underlying pathology (e.g., hyperkinetic ventricle in the course of mitral insufficiency or systolic dysfunction in the course of dilated cardiomyopathy). Eccentric hypertrophy can affect the left, right, or both sides of the heart (**figs. 19.15** and **19.16**). Concentric hypertrophy is secondary to increased afterload of the right or the left ventricle (e.g., pulmonic or aortic stenosis, pulmonary or systemic hypertension) or due to primary hypertrophic cardiomyopathy. It is characterized by an increased thickness of the ventricular walls with a preserved systolic function. The atria can be variably dilated due to elevated ventricular diastolic pressure. With time, concentric hypertrophy can evolve to a dilated hypokinetic form (afterload mismatch); at this stage, the hypertrophy is no longer evident (**figs. 19.17** and **19.18**).

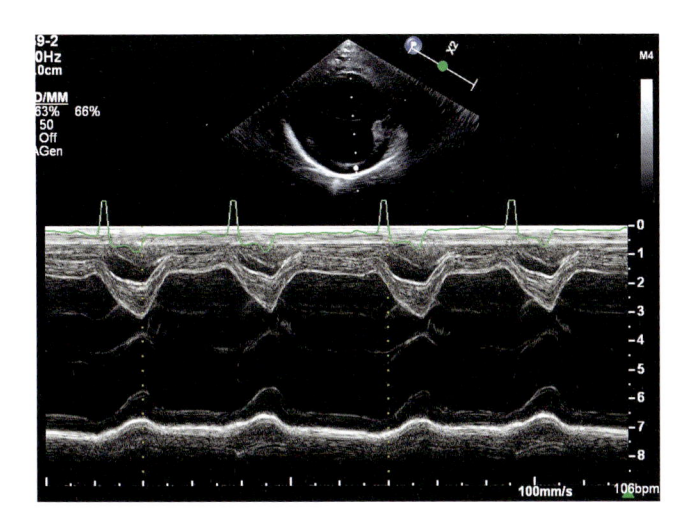

Fig. 19.15 Cavalier King Charles Spaniel affected by chronic degenerative mitral valve disease, ACVIM stage D. Right parasternal short axis view, M-mode at the level of the papillary muscles. Eccentric hypertrophy of the left ventricle with normal wall thickness. The systolic function is difficult to assess because the interventricular septum appears hyperkinetic due to the increased preload and the reduced afterload that characterize the disease.

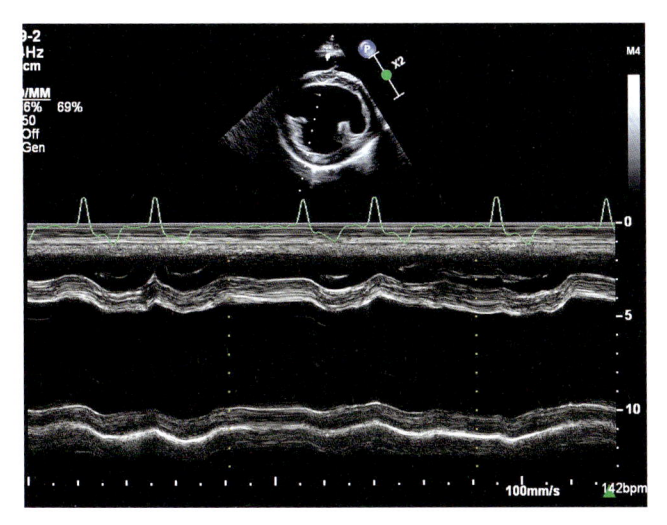

Fig. 19.16 Labrador Retriever affected by tachycardia-induced cardiomyopathy secondary to atrial fibrillation. Right parasternal short axis view at the level of the papillary muscles. Eccentric hypertrophy of the left ventricle associated to systolic dysfunction. The right ventricle appears normal in size. The atrial fibrillation is evident from the electrocardiographic monitoring for the absence of P waves and the irregularly irregular rhythm.

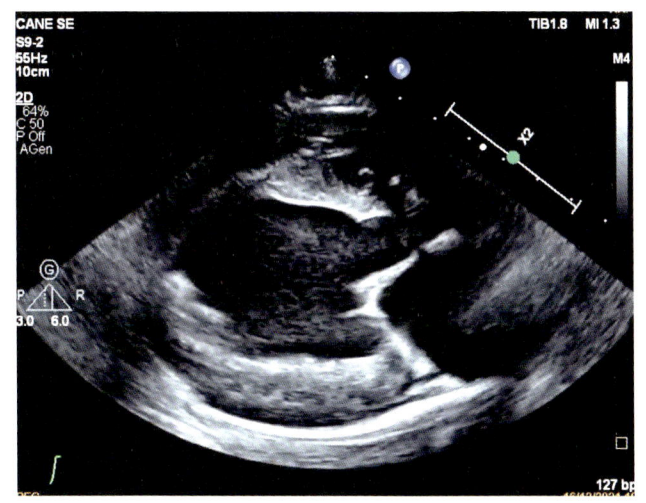

Fig. 19.17 A four-month-old Rottweiler affected by severe tunnel-like subaortic stenosis. Right parasternal long axis view. Concentric hypertrophy of the left ventricle; both interventricular septum and left ventricular free wall are thickened. The subendocardial myocardium appears hyperechoic due to the fibrosis. The right ventricle appears normal.

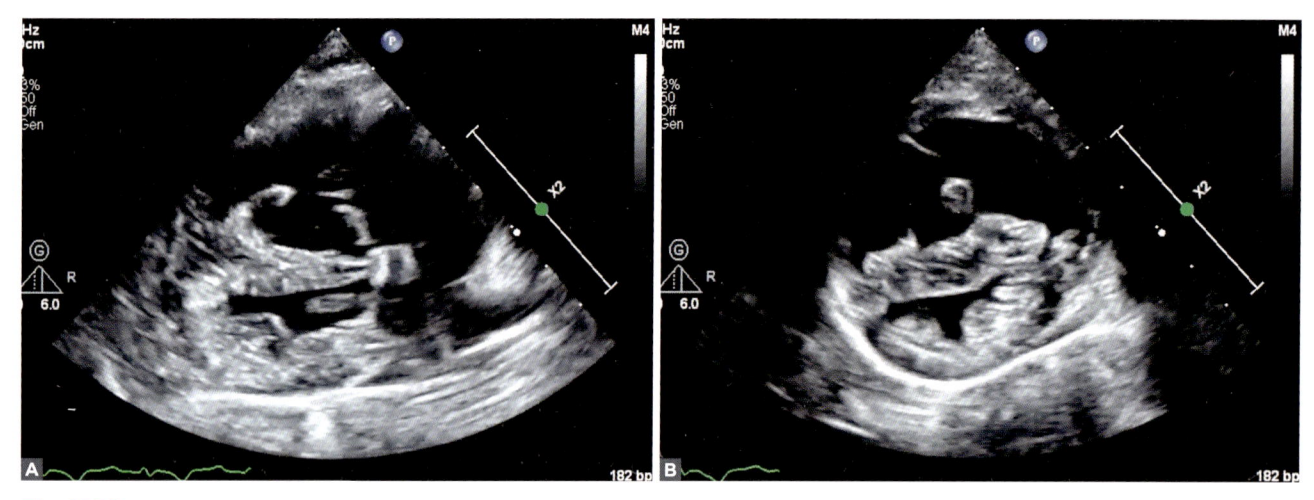

Fig. 19.18 Mongrel dog affected by pulmonary hypertension. (**A**) Right parasternal long axis view. Severe hypertrophy of the right ventricle and right atrial dilation; the thickening of the right ventricular walls is associated to right ventricular dilation. The right ventricular hypertrophy mimics a double apex heart. The left ventricle appears thick due to the reduced preload for severe pulmonary hypertension; this condition is called pseudohypertrophy. (**B**) Right parasternal short axis view. Right ventricular dilation and pseudohypertrophy of the left ventricle. The right ventricular pressure exceeds the left, causing the flattening of the interventricular septum and a triangular aspect of the left ventricle in diastole.

Radiographic appearance of right-sided cardiomegaly

Radiographically, right-sided cardiomegaly tends to cause the appearance of a wide heart on the lateral view and increased rounding of the right cardiac margin on the ventrodorsal/dorsoventral views. Bulges in the cardiac silhouette can be seen corresponding to the right atrium, right ventricle, or both according to the clock-face analogy. Numerous causes of right-sided cardiomegaly alone or in combination with left-sided cardiomegaly are summarized in **table 19.4**.

Right atrial enlargement will, if visible, cause an increase in soft tissue opacity between the cranial cardiac base and the cranial mediastinum on the lateral views (8:00-11:00 position). Most often, though, the orthogonal (VD or DV) view is more reliable in detecting right atrial enlargement as a bulge at the right cranial cardiac margin in the 9:00-11:00 position (**fig. 19.19**). Secondary to cardiac enlargement, the trachea will often be elevated, especially cranial to the hilus. On some occasions, especially with concurrent right ventricular enlargement, the cardiac apex will be displaced to the left on the ventrodorsal/ventrodorsal views. In general, right atrial enlargement is more evident on the ventrodorsal view. Right ventricular enlargement, when detectable, will cause an overall wide and rounded cardiac silhouette on the lateral view. Under normal circumstances, ⅔ the width of the heart on the lateral view should be located cranial to the hilus. An increase in this cranial proportion of the heart can be seen in cases having right ventriculomegaly. The heart may appear to contact a greater length of the sternum, referred to as increased sternal contact. However, this is an unreliable indicator that is often subject to overinterpretation of cardiomegaly, given the large variation in normal appearance related to thoracic conformation. This finding should be used with considerable caution and never as the sole indicator of cardiomegaly. On the VD view, a reverse D shape is caused by right ventriculomegaly when moderate or severe. The reverse D is non-specific for the underlying cause of right ventricular enlargement. A reverse D must not be mistaken for the normal right-sided cardiac margin on the ventrodorsal view. In a normal silhouette, the right atrium at the 9:00-11:00 position is the most peripheral part of the right cardiac margin, and then the heart begins to taper towards the apex. In a case having right ventricular enlargement, the cardiac margin in the 5:00-9:00 position on the ventrodorsal view protrudes and is rounded before angling towards the apex, creating the characteristic reverse D shape of right ventricular enlargement. These findings are shown in **figs. 19.20** and **19.21**.

CHAPTER 19 Congenital and acquired cardiac diseases

Table 19.4 Causes of right-sided cardiomegaly.

Right atrium	Right ventricle

▪ Chamber dilation only (eccentric hypertrophy)
  ▪ Volume overload due to:
    › Insufficient/dysplastic tricuspid valve
    › Atrial septal defect
  ▪ Pressure overload due to:
    › Stenotic tricuspid valve
▪ Right atrial mass
  ▪ e.g., hemangiosarcoma
	▪ Chamber dilation (eccentric hypertrophy)
	  ▪ Volume overload due to:
	    › Tricuspid valvular insufficiency
	    › Pulmonic valvular insufficiency
	    › Atrial septal defect
	    › Overhydration
	  ▪ Myocardial failure
	    › Cardiomyopathy (arrhythmogenic right ventricular cardiomyopathy)
	  ▪ Chronic anemia
	  ▪ Athletic heart
	  ▪ Cardiac conduction abnormalities
	▪ Wall thickening (concentric hypertrophy)
	  ▪ Pressure overload due to:
	    › Pulmonic stenosis
	    › Pulmonary hypertension (cor pulmonale)
	      – HW disease
	    › Tetralogy of Fallot
	  ▪ Cardiomyopathy (HCM)

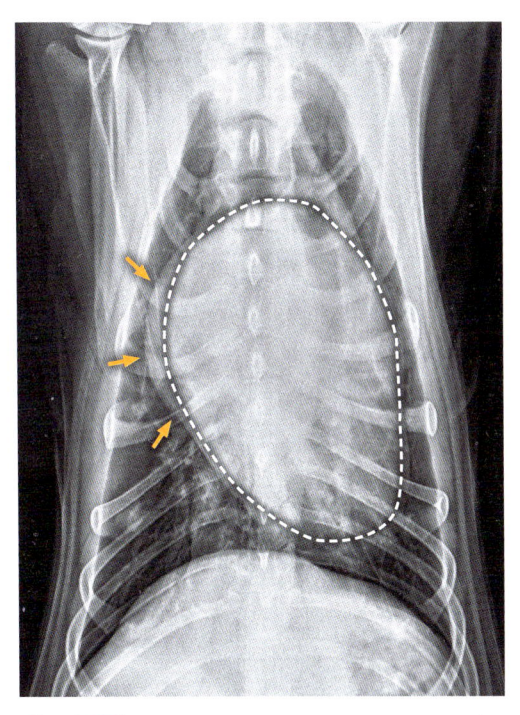

Fig. 19.19 Ventrodorsal of a 1.5-year-old Boxer dog having right atrial enlargement due to tricuspid dysplasia. A bulge is identified in the 9:00-11:00 position (orange arrows) consistent with the region of the right atrium/auricle on the clock face analogy, altering the shape of the heart from normal (dotted white tracing).

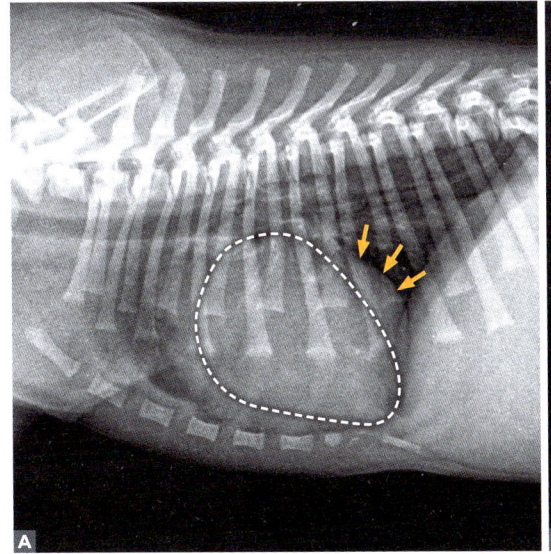

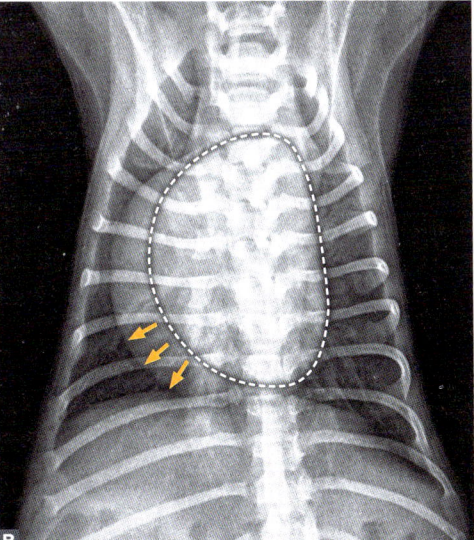

Fig. 19.20 Lateral and ventrodorsal views of a puppy having right ventricular enlargement due to severe pulmonic stenosis and pulmonic insufficiency. (**A**) The trachea is elevated, being parallel to the spine. The cardiac silhouette is subjectively wide on the lateral view encompassing over four intercostal spaces but, distinguishing this case from left-sided cardiomegaly, the caudal margin of the cardiac silhouette is very rounded on the lateral view (orange arrows). (**B**) The contour of the left margin of the cardiac silhouette is flat on the ventrodorsal view. The entire right cardiac margin is rounded with the ventricle (in the 5:00-9:00 position) being more peripheral than the atrium (orange arrows), creating a silhouette whose outline is reverse D in shape. The right ventricular enlargement alters the overall size and shape of the heart as compared to normal on both views (depicted as dotted line overlays in **A** and **B**).

SECTION IV THORAX

Fig. 19.21 Labrador Retriever with tricuspid valve dysplasia. Angled left parasternal apical view. Severe dilation of both right atrium and right ventricle.

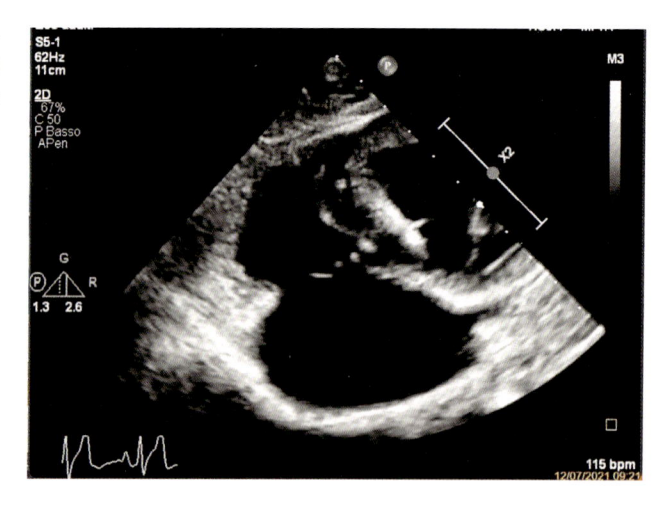

Radiographic appearance of left-sided cardiomegaly

Left-sided cardiomegaly tends to create the appearance of a tall heart on the lateral view with the tracheal elevation that can be identified in any cardiomegaly often being more pronounced with left-sided enlargement. Potential causes of left-sided cardiomegaly are summarized in **table 19.5**. Due to the prevalence of specific cardiac diseases in the canine and feline populations, left-sided cardiomegaly is far more common than right-sided. Additionally, most cardiomyopathies tend to preferentially cause left-sided cardiac remodeling, except for arrhythmogenic right ventricular cardiomyopathy (ARVC) in Boxer dogs.[11,12]

Left atrial enlargement will cause a bulge at the caudal dorsal aspect of the heart (12:00-3:00 position) on the lateral view. This changes the normal contour of the caudal dorsal aspect of the heart from convex to flat. In cats, the dilated left atrium appears as a rounded protrusion at the caudal dorsal

Table 19.5 Causes of left-sided cardiomegaly.

Left atrium	Left ventricle

▮ Chamber dilation only (eccentric hypertrophy)
  ▮ Volume overload due to:
    ▸ Insufficient/dysplastic mitral valve
    ▸ Left-to-right shunts
      – PDA
      – VSD
      – ASD
▮ Pressure overload
  ▸ Stenotic mitral valve
	▮ Chamber dilation (eccentric hypertrophy)
	  ▮ Volume overload due to:
	    ▸ Mitral valvular insufficiency
	    ▸ Aortic valvular insufficiency
	    ▸ Left-to-right shunts:
	      – PDA
	      – VSD
	      – ASD
	  ▸ Overhydration
	  ▮ Myocardial failure
	    ▸ Cardiomyopathy (dilated)
	  ▮ Chronic anemia
	  ▮ Athletic heart
	  ▮ Cardiac conduction disturbances
	▮ Wall thickening (concentric hypertrophy)
	  ▮ Pressure overload due to:
	    ▸ Aortic stenosis
	    ▸ Systemic hypertension
	  ▮ Cardiomyopathy (hypertrophic)

CHAPTER **19** Congenital and acquired cardiac diseases

margin of the heart. With severe dilation of the atrium, the heart may appear kidney-shaped on the lateral view. On the VD or DV view, the left atrium is superimposed on the caudal aspect of the cardiac silhouette between the mainstem bronchi. With moderate or severe dilation it can create a mass effect resulting in a "U-shaped" angle rather than the normal "V-shaped" angle between the bronchi on the DV/VD views. This appearance can also be created by an improperly centered view.[13] Sometimes, the caudal margin of an enlarged left atrium will create a well-defined rounded margin slightly cranial and parallel to the cardiac apex on the ventrodorsal view (**fig. 19.22**). An enlarged left atrial appendage protrudes from the cardiac silhouette on the ventrodorsal view at the 2:00-3:00 position.

Two objective measurements for left atrial size in dogs have been published, called the radiographic left atrial dimension (RLAD)[14] and the vertebral left atrial size (VLAS)[15] (**fig. 19.23**). These can be

Fig. 19.22 (**A**) Lateral and (**B**) ventrodorsal views of a dog having left atrial dilation due to mitral valvular endocardiosis. The trachea and mainstem bronchi are elevated. (**A**) The caudal cardiac margin is flat on the lateral view (white arrows). A bulge is visible in the caudal dorsal aspect of the heart (orange arrows). (**B**) On the ventrodorsal view, the angle between mainstem bronchi is widened (yellow arrows). The caudal margin of the enlarged left atrium is visible parallel to the caudal cardiac border (orange arrows). A left atrial appendage bulge is visible peripherally along the left cardiac margin (white arrows). These changes alter the overall shape and size of the cardiac silhouette from the expected normal (**A** and **B**, dotted white tracing).

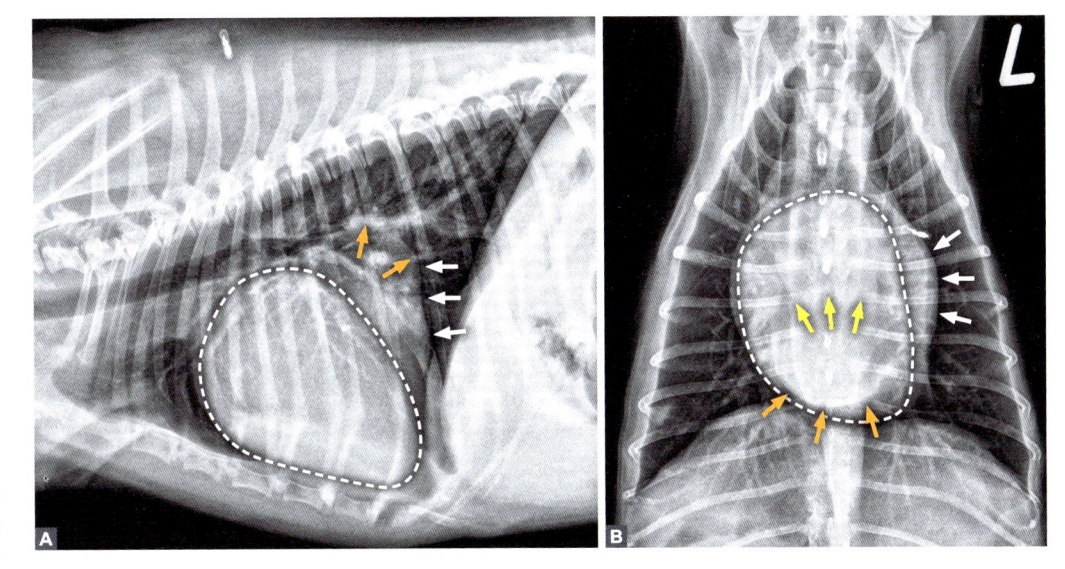

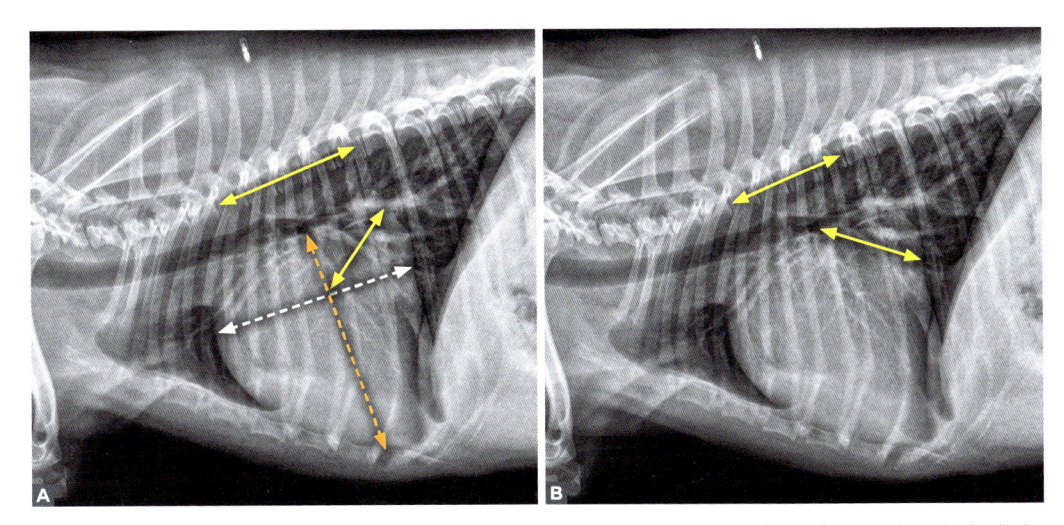

Fig. 19.23 Right lateral thoracic views of the same dog having left atrial enlargement due to degenerative mitral valvular disease. Measurement protocols for obtaining (**A**) the radiographic left atrial dimension (RLAD) and (**B**) the vertebral left atrial size (VLAS) are shown. (**A**) To obtain the RLAD, intersecting lines are drawn identical to those required to obtain a vertebral heart scale (VHS; see fig. 19.5; orange and white dotted arrows). Then an additional line is drawn bisecting the quadrant encompassed by the left atrium (yellow arrows). The length of this line is transposed onto the thoracic spine beginning at the cranial endplate of T4. The RLAD in this case measures 4.0 vertebrae. The optimal cutoff to distinguish normal from abnormal is reported to be 1.8 vertebrae,[14] indicating left atrial enlargement in this case. (**B**) To obtain the VLAS, a line is drawn from the most ventral aspect of the tracheal bifurcation to the caudal margin of the cardiac silhouette as it intersects with the dorsal aspect of the caudal vena cava (yellow arrows). The length of this line is transposed onto the thoracic spine beginning at the cranial endplate of T4. The VLAS in this case measures 3.75 vertebrae. A VLAS >2.3 vertebrae has been established as a predictor for left atrial enlargement in dogs.[15]

useful for confirming suspicion of left atrial enlargement and for objective assessment of change in size over time.

Left ventricular enlargement without concurrent left atrial enlargement is uncommon. Radiographic evaluation is insensitive for the detection of left ventricular enlargement occurring independently of left atrial enlargement. The heart, if visibly altered, will be tall encompassing greater than ⅔ the dorsoventral diameter of the thorax on the lateral view and elevating the caudal vena cava. The cardiac apex may be rounded and displaced towards the left on the ventrodorsal view.

Generalized cardiomegaly

The diagnosis of generalized cardiomegaly is reserved for cases that have evidence of both right- and left-sided enlargement, or when the silhouette is enlarged without definitive specific chamber enlargement such as with pericardial effusion. Recognizable dilation of the left atrium is usually present to some degree in cases of true cardiac enlargement, rather than pericardial disease (**fig. 19.26**). If the heart is markedly enlarged and globoid and a dilated left atrium is not seen, pericardial disease/effusion should be ranked first. Severe right-sided cardiomegaly can create a similar appearance to pericardial effusion. Differential diagnoses for generalized heart enlargement include any combination of diseases that can lead to right- or left-sided cardiomegaly, cardiomyopathy, ASD, chronic anemia, and cardiac conduction abnormalities. The heart often appears large in athletic canine animals, such as Greyhounds.

In cases of pericardial effusion, the echocardiographic exam is crucial because it helps define the etiology (e.g., cardiac mass, atrial rupture) and can confirm or exclude cardiac tamponade (**fig. 19.25**). Cardiac tamponade occurs when the pericardial pressure exceeds the pressures within the right heart. This causes diastolic collapse of the right atrium and, eventually, the right ventricle. The amount of effusion is not directly correlated to the presence of tamponade, because it depends also on the pericardial distensibility. The pericardium is fibrous and distends slowly in response to effusion. Rapid accumulation of quite small volume of fluid within the pericardium may elevate pressures sufficiently to cause tamponade.

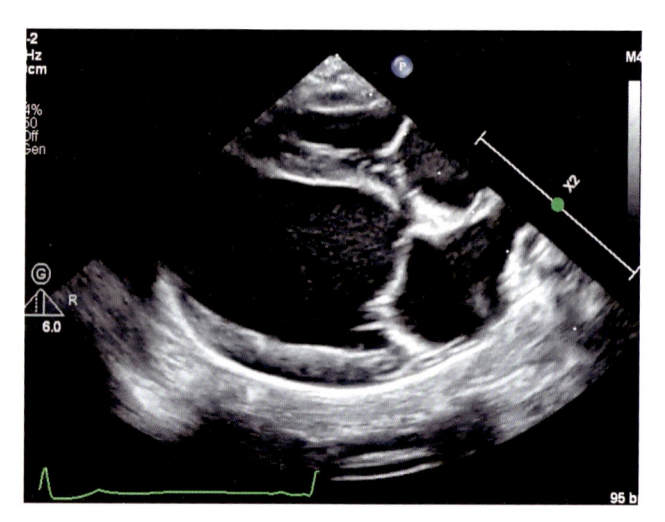

Fig. 19.24 Cavalier King Charles Spaniel with patent ductus arteriosus (PDA). The left ventricle looks rounded, with increased transverse diameters, due to the volume overload. The left atrium is normal in size, the pulmonary vein, visible at the insertion on the roof of the left atrium, is not dilated. A mild prolapse of the anterior leaflet of the mitral valve is evident. Right chambers are normal in size.

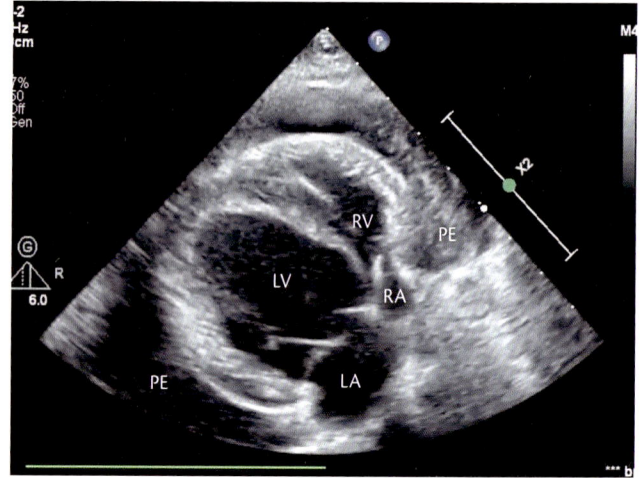

Fig. 19.25 Jack Russel terrier. Angled right parasternal view, late diastole. Pericardial effusion (PE), causing cardiac tamponade. The right atrium (RA) is collapsed. LA, left atrium; LV, left ventricle; RV, right ventricle.

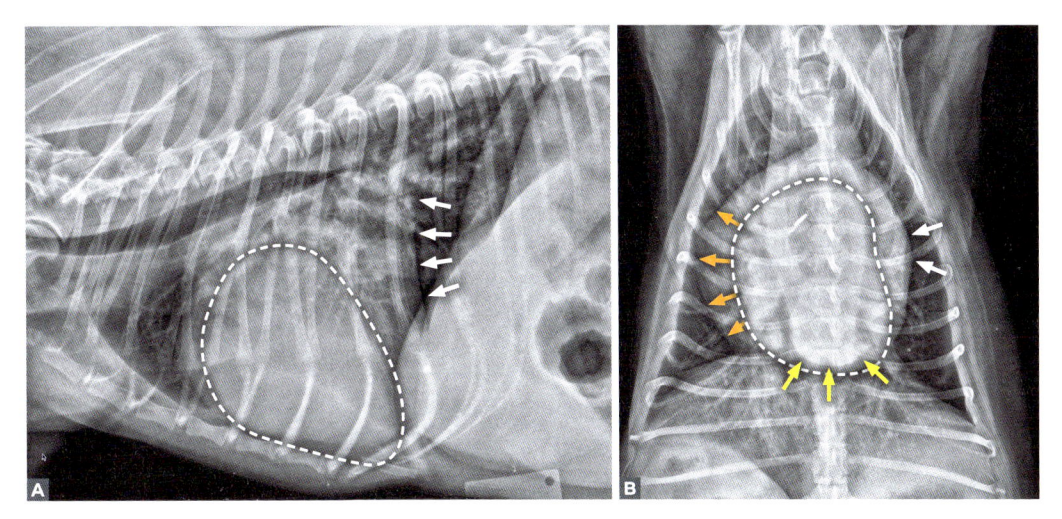

CHAPTER 19 Congenital and acquired cardiac diseases

Fig. 19.26 (**A**) Lateral and (**B**) ventrodorsal views of a nine-year-old Chihuahua having generalized (right- and left-sided) severe cardiomegaly due to concurrent tricuspid and mitral valvular degeneration. The heart is wide and tall as compared to the overlay of the expected cardiac size and shape (white dotted tracing). (**A**) The left atrium and atrial appendage are dilated indicated by a flat caudal cardiac margin on the lateral view (white arrows), (**B**) a well-defend line superimposed cranial to the cardiac apex on the ventrodorsal view (yellow arrows), and a mild bulge at the mid left cardiac margin on the ventrodorsal view (white arrows). The cardiac apex is rounded precluding assessment of left versus right ventricular dilation. The cranial and right cardiac borders are rounded consistent with dilation of the right heart.

Enlarged great vessels

Enlargement of the aorta and main pulmonary artery occurs subsequent to turbulent flow from a stenotic valve or vascular shunt or due to congestion. These vascular changes may or may not be accompanied by visible cardiomegaly or altered cardiac shape. Enlargement of the great vessels should prompt evaluation of the cardiac silhouette and pulmonary vessels.

Main pulmonary arterial enlargement is most readily identified on the ventrodorsal view and appears as a focal bulge of the left cranial heart in the 1:00-2:00 position, as shown in **fig. 19.27**. Dilation of the main pulmonary artery is caused by turbulent flow from pulmonic stenosis or patent ductus arteriosus, or from congestion associated with *Dirofilaria immitis* infection or acquired pulmonary hypertension. All causes of an enlarged main pulmonary artery can result in right-sided cardiomeg-

Fig. 19.27 (**A**) Lateral and (**B**) ventrodorsal radiographs of a dog having severe main pulmonary arterial dilation. (**A**) Though subtle, an increased convexity is present at the cranial cardiac border on the lateral view (arrows). (**B**) A large focal bulge is present at the left cranial cardiac margin on the ventrodorsal view in the region of the main pulmonary artery (1:00-2:00 position; arrows). In this case, the overall cardiac size is normal, but the MPA enlargement creates an altered shape compared to a normal dog (**A** and **B**, dotted tracings).

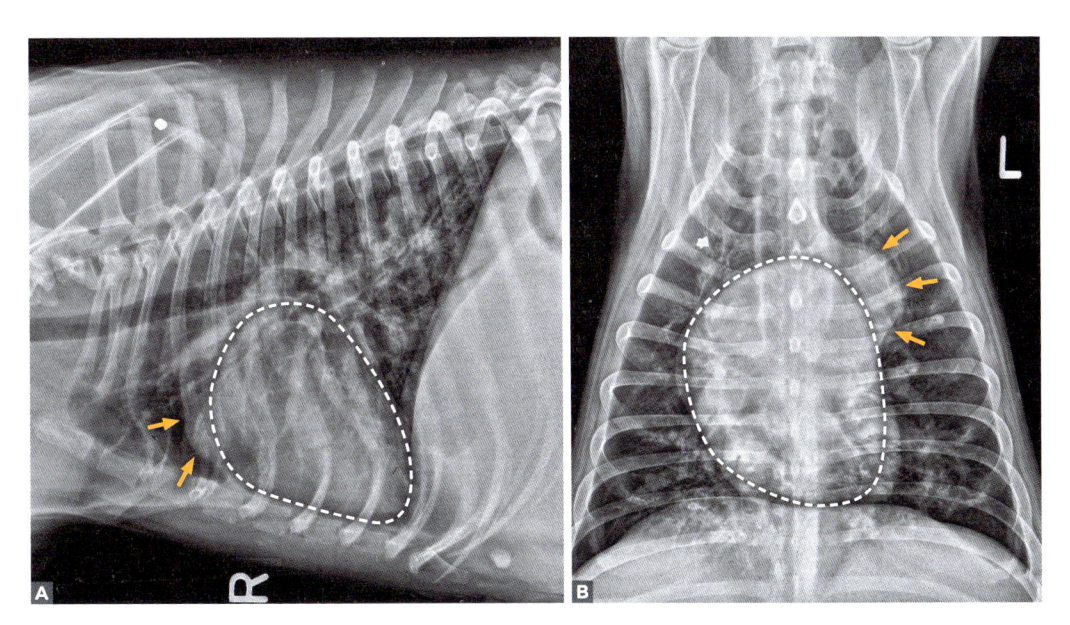

SECTION IV THORAX

aly. The main distinguishing factor among the differential diagnoses is the appearance of lobar pulmonary vasculature as shown in **fig. 19.28**. An enlarged aortic arch is located at the craniodorsal aspect of the heart (8:00-11:00 position) on the lateral view, similar to right auricular and main pulmonary arterial enlargement; however, the lateral view is insensitive to detection of aortic arch enlargement. Aortic arch enlargement is more readily detected on the VD or DV view and will appear as a bulge in the cranial cardiac margin within the caudal aspect of the cranial mediastinum. Enlargement of the aortic arch is most often caused by turbulent flow secondary to aortic stenosis as shown in **fig. 19.29**.

A second location of aortic enlargement occurs due to turbulent flow associated with a patent ductus arteriosus, located at the proximal descending aorta. Proximal descending aortic enlargement is pathognomonic for patent ductus arteriosus (left-to-right or reversed) and is most reliably visible on the ventrodorsal view (**fig. 19.30**).

Echocardiography is limited for assessment of the great vessels since only the proximal portions close to the heart are visible. Dilation of the pulmonary trunk and the main pulmonary arteries can be visible with pulmonary hypertension, post-stenotic dilation, or PDA (**figs. 19.31** and **19.32**). The ascending aorta can be dilated due to aortic/subaortic stenosis or systemic hypertension. The cranial and caudal venae cavae are distended in course of right congestive heart failure or obstruction to preload (e.g., intracavitary neoplasia or thrombi, cardiac tamponade). The evaluation of the caudal vena cava is more easily imaged by a subcostal approach through the liver.

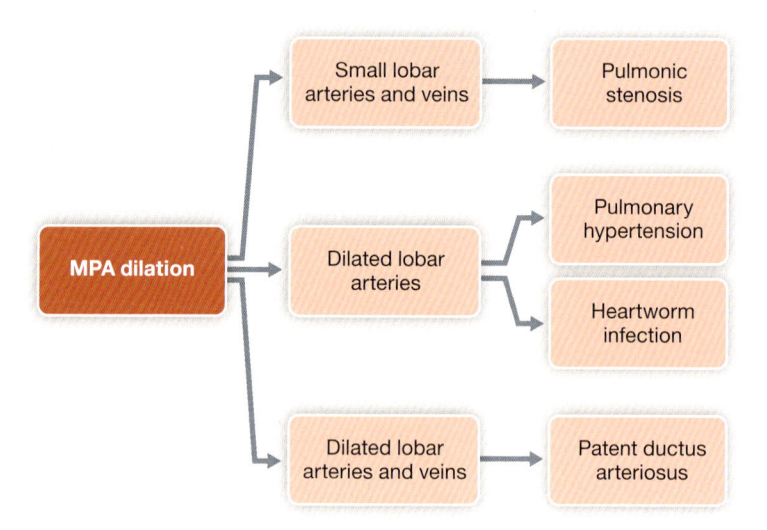

Fig. 19.28 Differential diagnoses for main pulmonary arterial (MPA) dilation.

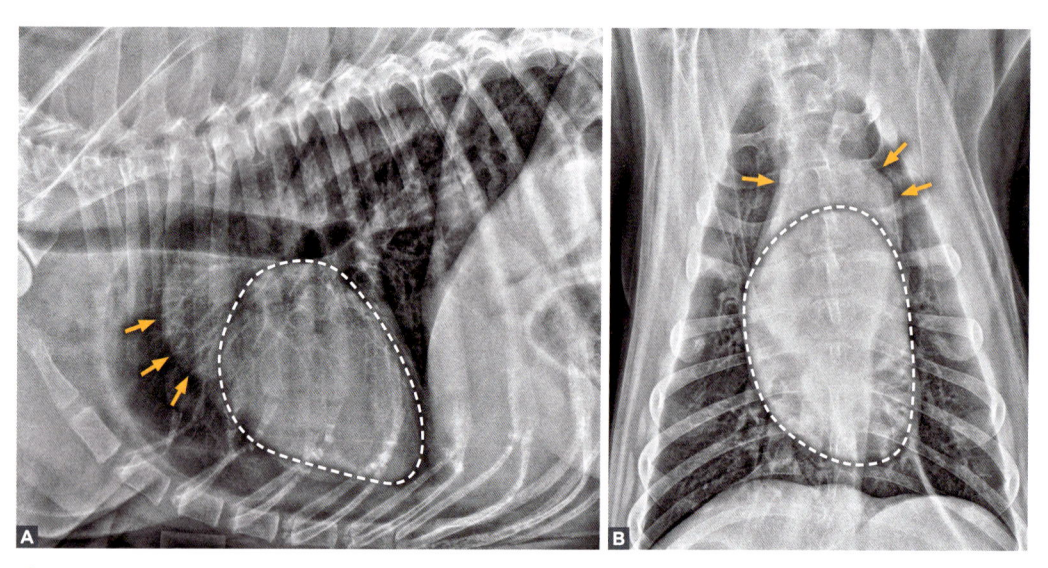

Fig. 19.29 (**A**) Lateral and (**B**) ventrodorsal views in a dog with post-stenotic dilation of the aorta from subaortic stenosis. (**A**) On the lateral view a focal bulge is seen at the cranial cardiac base (arrows). (**B**) On the ventrodorsal view, an increase in soft tissue opacity is seen at the caudal aspect of the cranial mediastinum at the 11:00-1:00 position of the cardiac silhouette (arrows). The cardiac size is normal; however, the shape of the cardiac silhouette reflects the typical appearance of aortic arch enlargement as compared to normal (**A** and **B**, dotted tracings).

CHAPTER **19** Congenital and acquired cardiac diseases

Fig. 19.30 Ventrodorsal radiograph of a dog with focal dilation of the proximal descending aorta from a patent ductus arteriosus (arrows). The proximal aspect of the descending aorta has a focal convexity at the level of the proximal descending aorta that increases the convexity of this region when compared to a normal proximal descending aorta (dotted tracing).

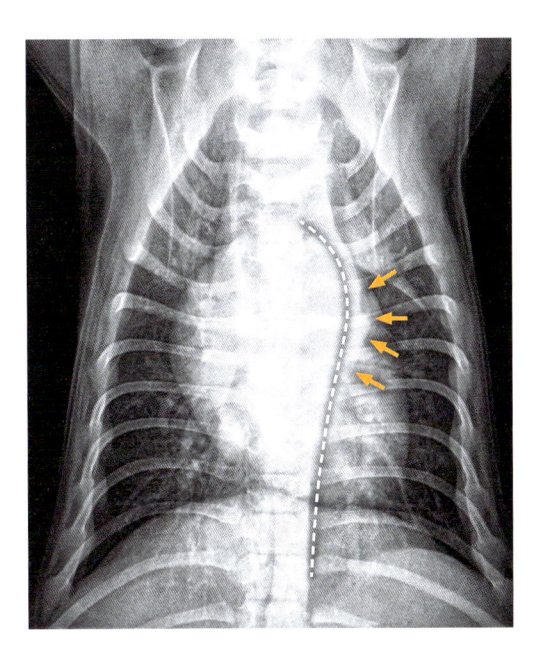

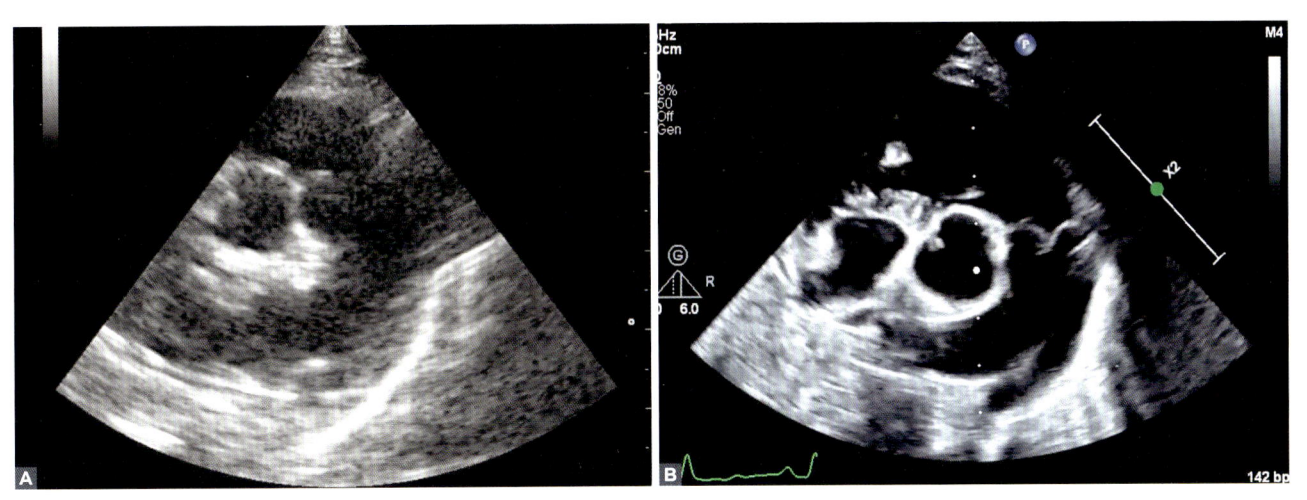

Fig. 19.31 (**A**) Domestic shorthair cat affected by left-to-right shunt ventricular septal defect. The pulmonary trunk and the right and left pulmonary arteries are distended due to the volume overload. The right ventricle is not dilated because the shunt flow, through the perimembranous defect, bypasses the right ventricle and enters directly into the right ventricular outflow tract and pulmonary artery. (**B**) Mongrel dog with type 3 pulmonary hypertension. The severe dilation of the pulmonary trunk and the right pulmonary artery is associated to the dilation of the right ventricle due to chronic pressure overload.

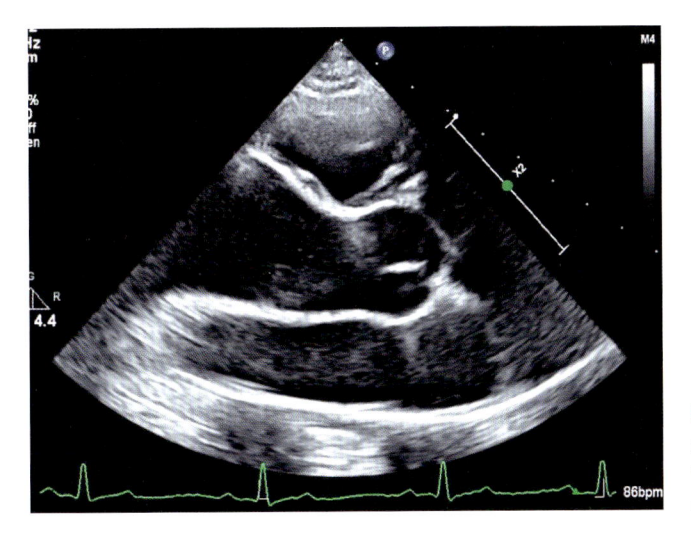

Fig. 19.32 Golden Retriever affected by subaortic stenosis. Left cranial aortic root view. The post stenotic dilation is evident downstream the senotubular junction.

Pulmonary vasculature

Initially, the pulmonary arteries and veins are closely apposed to the lobar bronchi creating a triad of artery, bronchus, and vein. With each branch of the vessels and bronchi, the bronchi become more closely associated with the pulmonary arteries until the final branching division creates pulmonary lobules where pulmonary bronchioles and arteries are central, and the vein is at the periphery. On the lateral view, the arteries are located dorsal to the bronchus, and veins are located ventral. The size of the cranial lobar vessels, assessed on the lateral views, should be similar in diameter to each other and no greater in size to the proximal aspect of the unmagnified fourth rib (**fig. 19.15**).[16, 17] The caudal lobar arteries and veins are best assessed on the ventrodorsal/dorsoventral view. The caudal lobar arteries are located lateral to the bronchi and veins. As such, the veins are centrally located and are said to be "central and ventral" within the triad of artery, bronchus, and vein. The size of the caudal lobar pulmonary arteries and veins should be similar to the diameter of the ninth ribs as they cross (**fig. 19.33**).

Pulmonary venous dilation occurs after a sustained elevation in left atrial pressure that results in congestion. The presence of pulmonary venous dilation usually indicates left-sided cardiac failure. Dilated pulmonary arteries occur due to increased pressure/obstruction downstream from the pulmonary arteries, i.e., at the distal artery, at the level of the capillaries, or post-capillary pressure elevations (e.g., chronically elevated left atrial pressure). In addition to the presence of pulmonary hypertension, myointimal proliferation and endothelial damage of the pulmonary artery can also directly cause enlargement of the artery in cases of *Dirofilaria immitis* infection from 3 months after inoculation.[18]

Concurrent dilation of pulmonary arteries and veins occurs from pulmonary overcirculation in congenital left-to-right cardiac shunting anomalies such as patent ductus arteriosus (PDA) and atrial or ventricular septal defects (ASD or VSD). Chronic left atrial pressure elevation from left-sided congestive cardiac failure may result in transmission of pressure elevation upstream from the capillary bed to the pulmonary arterial circulation causing dilation of both the pulmonary arteries and veins.[19] Generalized pulmonary vascular congestion may also occur from iatrogenic fluid overload.

Reduced size of the pulmonary arteries and veins can be caused by cardiac disease. Non-cardiac specific differential etiologies of hypovascularity are far more common, and include severe dehydration, hypovolemic shock, and rarely hypoadrenocorticism. The heart may also appear small.

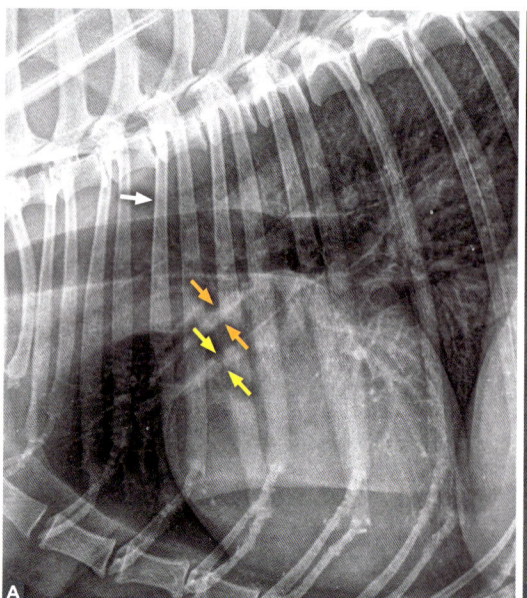

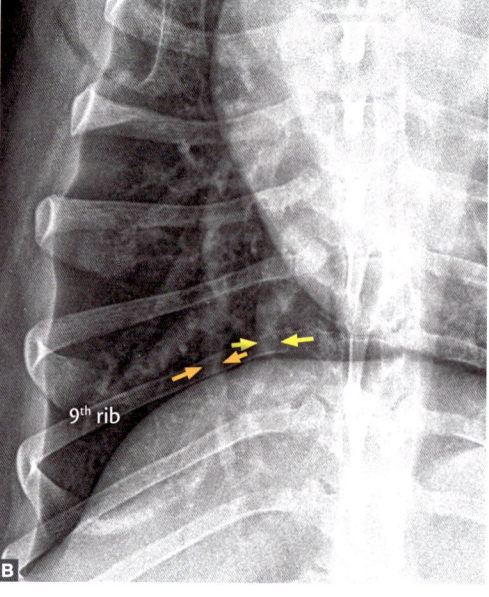

Fig. 19.33 (**A**) Lateral and (**B**) ventrodorsal views of a normal dog showing the diameters of normal lobar arteries and veins. The cranial and caudal lobar arteries (between orange arrows) and veins (between yellow arrows) should be similar in size to the proximal fourth rib (white arrow) and labeled ninth rib at the point of intersection (**B**), respectively.

Fig. 19.34 Differential diagnoses for pulmonary vascular dilation.

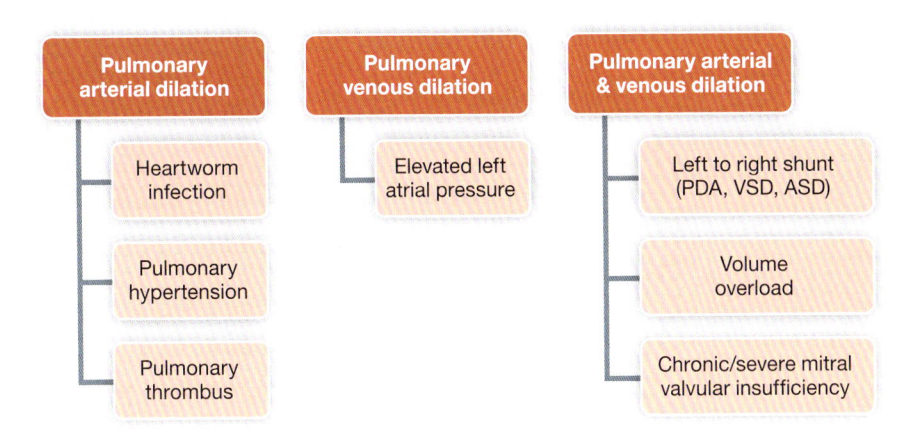

Pulmonary arterial dilation
- Heartworm infection
- Pulmonary hypertension
- Pulmonary thrombus

Pulmonary venous dilation
- Elevated left atrial pressure

Pulmonary arterial & venous dilation
- Left to right shunt (PDA, VSD, ASD)
- Volume overload
- Chronic/severe mitral valvular insufficiency

Congenital cardiac anomalies that can cause hypovolemia include severe pulmonic stenosis (causes decreased blood flow to pass into pulmonary circulation from the right ventricle), tricuspid dysplasia (decreased forward flow of blood to pulmonary arteries from right ventricle because of retrograde flow to right atrium), and right-to-left shunts (reverse PDA, reverse VSD, or tetralogy of Fallot causing systemic arterial circulation to receive blood that would normally go through pulmonary circulation). Pulmonary hypoperfusion may be caused by pericardial effusion and tamponade reducing cardiac output. Small pulmonary arteries and veins are also sometimes seen following diuretic treatment of congestive cardiac failure.

Peripheral pulmonary vascular abnormalities and radiographic changes of the cardiac silhouette are considered in combination to formulate a differential diagnosis list. **Figure 19.34** summarizes differential diagnoses for pulmonary arterial and/or venous enlargements.

Congestive heart failure

Cardiomegaly does not equal cardiac failure. Upon detection of cardiomegaly, every effort should be made to determine whether it is left- or right-sided (or rarely, generalized) and whether there is radiographic evidence of right- or left-sided failure. These findings must be correlated with the clinical status of the animal, as clinical signs of cardiac decompensation may develop before radiographic changes. Right-sided congestive heart failure causes congestion of the systemic venous system entering the right atrium (cranial vena cava, caudal vena cava, lymphatics) and slows the transmission of blood forward into the heart. It is the result of a sustained elevation in right atrial pressure. Once the compensatory mechanisms of the heart are overwhelmed, congestion occurs resulting in dilation of the caudal vena cava and hepatic veins, hepatic parenchymal congestion, and subsequent effusion (**figs. 19.35-19.37**).

Left-sided congestive heart failure occurs when sustained elevations in left atrial pressure overwhelm the compensatory mechanisms of the heart to accommodate an expansion of circulating vascular

Fig. 19.35 The typical order of findings associated with right heart failure is depicted. Often, these findings occur in combination with evidence of right-sided cardiomegaly or pericardial disease.

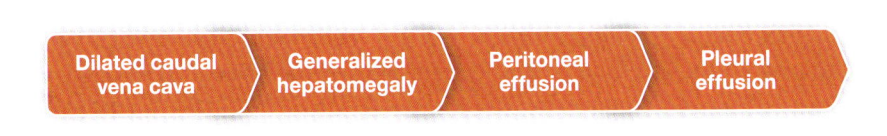

Dilated caudal vena cava → Generalized hepatomegaly → Peritoneal effusion → Pleural effusion

SECTION IV THORAX

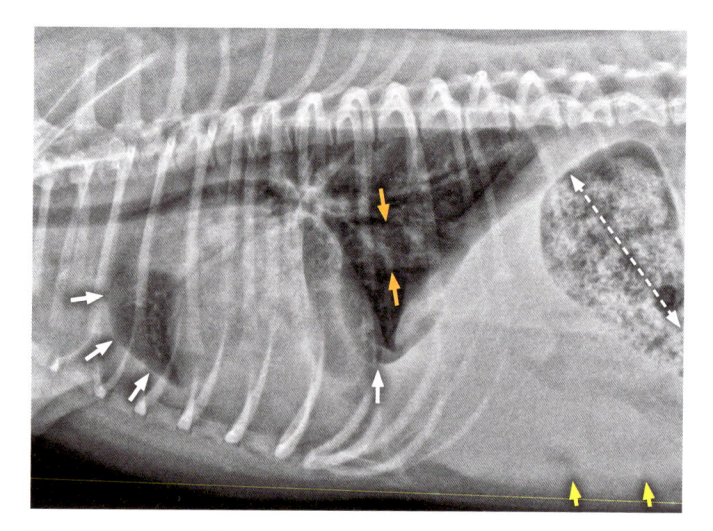

Fig. 19.36 Lateral thoracic radiograph in a dog with right-sided cardiac failure due to severe pulmonary hypertension. The caudal vena cava is congested and fails to taper towards the diaphragm (between orange arrows). The liver is enlarged, causing caudal displacement of the stomach (dotted white line). Peritoneal effusion is present, causing soft tissue opaque streaking and a decrease in visibility of the caudoventral liver margin (yellow arrows). Moderate separation of lungs from the thoracic wall by fluid is present (white arrows), indicating pleural effusion. These findings, combined with cardiomegaly, are indicative of right-sided heart failure.

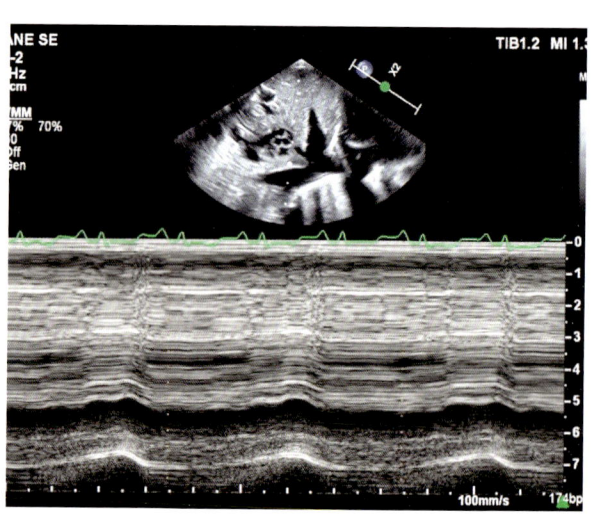

Fig. 19.37 Hepatic scan: M-mode of the caudal vena cava. In normal conditions, there is a variation of the internal diameter of the caudal vena cava with the respiration phase. The lack of excursion, named plethora cavale, depends on the increased central venous pressure.

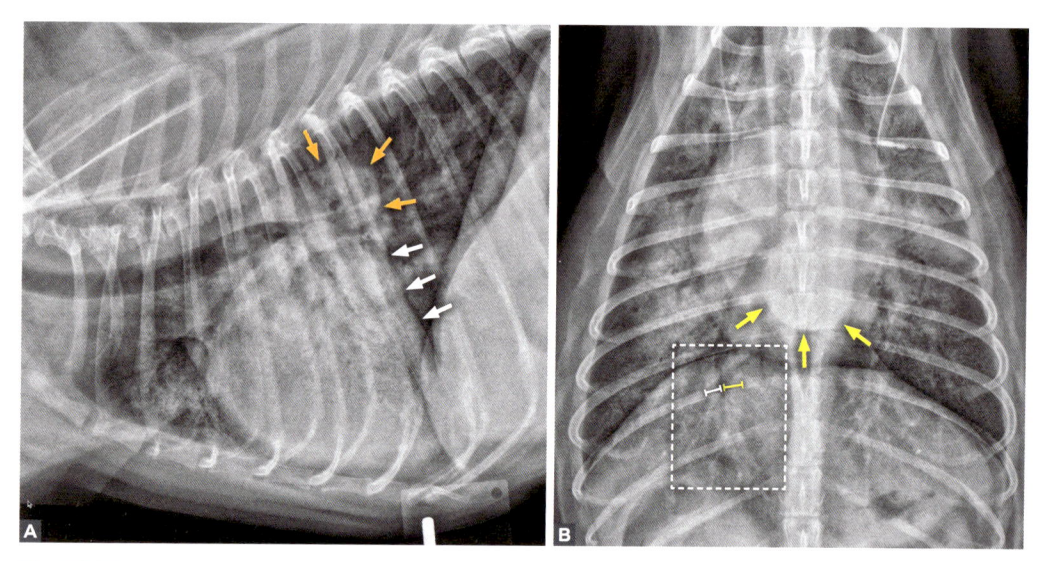

Fig. 19.38 (**A**) Lateral and (**B**) dorsoventral thoracic radiographs of a Pomeranian with left-sided cardiac failure due to mitral valvular endocardiosis. (**A**) The caudal cardiac margin is flat (white arrows). A bulge is present in the region of the left atrium that extends dorsal to the caudal lobar bronchi (orange arrows). (**B**) A well-defined margin is visible, representing the caudal edge of the left atrium on the ventrodorsal view (yellow arrows). The caudal lobar vessels are partially obscured by an increase in pulmonary opacity located in the hilar and middle zones that is more severe on the right side than the left. On the dorsoventral view of the thorax, the right caudal lobar vasculature is still faintly visible (inside dotted box). The right caudal lobar vein (yellow caliper) is dilated compared to the artery (white caliper) as they intersect the rib. There is also an interstitial pattern in both cranial lung lobes, more severe in the middle and peripheral zones. These findings are consistent with left-sided congestive cardiac failure and severe cardiogenic pulmonary edema.

volume returning via the pulmonary veins. With failure and the onset of pulmonary edema, the rate of extravascular fluid accumulation exceeds the rate of lymphatic removal. Visible indications of failure may include dilated pulmonary veins, although this is inconsistent, and cardiogenic edema is characterized in dogs by interstitial or alveolar pulmonary opacity having a perihilar/caudodorsal

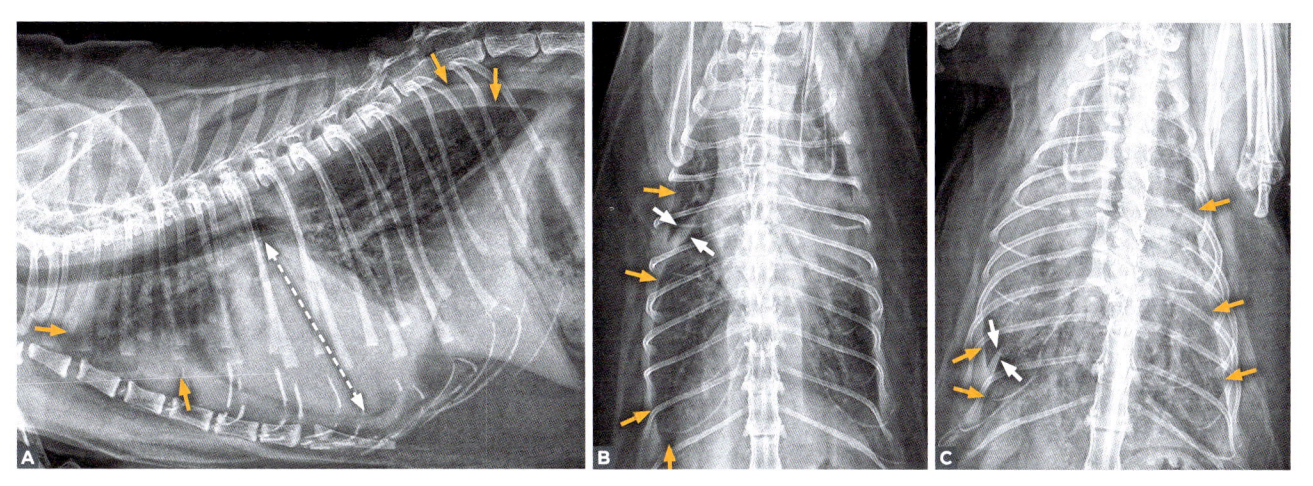

Fig. 19.39 (**A**) Lateral, (**B**) ventrodorsal, and (**C**) dorsoventral radiographs of a cat with left-sided congestive heart failure due to hypertrophic cardiomyopathy. The distribution of cardiogenic edema is multifocal and predominantly ventral, causing partial border effacement of the cardiac silhouette. (**A**) Cardiac enlargement causes dorsal elevation of the trachea and a tall cardiac silhouette (dotted line). Evidence of moderate pleural effusion is visible where lungs are retracted from the thoracic wall (**A**, **B**, and **C**, orange arrows), and small pleural fissure lines (**B** and **C**, between white arrows) are visible. Pleural fluid is a common finding in cats with left-sided cardiac failure, distinguishing features of left-sided heart failure found in dogs.

distribution (**fig. 19.38**). The edema is most often symmetrical but can be asymmetrically right-sided as well. A right-sided distribution, when present, occurs most often secondary to mitral valvular disease rather than dilated cardiomyopathy.[20] In cats, the distribution of cardiogenic edema is often less predictable in regional distribution and can be diffuse or multifocal (**fig. 19.39**) complicating the distinction between cardiogenic and noncardiogenic causes of increased pulmonary opacity. An important distinction between dogs and cats is that, although the mechanism is unclear, pleural effusion often accompanies cardiogenic edema in cases of left-sided failure in cats and is commonly present in small volumes.[21]

Congenital cardiac diseases

Numerous canine and feline congenital cardiac defects exist, and their radiographic appearances can be daunting to categorize without having a solid understanding of how the morphological abnormalities influence cardiac and vascular remodeling and resulting radiographic abnormalities. A few basic concepts such as cardiac shunting and alterations in blood flow that occur with many of the congenital cardiac defects and their influence on cardiac morphology as they apply to radiographic appearance are presented to assist in creating appropriate differential diagnoses.

Congenital cardiac diseases are morphological disorders that are present at birth. These disorders also include malformations of the great vessels in addition to the heart itself. The morphological abnormalities occur during heart formation, septation, and transformation of the six aortic arches during embryogenesis. The four cardiac chambers are created due to the formation of valves and the atrial and ventricular septa. The valves and the atrial and ventricular septa are in close proximity, and complex concurrent valvular and septal malformations can occur.

The specific etiology of congenital cardiac diseases is complex and incompletely understood. In dogs, genetic predispositions are known risk factors, since diseases like subaortic stenosis in the Newfoundland, pulmonic stenosis in the Beagle, patent ductus arteriosus in the Poodle, and conotruncal abnormalities (tetralogy of Fallot) in Keeshonds are known to have a hereditary basis.[22,23] Environmental factors that result in certain exposures during cardiac development are likely. A genetically determined increase in susceptibility to environmental triggers could similarly influence the formation of defects.[24] The reported ranking of the prevalence of various congenital diseases in dogs varies depending on the source, but consistently includes subaortic and pulmonic stenosis, patent ductus arteriosus, and ventricular septal defects.[25, 26] Atrioventricular valvular dysplasias are reported less commonly.

Congenital cardiac diseases in cats are uncommonly reported. Familial patterns of feline congenital cardiac diseases have been reported in several breeds. Siamese cats have been associated with aortic stenosis, atrioventricular valvular malformations, and endocardial fibroelastosis. Domestic shorthair cats are associated with ventricular septal defects and atrioventricular valvular malformations.[27] Ventricular septal defects are the most commonly reported feline congenital anomaly (50% of all congenital anomalies), followed by tricuspid dysplasia.[28, 29] A male sex predisposition has been recorded for several feline congenital cardiac anomalies.[27]

Shunting of blood

Several congenital cardiac defects result in shunting of blood. A septal defect (intracardiac) or communication between the arterial and venous systems (extracardiac) must be present to allow direct communication between the left and right-sided cardiac circulations. Blood traveling through a shunt always travels from a region of high pressure to a region of low pressure. As such, cardiac shunts are typically left-to-right, or oxygen-rich to deoxygenated. Right-to-left shunting of blood can occur but it requires two concurrent abnormalities to be present. First, a septal defect (intracardiac) or communication between arterial and venous systems (extracardiac) must be present. Second, an abnormality (acquired or congenital) resulting in elevated right-sided pressures that exceed those on the left side must be concurrently present. This can occur due to congenital pulmonic stenosis or due to pulmonary hypertension, for example.

The abnormality of increasing right-sided pressure must affect pressures distal to the shunt in order to cause flow reversal (i.e., right-to-left shunting). For example, a dog with concurrent pulmonary hypertension and patent ductus arteriosus can develop right-to-left shunting. However, a dog with pulmonic stenosis and patent ductus arteriosus would not have shunt reversal because pressure differences in the pulmonary arterial circulation at the site of shunting (distal to the stenosis) are normal and would result in a left-to-right anomalous flow configuration.

When shunting of blood occurs, the increased blood volume will cause enlargement of those chambers receiving the recirculated volume causing eccentric hypertrophy of the myocardium. In addition to cardiac enlargement, in cases of left-to-right shunt, pulmonary arteries and veins may be congested from recirculation of blood (pulmonary overcirculation) if a sufficiently large proportion of cardiac output is diverted through the shunt. In cases of right-to-left shunting, the pulmonary vessels appear normal, because recirculation of blood is not occurring through the lungs. If a large proportion of cardiac output is diverted through a right-to-left shunt, the lungs may appear underperfused.

Radiographic appearance of specific congenital cardiac diseases

In general, congenital diseases are more commonly diagnosed in dogs. The reported incidence of the most common congenital cardiac defects in dogs vary by institution but include patent ductus arteriosus, subaortic stenosis, ventricular septal defect, and pulmonic stenosis.[22, 23, 30] Each cardiac anomaly may cause specific alterations in the cardiac silhouette and vessels that can be used to make a presumptive diagnosis, in conjunction with cardiac auscultation. Echocardiography is almost always required to make a confirmed diagnosis. The most common cardiac congenital anomalies and their typical radiographic abnormalities are summarized in **table 19.6**. It cannot be overemphasized that many patients with congenital anomalies do not demonstrate some or all the expected radiographic changes. Radiographs do not provide a specific diagnosis in many cases, the echocardiographic exam remains the gold standard for the diagnosis of congenital heart disease. The degree of cardiomegaly can be used as a crude index of the severity of the anomaly. Radiographs are most helpful in confirming or excluding cardiac failure.

Table 19.6 Summary of radiographic changes seen with commonly reported congenital cardiac diseases.

Diseases causing left-to-right shunting

1) Patent ductus arteriosus (PDA)	■ Ductus bump in the proximal descending aorta (pathognomonic for PDA) ■ Different anatomical location than aortic arch enlargement due to post-stenotic dilatation from an aortic stenosis ■ Main pulmonary arterial enlargement ■ Left-sided cardiomegaly (eccentric hypertrophy) ■ Dilated pulmonary arteries and veins (pulmonary overcirculation)

2) Ventricular septal defect (VSD)	■ Usually left-sided cardiomegaly only (eccentric hypertrophy)
	  ■ VSD is usually small and located high in the interventricular septum resulting in blood flow directly into right ventricular outflow tract during systole rather than into the right ventricle
	  ■ Right ventricular enlargement occurs if VSD is in the muscular septum or is large
	■ Dilated pulmonary arteries and veins (pulmonary overcirculation)

3) Atrial septal defect (ASD)	■ Generalized cardiomegaly ■ Dilated pulmonary arteries and veins (pulmonary overcirculation)

Valvular obstructive diseases

1) Pulmonic stenosis (PS)	■ Enlarged right ventricle (concentric hypertrophy) ■ Main pulmonary arterial enlargement (post-stenotic dilatation) ■ Small to normal pulmonary arteries and veins
2) Subaortic stenosis (SAS)	■ Left-sided cardiomegaly (concentric hypertrophy) ■ Dilated aortic arch

Dysplasias of the atrioventricular valves

1) Tricuspid dysplasia (TD)	■ Right-sided cardiomegaly (eccentric hypertrophy) ■ Right atrial enlargement dominates ■ Small to normal pulmonary arteries and veins
2) Mitral dysplasia (MD)	■ Left-sided cardiomegaly (eccentric hypertrophy) ■ Left atrial enlargement dominates

Diseases causing right-to-left shunting

1) Tetralogy of Fallot (ToF)	■ Markedly enlarged right ventricle ■ Main pulmonary arterial enlargement (post-stenotic dilatation) ■ Small to normal pulmonary arteries and veins
2) Reverse PDA	■ Ductus bump in proximal descending aorta (pathognomonic for PDA) ■ Main pulmonary arterial enlargement ■ Right-sided cardiomegaly ■ Absence of pulmonary overcirculation

Diseases causing left-to-right shunting of blood

A patent ductus arteriosus (PDA) is caused by an extracardiac shunting of blood between the aorta and the main pulmonary artery. Blood from the high-pressure aorta flows into the main pulmonary artery creating a recirculation path from the aorta, through the pulmonary arteries, then veins, and back to the left atrium, as shown in **fig. 19.40**. Cardiovascular alterations occur within the parts of the heart and vasculature having abnormal flow in this altered pathway. Therefore, aneurysmal dilation is expected within the proximal descending aorta (in the location of the patent ductus arteriosus)

SECTION IV THORAX

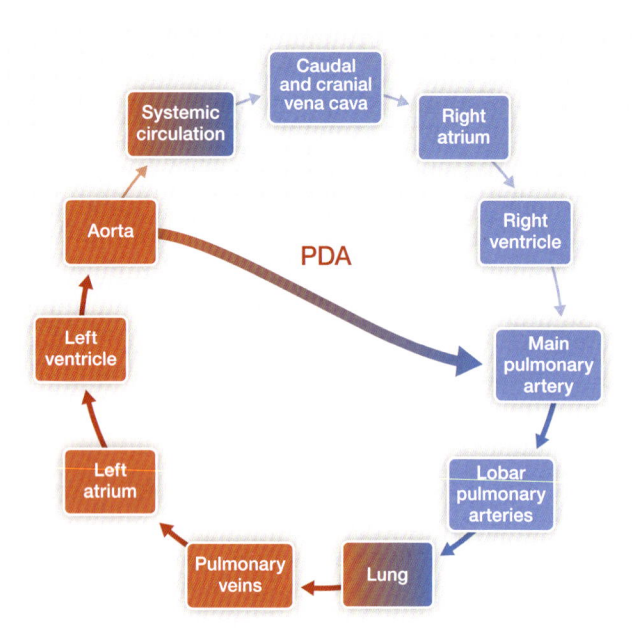

Fig. 19.40 Recirculation pathway caused by a patent ductus arteriosus. Cardiac enlargements occur in those structures receiving recirculated blood via the shunt including the pulmonary arteries and veins, the left atrium, and the left ventricle (eccentric hypertrophy). The main pulmonary artery and proximal descending aorta, in addition to receiving increased vascular volume, are subject to turbulent flow focal dilation of these structures.

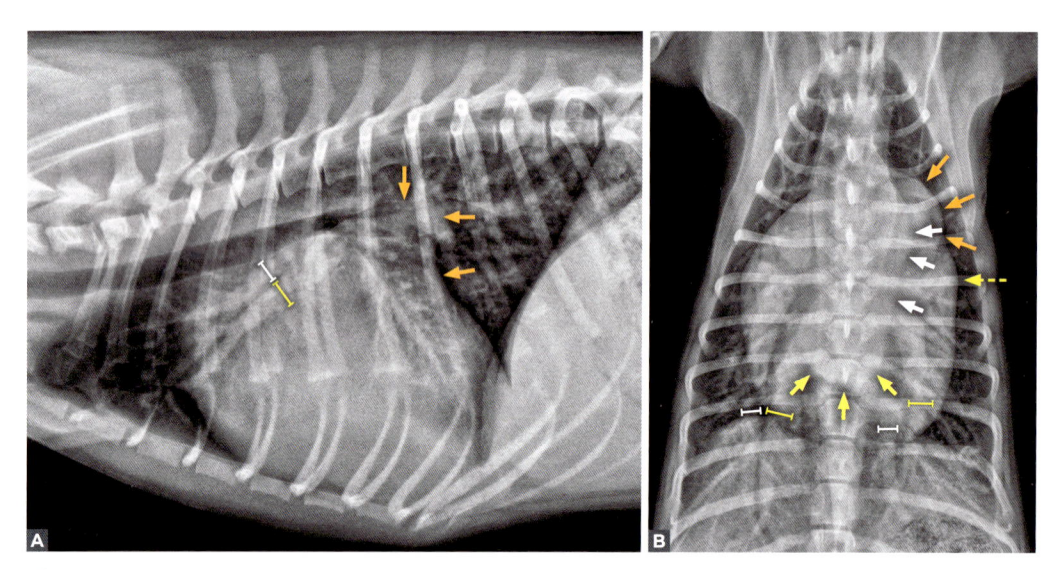

Fig. 19.41 (**A**) Right lateral and (**B**) ventrodorsal thoracic radiographs of a dog diagnosed with a patent ductus arteriosus (PDA). Left-sided cardiomegaly is present denoted by an enlarged left atrium identified on (**A**) the lateral view (orange arrows) that creates a visible caudal left atrial margin on (**B**) the ventrodorsal view (yellow arrows) and an enlarged left atrial appendage (dotted yellow arrow). The cardiac apex is rounded due to eccentric hypertrophy and increased volume of the left ventricle. The lobar pulmonary arteries and veins (white and yellow calipers, respectively) are both dilated, indicating pulmonary overcirculation. Finally, bulges are seen within the proximal descending aorta (white arrows) and the main pulmonary artery (orange arrows).

and/or main pulmonary artery from turbulent flow at the level of the ductus. Dilation of the aorta and main pulmonary artery is quite variable, and there may be dilation of one vessel only or none. The pulmonary arteries and veins are dilated if the shunt volume is large. Volume overload causes dilation and eccentric hypertrophy of the left ventricle and left atrial dilation (**fig. 19.41**). Right-to-left shunting through a PDA requires a concurrent elevation in main pulmonary arterial pressure to match or exceed aortic pressure that could occur due to acquired pulmonary hypertension secondary to chronic pulmonary overcirculation (Eisenmenger syndrome).

The echocardiographic exam allows the direct visualization of the ductus (**figs. 19.42** and **19.43**). The minimal ductal diameter (at the level of the insertion into the pulmonary artery) can be visual-

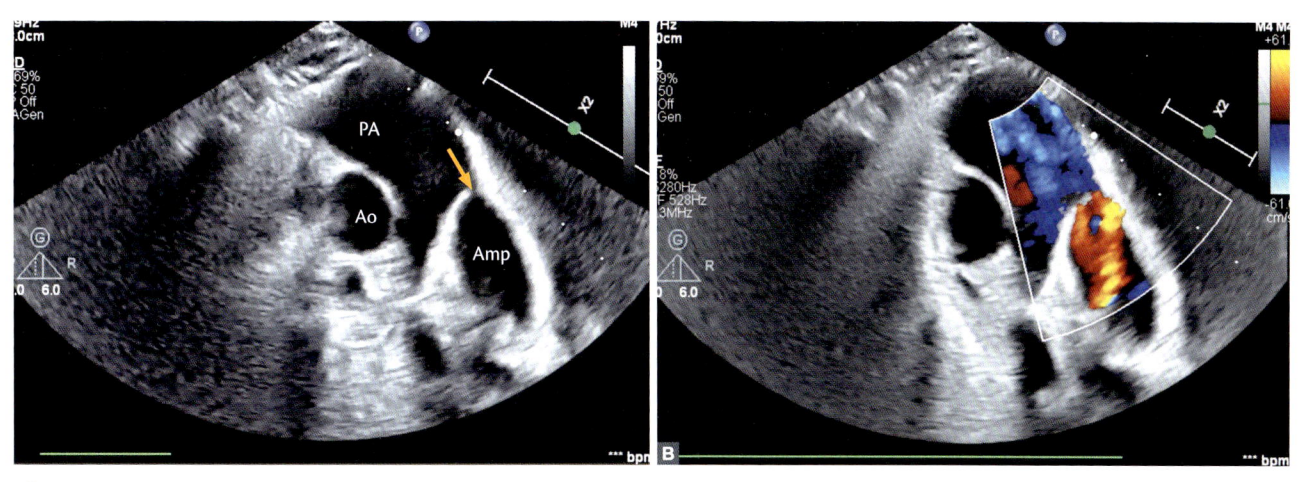

Fig. 19.42 Cavalier King Charles Spaniel with left-to-right shunt from a patent ductus arteriosus (PDA). (**A**) Left parasternal oblique view. The ductal ampulla is visible (Amp), and the point of insertion in the main pulmonary artery, the minimal ductal diameter (arrow). (**B**) Color Doppler of the shunt flow through the ductus. The dilation of the main pulmonary artery is evident. Ao, aorta; PA, pulmonary artery.

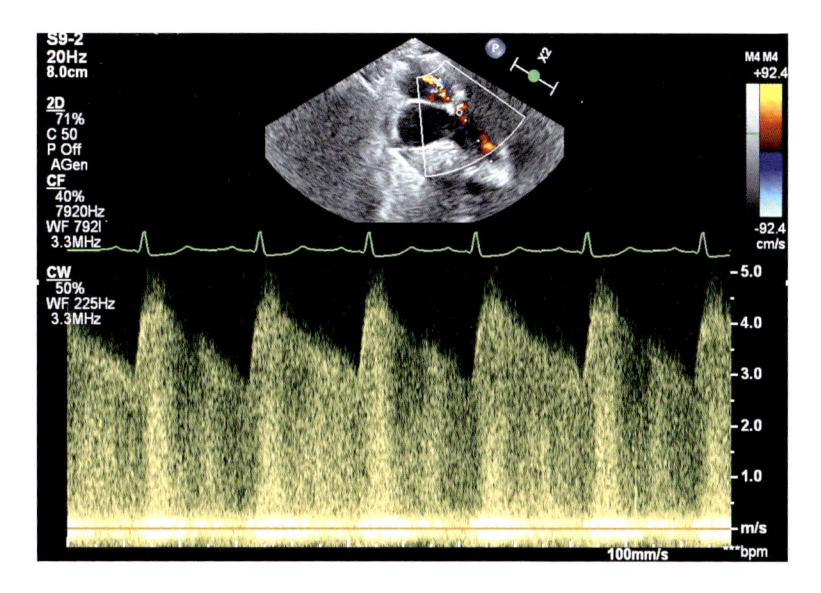

Fig. 19.43 Mongrel dog with left-to-right shunt PDA. Spectral Doppler of the continuous shunt flow. The velocity of the flow changes during the cardiac cycle with a peak in systole (4,8 m/s) and a lower velocity in diastole (3 m/s). The systolic pressure gradient through the ductus is 98 mmHg, suggesting normal pulmonary resistance.

ized and measured; however, for this purpose, transesophageal echocardiography is more accurate. Color and spectral Doppler allow evaluation of flow within the shunt: a normal left-to-right shunt shows continuous with an elevated velocity (systolic peak velocity around 5 m/s), which indicates a normal pressure gradient between the systemic and the pulmonary arterial circulations. When pulmonary resistance increases sufficiently to equal or exceed systemic pressures, the shunt becomes bidirectional or reverses to become right-to-left, with a decreased peak velocity.

A ventricular septal defect (VSD) creates intracardiac shunting of blood between the ventricles with the defect typically occurring at the basilar aspect of the interventricular septum, close to the cardiac valves, often called a "high" or a "membranous" VSD. Under many circumstances, the shunt is small in size, which limits the flow volume (referred to as restrictive), therefore maintaining normal pressure differences between the ventricles. With the most common configuration of VSD (membranous and restrictive), during systole, blood flowing from the high-pressure left ventricle enters directly into the right ventricular outflow tract due to the basilar location of the septal defect. Because of the location of the defect and flow orientation, volume and pressure overload of the right ventricle does not tend to occur with most VSDs. As with any shunt, the resulting cardiovascular changes occur in those structures receiving recirculated blood as shown in **figs. 19.44** and **19.45**. Given the blood flow pattern in membranous restrictive VSDs, the resulting cardiomegaly is often left-sided only with

SECTION IV THORAX

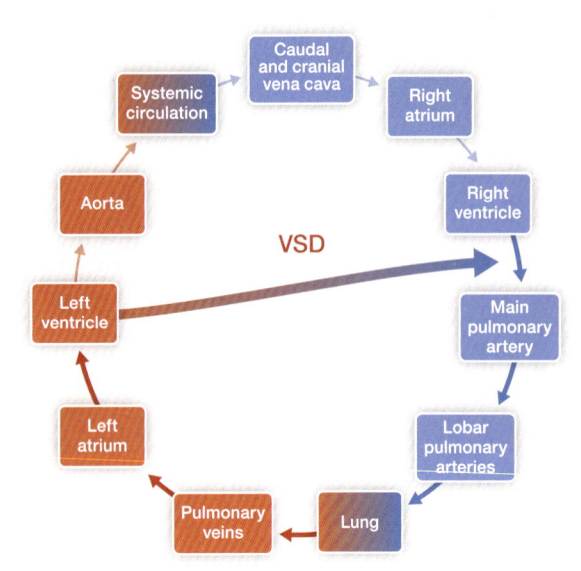

Fig. 19.44 Recirculation pathway caused by the most common configuration (membranous and restrictive to high-volume flow) of ventricular septal defect (VSD). Cardiac enlargements occur in those structures receiving recirculated blood due to the left-to-right shunt. As most VSDs are high within the interventricular septum, the blood flowing from the left ventricle tends to enter the right ventricular outflow tract directly, bypassing the right ventricle. As such, right ventricular enlargement is typically not a feature of VSDs. The excess vascular volume within the main pulmonary artery is often not sufficient to cause radiographically evident main pulmonary arterial enlargement.

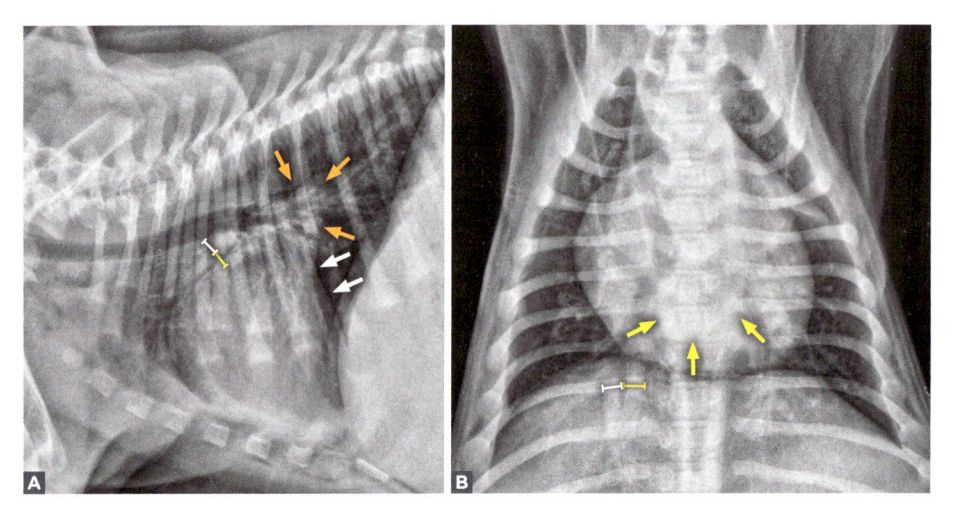

Fig. 19.45 (**A**) Right lateral and (**B**) ventrodorsal radiographs of a two-month-old Schnauzer having a membranous and restrictive ventricular septal defect. (**A**) The cardiac silhouette is tall on the lateral view and a flat caudal margin is evident (white arrows). A bulge is present in the region of the left atrium on the lateral view (orange arrows) and the caudal margin of the left atrial dilation is evident on (**B**) the ventrodorsal view (yellow arrows). Right cranial and caudal lobar arteries (white calipers) and veins (yellow calipers) are dilated consistent with pulmonary overcirculation occurring from left-to-right shunting of blood.

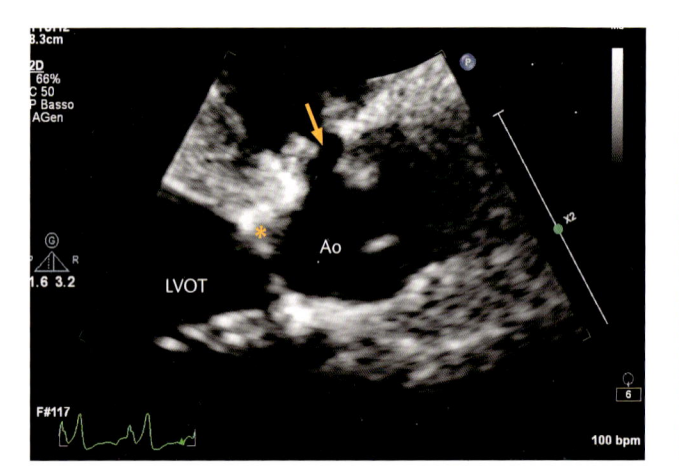

Fig. 19.46 German Shepherd affected by multiple congenital heart defects: left-to-right shunt from a ventricular septal defect, subaortic stenosis and double chamber right ventricle. Right parasternal long axis five chambers view; zoomed left ventricle outflow tract (LVOT). The subaortic fibrous ring (asterisk) is visible below the aortic leaflets (Ao). Above the fibrous ring a perimembranous ventricular septal defect is evident (arrow).

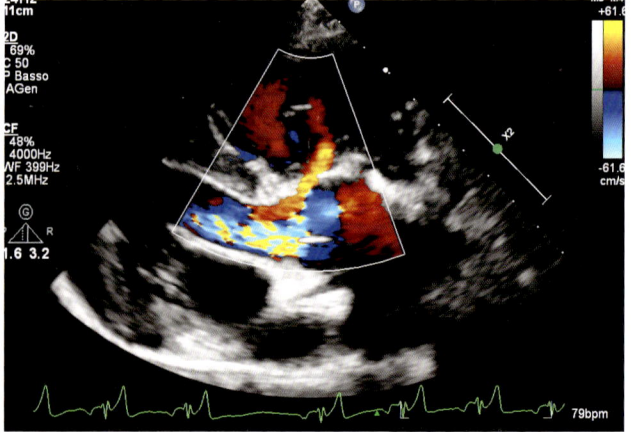

Fig. 19.47 German Shepherd affected by multiple congenital heart defects: left-to-right shunt from a ventricular septal defect (VSD), subaortic stenosis, and double chamber right ventricle. Right parasternal long axis five chambers view; color Doppler. A turbulent flow is evident in the left ventricle outflow tract below the subaortic fibrous ring. At the level of the perimembranous septum, a flow (red-orange colored) with left-to-right direction is evident through the VSD.

variable concurrent pulmonary overcirculation (dilated arteries and veins). The left heart enlargement and pulmonary overcirculation are similar to that of a PDA but there is no dilation of the proximal descending aorta. The membranous location of most VSDs and its proximity to the adjacent valves may give rise to more complex anomalies involving the aortic valve, resulting in concurrent aortic regurgitation. Ventricular septal defects that are large or occur in the muscular septum can result in concurrent right ventricular enlargement due to volume and pressure overload (**figs. 19.46-19.48**). Atrial septal defects result from a defect within the interatrial septum that allows blood to flow from the high pressure left atrium to the low-pressure right atrium. Recirculated blood travels throughout all chambers of the heart. If the defect causes diversion of a large proportion of cardiac output, generalized cardiomegaly (right and left-sided eccentric hypertrophy) can occur, and the pulmonary vascular overcirculation expected with left-to-right shunts may be visible, as shown in **figs. 19.49** and **19.50**. Most typically, though, the defect is small, and radiographs appear normal or are more detectable with increasing age.

The echocardiographic exam shows the localization of the defect (**figs. 19.51-19.53**). Based on that, the atrial septal defect is classified as: "septum primum", where the defect is in the lower part of the interatrial septum, close to the valvular plane; "septum secundum", where the defect is in the middle part of the interatrial septum; "patent foramen ovale", where the defect is in correspondence with the foramen ovale; this can be congenital or acquired; "coronary sinus" is associated to the lack of formation of the wall between the coronary sinus and the left atrium; "sinus venosus" is secondary to the abnormal attachment of the pulmonary vein to the cranial or caudal vena cava. The latter two are less common and more difficult to visualize.

Fig. 19.48 Domestic shorthair cat with a ventricular septal defect. Right parasternal short axis view at the level of the heart base; color Doppler. A turbulent flow going from the LVOT to the right ventricle is evident. The posiion of the defect, at 12:00 o'clock respect to the aorta, is typical od the perimembranous ventricular septal defect.

Fig. 19.49 Recirculation pathway caused by an atrial septal defect (ASD). Cardiac enlargements occur in all chambers as recirculated blood travels through each cardiac chamber and through pulmonary arteries and veins. Recirculated blood flowing through the main pulmonary artery and aorta do not cause dilation.

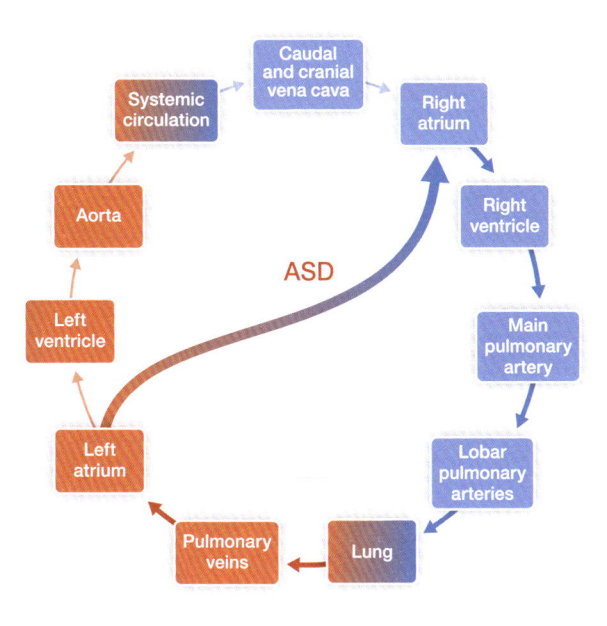

SECTION IV THORAX

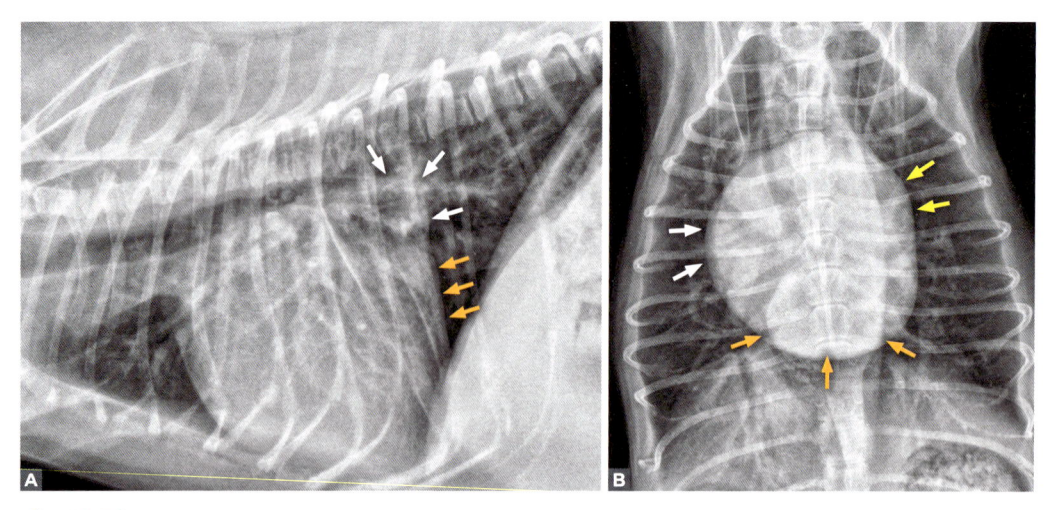

Fig. 19.50 (**A**) Left lateral and (**B**) ventrodorsal radiographs of a 15-year-old Yorkshire terrier having an atrial septal defect. (**A**) On the lateral view, the caudal cardiac margin is flat (orange arrows), and a bulge is present at the level of the left atrium (white arrows). The enlarged left atrium creates a visible caudal margin on (**B**) the ventrodorsal view (orange arrows). A shallow, broad-based protrusion is present in the region of the left auricle (yellow arrows). A broad bulge is also identified in the region of the right atrium (white arrows). Given the lack of visible pulmonary overcirculation and the age of the dog, atrioventricular valvular insufficiency would be a more likely differential for this radiographic appearance; however, due to the small size of the atrial septal defect, cardiac remodeling was delayed, and pulmonary overcirculation was not evident.

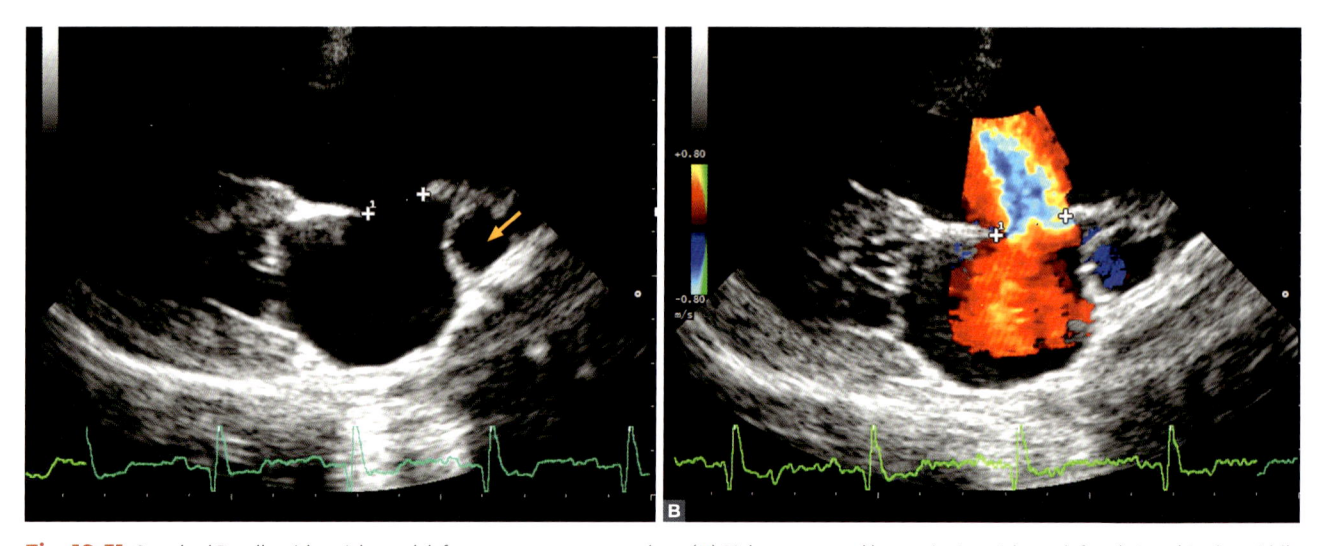

Fig. 19.51 Standard Poodle with atrial septal defect, type septum secundum. (**A**) Right parasternal long axis view. A large defect (14 mm) in the middle portion of the interatrial septum is evident. Volume overload of the right atrium and right ventricle; the right pulmonary artery is mildly distended due to the pulmonary overcirculation (arrow). The left side is normal in size. (**B**) Color Doppler showing a left-to-right shunt through the defect.

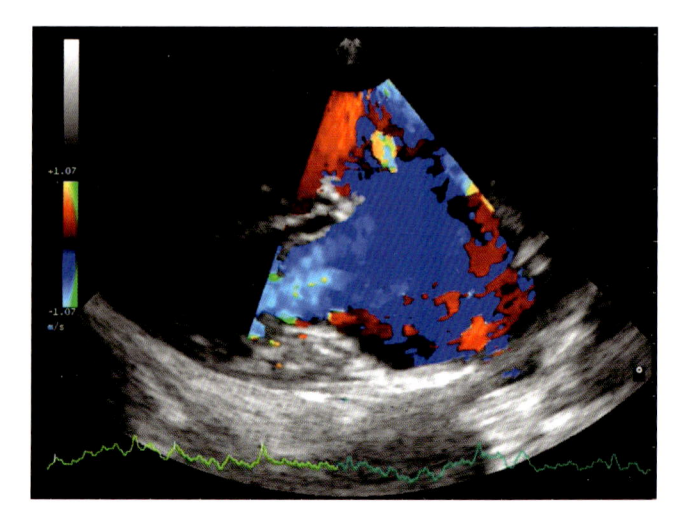

Fig. 19.52 Shih Tzu with degenerative mitral valve disease classified as ACVIM C. Right parasternal long axis view. Due to the increased left atrial pressure the foramen ovale opened, acting as a discharge valve. The color Doppler shows the diastolic flow from the left to the right atrium.

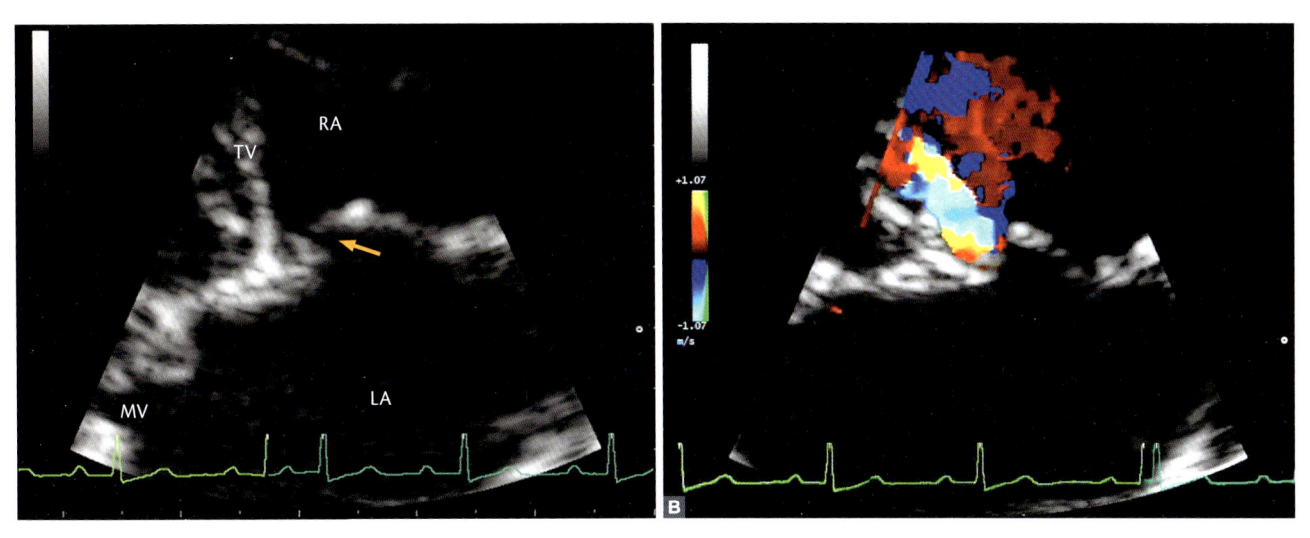

CHAPTER 19 Congenital and acquired cardiac diseases

Fig. 19.53 Close-up of fig. 19.52. (**A**) The arrow shows the loss of contrast at the level of the foramen ovale. TV, tricuspid valve; MV, mitral valve; RA, right atrium; LA, left atrium. (**B**) The color Doppler shows the direction of the shunting flow through the defect.

Diseases causing right-to-left shunting of blood

As previously mentioned, at least two concurrent abnormalities must be present in order for a shunt to be directed right-to-left. Congenital anomalies resulting in right-to-left shunts are rare. Any cardiac shunting anomaly can be reversed depending on the pressure differences between the right and left-sided circulation. If right-sided pressures match or exceed that of the left side, flow reversal will occur, resulting in deoxygenated blood mixing with oxygenated blood.

A reverse PDA is caused when the flow in a patent ductus arteriosus is directed from the pulmonary artery to the aorta. Reversal can occur after the development of pulmonary hypertension for any reason. Right-sided pressures elevate to exceed that of the systemic blood pressure and deoxygenated blood enters the aorta from the main pulmonary artery. This communication occurs distal to the origin of the brachiocephalic trunk and left subclavian, so that cyanosis is not seen within the cranial half of the animal but is present within the caudal half (i.e., differential cyanosis). Radiographically, a reverse PDA is distinct from a typical left-to-right PDA where pulmonary overcirculation is not present. Pulmonary hypertension causes concentric hypertrophy of the right ventricle resulting in right-sided cardiomegaly rather than left. A bulge in the proximal descending aorta often remains to alert the interpreter to the presence of a PDA. Main pulmonary arterial dilation is also typically present due to turbulent flow and concurrent pulmonary hypertension. A reverse PDA is shown in **fig. 19.54**.

The echocardiographic evaluation of the reverse PDA may be quite challenging due to the lack of an evident shunt flow through the ductus. Visualization of the ductus is the key for the diagnosis. Tetralogy of Fallot is a complex congenital anomaly that results in a right-to-left shunt. Three components of tetralogy of Fallot, a large VSD, a dextropositioned aorta that overrides the interventricular septum to communicate with the right and left ventricles, and pulmonic stenosis, cause marked right ventricular hypertrophy, which is the fourth component of the anomaly (**figs. 19.56** and **19.57**). The severity of the pulmonic stenosis influences the degree of cyanosis seen as resistance to flow from the right ventricle to the main pulmonary artery diverts deoxygenated blood into the aorta.[24] The main radiographic finding associated with tetralogy of Fallot is right-sided concentric hypertrophy that pushes the cardiac apex to the left on the VD or DV view. This creates an abnormal cardiac silhouette that can mimic that of a boot in shape, when severe, as shown in **fig. 19.55**. A post stenotic dilatation of the main pulmonary artery may or may not be visible. Mild cases of right ventricular concentric hypertrophy may not be radiographically visible.

SECTION IV THORAX

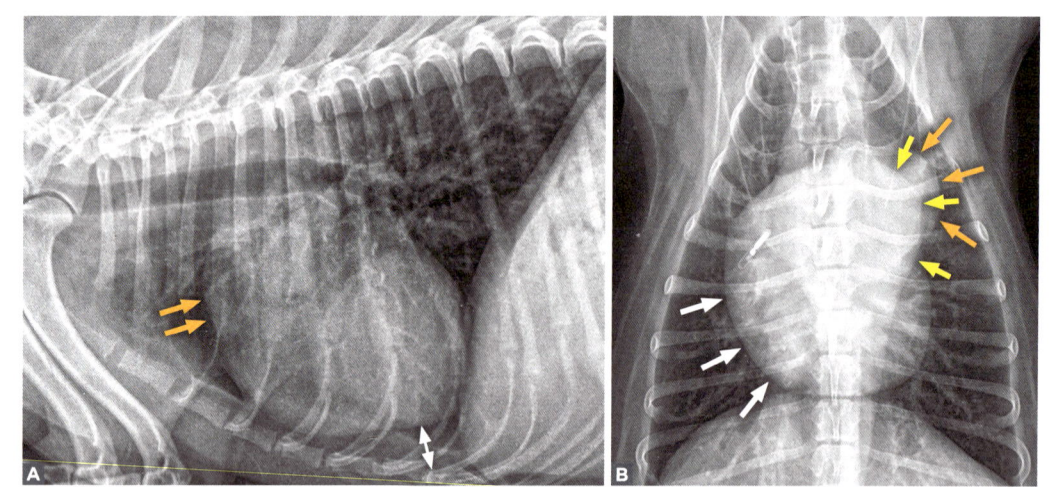

Fig. 19.54 (A) Right lateral and (B) ventrodorsal radiographs in a dog with a reverse PDA. (B) On the ventrodorsal view bulges are seen in the region of the main pulmonary artery (orange arrows) and the proximal descending aorta (yellow arrows). These findings indicate either a left-to-right or a right-to-left PDA. The key findings indicating a reverse PDA are the enlargement of the right ventricle rather than the left heart and lack of pulmonary overcirculation. (A) The apex is elevated from the sternum on the lateral projection, a finding most often seen with concentric hypertrophy of the right ventricle (double-sided white arrow). Also, the cranial cardiac edge is flat (orange arrows), indicating enlargement of the right atrium, main pulmonary artery and/or aortic arch (main pulmonary enlargement, in this case). (B) The right ventricle does not taper towards the apex giving the heart a reverse D shape (white arrows). There is no dilation of the pulmonary arteries and veins as pulmonary overcirculation ceases with flow reversal. In many instances, there is little evidence of the pulmonary hypertension (dilated pulmonary arteries) that results in the reversal of blood flow.

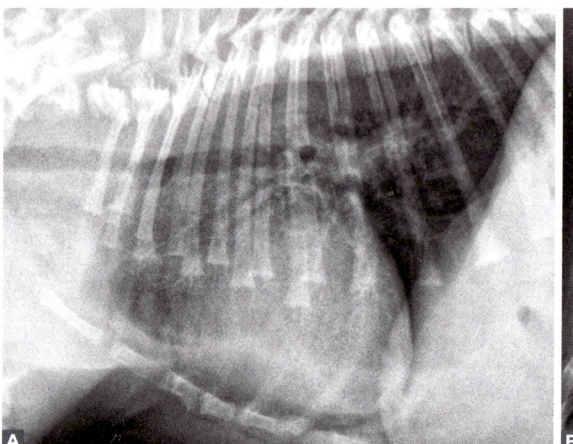

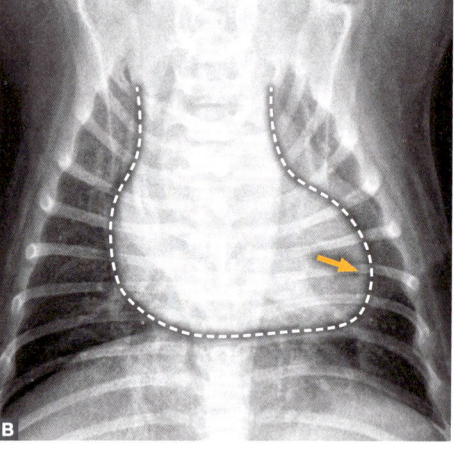

Fig. 19.55 (A) Right lateral and (B) ventrodorsal thoracic radiograph in a Bulldog puppy with tetralogy of Fallot. (B) The cardiac shape is abnormal due to severe right ventricular concentric hypertrophy that pushes the cardiac apex to the left of the midline (orange arrow) so that the overall heart shape mimics that of a boot (dotted white outline).

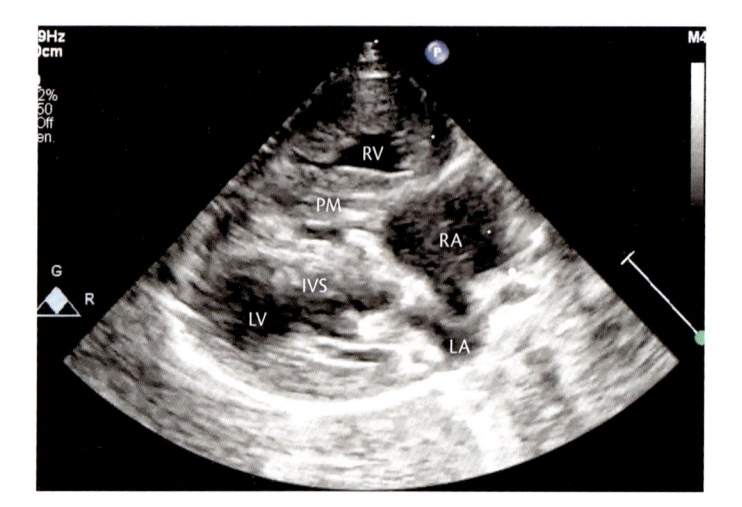

Fig. 19.56 A three-month-old Domestic shorthair cat with tetralogy of Fallot. Right parasternal long axis view. The massive hypertrophy of the right ventricle causes the displacement of the heart in the thorax. Both the interventricular septum (IVS) and the right ventricular free wall are very thick. The right papillary muscle (PM) is hypertrophic and seems to divide the ventricle in two chambers. The right atrium is dilated. The reduced preload of the left side causes a pseudohypertrophy of the left ventricle. LA, left atrium; LV, left ventricle; RA, right atrium; RV, right ventricle.

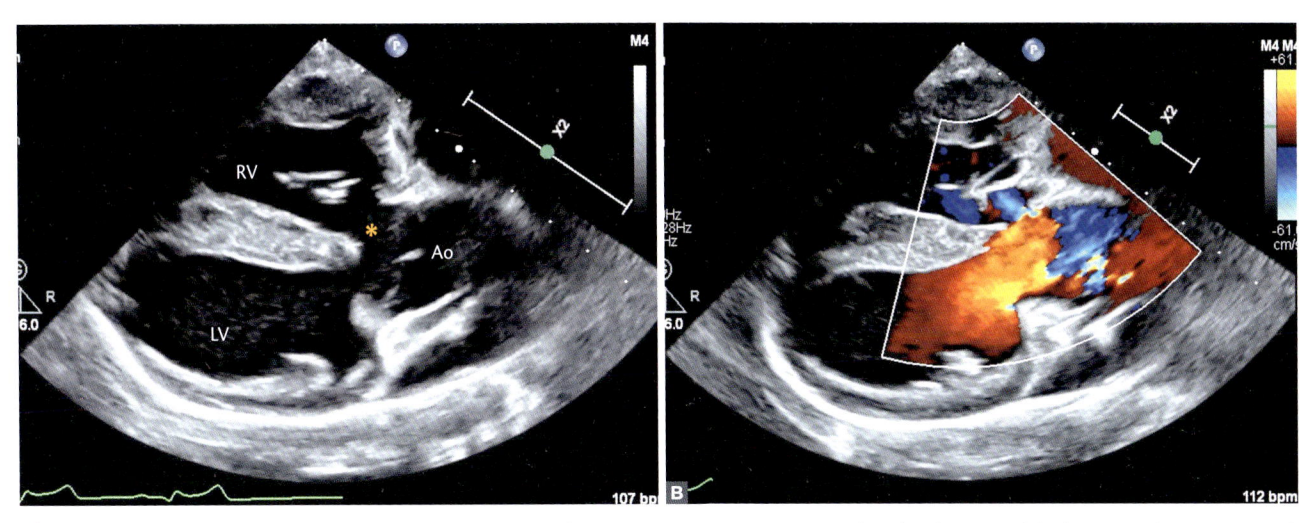

Fig. 19.57 A six-month-old German Shepherd with tetralogy of Fallot. Right parasternal long axis, five chambers view. (**A**) The aorta is dextrapositioned, dorsal to the interventricular septum, and a large septal defect (asterisk) is evident. (**B**) The color Doppler shows the systolic aortic flow coming from both the right (through the ventricular septal defect) and the left ventricle. Ao, aorta; LV, left ventricle; RV, right ventricle.

Congenital valvular obstructive diseases

Pulmonic stenosis most commonly originates from dysplasia of the valve leaflets and supporting tissues resulting in a fibrous ring. Subvalvular and supravalvular anomalies have also been reported but are rare. Concentric myocardial hypertrophy within the right ventricle occurs to compensate for the increased pressure required to transmit blood through the pulmonic valve into the main pulmonary artery. Decreased blood is expected in the pulmonary circulation, which can result in a decrease in size of the pulmonary arteries and veins when stenosis is severe. Stenosis of the pulmonary valve results in abnormal, turbulent flow in the main pulmonary artery immediately distal to the valve, resulting in an aneurysmal dilation of the main pulmonary artery. The morphologic changes include right ventricular enlargement, main pulmonary arterial enlargement, and small to normal peripheral pulmonary arteries and veins, as shown in **fig. 19.58**.

The staging and the classification of the pulmonic stenosis is performed with the echocardiographic exam (**figs. 19.59** and **19.60**). Visualization of the pulmonic valve, the right ventricular outflow tract,

Fig. 19.58 (**A**) Right lateral and (**B**) ventrodorsal views of a dog with moderate to severe pulmonic stenosis. (**A**) In the lateral view, the cardiac silhouette is wide, encompassing over four intercostal spaces. Increased sternal contact is present, also indicating right-sided cardiomegaly. A bulge is present at the cranial cardiac border (8:00-11:00 position) (orange arrows) giving the heart a flat rather than rounded shape cranially. (**B**) This bulge is clearly caused by an enlarged pulmonary artery in the 1:00-2:00 position on the ventrodorsal view (white arrows). The right ventricle is rounded and does not taper towards the apex (orange arrows) giving the heart a reverse D shape on the VD view. The pulmonary arteries (white calipers) and veins (yellow calipers) are thin, consistent with undercirculation.

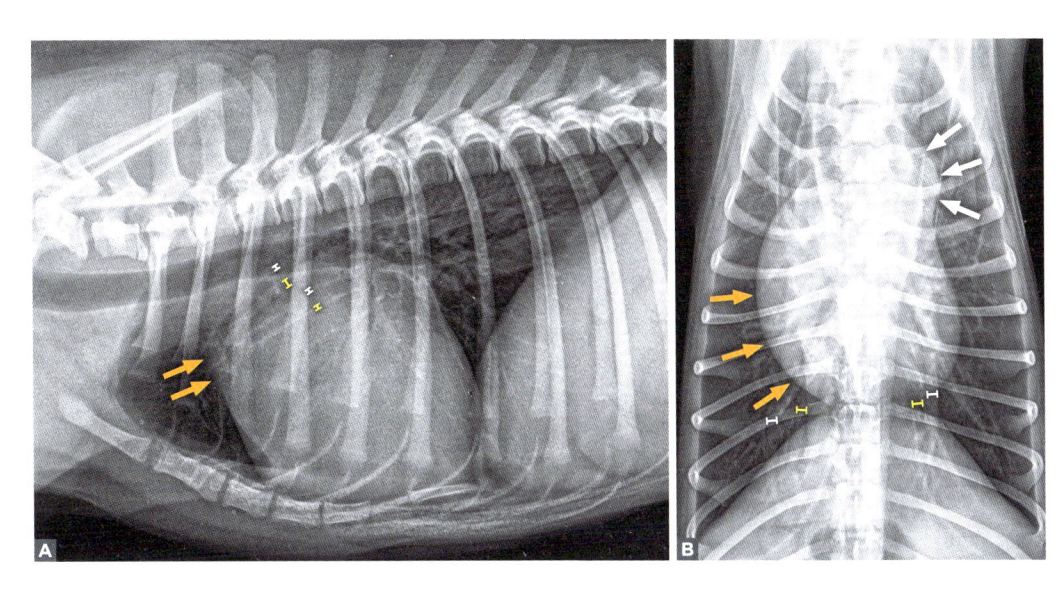

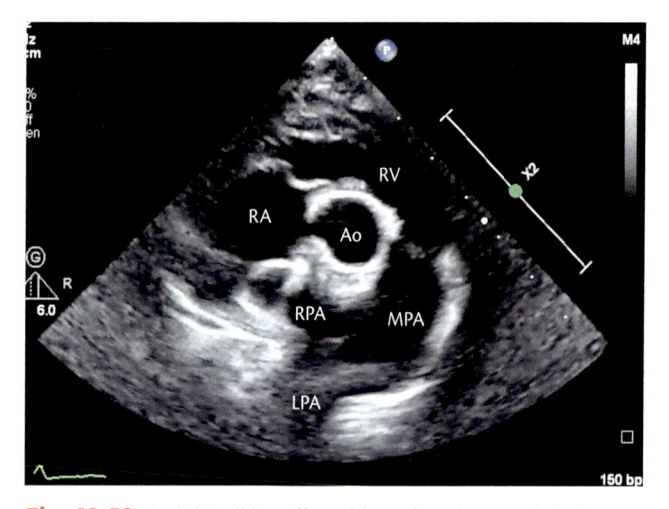

Fig. 19.59 English Bulldog affected by pulmonic stenosis. Right parasternal short axis view. The pulmonary leaflets appear thick and partially fused during systole. Severe post-stenotic dilation of the main pulmonary artery (MPA) and the left pulmonary artery (LPA). Ao, aorta; RPA, right pulmonary artery; RA, right atrium; RV, right ventricle.

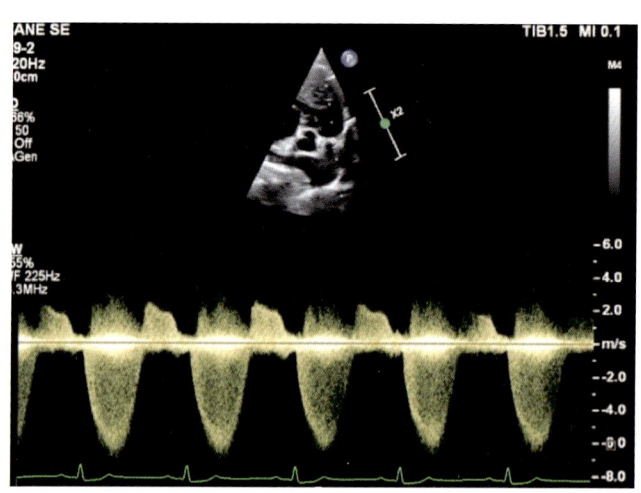

Fig. 19.60 Mongrel dog with pulmonic stenosis. Right parasternal short axis view, continuous Doppler of the pulmonic flow. The Doppler shows a high-velocity systolic flow (5.3 m/s), indicative of severe pulmonic stenosis; the diastolic regurgitant flow is visible.

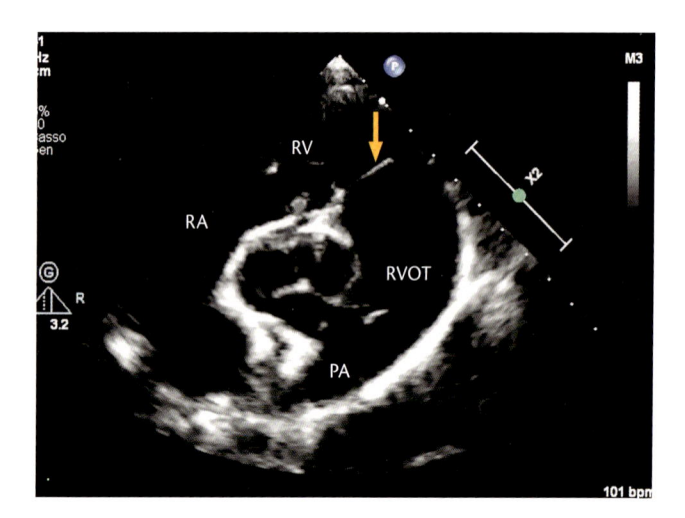

Fig. 19.61 German Shepherd affected by multiple congenital heart defects: left-to-right shunt ventricular septal defect (VSD), subaortic stenosis and double chamber right ventricle. Right parasternal short axis view at the level of the heart base. A membrane (arrow) divides the right ventricle in two chambers: a high-pressure chamber below the obstruction (RV) and a low-pressure chamber above the obstruction (RVOT). The pulmonary valve is normal. The double chamber right ventricle is a form of subvalvular pulmonic stenosis. RA, right atrium; PA, pulmonary artery.

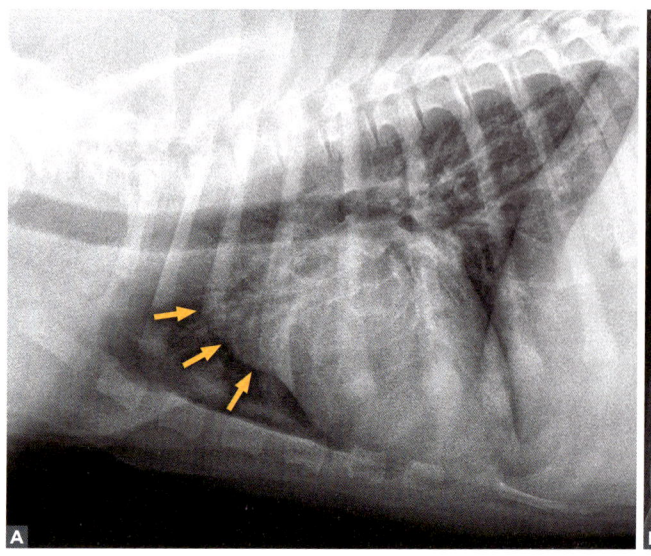

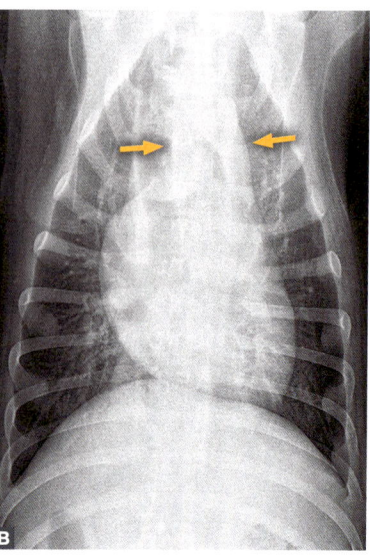

Fig. 19.62 (**A**) Right lateral and (**B**) ventrodorsal thoracic radiographs in a three-month-old Labrador Retriever with aortic stenosis. The overall cardiac size is unremarkable, typical of left ventricular concentric hypertrophy due to pressure overload, but enlargement of the aortic arch (arrows) due to post-stenotic dilation alters the cardiac silhouette. On the ventrodorsal view, the aortic arch enlargement often appears as a focal widening of the caudal aspect of the cranial mediastinum.

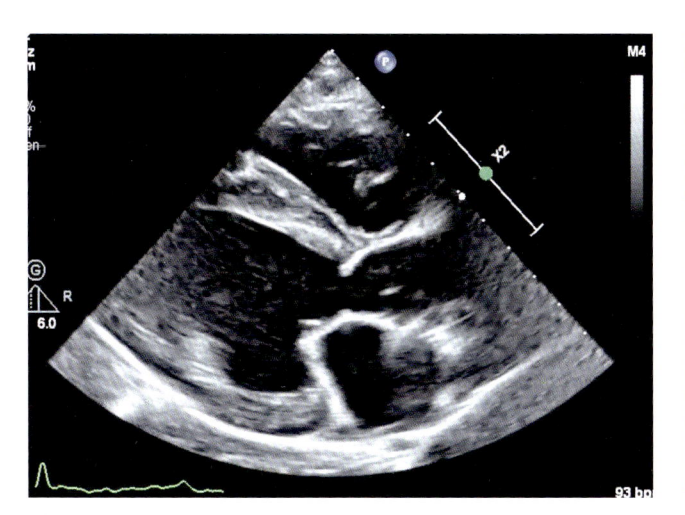

Fig. 19.63 Golden Retriever affected by subaortic stenosis grade 2. Right parasternal long axis five chambers view. The aortic leaflets are normal, and there is a subvalvular fibrous ring. The interventricular septum is mildly hypertrophic.

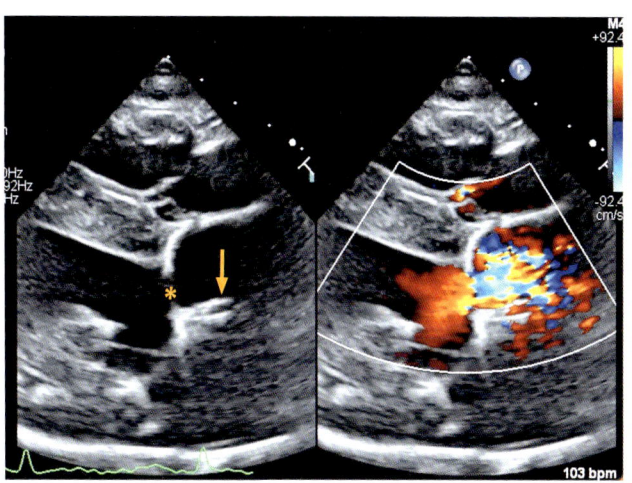

Fig. 19.64 Golden Retriever affected by subaortic stenosis grade 2. Right parasternal long axis five chambers view close-up of the left ventricle outflow tract in the systolic frame. (**A**) A subvalvular fibrous ring is visible (asterisk), and the aortic leaflets are open (arrow). (**B**) Color Doppler: systolic flow from the left ventricle that becomes turbulent at the level of the subvalvular ring.

and the pulmonary trunk allows the distinction between a valvular, subvalvular, or supravalvular stenosis (**fig. 19.61**). The severity of the stenosis is defined based on the pressure gradient (PG) across the narrowing: mild (PG <50 mmHg; moderate PG >50 mmHg and <75 mmHg; severe PG >75 mmHg). Right ventricular hypertrophy is present, especially when the stenosis is severe. When the right ventricular pressure exceeds the left ventricular pressure, flattening of the interventricular septum is evident.

Aortic stenosis is typically subvalvular in location, occurring from an accumulation of fibrous nodules or an obstructive ring of fibrous tissue.[24] The stenotic aortic valve increases the pressure required for the left ventricle to transmit blood into the aorta and results in compensatory concentric hypertrophy of the left ventricle. Radiographically, left ventricular enlargement may be seen when concentric hypertrophy is severe, but in most cases the left ventricle appears normal. Turbulent flow distal to the valve causes segmental dilation of the proximal aorta appearing as a bulge at the cranial aspect of the heart in the 8:00-11:00 position on the lateral view and in the 11:00-1:00 position (at the caudal aspect of the cranial mediastinum) on the ventrodorsal view as shown in **fig. 19.62**.

The morphologic classification of subaortic stenosis is based on the presence of a small nodule below the valvular plane (grade 1), a fibrotic ring (grade 2), or a fibrous, tunnel-shaped restriction of the left ventricular outflow tract (grade 3). The severity, similar to pulmonic stenosis, is defined by the pressure gradient across the obstruction as mild (PG <50 mmHg), moderate (PG >50 mmHg and <80-90 mmHg), and severe (PG >80-90 mmHg) (**figs. 19.63-19.65**).

Stenosis of atrioventricular valves (mitral and tricuspid) is uncommon; however, in such cases, dilation of the respective atria is expected. A component of valvular stenosis can be present with dysplasia of the atrioventricular valves discussed below.

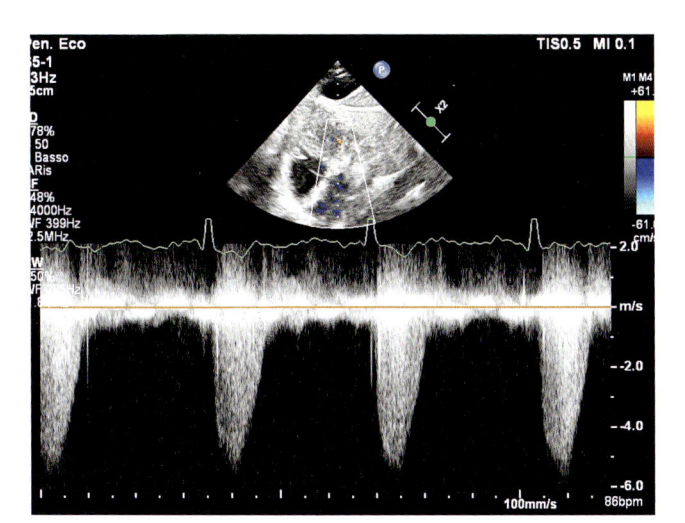

Fig. 19.65 Golden Retriever affected by subaortic stenosis grade 2. Subcostal view. Continuous Doppler of the aortic flow. The velocity of the flow (5,2 m/s) corresponds to 108 mmHg of pressure gradient, indicative of severe aortic stenosis.

SECTION IV THORAX

Dysplasia of the atrioventricular valves

Atrioventricular valvular dysplasia is uncommon, though, when present, most commonly affects the tricuspid valve. About one-third of dogs having tricuspid dysplasia have concomitant congenital anomalies as well.[31] Additionally, about one-third of cases having tricuspid dysplasia are considered severe, developing right-sided heart failure, reducing survival time. Insufficiency associated with the valve allows the vascular volume to return to the right atrium from the right ventricle during systole rather than flowing forward into the main pulmonary artery. This results in dilation of the right atrium that can be profound. Additionally, decreased vascular volume enters the lungs, which can create a visible decrease in the size of the pulmonary arteries and veins. An example of this is shown in **fig. 19.66**. Excessive volume recirculating through the right ventricle will result in right

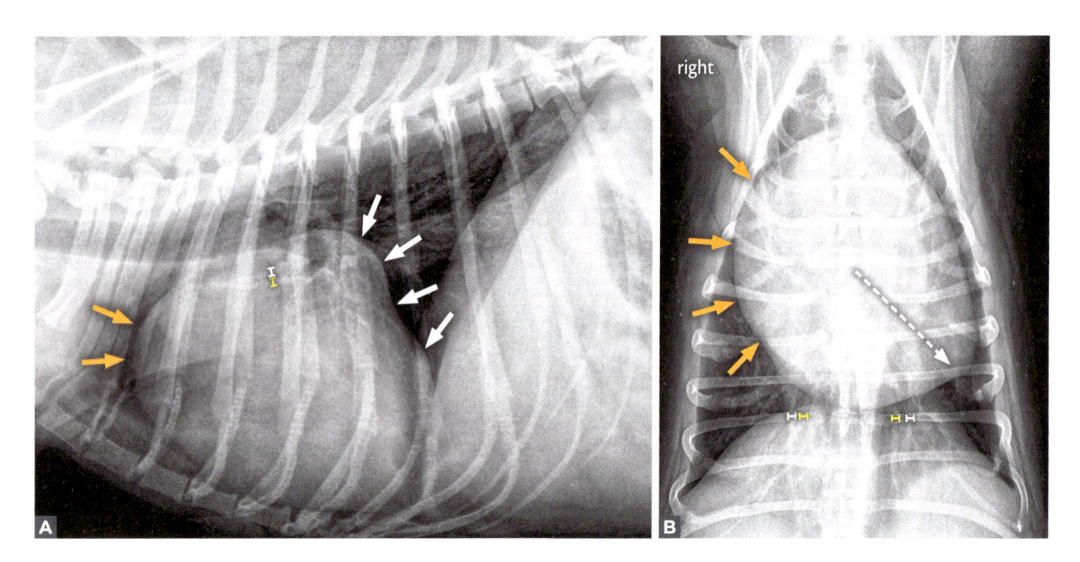

Fig. 19.66 (**A**) Right lateral and (**B**) ventrodorsal radiographs of a Dachshund with tricuspid dysplasia and right heart failure. The cardiac silhouette is large and rounded, but bulges remain evident, making severe pericardial effusion less likely. The cardiac silhouette is wide on the lateral view. (**A**) The cranial cardiac margin is rounded and protrudes (orange arrows). The caudal cardiac margin has a shallow dimple (white arrows) that mimics left atrium dilation. This occurs secondary to severe right atrial dilation as the chamber spans the cardiac silhouette. (**B**) A large broad-based protrusion is present in the region of the right atrium on the ventrodorsal view (orange arrows). The massive right atrium causes leftward displacement of the cardiac apex (dotted white arrow). Secondary to tricuspid regurgitation there is a reduction in right ventricular output, causing attenuation of the pulmonary arteries and veins (white and yellow calipers). In this case, the caudal vena cava is dilated, and abdominal detail is reduced due to ascites from right heart failure.

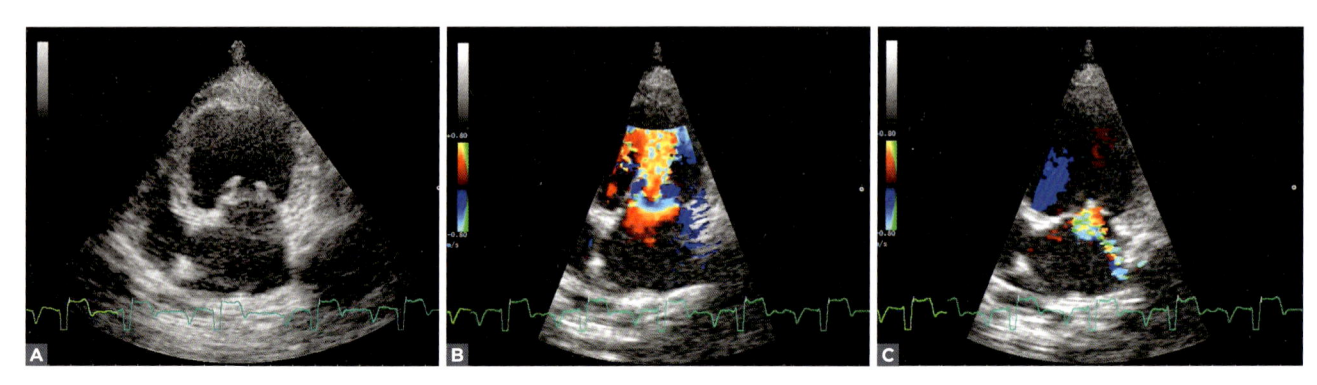

Fig. 19.67 Bull Terrier affected by mitral valve dysplasia. Left parasternal apical view. (**A**) Diastolic frame, the mitral valve is thick and partially fused. The left atrium and the left ventricle are dilated. (**B**) Color Doppler of the mitral valve, diastolic frame. The turbulent flow approaching the mitral valvular plane is indicative of valvular stenosis. (**C**) Color Doppler of the mitral valve, systolic frame. A regurgitant flow, posteriorly directed, is evident in the left atrium.

Fig. 19.68 Bull Terrier affected by mitral valve dysplasia. M-mode of the mitral valve. The reduced motility of the mitral valve leaflets hesitates in an EF slope, with the loss of the two distinct waves for the early diastolic and late diastolic opening (see fig. 19.67C).

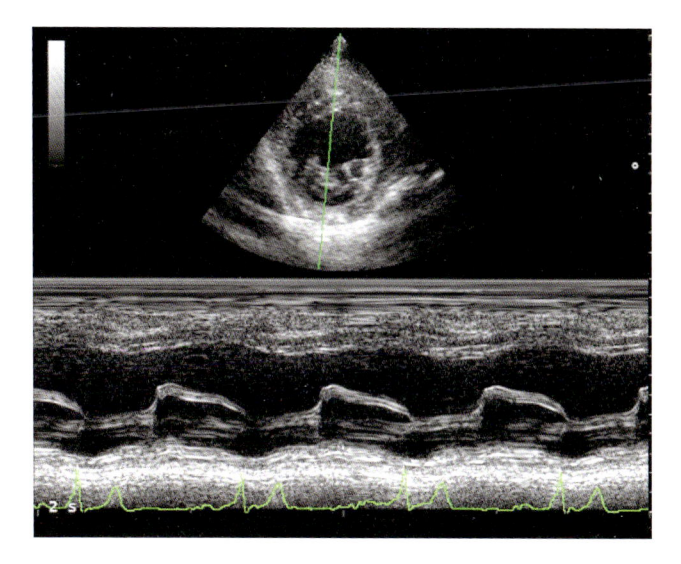

ventricular eccentric hypertrophy as well. Right ventricular enlargement is not often to the degree that right atrial enlargement is seen, especially in severe cases. A less common differential diagnosis for the radiographic appearance of tricuspid dysplasia would be cor triatrium dexter, which can occur as a common congenital comorbidity in cases having tricuspid dysplasia.[32]

Mitral valvular dysplasia is rare, being less common than tricuspid dysplasia but would result in an enlarged left atrium and ventricle, with the atrial enlargement being more profound (**figs. 19.67** and **19.68**).

Congenital cardiac diseases in cats

The common congenital cardiac diseases reported in cats vary by institution, but include atrioventricular valve dysplasia, ventricular septal defect, patent ductus arteriosus, and atrioventricular septal or endocardial cushion defects.[22,23,27,33] These diseases have the same radiographic features as those seen in dogs. A common atrioventricular canal or endocardial cushion defect is a failure of atrial and ventricular septa to fuse, which can create varying degrees of a common chamber. Given the proximity of valve formation and septal fusion during embryological formation, there is often concurrent AV valvular malformation. Radiographs commonly show marked generalized cardiomegaly with evidence of failure. Especially when left-to-right shunting of blood is severe due to larger septal defects, acquired pulmonary hypertension can be found at the time of diagnosis as well (**fig. 19.69**). Endocardial fibroelastosis is characterized by diffuse mural endocardial thickening by collagen and elastic tissue. It is inherited in Burmese cats.[27]

Peritoneal pericardial diaphragmatic hernia (PPDH) is an uncommon malformation but is the most common congenital pericardial anomaly in cats and dogs. Initial diagnosis is common in middle-aged and older pets, as the anomaly is clinically silent in half of the reported cases.[34] A communication between the pericardial sac and the peritoneal space allows passage of organs, including the liver, the spleen, the stomach, and the small intestine.[34] Cardiorespiratory signs are inconsistent and are related to the volume of the herniated abdominal organs or rarely associated with cardiac tamponade. Owners may report sporadic gastrointestinal signs, possibly from intermittent herniation. The increased volume within the pericardial space can theoretically result in poor filling of the right heart and secondary right-sided heart failure. The presence of adhesions between abdominal organs and the pericardium occurs somewhat commonly and can result in complications for surgical repair.[34] The overall prevalence is higher in cats (specifically, long-haired

SECTION IV THORAX

cats) compared to dogs. Weimaraners are at increased risk.[34,35] A PPDH is expected to cause varying degrees of cardiac silhouette enlargement which can be partially flat or angular rather than the rounded, globoid appearance of pericardial effusion. A key feature is the nonuniform opacity of the cardiac silhouette due to herniated mesentery or omentum. The presence of intestine containing gas makes the diagnosis straightforward, as shown in **fig. 19.70**. The cardiac and diaphragmatic outlines are contiguous. A decrease in abdominal organ volume is sometimes seen within the peritoneal space.

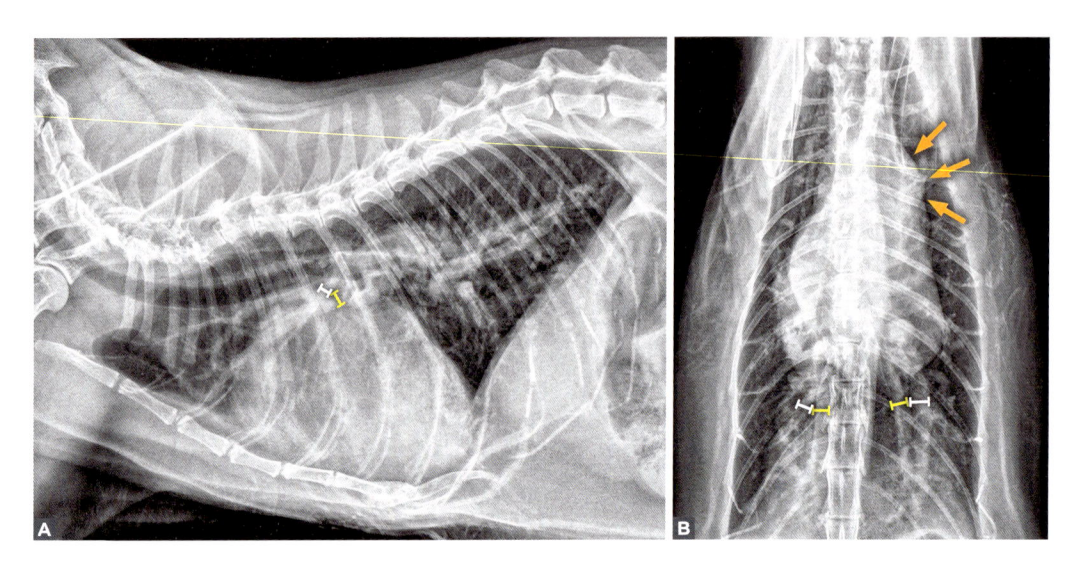

Fig. 19.69 (**A**) Right lateral and (**B**) ventrodorsal thoracic radiographs in a 14-year-old Domestic longhair cat presented for tachypnea. (**A**) The cardiac silhouette is markedly enlarged, being five intercostal spaces wide with a rounded shape on the lateral view. (**B**) On the ventrodorsal view, the left cardiac margin is flat and the right is rounded. A bulge is present in the region of the main pulmonary artery (orange arrows). The pulmonary arteries and veins are markedly dilated (white and yellow calipers, respectively). The cat was diagnosed with atrioventricular septal defect (or endocardial cushion defect) with acquired pulmonary hypertension thought to have occurred due to chronic pulmonary overcirculation.

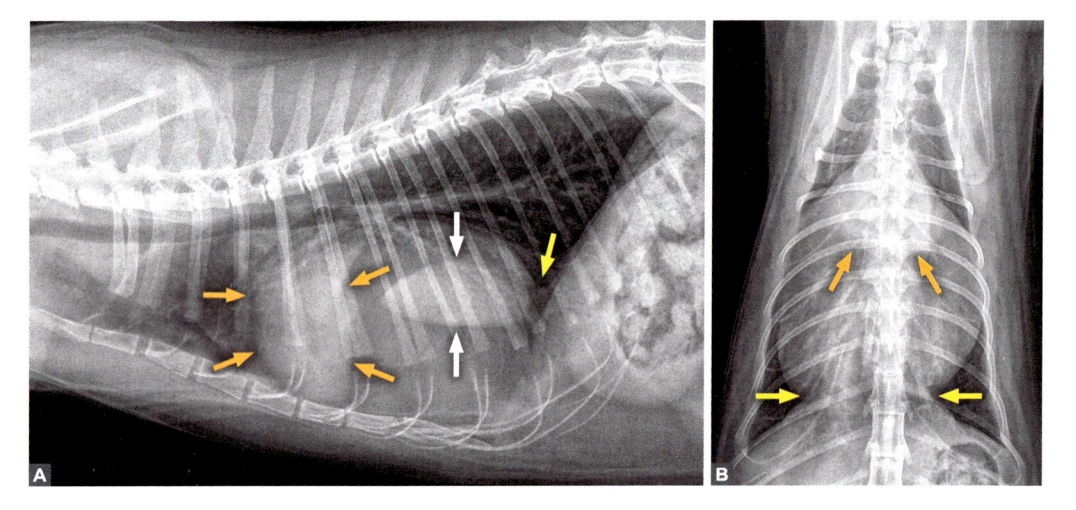

Fig. 19.70 (**A**) Lateral and (**B**) ventrodorsal views of a cat with a clinically silent peritoneal pericardial diaphragmatic hernia discovered on metastasis check. The cardiac silhouette is severely enlarged and is largely composed of fat. The heart, in this case, is displaced cranially within the pericardial sac with a somewhat recognizable shape outlined by fat (orange arrows). (**A**) An additional rounded soft tissue opacity structure is present (white arrows) surrounded by fat, likely representing either a liver lobe or the spleen. The cardiac silhouette and cupola of the diaphragm are contiguous (yellow arrows). The stomach is cranially positioned due to decreased intra-abdominal liver volume.

Acquired cardiac diseases

Acquired cardiac diseases are much more common than congenital lesions in dogs and in cats. A narrower range of differential diagnoses accounts for the vast majority of acquired cardiac disease. Most diseases fall into atrioventricular valvular insufficiency due to chronic valvular disease, cardiomyopathy, or heartworm infection.

Radiographic appearance of acquired cardiac diseases

Atrioventricular valvular endocardiosis, due to chronic myxomatous valvular degeneration, is the most common acquired cardiac disease in dogs with the mitral valve being the most commonly affected. The incidence of mitral valve involvement alone is slightly over 60%, while the incidence of combined mitral and tricuspid valvular involvement is nearly 30%, and the incidence of acquired disease in the tricuspid valve alone or in aortic and pulmonic valves is less than 10%.[36, 37] Most cases of acquired mitral valvular endocardiosis occur in small and toy breed dogs, usually 10 kg and smaller. The radiographic appearance of acquired mitral valvular disease is shown in **box 19.3** and **fig. 19.72**. Cardiac enlargement with mitral valvular disease is left-sided. During systole, blood within the left ventricle re-enters the left atrium through an incompetent mitral valve, causing volume overload of the left atrium, which then recirculates through the left ventricle. Left atrial enlargement is the predominant radiographic finding. Eccentric dilation due to volume overload in the left ventricle occurs. As left atrial pressure increases, pulmonary venous congestion and, eventually, cardiogenic edema, occur indicating left-sided heart failure. Pulmonary venous dilation is inconsistent and may not be present in all animals with cardiogenic edema. In cases where the tricuspid valve is additionally or solely affected, radiographic evidence of right-sided cardiomegaly may be seen but is quite rare. The typical echocardiographic appearance of chronic degenerative valvular disease is a thick and prolapsing mitral valve (**figs. 19.73-19.77**). The thickening can vary from mild to severe with vegetative proliferation of the valve leaflets. Both leaflets can prolapse, but the anterior leaflet is generally more affected. The chordae tendineae can be thickened as well, and sometimes these rupture. The tricuspid valve is often affected as well, but less severely than the mitral valve.

BOX 19.3 RADIOGRAPHIC APPEARANCE OF MITRAL VALVULAR DEGENERATION

Left-sided cardiomegaly

- Lateral view: flat caudal cardiac margin, bulge at the caudal cardiac base in the region of the left atrium (12:00-3:00 position)
- Ventrodorsal view: bulge creating separation between mainstem bronchi, bulge in the left cardiac margin in the region of the left auricle (2:00-3:00 position), rounded cardiac apex due to eccentric dilation of the left ventricle (3:00-5:00 position)

Left-sided cardiac failure, if present

- Pulmonary venous dilation
- Cardiogenic edema (perihilar or caudodorsal distribution of interstitial to alveolar pulmonary opacity)

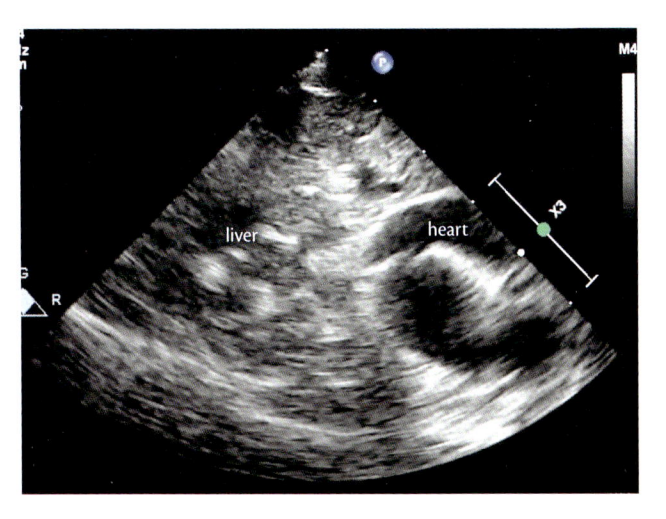

Fig. 19.71 Maine Coon cat. A peritoneal pericardial diaphragmatic hernia was an incidental finding during a breed screening echocardiography. The liver was herniated into the pericardial space and was visible close to the heart. The liver parenchyma was inhomogeneous with hyperechoic spots.

SECTION IV THORAX

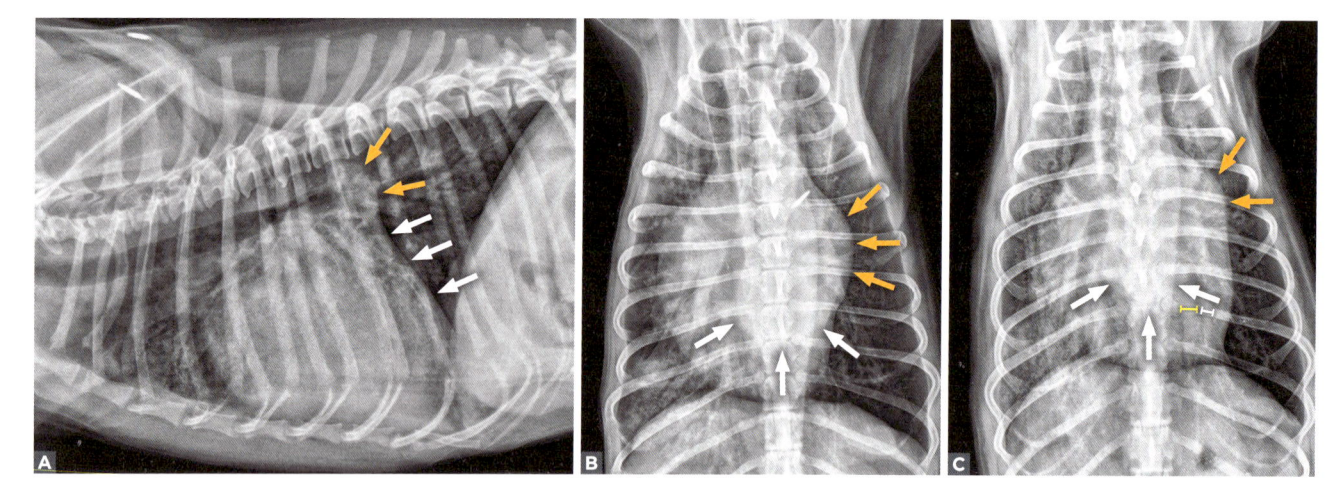

Fig. 19.72 (A) Right lateral, (B) ventrodorsal, and (C) dorsoventral radiographs of a 12-year-old Maltipoo with left-sided heart failure secondary to mitral valvular insufficiency. (A) The caudal cardiac margin is flat (white arrows), and a bulge is present at the caudal dorsal cardiac border, indicating dilation of the left atrium (orange arrows). (B, C) On the orthogonal views, the caudal border of the dilated left atrium is visible between the mainstem bronchi (white arrows). As expected, the cardiac silhouette is more elongated on the ventrodorsal view increasing the visibility of left auricular enlargement on that view (orange arrows) as compared to the dorsoventral view (orange arrows). A severe unstructured interstitial pattern is present in the right caudal lung lobe, right cranial lung lobe, and cranial subsegment of the left cranial lung lobe that reduces visibility of the pulmonary vessels. (C) The left caudal lung lobe has normal opacity, best seen on the dorsoventral view, where the left caudal lobar vein (yellow caliper) is mildly enlarged compared to the paired artery (white caliper).

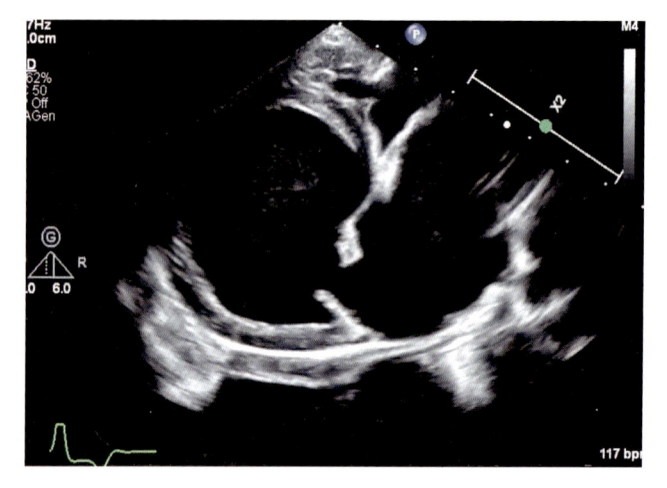

Fig. 19.73 Cavalier King Charles Spaniel affected by degenerative mitral valvular disease. Right parasternal long axis view. Severe eccentric hypertrophy of the left ventricle that appears rounded with an increased sphericity index. The left atrium is severely enlarged, and the interatrial septum is bulging toward the right side. The pulmonary vein draining into the left atrium is dilated. The mitral valve is moderately thickened and a severe prolapse of the anterior leaflet is evident.

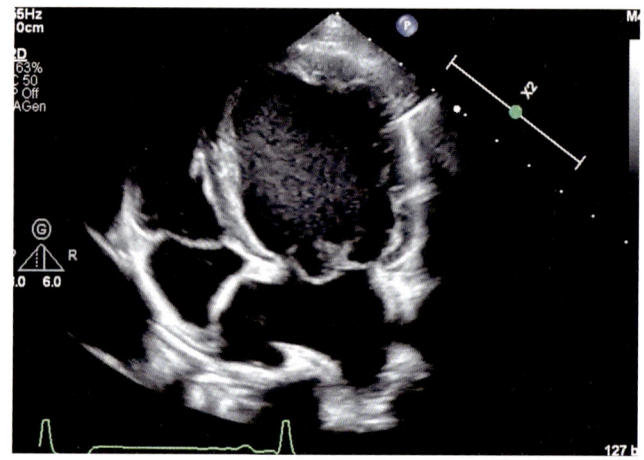

Fig. 19.74 Mongrel dog affected by degenerative mitral valvular disease. Left apical view. Both atrioventricular valves are degenerated. The septal leaflet of the tricuspid valve is prolapsing and mildly thickened. The alterations of the mitral valve are more evident, the valve is severely thickened and prolapsing. Eccentric hypertrophy of the left ventricle and dilation of the left atrium.

Dilated cardiomyopathy is a primary myocardial disorder of an unknown etiology resulting in ventricular dilation and reduced ventricular contractility (systolic dysfunction). It is more common in large and giant breed dogs with most commonly affected breeds including Doberman Pinschers, Boxers, and Great Danes. English Cocker Spaniels also have a predisposition.[38,39] The radiographic features of dilated cardiomyopathy are summarized in **box 19.4**. Some patients do not have appreciable cardiomegaly. Cardiomegaly, when present, ranges from minimal to severe and left-sided cardiomegaly tends to predominate. Left atrial dilation is a key feature as shown in **fig. 19.78**. Left atrial enlargement can be severe if mitral valve annular dilation results in secondary mitral insufficiency. The radiographic features of mitral valvular endocardiosis and dilated cardiomyopathy are

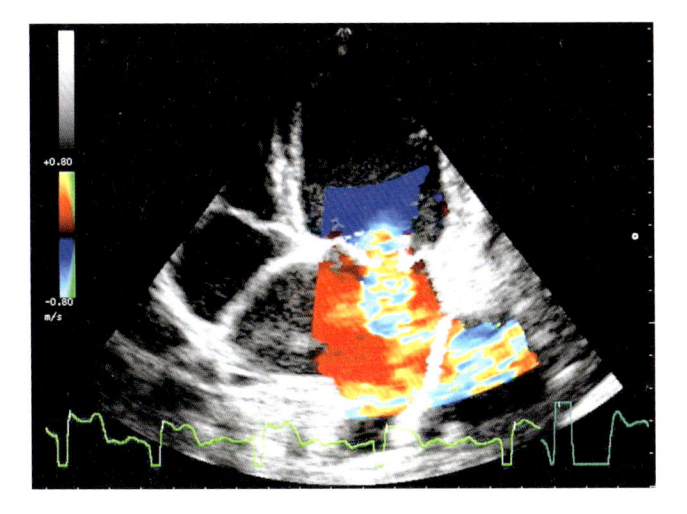

Fig. 19.75 Mongrel dog affected by degenerative mitral valvular disease. Left apical view, color Doppler. Turbulent regurgitant jet directed posteriorly and extending to the atrial roof. In course of degenerative mitral valve disease, the anterior leaflet is often the most affected and the regurgitant jet is eccentric.

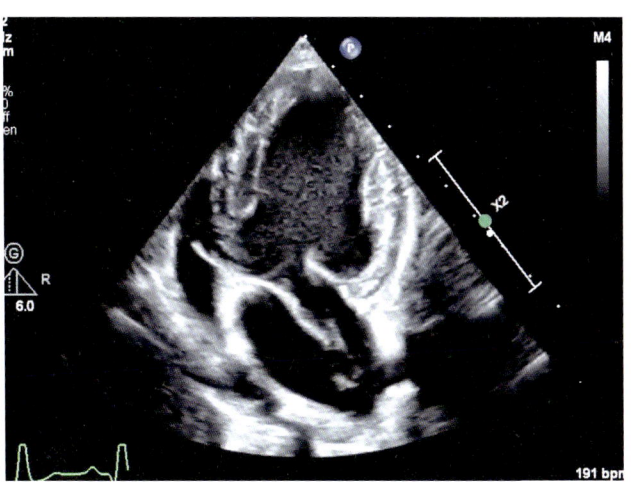

Fig. 19.76 Mongrel dog affected by myxomatous mitral valve disease. Left apical view. Dramatic prolapse of the mitral anterior leaflet due to the rupture of a primary chordae tendinae. The loss of structural support hesitates in a severe valve insufficiency.

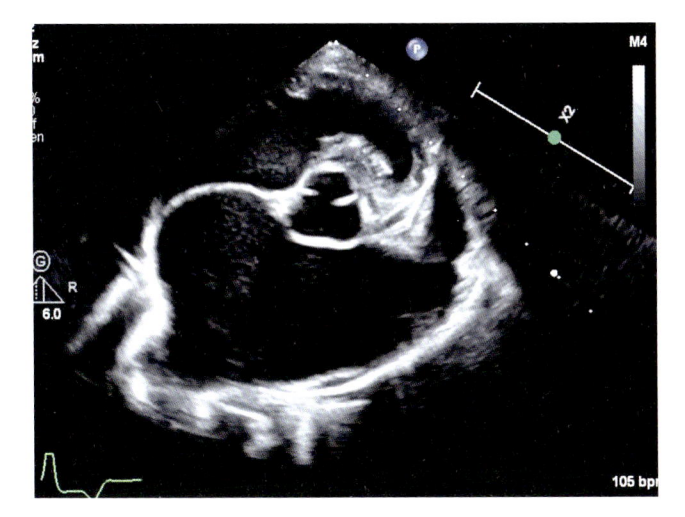

Fig. 19.77 Cavalier King Charles Spaniel affected by degenerative mitral valvular disease. Right parasternal view at the level of the aortic root. Severe atrial dilation and distension of the pulmonary vein entering the left atrium.

BOX 19.4 RADIOGRAPHIC APPEARANCE OF DILATED CARDIOMYOPATHY.

- If visibly enlarged, left-sided cardiomegaly often predominates
- Left-sided cardiac failure: more common
  - Congested pulmonary veins
  - Interstitial to alveolar pattern with hilar, peribronchial/perivascular, diffuse, or random distribution
- Right-sided cardiac failure
  - Congestion of the caudal vena cava
  - Generalized hepatomegaly
  - Peritoneal effusion
  - Pleural effusion

similar although the underlying pathogenesis differs. The affected populations are distinct although English Cocker Spaniels are affected by both conditions. The appearance of pulmonary edema in dilated cardiomyopathy is also quite variable, especially in Dobermans. The distribution of edema can follow the peribronchovascular interstitium creating an appearance that mimics a bronchial pattern as shown in **fig. 19.78**. Edema may affect the perihilar and central zones of the caudal lung lobes that can progress to a diffuse distribution with increasing severity. A random patchy or diffuse distribution may also be seen with some dogs having an apparent bronchial pattern as well. Dogs with DCM are at increased risk of concurrent rhythm disturbances, most commonly atrial fibrillation. Dogs with preclinical DCM are likely to progress towards left-sided failure; however, in cases having concurrent atrial fibrillation, there is increased risk of right-sided heart failure.[40]

In dilated cardiomyopathy the echocardiographic exam shows left ventricular hypertrophy, left atrial dilation, and severe systolic dysfunction (**figs. 19.79** and **19.80**). Mild mitral regurgitation is generally present due to the dilation of the valvular annulus.

SECTION IV THORAX

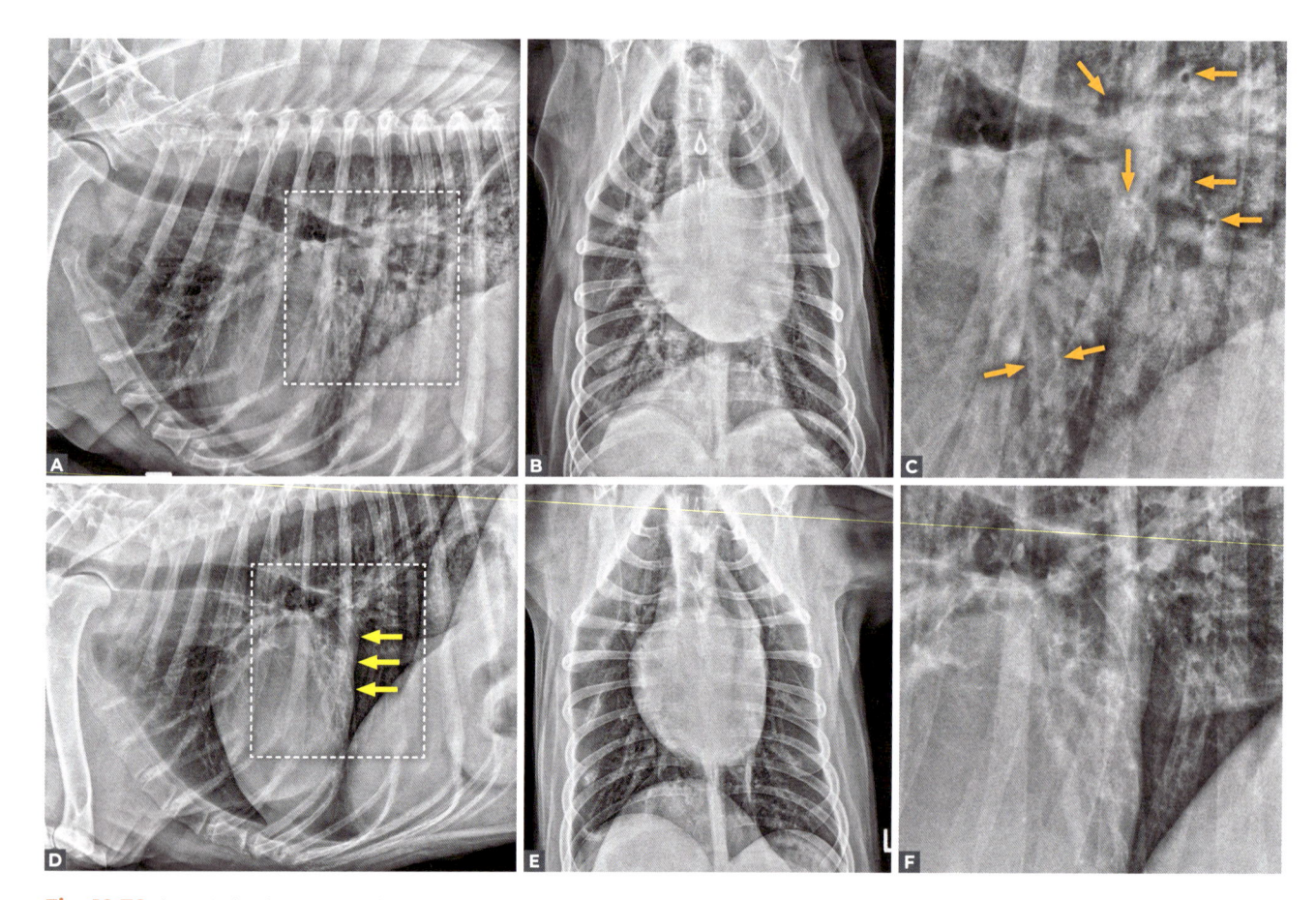

Fig. 19.78 (A and C) Left lateral and (B and D) ventrodorsal views of an eight-year-old Doberman Pinscher with dilated cardiomyopathy. (A, B, C) On initial presentation, an increase in pulmonary opacity limits the visibility of the cardiac margins and pulmonary vessels; some of the increased opacity conforms to the airways and vessels (A, dotted white inset showing magnified lungs; C, orange arrows). The peribronchial and perivascular edema mimics thickening of the airway walls. The trachea is elevated (as compared to normal Doberman Pinschers). (D, E, F) On views obtained following diuretic treatment, the cardiac silhouette is more visible and is somewhat enlarged. Most notable is the flat caudal cardiac margin indicative of left-sided cardiomegaly (yellow arrows). The vasculature is more visible following resolution of cardiogenic edema (D, dotted white inset showing magnified lungs in F).

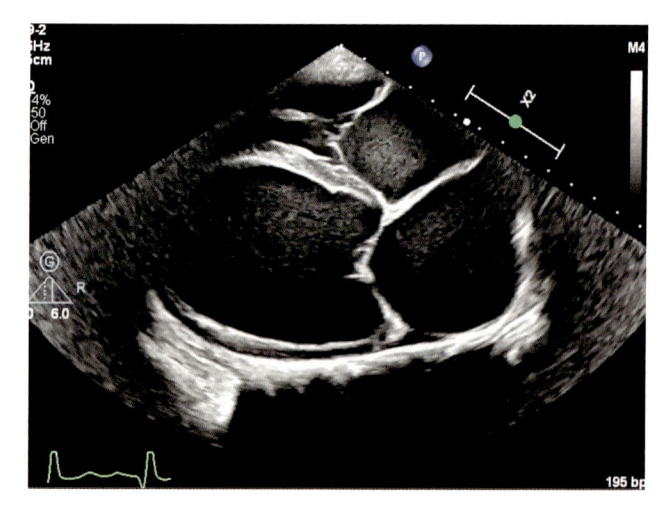

Fig. 19.79 Great Dane affected by dilated cardiomyopathy. Right parasternal long axis view. Severe eccentric hypertrophy of the left ventricle and dilation of the left atrium and the pulmonary vein. The right atrium and right ventricle are dilated too. Atrioventricular valves are normal.

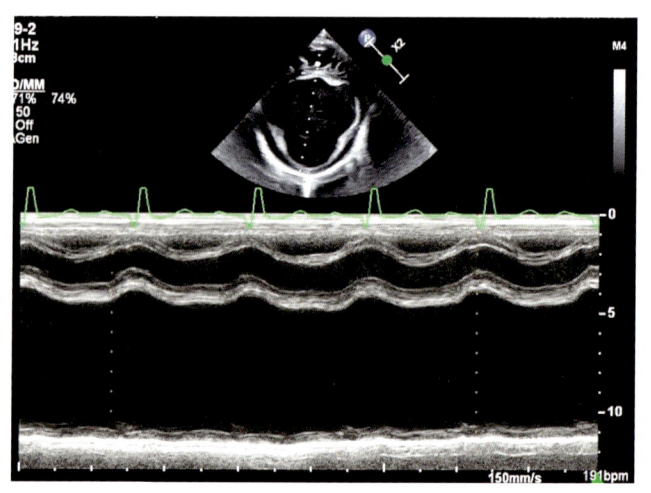

Fig. 19.80 Great Dane affected by dilated cardiomyopathy. M-mode of the left ventricle. Severe systolic dysfunction and dilation of both ventricles. The interventricular septum moves simultaneously with the right ventricular free wall, suggesting a passive shift instead of a contraction. The right ventricle is distended.

Hypertrophic cardiomyopathy is a feline primary myocardial disorder that results in myocardial hypertrophy and has no inciting cause (i.e., no evidence of chronic systemic hypertension or hyperthyroidism). Myocardial hypertrophy is usually concentric and uniform but may be geographic, affecting the interventricular septum, left ventricular free wall, and/or the papillary muscles. Concentric myocardial hypertrophy reduces luminal chamber volume, and resulting reduced myocardial compliance causes diastolic dysfunction is the primary factor causing clinical disease. The myocardial dysfunction is often predominantly left-sided. Chronically elevated left ventricular pressures caused by diastolic dysfunction are transmitted to the left atrium causing eccentric dilation. Radiographically, this produces the characteristic cardiac shape of atrial enlargement with a relatively normal ventricular silhouette (the so-called "valentine-shaped" heart) shown in **fig. 19.81**. Because concentric hypertrophy predominates within the ventricles (most commonly the left ventricle), affected cats may appear radiographically normal unless there is moderate or severe left atrial dilation. The radiographic findings of hypertrophic cardiomyopathy are summarized in **box 19.5** and the valentine-shaped heart created by a narrow cardiac apex and a widened base on the ventrodorsal view is predominantly caused by severe left atrial enlargement.[41] Echocardiographic evaluation of the diastolic thickening of the left ventricle is the key feature for the diagnosis of hypertrophic cardiomyopathy. The left atrium dilation is related to the severity of the disease, and it represents a risk factor for the development of thrombi.

Dirofilaria immitis or heartworm infection remains one of the top three acquired cardiac diseases in dogs in endemic regions. Infection also occurs in cats, although less frequently and with less severe

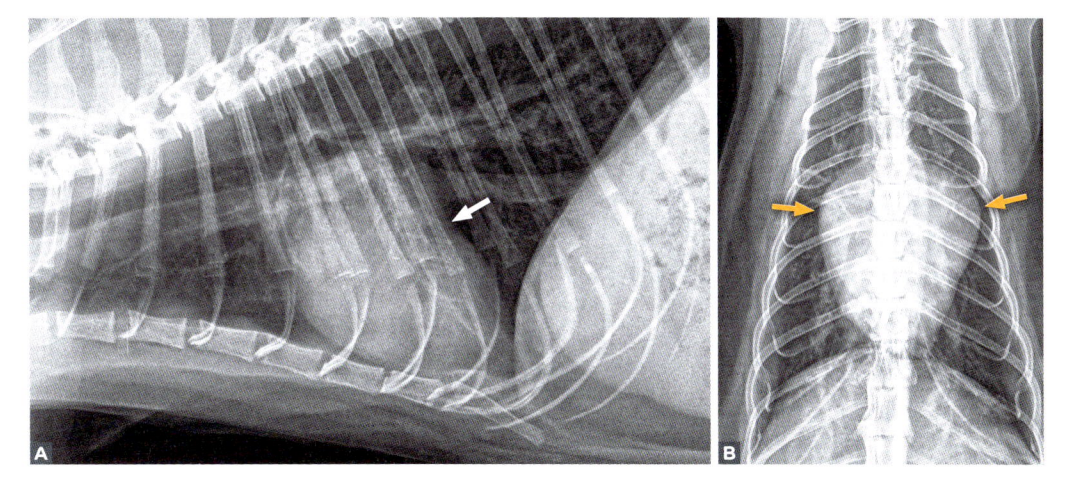

Fig. 19.81 (A) Lateral and (B) ventrodorsal thoracic radiographs of a cat with hypertrophic cardiomyopathy. The most notable feature is the change in shape of the cardiac silhouette. (A) A shallow indentation of the caudal cardiac margin can be seen at the junction between the left atrium and ventricle. (B) The cardiac apex is displaced slightly rightward to lie on midline; however, dilation of the left atrial appendage appears as a large bulge in the left lateral cardiac margin (orange arrows).

BOX 19.5 — RADIOGRAPHIC APPEARANCE OF HYPERTROPHIC CARDIOMYOPATHY.

- Left atrial or (rarely) biatrial enlargement
  - Concentric hypertrophy usually results in no radiographic enlargement of ventricles
  - Lateral view: kidney-shaped heart caused by a concavity at the caudal cardiac margin due to left atrial dilation
  - Ventrodorsal view: valentine-shaped heart caused by severely dilated left atrium or (rarely) right and left atrial enlargement combined
- Left-sided heart failure, most typically
  - Cardiogenic edema
    – Multifocal or patchy interstitial to alveolar pulmonary opacity
  - Small volume pleural effusion
  - Variable pulmonary venous congestion though often arteries and veins are affected

radiographic signs. Clinical signs are characterized by a combination of respiratory and cardiovascular effects with sudden death occurring more often in cats. The imaging features of heartworm infection are the result of changes induced in the pulmonary arteries by the parasites (**fig. 19.86**). The severity depends upon the parasite burden and chronicity of infection. The heartworms present in the pulmonary arteries initiate vascular damage proportional to their numbers, where endothelial damage, sloughing, and villous proliferation occur.[42] Thrombosis is a sequela to the physical presence of worms and alterations in the endothelial lining. The effects of heartworm infection on the heart are secondary to pulmonary hypertension. On some occasions, the direct presence of worms within the right atrium can affect valvular function, resulting in tricuspid incompetence in cases of overt caval syndrome. Radiographic signs associated with heartworm infection are shown in **box 19.6** and **fig. 19.85**. Pulmonary hypertension associated with heartworm infection causes concentric hypertrophy of the right ventricle. Main pulmonary arterial dilation occurs due to congestion. Peripheral pulmonary arteries can range from normal in size to markedly dilated, tortuous, and truncated. Unstructured pulmonary interstitial infiltrates representing eosinophilic inflammation associated with infec-

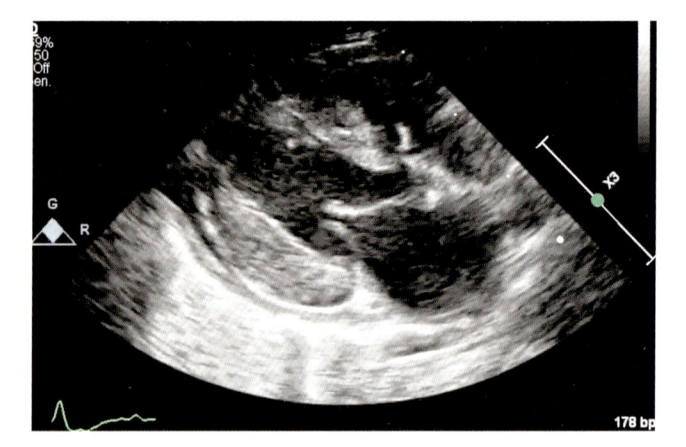

Fig. 19.82 Scottish Fold affected by hypertrophic cardiomyopathy. Right parasternal long axis view. Symmetric hypertrophy of the left ventricle. Mitral valve apparatus appears normal. A mild pericardial effusion is visible at the level of the apex.

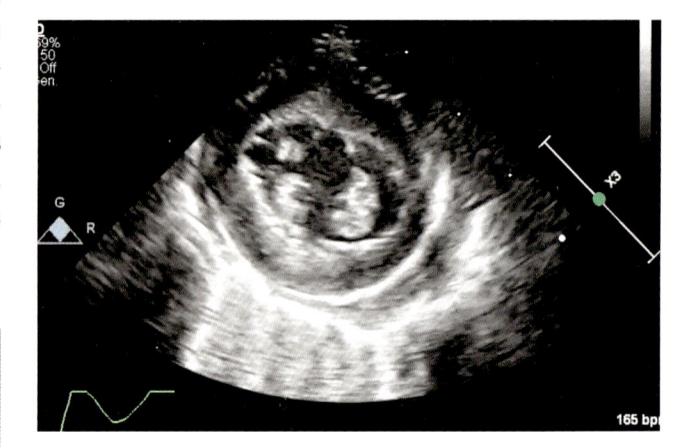

Fig. 19.83 Scottish Fold affected by hypertrophic cardiomyopathy. Right parasternal short axis view at the level of the papillary muscles. Symmetric hypertrophy of the left ventricle; hyperechogenicity of the papillary muscles and the subendocardial myocardium, suggestive of fibrosis/ischemia. Mild pericardial effusion.

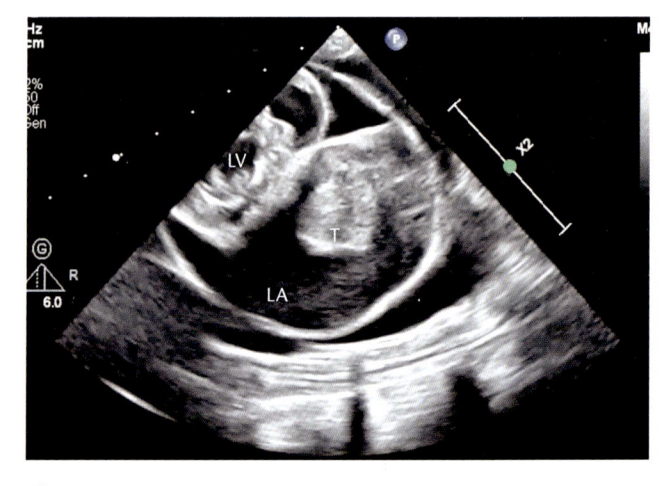

Fig. 19.84 Maine Coon affected by hypertrophic cardiomyopathy. Left cranial view oriented for the optimization of the left atrium (LA). A thrombus (T) is evident at the level of the left auricle. The left ventricle (LV) is cut off the image. A mild pleural effusion is evident around the heart.

BOX 19.6 RADIOGREIC APPEARANCE OF HEARTWORM INFECTION.

- Right ventricular enlargement
  - Concentric nature of hypertrophy makes radiographs insensitive for detection until severe
  - Lateral view: wide cardiac silhouette, increased sternal contact, elevated cardiac apex
  - Ventrodorsal view: bulge in 5:00-9:00 position at the right cardiac margin
- Main pulmonary arterial enlargement
  - Lateral view: bulge in the 8:00-11:00 position at the cranial cardiac base
  - Ventrodorsal view: bulge in the 1:00-2:00 position at the left cranial cardiac margin
- Peripheral pulmonary arterial enlargement
- Pulmonary eosinophilic inflammation
  - Peribronchial interstitial to alveolar pulmonary opacity
  - Multifocal nodular pulmonary pattern, in some cases
- Right-sided heart failure
  - Dilated caudal vena cava
  - Generalized hepatomegaly
  - Peritoneal effusion
  - Pleural effusion

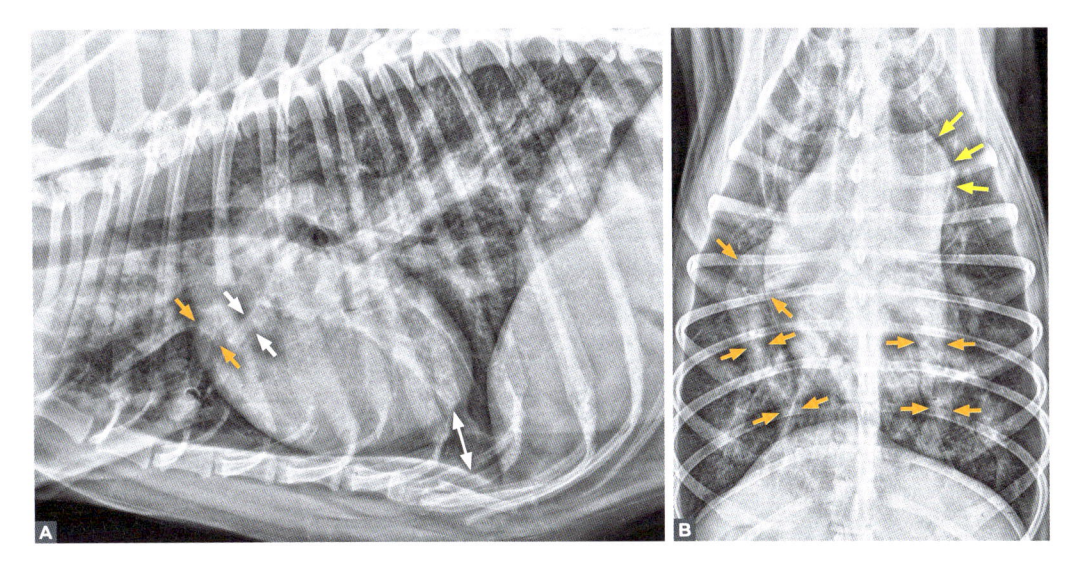

CHAPTER 19 Congenital and acquired cardiac diseases

Fig. 19.85 (A) Lateral and (B) ventrodorsal thoracic radiographs of a dog diagnosed with severe chronic *D. immitis* heartworm infection. The peripheral pulmonary arteries are markedly dilated, tortuous, and truncated (orange arrows). (A) Normal cranial lobar veins can be seen for comparison (white arrows). Right concentric ventricular hypertrophy is causing an elevated cardiac apex (double-headed white arrow). (B) Marked main pulmonary arterial dilation is seen (yellow arrows). Finally, increased unstructured interstitial pulmonary opacity within all lung lobes causes decreased delineation of pulmonary vessels consistent with eosinophilic infiltrates. Evidence of right-sided heart failure is not identified in this case.

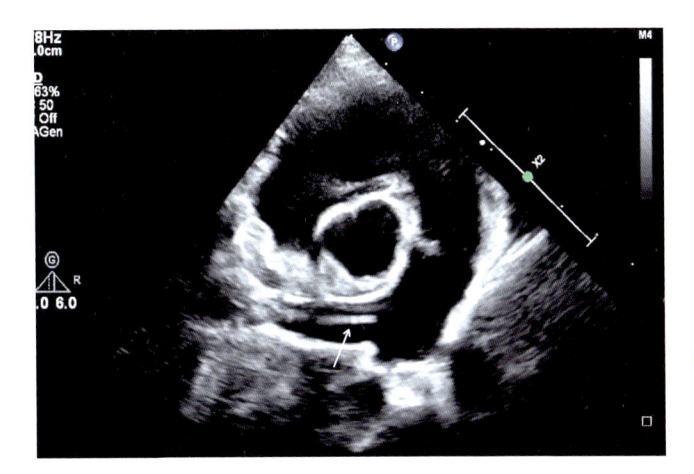

Fig. 19.86 Mongrel dog. Right parasternal short axis view. A heartworm is visible in the right pulmonary artery; it appears as two parallel hyperechoic lines (arrow).

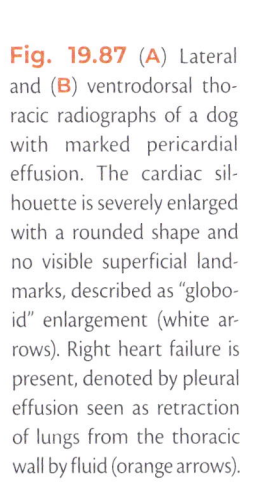

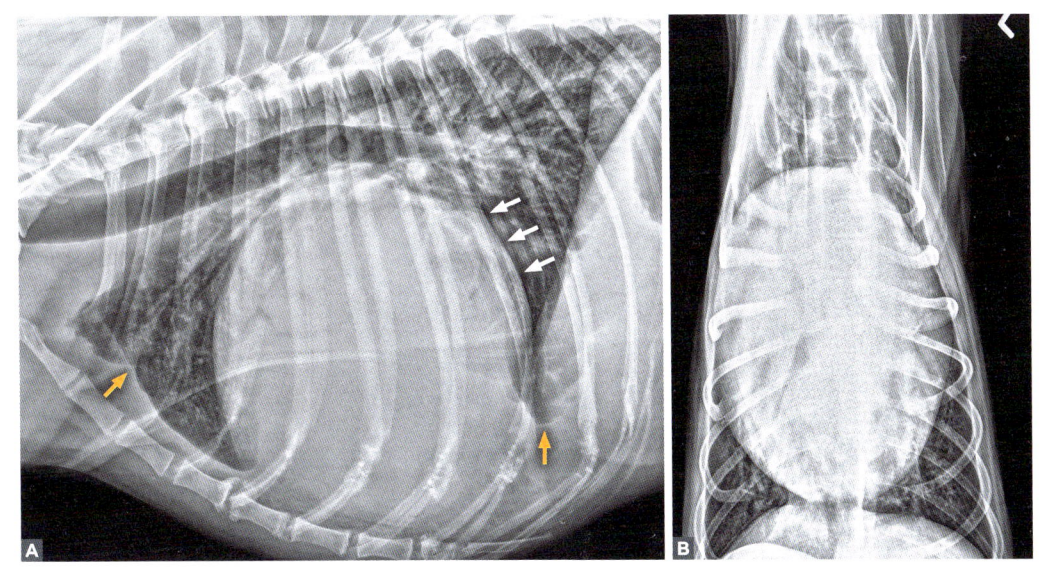

Fig. 19.87 (A) Lateral and (B) ventrodorsal thoracic radiographs of a dog with marked pericardial effusion. The cardiac silhouette is severely enlarged with a rounded shape and no visible superficial landmarks, described as "globoid" enlargement (white arrows). Right heart failure is present, denoted by pleural effusion seen as retraction of lungs from the thoracic wall by fluid (orange arrows).

311

tion are sometimes visible and may be the only radiographic change; changes are most often visible in caudal lung lobes and surrounding lobar bronchi leading to an apparent bronchial pulmonary pattern in some. A nodular pattern can also be seen due to eosinophilic granuloma formation.

Pericardial effusion is the most common acquired pericardial disease in dogs. Some cases are idiopathic. Intrapericardial neoplasia such as right atrial hemangiosarcoma, heart base chemodectoma, or mesothelioma are the most common differentials to rule out. Infectious pericarditis is rare in companion animals. Pericardial fluid increases the pressure within the pericardium and, once it equals or exceeds the right atrial and ventricular pressure, it causes these chambers to collapse, impairing diastolic filling. This is termed cardiac tamponade and leads to right-sided heart failure. Impaired diastolic filling of the right heart causes reduced right ventricular output and the pulmonary vessels may appear small. Radiographic signs associated with pericardial effusion are summarized in **box 19.7** and **fig. 19.87**. If there is a small volume of effusion the heart may appear normal. A moderate or large volume effusion within the pericardial space creates a globoid cardiac silhouette, with a smooth rounded outline on all projections. A key feature differentiating pericardial effusion from severe generalized cardiomegaly such as from dilated cardiomyopathy is the absence of visible left atrial dilation. Severe right-sided cardiomegaly and pericardial effusion can appear radiographically similar (**fig. 19.88**) with a predominantly left-sided cardiomegaly appearing distinctly different (such as with most dilated cardiomyopathies and acquired atrioventricular valvular degenerative disease). The pericardium is fibrous and relatively inelastic. Acute accumulation of a small volume of fluid such as from hemorrhage may

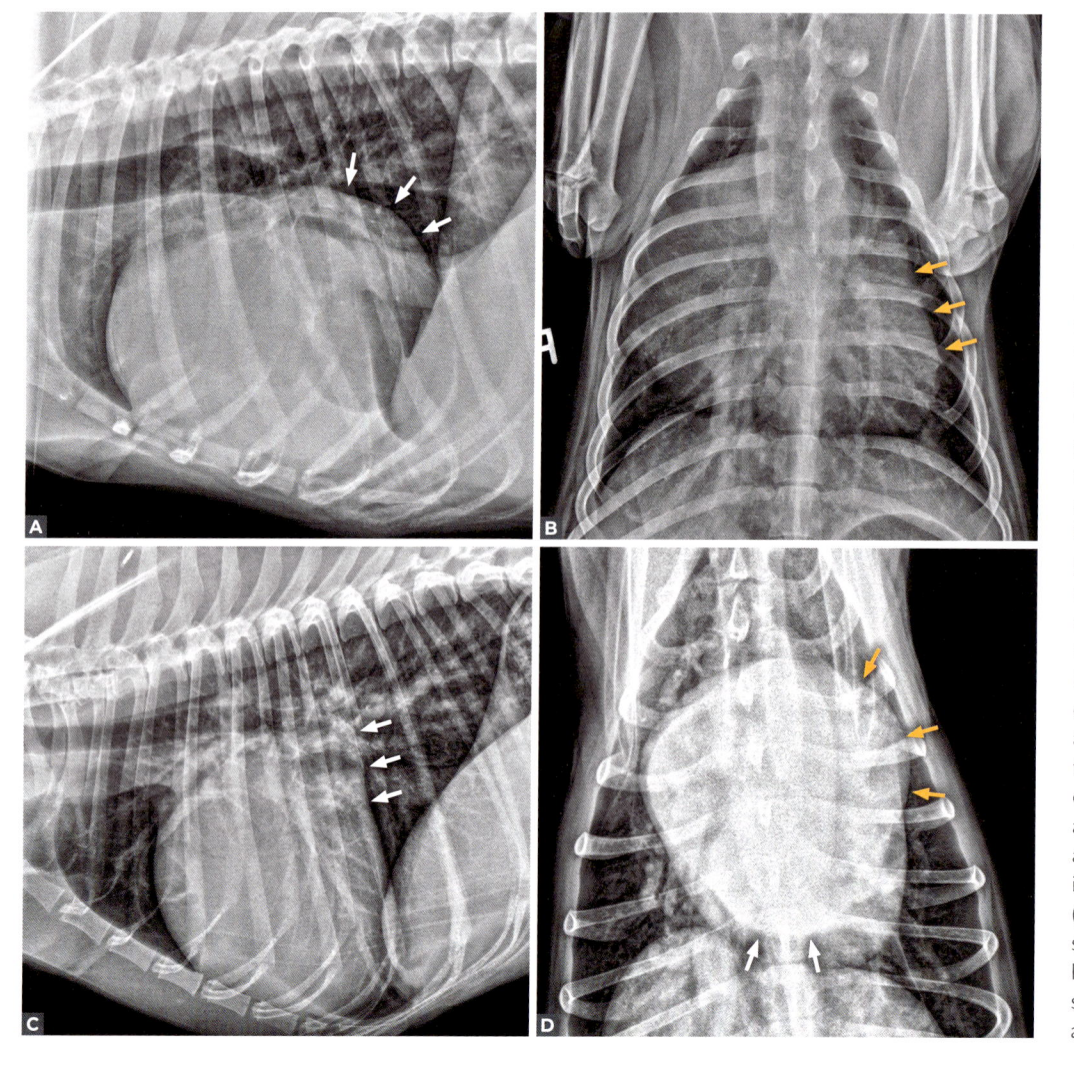

Fig. 19.88 Lateral and ventrodorsal radiographs in a dog having marked right-sided cardiomegaly due to concurrent tricuspid dysplasia and pulmonary hypertension (**A**, **B**) and in a dog having dilated cardiomyopathy (**C**, **D**). (**A**) The caudal cardiac margin is very convex and round in the dog having marked right-sided cardiomegaly (white arrows) that appears similar to the previous figure that had pericardial effusion (fig. 19.38). (**B**) The left cardiac margin on the VD view of this dog is moderately flat (orange arrows) which is useful in distinguishing the cardiomegaly as being right-sided versus secondary to pericardial effusion where this left margin would more typically be round. (**C**) In the dog having dilated cardiomyopathy, the caudal cardiac margin is flat (arrows), and (**D**) the caudal margin of the left atrium creates a well-defined line superimposed over the cardiac apex (white arrows). Additionally, a left auricular bulge is present in the 2-3 o'clock position (orange arrows) creating a set of findings distinctive for left-sided cardiomegaly versus right sided cardiomegaly or pericardial effusion.

cause cardiac tamponade without appreciable cardiomegaly on radiographs (**fig. 19.89**). Such cases may present for acute collapse and may not show signs of right-sided congestive cardiac failure. Signs of right-sided heart failure are usually seen at the time of diagnosis in patients with chronic pericardial effusion. Clinically significant pericardial effusion that is severe enough to cause right heart failure is rare in cats. Small volumes of pericardial effusion may be seen in cats presenting with myocardial disease such hypertrophic cardiomyopathy, feline infectious peritonitis, and multicentric lymphoma.[43] Microcardia is the term for reduced cardiac size from reduced circulating volume. The most common causes are hypovolemic shock, such as from acute hemorrhage and severe dehydration. Hypoadrenocorticism is an occasional etiology. The appearance may be mimicked by overinflated lungs and pneumothorax. Microcardia is often accompanied by a consistently small vena cava in addition to decreased size and number of visible pulmonary arteries and veins (**fig. 19.90**).

BOX 19.7 RADIOGRAPHIC APPEARANCE OF PERICARDIAL EFFUSION.

- Globoid cardiac silhouette
  - Cardiomegaly without radiographic evidence of specific chamber enlargements
- Right-sided heart failure
  - Pulmonary hypoperfusion
  - Dilated caudal vena cava
  - Generalized hepatomegaly
  - Peritoneal effusion
  - Pleural effusion

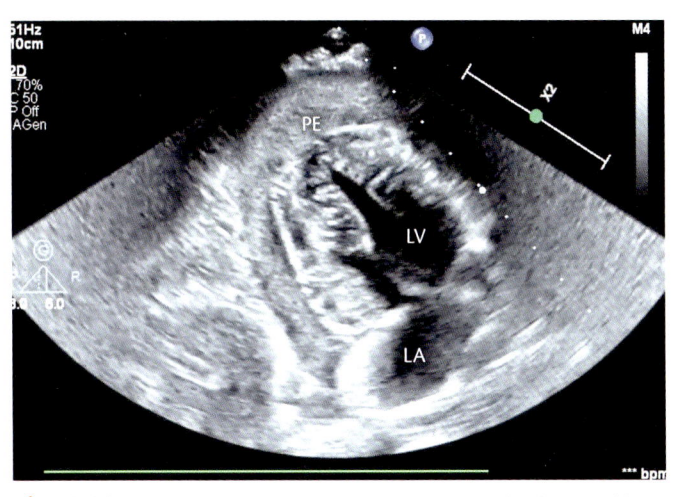

Fig. 19.89 Dachshund affected by myxomatous mitral valve disease. Oblique view obtained with the dog in standing position. Hyperechoic fluid in the pericardial sac (PE). The left ventricle looks (LV) thick because of the reduced preload (pseudohypertrophy) and the left atrium is smaller compared to the last echocardiographic exam. The dog had a left atrium (LA) rupture, because of the severe atrial dilation and elevated pressure. The pericardial fluid is hyperechoic because a clot is forming.

Fig. 19.90 (**A**) Lateral and (**B**) ventrodorsal thoracic radiograph of a Belgian Malinois presented for an Addisonian crisis. The heart is markedly reduced in size, spanning only two intercostal spaces, and is separated from the sternum. The pulmonary vessels are severely attenuated. The decreased vascular volume creates a hyperlucency within the lungs.

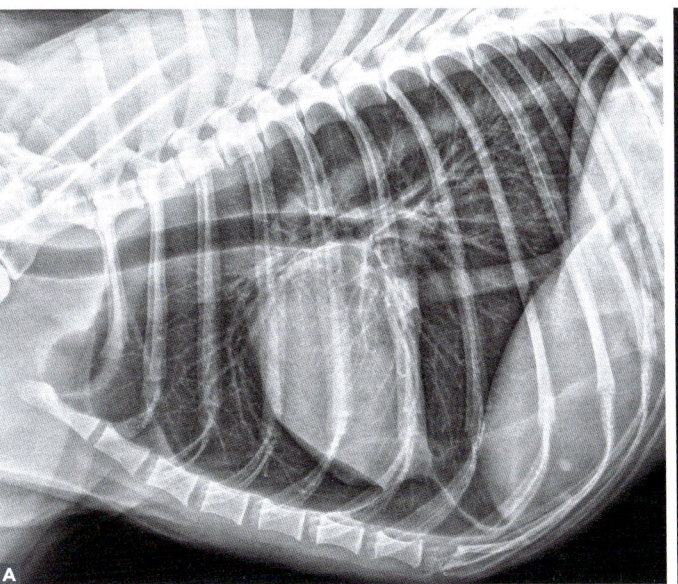

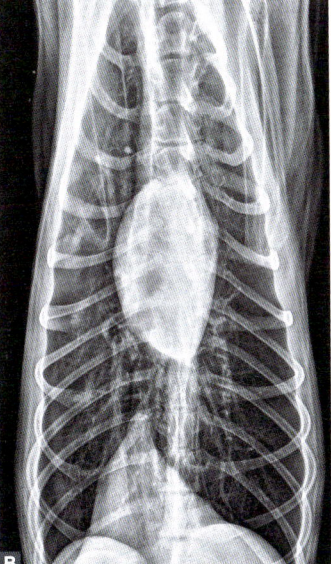

References

1. Ristic J. Clinical assessment of the dog with suspected cardiac disease. *In Practice* 26:192-199, 2004.
2. Buchanan JW, Bucheler J. Vertebral scale system to measure canine heart size in radiographs. *J Am Vet Med Assoc* 206: 194-199, 1995.
3. Litster AL, Buchanan JW. Vertebral scale system to measure heart size in radiographs of cats. *J Am Vet Med Assoc* 216:210-214, 2000.
4. Buchanan JW. Vertebral scale system to measure heart size in radiographs. *Vet Clin North Am Small Anim Pract* 30:379-393, 2000.
5. Bavegems V, Van Caelenberg A, Duchateau L, Sys SU, Van Bree H, De Rick A. Vertebral heart size ranges specific for whippets. *Vet Radiol Ultrasound* 46:400-403, 2005.
6. Jepsen-Grant K, Pollard RE, Johnson LR. Vertebral heart scores in eight dog breeds. *Vet Radiol Ultrasound* 54:3-8, 2013.
7. Kraetschmer S, Ludwig K, Meneses F, Nolte I, Simon D. Vertebral heart scale in the beagle dog. *J Small Anim Pract* 49:240-243, 2008.
8. Marin LM, Brown J, McBrien C, Baumwart R, Samii VF, Couto CG. Vertebral heart size in retired racing Greyhounds. *Vet Radiol Ultrasound* 48:332-334, 2007.
9. Lord P, Hansson K, Kvart C, Häggström J. Rate of change of heart size before congestive heart failure in dogs with mitral regurgitation. *J Small Anim Pract* 51:210-218, 2010.
10. Lord PF, Hansson K, Carnabuci C, Kvart C, Häggström J. Radiographic heart size and its rate of increase as tests for onset of congestive heart failure in Cavalier King Charles Spaniels with mitral valve regurgitation. *J Vet Intern Med* 25:1312-1319, 2011.
11. Fox PR. Canine myocardial disease. In Fox PR (editor). Canine and Feline Cardiology. New York, Churchill Livingstone, 1988, pp 467-493.
12. Meurs KM. Boxer dog cardiomyopathy: an update. *Vet Clin North Am Small Anim Pract* 34:1235-1244, 2004.
13. Le Roux A, Rademacher N, Saelinger C, Rodriguez D, Pariaut R, Gaschen L. Value of tracheal bifurcation angle measurement as a radiographic sign of left atrial enlargement in dogs. *Vet Radiol Ultrasound* 53:28-33, 2012.
14. Sanchez Salguero X, Prandi D, Llabres-Diaz F, Manzanilla EG, Bussadori C. A radiographic measurement of left atrial size in dogs. *Ir Vet J* 71:25, 2018.
15. Malcolm EL, Visser LC, Phillips KL, Johnson LR. Diagnostic value of vertebral left atrial size as determined from thoracic radiographs for assessment of left atrial size in dogs with myxomatous mitral valve disease. *J Am Vet Med Assoc* 253:1038-1045, 2018.
16. Thrall DE, Losonsky JM. A method for evaluating canine pulmonary circulatory dynamics from survey radiographs. *J Am Anim Hosp Assoc* 12:457-462, 1976.
17. Myer CW. Radiography review: the vascular and bronchial patterns of pulmonary disease. *Vet Radiol* 21:156-160, 1980.
18. Seiler GS, Nolan TJ, Withnall E, Reynolds C, Lok JB, Sleeper MM. Computed tomographic changes associated with the prepatent and early patent phase of dirofilariasis in an experimentally infected dog. *Vet Radiol Ultrasound* 51:136-140, 2010.
19. Serres FJ, Chetboul V, Tissier R, Carlos Sampedrano C, Gouni V, Nicolle AP, et al. Doppler echocardiography-derived evidence of pulmonary arterial hypertension in dogs with degenerative mitral valve disease: 86 cases (2001-2005). *J Am Vet Med Assoc* 229:1772-1778, 2006.
20. Diana A, Guglielmini C, Pivetta M, Sanacore A, Di Tommaso M, Lord PF, et al. Radiographic features of cardiogenic pulmonary edema in dogs with mitral regurgitation: 61 cases (1998-2007). *J Am Vet Med Assoc* 235:1058-1063, 2009.
21. Johns SM, Nelson OL, Gay JM. Left atrial function in cats with left-sided cardiac disease and pleural effusion or pulmonary edema. *J Vet Intern Med* 26:1134-1139, 2012.
22. Strickland KN. Congenital heart disease. In Tilley LP, Smith Jr FW, Oyama MA, Sleeper MM (editors). Manual of Canine and Feline Cardiology. St Louis, Elsevier, 2008, pp 215-239.
23. MacDonald KA. Congenital heart diseases of puppies and kittens. *Vet Clin North Am Small Anim Pract* 36:503-531, 2006.
24. Olivier NB. Congenital heart disease in dogs. In Fox PR (editor). Canine and Feline Cardiology. New York, Churchill Livingstone, 1988, pp 357-389.
25. Tidholm A. Retrospective study of congenital heart defects in 151 dogs. *J Small Anim Pract* 38: 94-98, 1997.
26. Oliveira P, Domenech O, Silva J, Vannini S, Bussadori R, Bussadori C. Retrospective review of congenital heart disease in 976 dogs. *J Vet Intern Med* 25:477-483, 2011.
27. Fox PR. Congenital feline heart disease. In Fox PR (editor). Canine and Feline Cardiology. New York, Churchill Livingstone, 1988, pp 391-408.
28. Tidholm A, Ljungvall I, Michal J, Häggström J, Hoglund K. Congenital heart defects in cats: a retrospective study of 162 cats (1996-2013). *J Vet Cardiol* 17:S215-219, 2015.
29. Riesen SC, Kovacevic A, Lombard CW, Amberger C. Prevalence of heart disease in symptomatic cats: an overview from 1998 to 2005. *Schweiz Arch Tierheilkd* 149:65-71, 2007.
30. Kittleson MD, Kienle RD. Cardiac embryology and anatomy. In Kittleson MD, Kienle RD (editors). Small Animal Cardiovascular Medicine. St. Louis, Mosby, 1998, pp 1-10.
31. Navarro-Cubas X, Palermo V, French A, Sanchis-Mora S, Culshaw G. Tricuspid valve dysplasia: a retrospective study of clinical features and outcome in dogs in the UK. *Open Vet J* 7:349-359, 2017.
32. Nadolny KE, Kellihan HB, Scansen BA, Tjostheim SS, Grint KA, Forrest LJ, et al. Cor triatriatum dexter in 17 dogs. *J Vet Cardiol* 23:129-141, 2019.
33. Roland R. Congenital Heart Disease. In August JR (editor). Consultations in Feline Internal Medicine. St. Louis, Elsevier, 2010, pp 421-429.
34. Banz AC, Gottfried SD. Peritoneopericardial diaphragmatic hernia: a retrospective study of 31 cats and eight dogs. *J Am Anim Hosp Assoc* 46:398-404, 2010.
35. Burns CG, Bergh MS, McLoughlin MA. Surgical and nonsurgical treatment of peritoneopericardial diaphragmatic hernia in dogs and cats: 58 cases (1999-2008). *J Am Vet Med Assoc* 242:643-650, 2013.
36. Buchanan JW. Chronic valvular disease (endocardiosis) in dogs. *Adv Vet Sci Comp Med* 21:75-106, 1977.
37. Häggström J, Pedersen HD, Kvart C. New insights into degenerative mitral valve disease in dogs. *Vet Clin North Am Small Anim Pract* 34:1209-1226, 2004.
38. Martin MW, Stafford Johnson MJ, Strehlau G, King JN. Canine dilated cardiomyopathy: a retrospective study of prognostic findings in 367 clinical cases. *J Small Anim Pract* 51:428-436, 2010.
39. O'Grady MR, O'Sullivan ML. Dilated cardiomyopathy: an update. *Vet Clin North Am Small Anim Pract* 34:1187-1207, 2004.
40. Ward J, Ware W, Viall A. Association between atrial fibrillation and right-sided manifestations of congestive heart failure in dogs with degenerative mitral valve disease or dilated cardiomyopathy. *J Vet Cardiol* 21:18-27, 2019.
41. Oura TJ, Young AN, Keene BW, Robertson ID, Jennings DE, Thrall DE. A valentine-shaped cardiac silhouette in feline thoracic radiographs is primarily due to left atrial enlargement. *Vet Radiol Ultrasound* 56:245-250, 2015.
42. Hoch H, Strickland K. Canine and feline dirofilariasis: life cycle, pathophysiology, and diagnosis. *Comp Contin Educ Vet* 30:133-140; quiz 141, 2008.
43. Davidson BJ, Paling AC, Lahmers SL, Nelson OL. Disease association and clinical assessment of feline pericardial effusion. *J Am Anim Hosp Assoc* 44:5-9, 2008.

CHAPTER 20

Lung: anatomy, techniques, and interpretation principles

John P. Graham and Juliette Besso

> **KEY POINTS**
>
> - Both left and right lateral radiographs, in addition to either a ventrodorsal or a dorsoventral radiograph, should be obtained in patients with suspected pulmonary disease.
> - The lung may appear hyperlucent, that is, with reduced opacity.
> - Increased lung opacity may be classified as bronchial, alveolar, nodular interstitial, and unstructured interstitial patterns.
> - Classification of pulmonary patterns is helpful but not absolute. Almost all pulmonary pathology will have a mix of two or more pulmonary patterns.
> - Acute pulmonary pathology can change quite quickly, often within hours, and serial radiographs are valuable for confirming a suspected diagnosis by progression or treatment response.
> - The distribution of lesions within the lung is important in formulating a differential diagnosis.

Obtaining radiographs

The air content of the lung makes it very suitable for radiographic evaluation. The conspicuity of pulmonary lesions is a result of the contrast between the soft tissue opacity lesion and adjacent aerated lung. However, even quite large lesions may be obscured by partial or complete atelectasis, as this removes the contrast between aerated lung and a lesion. In all patients, conscious, sedated, or anesthetized, some degree of atelectasis develops in the dependent part of the lung within minutes, particularly in the lung interposed between the heart or liver and body wall. In lateral recumbency, atelectasis affects the lung closer to the tabletop. In dorsal recumbency, atelectasis occurs in the middle and peripheral zones of the caudal lung lobes as these are compressed by gravity-induced cranial and dorsal shifting of the diaphragm, liver, and other abdominal viscera. There is minimal ventral peripheral atelectasis of the lungs from gravity and compression when a patient is positioned in sternal recumbency for a dorsoventral projection. Atelectasis of the dependent lung happens much more quickly and more severely when patients are sedated or anesthetized. Pulmonary lesions may only be visible when the lung containing the lesion is uppermost and well aerated.

General anesthesia should be avoided whenever possible for thoracic radiography patients, although it may be needed for patients that are particularly fractious or have severe pain, such as from traumatic orthopedic injury. If it cannot be avoided, anesthetic induction should be done immediately prior to radiography, and the patient ventilated to minimize atelectasis. Patients should be kept in sternal recumbency after induction and positioned in lateral recumbency immediately before taking

SECTION IV THORAX

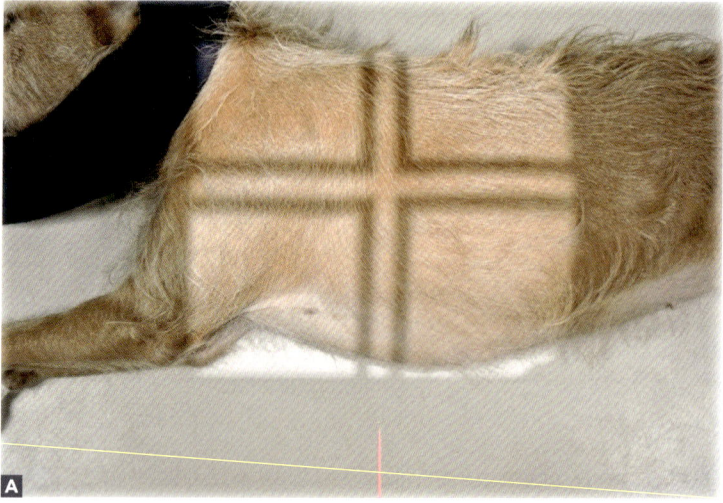

Fig. 20.1 Positioning of a canine patient for lateral and ventrodorsal radiographs of the thorax. The centering point is shown by the collimator crosshairs. This is at the level of the caudal margin of the scapula. On the lateral radiograph, the centering point is between one-third and one-half the distance from the ventral surface to the dorsal, depending on the shape of the thorax. Images courtesy of Ms. Danielle Mauragis, RVT.

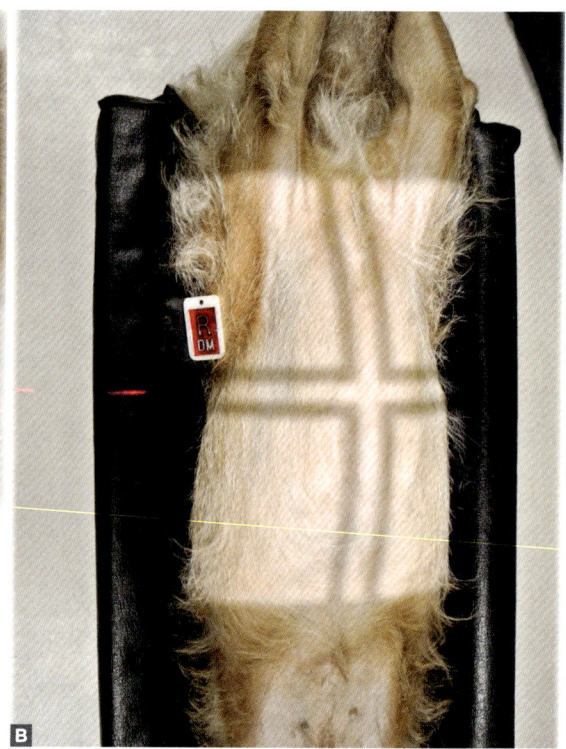

lateral radiographs and returned to sternal recumbency as quickly as possible afterward. Positive pressure ventilation is often required to achieve good pulmonary inflation.

Radiographs should be exposed at end inspiration as this will ensure maximum contrast in the lung, and there is usually a brief pause in respiratory motion at this point, which should eliminate or minimize motion artifact. Some sedation is helpful to optimize positioning and usually slows respiratory rate. Consistency of technique and positioning is fundamental to obtaining diagnostic quality radiographs and especially important for monitoring the progression or resolution of pathology. A technique chart should be used for consistency. Recording exposure parameters in the patient's medical record is quite helpful for serial examinations. In lateral recumbency, the thoracic limbs are extended cranially to eliminate superimposition. Radiolucent foam positioning wedges can be placed between the sternum and tabletop to ensure the thorax is not rotated so that the spine and sternum are equidistant from the tabletop. Placing foam wedges between the limbs may be helpful in larger dogs to prevent dropping of the upper limb, causing rotation of the thorax. For most dogs, the crosshairs of the collimator are centered at the caudal margin of the scapula and at a point approximately one-third to one-half of the distance from the ventral to dorsal skin surfaces (**fig. 20.1**). The centering point depends upon thoracic conformation, being relatively ventral in dogs with wide flat thoraxes and more dorsal in dogs with a deep narrow thorax. The collimated field should be extended to the level of the tip of the last floating rib, which will include the cranial lung fields. The beam is also centered at the caudal margin of the scapula and the exposure field extended to the tip of the last rib. The feline thorax is relatively longer than the canine, and the centering point is usually one to two finger widths caudal to the caudal margin of the scapula and at the midpoint between the dorsal and ventral skin surfaces. The same centering point is used for ventrodorsal (VD) or dorsoventral (DV) projections, and the exposure field is collimated as for canine patients.

When thoracic radiographs are primarily intended to assess for pulmonary disease, both left and right lateral projections and a VD or a DV should be obtained.[1] Radiographs are exposed at peak inspiration. Expiratory radiographs are seldom used to assess the lungs but may be helpful to document loss of pulmonary compliance from pathologies such as fibrosis or air trapping by demonstrating a

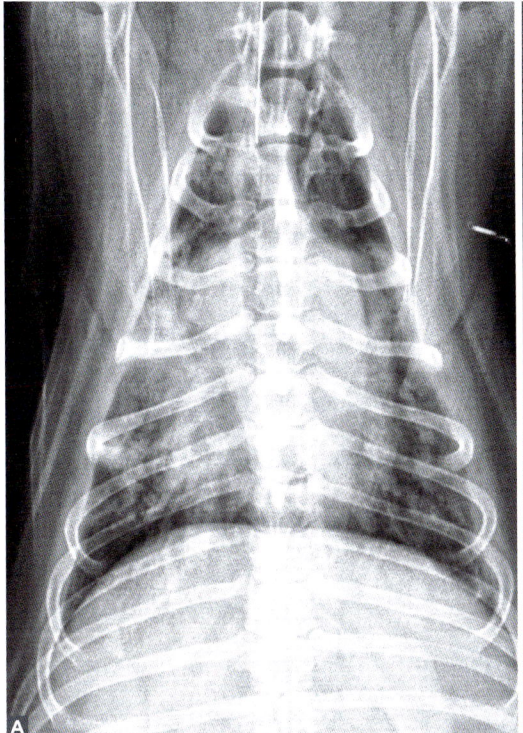

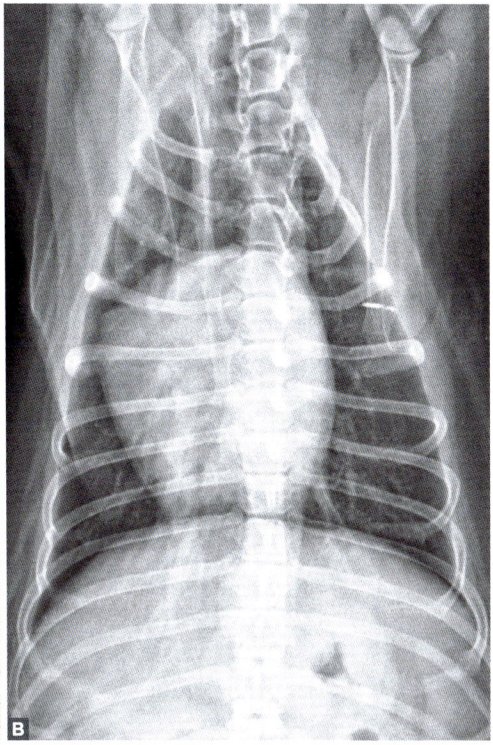

Fig. 20.2 (**A**) A ventrodorsal radiograph of a 12-year-old Jack Russell terrier radiographed following induction for general anesthesia after a mass was identified at the base of the tongue during intubation. The image shows multifocal increased opacity in all lung fields, resulting in near-complete effacement of the right cardiac border and partial effacement of the left cardiac border. The increased pulmonary opacity is a mix of alveolar and unstructured interstitial patterns. (**B**) A ventrodorsal radiograph of the same dog obtained approximately 2 hours after recovery from anesthesia. The overall lung volume is larger, and the lungs now have a normal uniform relatively dark opacity. Because the patient is now conscious there is slightly oblique positioning and some motion artifact.

consistent volume and overall appearance regardless of the respiratory phase. Expiratory radiographs may also help confirm a small volume of fluid or air in the pleural space. General anesthesia will result in atelectasis and increased opacity of the lung field to a varying and unpredictable degree. In such cases, it is not possible to reliably distinguish atelectasis from pathology. Similarly, pathologic lesions such as nodules may be readily obscured by atelectatic increased opacity (**fig 20.2**).

CT is well suited to the diagnosis of pulmonary pathology as lesion contrast with aerated lung is even better than on radiographs, and superimposition is essentially eliminated. For most cases, sternal recumbency is preferred to avoid atelectasis. Some patients can be scanned without chemical restraint but, unlike humans, small animals cannot be instructed to hold a breath and respiratory motion artifact is a problem. Several scans may be required to ensure the entire thorax is imaged without motion artifact. Sedation is often helpful to minimize patient stress and slow the respiratory rate. General anesthesia is less problematic than with radiography as patients can be ventilated to enforce a breath hold.

Normal lung

The anatomy of the lungs is similar in cats and dogs. The left lung comprises a cranial lobe, which has incompletely separated cranial and caudal subdivisions, and a caudal lobe. The apex of the left cranial lobe often extends cranial to the first rib and just to the right of the midline. The division between the two lobes is oriented obliquely from craniodorsal to caudoventral. The caudal ventral margin of the cranial lobe extends to the diaphragm in many dogs. The right lung comprises four lobes. The cranial, middle, and caudal lobes fill the right hemithorax. The accessory lung lobe is interposed between the heart and diaphragm, extends to the left of the midline, and partly encases the caudal vena cava.

The normal lung is predominantly comprised of air with a relatively small volume of soft tissue and blood and should appear relatively dark. The walls of larger bronchi are visible in the hilar part of the lung in dogs and sometimes in cats. Normal bronchial walls may be visible in the middle zone of the

SECTION IV THORAX

Fig. 20.3 (**A**) Right lateral and (**B**) ventrodorsal radiographs of a ten-year-old female neutered Golden Retriever and (**C**) close-up lateral image of a six-year-old mixed breed dog. The radiographs are normal. Notice the relatively radiolucent appearance of the lungs. Normal vessels are clearly visible extending from the region of the heart base to the periphery of the lung (white arrows). The bronchial walls are visible in the hilar segment of the lung only (orange arrows). The close-up image (**C**) shows normal smaller pulmonary vessels in the periphery of the lung. The visibility of small pulmonary vessels in the middle and peripheral zones of the lung is a useful internal control to confirm or exclude the presence of an unstructured interstitial pattern. Relatively small vessels should be visible in the normal lung on good quality radiographs.

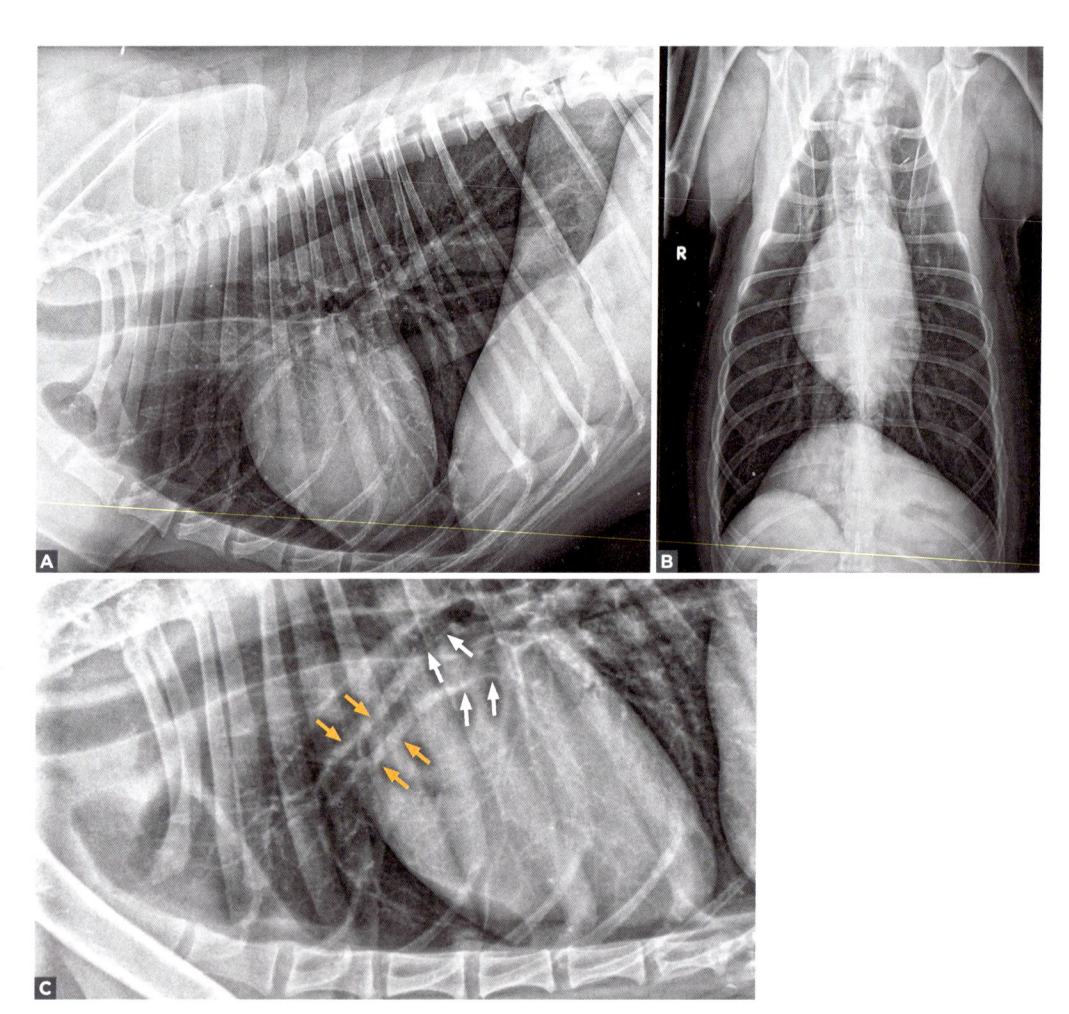

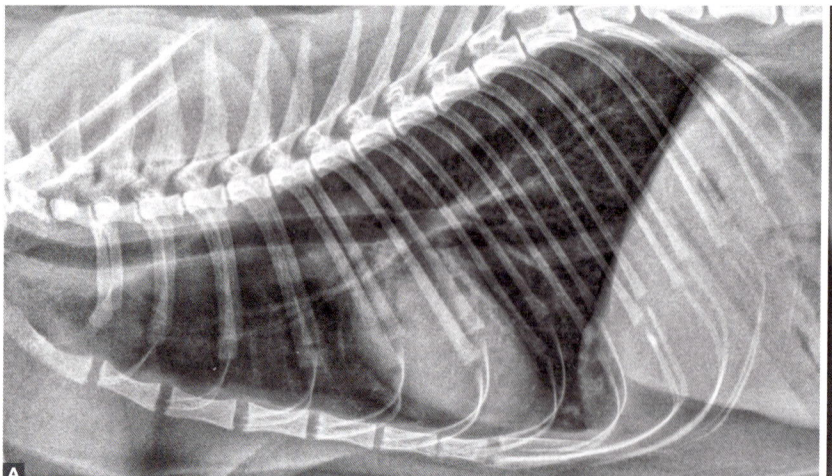

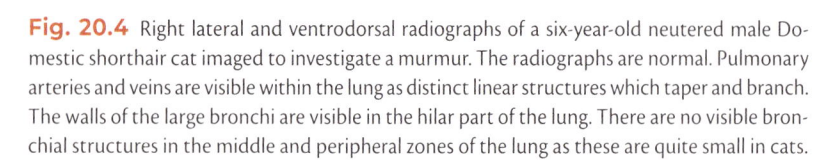

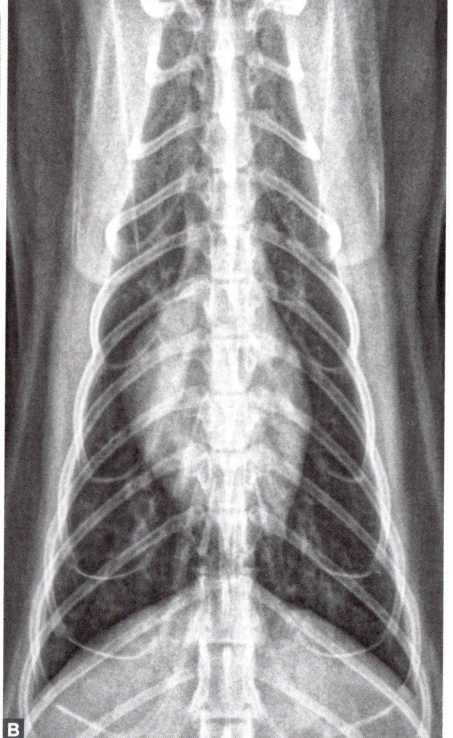

Fig. 20.4 Right lateral and ventrodorsal radiographs of a six-year-old neutered male Domestic shorthair cat imaged to investigate a murmur. The radiographs are normal. Pulmonary arteries and veins are visible within the lung as distinct linear structures which taper and branch. The walls of the large bronchi are visible in the hilar part of the lung. There are no visible bronchial structures in the middle and peripheral zones of the lung as these are quite small in cats.

lung in medium and larger dogs. The airways in the periphery of the lung in dogs and cats are quite small and not visible on radiographs when normal. Pulmonary arteries and veins are visible and small vessels can be traced almost to the periphery of the lung (**figs. 20.3** and **20.4**).

On CT normal bronchial walls and pulmonary vessels are clearly visible. As these structures are seldom oriented parallel to the image plane, they are usually seen in oblique cross-section. Bronchial walls and vessels are visible to the mid zone of the lung but are too small to resolve in the periphery of the lung. The tissues of the alveolar walls, interstitium, and capillary bed contribute to an overall hazy opacity when the display parameters are suitably adjusted. When CT images are adjusted to display detail of soft tissue structures such as vessels or the mediastinum, normal lung appears almost black with only the larger vessels and airways being visible (**fig 20.5**).

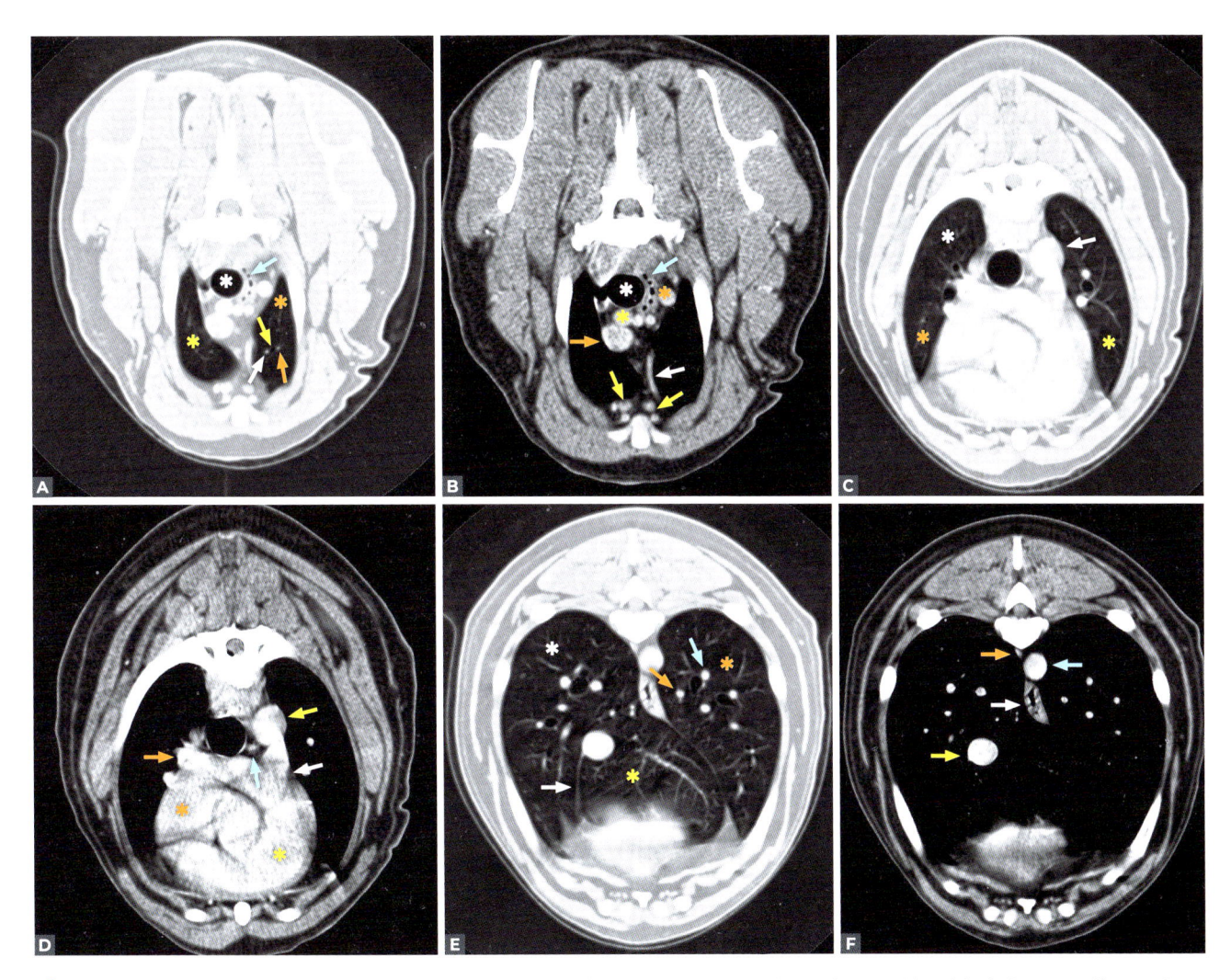

Fig. 20.5 (**A**) Transverse computed tomography image of the cranial mediastinum lung window. Right cranial lung lobe (yellow asterisk), cranial portion of the left cranial lung lobe (orange asterisk). Pulmonary vein of left cranial lung lobe (white arrow), pulmonary artery of left cranial lung lobe (orange arrow), lobar bronchus to left cranial lung lobe (yellow arrow). (**B**) Transverse computed tomography image of the cranial mediastinum soft tissue window post-contrast. Trachea (white asterisk), esophagus, cranial vena cava (orange arrow), right subclavian artery (yellow asterisk), right subclavian artery (orange asterisk), thymus (white arrow), sternal lymph nodes (yellow arrows). (**C**) Transverse computed tomography image of the middle mediastinum lung window. Right cranial lung lobe (white asterisk), right middle lung lobe (orange asterisk), and caudal portion of the left cranial lung lobe (yellow asterisk). (**D**) Transverse computed tomography image of the middle mediastinum soft tissue window post-contrast. Thoracic aorta (yellow arrow), left pulmonary artery (white arrow), right pulmonary artery (orange arrow), right atrium (orange asterisk), right ventricle (yellow asterisk), left tracheobronchial lymph nodes (blue arrow). (**E**) Transverse computed tomography image of the caudal mediastinum lung window. Right caudal lung lobe (white asterisk), caudal left lung lobe (orange asterisk), accessory lung lobe (yellow asterisk), pulmonary vein of left caudal lung lobe (orange arrow), pulmonary artery of left caudal lung lobe (blue arrow), a fold of vena cava (white arrow). (**F**) Transverse computed tomography image of the caudal mediastinum soft tissue window post-contrast. Thoracic aorta (blue arrow), azygos (orange arrow), esophagus (white arrow), and caudal vena cava (yellow arrow).

Interpretation of pulmonary pathology

The basic radiologic interpretation principle of assessing changes in size, shape, number, position, and opacity applies to the lungs.[2] In most cases, pulmonary pathology is manifested by a change in opacity, occasionally decreased but usually increased. Essentially, the first assessment is to decide if the lungs appear normal, less opaque, or more opaque than normal. If the lungs are abnormal, one must decide the type or types of pattern present and the distribution of the changes. Bronchial, alveolar, and nodular interstitial patterns have features that usually allow their identification with a fair degree of confidence. Unstructured interstitial patterns have fewer distinctive features and can be thought of like the "if I can't call it anything else" diagnosis. The compartmentalized approach to interpreting pulmonary pathology is helpful but should be used flexibly as most diseases will show a mixed pattern of two or more components. The pulmonary abnormalities combined with any additional imaging findings, history, and clinical data are used to formulate a diagnosis or differential diagnosis. Pulmonary radiographic abnormalities may change quickly, sometimes within minutes or hours. In patients with peracute signs, radiographic abnormalities may not have had sufficient time to become evident, such as from bacterial bronchopneumonia, aspiration pneumonia, or traumatic pulmonary contusions. Serial radiographs obtained over hours or days to evaluate progression and response to treatment are often very helpful. Radiographic resolution of pulmonary changes may be slower than clinical response, and both should be used when assessing the efficacy of treatment.

Reduced pulmonary opacity

Hyperlucent is the descriptive term for a lung that is relatively darker than normal, i.e., has reduced radiographic opacity. This assessment is largely subjective and depends on familiarity with the appearance of images from a particular system or clinic.

This may be a normal appearance in very thin, athletic, or cachectic patients, as the lack of body fat causes relative overexposure. True overexposure can also cause this appearance, although digital imaging systems are less susceptible than film. Relative overexposure of the cranial ventral lung field on lateral radiographs of large deep-chested dogs can occur as this is the thinnest part of the thorax.

In patients with generalized hyperlucency of the lungs, the lung appears darker than normal, and the periphery of the lung may appear devoid of normal small vessels. Adjusting the zoom and displaying the gray scale will usually show some small peripheral vessels. At first glance, and especially in patients with reduced cardiac size (microcardia), the appearance may be mistaken for pneumothorax.

Generalized hyperlucency is most often from severe dehydration or hypovolemic shock, where depleted volume in the pulmonary circulation reduces the overall opacity of the lung (**fig. 20.6**). Common etiologies are severe hemorrhagic gastroenteritis, blunt trauma such as a motor vehicle accident, and severe acute hemorrhage such as from a ruptured splenic hematoma or neoplasm. The pulmonary vessels are smaller than normal in these patients, and in severe cases the heart is also small. Generalized hyperlucency is an occasional but inconsistent manifestation of Addison's disease, also as a result of reduced circulating volume, and the heart and the pulmonary vessels may also be small.

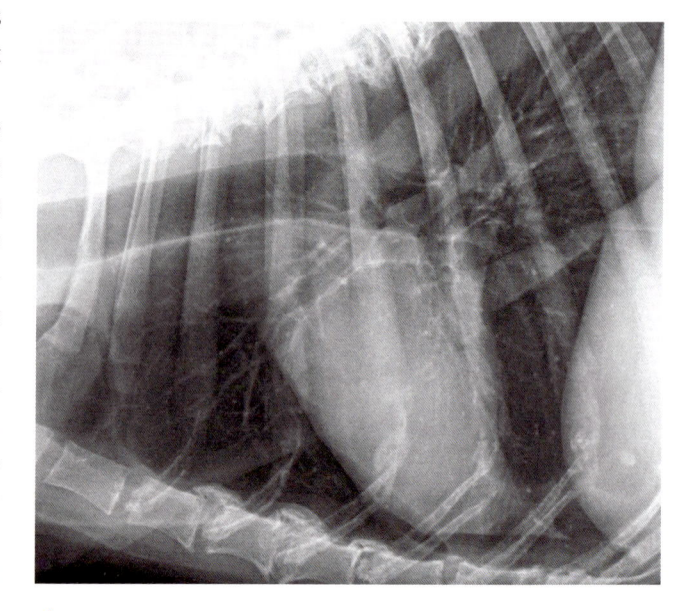

Fig. 20.6 Right lateral radiograph of a ten-year-old neutered male German Shepherd. The patient presented with acute intraperitoneal hemorrhage from a splenic mass. The heart and pulmonary vessels are much smaller than normal and pulmonary vessels are not visible in the periphery of the lung. The lung appears diffusely hyperlucent, darker than expected, because of the reduced volume of blood in the pulmonary circulation. These findings come from hypovolemic shock.

CHAPTER 20 Lung: anatomy, techniques, and interpretation principles

Overinflation caused by obstructive small airway disease and air trapping is relatively common in cats with feline asthma (**fig 20.7**). In some patients, overinflation makes the lungs appear darker than normal as it effectively "dilutes" any increase in bronchial or interstitial opacity. More often, affected patients show some bronchial thickening and an unstructured interstitial pattern. The overall lung volume is increased, and the thorax appears barrel-shaped rather than the normal elongated triangular shape. On lateral projections, there is increased separation of the diaphragm and heart, and the diaphragm is displaced caudally and flattened. On VD or DV projections, the ribs are oriented almost perpendicular to the spine. Inspiratory and expiratory radiographs of these patients often show little change in overall lung volume.

One lung may be hyperinflated and hyperlucent if there is unilateral atelectasis and compensatory overinflation of the contralateral lung. This is most often iatrogenic in patients with recumbent atelectasis from anesthesia or sometimes from the use of a long endotracheal tube resulting in selective bronchial intubation (**fig 20.8**). The appearance is also common in patients in prolonged recumbency from paralysis or pain related to trauma or major surgery. Obstruction of a bronchus by an inhaled foreign object usually causes atelectasis of the associated lobe. In rare cases, the foreign object acts as a one-way valve, allowing inflow of air but blocking outflow, and causes overinflation of a lobe of one lung. Depending on the severity of overinflation, there may be atelectasis of the unaffected lung.

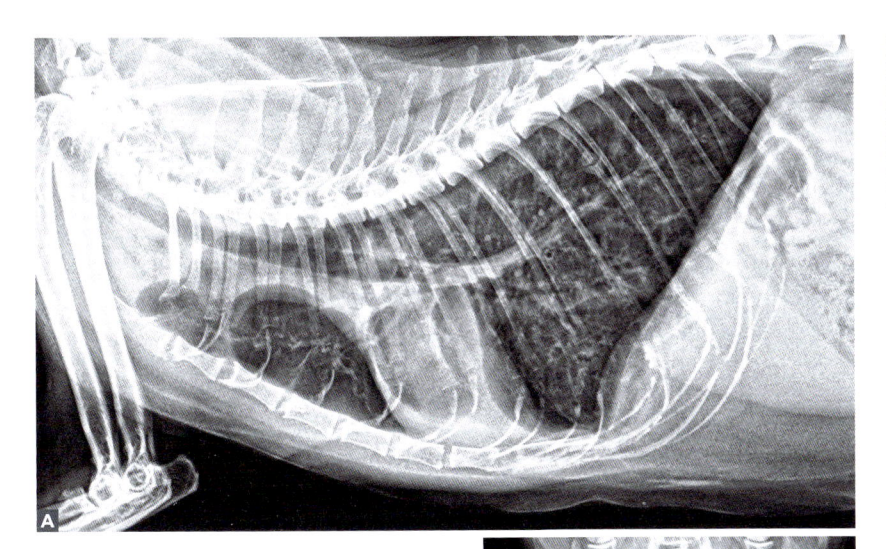

Fig. 20.7 Lateral and ventrodorsal radiographs of an 11-year-old Siamese cat with a chronic history of cough with recent-onset dyspnea. (**A**) The lung field is overexpanded with caudal displacement and flattening of the diaphragm. The lungs are slightly hyperlucent, overall appearing darker than normal, but closer examination shows numerous bronchial markings visible as "doughnuts" and "tram lines". The severity of the pulmonary changes is effectively diluted by the overinflation. (**B**) There is complete collapse of the right middle lung lobe, seen as a well-defined triangular structure adjacent to the right cardiac border. The overinflation of the lung and collapse of the right middle lung lobe is both a result of obstruction of small airways. There are also fractures of the right ninth through 12th ribs with some callus formation. These represent chronic stress fractures from loss of pulmonary compliance rather than traumatic injuries.

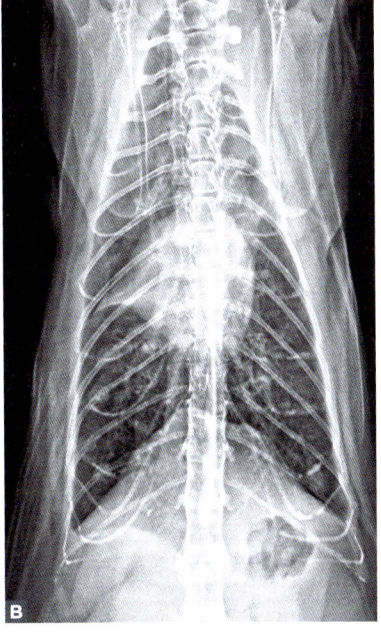

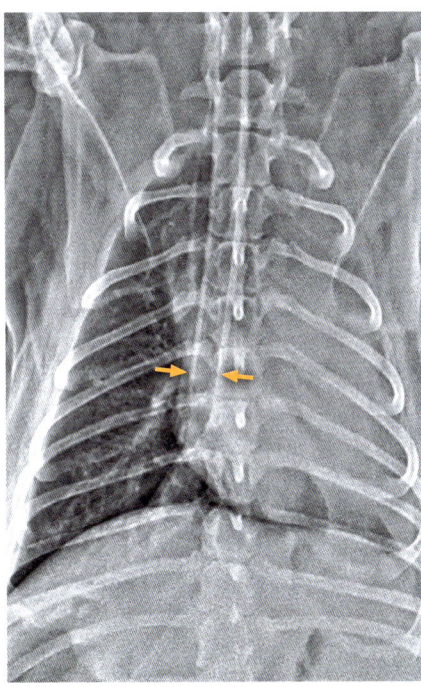

Fig. 20.8 A ventrodorsal radiograph of an 11-year-old Bichon Frisé. An endotracheal tube has been placed with the tip located in the right caudal lobar bronchus (arrows). This prevents ventilation of the left lung with complete, secondary atelectasis. The left lung is uniform soft tissue opacity, completely obscuring the cardiac and diaphragmatic outlines and intrapulmonary vascular structures. The heart and mediastinum are displaced toward the left thoracic wall, a mediastinal shift, from atelectasis.

Hyperlucency affecting a lobe or lobes or segment of a lobe is less common than generalized hyperlucency. Bullae are thin-walled air-filled hyperlucent structures that may be congenital or a sequel to traumatic laceration of the lung. On radiographs, these appear as discrete soap bubble-like structures (**fig 20.9**). Relatively rare causes of lobar or segmental hyperlucency include lobar emphysema and pulmonary thromboembolism (**fig 20.10**).

Increased pulmonary opacity

Most pulmonary pathology results in increased soft tissue opacity. Interpretation of pulmonary changes is complex and may appear overwhelming, but fortunately lends itself to a systematic, iterative approach. Increased opacity is classified according to the anatomic components affected, i.e., bronchi, alveoli, and interstitium. The classification system is simplified as the notional anatomic components are not truly separate. For example, the interstitium of the lung is contiguous with the

Fig. 20.9 Left lateral thoracic radiograph of a geriatric Pit Bull Terrier. A thin-walled air-filled bulla is present superimposed on the central part of the cardiac silhouette (white arrows). A second fluid-filled bulla is present in the cranial ventral lung field (orange arrows), appearing as a discrete spherical soft tissue opacity structure, mimicking a nodule. These were incidental findings, and the patient had no respiratory signs.

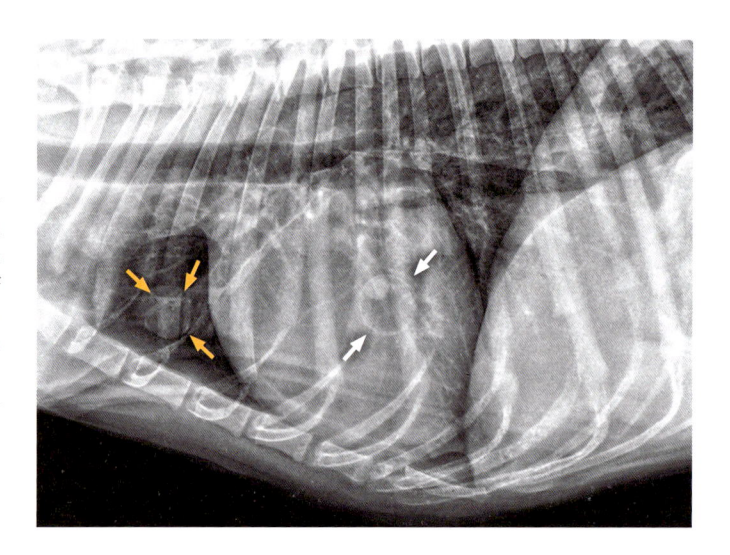

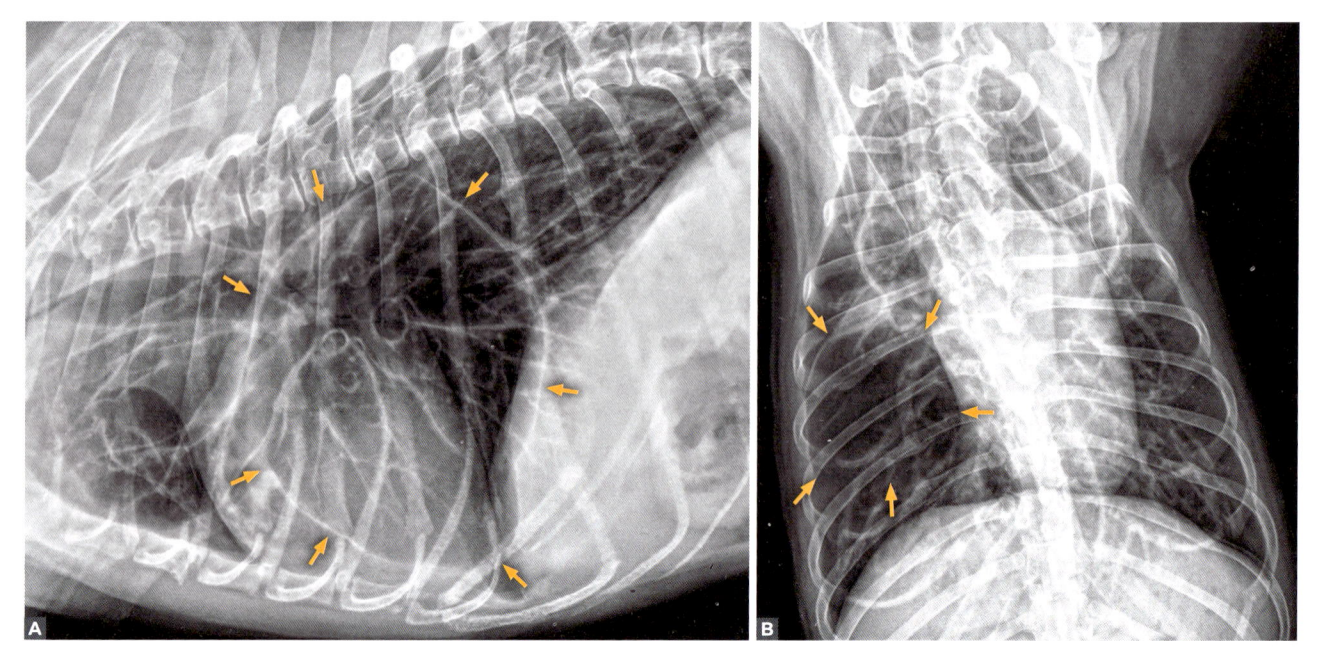

Fig. 20.10 Right lateral and ventrodorsal radiographs of a 12-year-old mixed breed dog with a history of chronic coughing unresponsive to treatment. A large air-filled structure with a discrete soft tissue wall occupies most of the right mid thorax (arrows). This structure is devoid of the normal vessels and airways which should be visible in the lung. The lesion represents either a large bulla or emphysema of the right middle lung lobe. There is also severe uniform dilation of multiple bronchi in all lung lobes consistent with severe diffuse tubular bronchiectasis, and the bronchial walls are thickened. The bullous lesion is a sequel to chronic severe bronchial disease.

interstitial spaces around the bronchi and vessels, and a process affecting the interstitium may affect the peribronchial tissues and give the impression of bronchial thickening. Most pathologic processes show mixed patterns, exhibiting at least two components. The effect of increased opacity in the lung on the appearance of normal pulmonary vessels and cardiac and diaphragmatic outlines are important built-in controls, as is the contrast between abnormal and normal lung.

The distribution of lesions within the lung is important in formulating a differential diagnosis. The lobe or lobes and the region within the lung affected should be noted. For descriptive purposes, the lung is roughly divided into three concentric zones: hilar, middle, and peripheral. Keep in mind that we are using two-dimensional images to assess complex three-dimensional anatomy, and lesion location should be confirmed on orthogonal projections.

Bronchial pattern

A bronchial pattern may be caused by increased luminal secretions, mucosal infiltration, peribronchial edema or cellular infiltrates, or a combination of these. On radiographs and CT this appears as a thickening of the bronchial walls.

Thickened bronchi appear as converging soft tissue opacity lines when oriented perpendicular to the X-ray beam, described as train tracks or tram lines (**fig 20.11**). The bronchi appear as circular soft tissue opacity structures with a lucent center when oriented parallel to the beam, described as doughnuts or ring shadows. A bronchial pattern makes smaller airways in the middle and peripheral zones of the lung visible. Thickening of the normally visible bronchial walls in the hilar part of the lung is reported to be the most common abnormality in dogs with chronic bronchitis.[3] However, this assessment is subjective and depends upon experience and availability of comparison radiographs. In normal medium and large dogs, bronchi are usually visible in the hilar and middle zones. In smaller dogs and cats, bronchi may be visible in the hilar part of the lung but may be too small to resolve in some patients. Bronchi in the periphery of the lung are small and not visible when normal. Visible bronchial markings in the periphery of the lung are a reliable sign that the patient has bronchial disease (**fig 20.12**).

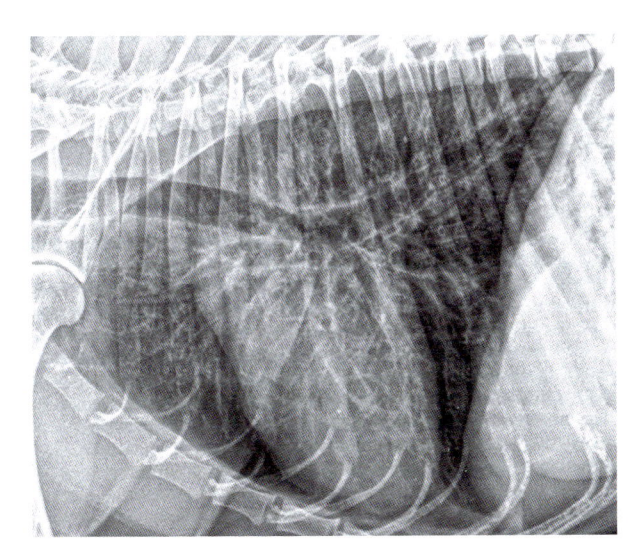

Fig. 20.11 Radiograph of an eight-year-old German Shepherd cross with a history of chronic coughing from chronic bronchitis. There is diffuse increased opacity of the lung fields. The walls of the major bronchi are thicker than normal and visible further into the periphery of the lung than normal. Bronchi are visible in the middle and peripheral parts of the lung as converging, thick, soft tissue opacity lines. There are also a number of end-on bronchi that appear as "doughnuts" or soft tissue opacity rings in the caudal lung fields, best seen just caudal to the heart and dorsal to the caudal vena cava.

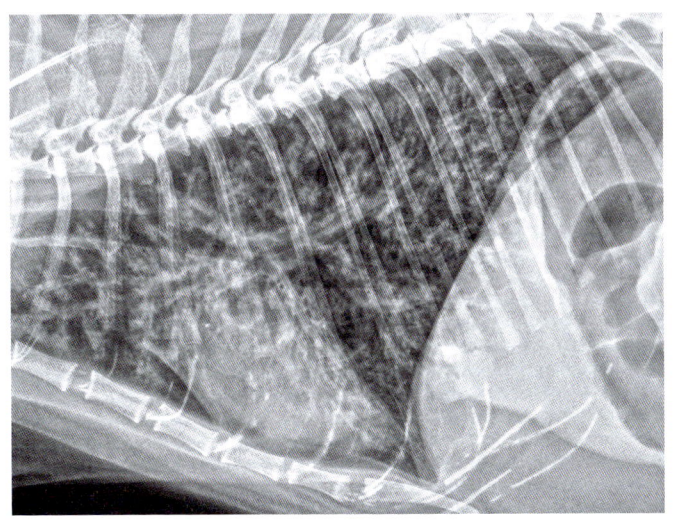

Fig. 20.12 Left lateral radiograph of a nine-year-old Domestic longhair cat with a chronic history of coughing. There is diffuse increased opacity of the lungs. Numerous thickened bronchi are visible as doughnut-type shadows dispersed throughout the lung. There is also marked thickening of the bronchial walls visible as converging soft tissue opacity linear markings throughout the lung. Some of the abnormal bronchi appear filled with soft tissue opacity material and bronchial plugs. There is also a diffuse increase in unstructured interstitial opacity in the lung, with reduced visibility of normal vascular markings. The patient was diagnosed with chronic, severe feline asthma.

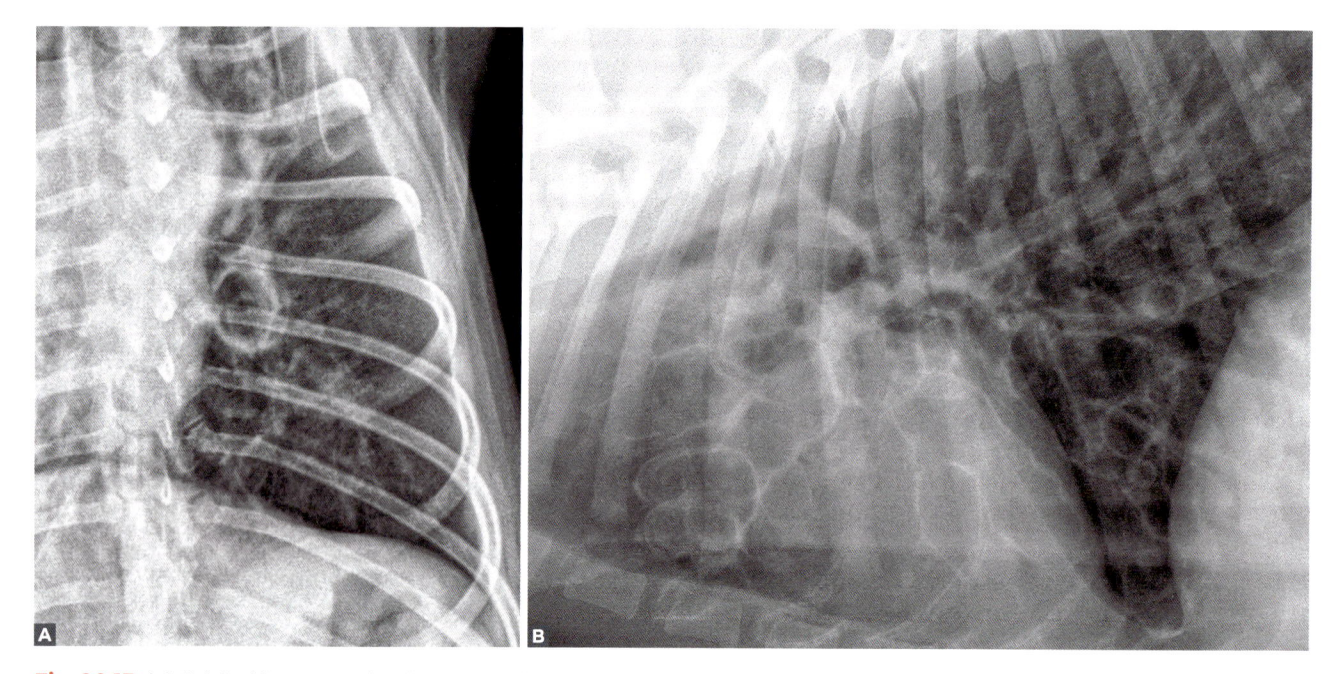

Fig. 20.13 (**A**) Slightly oblique ventrodorsal radiograph of an eight-year-old Cocker Spaniel with a history of chronic coughing. The bronchus for the caudal subsegment of the left cranial lung lobe is seen end-on and is moderately dilated and has moderate thickening of the bronchial wall, appearing as a thick-walled soft tissue opacity ring structure adjacent to the left cardiac border. This is tubular bronchiectasis. (**B**) A right lateral radiograph of a seven-month-old dog with a history of chronic, recurrent pneumonia and chronic cough. There is dilation of the bronchi throughout the ventral part of the thorax. Multiple thick-walled sac-like dilations of the airways are visible in the cranial ventral thorax, consistent with severe saccular bronchiectasis. There are also multiple sac-like dilations of the bronchi with less severe thickening of the walls in the caudal ventral thorax, seen between the heart, caudal vena cava, and liver.

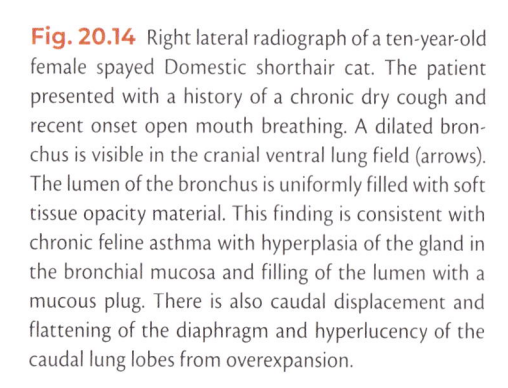

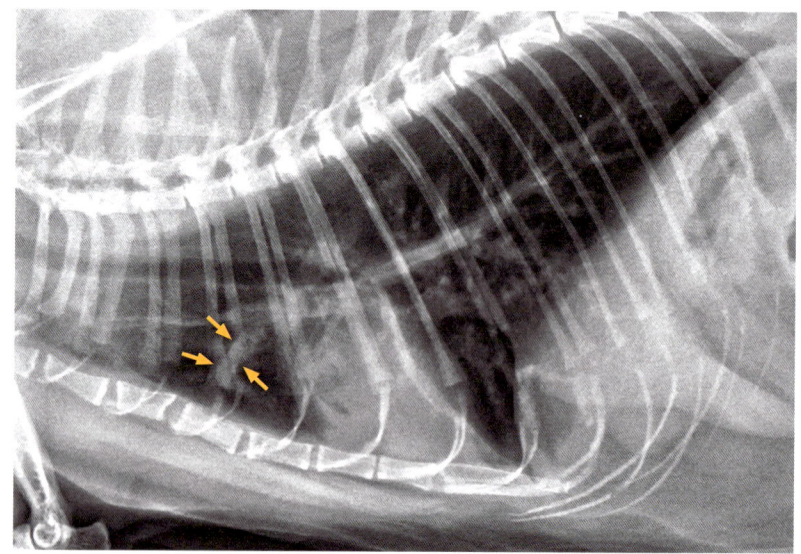

Fig. 20.14 Right lateral radiograph of a ten-year-old female spayed Domestic shorthair cat. The patient presented with a history of a chronic dry cough and recent onset open mouth breathing. A dilated bronchus is visible in the cranial ventral lung field (arrows). The lumen of the bronchus is uniformly filled with soft tissue opacity material. This finding is consistent with chronic feline asthma with hyperplasia of the gland in the bronchial mucosa and filling of the lumen with a mucous plug. There is also caudal displacement and flattening of the diaphragm and hyperlucency of the caudal lung lobes from overexpansion.

Mineralization of the bronchial cartilages is normal and a common finding in middle-aged and older dogs. These appear as thin, quite radiopaque, well-defined converging lines and rings in the hilar and middle zones of the lung. Pulmonary arteries and veins are closely apposed to the bronchi and should not be mistaken for airway walls.

Bronchiectasis is dilation of the bronchi and may be congenital but is usually a sequel to chronic bronchial and pulmonary parenchymal disease. The bronchus does not taper as normal and is usually dilated to some degree, and the bronchial walls are thickened. The dilation is described as tubular when the dilated bronchus has a mostly uniform diameter. Multiple segmental nonuniform dilations of the bronchi are described as saccular bronchiectasis. Several confluent bronchi with saccular dilation can appear as thick-walled soap bubble-like structures or "bunch of grapes" (**fig. 20.13**). Patients with recurrent pneumonia and bronchiectasis often have a local or systemic immune deficiency. Peripheral tubular bronchiectasis is reported in cats with chronic feline asthma, and the dilated bronchi are more visible when filled with hyperplastic tissue and inspissated secretions (plugs) and appear as branching soft tissue opacity structures. This has been described as resembling a "hand in glove" (fig 20.14).

Alveolar pattern

With an alveolar pattern, the air which normally fills the alveoli is replaced by fluid (blood, pus, or edema) or displaced from the alveoli by collapse in the case of atelectasis. The radiographic features of an alveolar pattern derive from this increased opacity and its effect on the appearance of intrapulmonary structures, heart, and diaphragm.

With an alveolar pattern, the affected region of the lung becomes soft tissue opacity, comparable to the heart or liver. The air bronchogram can be considered the "gold standard" sign for an alveolar pattern. An air bronchogram represents an air-filled bronchus surrounded by homogeneous soft tissue opacity lung parenchyma. The pulmonary vessels adjacent to the bronchus are used to double-check this finding, as these will be hidden by the alveolar pattern. This is analogous to the liver, which contains numerous blood vessels, all completely invisible on radiographs. Conversely, if the pulmonary vessels remain visible, there is no alveolar pattern. Air bronchograms are usually better seen on lateral projections as the airways are oriented perpendicular to the X-ray beam and appear as branching lucent lines within the abnormal lung (fig. 20.15).

The "silhouette" sign, better described as border obliteration or border effacement, occurs when two objects of the same opacity are in contact rendering their edges at the point of contact invisible. This occurs when a segment of the lung with an alveolar pattern contacts the heart or diaphragm

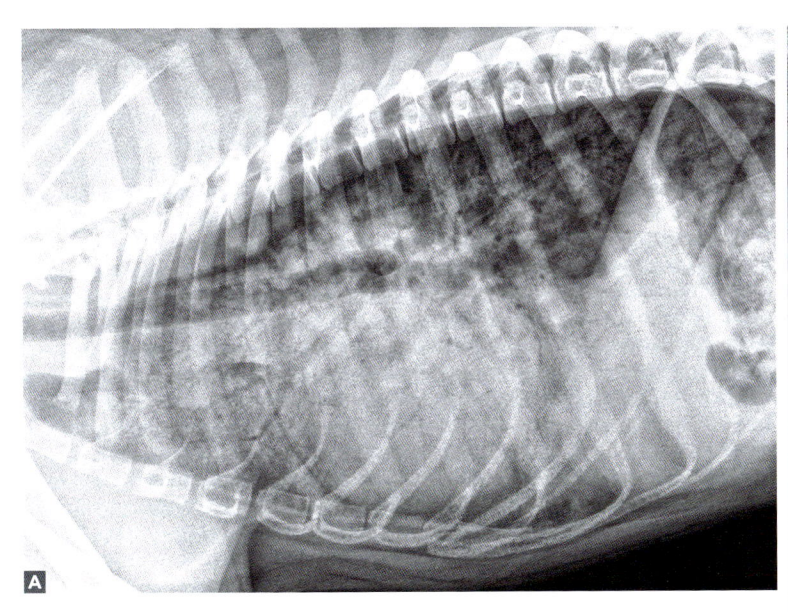

Fig. 20.15 Left lateral and ventrodorsal radiographs of a ten-month-old Retriever cross. The patient presented with acute severe cough and hemoptysis. (**A**) There is marked increased opacity of the ventral lung field. An air bronchogram is visible as a branching radiolucent structure extending from the tracheal bifurcation to the cranial ventral periphery of the lung. (**B**) There is uniform soft tissue opacification of the right lung with effacement of the cardiac and diaphragmatic outlines. The vessels within the lung are also completely effaced and there are multiple air bronchograms. There is increased soft tissue opacity in the left cranial lung lobe with air bronchograms and effacement of the left cardiac border. The left caudal lung lobe appears spared with normal visible vessels, and the left hemidiaphragm remains clearly visible. These changes represent hemorrhage from anticoagulant rodenticide intoxication.

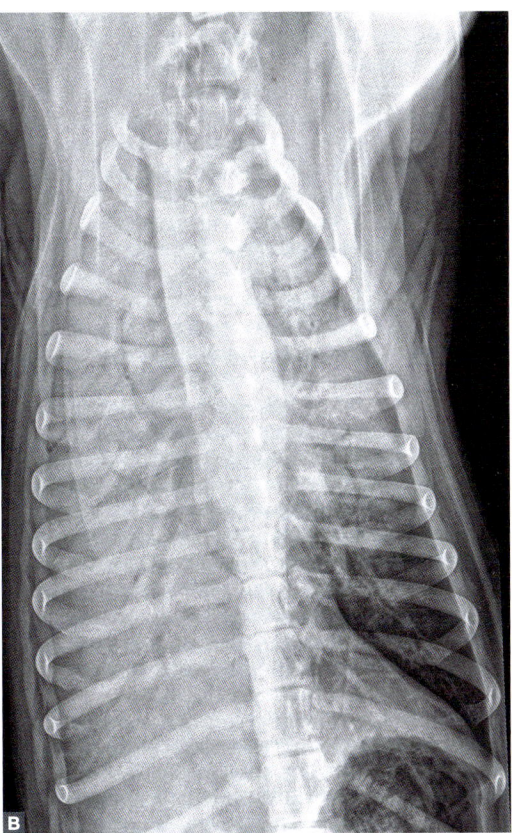

and effaces the outline. This finding is more easily seen on the VD or DV projection when part of the cardiac or diaphragmatic margins are effaced and partially preserved. The silhouette sign or border effacement may also occur with a pulmonary, pleural, or mediastinal mass or pleural fluid and should not be used as the sole basis for diagnosing an alveolar pattern.

A lobar sign occurs when a lobar or segmental alveolar pattern abuts the pleural division between lobes or between the subsegments of the left cranial lung lobe (**fig 20.16**). A discrete curvilinear border is visible at the junction of the infiltrated and aerated lung. This sign is only visible if the X-ray beam is oriented parallel to the division, so it usually distinctly visible in one projection and not seen in others. For example, with an alveolar pattern throughout the right middle lung lobe, a lobar sign at the cranial aspect of the lobe appears as a discrete curvilinear border on the VD projection but is not seen on lateral projections. A lobar sign is seen at the caudal border of the right middle lung lobe and is visible on lateral projections but not on VD projections.

Nodular interstitial pattern

Nodular interstitial patterns are characterized by soft tissue nodules varying in size from 4-5 mm to 2 cm. Solid soft tissue lesions greater than 2 cm are termed masses. This classification is entirely arbitrary

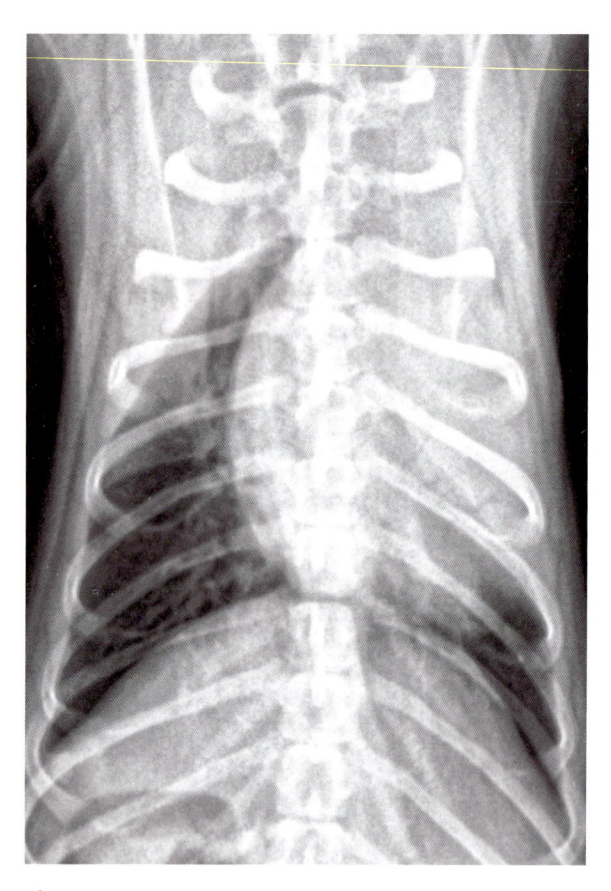

Fig. 20.16 Ventrodorsal radiograph of a nine-month-old mixed breed dog with recent onset productive cough, fever, depression, and anorexia. There is uniform soft tissue opacification of the right cranial lung lobe, which has a distinct concave caudal border abutting the right middle lung lobe. There is also diffuse increased opacity in the right middle lung lobe, which highlights the lobar border at the right caudal lung lobe. The cranial margin of the right caudal lung is more cranial than normal, indicating partial atelectasis of the cranial and middle lobes. Uniform increased opacity is also present throughout both subsegments of the left cranial lung lobe with complete effacement of the left cardiac border. The caudal margin of the left cranial lung lobe is not distinct as this is oriented obliquely to the X-ray beam. These changes indicate alveolar opacification of the right cranial and left cranial lung lobes and a severe interstitial pattern in the right middle lung lobe. The diagnosis was bacterial bronchopneumonia.

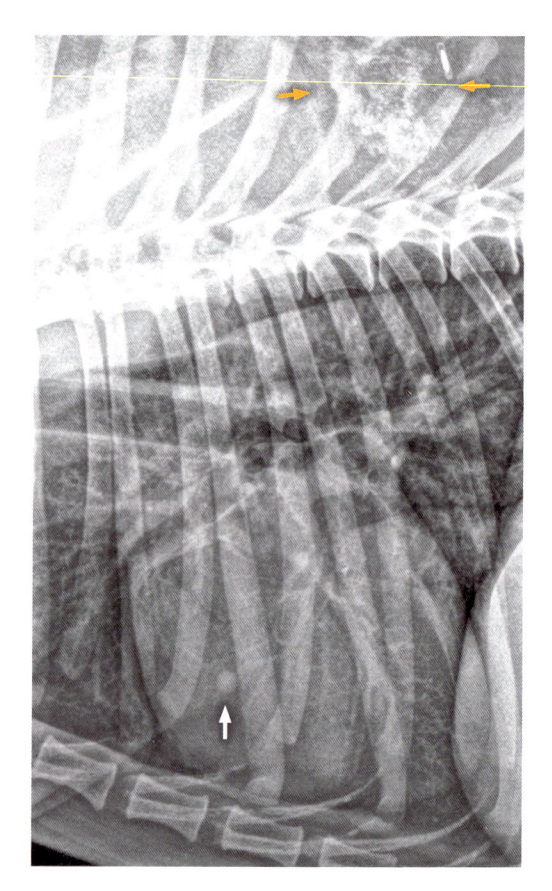

Fig. 20.17 Left lateral thoracic radiograph of a ten-year-old male neutered Husky with a firm mass lesion between the shoulder blades. Amorphous coarse granular mineralization is noted superimposed on the spinous processes in the mid-thoracic spine (white arrows). There is complete destruction of the dorsal half of the spinous process of T5. A single soft tissue opacity well-defined nodule is present overlying the cranial ventral aspect of the heart (orange arrow). Notice that the nodule has a larger diameter than adjacent blood vessels. The lesion of the spinous process is consistent with primary malignant osseous neoplasia such as osteosarcoma. The solitary pulmonary nodule most likely represents a metastatic lesion.

and should be employed flexibly, a 1.5 cm lesion is relatively larger in a 3 kg dog versus a 50 kg dog. Pulmonary nodules are roughly spherical, homogeneous soft tissue lesions that have well or poorly defined margins (figs. 20.17 and 20.18). Most nodular lesions are hematogenous in origin and are more common in the periphery of the lung. Numerous very small nodules (1-3 mm) are termed a miliary nodular pattern (from the appearance of millet seeds) and when severe, superimposition of the nodules can create a "snowstorm" effect with a diffuse, inhomogeneous increase in soft tissue opacity. In these patients, individual nodules are often difficult to distinguish. These are more easily discerned in thinner parts of the lungs, where there is less superimposition, such as in the ventral periphery of the lung overlying the heart or liver (fig. 20.19).

Nodules may be mimicked by normal structures. End-on projections of pulmonary blood vessels appear as well-defined round soft tissue structures and can be mistaken for nodules (fig. 20.20). A

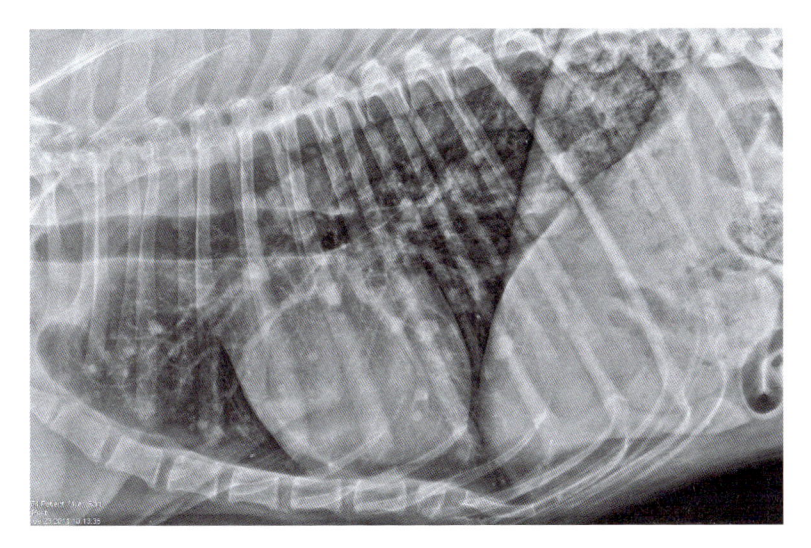

Fig. 20.18 Left lateral thoracic radiograph of a 12-year-old mixed breed dog diagnosed with prostatic carcinoma 2 months earlier. The radiograph shows numerous well-defined soft tissue opacity nodules of variable size dispersed throughout the lung. These represent pulmonary metastases.

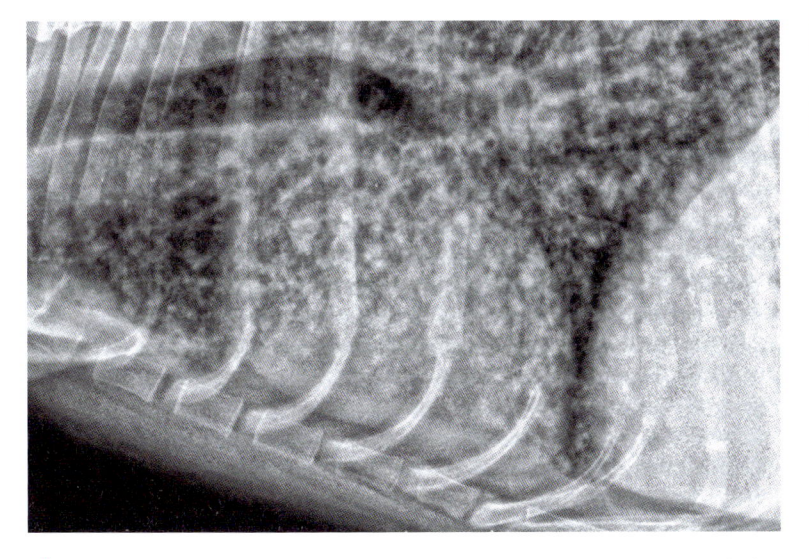

Fig. 20.19 Lateral radiograph of a 12-year-old dog that had had a splenectomy for hemangiosarcoma six months earlier. There is generalized increased opacity of the lung field, which has a coarse mottled appearance. This is a miliary nodular pattern, and nodules can be more readily distinguished in the ventral periphery of the lung. The pulmonary change represents diffuse metastasis.

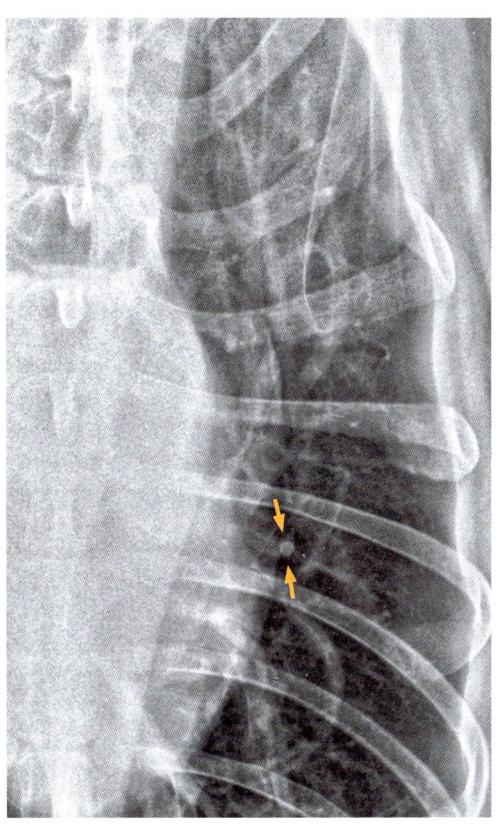

Fig. 20.20 Ventrodorsal radiograph of an eight-year-old mixed breed dog radiographed for investigation of a heart murmur. A normal end-on blood vessel is visible in the left mid thorax adjacent to the left cardiac border (arrows) and appears relatively more opaque than side-on pulmonary vessels visible cranial and caudal to the structure. The greater opacity of the structure in relation to side-on vessels indicates this is a vessel and not a parenchymal nodule. The close association of the nodular-like structure to the bronchus is also an important clue that this represents a vessel rather than a true nodule. End-on vessels are usually seen in the hilar part of the lung, where the vessels are larger. In contrast, most pulmonary nodules are hematogenous lesions and more common in the periphery of the lung.

number of features assist in differentiating the two. In geometric terms, vessels are cylinders, while nodules are spheres. Vessels projected side-on and nodules of the same diameter will have the same opacity as the X-ray beam passes through the same amount of tissue. End-on vessels appear more opaque than side-on vessels or nodules of similar diameter as the X-ray beam passes through more tissue along the length of the cylinder. The opacity of any suspected nodule should be compared to that of a side on a vessel of similar size in the same region of the lung. True nodules will have similar opacity to the side-on vessel, while end-on vessels appear more opaque. End-on vessels are more commonly seen in the hilar zone of the lung, as vessels are larger in this region of the lung. On closer examination, a bronchus may be visible immediately adjacent to the "nodule".

Many middle-aged and older dogs have pulmonary osteomas, small (2-5 mm), irregularly shaped, well-defined, mineralized foci of heterotopic bone (**fig. 20.21**). These are more opaque than adjacent vessels of similar size and may have an irregular outline. The number present is quite variable. Some cats with chronic bronchial disease develop mineralization in hyperplastic bronchial glands, which may resemble canine pulmonary osteomas. Mineralized pulmonary nodules from metastases or systemic fungal infection are extremely rare.

Structures that protrude from the skin surface, such as nipples, warts, cutaneous masses, and engorged ticks, when outlined by air, can mimic pulmonary nodules. The cutaneous "pulmonary" lesion may have one poorly defined border where it blends with the skin surface. Examination of the patient usually confirms the "nodule" is an artifact. If in doubt, barium paste can be applied to the suspicious skin structure or a paperclip placed over it, and the radiograph repeated for confirmation (**fig. 20.22**).

Many pulmonary nodules in companion animals are primary or metastatic neoplastic lesions. Abscesses and granulomas are the primary differential diagnoses. Segmental dilation of pulmonary arteries from *Dirofilaria immitis* infection and bronchial plugs can also mimic parenchymal nodules.

Unstructured interstitial pattern

An unstructured interstitial pattern is present if the lung appears more radioopaque than normal and other pulmonary patterns have been excluded; in essence, this is the diagnosis of last resort. This pattern appears as a hazy amorphous increase in opacity, resembling cotton candy (or candy floss). The effect is to increase the overall opacity in the lung and partly obscure pulmonary vessels (**fig. 20.23**). Increasing severity of the pattern will result in larger vessels being obscured. The larger lobar vessels almost always remain visible, although they may be difficult to discern clearly when

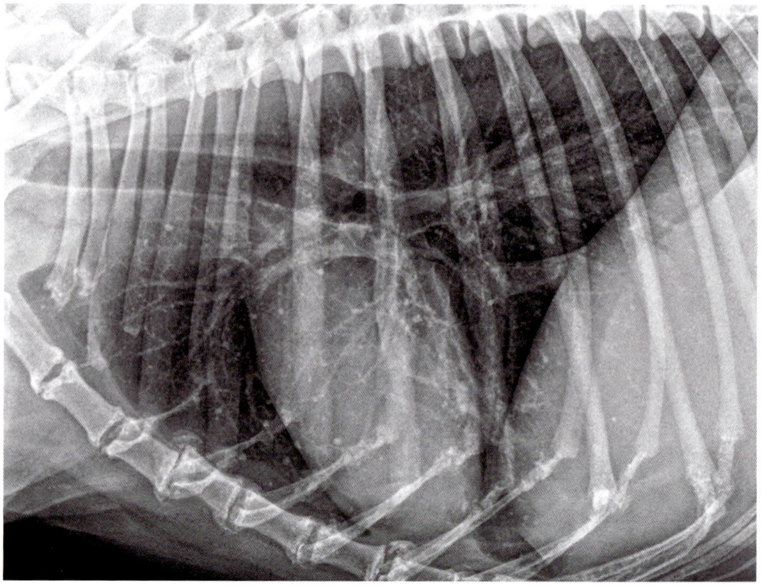

Fig. 20.21 Lateral radiograph of a 14-year-old mixed breed dog imaged to screen for metastasis after diagnosis of a hepatic mass lesion. There are numerous small, well-defined radiopaque nodular structures distributed within the lung, best seen in the cranial ventral lung field. These are more opaque than adjacent vessels indicating the structures are mineral opacity and represent so-called osteomas or heterotopic bone formation. These are common, incidental, clinically insignificant findings in middle-aged and older patients.

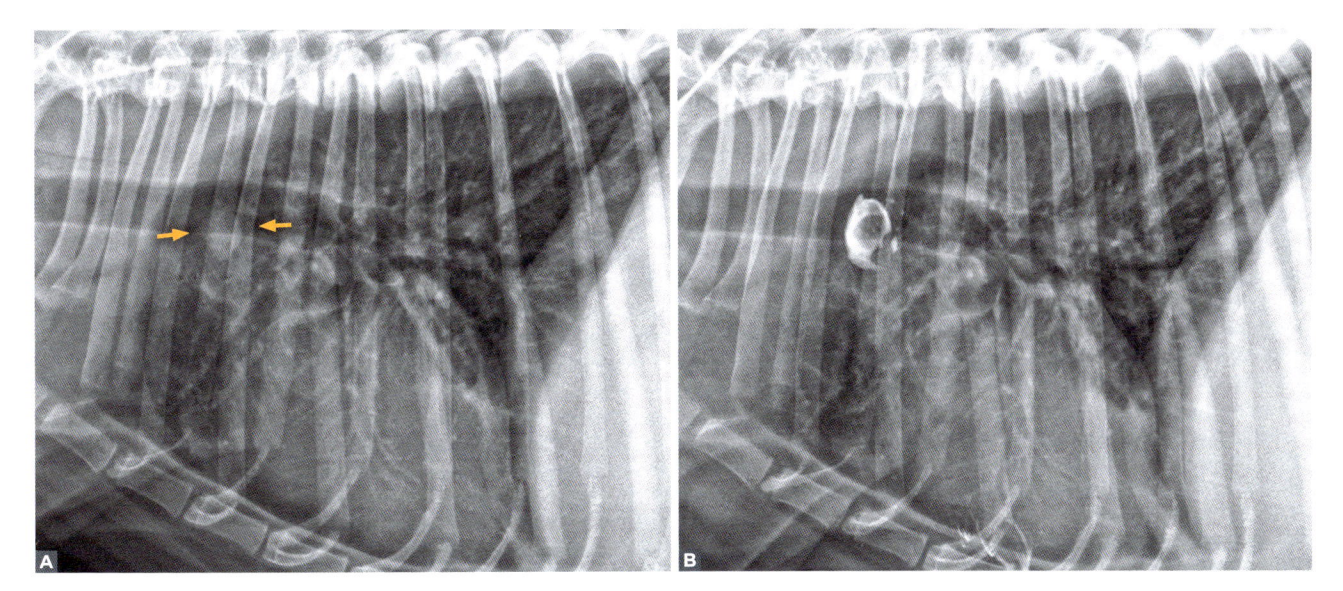

Fig. 20.22 Lateral thoracic radiographs of a ten-year-old Beagle with a history of a chronic cough. A nodular soft tissue opacity structure is present superimposed on the ventral margin of the trachea at the level of the heart base on the initial lateral radiograph (arrows). The cranial and dorsal margins of this structure are slightly less distinct than expected. A skin tag was found in this area when the patient was examined, and radiographs were repeated after application of barium paste to the skin tag. The repeat radiograph shows the "nodule" is now coated with barium paste, indicating this is not a pulmonary lesion.

the pattern is severe. The visibility of pulmonary vessels is a key control feature when considering a diagnosis of an unstructured interstitial pattern. If small pulmonary vessels are visible in the "abnormal" lung, a conclusion of an unstructured interstitial pattern is most likely a result of overzealous interpretation than real pathology.

An artifactual unstructured interstitial pattern is readily created by underexposure, limited inspiration, obesity, or a combination of these factors. Employing a broad dynamic range and excessive edge enhancement may also create an artifactual unstructured interstitial pattern. Unstructured interstitial patterns are a common overdiagnosis in clinical practice, and such a conclusion should always be double-checked. As indicated above, visibility of small vessels is the internal control used to determine if a suspected unstructured interstitial pattern is real or artifactual.

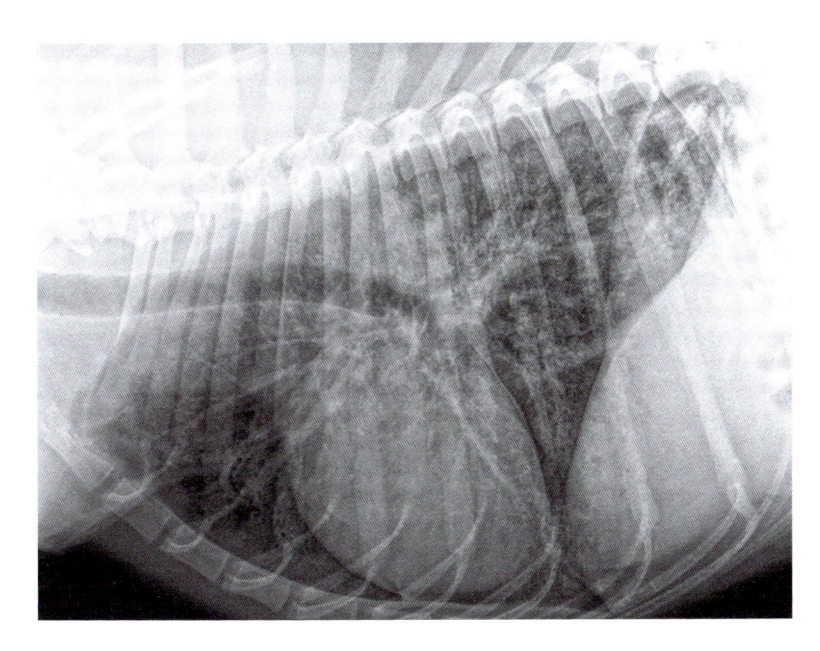

Fig. 20.23 Left lateral thoracic radiograph of a five-year-old mixed breed female spayed dog with multicentric lymphoma. There is generalized increased opacity of the lungs. This appears as a fine diffuse hazy increase in opacity. The cardiac and diaphragmatic outlines and larger pulmonary vessels are visible, but the peripheral pulmonary vessels are obscured. This is compatible with a severe generalized unstructured interstitial pattern from pulmonary lymphoma. There is also more marked poorly defined increased opacity caudal and dorsal to the tracheal bifurcation consistent with enlargement of the tracheobronchial lymph nodes.

Mixed patterns

Many patients with pulmonary disease have features of several pulmonary patterns. For example, a patient diagnosed with bacterial bronchopneumonia in the periphery of the right middle lung lobe shows a peripheral alveolar pattern and an unstructured interstitial pattern at the transition to the aerated lung. There is likely to be a bronchial pattern in the aerated lung from associated bronchitis. Patients with chronic bronchitis usually have a combination of bronchial and unstructured interstitial patterns. The term "broncho-interstitial" is widely used to describe such pulmonary infiltrates, but it is recommended to assess the relative contributions of each component.

Differential diagnoses of pulmonary patterns

The type, severity, and distribution of pulmonary radiographic abnormalities are key components for formulating a diagnosis. Other radiographic changes such as cardiomegaly, lymph node enlargement, and traumatic injuries are also used in synthesizing a diagnosis. Patient history, geographic location (including travel), and laboratory results such as hematology and serum chemistry should also be considered if available. For example, a finding of an alveolar pattern throughout the right middle lung lobe in a young adult dog suggests differential diagnoses of pneumonia or hemorrhage. A history of recent onset cough, fever, and leukocytosis supports the former diagnosis. A history of access to anticoagulant rodenticide, cutaneous ecchymoses, and prolonged coagulation times support a diagnosis of hemorrhage from coagulopathy. The viewer should also be familiar with regionally endemic diseases (**table 20.1**).

Bronchial

A bronchial pattern can be the result of exudate, transudate, or hemorrhage within the airway lumen and edema, cellular infiltration, or hemorrhage within the mucosa or peribronchial tissues.

A bronchial pattern may be seen in some patients with severe canine infectious tracheobronchitis, but affected patients often appear radiographically normal, and this is a diagnosis of exclusion. Chronic nonspecific bronchitis in dogs and chronic asthma in cats are common diagnoses. *D. immitis* heartworm-associated airway disease is the major differential diagnosis for cats in endemic regions.[4] Radiographic changes with these diagnoses do not correlate well with the severity of signs, and some affected patients appear normal, and clinically normal patients may have abnormal radiographs. A severe bronchial pattern in young and middle-aged dogs with acute onset signs is suspicious for eosinophilic bronchopneumopathy. This disease may also present with multifocal randomly distributed alveolar infiltrates and poorly defined nodules or masses.

Alveolar

An alveolar pattern may occur from complete atelectasis. The degree of volume loss required to create uniform soft tissue opacity is quite marked, in excess of 80%, as normal lung is mostly comprised of air. There is compensatory overinflation of normal lung and sometimes a mediastinal shift towards the affected side. Some degree of atelectasis occurs with pathologies causing an alveolar pattern, from reduced perfusion and ventilation. The viewer should decide if the degree of volume loss is sufficient to account for the increased opacity from atelectasis alone. If not, the alveolar pattern must be accounted for by the presence of fluid in the airspaces or cellular infiltration in the lung.

An alveolar pattern most often occurs from flooding of the alveoli with pus, blood, edema fluid, or rarely neoplastic cells. The major differential diagnoses for an alveolar pattern are bacterial pneumonia, aspiration pneumonia, hemorrhage from trauma or coagulopathy, cardiogenic edema, and non-cardiogenic edema. The presenting history, clinical findings, and available laboratory results

CHAPTER 20 Lung: anatomy, techniques, and interpretation principles

Table 20.1. Differential diagnoses of pulmonary patterns.

Pulmonary pattern	Common	Occasional	Rare	Regional
Generalized pulmonary hyperlucency	Artifact from cachexia/body condition Severe dehydration Hypovolemic shock Feline asthma, air-trapping	Addison's disease		
Focal pulmonary hyperlucency	Bulla Traumatic pneumatocele	Lobar emphysema Bronchial obstruction by a foreign body or mass	Pulmonary thromboembolism	
Alveolar	Bacterial bronchopneumonia Aspiration pneumonia Cardiogenic edema Traumatic contusion Coagulopathy, hemorrhage Atelectasis	Noncardiogenic pulmonary edema Lung lobe torsion	Lymphoma Primary pulmonary neoplasm Pulmonary thromboembolism/infarction Smoke inhalation	*Blastomyces* *A. vasorum*
Bronchial	Nonspecific bronchitis (C) Feline asthma	Pulmonary infiltrate with eosinophilia/eosinophilic bronchopneumopathy		Canine *D. immitis* infection Feline *D. immitis*-associated airway disease Feline *A. abstrusus* infection
Nodules and mass	Metastatic neoplasia Primary pulmonary neoplasia	Abscess Granuloma Hematocele	Pulmonary infiltrate with eosinophilia/eosinophilic bronchopneumopathy	*Blastomyces* *Coccidioides* *Histoplasma* *Cryptococcus*
Unstructured interstitial	Artifact: underexposure, exposure at expiration, image processing Nonspecific bronchitis Feline asthma Idiopathic pulmonary fibrosis Disease in transition	Viral pneumonitis Lymphoma Uremic pneumonitis Diffuse mineralization from chronic Cushing's syndrome	Metastatic carcinoma Smoke inhalation	*Blastomyces* *Histoplasma* Canine *D. immitis* infection Feline *D. immitis* infection Feline *A. abstrusus* infection *A. vasorum*

often suggest a diagnosis before imaging or help confirm a presumptive imaging diagnosis. The distribution of the alveolar pattern within the lung is the key factor in deciding a radiologic diagnosis. It is not possible to distinguish between bacterial and aspiration pneumonia based on the radiographic appearance. Both bacterial and aspiration pneumonia affect the dependent parts of the right cranial, right middle, and left cranial lung lobes, extending from the periphery to the hilus with increasing severity. In early cases the infiltrates sometimes show a peribronchial distribution that progresses to more diffuse opacification. The right middle lung lobe is most commonly affected, because of the origin of the lobar bronchus and the long, thin shape which limits collateral air circulation within the lobe. Alveolar infiltrates may extend to the ventral periphery of the caudal lung lobes in severe cases. The distribution of pneumonia in patients who aspirate while anesthetized or obtunded depends upon how the patient was positioned when the event occurred and may be bizarre, e.g., distribution in the caudal lobes if the patient was in dorsal recumbency.

SECTION IV THORAX

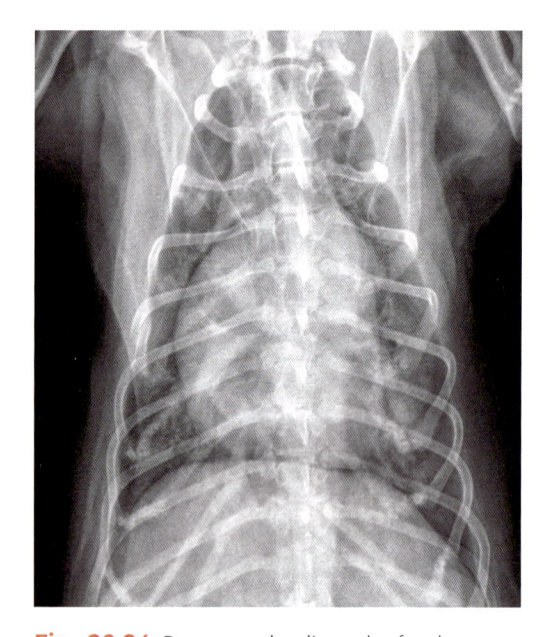

Fig. 20.24 Dorsoventral radiograph of a three-year-old dog hit by a car approximately 2 hours earlier. There is poorly defined increased opacity in the left lung adjacent to the left cardiac border. The left cardiac border is partly obscured, as are the pulmonary vessels in the affected part of the lung. The increased opacity is a mix of alveolar and unstructured interstitial patterns. This finding indicates traumatic pulmonary contusion. There is also a fracture of the right fifth rib with overriding of the fracture ends, also from trauma.

The distribution of pulmonary hemorrhage is quite random regardless of the etiology[5] (**fig. 20.24**). The distribution can mimic diagnoses such as pneumonia or cardiogenic edema, and the diagnosis is often suggested by the history and laboratory results. Other traumatic injuries such as rib and long bone fractures, pneumothorax, pneumomediastinum, or pleural hemorrhage support a diagnosis of traumatic contusion. The full extent of traumatic contusions may not be evident until several hours after injury. Patients with hemorrhage from coagulopathy may show concurrent pleural, mediastinal, or tracheal mucosal hemorrhage.

The distribution of cardiogenic edema from left-sided congestive cardiac failure shows some variation[6] (**figs. 20.25** and **20.26**). In dogs with degenerative valvular disease, edema is usually relatively symmetrical in the caudal lung lobes, initially present at the hilus and extending towards the periphery with increasing severity. A similar distribution of edema is seen with severe iatrogenic fluid overload. In patients with acute decompensation, unilateral edema affecting the right caudal lung lobe occurs relatively commonly and rarely in the left caudal lung lobe. Patients with severe congestive cardiac failure may have unstructured interstitial pattern (edema) in the ventral periphery of both cranial lung lobes.

Cardiogenic edema sometimes follows a similar pattern of distribution in patients with degenerative valvular disease in dogs with dilated cardiomyopathy (DCM) and in cats with cardiomyopathy. More often, dogs with DCM and cats with cardiomyopathy show a diffuse nonuniform mixed alveolar and unstructured interstitial or random alveolar pattern. Some cats with cardiogenic edema from cardiomyopathy have a predominantly

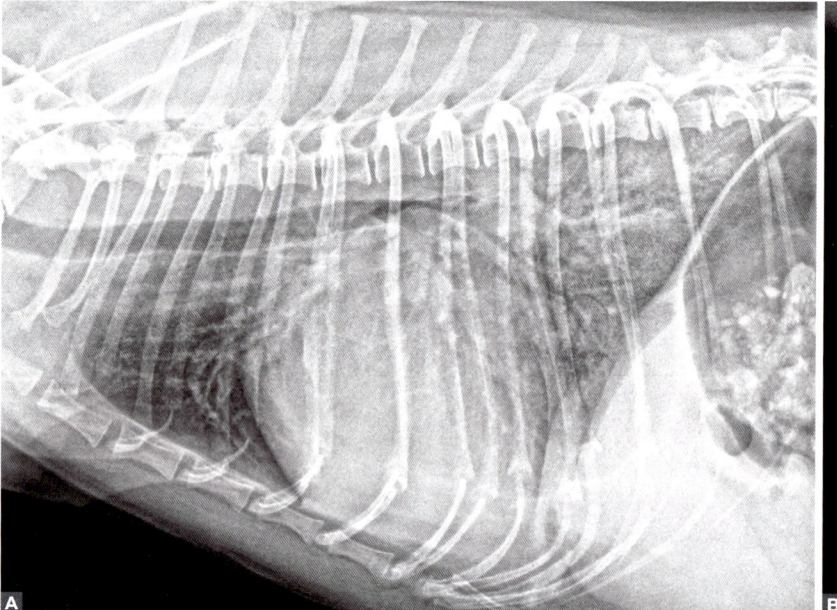

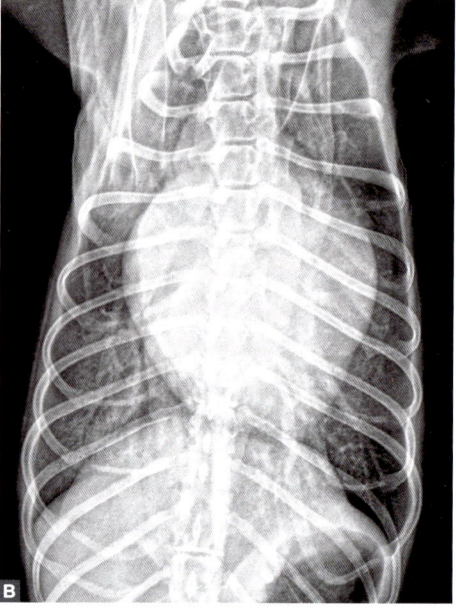

Fig. 20.25 Lateral and ventrodorsal radiographs of a ten-year-old neutered male miniature Poodle. The patient has a history of chronic mitral valve endocardiosis with recent-onset dyspnea, tachypnea, and cough. The heart is severely enlarged on both projections. (**A**) There is severely increased opacity in the caudal lung lobes which obscure the caudal dorsal cardiac border. (**B**) The increased opacity in the caudal lung lobes is nonsymmetrical. There is greater increased opacity in the right caudal lung lobe which extends to the periphery. The vessels in the right caudal lung lobe are almost completely obscured. The increased opacity in the left caudal lung lobe affects the hilar and middle zones, sparing the periphery. The pulmonary opacity is an example of a severe interstitial pattern transitioning to an alveolar pattern and represents severe cardiogenic edema from left-sided congestive cardiac failure.

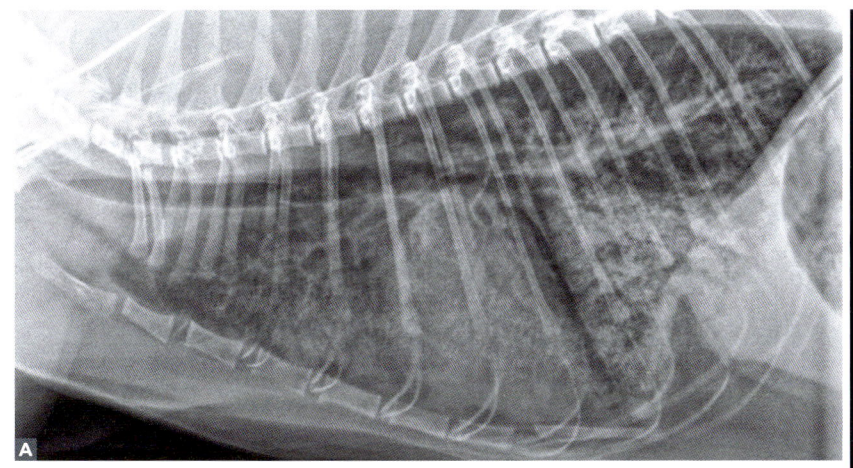

Fig. 20.26 Lateral and ventrodorsal radiographs of an eight-year-old cat presented with acute collapse, tachypnea, and dyspnea. The heart is partly obscured on both images, limiting evaluation. The heart is increased in height on the lateral projection and is also widened on the ventrodorsal projection. There is nonuniform soft tissue opacity in both caudal lung lobes that obscures the cardiac and diaphragmatic outlines and the pulmonary vessels. (**A**) The dorsal part of the caudal lung field is relatively spared. The lateral radiograph also shows similarly increased opacity in the cranial ventral lung field, obscuring the cranial cardiac border and the vessels within the lung. The pulmonary pattern is consistent with severe cardiogenic edema from left-sided congestive cardiac failure.

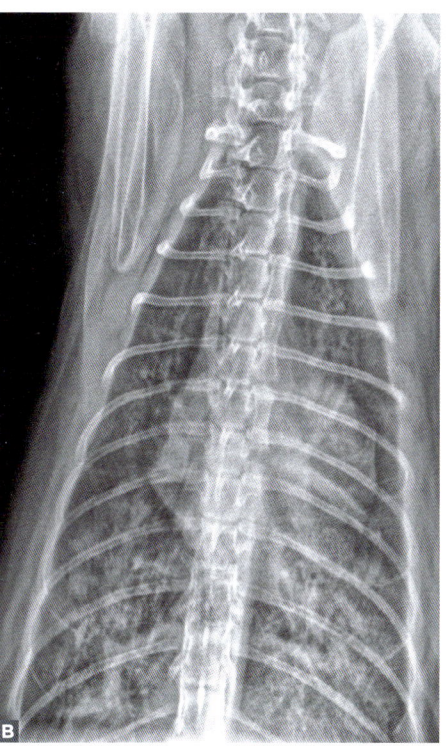

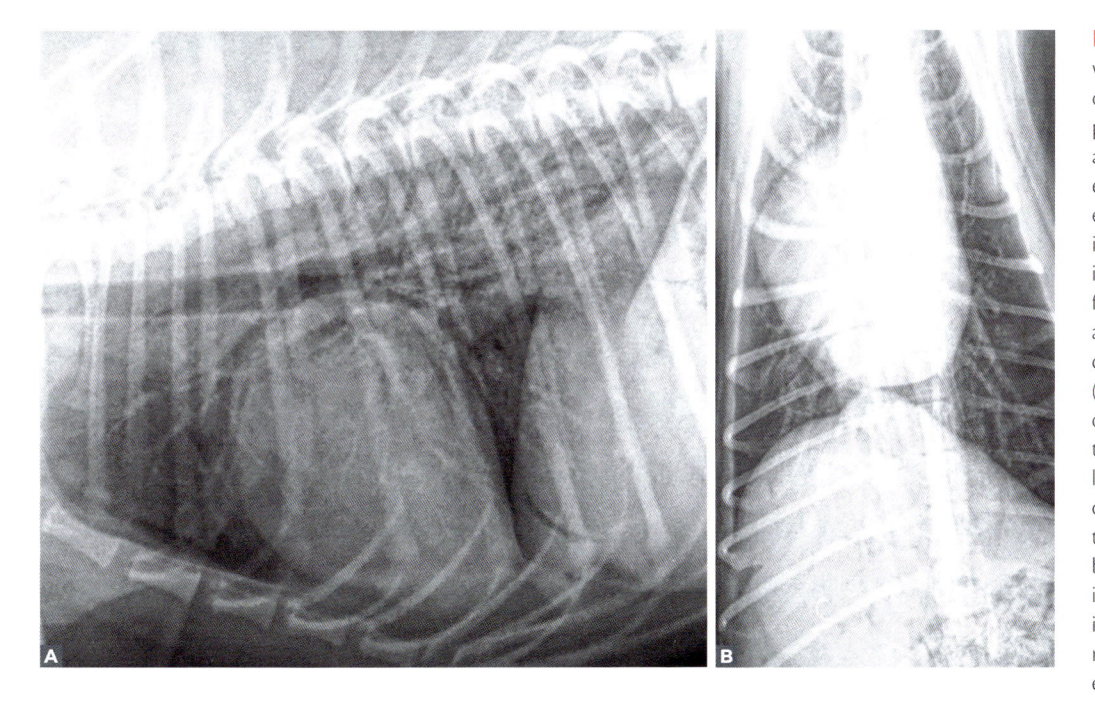

Fig. 20.27 Lateral and ventrodorsal radiographs of a Golden Retriever puppy that developed dyspnea after chewing through an electrical cord and being electrocuted. (**A**) There is increased soft tissue opacity in the caudal dorsal lung field, obscuring the vessels and almost obscuring the diaphragmatic outline. (**B**) The ventrodorsal radiograph is obliquely positioned. There is an alveolar pattern and the right caudal lung lobe, overlying the liver/diaphragm. Air bronchograms are visible in the affected lung, superimposed on the liver. This represents noncardiogenic edema from electrocution.

ventral distribution, mimicking severe pneumonia. While clinical response to treatment may be quite rapid, radiographic improvement takes at least 12 hours and is more reliably seen after 24 hours of treatment.

Noncardiogenic edema has numerous potential etiologies, including near-drowning, transient airway occlusion, seizures, traumatic brain injury, and vasculitis[7] (**fig. 20.27**). The distribution is usually symmetrical in the middle and peripheral zones of the caudal lung lobes, extending to the hilar zone when severe. Severe cases may also show random, patchy alveolar or interstitial infiltrates in the other lung lobes. Patient history will often suggest the diagnosis.

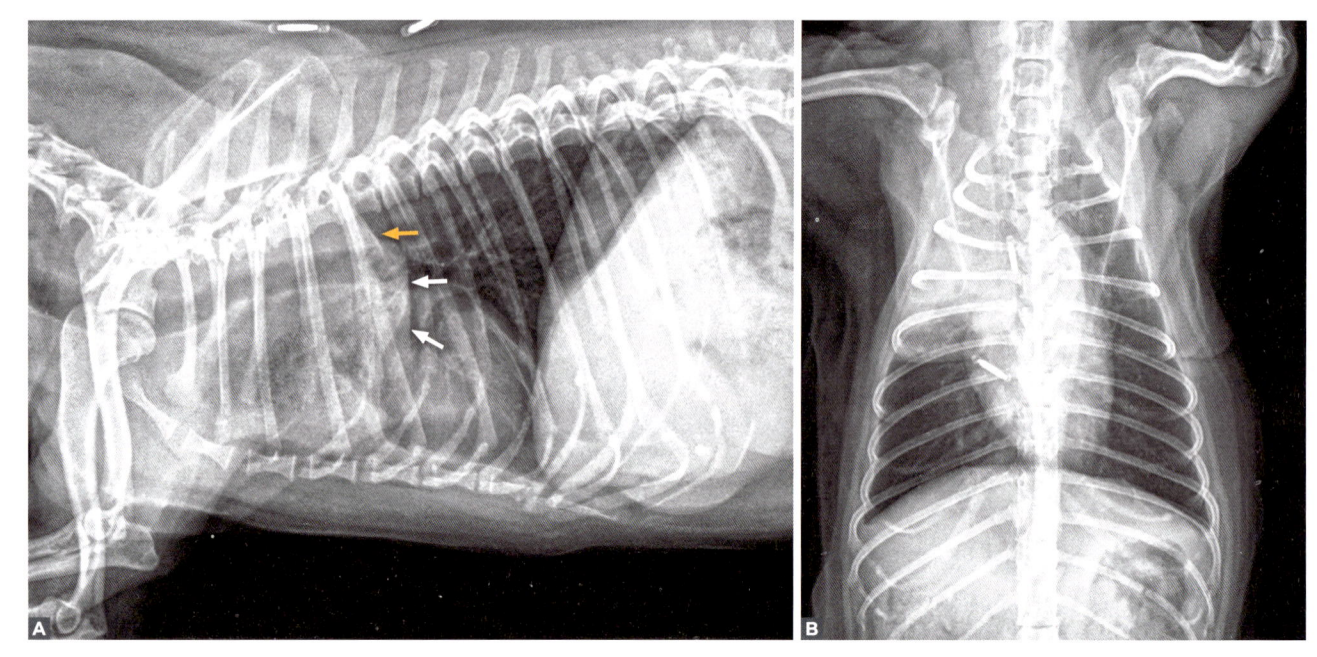

Fig. 20.28 Left lateral and ventrodorsal radiographs of a nine-year-old Shih Tzu. The patient presented with a history of a cough of 2 weeks duration and recent onset dyspnea. There is diffuse soft tissue opacification of the right cranial lung lobe, completely obscuring the vessels within this lung lobe and the adjacent right cranial aspect of the cardiac border. Small pinpoint pockets of gas are visible in the cranial ventral part of the lung lobe on the lateral projection. This has been described as a vesicular pattern and occurs when there are air and fluid-filled adjacent pulmonary acini. The soft tissue opacification extends to the dorsal margin of the lobe, and the caudal dorsal margin of the lobe appears as a distinct interface dorsal to the tracheal bifurcation in the fifth intercostal space (orange arrow). On the lateral radiograph the right cranial lung lobe has an abnormal convex caudal border (white arrows). A diagnosis of torsion of the right cranial lung lobe was confirmed by CT.

Lung lobe torsion presents as an alveolar pattern affecting a single lung lobe or rarely two lobes[8] (**fig. 20.28**). Large breed, deep-chested dogs are predisposed, but the condition also occurs in small breed dogs and rarely in cats. Occlusion of the pulmonary arteries, veins, and lymphatic drainage at the hilus of the lung lobe result in congestion, edema, and infarction. The lobar bronchus proximal to the torsion may have an abnormal orientation, resembling a "pigtail" or "corkscrew". In most patients, the lobar bronchus is filled with fluid, and air bronchograms are not visible. In patients with relatively recent torsion, the lung lobe may show diffuse soft tissue opacity with numerous small interspersed gas pockets, which has been referred to as a vesicular pattern. In more chronic cases, the affected lobe is usually uniform soft tissue opacity. The abnormal lung lobe is larger than normal from congestion and edema and may have a rounded shape with a mass effect causing displacement of adjacent normal aerated lung. The abnormal lobe may be obscured if there is concurrent pleural effusion. The right middle lung lobe and left cranial lung lobe are most commonly affected. Torsion has also been reported in the right cranial, left caudal, and accessory lung lobes.

Primary pulmonary neoplasia and pulmonary lymphoma are uncommon causes of alveolar patterns. The distribution is random but can mimic pneumonia or edema.

Nodules and masses

Solitary mass lesions most likely represent primary neoplasia in both dogs and cats. Primary pulmonary neoplasms appear to have a predilection for the caudal lung lobes in cats. Mycotic granuloma such as from *Blastomyces* or *Coccidioides* infection is also a potential etiology in dogs and rarely in cats. Repeat radiographs after 4 weeks and 12 weeks can be obtained if surgery or sampling of the lesion is not performed. Increasing size of the lesion after 4 weeks substantially increases suspicion of malignant neoplasia. Static lesion size after 12 weeks most likely indicates the lesion is an abscess or granuloma but may be noted with indolent primary neoplasms in cats.

CHAPTER 20 Lung: anatomy, techniques, and interpretation principles

In a patient with a known malignant neoplasm, pulmonary nodules should be assumed to represent metastasis. In patients without a confirmed diagnosis of malignant neoplasia, metastasis remains likely, but inflammatory granulomas and abscesses are also diagnostic considerations (**figs. 20.29** and **20.30**). Malignant histiocytic sarcoma and less often lymphoma can also present with multiple

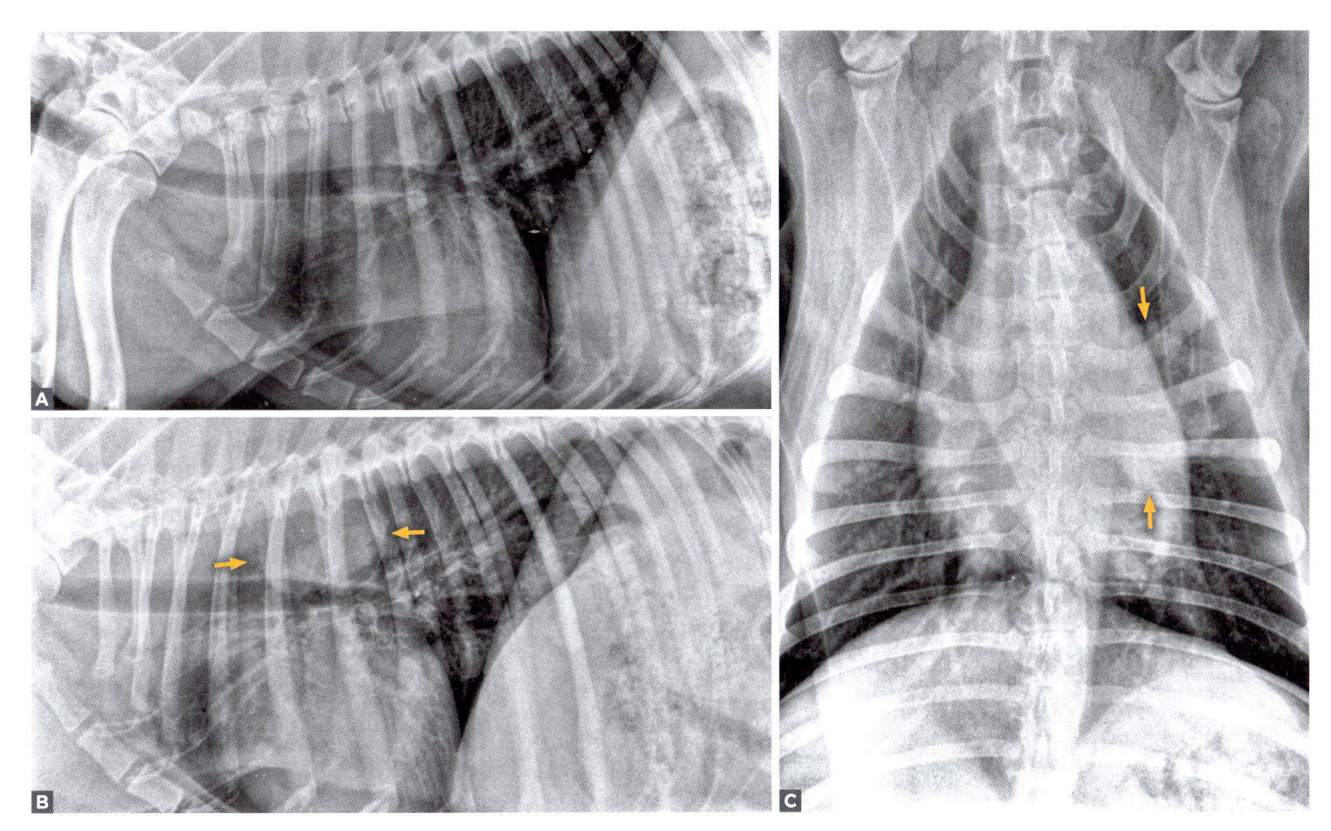

Fig. 20.29 Right lateral, left lateral and ventrodorsal radiographs of the thorax of a 12-year-old mixed breed dog with a chronic cough. (**A**) On the right lateral projection a spherical soft tissue opacity mass lesion is clearly visible in the cranial dorsal thorax overlying the caudal intrathoracic trachea. (**B**) The lesion is faintly visible on the left lateral projection immediately dorsal to the tracheal bifurcation (arrows) but far less conspicuous than on the right lateral projection. This is because of partial atelectasis of the dependent left lung in this projection. (**C**) On the ventrodorsal projection the lesion is also less conspicuous and is visible overlying the left border of the heart and superimposed on the left fourth, fifth, and sixth ribs (arrows). The reduced conspicuity of the lesion on the ventrodorsal image is also from partial atelectasis of the dorsal part of the lung, as the patient is positioned in dorsal recumbency. A carcinoma was confirmed by fine-needle aspiration.

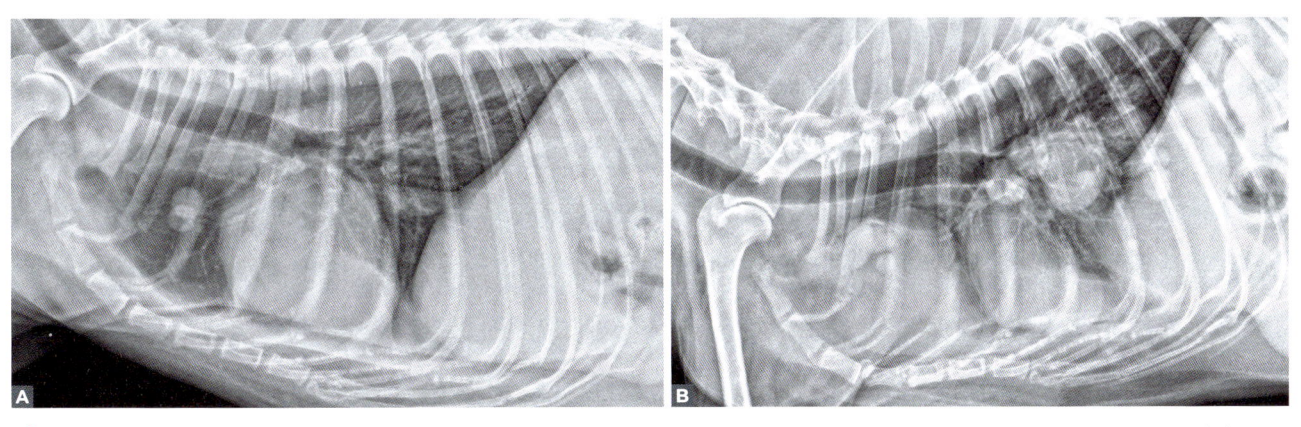

Fig. 20.30 Lateral thoracic radiographs of a ten-year-old mixed breed dog that had had a thoracic limb amputation for osteosarcoma. (**A**) Image obtained 2 months after amputation; there are two well-defined spherical soft tissue opacity nodules in the cranial thorax, seen in the intercostal space approximately halfway between the trachea and sternum. No additional lesions were identified on other thoracic radiographs at that time. (**B**) Image obtained 6 months after amputation. There is a large mass occupying most of the cranial thorax and obscuring the cardiac border. Multiple large nodules are present throughout the lung. Progression of pulmonary nodules or masses over time can be used to make a presumptive diagnosis of malignant neoplasia if confirmation of the diagnosis is not available by other means.

pulmonary nodules or masses. Imaging of the abdomen by radiographs, ultrasound and/or CT should be performed to screen for a primary lesion. Similar to solitary lesions, increasing size and/or number of the nodules on repeat radiographs after 4 weeks would make a diagnosis of metastatic malignant neoplasia far more likely.

Unstructured interstitial pattern

The differential diagnosis for an unstructured interstitial pattern is extremely broad. Some interstitial infiltrates are present in many patients with nonspecific chronic bronchial disease. A diffuse mild to moderate unstructured interstitial pattern is relatively common in middle-aged and older dogs, often described as age-related change and likely represents a combination of scarring, fibrosis, and subclinical chronic airway disease. Potential etiologies of a diffuse unstructured interstitial pattern include fibrosis, acute viral pneumonitis, lymphoma, disseminated metastasis, uremic pneumonitis, and diffuse mineralization from chronic hyperadrenocorticism. Focal or multifocal random unstructured interstitial infiltrates can be caused by *D. immitis* infection, *Angiostrongylus vasorum* infection, leptospirosis, and early *Blastomyces* infection. Idiopathic pulmonary fibrosis of West Highland White Terriers shows a severe nonuniform diffuse interstitial pattern. Most diseases presenting with an interstitial pattern will also have a bronchial component.

Computed tomography of pulmonary disease

CT is well suited to the diagnosis of pulmonary disease. In comparison to radiography, the lack of superimposition, much greater image contrast, and good spatial resolution result in improved sensitivity and specificity (**fig. 20.5**).[9, 10] The entire thorax can be imaged in a few seconds by multi-slice scanners obviating the need for anesthesia in many patients. Imaging can often be performed with sedation, and some patients can be imaged conscious. Bronchi and vessels are readily assessed and traced to the periphery of the lung. There are published normal values for relating bronchial wall to vessel size used for the diagnosis of bronchial disease. High-resolution CT, that is, image slices acquired at 1 mm thickness or less, high mAs, and axial technique, provides a much more detailed assessment of the severity and extent of bronchial and interstitial infiltrates in diseases such as feline asthma. CT is superior to radiographs for assessment of the severity and extent of interstitial infiltrates. The distribution in relation to the airways, vessels, and affected regions within lung lobes can be assessed. CT of the thorax is most valuable for diagnosis and staging of oncologic patients and is the preferred imaging modality for this purpose where it is available. CT can be used to confirm the precise anatomic location of intrathoracic masses, such as determining if a mass lesion in the cranial thorax is of pulmonary or mediastinal origin. CT is also more sensitive and specific than radiographs for the detection of pulmonary nodules, frequently identifying lesions that are not visible on radiographs. CT is also significantly more sensitive than radiographs for the detection of enlargement of the tracheobronchial lymph nodes.

Ultrasound of pulmonary disease

Ultrasound is of relatively limited value for the investigation of pulmonary disease (**fig. 20.31**), as air within the lung will reflect the ultrasound beam, and ultrasound is only of value when the lesion extends to the visceral pleural surface at the thoracic wall. As with many abdominal lesions, the ultrasound features of pulmonary masses are nonspecific. Ultrasound does facilitate guided diagnostic sampling of lesions for cytologic or histologic diagnosis. A pathology that is characterized

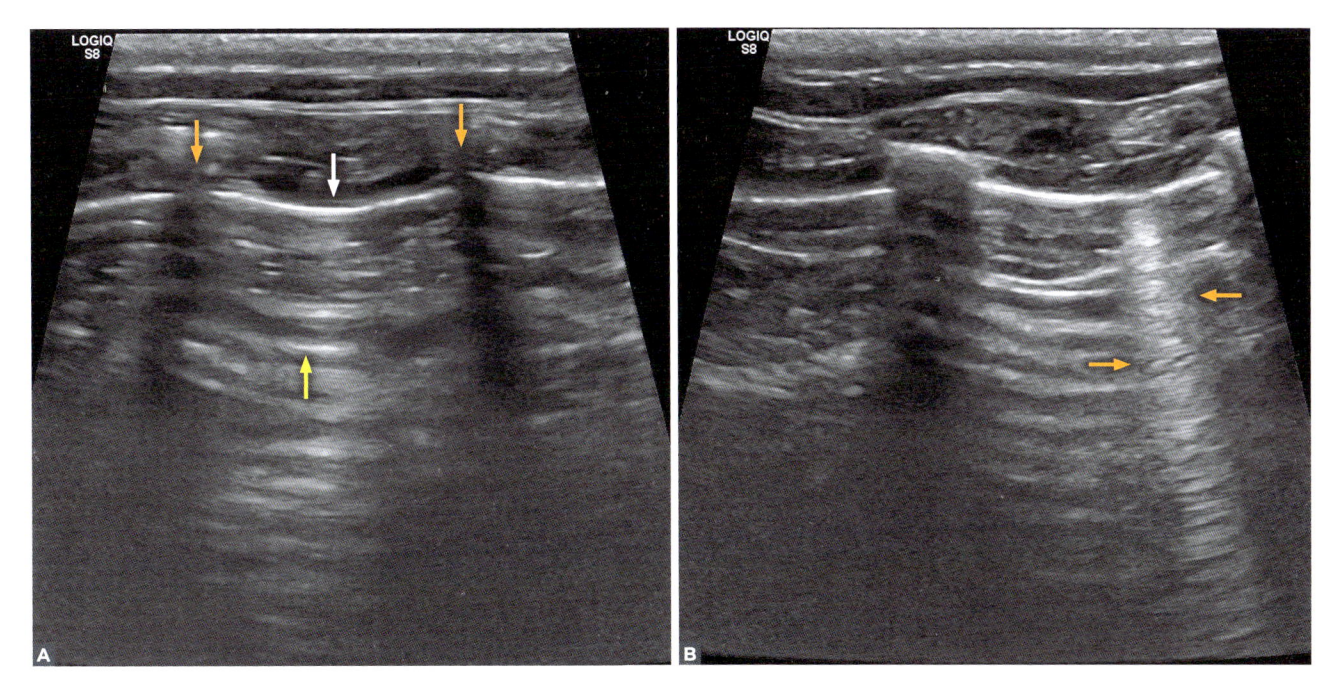

CHAPTER 20 Lung: anatomy, techniques, and interpretation principles

Fig. 20.31 Ultrasound of the lung. (**A**) A three-year-old castrated male cat. Normal appearance of the intercostal space in a longitudinal scan: shadowing of ribs (orange arrow) which helps identify the hyperechoic pleural line (white arrow) formed by the parietal and visceral pleura. A-lines (yellow arrow) are horizontal hyperechoic reverberation artifacts, parallel and equidistant to pleural line. (**B**) A three-year-old male healthy cat. Isolated B-lines (orange arrows) appear as vertical hyperechoic artifacts arising from the pleural surface and extending to the far-field of the image, obscuring A-lines. Courtesy of Dr. Giovanni Aste DVM, PhD.

by alveolar infiltrates on radiographs can also be assessed using ultrasound if this extends to the visceral pleural surface. Pneumonia, hemorrhage, or edema usually cause lung parenchyma to have relatively uniform echogenicity. Larger pulmonary veins and arteries may be visible within the lung. The air-filled bronchi appear as linear hyperechoic structures with acoustic shadowing if air-filled. The bronchi may appear similar to vessels if filled with blood, exudate, or edema fluid. Ultrasound can be used for a crude assessment of diffuse interstitial pulmonary pathology, as infiltrates which extend to the visceral pleural surface result in linear streaks from reverberation artifacts. However, radiographs are more sensitive and specific for this assessment.

References

1. Biller DS, Meyer CW. Case examples demonstrating the clinical utility of obtaining both right and left lateral thoracic radiographs in small animals. *J Am Anim Hosp Assoc* 23:381, 1987.
2. Suter PF, Lord PF. Thoracic radiography: a text atlas of thoracic disease in the dog and cat. Wettswil, Switzerland, 1984.
3. Mantis P, Lamb CR, Boswood A. Assessment of the accuracy of thoracic radiography in the diagnosis of canine chronic bronchitis. *J Small Anim Pract* 39:518-520, 1998.
4. Garrity S, Lee-Fowler T, Reinero C. Feline asthma and heartworm disease: clinical features, diagnostics and therapeutics. *J Feline Med Surg* 21:825-834, 2019.
5. Berry CR, Gallaway A, Thrall DE, Carlisle C. Thoracic radiographic features of anticoagulant rodenticide toxicity in fourteen dogs. *Vet Radiol Ultrasound* 34:391-396, 1993.
6. Diana A, Guglielmini C, Pivetta M, Sanacore A, Di Tommaso M, Lord PF, et al. Radiographic features of cardiogenic pulmonary edema in dogs with mitral regurgitation: 61 cases (1998-2007). *J Am Vet Med Assoc* 235:1058-1063, 2009.
7. Bouyssou S, Specchi S, Desquilbet L, Pey P. Radiographic appearance of presumed noncardiogenic pulmonary edema and correlation with the underlying cause in dogs and cats. *Vet Radiol Ultrasound* 58:259-265, 2017.
8. Gicking J, Aumann M. Lung lobe torsion. *Comp Contin Educ Vet* 33:E4, 2011.
9. Lamb CR, Whitlock J, Foster-Yeow ATL. Prevalence of pulmonary nodules in dogs with malignant neoplasia as determined by CT. *Vet Radiol Ultrasound* 60:300-305, 2019.
10. Masseau I, Reinero CR. Thoracic computed tomographic interpretation for clinicians to aid in the diagnosis of dogs and cats with respiratory disease. *Vet J* 253:105388, 2019.
11. Dicker SA, Lisciandro GR, Newell SM, Johnson JA. Diagnosis of pulmonary contusions with point-of-care lung ultrasonography and thoracic radiography compared to thoracic computed tomography in dogs with motor vehicle trauma: 29 cases (2017-2018). *J Vet Emerg Crit Care* 30:638-46, 2020.

CHAPTER 21

Trachea

Chiara Mattei

KEY POINTS

- Tracheal hypoplasia mainly affects young brachycephalic dogs and is radiologically characterized by a static uniform narrowing of the tracheal diameter.
- Dynamic tracheal collapse results from weakening and deformity of the cartilaginous rings. Radiography shows a dorsoventral luminal flattening and invagination of the dorsal tracheal membrane into the lumen.
Fluoroscopy or bronchoscopy are more sensitive for diagnosis of tracheal collapse and to determine severity and extent.
- Rupture may occur anywhere in the trachea, but commonly affects the cervical segment and radiographs show fascial and subcutaneous emphysema and pneumomediastinum.
- Coumarin rodenticide intoxication can cause tracheal submucosal hemorrhage, with variable narrowing of the lumen.

Hypoplasia

Hypoplasia is a congenital generalized narrowing of the tracheal diameter caused by abnormal overlapping or complete cartilage rings and negligible dorsal tracheal membrane (DTM).
It is most often diagnosed in brachycephalic dogs, and is part of the brachycephalic obstructive airway syndrome (BOAS).[1] Affected animals present with respiratory distress, coughing, and recurrent respiratory infections.[1]
With radiographs and fluoroscopy, the hypoplastic trachea appears uniformly narrowed with no variation in breathing (**fig. 21.1**).[1]
Two objective radiographic methods[1,2] have been reported to diagnose tracheal hypoplasia, but the agreement between them and with the endoscopic findings is poor and their utility is questionable:[3,4]

- The mid-thoracic tracheal luminal diameter/width of the proximal third of the third rib ratio (TT/3R). Values <2.0 or <3.0 define tracheal hypoplasia.
- The tracheal luminal diameter/thoracic inlet distance ratio (TD:TI) (**fig. 21.2**). The mean ratios of <0.13 in English Bulldogs (with the smallest ratio in asymptomatic dogs being 0.09), <0.16 in non-Bulldog brachycephalic breeds, and <0.20 for other dogs' conformation are used to define hypoplasia.

These numerical values support the diagnosis, but the condition may be asymptomatic in the absence of concurrent pulmonary disease and congenital defects. If tracheal hypoplasia is suspected in a juvenile, the airway should be reassessed after maturity as the severity of narrowing often improves.

SECTION IV THORAX

Fig. 21.1 Lateral radiograph of a two-month-old dyspneic English Bulldog. The included trachea is uniformly severely narrowed, raising the suspicion of hypoplasia. The mainstem bronchi have a relatively larger diameter. No concurrent pneumonia was detected. The finding can be part of the brachycephalic obstructive airway syndrome. Repeated radiographs should be obtained at maturity as the apparent severe narrowing often improves.

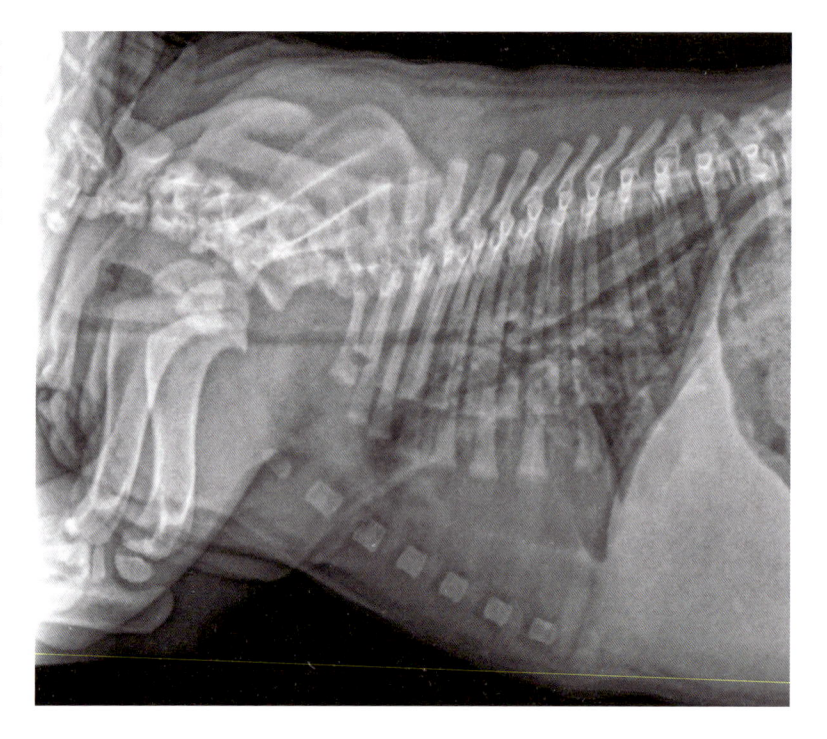

Fig. 21.2 Lateral thoracic radiograph of a five-year-old mesocephalic mixed breed dog, imaged for resolving pneumonia. The tracheal luminal diameter/thoracic inlet distance ratio (TD:TI) is shown. The luminal diameter (blue line) is measured perpendicularly to the tracheal long axis at the thoracic inlet; the thoracic inlet distance (orange line) from the ventral aspect of the midpoint of the first thoracic vertebra to the dorsal surface of the manubrium at its thinnest point. The ratio is >0.2, which is normal.

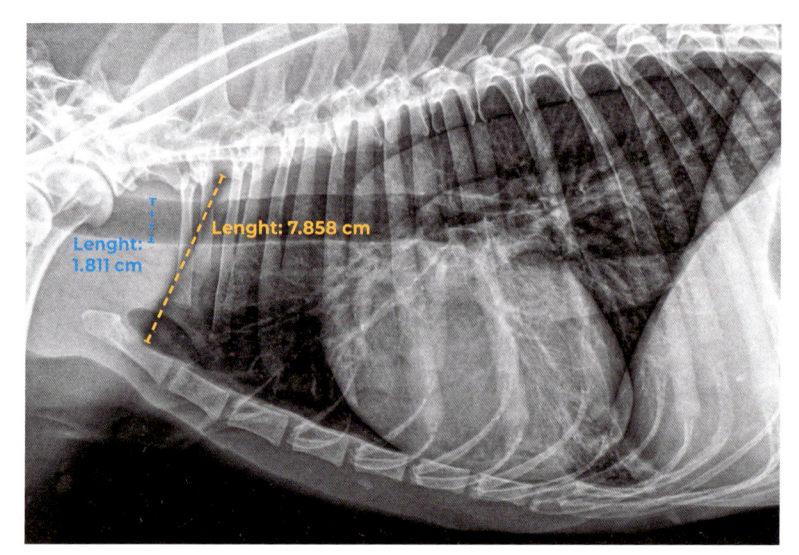

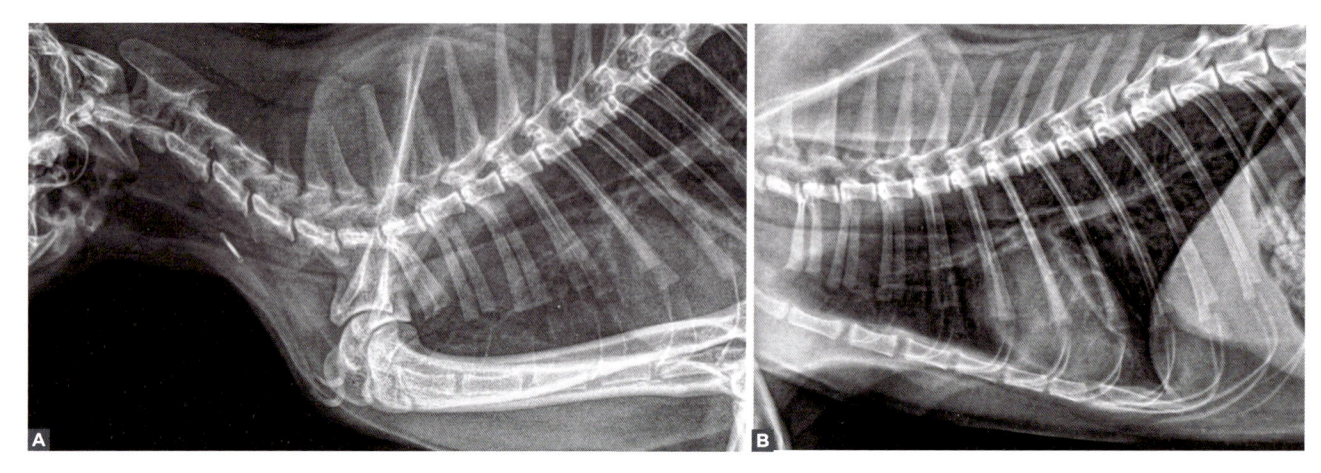

Fig. 21.3 Lateral cervical (**A**) and thoracic (**B**) radiographs of a 1.5-year-old cat with respiratory distress. There is a consistent moderate-severe narrowing of the caudal cervical and intrathoracic trachea. A primary tracheal collapse in cats is rare and an upper airway problem should always be excluded.

340

Dynamic collapse

Tracheal collapse results from softening of the cartilages and inability to maintain functional rigidity. It is characterized by dorsoventral ring flattening, stretching and luminal protrusion of the DTM, and variable luminal narrowing.[5] It is commonly a dynamic process, but can also be static. It affects middle-aged small breed dogs, presented for a progressive cough. Tracheal collapse in cats is rare and usually secondary to an upper airway obstruction (**fig. 21.3**).[6]

Radiography and fluoroscopy are complementary techniques for diagnosing tracheal collapse.[7]

Lateral cervical/thoracic radiographs extending from the pharynx to caudal to the carina should be obtained at end inspiration and expiration. These may show a dorsoventral luminal flattening affecting a segment of the trachea or most of the length, and invagination of the DTM into the lumen (**fig. 21.4**).

This latter should be differentiated from DTM redundancy, seen in clinically normal dogs (**fig. 21.5**).[7,8] An increased dorsoventral height can be also seen on lateral radiographs (**fig. 21.6**).[9]

This is caused by axial rotation of the collapsed trachea, with the perceived dorsoventral luminal dimension on radiography representing the laterolateral dimension on CT.[9] A skyline projection of the trachea may be helpful to show collapse. This is obtained with the patient in sternal recumbency and with dorsiflexion of the head and neck. The X-ray beam is oriented slightly cranial to caudal and centered at the thoracic inlet. The skyline radiographic view may show a crescent to slit-like shape and asymmetric narrowing. CT of the neck and thorax better demonstrates the severity and extent of narrowing of the trachea (**fig. 21.7**).

Possible concurrent radiographic findings include bronchial collapse and bronchiectasis. Intermittent end-expiratory cervical lung herniation can be seen with intrathoracic tracheal collapse and extrathoracic tracheal kinking (**fig. 21.8**).[5]

Radiography significantly underestimates the frequency and degree of tracheal collapse compared to fluoroscopy, even with inspiratory and expiratory views, and normal radiographs do not exclude this diagnosis.[7] Fluoroscopy is the modality of choice because it allows a real-time study during the entire respiratory cycle, normal respiration, and forceful cough-induced expiration.[5,7] Due to the pressures developed during the respiratory cycle, fluoroscopy shows the dynamic nature of tracheal collapse, affecting the extrathoracic part during inspiration, and the intrathoracic segment during expiration (**fig. 21.9** and **videos 21.1-21.3**).[7]

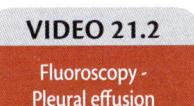

VIDEO 21.1 Fluoroscopy - Spontaneous contrast

VIDEO 21.2 Fluoroscopy - Pleural effusion

VIDEO 21.3 Fluoroscopy - Pericardial effusion

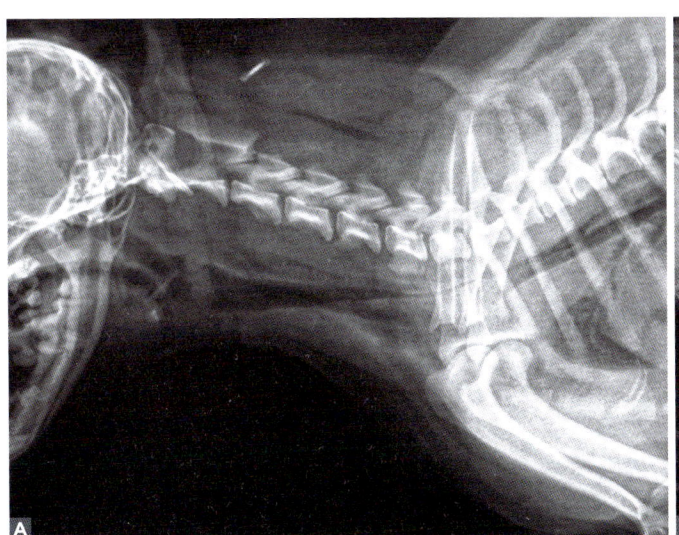

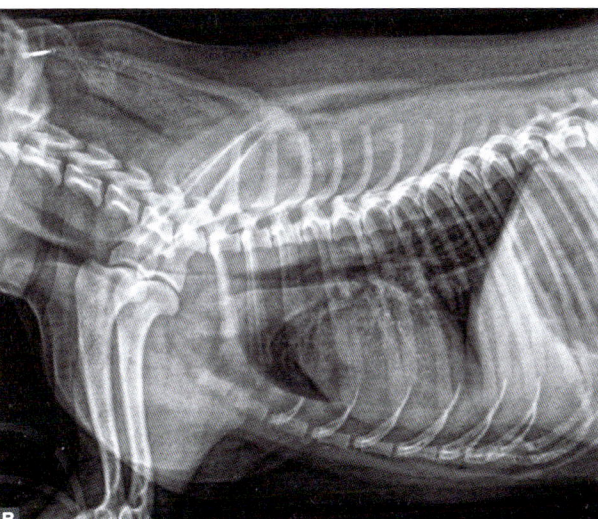

Fig. 21.4 Lateral cervical (**A**) and thoracic (**B**) radiographs of a two-year-old Spitz dog presented with cough. There is effacement of the tracheal lumen at the thoracic inlet in all images, due to a static collapse of the lumen. A grade 4 (100%) tracheal collapse was confirmed at the thoracic inlet with endoscopy.

SECTION IV THORAX

Fig. 21.5 Lateral cervical and thoracic radiograph of a 1.5-year-old Golden Retriever with no reported respiratory signs. A soft tissue opacity (white arrows) is seen along the dorsal margin of the tracheal lumen in the caudal cervical segment and at the thoracic inlet. The dorsal aspect of the trachea can be clearly delineated (orange arrows). This represents a DTM redundancy rather than collapse of the rings.

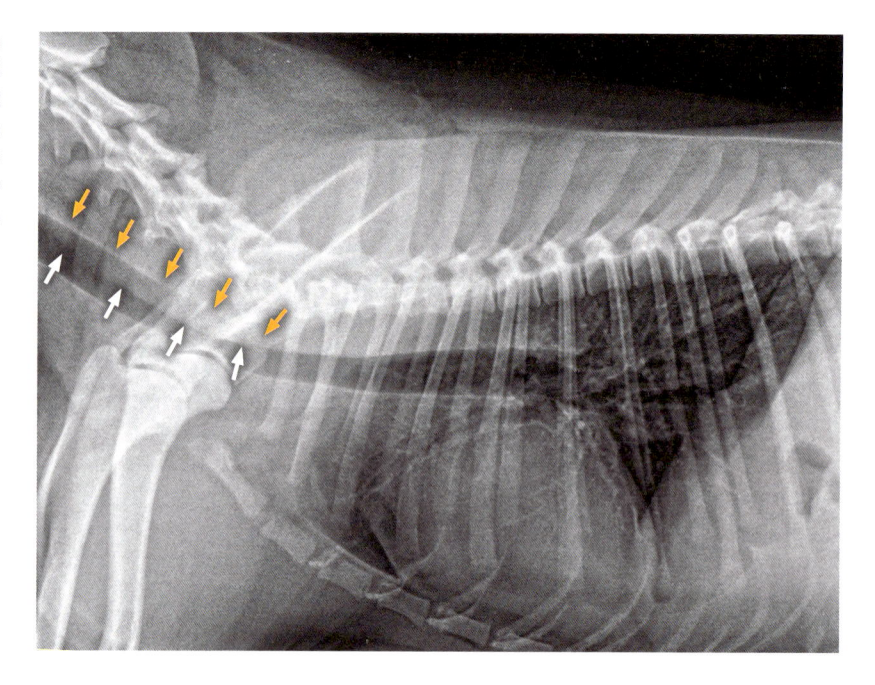

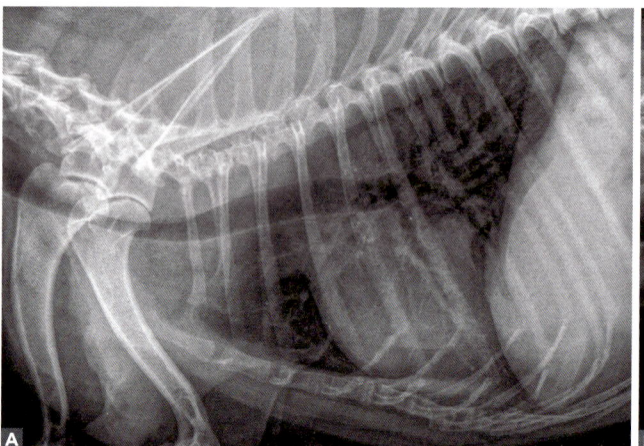

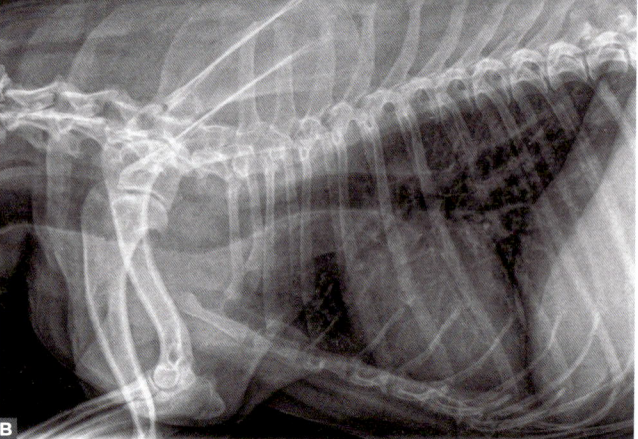

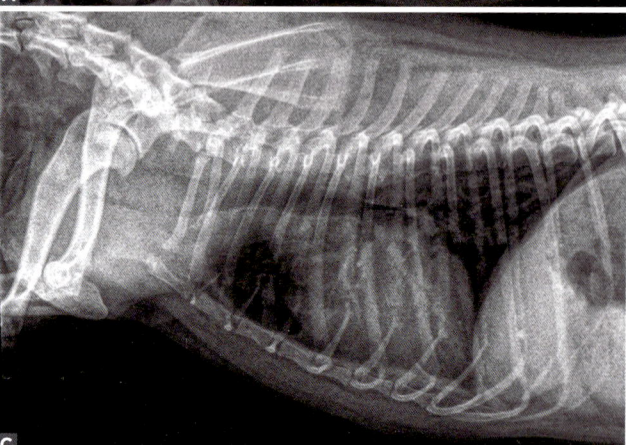

Fig. 21.6 (A-B) Lateral thoracic radiographs of a 13-year-old Terrier mixed dog with cough. There is segmental collapse of the tracheal lumen at the thoracic inlet, indicating a lack of rigidity of the tracheal rings. (C) Lateral thoracic radiograph of a 13-year-old Yorkshire Terrier presented for respiratory distress. There is an increased dorsoventral height of the cervical trachea to the thoracic inlet, with an intraluminal tubular soft tissue opacity outlined by air dorsally and ventrally. This is caused by axial rotation of the collapsed trachea. Image courtesy of Antech Imaging Services, Fountain Valley, CA, USA.

CHAPTER 21 Trachea

Fig. 21.7 A seven-year-old Spitz underwent a CT study for tracheal collapse for suspicion of tracheal and bronchial collapse. (**A-C**) Represent the transverse section of the cervical trachea with soft tissue window at different levels corresponding to the color line in (**D**). (**B**) Shows a moderate to severe tracheal collapse. (**E**) Highlights the collapse of the main left bronchus, also proved with endoscopy.

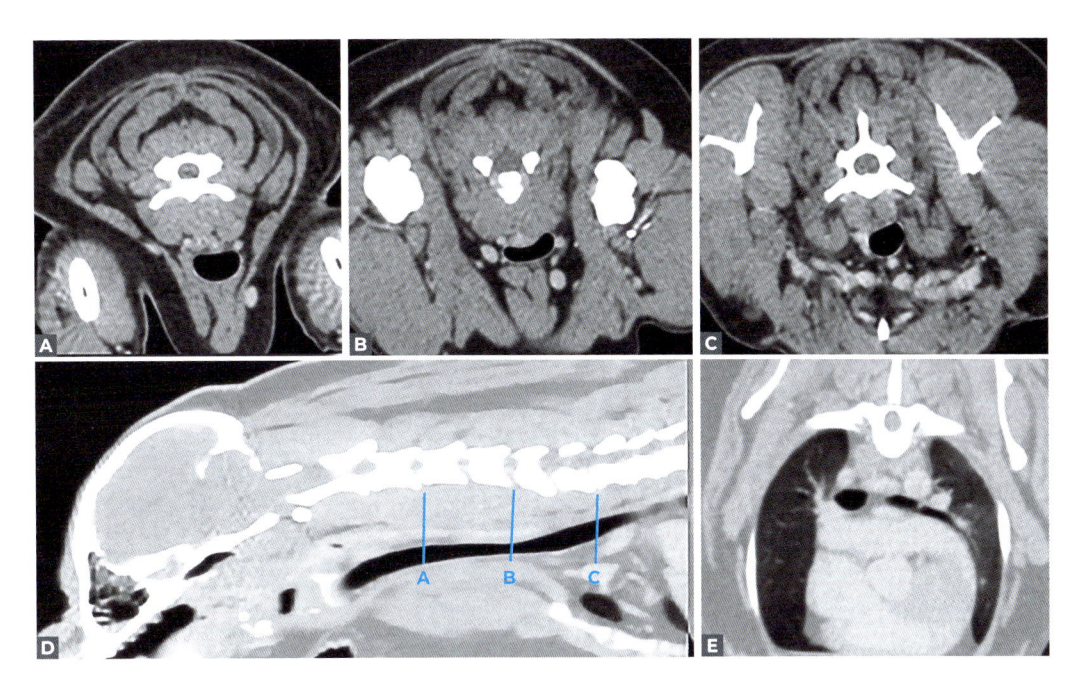

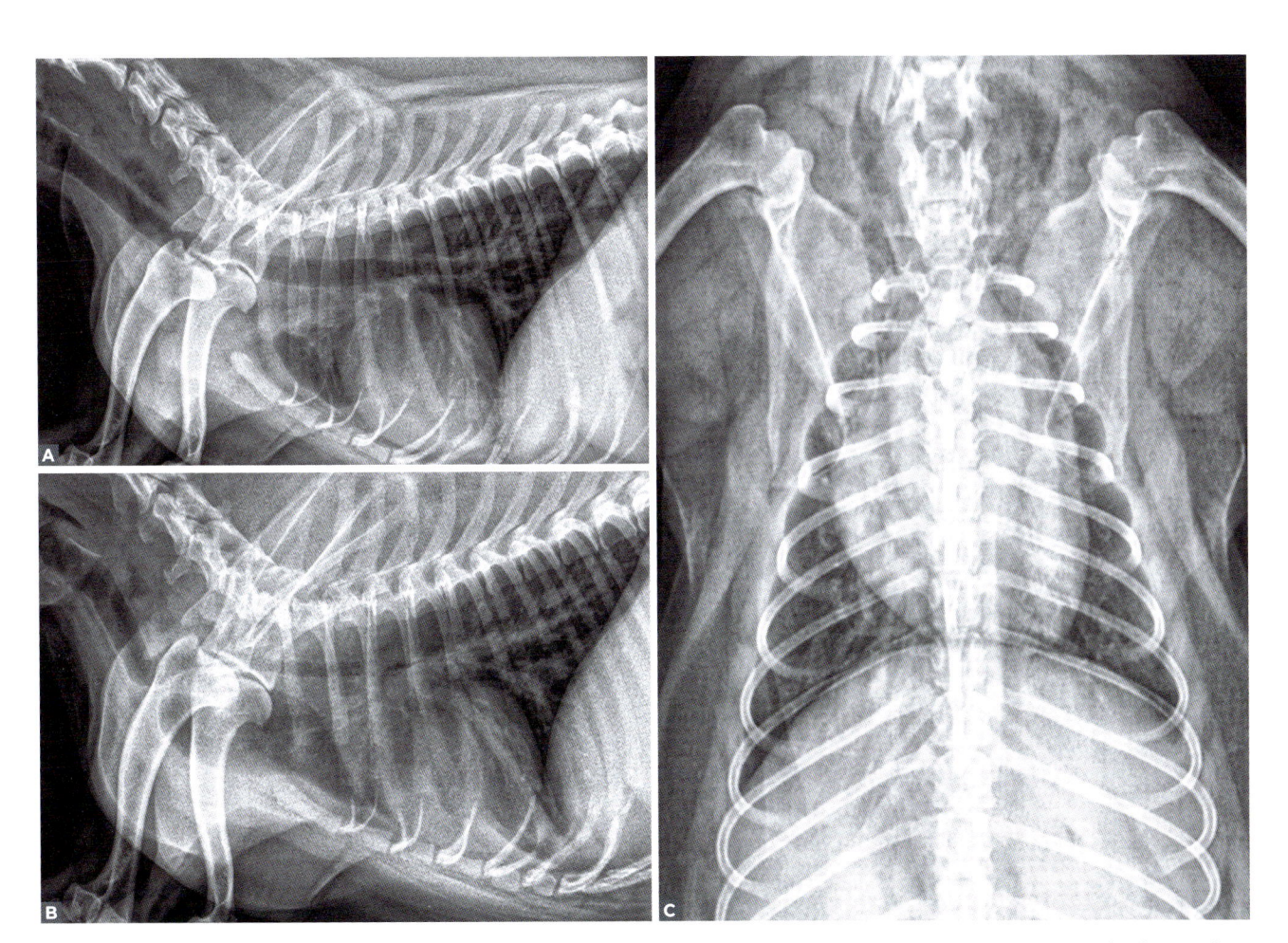

Fig. 21.8 Lateral thoracic radiographs of a nine-year-old Chihuahua with a history of a chronic cough. In (**A**) the intrathoracic trachea has a uniform diameter and the lungs are in a normal position. At expiration during coughing (**B**), the intrathoracic trachea, carina, and major bronchi are collapsed and displaced cranially. Kinking of the extrathoracic trachea is present. The cranial lung lobes are herniated cranially into the cervical region. A similar lung herniation is confirmed for both cranial lung lobes in the ventrodorsal thoracic radiograph (**C**).

SECTION **IV** THORAX

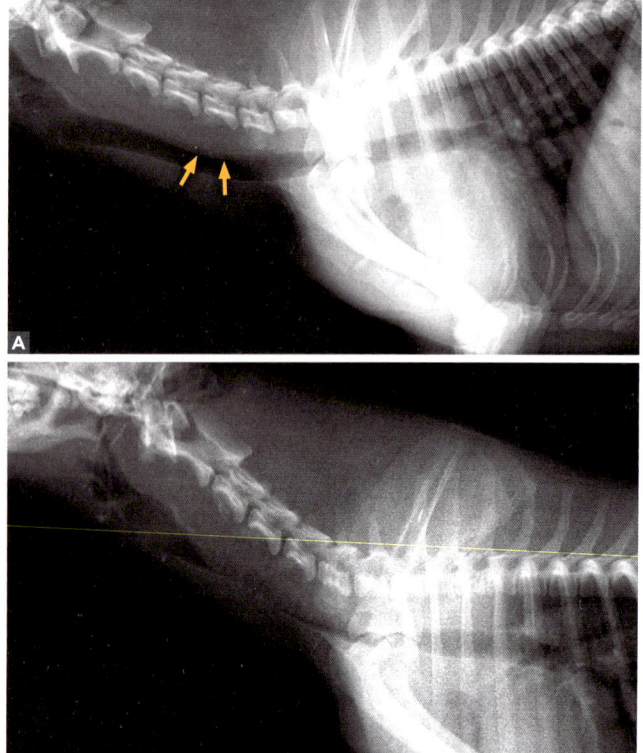

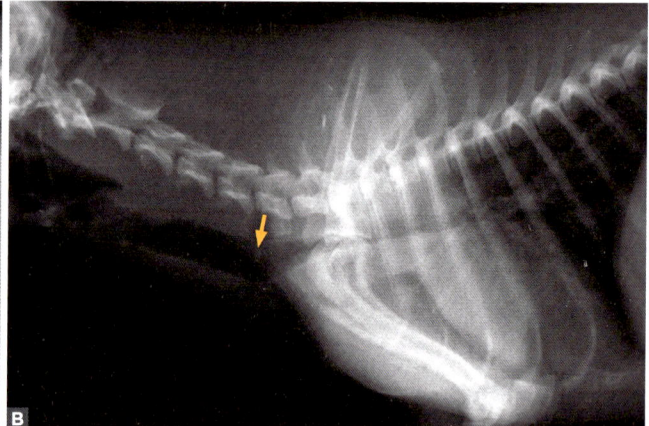

Fig. 21.9 Fluoroscopic study and derived images of a three-year-old mixed breed dog presented for a progressive cough and respiratory distress. During a normal respiratory phase (video 21.1 and fig. 21.9A), the lumen of the trachea has an abnormal uniform diameter, with a minor invagination of the DTM at the level of C4-C5 (orange arrows in image **A**). When stimulating the trachea to provoke a cough (video 21.2 and corresponding image 21.9B), the intrathoracic trachea completely collapses, the cervical part widens and there is a tracheal kinking with a visible fold dorsally at C6 (orange arrow in image **B**). When closing the nostrils to force inspiration (video 21.3 and corresponding image 21.9C), complete collapse of the cervical trachea is seen, followed by its widening. Image courtesy of SLU University Animal Hospital, Uppsala, Sweden.

Trauma and stenosis

Traumatic injury of the trachea may cause rupture or avulsion. Rupture refers to full-thickness wall disruption, typically affecting the cervical trachea from causes such as bite wounds, choke chains, and endotracheal intubation.[10] Avulsion is described in cats, secondary to blunt trauma-induced hyperextension of the neck, causing separation of the thoracic tracheal rings usually at the second to fourth thoracic vertebrae, with intact adventitia or mediastinal tissue temporarily maintaining the integrity of the airway.[11]

Tracheal rupture is rarely diagnosed on radiographs, the actual injury of the tracheal wall being invisible; the shape of the trachea may be altered, with irregular walls, and focal malalignment of the rings and lumen. More readily identifiable secondary features are subcutaneous or fascial emphysema, pneumomediastinum, and occasionally pneumoretroperitoneum and pneumothorax (**fig. 21.10**).[10] Acute avulsion may cause dyspnea but some patients show no acute signs; radiographic features include focal disruption or narrowing of the intrathoracic trachea, luminal effacement, and pneumomediastinum.[11]

In chronic avulsion, a complete circumferential tracheal discontinuity with a well-defined spherical gas dilation surrounded by thin soft tissue margins is seen in some cases. The segmental ballooning, termed pseudoairway, is formed by the tracheal adventitia and mediastinal connective tissues. Progressive circumferential stenosis of the ruptured tracheal ends causes gradual onset and progressive dyspnea (2-3 weeks after trauma).[11]

CHAPTER 21 Trachea

Severe stenosis affecting a short segment of the trachea may also occur as a sequel to trauma if there is no distraction of the ruptured trachea. Pneumomediastinum is not present (**fig. 21.11**).[11]

CT may show a tear of the tracheal wall, with better definition of the location and extent of the laceration (**figs. 21.12** and **21.13**). Reported features include misshapen tracheal lumen, discontinuous wall with lack of rings, and localized or extensive emphysema or pneumomediastinum. In chronic cases there may be circumferential contrast enhancing thickening of the surrounding tissue with segmental stenosis of the tracheal luminal diameter.

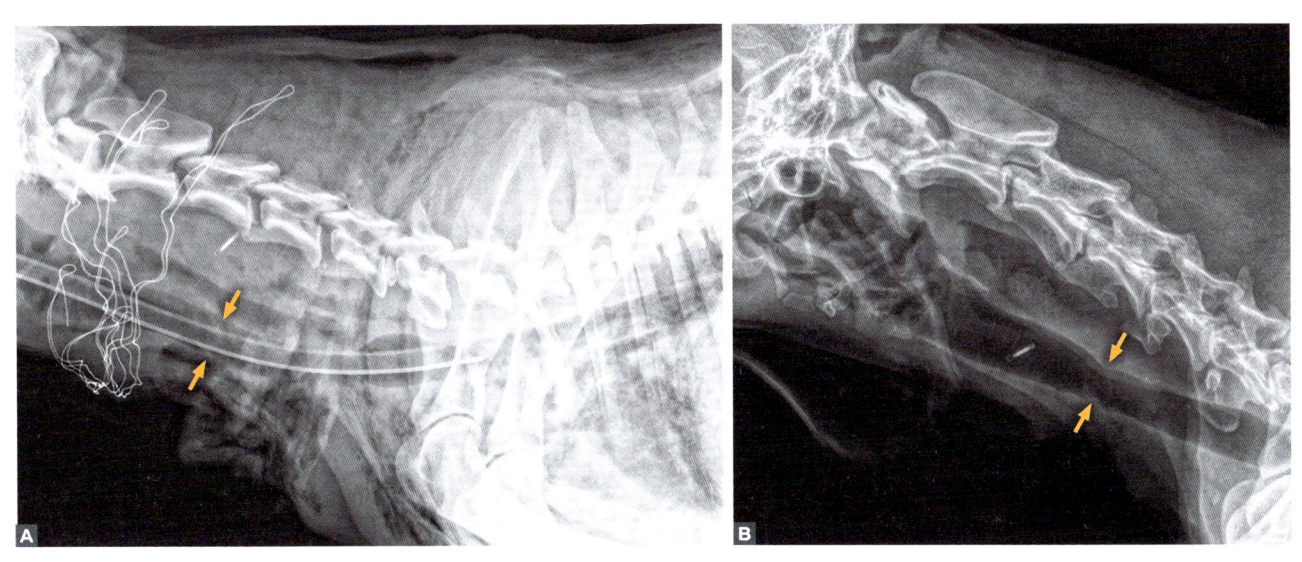

Fig. 21.10 Lateral cervical radiographs of a six-year-old mixed breed dog. (**A**) The dog presented with cervical bite wounds after a fight with another dog. There is a mild irregularity of the dorsal and ventral tracheal walls at the level of C3-C4, where a soft tissue line is visualized (arrows). Between this area and the endotracheal tube cuff, there is reduced visualization of the tracheal walls and air column. The actual wall lesion is difficult to identify, but the concomitant emphysema and pneumomediastinum raise the suspicion of an upper airway rupture. A cervical tracheal rupture was surgically identified and repaired. The radiopaque thread is part of a bandage positioned around the neck. (**B**) Same dog six months after trauma. A static mild circumferential narrowing of the tracheal lumen (arrows) is visualized in the surgical area, compatible with mild stenosis.

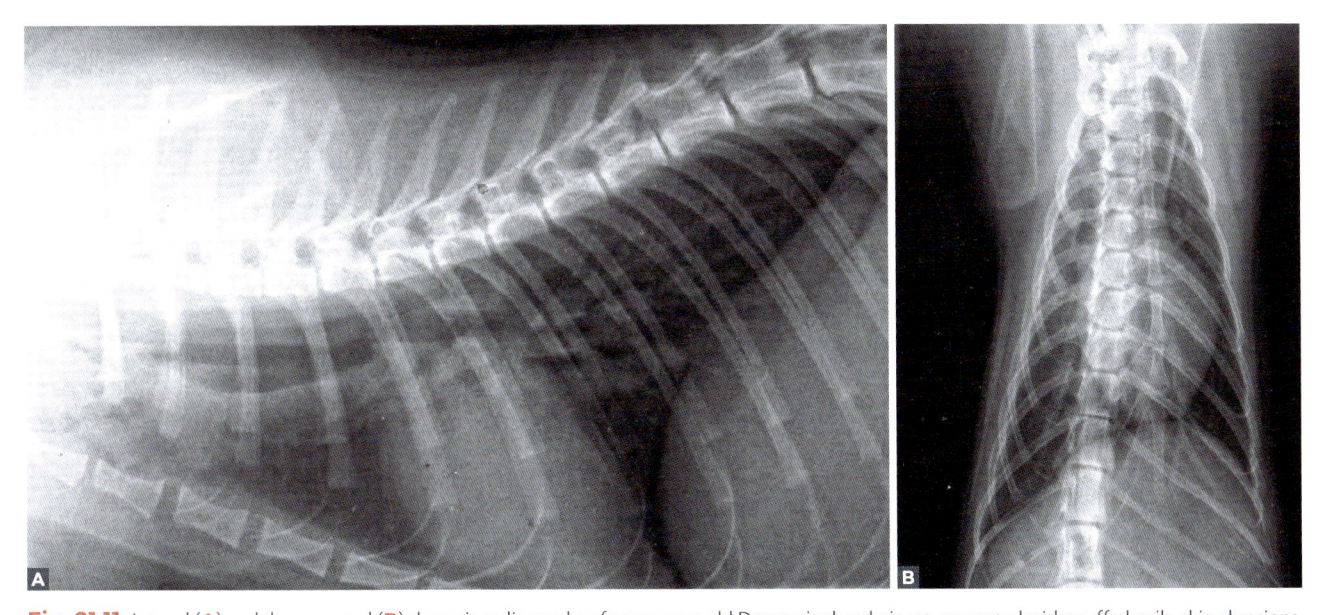

Fig. 21.11 Lateral (**A**) and dorsoventral (**B**) thoracic radiographs of a two-year-old Domestic shorthair cat, presented with scuffed nails, skin abrasions, and marked dyspnea. A road traffic accident was suspected. A tubular gas lucency is seen overlying and to the left of the intrathoracic trachea, from the second to the fourth intercostal spaces. The ventral wall of the trachea in this region is not clearly identified, and the dorsal wall is deviated ventrally. A tracheal avulsion with pseudoairway formation is the likely diagnosis. Image courtesy of Dr. Paul Mahoney.

SECTION IV THORAX

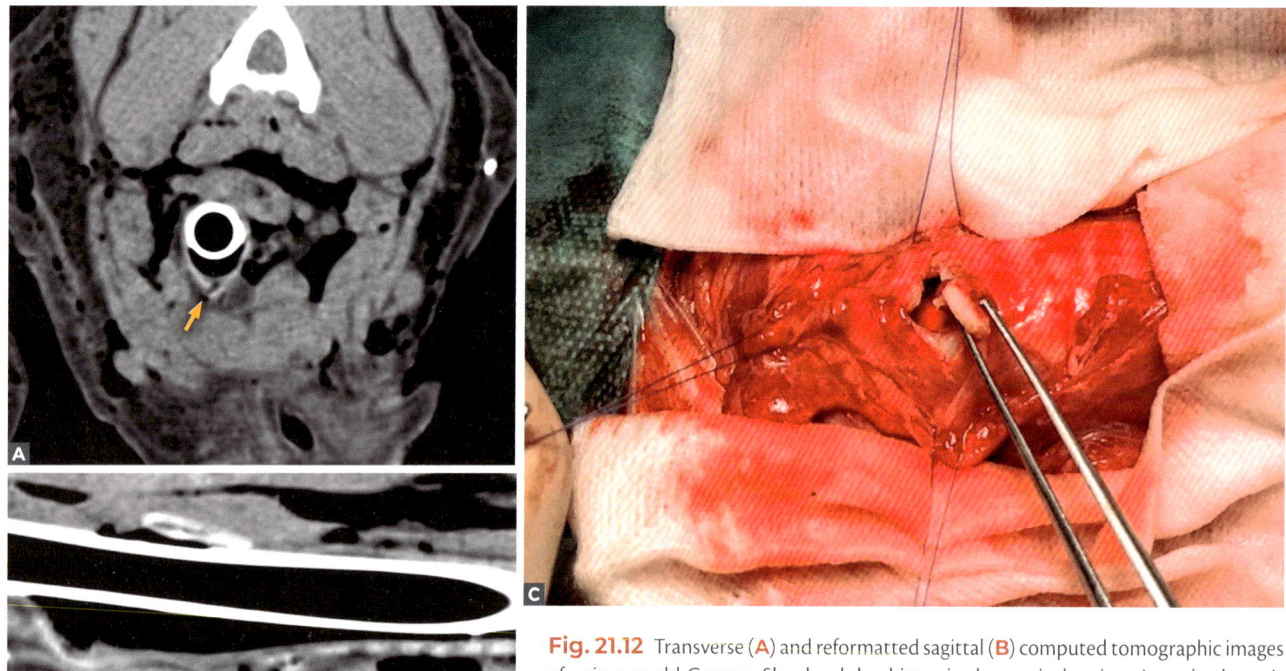

Fig. 21.12 Transverse (**A**) and reformatted sagittal (**B**) computed tomographic images of a six-year-old German Shepherd dog bitten in the cervical region. A tracheal tear is present, characterized by disruption of the ventral cervical tracheal wall and discontinuity of the tracheal rings. Small pockets of air are present in the tracheal wall adjacent to the laceration (arrows) and there is extensive dissecting emphysema. The tracheal rupture was surgically confirmed (**C**). Images courtesy of Dr. Eduard Anadón, Hospital Veterinari Glòries, Barcelona, Spain.

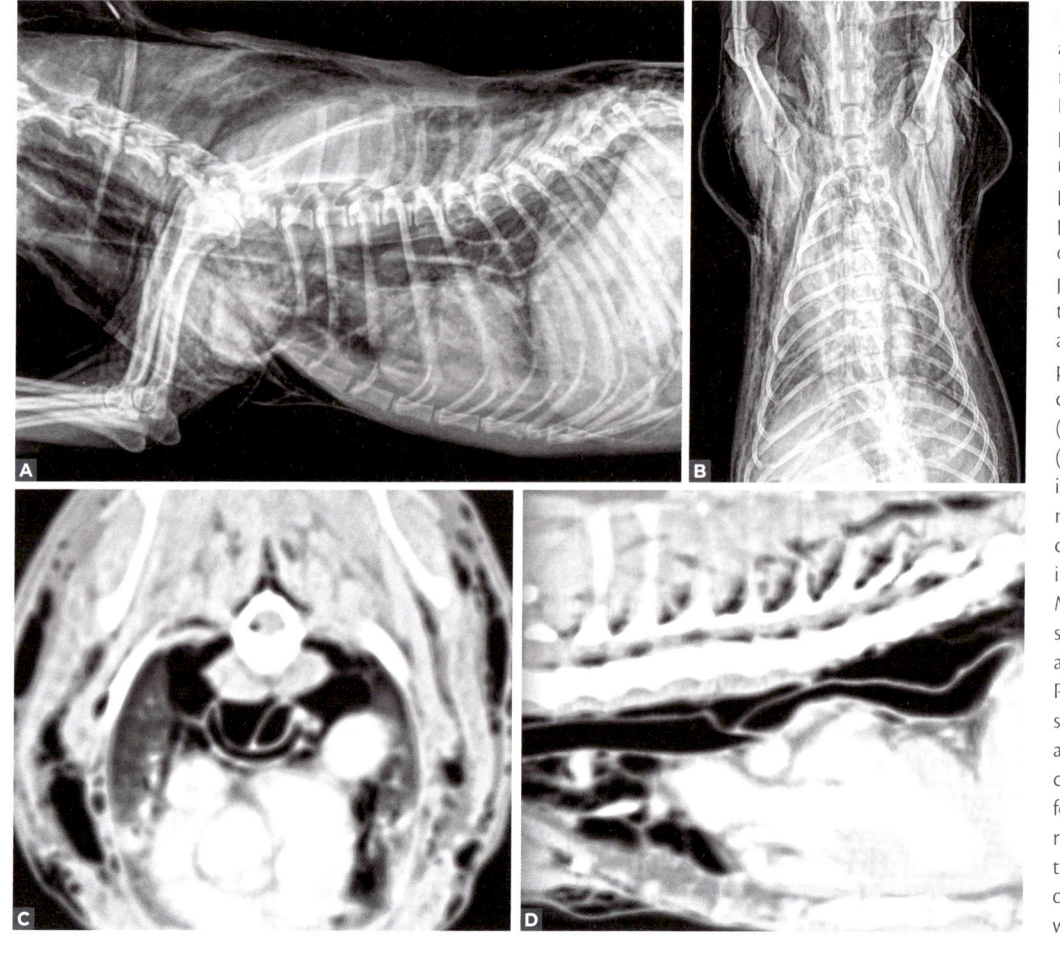

Fig. 21.13 Left lateral (**A**) and dorsoventral (**B**) thoracic radiographs of an 11-year-old Bichon Frisé that developed progressive severe subcutaneous emphysema and respiratory distress after a dental procedure. A large amount of air is seen in the fascial planes and subcutaneous tissues of the neck, thorax, and forelimbs, and there is pneumomediastinum. In the cranial thorax on transverse (**C**) and reformatted sagittal (**D**) computed tomographic images, the trachea is abnormally shaped, flattened dorsoventrally, and widened in laterolateral direction. Marked infolding of the dorsal tracheal membrane and adjacent esophagus is seen. Pneumomediastinum and subcutaneous emphysema are confirmed. On endoscopy, a tracheal rupture was found in the caudal intrathoracic trachea extending to the bifurcation. Invagination of the esophagus into the tear was also found.

Coumarin hemorrhage

Ingestion of coumarin-based rodenticides is the most common cause of vitamin K-deficient coagulopathy in small animals. Hemorrhage can occur anywhere in the body and signs depend on the site, amount, and duration of hemorrhage; dyspnea, lethargy, coughing, hemoptysis, pallor, and epistaxis are frequently reported.[12]

Diffuse thickening of the tracheal wall from submucosal hemorrhage, causing variable luminal narrowing, is a characteristic imaging feature of rodenticide intoxication and is readily identified on lateral cervical and thoracic radiographs.[12,13] Unlike dynamic collapse the narrowing is static and the appearance is consistent on serial radiographs.[13] Both the intrathoracic and extrathoracic trachea can be affected, with the luminal narrowing being focal or diffuse.[12,13] This finding resolves with therapy.[12] Other commonly associated thoracic radiographic findings include mediastinal, pleural, and pulmonary hemorrhage (**figs. 21.14** and **21.15**).[12]

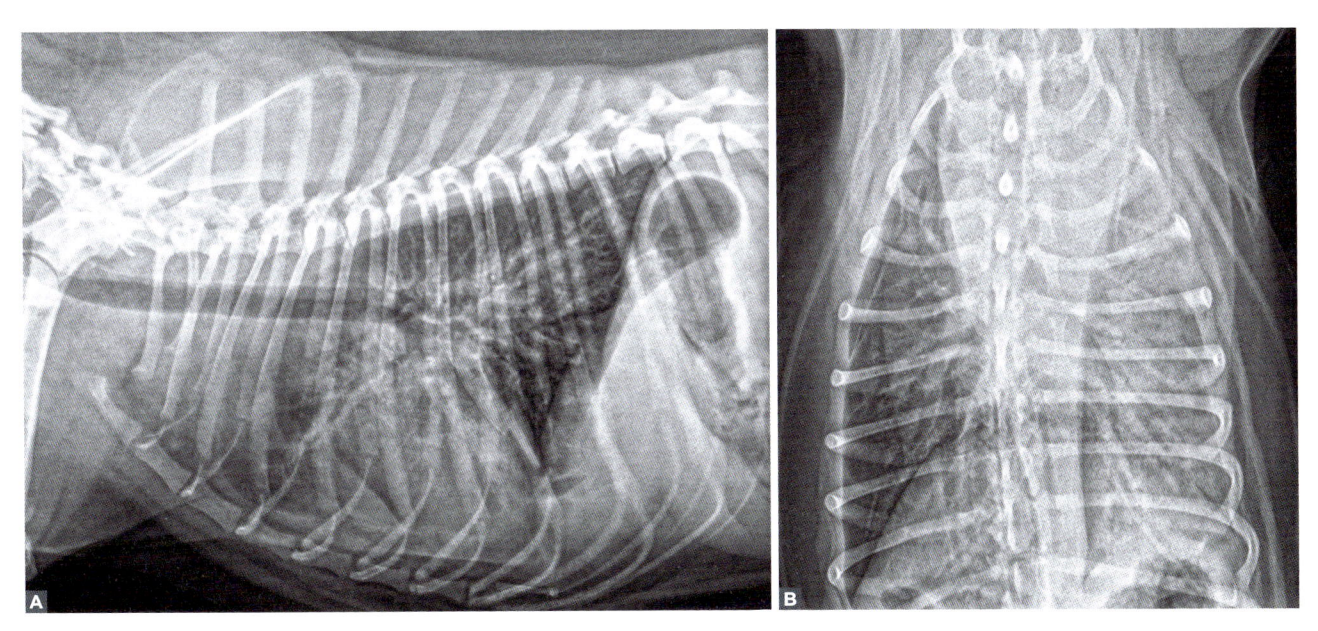

Fig. 21.14 Right lateral (**A**) and ventrodorsal (**B**) thoracic radiographs of a 1.5-year-old Golden Retriever presented for lethargy, sporadic cough, and epistaxis. There is mild narrowing of the trachea from thickening of the dorsal tracheal membrane. There is also bilateral pleural effusion, soft tissue widening of the cranial mediastinum, and mixed interstitial-alveolar opacification of the left cranial lung lobe. Coagulation was prolonged and anticoagulant rodenticide intoxication was suspected. The dog responded to vitamin K treatment.

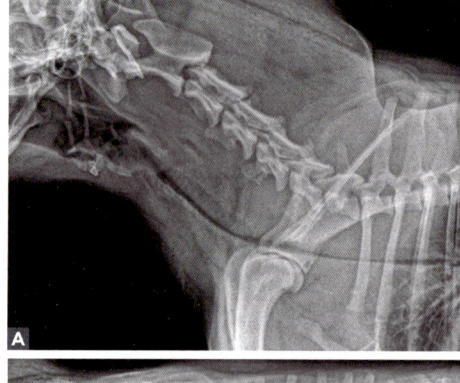

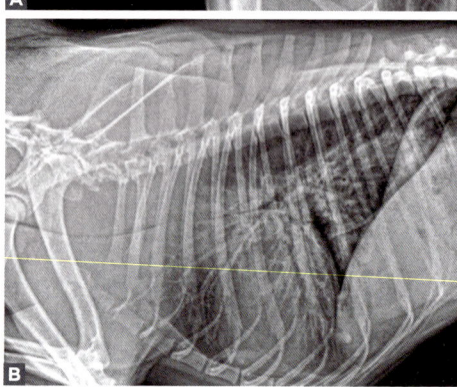

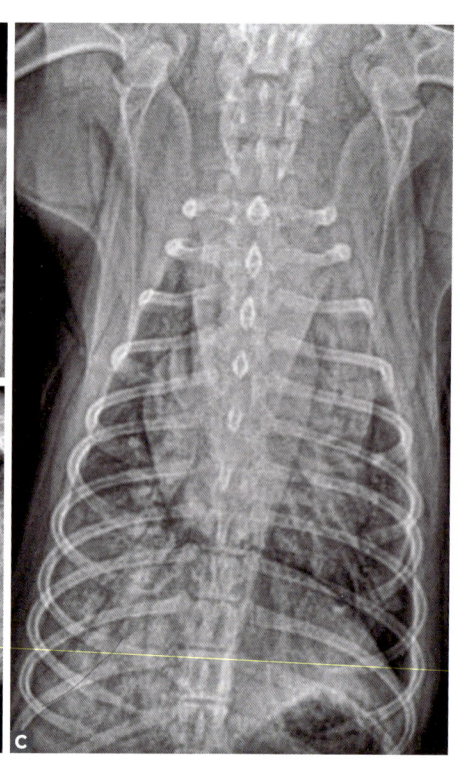

Fig. 21.15 A two-year old Labrador mix dog with lethargy, anorexia, and dry hacking cough. The lateral radiograph of the neck (**A**) shows a diffuse thickening of the tracheal wall and severe generalized narrowing of the lumen. A broad-based swelling of the superficial soft tissues of the dorsal aspect of the neck is also seen, likely representing an injection-related hematoma. The left lateral (**B**) and ventrodorsal (**C**) thoracic radiographs of the same dog confirm a similar severe static narrowing of the intrathoracic trachea, and show a non-uniform alveolar opacity in the right caudal and cranial subsegment of the left cranial lung lobes, and a widened soft tissue opaque cranial mediastinum. The tracheal changes are characteristic of hemorrhage from coumarin intoxication. The findings also indicate multifocal pulmonary hemorrhage and mediastinal hemorrhage. Coagulation parameters were prolonged, and exposure to anticoagulant rodenticide was confirmed by the owner. Image courtesy of Dr. John Graham.

References

1. Coyne BE, Fingland RB. Hypoplasia of the trachea in dogs: 103 cases (1974-1990). *J Am Vet Med Assoc* 201:768-772, 1992.
2. Harvey CE, Fink EA. Tracheal diameter: analysis of radiographic measurements in brachycephalic and nonbrachycephalic dogs. *J Am Anim Hosp Assoc* 18:570-576, 1982.
3. Ingman J, Näslund V, Hansson K. Comparison between tracheal ratio methods used by three observers at three occasions in English Bulldogs. *Acta Vet Scand* 56:79, 2014.
4. Kaye BM, Boroffka SAEB, Haagsman AN, Haar GT. Computed tomographic, radiographic, and endoscopic tracheal dimensions in English Bulldogs with grade 1 clinical signs of brachycephalic airway syndrome. *Vet Radiol Ultrasound* 56:609-616, 2015.
5. Lee J, Yun S, Lee I, Choi M, Yoon J. Fluoroscopic characteristics of tracheal collapse and cervical lung herniation in dogs: 222 cases (2012-2015). *J Vet Sci* 18:499-505, 2017.
6. Fujita M, Miura H, Yasuda D, Hasegawa D, Orima H. Tracheal narrowing secondary to airway obstruction in two cats. *J Small Anim Pract* 45:29-31, 2004.
7. Macready DM, Johnson LR, Pollard RE. Fluoroscopic and radiographic evaluation of tracheal collapse in dogs: 62 cases (2001-2006). *J Am Vet Med Assoc* 230:1870-1876, 2007.
8. Lindl Bylicki BJ, Johnson LR, Pollard RE. Comparison of the radiographic and tracheoscopic appearance of the dorsal tracheal membrane in large and small breed dogs. *Vet Radiol Ultrasound* 56:602-608, 2015.
9. Heng HG, Lim CK, Gutierrez-Crespo B, Guptill LF. Radiographic and computed tomographic appearance of tracheal collapse with axial rotation in four dogs. *J Small Anim Pract* 59:53-58, 2018.
10. Basdani E, Papazoglou LG, Patsikas MN, Kazakos GM, Adamama-Moraitou KK, Tsokataridis I. Upper airway injury in dogs secondary to trauma: 10 dogs (2000-2011). *J Am Anim Hosp Assoc* 52:291-296, 2016.
11. White RN, Burton CA. Surgical management of intrathoracic tracheal avulsion in cats: long-term results in 9 consecutive cases. *Vet Surg* 29:430-435, 2000.
12. Berry CR, Gallaway A, Thrall DE, Carlisle C. Thoracic radiographic features of anticoagulant rodenticide toxicity in fourteen dogs. *Vet Radiol Ultrasound* 34:391-396, 1993.
13. Lawson C, O'Brien M, McMichael M. Upper airway obstruction secondary to anticoagulant rodenticide toxicosis in five dogs. *J Am Anim Hosp Assoc* 53:236-241, 2017.

CHAPTER 22

Infectious pulmonary disease

John P. Graham

KEY POINTS

- Both left and right lateral radiographs should be obtained in addition to a ventrodorsal or dorsoventral view.
- Pneumonia may be caused by primary bacterial infection or aspiration of food, vomitus, or other material
- The ventral/dependent lung fields are primarily affected, and alveolar infiltrates are the characteristic radiographic feature.
- Radiography is a useful tool to assess therapeutic efficacy, but improvement may be slower than clinical response.
- Most mycotic infections are endemic to specific regions.
- Mycotic infections show a broad range of abnormalities that often overlap those of pulmonary, pleural, or multicentric neoplasia.

Infectious pulmonary disease is a relatively common clinical entity in companion animals. As with other pulmonary diseases, both left and right lateral radiographs should be obtained as abnormalities in the dependent lung, that is, the lung closest to the radiography table may be completely obscured by partial atelectasis, even in unsedated patients. A ventrodorsal or dorsoventral radiograph should also be obtained, as this more readily facilitates comparison of the left and right lungs. A single dorsoventral radiograph can be obtained in patients with severe dyspnea, as such patients are more stable and comfortable in sternal recumbency. This projection will allow an overview of the lungs, pleural space, and cardiovascular structures and may provide sufficient information for a tentative diagnosis and treatment plan.

Bacterial pneumonia and aspiration pneumonia are the most common infectious or inflammatory pulmonary diseases diagnosed in companion animals. In most cases, the diagnosis is usually suspected before radiography based on the history and clinical signs. Most mycotic infectious agents are endemic to specific regions, and geographic location combined with clinical signs usually suggests the diagnosis before radiography. However, occasional cases are identified outside typical endemic regions in pets that travel with owners or in rescued pets of uncertain geographic origin. Sporadic cases of mycotic infection, particularly blastomycosis, can also occur outside the endemic regions. Local health agencies such as the Centers for Disease Control in the USA publish maps showing the known distribution of mycotic infectious agents. It is possible that climate change may alter the geographic distribution of some of these diseases.

Bacterial pneumonia and aspiration pneumonia

Common etiologies of pneumonia in companion animals are bacterial infection and aspiration of food, vomitus, and/or gastrointestinal secretions.[1,2] In juvenile canine patients, bacterial pneumonia may be a sequel to viral pneumonitis. The radiographic changes are similar no matter the underlying etiology, and diagnosis is based on a combination of patient history, clinicopathologic data, and thoracic radiography. Pneumonia is more commonly diagnosed in dogs than in cats, but the features are similar in both species. Patients with bacterial pneumonia may present with either acute signs or a history of chronic waxing and waning illness. Respiratory signs include nasal discharge, cough, and tachypnea and systemic signs include fever, lethargy, anorexia, and weakness.[1-3]

Patients with aspiration pneumonia usually have an acute presentation with a history of dysphagia, regurgitation, vomiting, or force-feeding. Pre-existing conditions which predispose to the development

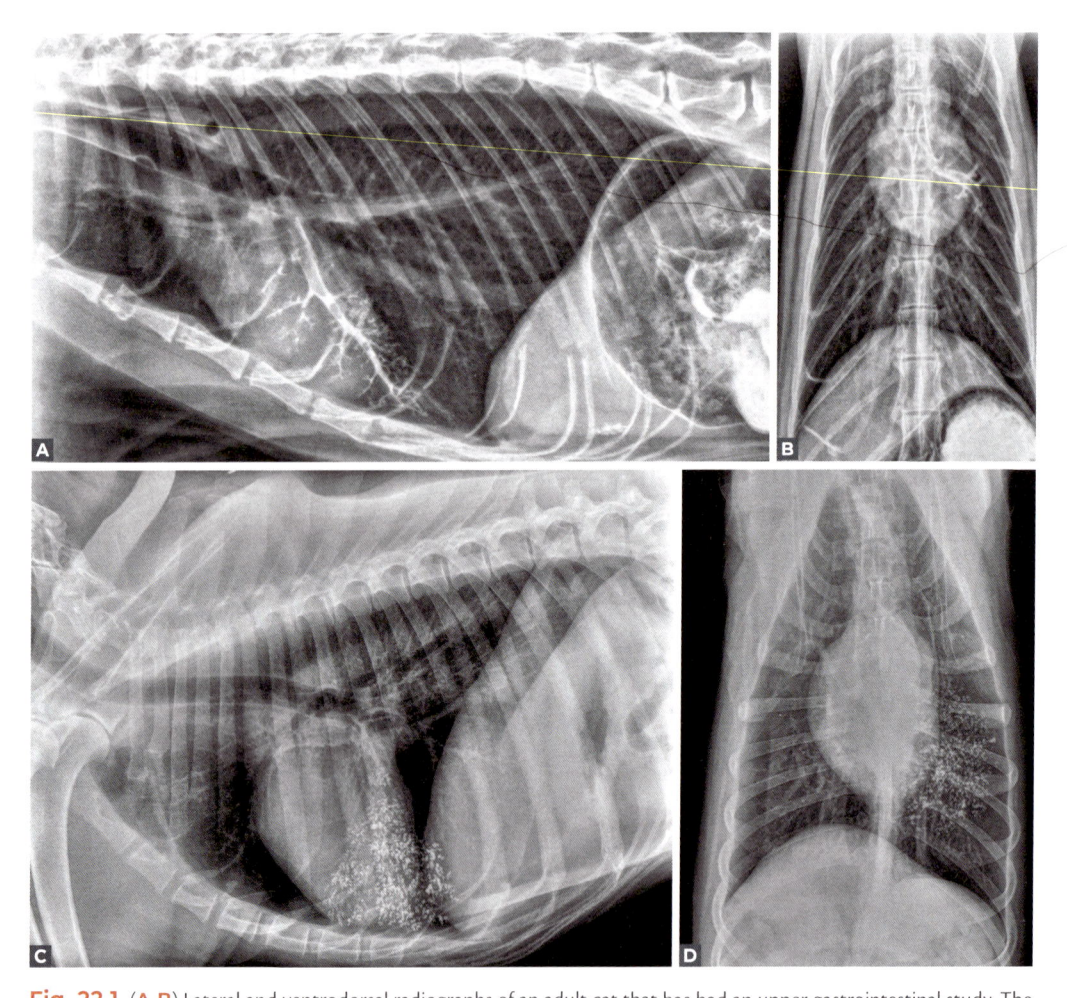

Fig. 22.1 (**A-B**) Lateral and ventrodorsal radiographs of an adult cat that has had an upper gastrointestinal study. The lateral radiograph shows a small volume of barium contrast within the thoracic tracheal lumen. There is also a small volume of barium contrast within the esophagus immediately dorsal to the trachea. Aspirated barium contrast is noted within the bronchus of the caudal subsegment of the left cranial lung lobe, overlying the cardiac silhouette on the lateral projection and superimposed on the left border of the heart on the ventrodorsal projection. Aspiration of barium may be the result of abnormal pharyngeal or esophageal function but can occur in normal patients with excessively vigorous force-feeding of contrast. The radiographs show the distribution of contrast within the major bronchus and also within the smaller bronchi to the periphery of the lung. (**C-D**) Lateral and ventrodorsal radiographs of the thorax of an adult mixed breed dog. Mottled mineral opacity is seen throughout the caudal subsegment of the left cranial lung lobe. This is consistent with barium suspension located within the airspaces of the lung. The barium aspiration was an incidental finding attributed to an upper gastrointestinal study the patient had had some years earlier. The patient had no respiratory signs. The radiographs show the destination of aspirated material such as vomitus and show the expected distribution of aspiration pneumonia.

of aspiration pneumonia include esophageal dysfunction, refractory vomiting, seizures, and laryngeal dysfunction. Aspiration pneumonia can also occur as a complication of an anesthetic procedure in otherwise healthy patients. This diagnosis should be suspected in patients with the above-mentioned risk factors who develop acute respiratory signs. The severity of response depends on the type and volume of aspirated material. At first, there is chemical pneumonitis that may be followed by septic inflammation, particularly if food is aspirated or there is a preexisting pulmonary disease.[1-3]

Barium sulphate suspension is inert, and although aspiration can result in impressive radiographic changes, affected patients do not usually show any clinical ill effects. Barium suspension may be seen in the trachea and bronchi if radiographs are taken immediately following aspiration (**fig. 22.1**). Barium in the airways is cleared quickly by the mucociliary elevator and coughing. Barium that reaches the alveoli appears as a mottled mineral opacity from alternating air and barium-filled clusters of alveoli and is cleared by a combination of coughing and phagocytosis by alveolar macrophages. Barium that is phagocytosed is transported to the tracheobronchial lymph nodes. Aspirated barium may persist in the alveoli and tracheobronchial lymph nodes for years after the aspiration event. Radiographic changes in these patients are frequently quite striking, but there are usually no associated respiratory signs. Aspiration of barium mixed with food or vomitus causes pneumonia just as aspiration of food or vomitus alone would. Water-soluble iodinated contrast for gastrointestinal contrast studies should be avoided in patients at risk of aspiration as these agents are markedly hyperosmotic at concentrations used for diagnosis and cause severe, potentially lethal pulmonary edema.

Radiologic features of bacterial and aspiration pneumonia

Radiographic changes may lag behind the onset of clinical signs by 12-24 hours in some patients but progress quickly. In patients with acute onset signs of less than 24 hours duration and normal radiographs or tenuous radiographic changes, repeat imaging after 24 hours will usually demonstrate progression to confirm the diagnosis. Most patients have radiographic abnormalities at the time of presentation. In early cases, the pulmonary infiltrates have a peribronchial distribution in the peripheral and middle zones of the lung and are characterized by an unstructured interstitial pattern that may coalesce to foci of alveolar opacification (**fig. 22.2**), adjacent to the bronchi or in the ventral periphery of the lung.

Most patients show segmental or lobar alveolar infiltrates at the time of diagnosis (**fig. 22.3**). Air bronchograms are usually visible in the infiltrated lung and are most readily identified when the bronchi are oriented perpendicular to the path of the X-ray beam. The alveolar pattern obscures pulmonary vessels in the affected pulmonary segment. The interface between an abnormal lung lobe and an adjacent normal or less severely affected lung lobe will appear as a discrete curvilinear margin if the X-ray beam is oriented parallel to the interlobar division, referred to as a lobar sign. If the infiltrated lung is in contact with the heart or diaphragm, the border is effaced, also referred to as a "silhouette sign".

Fig. 22.2 Lateral and ventrodorsal radiographs of a four-year-old Labrador with weakness, fever, and productive cough of approximately 12 hours duration. There is increased unstructured interstitial opacity in the left cranial lung lobe and right middle lung lobe. On the lateral projection, there is moderate to severe thickening of the bronchial walls of the right middle lung lobe (arrows). The interstitial pattern has a patchy peribronchial distribution in the middle and peripheral zones of the right middle lung lobe, overlying the cardiac silhouette on this projection. These changes are consistent with early bacterial bronchopneumonia or aspiration pneumonia.

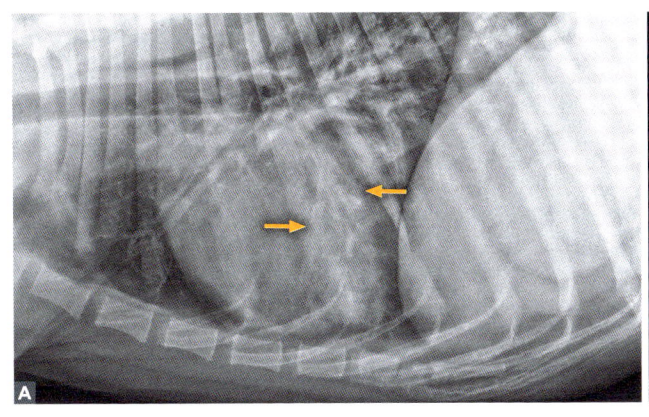

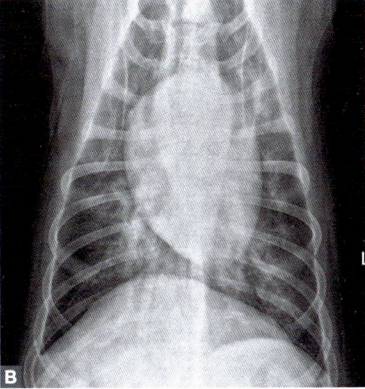

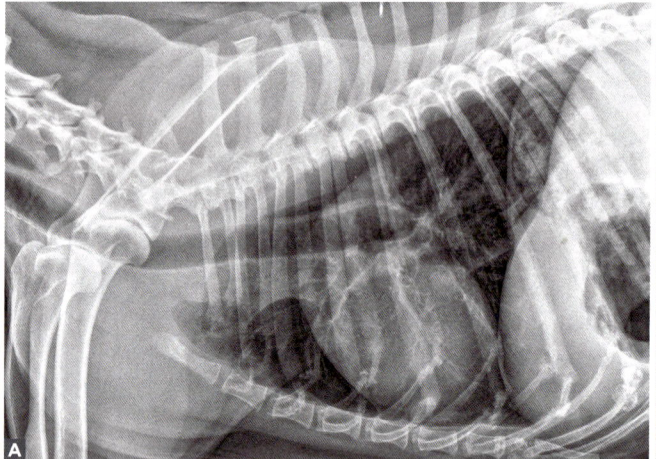

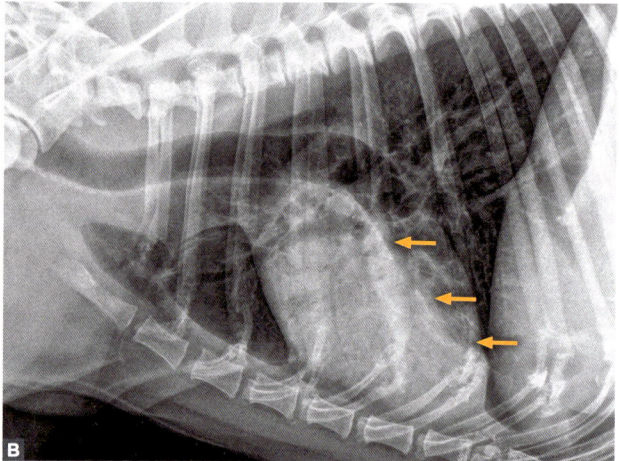

Fig. 22.3 Left lateral, right lateral, and ventrodorsal radiographs of the thorax of a ten-year-old mixed breed dog with bacterial pneumonia. No pulmonary parenchymal changes are evident on the left lateral projection. On the right lateral projection, air bronchograms are visible in the cranial and caudal subsegment of the left cranial lung lobe, best seen overlying the heart. The caudal border of the lung lobe is visible as a discrete curvilinear margin overlying the heart (arrows). The ventrodorsal projection confirms the alveolar pattern in the left cranial lung lobe, resulting in effacement of part of the left cardiac border. There is also partial volume loss of the left cranial lung lobe with resulting displacement of the heart and mediastinum toward the left thoracic wall. This is the result of reduced perfusion and ventilation of the pneumonic lung lobe.

The most common sites for pneumonia are the dependent, ventral parts of the left cranial, right cranial, and right middle lung lobes (**figs. 22.4A** and **22.4B**). With increasing severity, the infiltrates extend toward the hilus of the lung and opacify the entire lobe. In patients with severe disease, the accessory lung lobe and ventral periphery of the caudal lung lobes may also be involved (**figs. 22.4C** and **22.4D**). The right middle lung lobe is most commonly affected by both bacterial and aspiration pneumonia in part because of the origin of the lobar bronchus. The long, thin shape of the lobe, which limits collateral air circulation within the lobe, also makes it more vulnerable to pneumonia and atelectasis.[5] The distribution of aspiration pneumonia can vary from this pattern in patients who were unconscious or obtunded, depending on how the patient was positioned when aspiration occurred.

Pneumonic infiltrates in the ventral periphery of the lung may be visible only on the lateral projection where the affected lung is uppermost, e.g., pneumonia in the ventral periphery of the right lung may be visible on a left lateral recumbent projection only. This is especially true for pneumonia in the periphery of the right middle lung lobe and caudal subsegment of the left cranial lung lobe, which is readily obscured by the heart. When attempting to confirm or exclude pneumonia, both right and left lateral projections should be obtained in addition to a ventrodorsal or dorsoventral projection.[4]

Unstructured interstitial infiltrates are usually present in the transition zone between alveolar infiltrates and normal lung, which is usually broad and relatively indistinct. There may be visible thickening of the walls of major bronchi in the pneumonic lobes.

Pneumonia usually results in some degree of atelectasis from reduced ventilation and perfusion of the affected segments or lobe/lobes. If the disease is unilateral or asymmetrically distributed, this may result in a mediastinal shift towards the more severely affected lung. The severity of atelectasis is insufficient to account for the severity and extent of increased pulmonary opacity in these patients, which helps to distinguish atelectasis associated with pneumonia from uncomplicated atelectasis. The distribution of pulmonary changes in aspiration pneumonia is usually the same as with bacterial pneumonia (**fig. 22.5**). Aspiration pneumonia may have an atypical focal or multifocal

CHAPTER 22 Infectious pulmonary disease

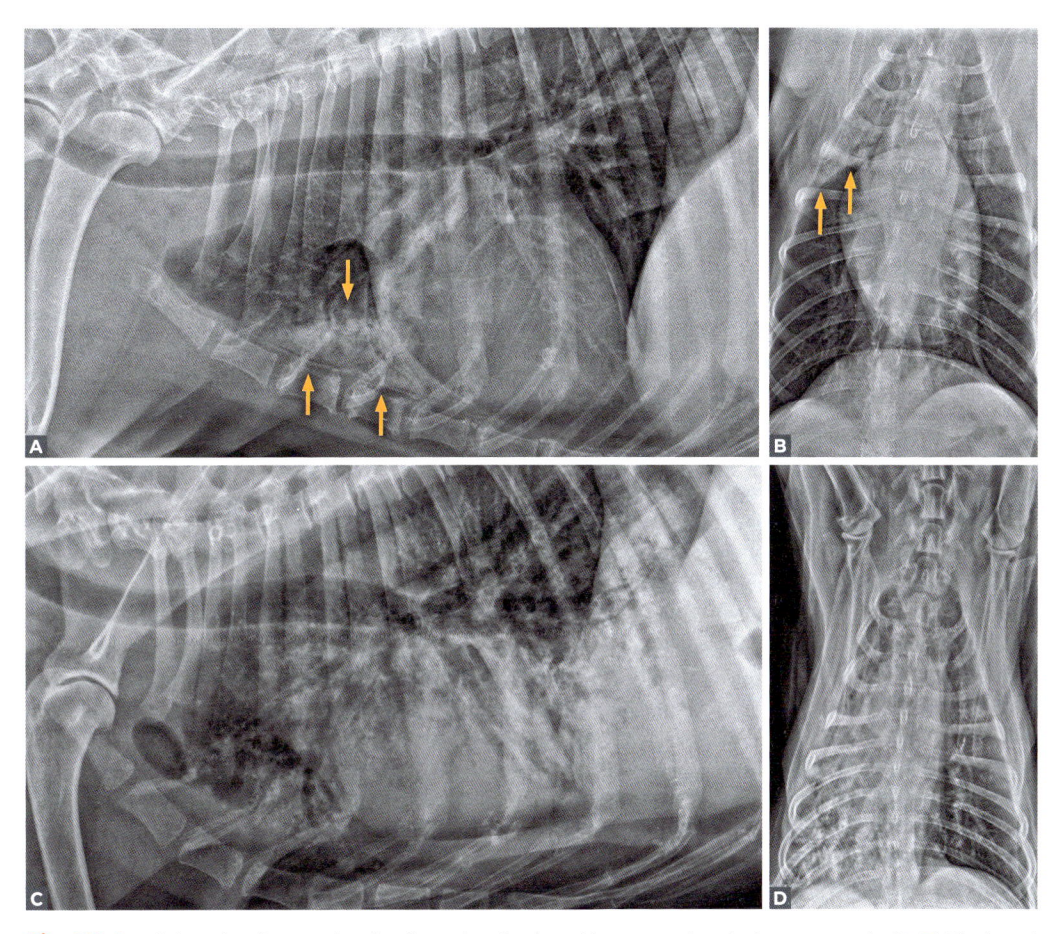

Fig. 22.4 Left lateral and ventrodorsal radiographs of a dog with suspected aspiration pneumonia. (**A-B**) The lateral radiograph shows focal alveolar opacity in the cranial ventral periphery of the lung, seen interposed between the heart and sternum (arrows). Air bronchograms are visible within the segment of the lung. There is hazy unstructured interstitial opacity dorsal to the region of alveolar opacity, representing the transition zone to normal lung. The ventrodorsal radiograph shows increased soft tissue opacity in the right cranial lung lobe compared to the left cranial lung lobe. There is also an example of a lobar sign, as the junction of the right cranial and right middle lung lobes forms a curved well-defined interface (arrows). (**C-D**) Left lateral and ventrodorsal radiographs of a dog with severe right-sided pneumonia. The lateral projection shows nonuniform increased opacity throughout the ventral thorax with multiple air bronchograms. The caudal cardiac border, caudal vena cava, and cupola of the diaphragm are obscured, indicating that pneumonia affects the accessory lung lobe and ventral periphery of the right caudal lung lobe. On the ventrodorsal projection, there is diffuse increased opacity in the right lung resulting in effacement of the cardiac and diaphragmatic outlines. This patient also demonstrates a rightward mediastinal shift from partial atelectasis of the right lung. The left lung appears normal.

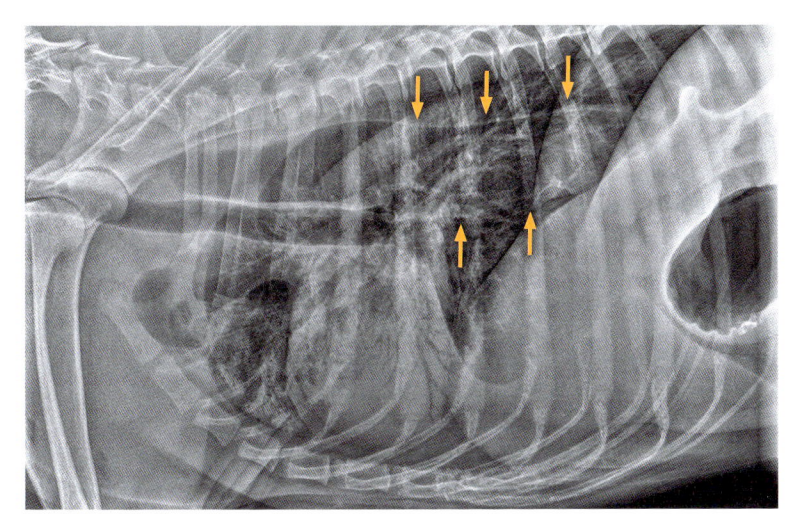

Fig. 22.5 Left lateral thoracic radiograph of a five-year-old Great Dane. The patient has a 180-degree gastric volvulus without dilation and secondary aspiration pneumonia. The pyloric antrum is gas-filled and positioned in the cranial dorsal abdomen caudal to the left diaphragmatic crus. The gastric fundus is also gas-filled and identified by the presence of rugal folds. There is moderate generalized dilation of the esophagus, secondary to occlusion of the gastroesophageal junction (arrows). The patient has aspiration pneumonia with increased opacity throughout the ventral lung fields. Multiple air bronchograms are present superimposed on the caudal half of the cardiac silhouette indicating an alveolar pattern throughout the right middle lung lobe. There is also a lobar sign highlighting the caudal border of this lung lobe. Increased opacity is also present in the middle and peripheral zones of the right cranial lung lobe. This appears to be a severe interstitial pattern coalescing to an alveolar pattern in the periphery of the lung.

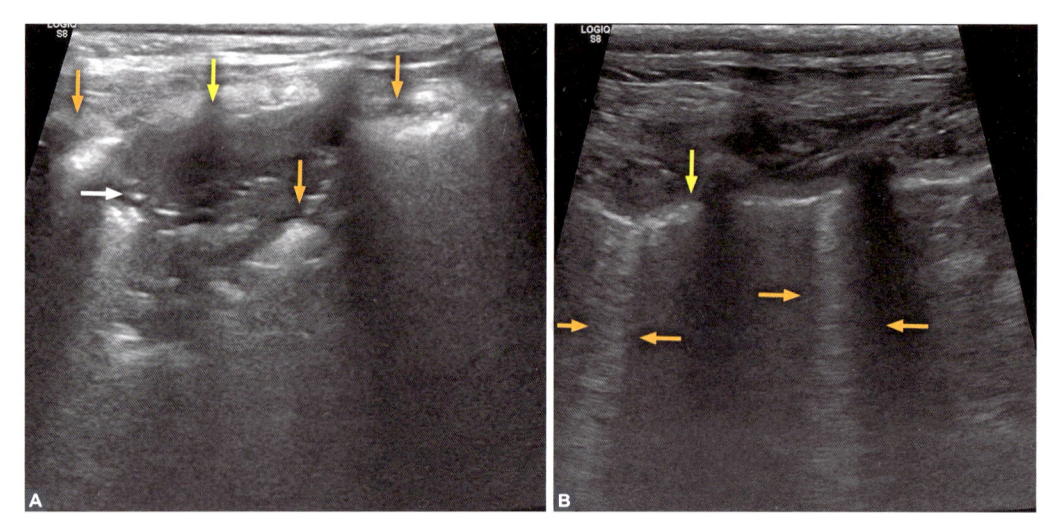

Fig. 22.6 (**A**) A 13-year-old Maltese dog with bacterial pneumonia. Lung consolidation: substantial alveolar consolidation without air bronchograms (liver-like pattern) (yellow arrow), air bronchogram shown longitudinally (orange arrows), and B-lines arising from bronchi (white arrow). The small white punctate foci are transverse ("end on") air-filled bronchi. (**B**) A 14-year-old Maltese dog with partly resolved bacterial pneumonia. Irregular pleural lines (yellow arrow) with isolated B-lines (orange arrows) that appear as vertical hyperechoic artifacts arising from the pleural line and extending to the far-field of the image, deleting A-lines. Courtesy of Dr. Giovanni Aste, DMV, PhD.

distribution if the patient was anesthetized, obtunded, or unconscious when aspiration occurred, for example, with regurgitation during recovery from general anesthesia. Aspirated material will distribute to the lung that was dependent when the event occurred. In such patients, pneumonia may be present in the caudal lung lobes or have a bizarre multifocal distribution if there were several aspiration events.

Dilation of the esophagus should increase suspicion of acquired megaesophagus and aspiration pneumonia, particularly if there is a history of dysphagia or regurgitation. However, some patients with dyspnea from pneumonia may exhibit transient esophageal dilation from aerophagia. In patients with esophageal dilation, pneumonia and dyspnea, radiographs should be repeated once the patient is stable and eupneic to document persistence or resolution of esophageal dilation. A diagnosis of megaesophagus should be reserved until dyspnea and tachypnea have resolved, and there is persistent esophageal dilation.

The radiographic features of pneumonia are relatively characteristic, and the diagnosis is usually straightforward based on radiographic changes and clinical data. While the distribution of pulmonary hemorrhage from coagulopathy or trauma can mimic pneumonia, the history and clinical data can usually be used to confirm the more likely diagnosis. In rare cases, primary pulmonary neoplasia or pulmonary lymphoma can mimic pneumonia and the clinical presentation can mimic chronic pneumonia. Lack of clinical and radiographic response to treatment should prompt a reassessment of the diagnosis and additional diagnostic testing such as percutaneous sampling of the lung with ultrasound guidance.

Ultrasound can be used as a screening tool in patients with suspected pneumonia. Pneumonic exudates in the airspaces allow the ultrasound beam to pass through the lung (**fig. 22.6**). The echogenicity of the affected lung is quite variable and ranges from quite hypoechoic to hyperechoic, usually with a heterogeneous echotexture. Pneumonic lung frequently resembles liver or spleen on ultrasound. Air-filled bronchi appear as linear hyperechoic structures within the consolidated lung. The transition from consolidated to aerated lung usually appears as a hyperechoic, ragged margin. Serial ultrasound studies can be used to estimate the progression or treatment response of suspected pneumonia and are easier to perform than radiographs in patients that are unstable or oxygen-dependent.

CHAPTER 22 Infectious pulmonary disease

Fig. 22.7 Left lateral and ventrodorsal thoracic radiographs of an eight-year-old Beagle with a history of chronic nonspecific illness and weight loss. An alveolar pattern is present in the right middle lung lobe, resulting in effacement of part of the right cardiac border on the ventrodorsal projection. There is a generalized increase in pulmonary soft tissue opacity. This is from diffuse severe thickening of the bronchial walls, which also show diffuse moderate tubular dilation (arrows). These changes are consistent with chronic pneumonia and severe generalized tubular bronchiectasis.

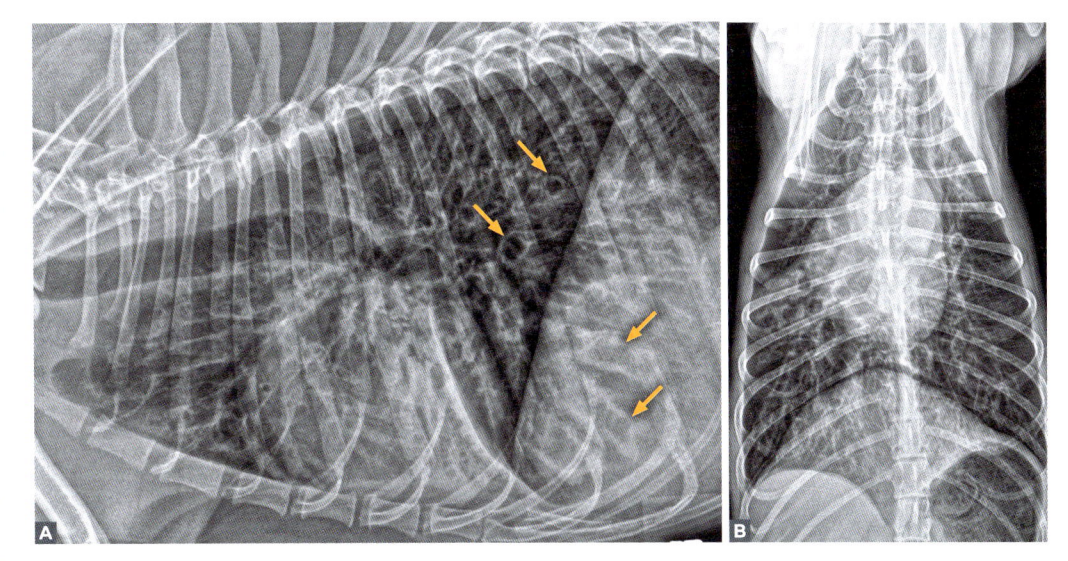

Bronchiectasis is a rare sequel to pneumonia and, in turn, predisposes to recurrent infection. Bronchiectasis may result in either tubular or saccular dilation of the bronchi (**fig. 22.7**). Bronchiectasis and recurrent or chronic pneumonia likely indicate either local or systemic immune deficiency.[6,7] Radiographs are routinely used to assess treatment response. Some patients show clinical response to therapy before radiographic improvement is evident, and the initial assessment of therapeutic efficacy may depend more on clinical impression than radiographic changes. Time to resolution of radiographic changes is variable, but for most patients, substantial improvement or resolution of radiographic changes would be expected after 10-14 days of treatment. Radiographs may return to normal but persistent foci of alveolar infiltration, unstructured interstitial infiltrates, and bronchial thickening may be seen in some patients. These changes may represent incompletely resolved disease or scarring/fibrosis. The latter diagnosis is more likely if there is no appreciable alteration in the appearance of the lung on serial convalescent radiographs.[1,3,8]

Blastomycosis

Blastomyces dermatitidis is an opportunistic yeast that has been recorded in many parts of North America but is most common in the eastern and mid-western regions of Canada and the USA. The lungs are infected initially, followed by systemic spread. Clinical signs include anorexia, weight loss, fever, cough, dyspnea, and lymphadenopathy. The infection affects the lungs and tracheobronchial lymph nodes and may extend to the pleurae and mediastinum. Skeletal, central nervous system, and abdominal visceral lesions also occur with systemic spread.[3,9] Confirmation of the diagnosis is usually based on identifying the yeast organisms by cytology or histology.

Blastomyces infection has a broad range of radiographic manifestations, and the diagnosis may be challenging. Unstructured interstitial infiltrates are commonly reported and have a random or diffuse distribution (**figs. 22.8A** and **22.8B**). In more chronic infections, the pulmonary infiltrates coalesce to form segmental or lobar alveolar infiltrates, nodules, and masses (**fig. 22.9**). Enlargement of the tracheobronchial lymph nodes appears as relatively indistinct increased opacity adjacent to the tracheal bifurcation. With severe enlargement of these lymph nodes, a discrete mass may become apparent with displacement and compression of the major bronchi. Pleural effusion, mediastinal effusion or a mediastinal mass are occasional features. *Blastomyces* infection can mimic diagnoses such as pneumonia, primary pulmonary neoplasia, and lymphoma. Skeletal lesions usually occur

SECTION IV THORAX

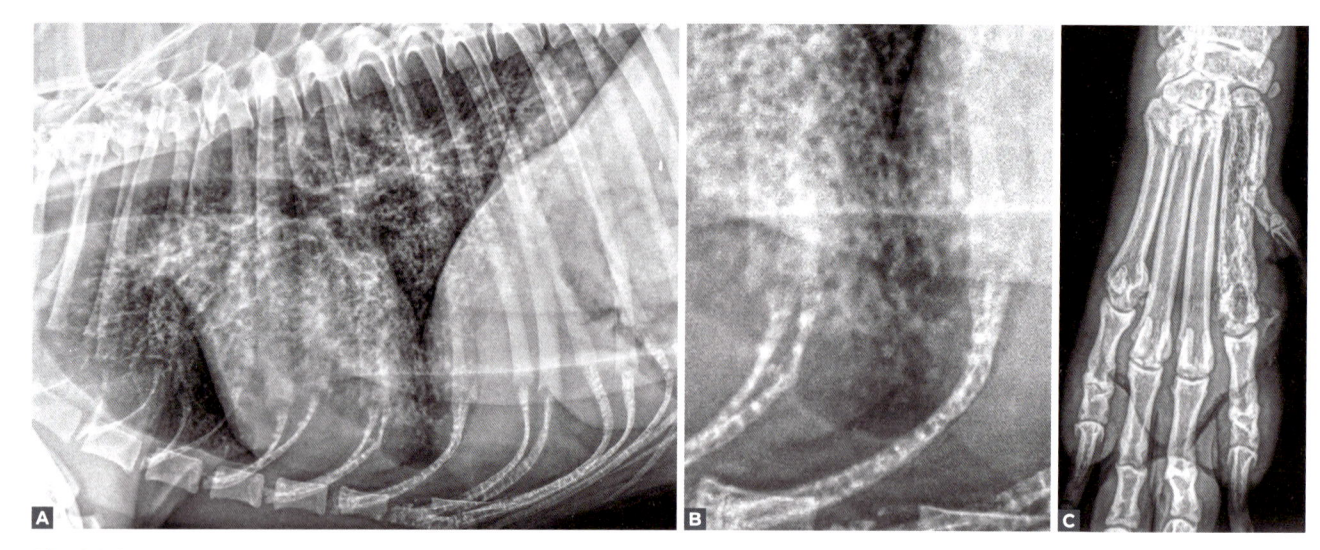

Fig. 22.8 Lateral thoracic radiographs, close-up images of the caudal ventral lung field, and dorsopalmar radiograph of the left metacarpal region of a three-year-old mixed breed dog. The patient presented with swelling of the left thoracic limb, lethargy, and occasional cough. There is generalized increased opacity in the lungs characterized by a severe unstructured interstitial pattern. Small, poorly defined nodules are also present dispersed throughout the lungs, best seen in the thinner peripheral parts of the lung. There is diffuse swelling of the carpus and foot. Foci of moth-eaten lysis are present throughout the second metacarpal bone with extensive destruction of the cortices and trabecular bone of the medullary cavity. There is smooth, relatively well-defined periosteal new bone on the medial and lateral cortices of the metacarpal diaphysis. The changes do not appear to extend to affect the adjacent third metacarpal or phalanges of the first digit. Blastomyces pneumonia and osteomyelitis were confirmed by identification of *Blastomyces* antigen.

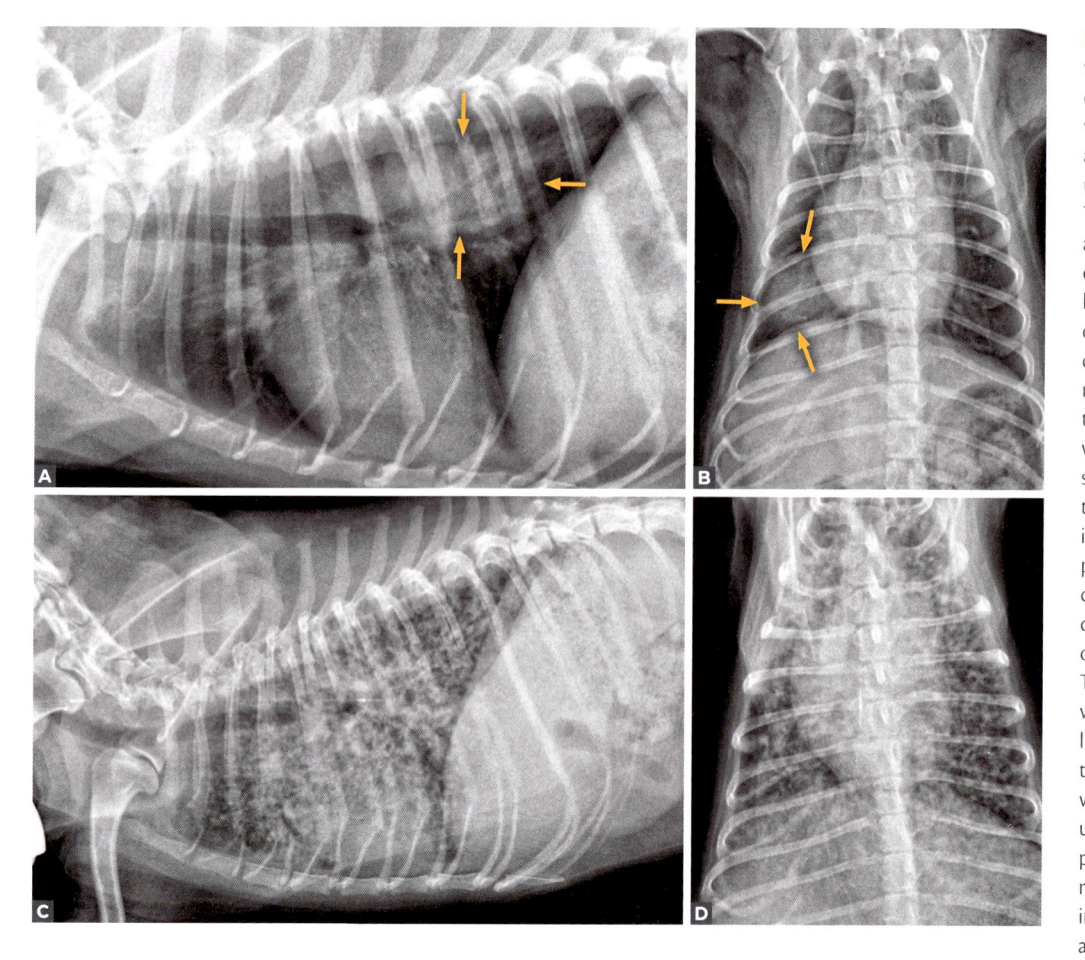

Fig. 22.9 Lateral and ventrodorsal radiographs of a ten-year-old Shih Tzu with a history of dyspnea and cough that have been unresponsive to treatment. The initial radiographs show a poorly defined homogeneous soft tissue opacity mass lesion in the hilar and middle zones of the right caudal lung lobe (arrows). The mass lesion is not evident on the follow-up radiographs, which show a generalized severe unstructured interstitial pattern affecting all lung lobes. Primary pulmonary neoplasia was considered the most likely diagnosis for the mass lesion on the initial radiographs. The patient was treated with corticosteroids to palliate clinical signs based on this presumptive diagnosis which may have contributed to the relatively rapid progression of the pulmonary infiltrates. *Blastomyces* infection was confirmed after the second set of radiographs was obtained.

in the metaphyses and adjacent diaphyses of the long bones (**fig. 22.8C**). The lesions exhibit both lytic and productive osseous remodeling. The radiographic features are similar to malignant osseous neoplasia, such as osteosarcoma. The presence of multiple lesions or lesions at atypical sites for osteosarcoma should increase suspicion of this diagnosis. Cytological or histological evaluations are required to confirm the diagnosis. Involvement of the CNS can be confirmed by CRT or MRI.

Coccidioides mycosis

Coccidioides spp. are soil-borne opportunistic fungal pathogens with widespread distribution in arid and semi-arid regions of North and South America and are most often diagnosed in the southwestern USA.[3, 10, 11] Infection occurs by inhalation, and initial lesions develop in the lung and subsequently the tracheobronchial lymph nodes. Systemic spread to the bone, CNS, and abdominal viscera can occur. Clinical signs may include cough, intermittent fever, lethargy, hyporexia, and weight loss, often with a chronic waxing and waning course. Detection of organisms in samples from affected organs confirms the diagnosis, but in many cases, a presumptive diagnosis is made based on clinical signs, clinicopathological results, positive antibody titers, and response to antifungal treatment.

Radiographs are often normal in infected patients with recent onset or mild clinical signs. Radiographic changes are more likely to be identified in patients with chronic or recurrent relatively severe clinical signs (**figs. 22.10** and **22.11**). Enlargement of the tracheobronchial lymph nodes is

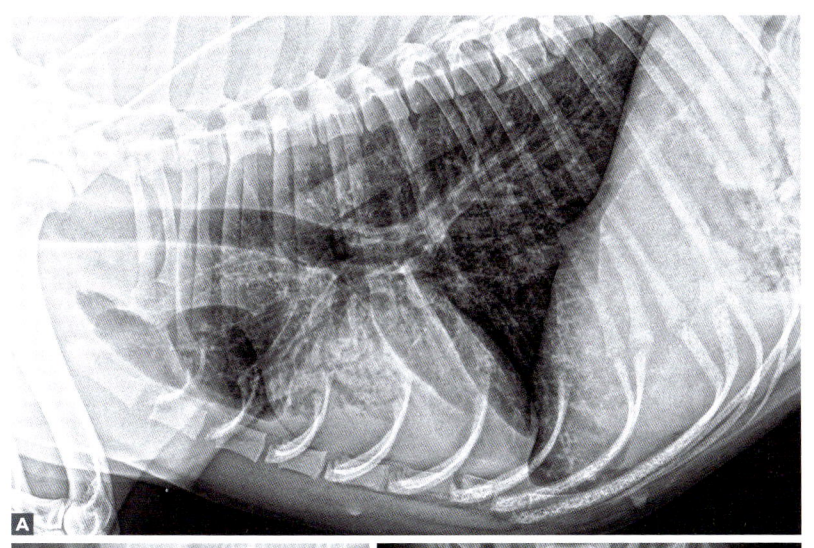

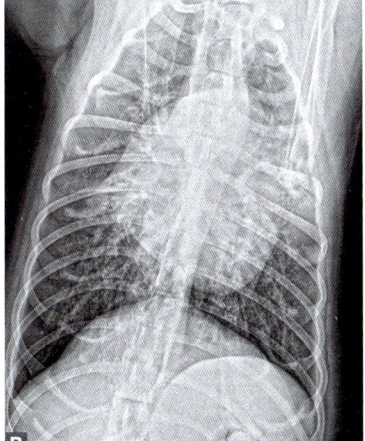

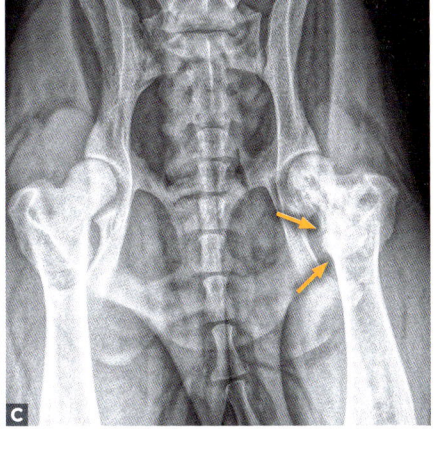

Fig. 22.10 Thoracic and pelvic radiographs of a two-year-old medium-sized mixed breed dog with a history of a productive cough of several weeks duration and severe left pelvic limb lameness from *Coccidioides* infection. The thoracic radiographs show alveolar opacity in the right middle and left cranial lung lobes with several visible air bronchograms and effacement of the cardiac border. A generalized increase in unstructured interstitial opacity is present throughout the remaining lung fields. The pulmonary changes are from *Coccidioides* infection but could also have been attributed to pneumonia. There is well-defined well-mineralized proliferative new bone along the ventral margin of T9. The new bone formation is more extensive than occurs with spondylosis deformans, which would also be unlikely in a patient of this age. This likely represents a *Coccidioides* osteomyelitis lesion. Poorly defined osteolytic foci are present within the left femoral head and neck. There is also well mineralized new bone formation with a somewhat poorly defined border along the medial aspect of the femoral neck and adjacent proximal femoral metaphysis (arrows), consistent with chronic *Coccidioides* osteomyelitis. There is no appreciable extension to affect the left acetabulum. The right hip is normal. Systemic mycotic infections have a broad range of clinical and radiographic presentations, and the radiographic changes can mimic primary pulmonary or osseous neoplasia or multicentric neoplasia.

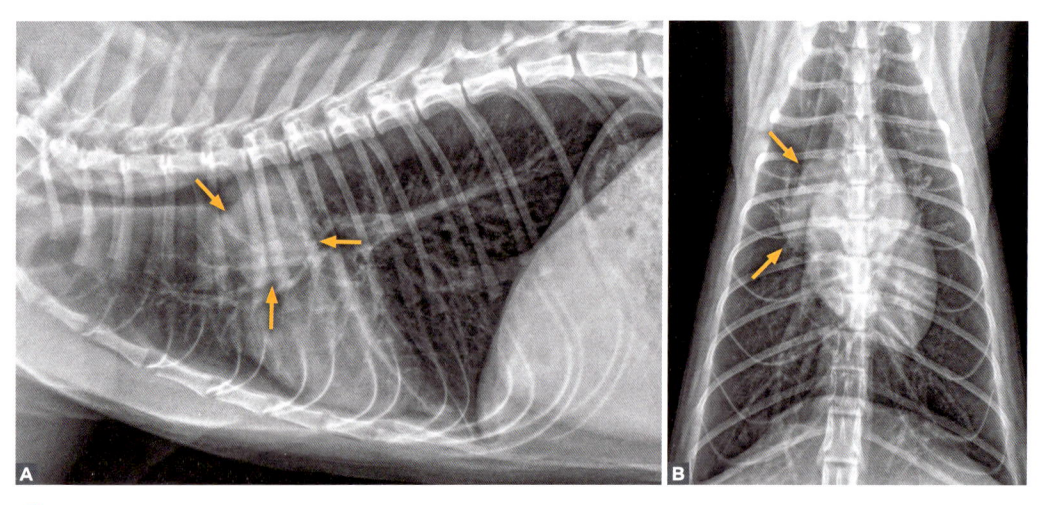

Fig. 22.11 Lateral and ventrodorsal radiographs of a six-month-old Domestic shorthair cat with *Coccidioides* infection. The patient had a presenting history of dyspnea, cough, and lethargy. On the lateral radiograph, a lobulated well-defined homogeneous soft tissue opacity mass lesion is noted overlying the region of the heart base, causing dorsal displacement of the trachea just cranial to the bifurcation (arrows). On the ventrodorsal projection, the mass lesion can be seen overlapping the right cranial cardiac border (arrows). This is consistent with severe enlargement of tracheobronchial lymph nodes.

the most common thoracic radiographic abnormality. In most patients, this is subtle and less severe than seen with lymphoma. Pulmonary abnormalities include focal or multifocal unstructured interstitial infiltrates. Osseous lesions may also be present from systemic spread affecting both the axial and appendicular skeleton and may be solitary or multiple. Most osseous lesions are characterized by proliferative rather than destructive changes. Systemic dissemination may result in infection of the CNS in some patients. MRI can be used to confirm infection and monitor response to treatment.

Other infectious pneumonia

Granulomatous pneumonia may also be caused by a range of pathogens in both canine and feline patients, including *Histoplasma capsulatum*, *Cryptococcus* spp., *Aspergillus* spp., and *Mycobacterium* spp. *Histoplasma* occurs throughout the Americas. *Cryptococcus*, *Aspergillus*, and *Mycobacterium* have a global distribution. These agents can cause both pulmonary and systemic infections.[3] The radiographic changes seen with these infections are quite variable, with changes including unstructured interstitial infiltrates, segmental and lobar alveolar infiltrates, nodules, mass lesions, and thoracic lymph node enlargement (**figs. 22.12** and **22.13**). As infections are sporadic and do not have characteristic imaging features, sometimes mimicking primary, metastatic, or multicentric neoplasia, confirmation of a diagnosis depends upon identifying infectious organisms in diagnostic samples from the airways or lung parenchyma. Both tuberculous and nontuberculous mycobacterial species can cause pulmonary infections in canine and feline patients. If infection by a tuberculous *Mycobacterium* is confirmed, the local public health authorities should be consulted, as infection may be from contact with an infected human, and treatment of infected animals may be proscribed by local regulations.

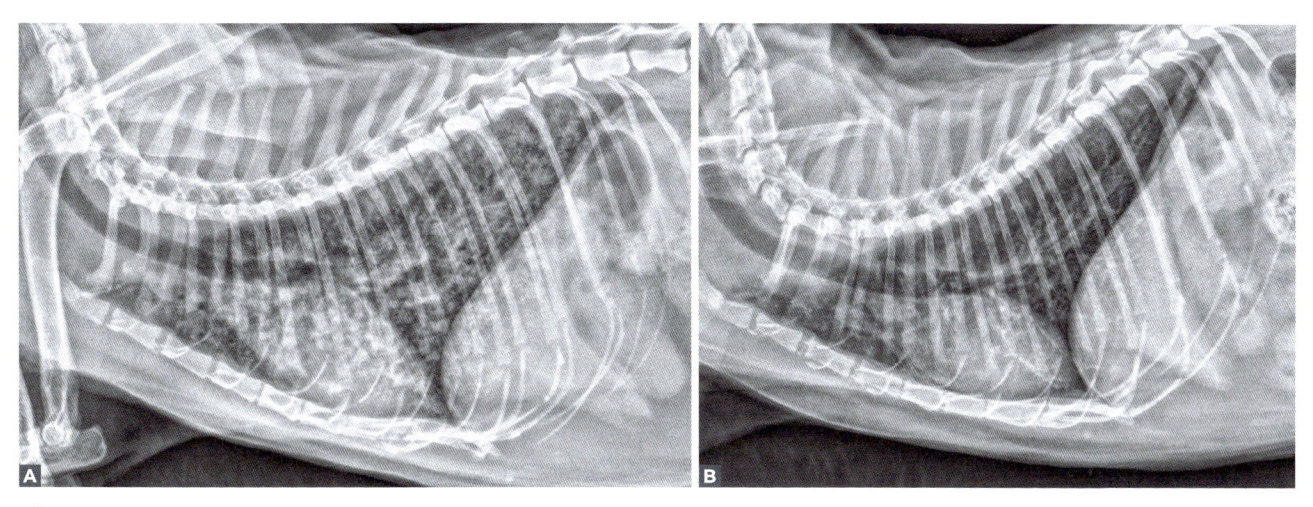

Fig. 22.12 Lateral thoracic radiographs of a two-year-old Domestic shorthair cat with *Histoplasma* pneumonia. The initial radiograph shows a generalized increase in pulmonary soft tissue opacity. This is characterized by a severe unstructured interstitial pattern, almost completely obscuring the pulmonary vessels. The second radiograph was obtained after 10 weeks of antifungal therapy and shows marked improvement in the appearance of the lung with some persistent interstitial opacity. The persistently increased opacity could represent chronic infection or scarring and fibrosis. The pulmonary changes are relatively nonspecific, and potential differential diagnoses include severe feline asthma, severe heartworm-associated airway disease, disseminated multicentric or metastatic neoplasia, and fibrosis.

Fig. 22.13 Lateral and ventrodorsal radiographs of a two-year-old cat with confirmed *Mycobacterium avium* infection. The radiographs show a generalized severe unstructured interstitial pattern with all lung lobes affected. There are more opaque foci in the periphery of the lung on the ventrodorsal projection, representing regions of alveolar opacification. These changes are nonspecific and additional testing such as airway sampling for cytology and culture would be required to obtain a confirmed diagnosis.

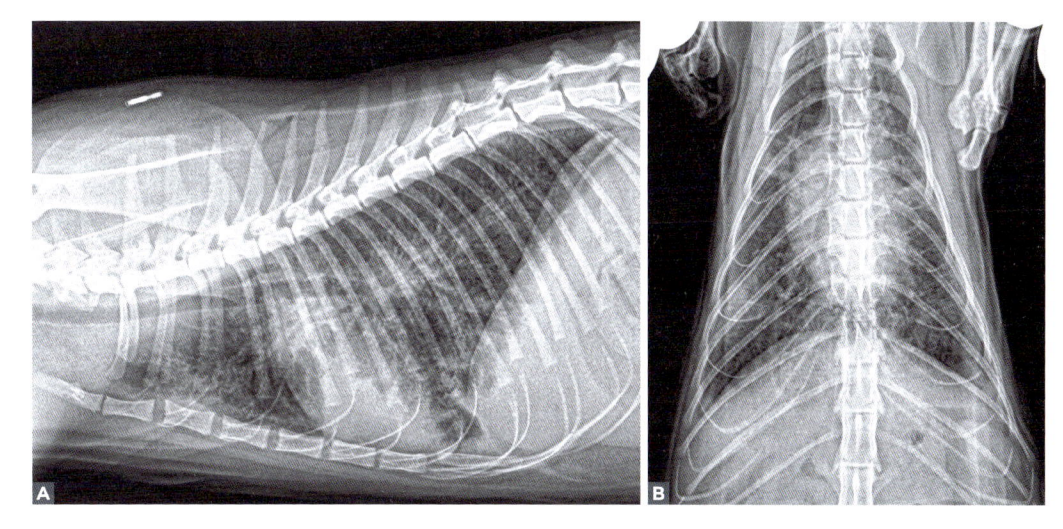

Aelurostrongylus abstrusus infection

Aelurostrongylus abstrusus is a nematode parasite of the airways in cats with global distribution.[3, 12] Infection occurs from consumption of intermediate hosts. Infected patients may be clinically normal or present with a history of chronic cough and intermittent dyspnea, similar to patients with feline asthma/bronchitis. In patients with severe infection, there may also be hemoptysis. The radiographic changes are variable, depending upon the parasite burden and chronicity of infection, and some infected patients appear radiographically normal. Radiographic changes range from bronchial wall thickening, and patchy unstructured interstitial infiltrates to multifocal or diffuse alveolar infiltrates in patients with severe infection (**fig. 22.14**). Confirmation of the diagnosis requires the identification of larvae in samples obtained from the airway or by fecal flotation. Pulmonary abnormalities usually resolve within a few weeks in response to treatment.

SECTION IV THORAX

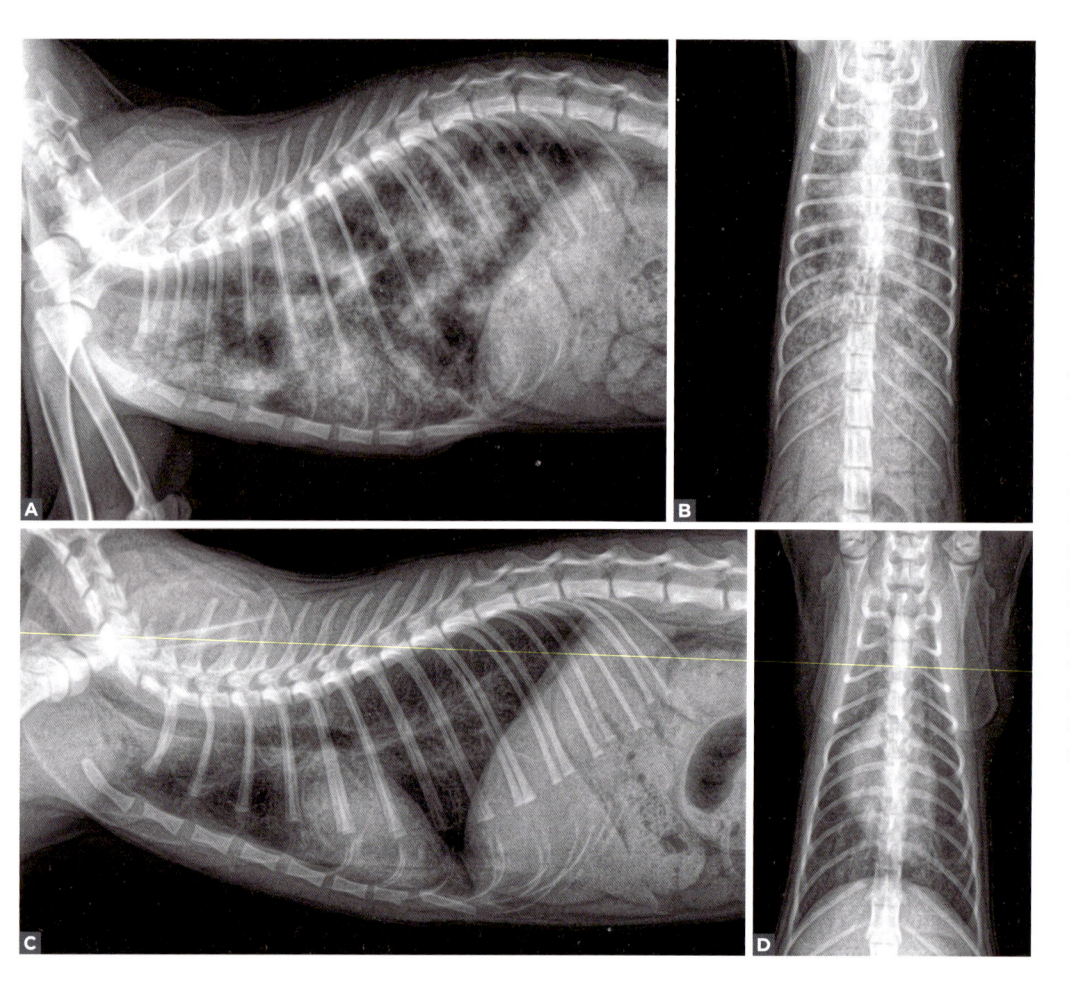

Fig. 22.14 Lateral and ventrodorsal radiographs of a five-month-old cat with confirmed lungworm infection with presenting signs of fever, cough, and lethargy. The initial lateral and ventrodorsal radiographs show generalized increased opacity in the lung fields, completely obscuring the pulmonary vessels and partly obscuring the cardiac silhouette. The pulmonary opacity is characterized by a severe unstructured interstitial pattern with random, poorly defined foci of alveolar opacification. The radiographs obtained 8 weeks after anthelminthic treatment show complete resolution of the pulmonary abnormalities.

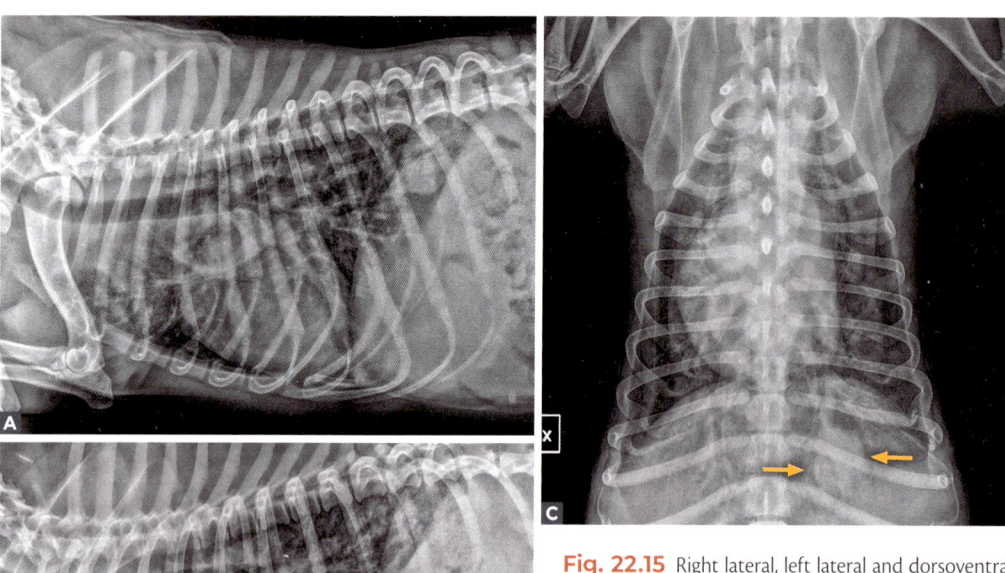

Fig. 22.15 Right lateral, left lateral and dorsoventral radiographs of a three-year-old mixed breed dog with confirmed A. vasorum infection. There is a moderate diffuse increase in unstructured interstitial opacity and diffuse thickening of the bronchial walls. On both lateral projections, there is severely increased interstitial opacity in the cranial lung fields. The left lateral projection also shows a severe increase in interstitial opacity in the caudal dorsal periphery of the right caudal lung lobe, which partly blurs the outline of the diaphragmatic crus. A soft tissue opacity mass-like lesion is present in the caudal dorsal periphery of the left caudal lung lobe, adjacent to the pulmonary artery. This is best seen superimposed on the liver on the dorsoventral projection (arrows). This lesion is consistent with an inflammatory granuloma. Courtesy of Dr. Rossella Terragni, DVM, PhD, SPCAA.

Angiostrongylus vasorum infection

Angiostrongylus vasorum is a nematode parasite of foxes and dogs which is endemic in Europe, Africa, and South America. Sporadic cases have also been recorded on the East Coast of Canada and the United States.[3] The parasite has an indirect life cycle, with dogs acquiring infection by consumption of intermediate gastropod hosts. The adult parasites live in the right heart and pulmonary arteries of the host. Larvae hatch from eggs laid by the females and penetrate the airway walls, and are expectorated, swallowed, and then passed in feces. Clinical signs in affected patients are quite variable. Similar to *Dirofilaria immitis* infection, the presence of lungworms in the pulmonary arteries may result in impaired flow and hypertension. There are also inflammatory changes in the lungs from the presence of adult worms and migrating larvae. The parasites may cause coagulopathy in some patients with hemorrhage in the lungs or at any site in the body. Cardiopulmonary signs such as cough and dyspnea are most common. Patients may also show signs of coagulopathy with hemoptysis, epistaxis, petechiae, or ecchymoses. The diagnosis is confirmed by detection of larvae in feces or by a serum PCR antigen test.

The radiographic changes are quite variable, and some affected patients appear radiographically normal. Pulmonary changes are usually the result of inflammatory reactions and hemorrhage (**fig. 22.15**). These are characterized by bronchial thickening, diffuse increased unstructured interstitial opacity, or random focal or multifocal unstructured interstitial infiltrates.[13] Severe hemorrhage may result in multifocal or peripheral alveolar opacification. In chronic severe cases, acquired pulmonary hypertension may result in right side cardiomegaly, dilation of the main pulmonary artery, and dilation and/or tortuosity of the peripheral pulmonary vessels. Interstitial and alveolar infiltrates surrounding inflammatory granulomas have been reported on CT evaluation of infected individuals.

References

1. Dear JD. Bacterial pneumonia in dogs and cats. *Vet Clin North Am Small Anim Pract* 44:143, 2014.
2. MacDonald ES, Norris CR, Berghaus RD, et al. Clinicopathologic and radiographic features and etiologic agents in cats with histologically confirmed infectious pneumonia: 39 cases (1991-2000). *J Am Vet Med Assoc* 223:1142, 2003.
3. Cohn LA. Diseases of the pulmonary parenchyma. In Ettinger SJ, Feldman EC, Côtè E (editors). Textbook of Veterinary Internal Medicine 8th edition. St Louis, Elsevier, 2017, pp 2730-2806.
4. Biller DS, Meyer CW. Case examples demonstrating the clinical utility of obtaining both right and left lateral thoracic radiographs in small animals. *J Am Anim Hosp Assoc* 23:381, 1987.
5. Lord PF, Gomez JA. Lung lobe collapse: pathophysiology and radiologic significance. *Vet Radiol* 26:187, 1985.
6. Myer CW, Burt JK. Bronchiectasis in the dog: its radiographic appearance. *J Am Vet Radiol Soc* 14:3, 1973.
7. Norris CR, Samii VF. Clinical, radiographic, and pathologic features of bronchiectasis in cats: 12 cases (1987-1999). *J Am Vet Med Assoc* 223:1628, 2003.
8. Wayne A, Davis M, Sinnott VB, Bracker K. Outcomes in dogs with uncomplicated, presumptive bacterial pneumonia treated with short or long course antibiotics. *Can Vet J* 58:610, 2017.
9. Brömel C, Sykes JE. Epidemiology, diagnosis, and treatment of blastomycosis in dogs and cats. *Clin Tech Small Anim Pract* 20:233-239, 2005.
10. Graupmann-Kuzma A, Valentine BA, Shubitz LF, Dial SM, Watrous B, Tornquist SJ. Coccidioidomycosis in dogs and cats: a review. *J Am Anim Hosp Assoc* 44:226-235, 2008.
11. Johnson LR, Herrgesell EJ, Davidson AP, Pappagianis D. Clinical, clinicopathologic, and radiographic findings in dogs with coccidioidomycosis: 24 cases (1995-2000). *J Am Vet Med Assoc* 222:461-466, 2003.
12. Febo E, Crisi PE, Traversa D, Luciani A, Di Tommaso M, Pantaleo S, Santori D, Di Cesare A, Boari A, Terragni R, Vignoli M. Comparison of clinical and imaging findings in cats with single and mixed lungworm infection. *J Feline Med Surg* 21:581-589, 2019.
13. Boag AK, Lamb CR, Chapman PS, Boswood A. Radiographic findings in 16 dogs infected with *Angiostrongylus vasorum*. *Vet Rec* 154:426-430, 2004.
14. Dennler M, Makara M, Kranjc A, Schnyder M, Ossent P, Deplazes P, Ohlerth S, Glaus TM. Thoracic computed tomography findings in dogs experimentally infected with *Angiostrongylus vasorum*. *Vet Radiol Ultrasound* 52:289-294, 2011.

CHAPTER 23

Pulmonary infiltrations

Margareta Uhlhorn, Carolina Carlsson Nilemo and Jessica Ingman

KEY POINTS

- Pulmonary disease sufficient to cause respiratory signs can occur in the absence of radiographic changes.
- Different pulmonary diseases may have overlapping radiological appearances, and it is crucial to interpret imaging findings in light of history and other clinical data.
- Both cats and dogs can be affected by fibrotic interstitial lung disease.
- Radiologically air-filled lung lesions are often difficult to distinguish from each other and names are often used interchangeably.
- Noncardiogenic edema has multiple etiologies but the radiographic appearance is similar for all.
- Primary pulmonary neoplasia is the most likely diagnosis for a single mass in both dogs and cats.
- Pulmonary histiocytic sarcoma often presents as several pulmonary masses.

Feline bronchial disease and feline asthma

Feline asthma and feline chronic bronchitis are idiopathic inflammatory airway diseases with small airway obstruction, causing a chronic cough. The broader term feline lower airway disease encompasses both inflammatory and noninflammatory bronchial diseases.

It is challenging to discriminate feline asthma from chronic bronchitis because of overlapping clinical and radiological findings. Feline asthma is described as an allergic condition with eosinophilic airway inflammation, whereas chronic bronchitis has neutrophilic airway inflammation; however, mixed inflammation is commonly seen in bronchoalveolar lavage.[1]

Affected cats are often young to middle-aged. Chronic cough is the most common clinical sign. Other symptoms are wheezing, increased respiratory effort, tachypnea, nasal discharge and sneezing.[1,2]

Radiological findings vary depending on the severity and duration of the disease. Radiographs may be normal and the absence of changes does not rule out feline lower airway disease. A bronchial pattern is most commonly seen with thickened bronchial walls, in transverse seen as doughnuts and in longitudinal as tramlines (**fig. 23.1**). In addition, a diffuse or patchy unstructured interstitial pattern is commonly seen, and areas with alveolar pattern can be present.[1,3] *Dirofilaria immitis*-associated airway disease may have similar changes and is the major differential diagnosis in endemic regions. Similar to radiography, bronchial thickening, increased peribronchovascular interstitial opacity, and ground-glass opacity can be seen on CT.[2]

SECTION IV THORAX

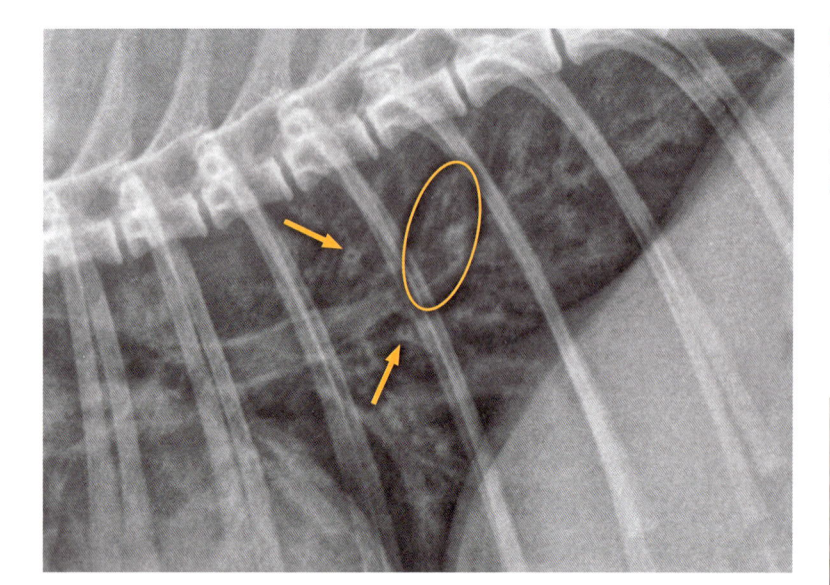

Fig. 23.1 Close-up left lateral recumbency thoracic radiograph of a one-year-old Domestic shorthair cat illustrating a generalized bronchial pattern. The bronchial walls are moderately thickened and multiple doughnuts (bronchi in transverse, arrows) and tramlines (parallel lines of bronchi in longitudinal, encircled) are seen.

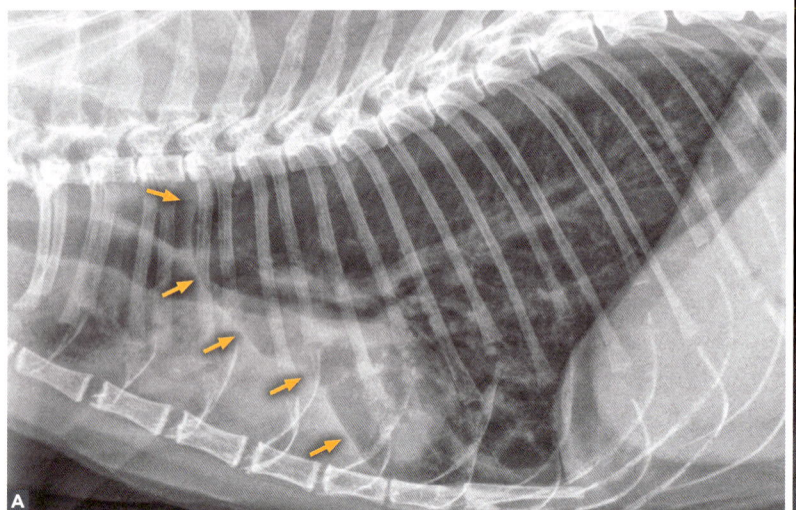

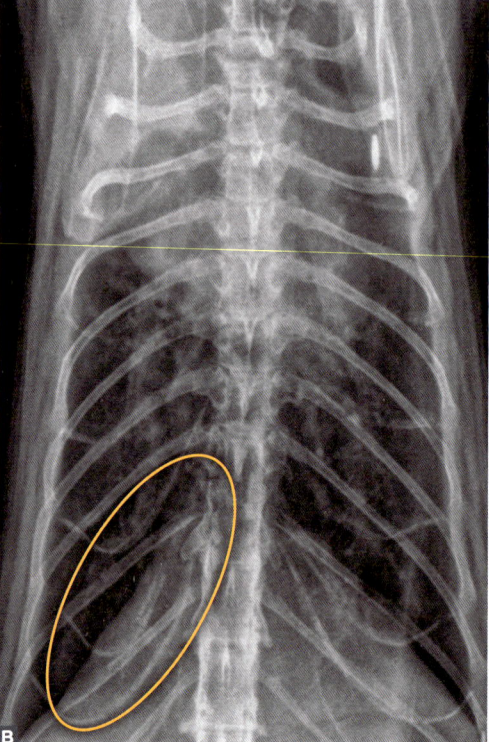

Fig. 23.2 Thoracic left lateral recumbency (**A**) and ventrodorsal (**B**) radiographs of an 11-year-old Siamese cat with feline asthma and recent worsening cough, tachypnea, wheezing breathing sounds and breathing with increased abdominal effort. A mild generalized bronchial pattern and pulmonary hyperinflation can be seen. (**A**) The right caudal lung lobe is hyperinflated and extends further cranial (arrows) and caudal than normally. The diaphragm is flattened and caudally displaced causing an increase in distance between the cardiac silhouette and the diaphragm. (**B**) Tenting of the diaphragm is seen predominantly in the right hemithorax (encircled). The diaphragm is pushed caudally by the hyperinflated lung causing tension at the diaphragmatic insertion points on the rib cage. The mild asymmetry of the diaphragm can be explained by a more severe right sided hyperinflation. The right cranial lung lobe and possibly also the right middle lung lobe are of soft tissue opacity and small air bronchograms can faintly be seen in the LLR projection. The appearance of the right cranial and possibly right middle lung lobe is consistent with collapse secondary to mucus plugs or, less likely, bronchopneumonia.

Air-trapping from small airway obstruction is often present, causing pulmonary hyperinflation with an enlarged radiolucent lung. This causes an increased distance between the cardiac silhouette and the diaphragm and flattening of the diaphragm.[1] On the ventrodorsal or dorsoventral view the ribs are oriented perpendicular or almost perpendicular to the spine and the thorax loses its normal triangular shape. In severe cases there may be tenting of the diaphragm. Tenting of the diaphragm is more easily seen in the ventrodorsal or dorsoventral projection (**fig. 23.2**). A mosaic pattern (patchy areas of variable attenuation) may be seen in areas of air-trapping in CT.[4]

Another commonly recognized finding in feline asthma is atelectasis of the right middle lung lobe secondary to mucoid plugging and bronchial obstruction. The collapsed lobe appears small

CHAPTER 23 Pulmonary infiltrations

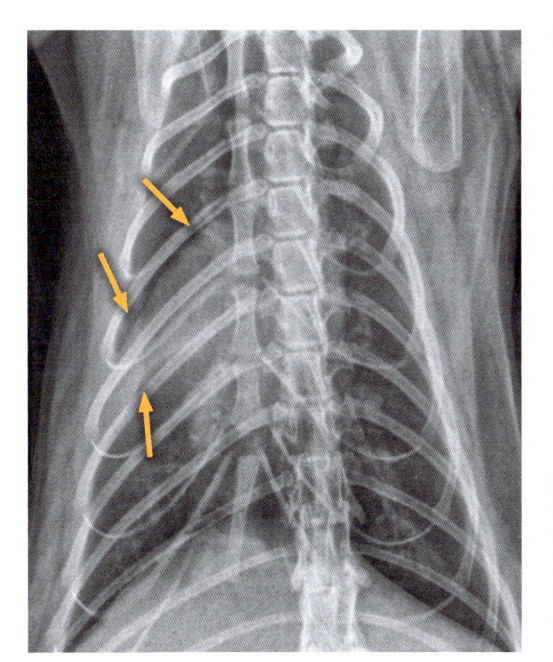

Fig. 23.3 Ventrodorsal thoracic radiograph of a seven-year-old Siamese cat with a history of treatment for feline asthma. The right middle lung lobe is collapsed with a homogeneous soft tissue opacity and distinct margins causing a lobar sign towards the aerated cranial and caudal lung lobes (arrows). The right middle lung lobe is causing border effacement with the cardiac silhouette. Mild right mediastinal shift of the cardiac silhouette towards the atelectatic lung. A generalized bronchial pattern is also present.

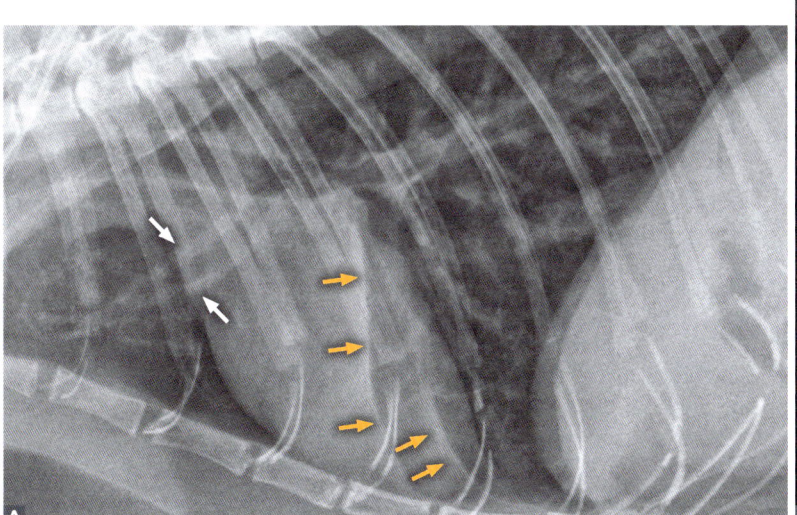

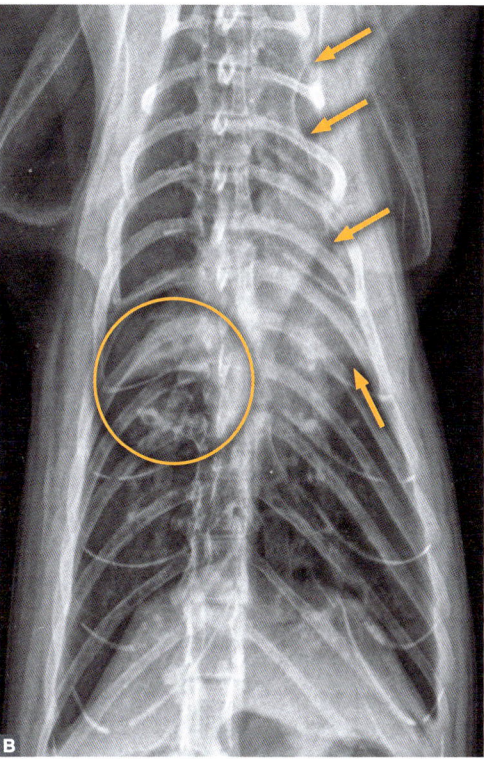

Fig. 23.4 Thoracic left lateral recumbency (**A**) and ventrodorsal (**B**) radiographs of a 14-year-old Domestic shorthair cat diagnosed with feline asthma for the last five years and recent increase in coughing. A generalized bronchial pattern is present. (**B**) The right middle lung lobe is collapsed and small, with a triangular shape (encircled). A lobar sign is seen between the right middle lung lobe and the right cranial and caudal lung lobes. The left cranial lung lobe is also collapsed (arrows) causing a leftward mediastinal shift of the cardiac silhouette. (**A**) Two slightly curved soft tissue lines are superimposed on the cardiac silhouette (arrows). These represent the caudal borders of the collapsed right middle and left cranial lung lobes. Only one pair of pulmonary vessels are seen in the cranial thorax (white arrows). The vessels to the collapsed left cranial lung lobe are surrounded by soft tissue opacity and obscured. The increased opacity of the collapsed left cranial lung lobe cannot be seen in the left lateral recumbency projection because of hyperinflation of the right cranial lung lobe. Hyperinflation of the caudal lung lobes causes flattening of the diaphragm and increased distance between the caudal cardiac silhouette and the diaphragm. Slight rotation of the thorax in (**B**) causes artifactual asymmetry of the caudal lobes.

and triangular and has a homogeneous soft tissue opacity (**figs. 23.3** and **23.4**). Less commonly, there is atelectasis of the right cranial or left cranial lung lobes. Bronchial mucus accumulation or plugs may also create a nodular-like pattern. Secondary broncholithiasis and bronchiectasis may be present in chronic cases. Filling of dilated bronchi with hyperplastic mucosa and mucus may be seen on radiographs in chronic severe cases, appearing as branching linear soft tissue opacity structures. This is sometimes described as a finger in glove pattern and is analogous to the tree-in-bud pattern of CT.[1,2]

SECTION IV THORAX

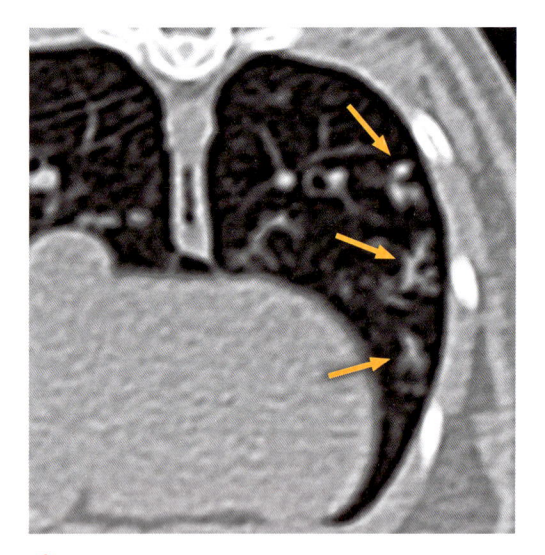

Fig. 23.5 Close-up transverse CT image displayed in a lung window of an 11-year-old Domestic shorthair cat, illustrating the tree-in-bud pattern. In the periphery of the left caudal lung lobe, soft tissue structures can be seen with a mix of linear and nodular shapes resembling a budding tree (arrows).

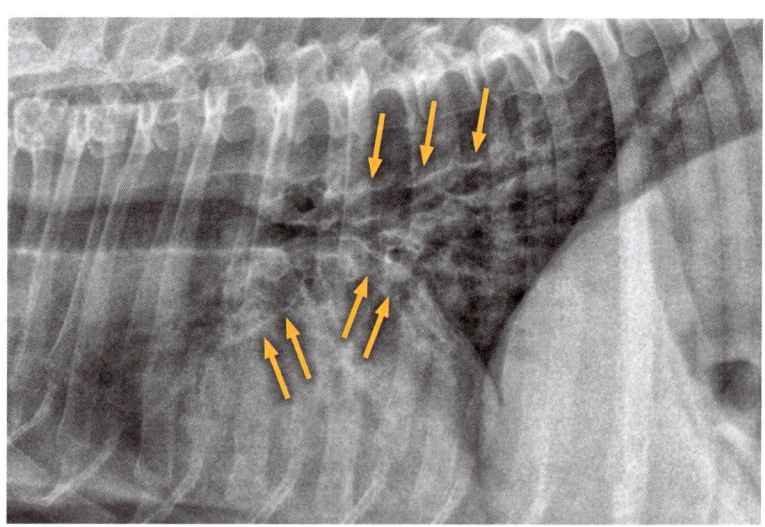

Fig. 23.6 Thoracic left lateral recumbency radiograph of a 15-year-old West Highland White Terrier, illustrating mineralized bronchial walls (arrows). The dog had a history of chronic cough and bronchial pattern on multiple radiographs in the preceding three years and was diagnosed with chronic bronchitis, possibly in combination with pulmonary fibrosis. The mineralized bronchi may be an age-related change or secondary to chronic bronchitis.

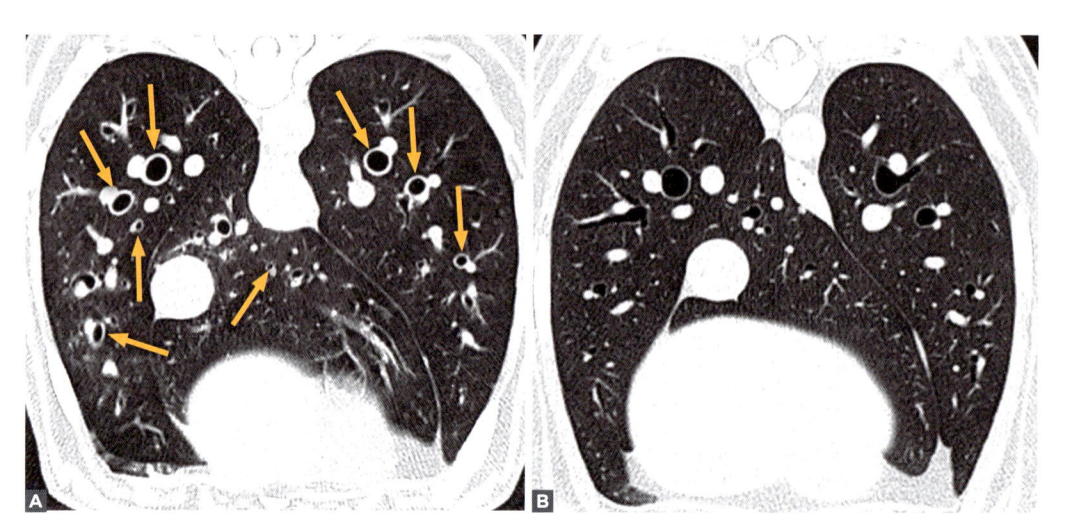

Fig. 23.7 Transverse CT images displayed in a lung window of two adult dogs to illustrate thickened bronchial walls (arrows in [A]) in comparison with normal bronchial walls (B) on CT.

Fig. 23.8 Close-up image of the accessory lung lobe area in a right lateral recumbency thoracic radiograph of a five-year-old spayed female Cavalier King Charles Spaniel. Diagnosed as eosinophilic bronchopneumonia based on bronchoalveolar lavage, marked blood eosinophilia, and radiographic appearance. There is diffuse thickening of bronchial walls. Bronchi with thickened walls, projected end-on in cross-section, are seen as doughnuts. Similar bronchi projected *en face* appear as converging lines or tramlines.

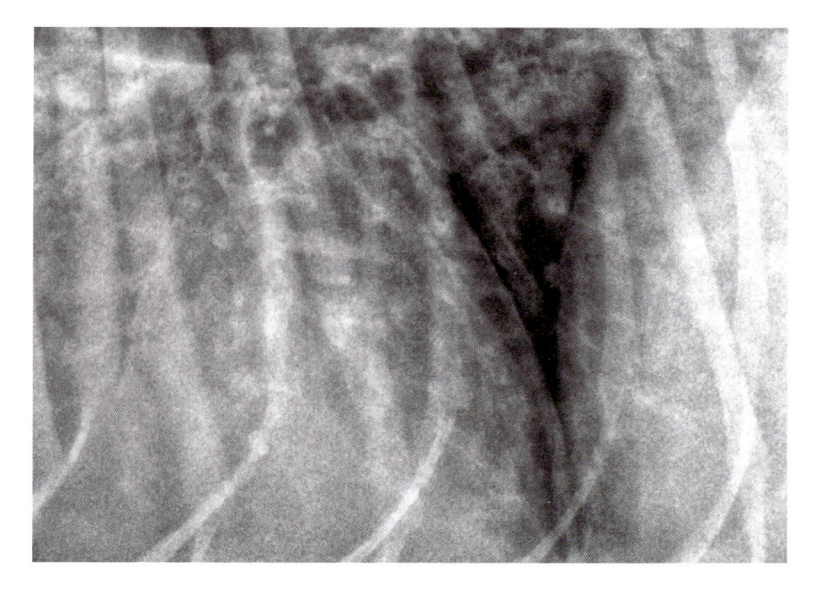

CT tree-in-bud pattern (**fig. 23.5**) is seen when the dilated small branching airways are filled with secretions and hyperplastic tissue and the pattern resembles a budding tree.[2,4] The shape can be branching V or Y lines, nodular or both.[2] Spontaneous rib fractures may occur secondary to severe coughing, loss of lung compliance and increased respiratory effort. It is more commonly seen in the midportion of the caudal ribs, and multiple rib fractures with different stages of healing may be present.[1]

Canine bronchial disease

Canine chronic bronchitis is defined as an inflammatory chronic lower airway disease, causing harsh cough almost daily for at least two months. The diagnosis is sometimes by exclusion. It occurs frequently with diseases with overlapping signs including tracheal collapse and myxomatous mitral valve disease (MMVD), since the predisposed patients are middle-aged to older small breed dogs and some patients with a chronic cough have several contributing etiologies.[5]

Radiographs are relatively insensitive for the diagnosis of chronic bronchitis in dogs and a significant proportion of patients appear normal. On thoracic radiographs, a bronchial pattern with an increased amount of both doughnuts (also called ring shadows) and tramlines can be seen caused by thickening of the bronchial walls (**figs. 23.1** and **23.8**). Cellular or fluid infiltrations in the immediate peribronchial interstitium may also contribute to a bronchial pattern. This is sometimes referred to as peribronchial cuffing but the distinction is quite tenuous on survey radiographs. Secondary bronchiectasis and hyperinflation may be present.[5]

Bronchial mineralization is a common, age-related, clinically insignificant change especially in smaller dogs (**fig. 23.6**) and is an uncommon change secondary to chronic bronchitis. Bronchial mineralization can also be related to hyperadrenocorticism.[3]

The findings in chronic bronchitis in CT examinations are similar to those in thoracic radiographs, with thickened walls (**fig. 23.7**). Occasionally mucus plugs may be identified. Just as chronic bronchitis cannot be ruled out based on normal radiographs some affected patients have a normal CT examination.

Radiographic and CT examinations may not demonstrate abnormalities in some patients with chronic bronchitis but are useful for confirming or excluding other etiologies of a chronic cough.

Eosinophilic bronchopneumopathy

Eosinophilic bronchopneumopathy (also called pulmonary infiltrate with eosinophilia) in dogs is a disease complex characterized by eosinophilic infiltration of bronchial walls and pulmonary parenchyma. Eosinophilic bronchopneumopathy is considered idiopathic, but eosinophilic infiltration of the lung can also occur from parasitic, fungal or neoplastic etiologies with similar radiographic changes. The radiographic findings have a multifocal or generalized distribution. Reported abnormalities include moderate to severe bronchointerstitial patterns (**figs. 23.8-23.10**), areas of alveolar pattern (**fig. 23.11**) and thickened bronchial walls. Chronic cases may have bronchiectasis. Reported computed tomographic changes are interstitial pulmonary parenchymal infiltrates, bronchial wall thickening, bronchial plugging by mucus and debris, and bronchiectasis[6] (**figs. 23.12** and **23.13**). Rare cases may have nodules and masses in the pulmonary parenchyma, referred to as eosinophilic granulomatous pneumonia.[7]

SECTION IV THORAX

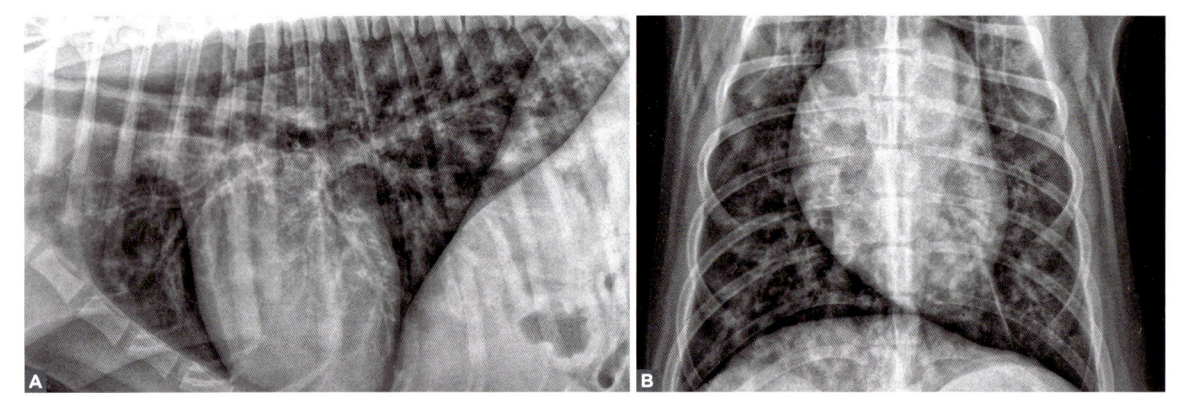

Fig. 23.9 Thoracic radiographs, left lateral recumbency (**A**) and ventrodorsal (**B**) projections of a three-year-old female Standard Poodle. She had severe circulating eosinophilia, 60% eosinophils on bronchoalveolar lavage cytology and was diagnosed with eosinophilic bronchopneumopathy. There is a generalized bronchointerstitial pattern throughout all lung lobes. In some areas, the interstitial component becomes slightly patchy.

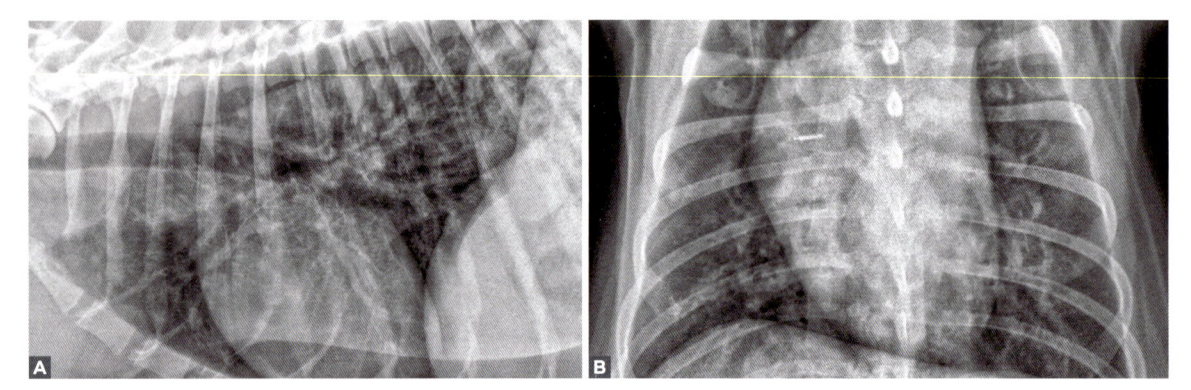

Fig. 23.10 An eight-year-old female castrated English Springer Spaniel. Left lateral recumbency (**A**) and close-up ventrodorsal (**B**) projections of the thorax. There is a generalized mixed bronchial and unstructured interstitial pattern from eosinophilic bronchopneumopathy. This dog has a somewhat greater interstitial component and in the caudal lung lobes this partly obscures the margins of the pulmonary vasculature and aorta.

Fig. 23.11 (**A**) Right lateral recumbency, (**B**) left lateral recumbency and (**C**) ventrodorsal projections of the thorax of an eight-year-old male Dachshund. This dog was diagnosed with eosinophilic bronchopneumopathy based on hematology, bronchoalveolar lavage and radiography. Soft tissue opacity obscures the vascular margins and creates a faint air bronchogram in the left caudal lung lobe. This is consistent with a severe unstructured coalescing to alveolar pattern.

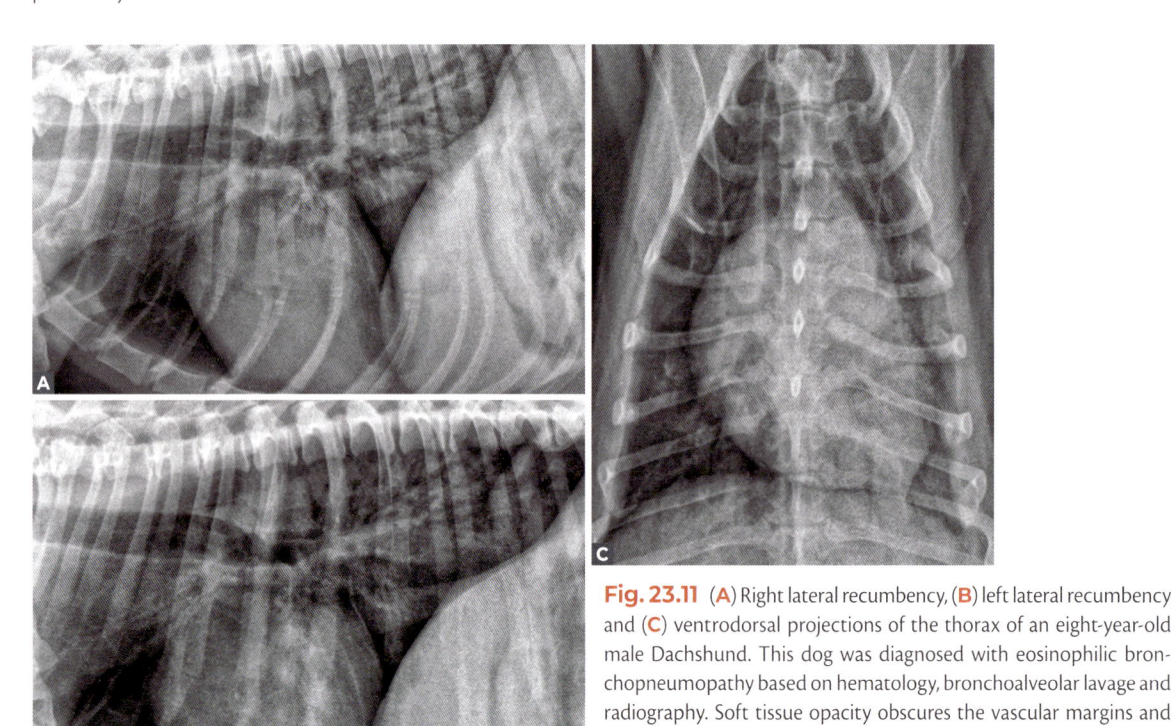

CHAPTER 23 Pulmonary infiltrations

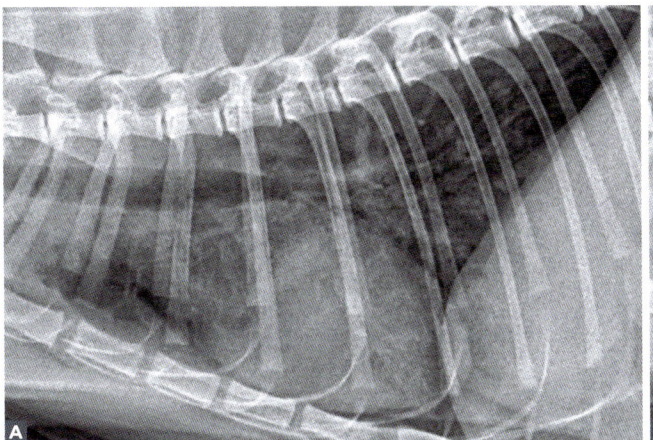

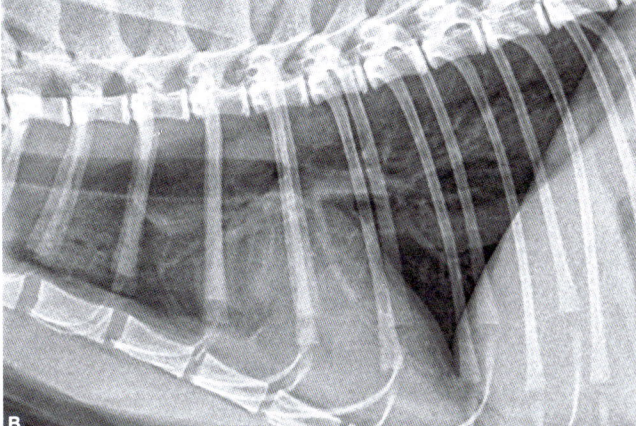

Fig. 23.12 A two-year-old castrated male Abyssinian cat. (**A**) Left lateral recumbency thoracic radiograph of the thorax at initial presentation for sudden onset of coughing. There is a moderate interstitial pattern in the accessory lung lobe area. The opacity is obscuring the borders of the caudal vena cava. The cat was diagnosed with eosinophilic bronchopneumopathy, and treatment was initiated. (**B**) Left lateral recumbency thoracic radiograph of the same cat nine months later. (**C**) A transverse CT reconstruction of the cat's lungs at initial presentation. The image is windowed for lungs and shows the thorax at the level of the caudal and the accessory lung lobes. Changes were seen in all lung lobes, but more marked in the caudal lobes. There is a mix of patterns: multifocal distinctly outlined areas of interstitial pattern (ground-glass opacity) interspersed with a reticular pattern and normal-appearing lung tissue. There is also multifocal moderate thickening of bronchial walls. The CT appearance is non-specific but shows more severe changes and extensive changes than apparent on radiograph (**A**), obtained at the same time.

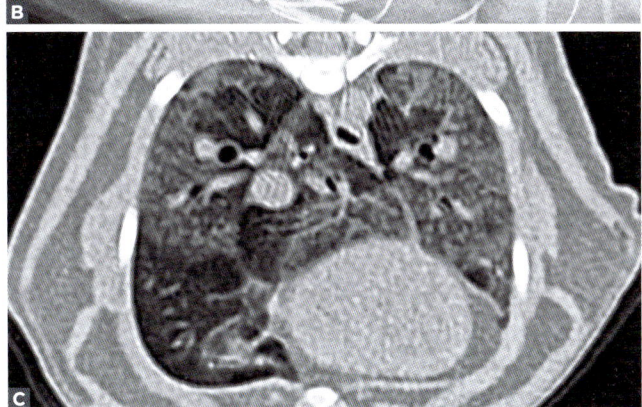

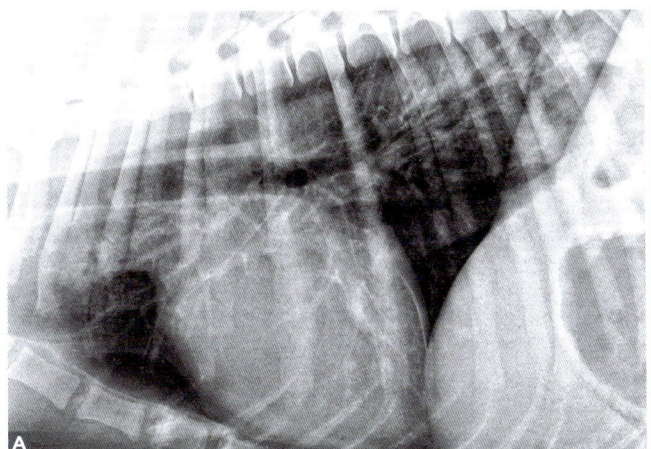

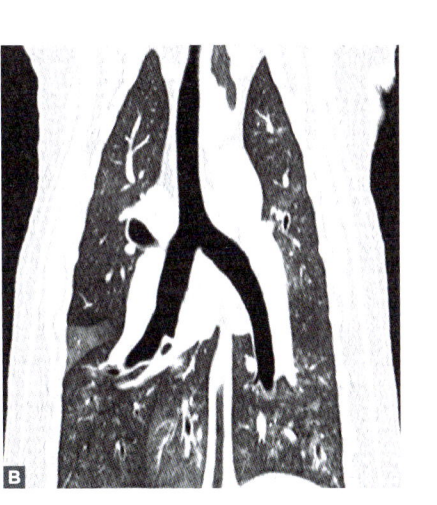

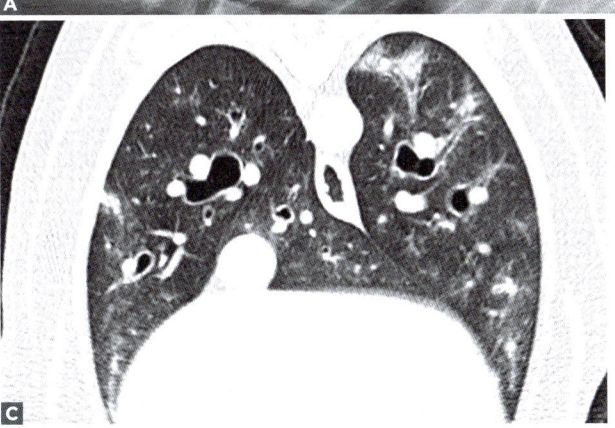

Fig. 23.13 An 11-year-old castrated male Golden Retriever that had been coughing for one month. A left lateral recumbency radiograph (**A**) and two CT images with lung windowing reconstructed in dorsal (**B**) and transverse (**C**) planes of the thorax. (**A**) There are patches of moderate unstructured interstitial pattern in the caudodorsal lung field. In the CT images, changes are seen in more detail and seem more severe. In the dorsal reconstruction (**B**), a difference in attenuation is seen between the cranial and caudal lung fields. The caudal lung fields have a higher attenuation (are opaquer), a so-called ground-glass opacity. The cranial lung lobes appear more normal. In the transverse CT image (**C**), except for the general ground-glass opacity, there are also foci with even higher attenuation and bronchial thickening. Bronchoalveolar lavage showed severe eosinophilia. The diagnosis was eosinophilic bronchopneumopathy.

Bronchiectasis

Bronchiectasis is an irreversible and progressive dilation of the bronchi secondary to chronic airway inflammation and bronchial obstruction by inflammatory exudate, causing destruction of the normal bronchial wall and impaired respiratory secretion clearance. It leads to a vicious cycle of pooling of mucus and exudate in the bronchial lumen predisposing to repeat infection, inflammatory response and further damage and weakening of the bronchial wall.

Thus, bronchiectasis is a sequel or complication of other airway diseases such as pneumonia (including infectious, aspiration, foreign body or interstitial), eosinophilic bronchopneumopathy, inflammatory airway diseases such as chronic bronchitis, or ciliary dyskinesia.[8] In cats, the underlying diseases are commonly chronic bronchitis, obstructive neoplasia, or bronchopneumonia.[9] Middle-aged to older dogs and older male cats are more often affected. Multiple dog breeds have been reported with bronchiectasis and a predilection in Cocker Spaniels has been proposed.[8,10]

Coughing is the most common clinical sign, but the clinical signs are related to the underlying disease. Bronchiectasis has also been diagnosed in patients without clinical symptoms from the respiratory tract. Bronchiectasis can be diagnosed with radiology, bronchoscopy or computed tomography (CT). It can be missed on radiographs in early or mild cases in both dogs and cats. In one study, the sensitivity of detecting bronchiectasis in dogs was 60% on radiography, 92% at bronchoscopy, and 100% in CT.[8] In affected patients, the bronchi are visible further peripheral than usual on radiographs. Bronchiectasis in dogs and cats is described as tubular and saccular. Tubular bronchiectasis (**fig. 23.14**) is the most common type in both dogs[3,9-11] and cats,[9] and has relatively uniform dilation without peripheral tapering. In saccular bronchiectasis (**fig. 23.15**), the bronchi show multifocal balloon or sac like dilations and it has been compared with a cluster of grapes. Fluid filling of peripheral saccular dilations may appear as nodular-like lesions. Both types can be present in one patient.

The distribution of bronchiectasis may be generalized, multifocal, lobar or focal. Generalized and multifocal bronchiectasis is described as most commonly seen in dogs.[8,10,11] Focal, lobar or multifocal disease more often affects one or both of the right cranial and right middle lung lobes (**fig. 23.16**).

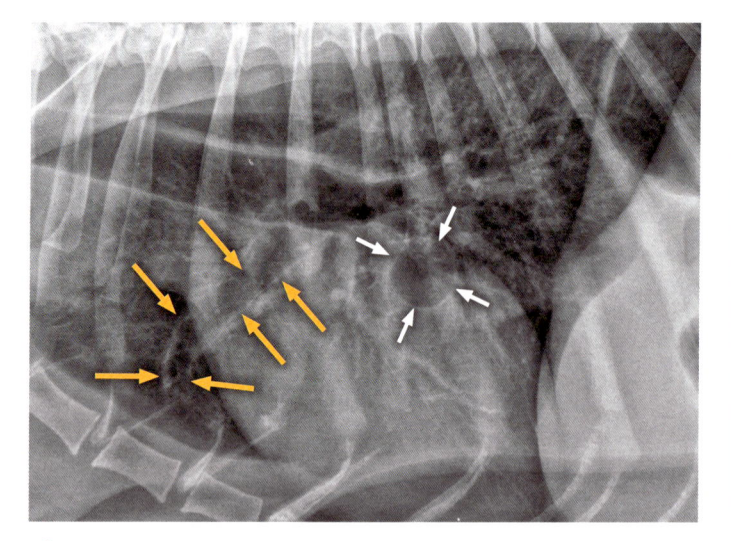

Fig. 23.14 Left lateral recumbency thoracic radiograph of a 12-year-old Australian Shepherd with a cough of several months that had worsened recently. The bronchus to the right cranial lung lobe is widened with thin relatively parallel bronchial walls that can be followed further peripheral than normally seen. This represents the tubular type of bronchiectasis (orange arrows). A round thin-walled radiolucent lesion is superimposed on the caudodorsal cardiac border, representing a bullae and may be related to a chronic airway disease but equally may be an incidental finding (white arrows).

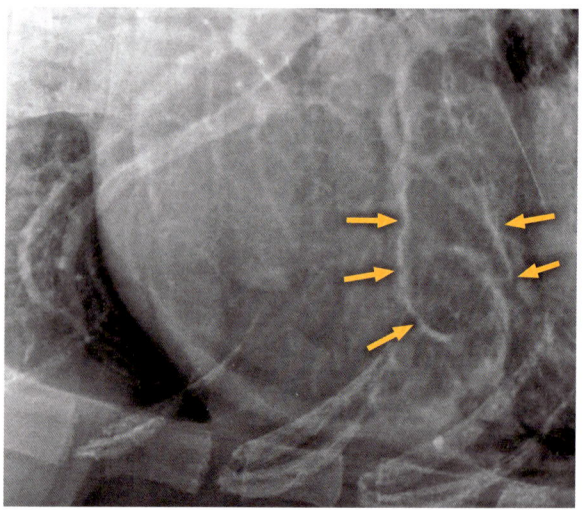

Fig. 23.15 Close-up thoracic left lateral recumbency radiograph of a dog illustrating saccular bronchiectasis in the right middle lung lobe. The bronchi are dilated in the periphery of the lung and the bronchial walls are thick, irregular and wavy in shape (arrows).

CHAPTER 23 Pulmonary infiltrations

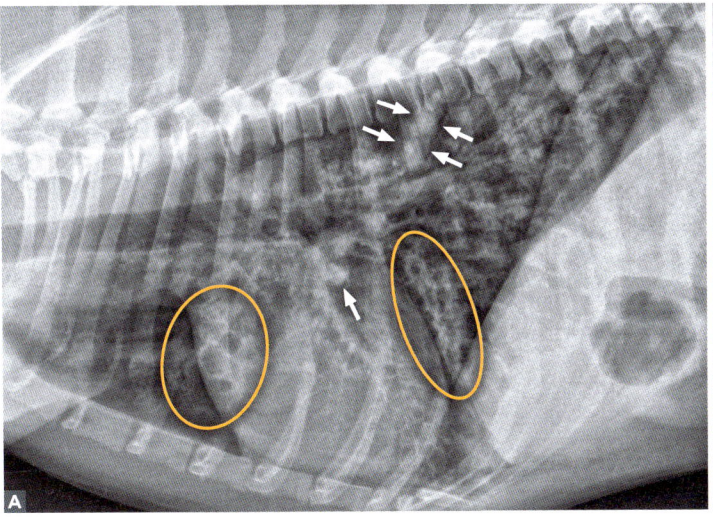

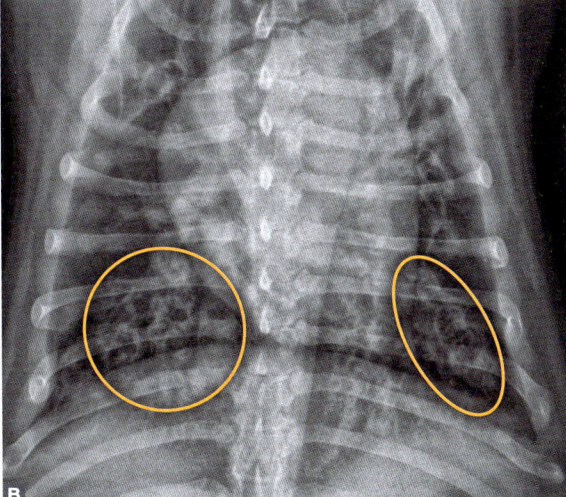

Fig. 23.16 Left lateral recumbency and ventrodorsal radiographs of the thorax of a six-year-old Glen of Imaal Terrier with generalized saccular bronchiectasis. (A, B) The bronchi are thickened in all lung lobes and have a cystic and saccular shape and can be followed to the periphery of the lung (encircled). (A) Multiple nodular and confluent foci of soft tissue opacity are seen in the dorsal aspect of the lung (white arrows). These areas corresponded to accumulations of mucus and pus confirmed on bronchoscopy. The dog was presented with chronic cough and recurring bacterial pneumonia for at least one year. Necropsy revealed a chronic peribronchiolitis and acute multifocal to confluent fibrinopurulent and necrotizing bronchopneumonia with bacteria.

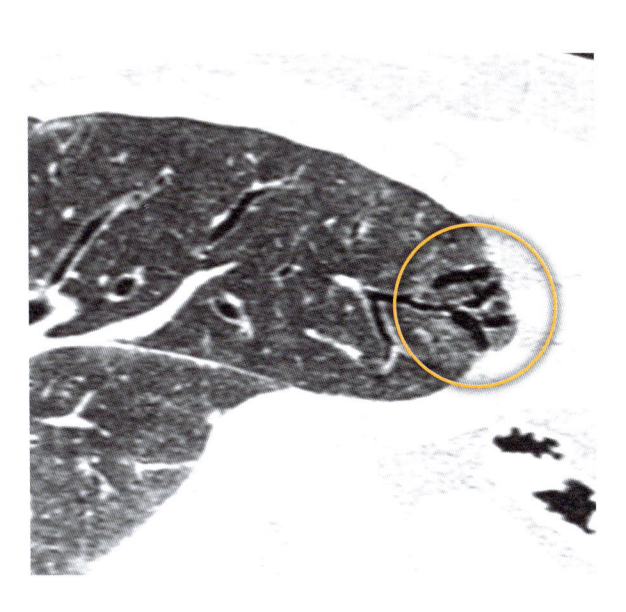

Fig. 23.17 CT image displayed in a lung window of a seven-year-old Bullmastiff with focal peripheral bronchiectasis. Several dilated bronchial segments are present in the caudal dorsal periphery of the right caudal lung lobe (encircled).

In cats, it is more often the caudal or middle lobes that are affected.

Bronchiectasis is more easily recognized in CT because of the lack of summation. The dilated bronchi are wider than the adjacent vessels, and the dilation may extend to the periphery of the lung tissue (**fig. 23.17**). The bronchoarterial ratio threshold (bronchial lumen to pulmonary artery diameter) in normal dogs is suggested to be <2.0, although this will exclude some patients with mild disease.[11] Other concurrent CT findings include pulmonary consolidation, bronchial wall thickening and occasionally bronchial luminal occlusion.

Pulmonary fibrosis

Idiopathic pulmonary fibrosis belongs to a heterogeneous group of interstitial lung diseases that affect humans, cats and dogs. Pulmonary fibrosis has varying etiologies, but in the majority of cases the etiology remains unknown. Canine idiopathic pulmonary fibrosis mainly affects West Highland White Terriers, but other breeds can be affected as well. Canine idiopathic pulmonary fibrosis is usually diagnosed in older dogs. Cats can be affected at any age.

The commonly reported radiographic appearance in dogs is a generalized moderate to severe mixed

SECTION IV THORAX

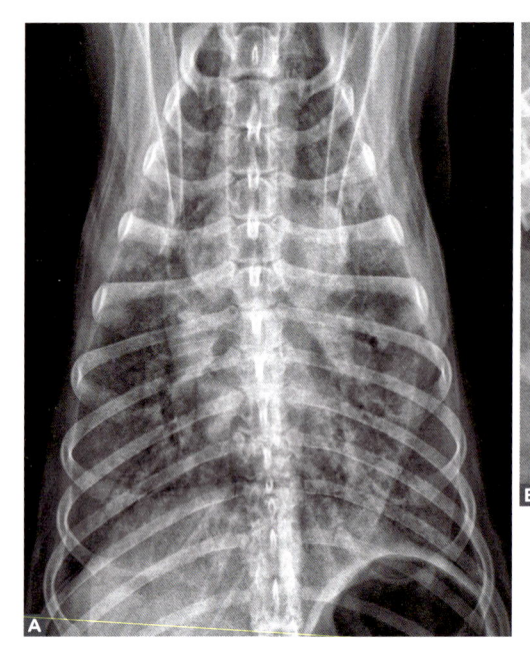

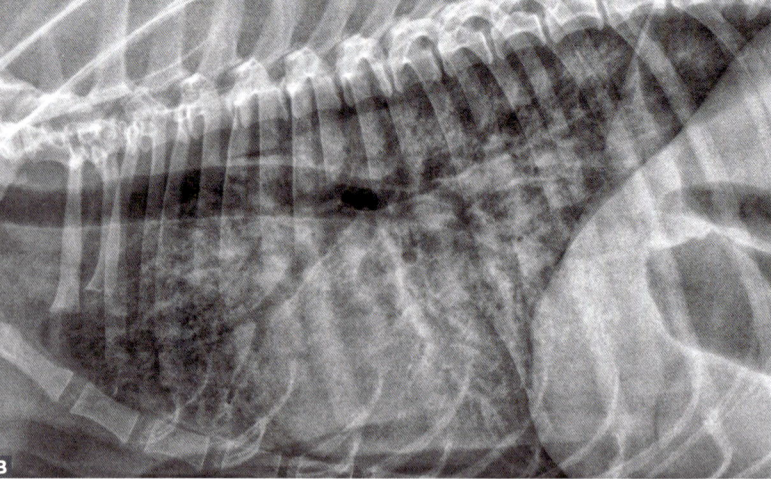

Fig. 23.18 (**A**) Ventrodorsal and (**B**) left lateral recumbency thoracic radiographs of a 13-year-old female Nova Scotia Duck Tolling Retriever. All lung lobes are abnormal, there is a diffuse nonuniform severe unstructured interstitial pattern with a bronchial component. (**B**) There is also border effacement affecting the caudal cardiac border, caudal vena cava and diaphragm, indicating an alveolar pattern in the accessory lung lobe. This dog had chronic interstitial pneumonia confirmed on pathology.

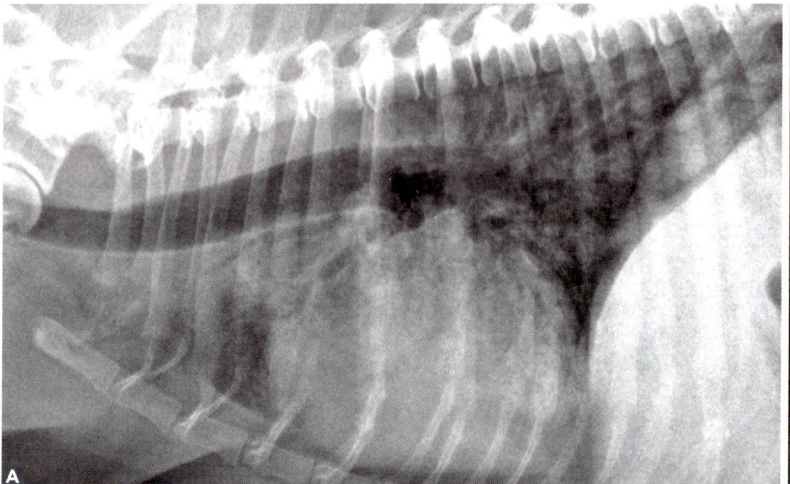

Fig. 23.19 Thoracic radiographs with left lateral recumbency (**A**) and ventrodorsal (**B**) projections of a 13-year-old female West Highland White Terrier with histopathologically confirmed canine idiopathic pulmonary fibrosis. There is a severe hazy soft tissue opacity throughout the lung field partly obscuring the pulmonary vessels, characterized as a severe unstructured interstitial pattern. The lung field is small in all projections despite several attempts to take them on inspiration, suggesting reduced lung compliance. There is also right-sided cardiomegaly, seen in the left lateral recumbency projection (**A**) by the cardiac silhouette having an increased length of sternal contact, and in the ventrodorsal projection (**B**) by the cardiac silhouette having a rounded right border. The combination of right-sided cardiomegaly and the pulmonary changes are strongly suspicious for acquired pulmonary hypertension.

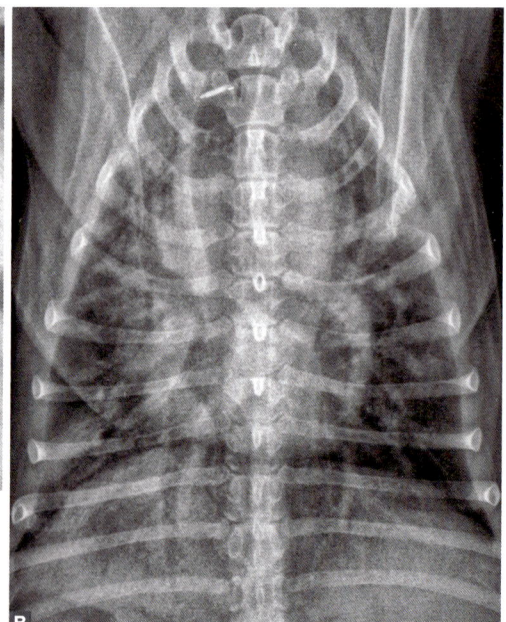

bronchial and unstructured interstitial pattern or unstructured interstitial pattern (**fig. 23.18**). Due to loss of compliance of the fibrotic lungs, they may have a reduced volume, and the size of the lung may not differ between inspiratory and expiratory radiographs (**fig. 23.19**). The most frequent finding on computed tomography studies is a generalized hazy increased opacity (ground-glass opacity) in the lungs.[12] Many dogs with canine idiopathic pulmonary fibrosis develop secondary pulmonary hypertension. In chronic severe pulmonary hypertension cases, there may be right-sided cardiomegaly; however, some affected patients do not show appreciable cardiomegaly. Echocardiography is more sensitive for diagnosis and can also be used to quantify severity of hypertension (**fig. 23.19**).

Radiographic changes in cats with idiopathic pulmonary fibrosis vary significantly and can therefore mimic other pulmonary diseases, making the diagnosis difficult. One or any combination of the following patterns have been described in cats: bronchointerstitial pattern, interstitial (both structured and unstructured) pattern, alveolar patterns, pulmonary masses, bulla formation, emphysematous changes and pleural effusion (**figs. 23.20** and **23.21**). The localization of the findings can also vary from generalized to multifocal with different lung lobes involved. Secondary pulmonary hypertension has also been reported in cats with idiopathic pulmonary fibrosis but is better diagnosed through echocardiography as radiographs often show no cardiac changes.[13]

The imaging findings in dogs and cats with idiopathic pulmonary fibrosis are not pathognomonic for the condition, and the radiographic appearance must be interpreted in the light of other clinical data. Pulmonary fibrosis can only be confirmed by histologic examination of lung tissue.

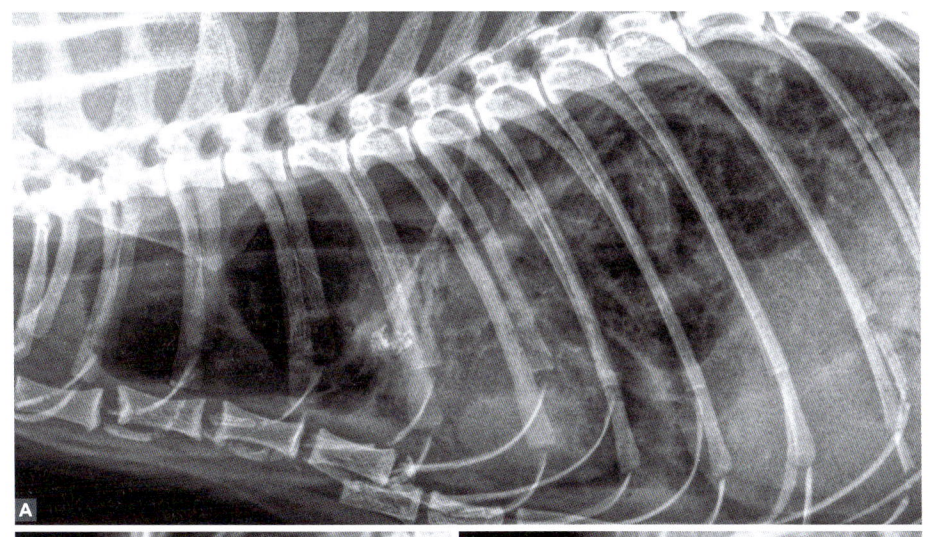

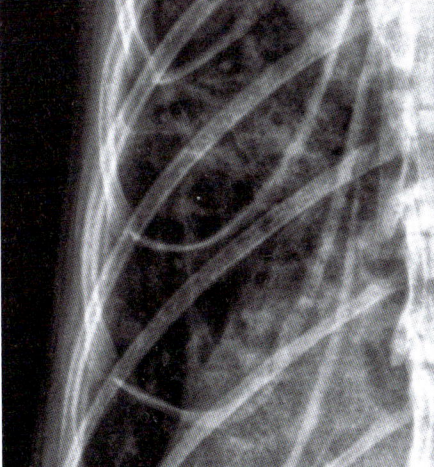

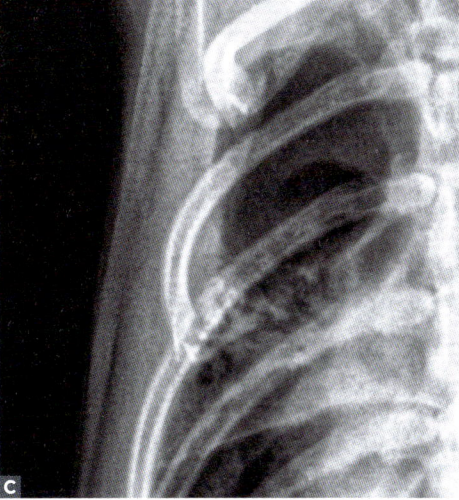

Fig. 23.20 A 15-year-old Domestic shorthair cat with history of respiratory signs for several years. A presumptive diagnosis of a pulmonary fibrosis was made after exhaustive testing to exclude infectious or inflammatory disease. (**A**) Left lateral recumbency thoracic radiograph, and close-up ventrodorsal projections of the right caudal (**B**) and right cranial thorax (**C**). All lungs are abnormal, with a mixture of different patterns. There is mainly a severe mixed bronchial and interstitial pattern, partly obscuring the pulmonary vasculature margins. But there are also areas with numerous thin, distinct, soft tissue opaque lines that traverse the pulmonary parenchyma in haphazard directions (**A**, **B**). Some of these lines radiate to the pleural surface, creating corresponding indentations in the lung surface (**A**). The lung lobes also have abnormal lobulated margins. These findings are consistent with fibrosis and contracture. The left lateral recumbency (**A**) and ventrodorsal (**C**) projections show that the cranial lung lobes are hyperlucent, without any visible bronchial or vascular structures, consistent with emphysematous changes. In the right cranial thorax (**A**, **C**), there are also some small focal areas of amorphous mineral opacity. As an incidental finding, the cat has a chronic subluxation of the sternum.

Fig. 23.21 (**A**) Ventrodorsal, (**B**) right lateral recumbency, and (**C**) close-up right lateral recumbency projections of a ten-year-old Domestic shorthair cat with a history of altered breathing for several months. After extensive testing to exclude other diagnoses, a presumptive diagnosis of pulmonary fibrosis was made. There is a generalized severe bronchointerstitial pattern in all lung lobes. Many small round radiolucencies are seen in the periphery of the lung and are too large and close to each other to represent normal bronchi. These likely represent emphysematous changes and bronchiectasis.

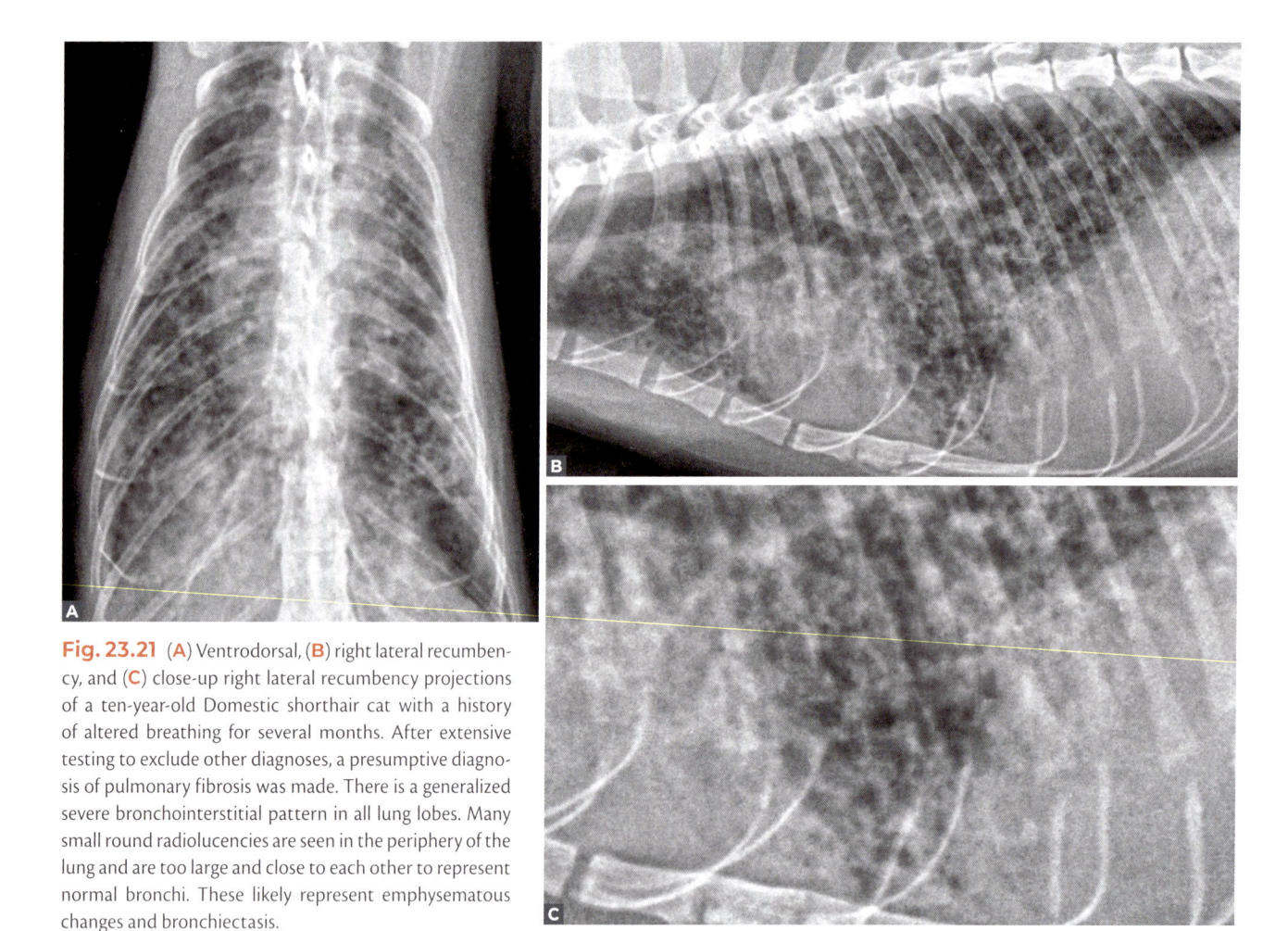

Pulmonary emphysema

Pulmonary emphysema is an irreversible condition with dilation and rupture of alveoli and is rare in dogs and cats. The acquired form can occur as a sequel to chronic bronchitis. There are several reports of congenital pulmonary emphysema in dogs, and in some cases combined with pulmonary or bronchial hypoplasia.[14]

The imaging findings are focal or lobar increased radiolucency (on radiographs) and decreased attenuation (on CT) from hyperinflation and loss of parenchyma, and increased lung volume with caudal displacement of the diaphragm. In patients with lobar or unilateral disease, there may be a contralateral mediastinal shift and partial or complete atelectasis of unaffected lobes. Spontaneous pneumothorax may occur[3] (**figs. 23.22-23.24**).

Radiologically it can be almost impossible to distinguish the reversible conditions of overinflation and air-trapping in bronchial disease from irreversible pulmonary emphysema. Therefore, the radiological findings need to be interpreted with care and together with the patient's total clinical picture.

When performing both inspiratory and expiratory radiographs, the hyperlucent emphysematous lung lobe will stay unchanged. On horizontal beam dorsoventral or ventrodorsal projections with the suspected affected lobe recumbent, the emphysematous lobe will not collapse as expected on a normal lung lobe.[3]

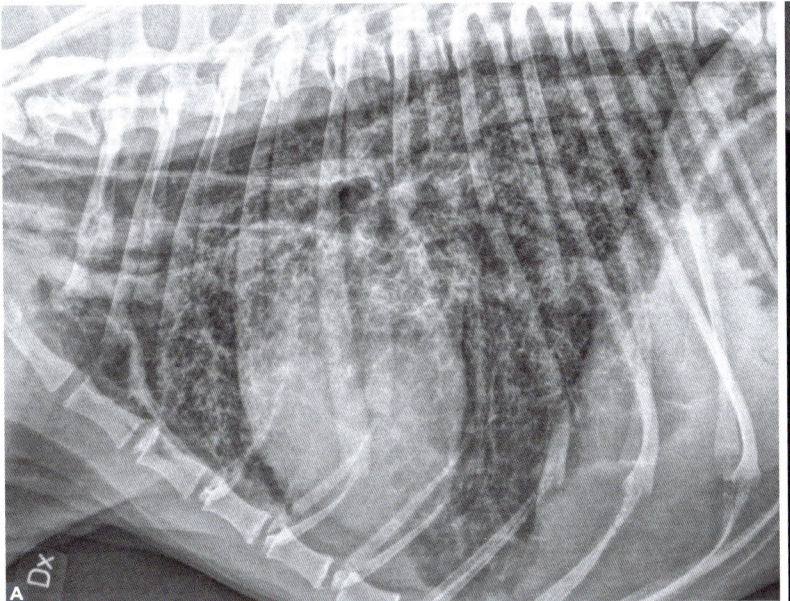

Fig. 23.22 A seven-year-old male Standard Poodle presented with lethargy and forced breathing. Thoracic radiographs with right lateral recumbency (**A**) and ventrodorsal (**B**) projections. The lung field is generally enlarged, and the diaphragm is flattened, indicating hyperinflation. There is a generalized severe bronchointerstitial pattern with a reticular appearance. The large vessels, esophagus and trachea in the cranial mediastinum are clearly outlined by gas indicating a pneumomediastinum. Chronic bronchitis and bronchointerstitial pneumonia with emphysema was the primary differential with infiltrative neoplasia, with emphysema considered less likely. The dog responded to steroid treatment, but on repeat radiographs two months later, the findings were identical supporting the initial suspicion of chronic bronchitis and emphysema.

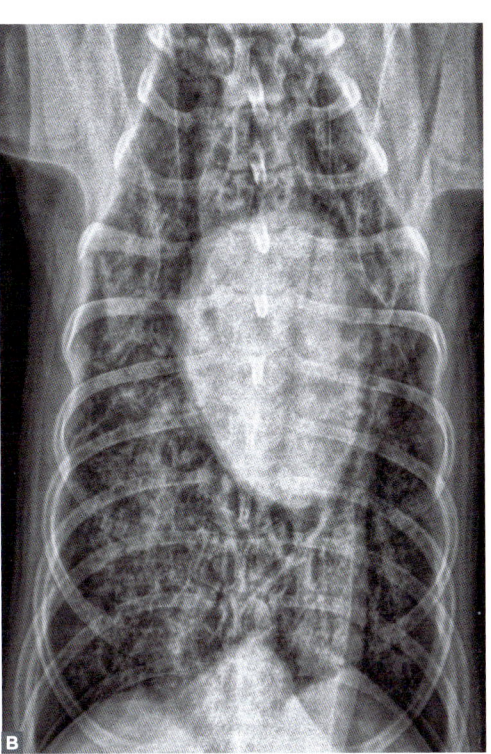

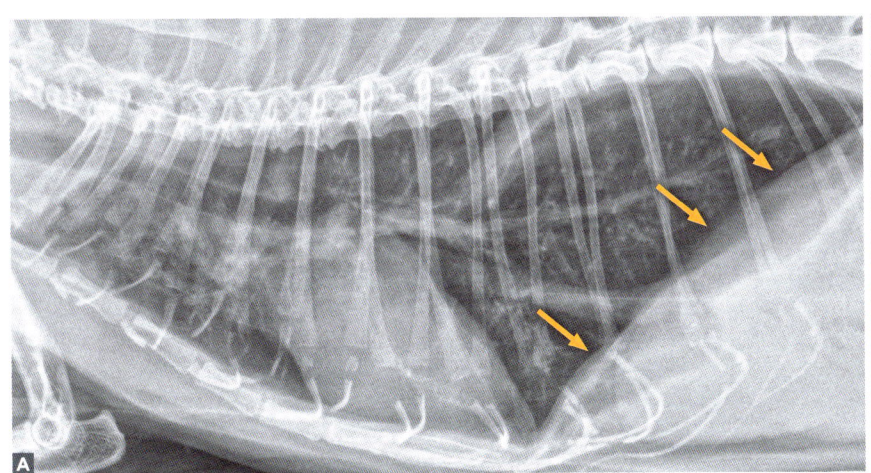

Fig. 23.23 Left lateral recumbency (**A**) and ventrodorsal (**B**) projections of a 12-year-old Domestic shorthair cat. The lung field is enlarged with a flattened and caudally displaced diaphragm (arrows). Both caudal lung lobes are hyperlucent. There is a generalized increased bronchointerstitial pattern. The cardiac silhouette is shifted towards the right side. A soft tissue band extending caudodorsally from the hilar region in the left lateral recumbency projection was interpreted as thickened pleura possibly combined with peripheral atelectasis. The presumed diagnosis was a chronic inflammatory process (bronchitis/feline asthma/fibrosis) with lobar emphysema in both caudal lung lobes in combination with a thickened pleura.

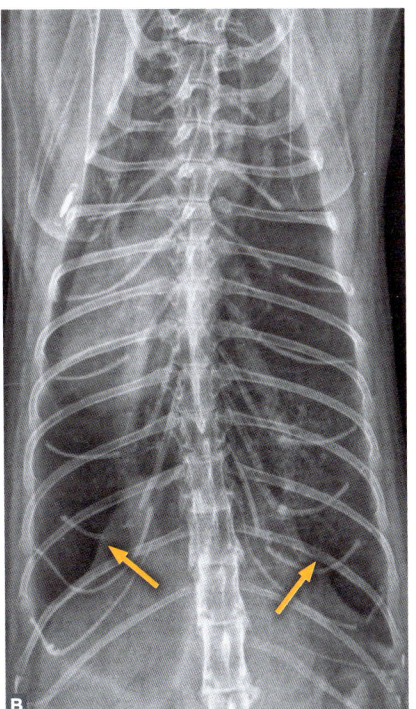

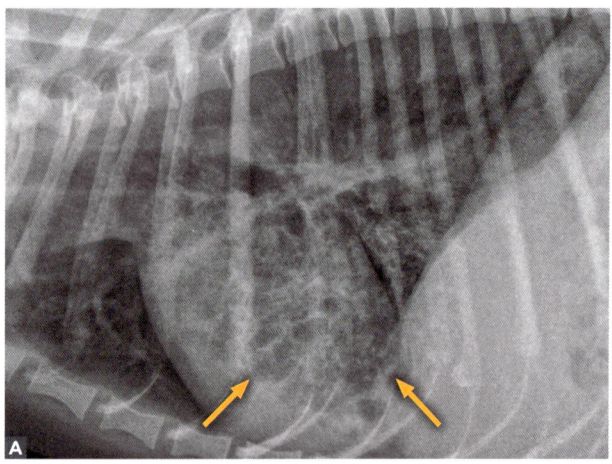

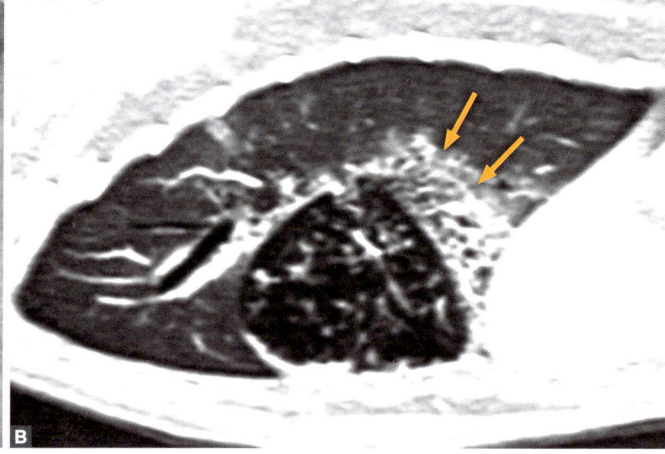

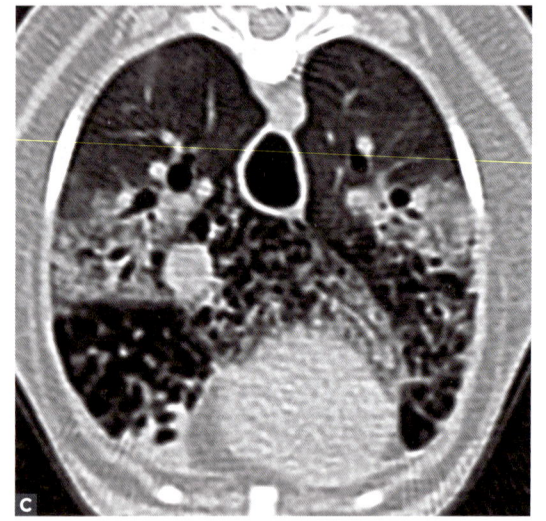

Fig. 23.24 A six-year-old Chihuahua presented with recurrent cough. The thoracic left lateral recumbency projection (**A**) shows a multilobular radiolucent area (arrows) in the ventral part of the right middle lung lobe with moderate increased interstitial pattern dorsal to this. In the parasagittal reconstruction from the CT examination (**B**) of the thorax optimized for evaluating the lungs, the hypoattenuating right middle lung lobe appears enlarged with a rounded shape indicative of emphysema. The cranioventral aspect of the right caudal lung lobe is diffusely hyperattenuating (arrows), most likely caused by focal atelectasis. The transverse reconstruction (**C**) just caudal to the heart shows the hypoattenuating part of the right middle lung lobe with a honeycomb pattern and a similar appearance in the included part of the accessory lung lobe and the cranioventral aspect of the left caudal lung lobe. Adjacent to the hypoattenuating regions there are hyperattenuating areas of ground-glass appearance to more homogenous attenuation compatible with a combination of atelectasis and inflammation, fibrosis or edema.

Traumatic hematocele and pneumatocele and pulmonary bullae

Radiologically air-filled lung lesions are difficult to distinguish from each other and names are often used interchangeably. On CT, it is easier to see the exact location of the lesion but there are still overlapping features. CT is also more sensitive in detecting the lesions than radiography. Terms like cavity, bulla, pneumatocele, bleb, pseudocyst and cyst have all been used and are nonspecific.

Bullae may be congenital or secondary to trauma or inflammation. They are spherical air-filled structures with a thin wall (less than 1 mm) located anywhere in the lung parenchyma. Some are accompanied by signs of the primary lesion (areas of increased opacity or attenuation), but many are incidental with no other pulmonary disease. Sometimes the lesion is filled with fluid and may mimic a solid nodule or mass. Traumatic bullae are often called pneumatoceles. These may be partly or completely filled with fluid, presumed to be blood, and are referred to as hematocele or pulmonary hematoma. Pneumatoceles and hematoceles are usually transient lesions and most resolve in weeks to months. Necrosis in the central part of a pulmonary neoplasm or abscess can result in an air-filled cavity if there is communication with an airway. However, in such lesions the wall usually appears quite thick and has an irregular inner contour (**fig. 23.25**).

When several bullae coalesce to affect a segment of lung, a lobe or multiple lobes the term bullous emphysema is used. Bullae are often located in the periphery of the lung. The term bleb is sometimes used for a subpleural bulla (**fig. 23.26**).

CHAPTER 23 Pulmonary infiltrations

Although bullae can be an incidental finding (**figs. 23.14** and **23.27**), rupture of these superficial air-filled bullae is a common cause for spontaneous pneumothorax (**fig. 23.28**). CT is more sensitive in detecting air-filled bullae than radiography, but the sensitivity for detecting the etiologic lesion in spontaneous pneumothorax cases is limited as the ruptured bulla collapses.[15] Using both sternal and dorsal recumbency in CT studies of patients with spontaneous pneumothorax can somewhat improve the sensitivity but confirmation of the source of spontaneous pneumothorax by CT is sometimes not possible.[15]

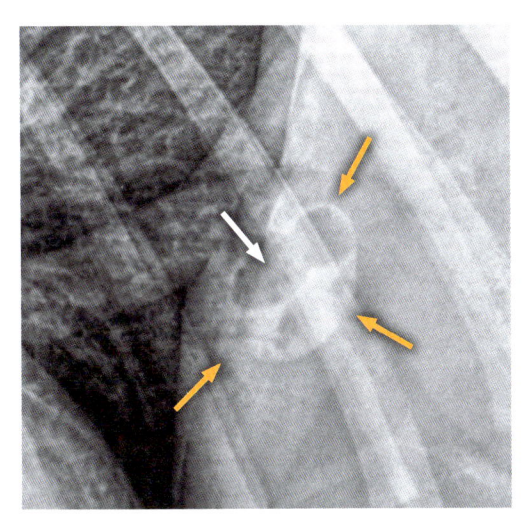

Fig. 23.25 Close-up view of a right lateral recumbency projection of the thorax of a six-month-old Siberian Husky that was hit by a car the day before. An oval shaped soft-tissue opacity structure (orange arrows) with two asymmetrically positioned gas filled pockets (white arrow) is present superimposed on the liver ventral to the caudal vena cava. The appearance together with the presenting history is consistent with a traumatic hemato-pneumatocele.

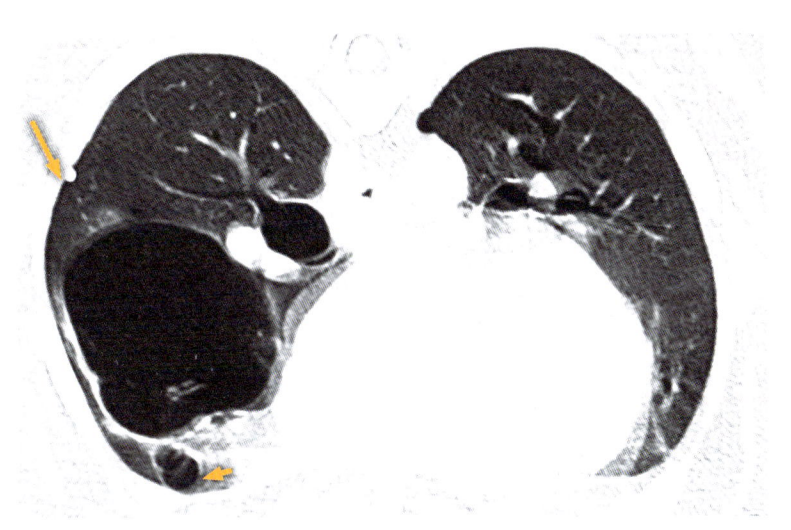

Fig. 23.26 Transverse CT reconstruction of the lungs at the level of the heart of a five-year-old Bernese Mountain dog showing a 6 cm large, thin-walled gas attenuating bulla in the ventral half of the right middle lung lobe and a small subpleural bulla (bleb) ventral to that (arrowhead). The dog was presented initially with right-sided pneumothorax and a pleural drain is seen lateral to the lung (arrow).

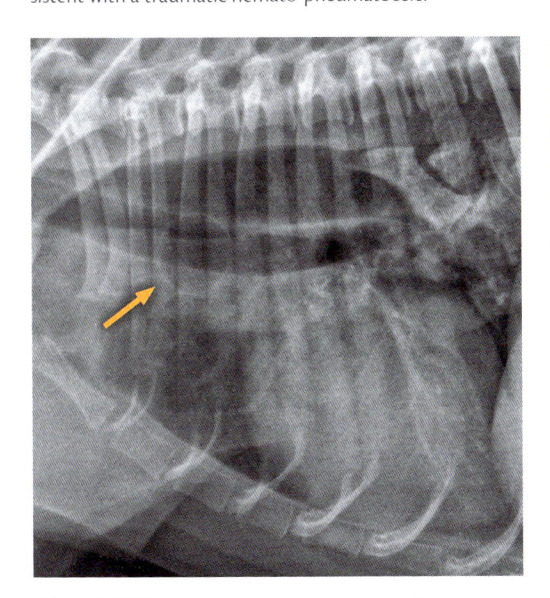

Fig. 23.27 A left lateral recumbency projection of an eight-year-old German Hunting Terrier with several bone foreign bodies in the caudal thoracic esophagus, with a gas-filled dilated esophagus in the cranial mediastinum. There is an incidental 2 cm in diameter, thin-walled, air-filled bulla superimposed on the cranial mediastinum (arrow).

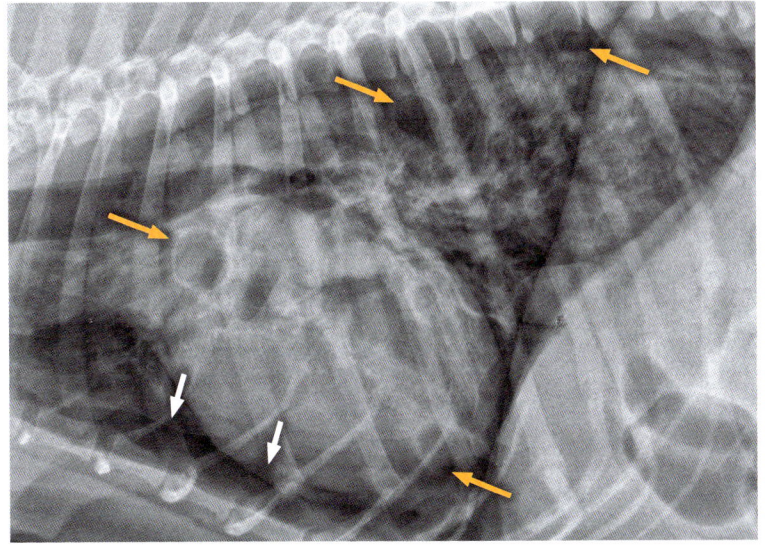

Fig. 23.28 A 14-year-old mixed breed dog was radiographed because of acute respiratory distress and cough. The left lateral recumbency projection shows multiple rounded, lucent bullae of varying size from 8-20 mm in diameter with a thin soft-tissue wall (orange arrows). Gas is interposed between the heart and sternum, indicating pneumothorax (white arrows). A ruptured bulla was the most likely cause of the pneumothorax.

Pulmonary hemorrhage

Hemorrhage in the lungs of small animals is commonly caused by trauma but is also seen with coagulopathies from etiologies including thrombocytopenia, disseminated intravascualr coagulation and anticoagulant rodenticide intoxication.

The radiographic features of pulmonary hemorrhage include alveolar, interstitial or mixed patterns with focal, patchy, or often random distribution. Concurrent pleural and mediastinal hemorrhage can be seen. Narrowing of the tracheal lumen due to mucosal, submucosal or extratracheal bleeding is a relatively characteristic feature of anticoagulant intoxication[16] (**fig. 23.29**).

In traumatic injuries, the pulmonary changes are sometimes combined with traumatic thoracic wall lesions, such as fractured ribs and hemo- or pneumothorax (**fig. 23.30**).

Radiographic changes from acute traumatic contusion may be delayed up to 24 hours, and there is a risk of underestimating lung lesions if the examination is performed directly in the acute phase. CT is more accurate in detecting contusions as well as grading the severity of the lesions compared to radiography, but the difference has not been shown to affect the management or clinical outcome (**fig. 23.31**).

Ultrasound of the thorax can help monitor the progression of contusions in critical care patients as long as the lesions are situated in the periphery of the lungs.[17]

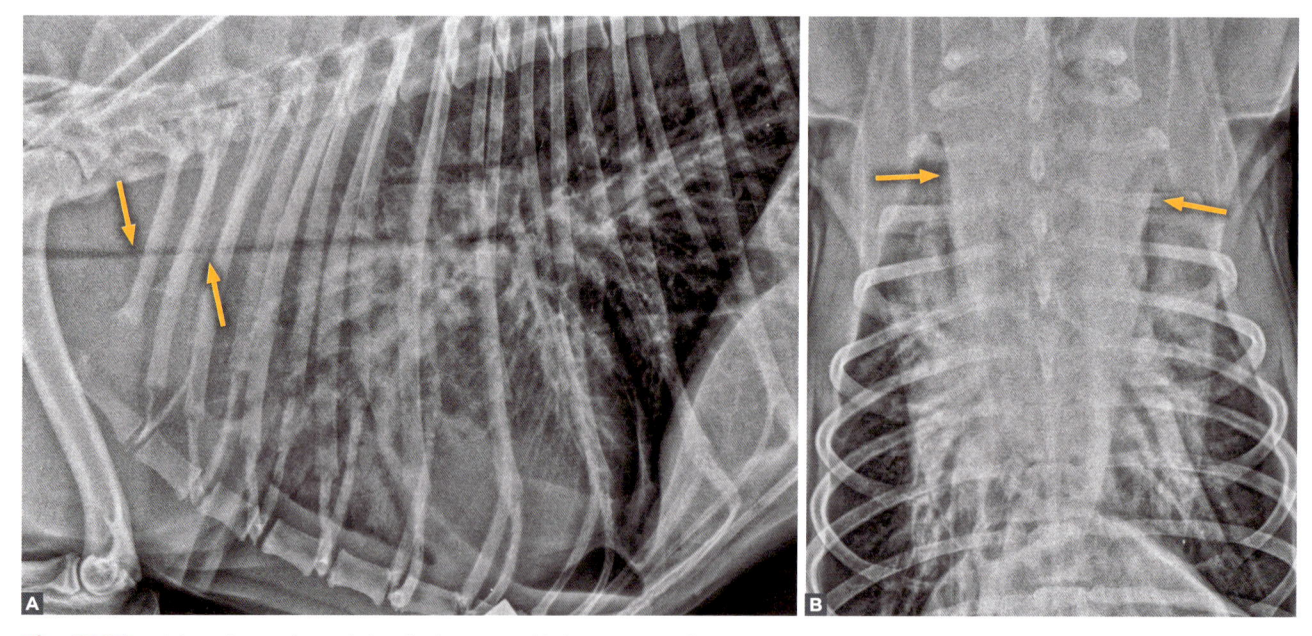

Fig. 23.29 Left lateral recumbency (**A**) and a dorsoventral (**B**) projections of a Labrador Retriever with coagulopathy due to rodenticide (coumarin) poisoning. The uniformly severely narrowed tracheal lumen (arrows) is from hemorrhage into the tracheal ligament, a characteristic feature of coumarin intoxication. Patchy interstitial to alveolar pattern in the cranial lung lobes and a widened cranial mediastinum (arrows) indicate concurrent pulmonary and mediastinal hemorrhage. The lung lobes are mildly separated from each other and the thoracic wall by soft-tissue opacity, and in the dorsoventral projection the cardiac silhouette is obscured, indicating there is also pleural hemorrhage.

CHAPTER 23 Pulmonary infiltrations

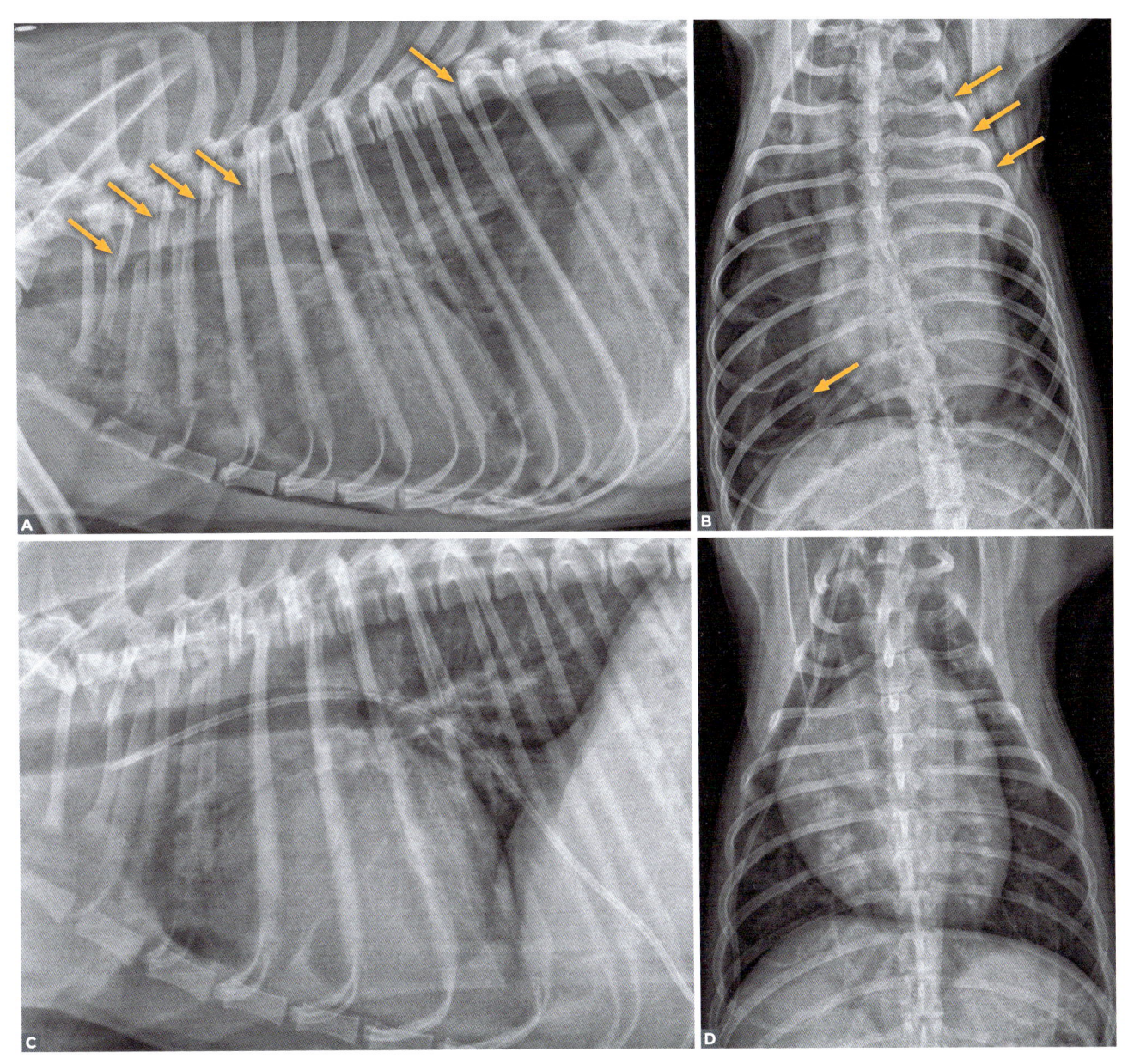

Fig. 23.30 A three-year-old mixed breed dog was hit by a car and right lateral recumbency (**A**) and dorsoventral (**B**) radiographs of the thorax were taken two hours after the accident. Initial radiographs reveal fractured 2nd-5th ribs on the left side (arrows), in combination with mild focal fascial emphysema, and an alveolar pattern in the left cranial lung lobe, indicating hemorrhage. An interstitial to an alveolar pattern is also present in the right cranial lung lobe. On the dorsoventral view, the periphery of the thorax is hyperlucent from air interposed between the lungs and the thoracic wall. The rest of the lung field has an interstitial pattern attributed to mild atelectasis from the bilateral pneumothorax. In the dorsal aspect of the right caudal lung lobe, an oval thin-walled air-filled cavity is noted, a traumatic bullae (arrow). Repeated right lateral recumbency (**C**) and ventrodorsal (**D**) radiographs four days after the accident show a marked improvement of the contusions and the pneumothorax. The air-filled cavity in the right caudal lung lobe is no longer seen and interpreted as a resolved traumatic pneumatocele. A pleural drain is seen in the images. Note the difference in the size of the heart between the examinations. Initially it is smaller due to hypovolemic shock and later normal when the patient was stabilized.

SECTION IV THORAX

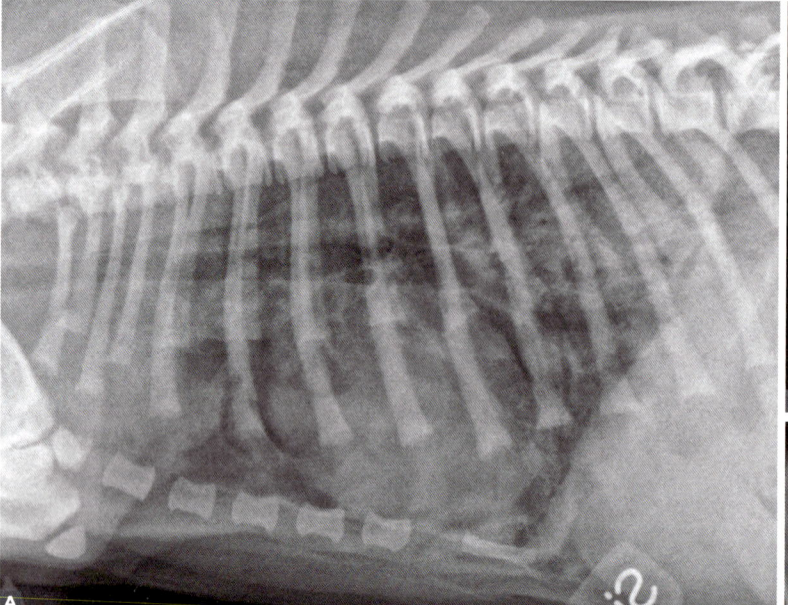

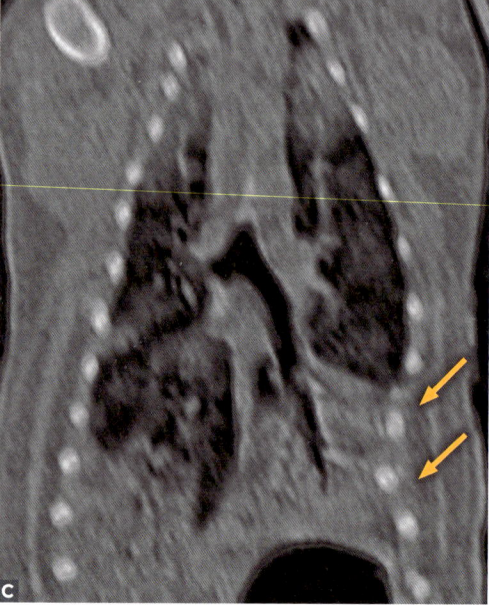

Fig. 23.31 A three-month-old Jack Russell Terrier was hit by a car, and on presentation the clinical condition only permitted a single left lateral recumbency (A) projection of the thorax. A moderate to severe interstitial to alveolar pattern is seen mostly in the caudodorsal and cranioventral lung field and the dorsal aspect of the diaphragm is obscured by the opacity. There is no detectable pleural fluid, pleural air or fractured ribs. The puppy underwent a CT examination awake in a "mouse-trap" immediately following the radiographic examination. A transverse (B) and a dorsal (C) reconstruction in bone window show mildly displaced fractures of the 8th and 9th (arrows) left ribs with a focal hyperattenuation of the left caudal lung lobe indicating traumatic hemorrhage. There is also marked increased attenuation in the middle and peripheral regions of the right caudal lung lobe also representing contusion. Additional patchy hyperattenuation is seen in both cranial lung lobes, again indicating contusion.

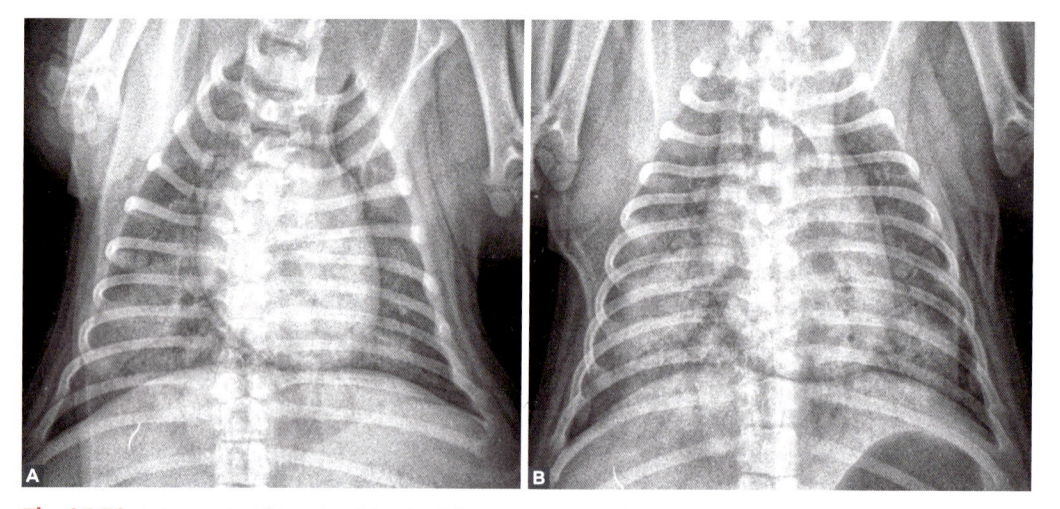

Fig. 23.32 A six-month-old French Bulldog that fell in a swimming pool presented with near-drowning and development of noncardiogenic edema. A ventrodorsal projection (A) taken immediately on arrival to the clinic showed only moderate interstitial opacities in the right and left caudal lung lobes and the right middle lung lobe. However, after two hours a dorsoventral projection (B) shows an increasing opacity with air bronchograms partly obscuring the cardiac silhouette and the diaphragm consistent with a nonuniform alveolar pattern. In acute situations, there may be a delay in the radiographic development of edema or hemorrhage in the lungs and if there is a mismatch between clinical assessment and initial radiographic findings, repeated examination should always be considered.

Pulmonary edema

Pulmonary edema is a pathologic accumulation of extravascular fluid in the lung that occurs secondary to other primary disease conditions causing an increased vascular hydrostatic pressure, increased vascular permeability, decreased plasma oncotic pressure or decreased lymphatic drainage.[18,19] Pulmonary edema is one of the most common causes of respiratory distress in dogs and is classified into cardiogenic or noncardiogenic edema.[19] Differentiating the two types of edema is vital since the treatment strategies differ.

The patient often presents with an acute onset of respiratory distress, and the clinical assessment is used to determine if radiology can be performed safely. As with pulmonary hemorrhage, the radiological changes may not be evident in the acute phase but develop within 24 hours (**fig. 23.32**). The radiological presentation is not specific, and as for many situations with lung pathology, edema is one of several possibilities on the list of differentials that needs to be confirmed or excluded through the entire clinical picture of the patient. The pulmonary pattern, distribution and extent reflects the severity of the edema. Radiology is especially valuable in assessing response to treatment, which may be helpful in confirming a diagnosis (**figs. 23.33** and **23.36**).

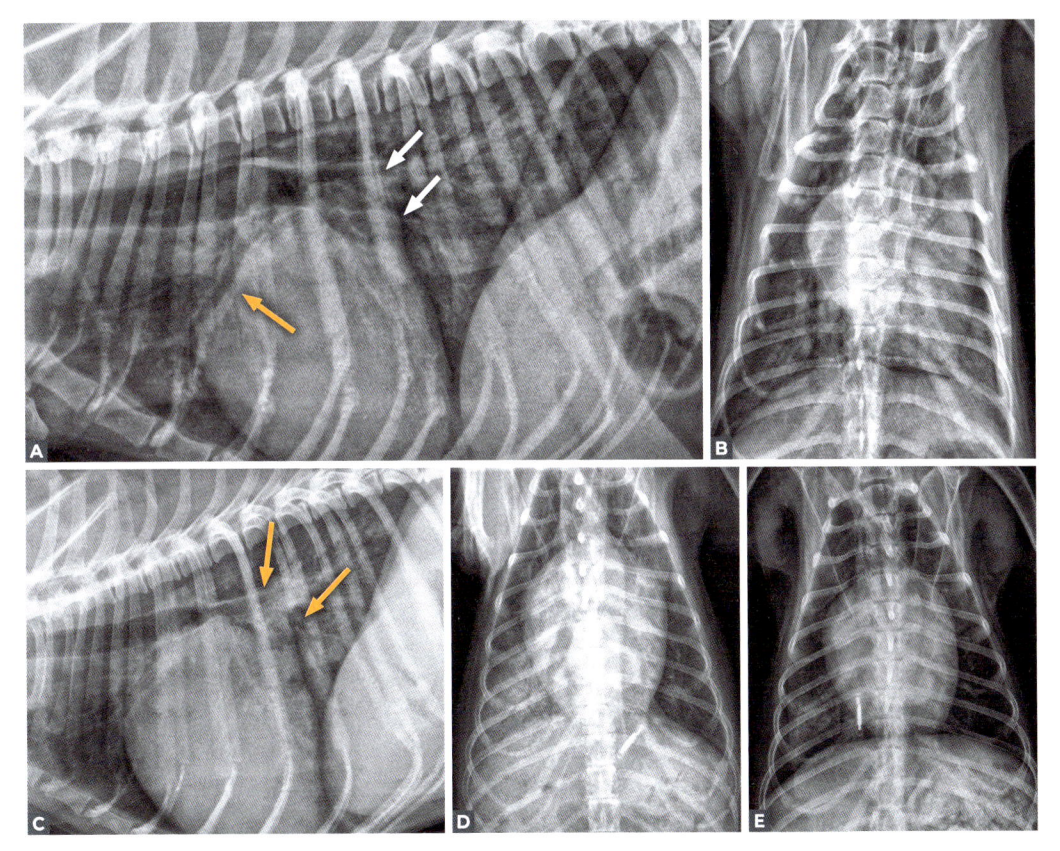

Fig. 23.33 Left lateral recumbency (**A**) and ventrodorsal (**B**) projections of an eight-year-old Dachshund with myxomatous mitral valve disease showing a classic presentation of left-sided heart failure and cardiogenic pulmonary edema. There is cardiomegaly with a left atrial enlargement (white arrows in image **A**) and pulmonary venous congestion (arrows) together with an interstitial coalescing to alveolar opacity fairly symmetrically distributed in both caudal lung lobes. Images (**C**) and (**D**) show a ten-year-old Chihuahua, also with myxomatous mitral valve disease and signs of acute left-sided congestive cardiac failure. Left lateral recumbency (**C**) and ventrodorsal (**D**) projections were taken in the acute stage. Compared to the previous dog (**A**, **B**) with the same disease, this dog shows a clearly asymmetrical distribution of the lung edema seen as an alveolar pattern in the entire right caudal lung lobe. In the left lateral recumbency (**C**) projection the left caudal lobar bronchus is dorsally displaced and partly compressed by the dilated left atrium (arrows in image **C**) protruding at the caudodorsal aspect of the heart. A ventrodorsal projection (**E**) taken two days later after one treatment with diuretics shows the alveolar pattern in the right caudal lung lobe is clearly improved with a moderate interstitial pattern and the cardiac and diaphragmatic outlines are now visible. Cardiogenic edema will usually improve in response to treatment within 24-48 hours, although clinical improvement may be apparent sooner.

SECTION IV THORAX

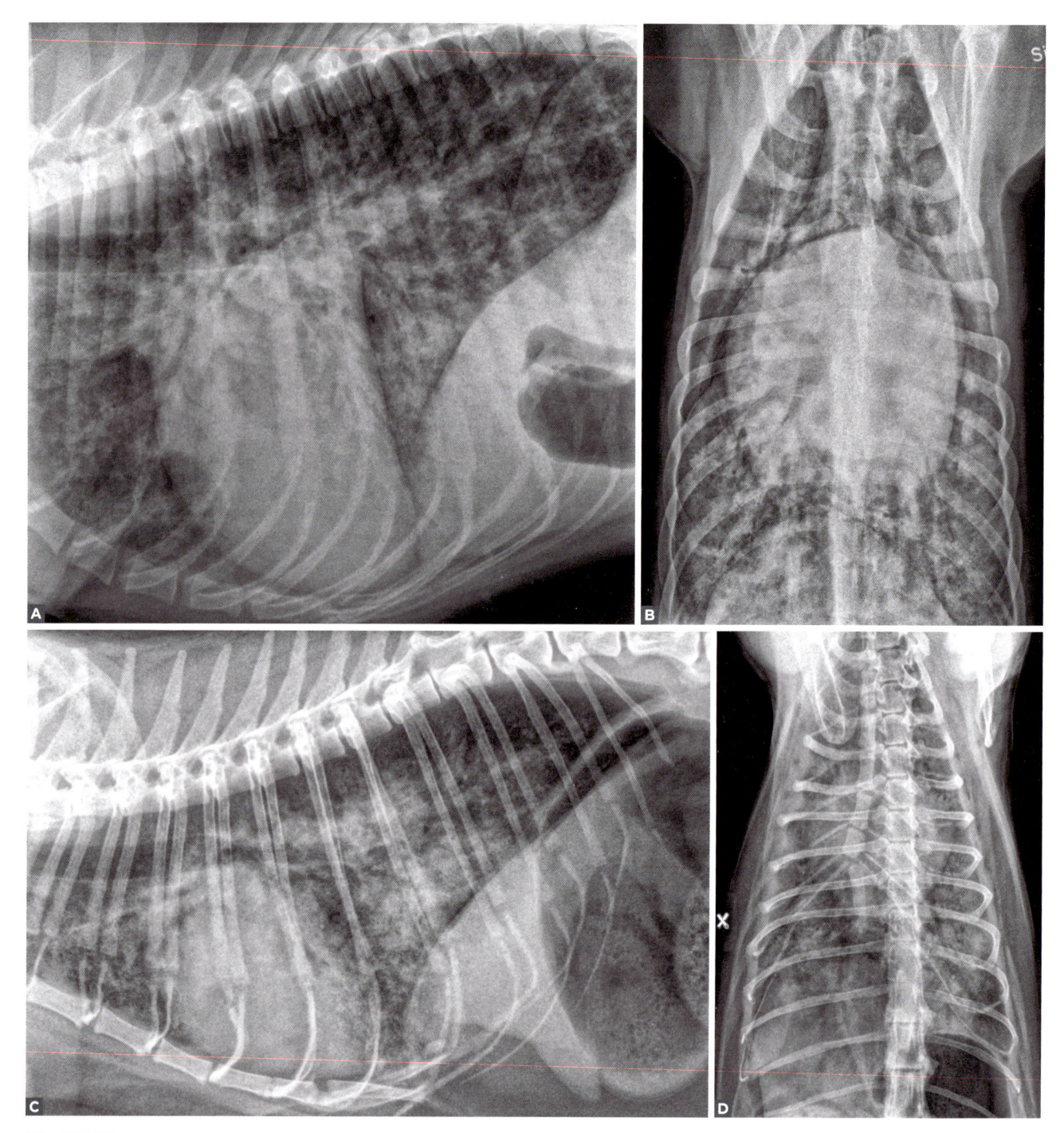

Fig. 23.34 A four-year-old Dobermann Pinscher with dilated cardiomyopathy and acute left-sided heart failure. Left lateral recumbency (A) and ventrodorsal (B) projections were obtained. There is a generalized increased opacity in the lungs with a mixed pattern, including severe unstructured interstitial component that in the ventral parts of the lung field coalesces to foci alveolar opacity with air bronchograms. The heart is tall with a straight caudodorsal margin indicating a left atrial dilation and the pulmonary veins are dilated indicating congestion. Images (C) and (D) were taken from a ten-year-old Birman cat diagnosed with a restrictive type of cardiomyopathy and acute left-sided heart failure. The edema has a somewhat more ventral distribution compared to the mitral insufficiency cases presented in previous fig. 24.33. There is a patchy mostly alveolar pattern in most of the lung with sparing of the caudodorsal periphery. The distribution of the lesions is symmetrical. The heart is enlarged and kidney-shaped in the left lateral recumbency (C) projection indicating dilation of the left atrium. Obliquity of the dorsoventral projection precludes accurate assessment of cardiac size but the image is adequate to assess the lungs. The pulmonary vessels are obscured by the edema. Note the gas-filled stomach indicative of aerophagia.

Cardiogenic edema

Cardiogenic edema develops due to increased hydrostatic pressure seen with left-sided heart failure and is also discussed in chapter 20.

The most common cause for cardiogenic edema in dogs is left-sided congestive heart failure seen with myxomatous mitral valve disease (MMVD or mitral valve endocardiosis), and the typical appearance of the pulmonary edema is increased soft tissue opacity with symmetrical distribution in the hilar region of the caudal lung lobes. The pattern can range from mild unstructured interstitial to uniform alveolar opacification depending on the severity of edema and is often mixed, especially in the transition zone between affected and normal lung. In approximately 30% of dogs with pulmonary edema due to MMVD, the distribution is asymmetrical with predominantly the right caudal lung lobe being affected exclusively or more severely[19] (**fig. 23.33**). Cardiomegaly with left atrial enlargement supports a diagnosis of cardiogenic edema. However, depending on the primary cause of heart failure, the heart may not be appreciably enlarged.

In dogs with dilated cardiomyopathy (DCM) and in cats with cardiomyopathy (often hypertrophic) causing congestive heart failure the distribution of the pulmonary edema can be more ventral in the lung field often with a patchy mixed pattern and occasionally also with a pleural effusion (**fig. 23.34**). In dogs with cardiomegaly and moderate or severe dilation of the left atrium, the left mainstem bronchus is often compressed by the atrium, causing reduced ventilation. The degree of inspiration also affects the opacity of the caudal lung lobes and any suspected interstitial opacity seen on lateral projections should always be confirmed in ventrodorsal or dorsoventral projections to avoid a false-positive diagnosis of pulmonary edema (**fig. 23.35**).

Noncardiogenic edema

Noncardiogenic edema has multiple etiologies, but all present with similar radiographic changes. Neurogenic pulmonary edemas can be seen with trauma to the head and other causes for increased intracranial pressure, seizures, electrocution, and hypoglycemia. It is thought to be caused by massive

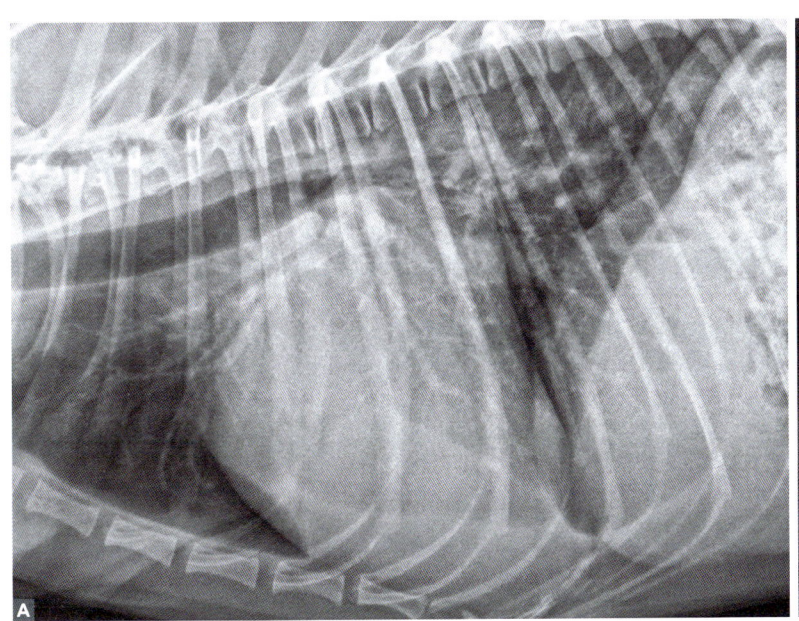

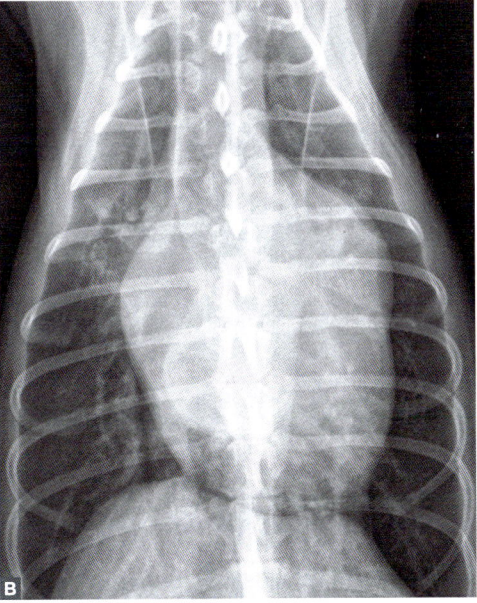

Fig. 23.35 An eight-year-old Tibetan Spaniel radiographed with a known diagnosis of myxomatous mitral valve disease. Both the right lateral recumbency (**A**) and the ventrodorsal (**B**) projections show severe cardiomegaly with a dilated left atrium compressing the bronchi of the caudal lung lobes. The pulmonary vessels are normal. In the right lateral recumbency projection, the hilar area and the entire caudal lung field have a moderately increased opacity, but this is not confirmed in the ventrodorsal projection. A combination of expiration, compressed main stem bronchi causing reduced ventilation of caudal lung lobes, and the enlarged left atrium contributing to an increased opacity in the hilar region, can give a false impression of increased opacity in the lung.

catecholamine release. Swedish Drevers (hunting dogs) have been described to develop neurogenic edema during hunting[20] (**figs. 23.36** and **23.37**).

Post-obstructive pulmonary edema is seen with near-drowning, strangulation, pharyngeal or laryngeal obstruction, brachycephalic obstructive airway syndrome or other causes for upper airway obstruction (**fig. 23.38**).

Toxic inhalants (smoke or toxic gases) and heat stroke cause direct local damage in the lung with increased vascular permeability. Toxins, sepsis, uremia, pancreatitis, and acute respiratory distress syndrome (ARDS) cause indirect damage in the lungs due to inflammatory reaction increasing the vascular permeability. Altitude sickness, iatrogenic fluid overload, blood transfusion-related acute lung injury and anaphylaxis are other reported causes of noncardiogenic edema (**fig. 23.32**).

The most common radiographic features of noncardiogenic pulmonary edema in dogs and cats are bilateral, symmetric, unstructured interstitial to alveolar patterns in the caudal lung lobes, usually affecting the middle and peripheral zones[18] (**figs. 23.36-23.38**). In severe cases the edema may affect all of the caudal lung lobes with patchy edema in other lobes. As in many situations in radiology, the diagnosis cannot be made solely on the radiographic appearance. The history is a key component in the diagnosis in combination with excluding other causes such as cardiogenic pulmonary edema, hemorrhage and inflammatory processes.

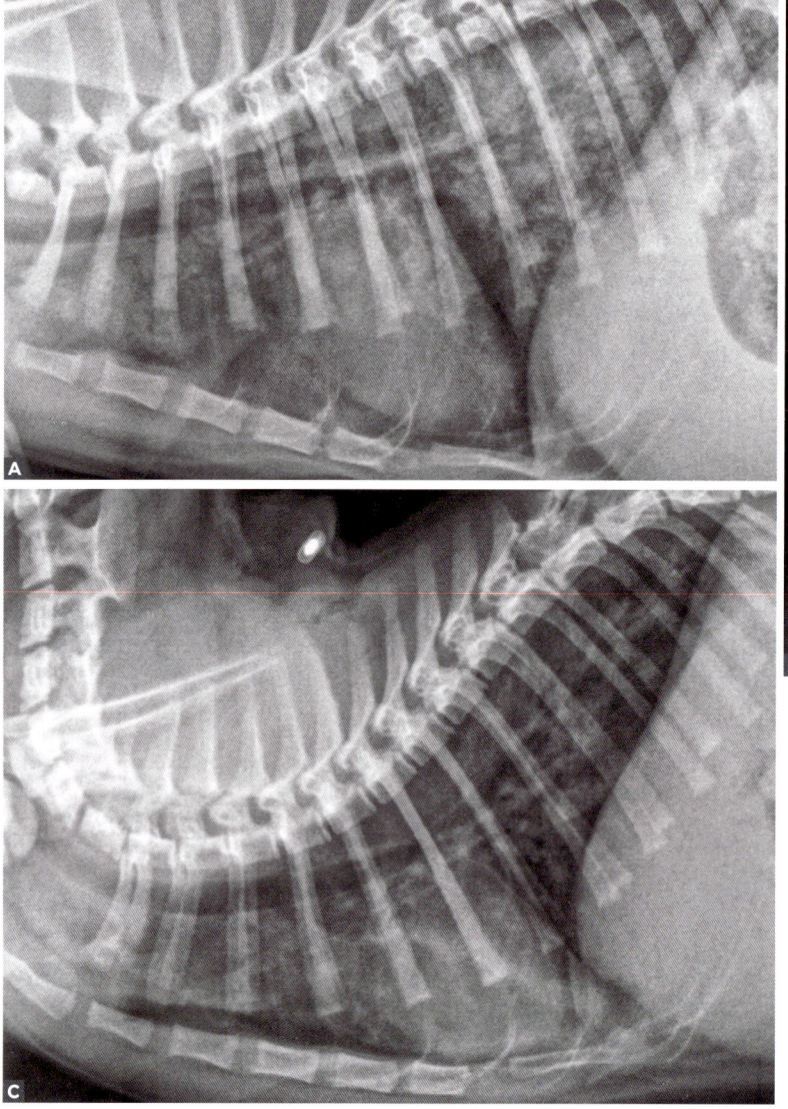

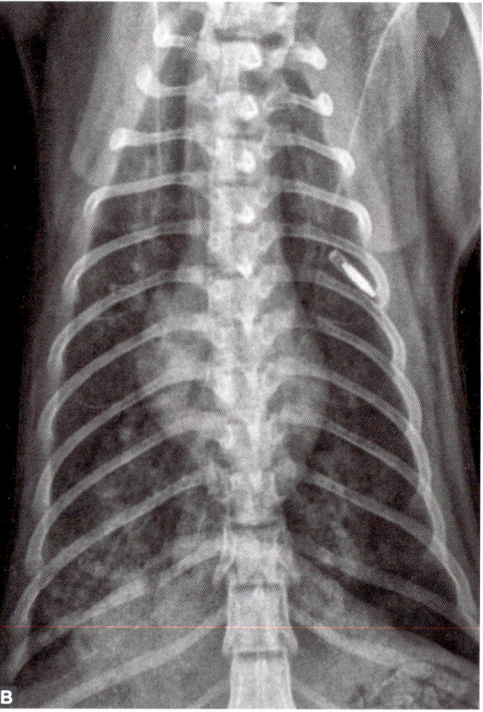

Fig. 23.36 A three-month-old Ragdoll kitten was electrocuted after chewing on an electric cord and arrived at the clinic in shock. Right lateral recumbency (**A**) and ventrodorsal (**B**) projections of the thorax shows a patchy alveolar pattern asymmetrically distributed in the caudal lung lobes, more severe on the right, indicating noncardiogenic edema. Follow-up radiographs three days later, after medical treatment and clinical improvement, shows a reduced now mostly interstitial opacity in the caudodorsal lung field on the right lateral recumbency projection (**C**).

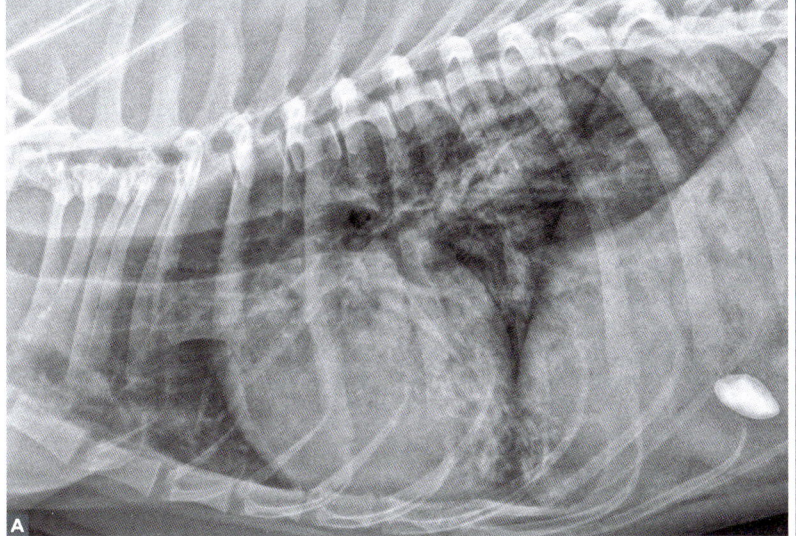

Fig. 23.37 A two-year-old Drever (Swedish hunting dog) arrived at the clinic with respiratory distress that developed while hunting. A left lateral recumbency (**A**) and a dorsoventral (**B**) projection of the thorax shows a patchy severe interstitial to alveolar opacity in the caudal lung lobes, and partly in the right middle lung lobe. The heart and pulmonary vessels are normal in size for the breed. A stone foreign body is present in the stomach as an incidental finding. The clinical presentation, in combination with the radiographic findings, is indicative of a neurogenic noncardiogenic edema that has been described in this breed.

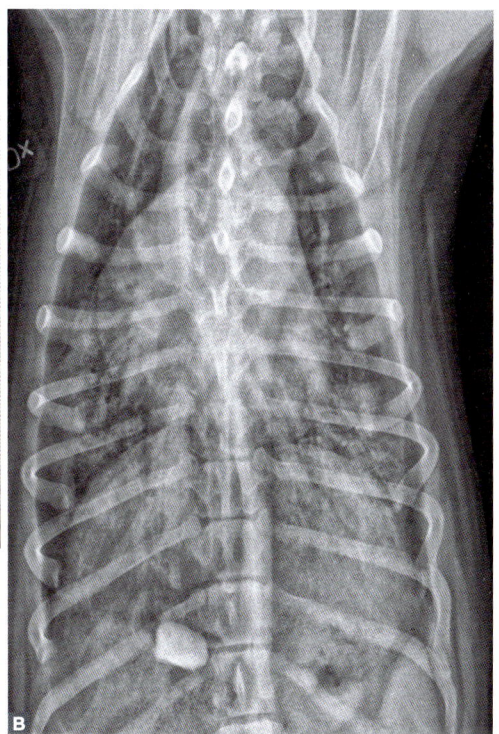

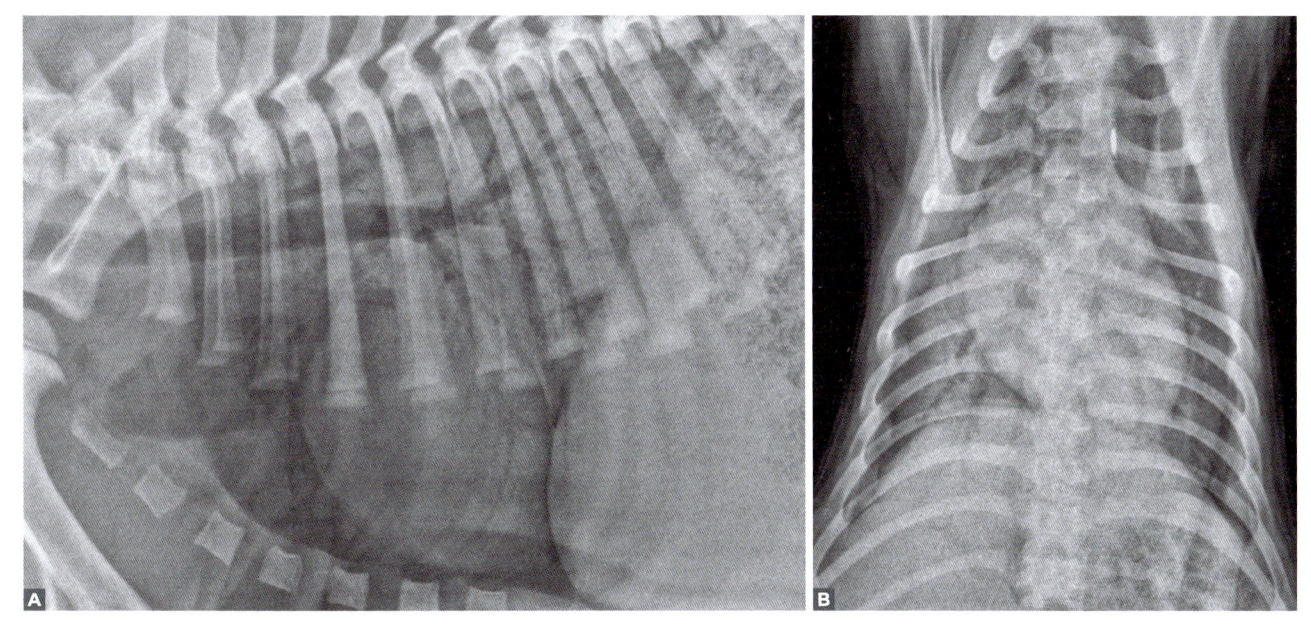

Fig. 23.38 Noncardiogenic edema secondary to upper airway obstruction by a bone foreign body in a nine-week-old Boxer puppy. Left lateral recumbency (**A**) and ventrodorsal (**B**) projections show an alveolar pattern in the caudal lung lobes with an asymmetrical distribution more severely affecting the right caudal lung lobe but also the left caudal and the right middle lung lobe.

Lymphoma

Lymphoma is a group of several neoplastic diseases of several subtypes arising from lymphoreticular cells. Multicentric lymphoma is the most common form in the dog, with simultaneous pulmonary involvement commonly seen. Primary pulmonary lymphoma has not yet been described in the dog.[21] There is wide variability in the thoracic radiographic changes in dogs and cats with pulmonary lymphoma. An unstructured interstitial pattern is the most commonly reported pattern in dogs. Mixed patterns, nodules and masses, alveolar pattern, bronchial pattern, lymphadenopathy (tracheobronchial, sternal, cranial mediastinal) and pleural effusion also occur. The thorax may be normal in some cases (**figs. 23.39** and **23.40**).

In cats, pulmonary masses and nodules and a bronchial infiltrate have been the most commonly described patterns, but unstructured interstitial and alveolar patterns have also been reported.[21] In cats, a mediastinal form of lymphoma can involve the thymus, mediastinal, and sternal lymph nodes. Pleural effusion is frequent (**fig. 23.41**).

Imaging is an aid in making the diagnosis, and for staging and to characterize the response to treatment.

Nodules and mass lesions

A structured interstitial pattern refers to nodular or mass lesions in the pulmonary parenchyma. The distinction between a nodule and a mass is purely dependent on size, but the distinction is arbitrary. Nodules are roughly spherical lesions, which measure ≤2 cm in diameter. Lesions >2 cm in diameter are called masses, and lesions <3 mm may be more readily detected on CT and are referred to as micronodules. These distinctions are arbitrary, as 1 cm lesions are relatively larger in a dog weighing 3 kg than in a dog weighing 45 kg.

Nodules and masses can be caused by any abnormal tissue, benign or malignant. Potential etiologies include inflammation, infection, atelectasis, tumor, granuloma, abscess, hematoma, mucus-filled

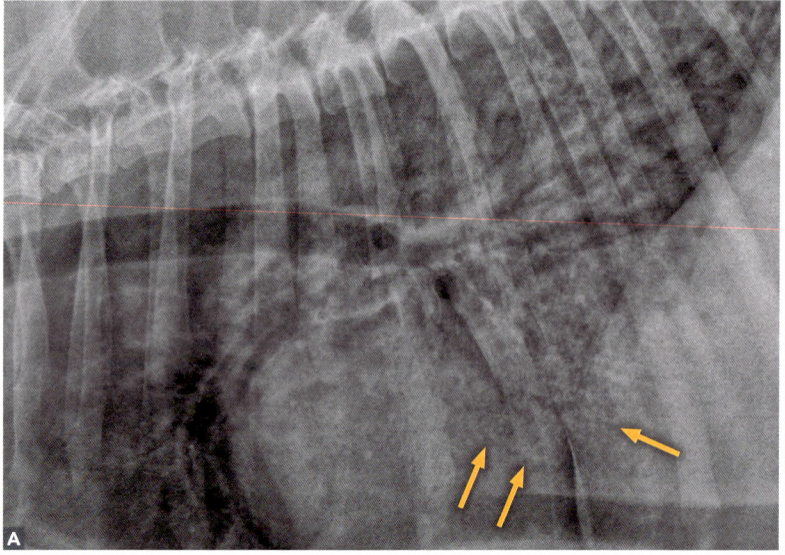

Fig. 23.39 An 11-year-old Rottweiler. Right lateral recumbency (**A**) and dorsoventral (**B**) projections of the thorax. Abnormal opacity which is mainly a severe unstructured interstitial pattern is distributed diffusely in all lung lobes, although sparing the cranial periphery of both lungs. (**A**) There is effacement of the caudal cardiac border, caudal vena cava and cupola of the diaphragm and air bronchograms indicating an alveolar pattern within the accessory lung lobe. Fine-needle aspirates from several peripheral lymph nodes showed abnormal lymphoid cells confirming a diagnosis of multicentric lymphoma.

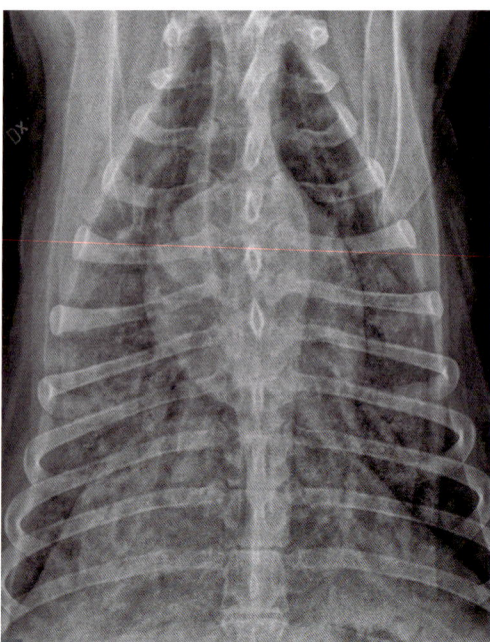

CHAPTER 23 Pulmonary infiltrations

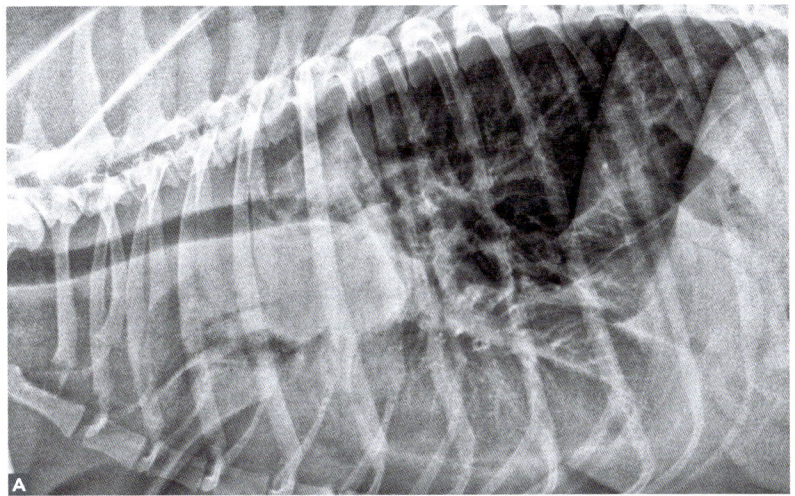

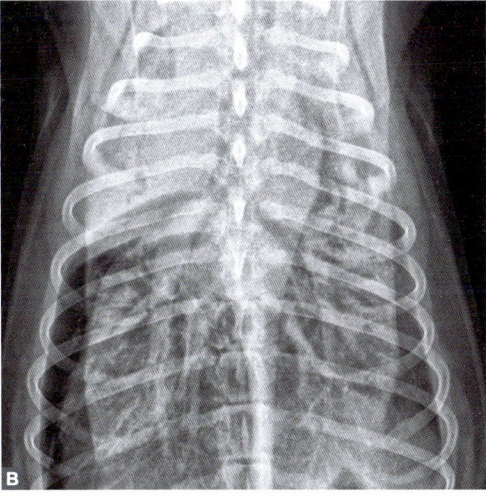

Fig. 23.40 Radiographic and ultrasound images of the thorax of a seven-year-old mixed breed female dog. In the left lateral recumbency projection (A) there is a soft tissue mass overlying the trachea and cranial aspect of the heart, and displacing the trachea dorsally. Within the mass, an air bronchogram extends in a cranial direction, indicating that parts of the mass involve the right cranial lung lobe. Due to its hilar location, at least some of the mass likely represents enlarged tracheobronchial lymph nodes. The bronchus of the right middle lung lobe has an abnormal caudal orientation from displacement, and the soft tissue mass obscures its hilar region. In the ventrodorsal projection (B) the entire right cranial lung lobe has an alveolar pattern, with a few air bronchograms. The alveolar pattern creates a lobar sign at the junction with the aerated right middle lung lobe. Image (C) shows an ultrasound guided FNA procedure using an intercostal approach in the right cranial thorax using a 11 MHz linear transducer. The needle (arrows) penetrates the thoracic wall into a focal hypoechoic lesion within the right cranial lung. The cytology from the lesion revealed a lymphoma.

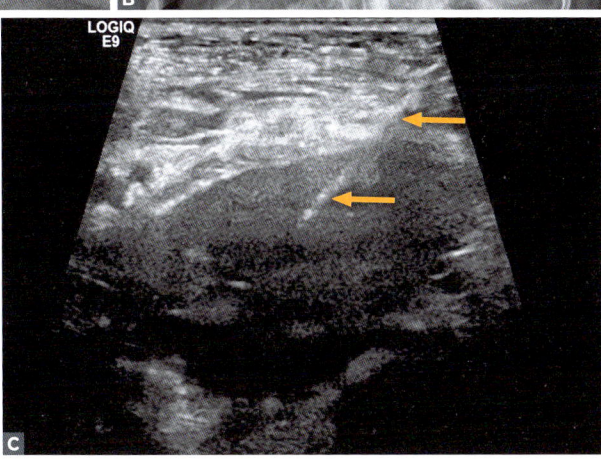

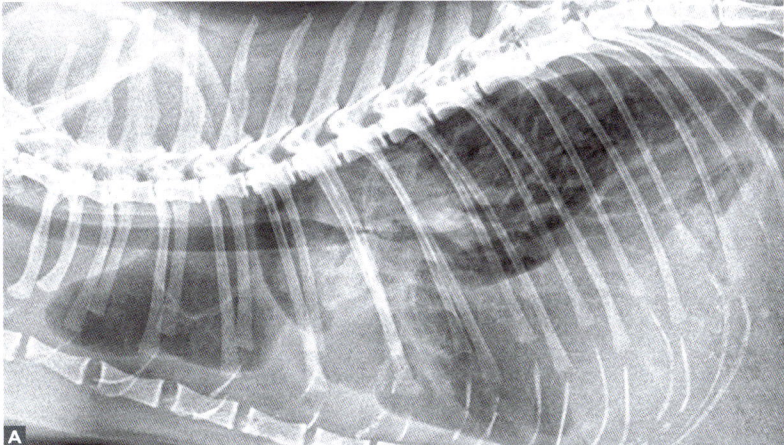

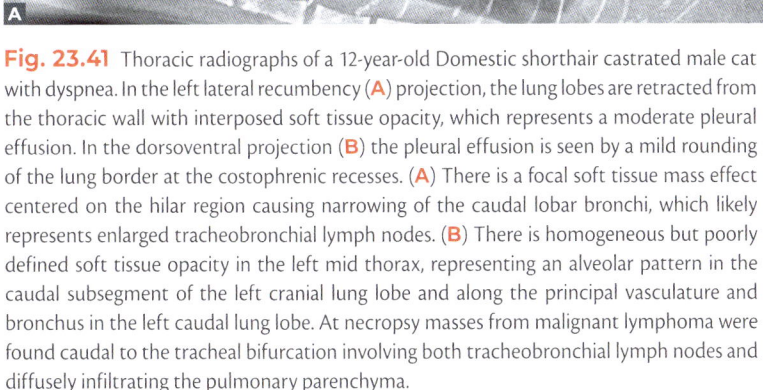

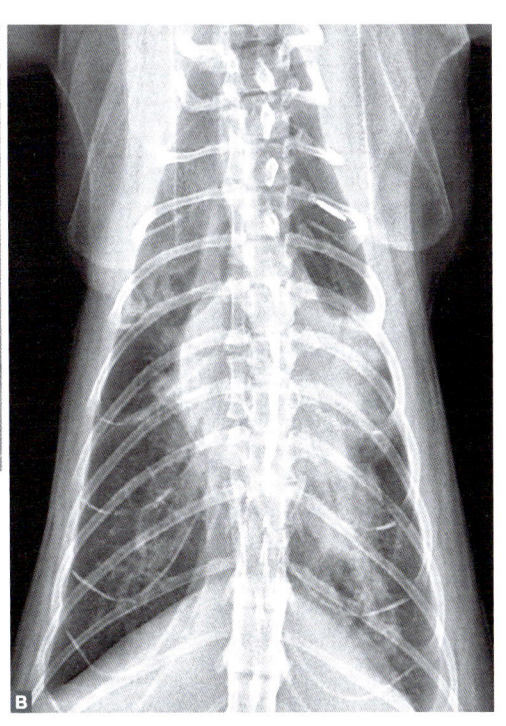

Fig. 23.41 Thoracic radiographs of a 12-year-old Domestic shorthair castrated male cat with dyspnea. In the left lateral recumbency (A) projection, the lung lobes are retracted from the thoracic wall with interposed soft tissue opacity, which represents a moderate pleural effusion. In the dorsoventral projection (B) the pleural effusion is seen by a mild rounding of the lung border at the costophrenic recesses. (A) There is a focal soft tissue mass effect centered on the hilar region causing narrowing of the caudal lobar bronchi, which likely represents enlarged tracheobronchial lymph nodes. (B) There is homogeneous but poorly defined soft tissue opacity in the left mid thorax, representing an alveolar pattern in the caudal subsegment of the left cranial lung lobe and along the principal vasculature and bronchus in the left caudal lung lobe. At necropsy masses from malignant lymphoma were found caudal to the tracheal bifurcation involving both tracheobronchial lymph nodes and diffusely infiltrating the pulmonary parenchyma.

SECTION IV THORAX

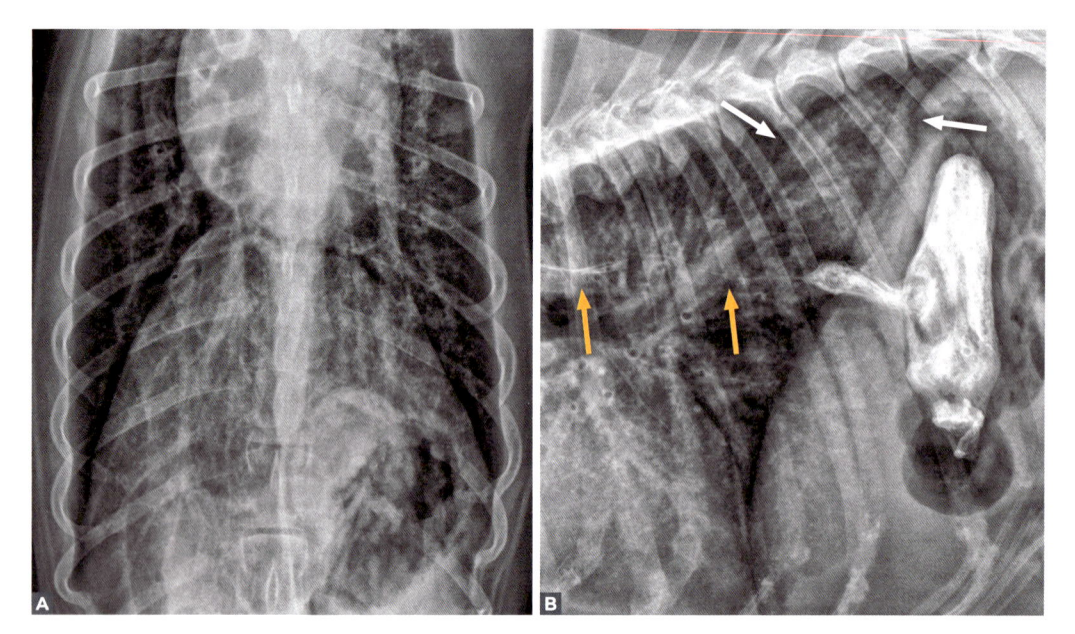

Fig. 23.42 A 13-year-old mixed breed male dog. In the initial plain thoracic right lateral recumbency (image is not shown) and dorsoventral (A) projections, an oval soft tissue mass outlined by aerated pulmonary parenchyma was seen, slightly to the left of the midline in the caudodorsal periphery of the thorax. There was some uncertainty whether the mass could involve the mediastinum and esophagus. A barium esophagogram with a right lateral recumbency projection (B) was made to investigate whether the mass involved the esophagus. The normal esophageal lumen is outlined by a thin line of barium contrast (orange arrows), and the soft tissue mass is dorsal to and separate from the esophagus (white arrows) and was determined to be of pulmonary origin. A definitive diagnosis was not obtained, but the mass was assumed most likely to represent primary neoplasia within the left caudal lung lobe. There is a generalized moderate to severe mixed bronchial and interstitial pattern.

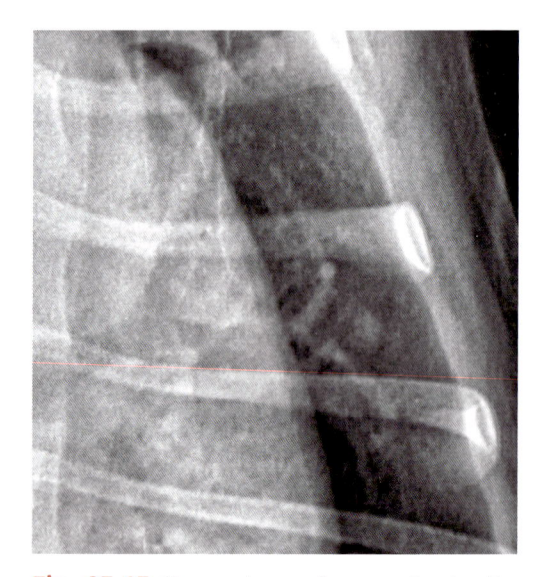

Fig. 23.43 Close-up image of a ventrodorsal radiographic projection of the thorax showing the left cranial lung lobe. The image shows a round distinctly outlined soft tissue structure that measured 1.5 mm in diameter. The structure and the longitudinally oriented vessel crossing it have the same diameter but the round structure is opaquer, indicating it is an end-on vessel.

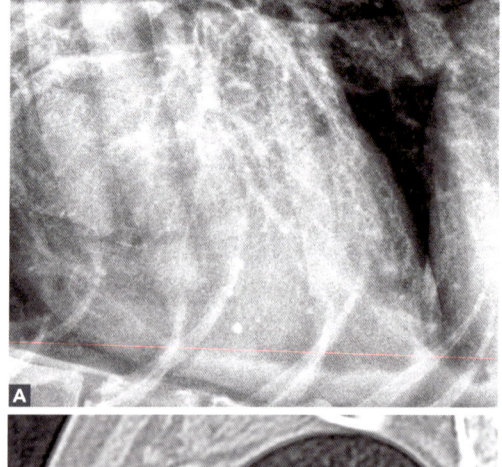

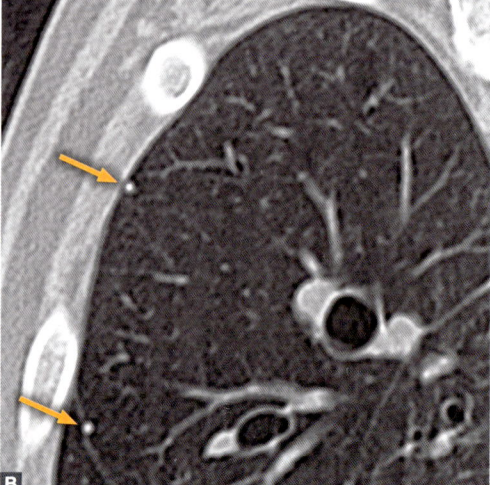

Fig. 23.44 Close-up of a right lateral recumbency thoracic radiograph (A) of a ten-year-old Rottweiler with pulmonary osseous metaplasia. Several small mineral opacity structures are seen in the ventral thorax in the lung superimposed on the cardiac silhouette. These range in size between 1-3 mm, which is smaller than the detection limit for soft tissue nodules, and these are visible because they are mineralized. These do not have a connection with the visible vascular tree and are therefore not end-on vessels. A close-up of a transverse CT image (B) in lung window of the right caudal lung lobe in the same dog. Two very small (<2 mm in diameter) mineral attenuating lesions (arrows) are visible close to the visceral pleural surface of the lung. These represent pulmonary osseous metaplasia as seen in the radiograph (A).

bronchus, fluid-filled bullae, cyst, or even a vascular malformation. Therefore, their interpretation must be considered together within the entire clinical context, and never solely on the radiological appearance. For instance, a pulmonary nodule in a patient with a proven malignant neoplasm is more likely to be a metastatic lesion than a nodule found in a patient being assessed for cardiac disease. Masses in the lung may be suitable for ultrasound-guided fine-needle aspirate if the lesion reaches the visceral pleural surface of the lung, adjacent to the thoracic wall (without any interposed gas). The patient usually needs to be sedated or anesthetized to minimize the risk of iatrogenic pneumothorax or hemothorax. A barium esophagogram can in some instances help to distinguish if a mass is associated with the esophagus (**fig. 23.42**).

There is the potential for erroneous overdiagnosis of nodules. It is crucial to recognize that pulmonary vessels seen end-on, can mimic soft tissue nodules. Soft tissue nodules smaller than 5-10 mm are usually not visible on conventional radiographs and any distinctly visible soft tissue opacity nodular structure smaller than 5 mm is likely to be an end-on vessel. Pulmonary vessels are so clearly visible when they are projected end-on, because the structure is a cylinder rather than a sphere and therefore opaquer than comparably sized nearby side-on vessels. End-on vessels are of similar or smaller diameter as nearby side-on blood vessels. End-on vessels are of larger diameter at the hilus and smaller in the periphery since the branching vessels in the vascular tree gradually taper (**fig. 23.43**). Pulmonary osseous metaplasia (also called pulmonary osteomas, subpleural osteomas, heterotopic bone, pneumoliths, and calcified pleural plaques), is a form of dystrophic mineralization in the pleura and lung parenchyma and is common benign incidental finding in older dogs. It is essential not to mistake these with pulmonary soft tissue nodules (**fig. 23.44**). Pulmonary osseous metaplasias are small, often only a few millimeters in diameter. They are extremely opaque (mineral opacity) for their small size, often irregular in shape, and have a predominantly ventral distribution. In spite of their small size, they are visible because of their mineral content, and are usually opaquer than adjacent larger side-on vessels. Mineralization in metastatic or inflammatory pulmonary lesions is relatively rare.

Metastatic neoplasia

Screening for pulmonary metastases should include a minimum of ventrodorsal or dorsoventral, left, and right lateral recumbent projections, since the atelectasis that occurs in dependent parts of the lung can prevent identification of nodules and masses. While radiographs are a good screening tool for nodules, lesions less than 5-10 mm in size may go undetected. CT has proven significantly more sensitive than radiographs for the detection of pulmonary soft tissue nodules in dogs. CT can detect smaller nodules and identifies more nodules. CT is preferred to radiographs if any evidence of metastasis will substantially alter treatment or prognosis of a cancer patient. However, the higher sensitivity for detecting nodules on CT can also be problematic, since not all small nodules or micronodules are neoplastic. Serial studies may be required to determine if lesions progress or are inactive.

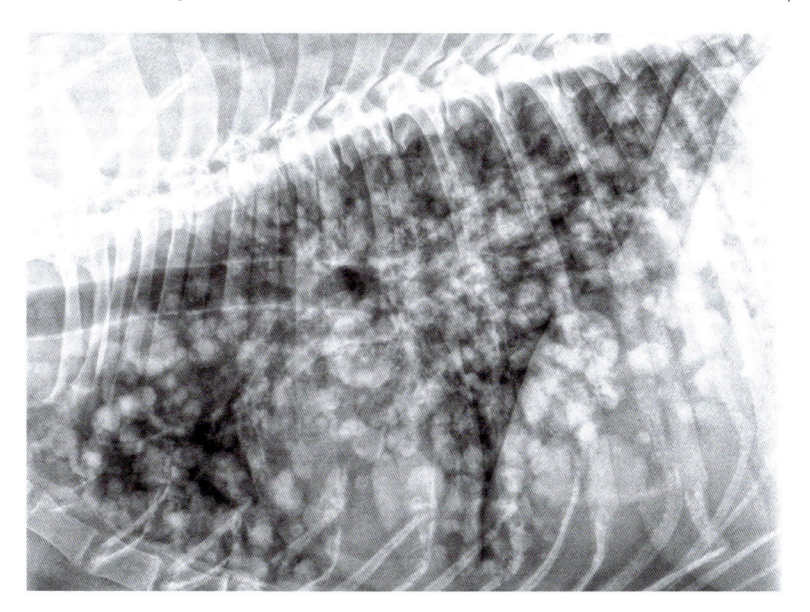

The radiological appearance in metastatic neoplasia varies greatly. The typical pattern is of a few or multiple soft tissue nodules in multiple lung lobes. They are often of different sizes owing to multiple episodes of tumor embolism (**fig. 23.45**). The term miliary pattern is sometimes used when describing numerous very small nodules, which may coalesce making it difficult to discern individual nodules (**fig. 23.46**). Individual nodules may be more readily distinguished in ventral periphery of

Fig. 23.45 Right lateral recumbency thoracic radiograph of a nine-year-old female German Shepherd dog. Multiple variably sized soft tissue nodules (structured interstitial pattern) are present throughout all lung lobes. A few are larger mass lesions, greater than 3 cm in diameter. The dog had an anal gland adenocarcinoma that had metastasized to the lungs.

the lung overlying the heart or liver where the lung is thinner. Metastases can also present as a generalized bronchointerstitial pattern, unstructured interstitial pattern (**fig. 23.47**) or random alveolar pattern (**fig. 23.48**), or as a solitary nodule or mass. Metastatic neoplasia can also appear as a generalized unstructured interstitial pattern, in cases where neoplastic cells infiltrate and block lymphatic vessels.

Primary lung neoplasia

Primary lung neoplasia affects both dogs and cats, although it is rare. They are more often malignant, with reported types including bronchoalveolar carcinoma, adenocarcinomas, adenosquamous carcinoma, and squamous cell carcinomas. Adenocarcinomas are most common in both cats and dogs. The most common radiographic appearance of a primary pulmonary tumor is a single, distinctly well circumscribed mass or nodule, located peripherally in a lung lobe.

The appearance and location of lesions can, however, vary significantly (partly related to tumor type), and varies more in the cat than in the dog. The more common adenocarcinomas tend to be located in the peripheral lung regions, and more so in caudal lung lobes in both dogs[22] and cats[23] (**fig. 23.49**). Bronchioloalveolar carcinomas tend to be located more in the middle or peripheral regions, and squamous cell carcinomas are more often perihilar.[24] In addition to a mass lesion, findings in cats can include pleural effusion (**fig. 23.50**), and tracheobronchial lymphadenopathy.[23] Rarely a primary carcinoma may have a lobar or segmental bronchointerstitial pattern (**fig. 23.51**). In dogs, CT is more sensitive than radiographs in showing tracheobronchial lymphadenopathy with pulmonary neoplasia, which is an important prognostic factor if surgical resection is contemplated. Primary tumors may be cavitated, i.e., contain varying amounts of air, if the center is necrotic and communicates with an airway (**fig. 23.50**), and they may or may not be calcified (**fig. 23.52**). Cavitation is usually not seen with metastatic disease.[23] Superficial lesions may be accessible for ultrasound guided sampling. If this is not feasible or is declined, serial radiographs at 4-6 week intervals are recommended for monitoring progression if surgical excision is not elected. If the lesion has a static appearance after 2-3 months, malignant neoplasia is unlikely.

CT studies describing the appearance of primary lung tumors in cats and dogs agree that single mass lesions in peripheral lung regions are most common. They also show that masses tend to be bronchocentric, contain internal air bronchograms, have intratumoral mineralizations and tracheobronchial lymphadenopathy. Some dogs have additional pulmonary nodules, which is interpreted as nodular metastasis from the primary pulmonary tumor. Because CT is more sensitive for evaluating tracheobronchial lymph node enlargement and intrapulmonary metastases, CT should be considered part of the staging process in primary lung tumors.[24]

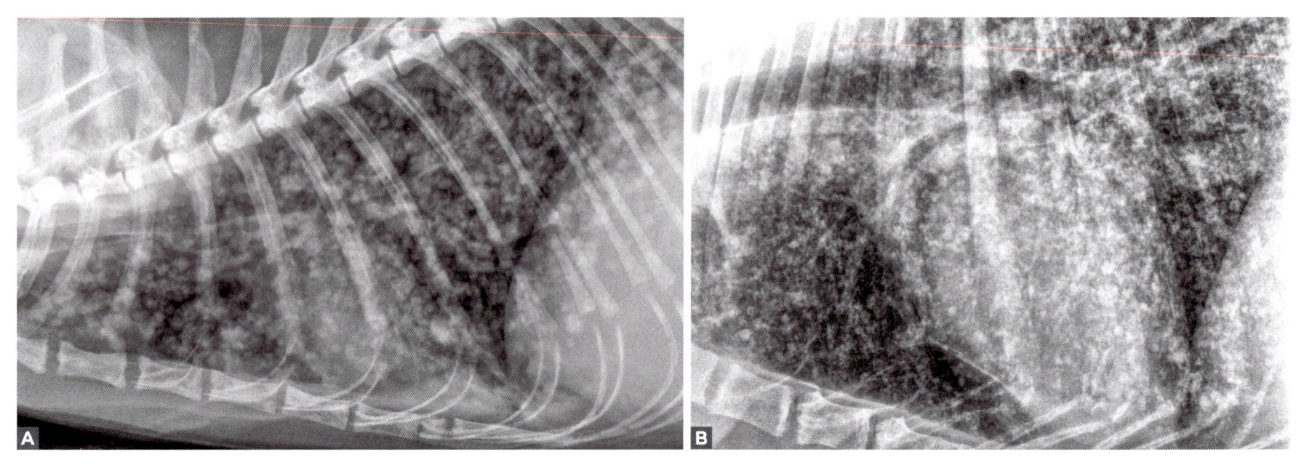

Fig. 23.46 Lateral thoracic radiographs of an eight-year-old castrated male Domestic shorthair cat (**A**) and of an eight-year-old German Shepherd dog (**B**). Both have numerous small nodular soft tissue opacity lesions throughout the lung field. This can be described as a miliary pattern due to its resemblance to millet seeds. (**A**) The lesions were thought to be metastases from a diffuse iris melanoma. (**B**) The metastases to the lungs were thought to originate from a soft tissue neoplasia in a hindlimb.

CHAPTER 23 Pulmonary infiltrations

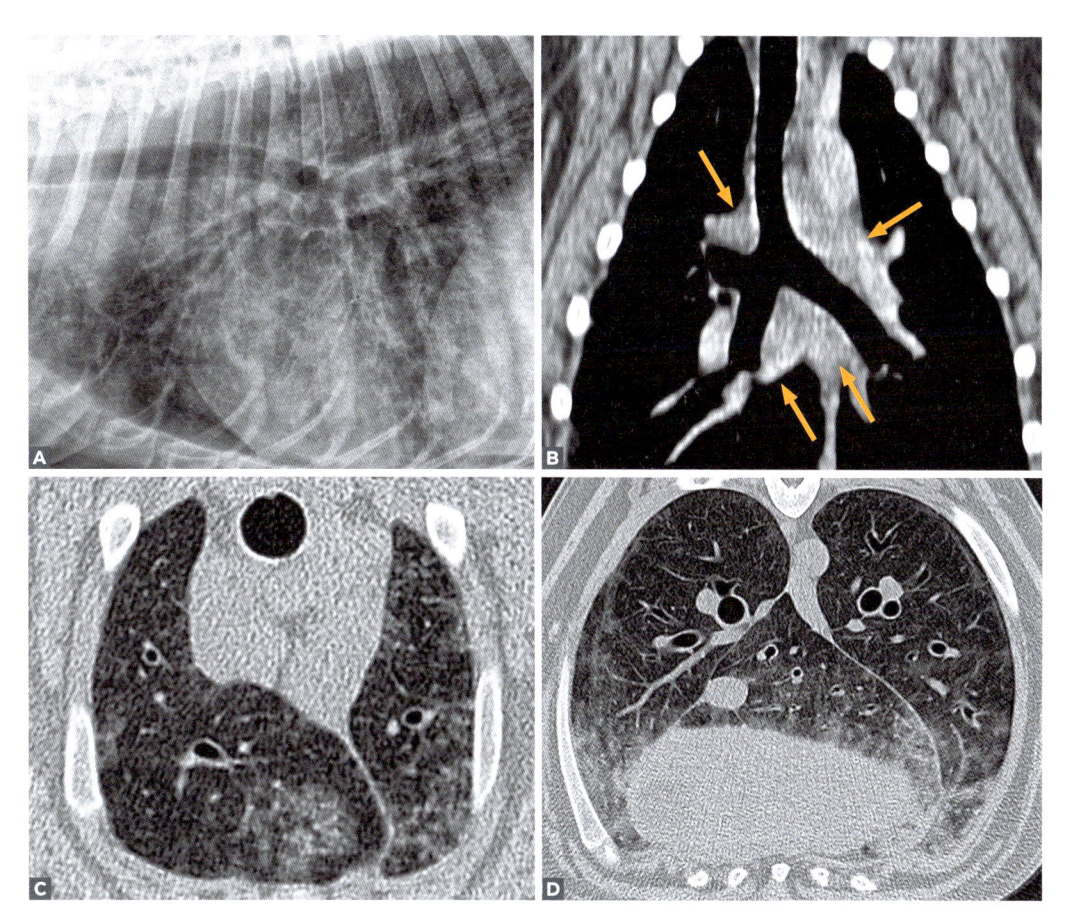

Fig. 23.47 A seven-year-old female castrated Bullmastiff where neoplastic cells consistent with carcinoma were found on a bronchoalveolar lavage. In the initial right lateral recumbency thoracic radiograph (A) a severe patchy unstructured interstitial pattern is seen in the ventral lung field. A CT of the thorax (B-D) was performed a few days after radiography. (B) A dorsal plane soft tissue reconstruction after intravenous contrast injection. It shows a significant enlargement of multiple lymph nodes around the tracheal bifurcation (arrows), which are not visible on the radiograph. (C, D) Transverse reconstructions windowed for lung at the level of the cranial lung lobes (C), and caudal lung lobes (D). There are patches of ground-glass attenuation mainly in the ventral parts of the lung lobes, but there are also areas of increased attenuation in the dorsal subpleural parts of the lungs. Some larger bronchi have thickened walls. The origin of the neoplasia could not be determined.

Fig. 23.48 Dorsoventral (A) and left lateral recumbency (B) thoracic radiographs of a nine-year-old male Malinois. There is a generalized increased pulmonary opacity. An alveolar pattern with air bronchograms and border effacement of the cardiac silhouette is present throughout the ventral lung field. A patchy severe interstitial pattern is visible in the caudodorsal lung field. At necropsy, 70-80% of the pulmonary volume was occupied by neoplastic tissue, confirmed as hemangiosarcoma.

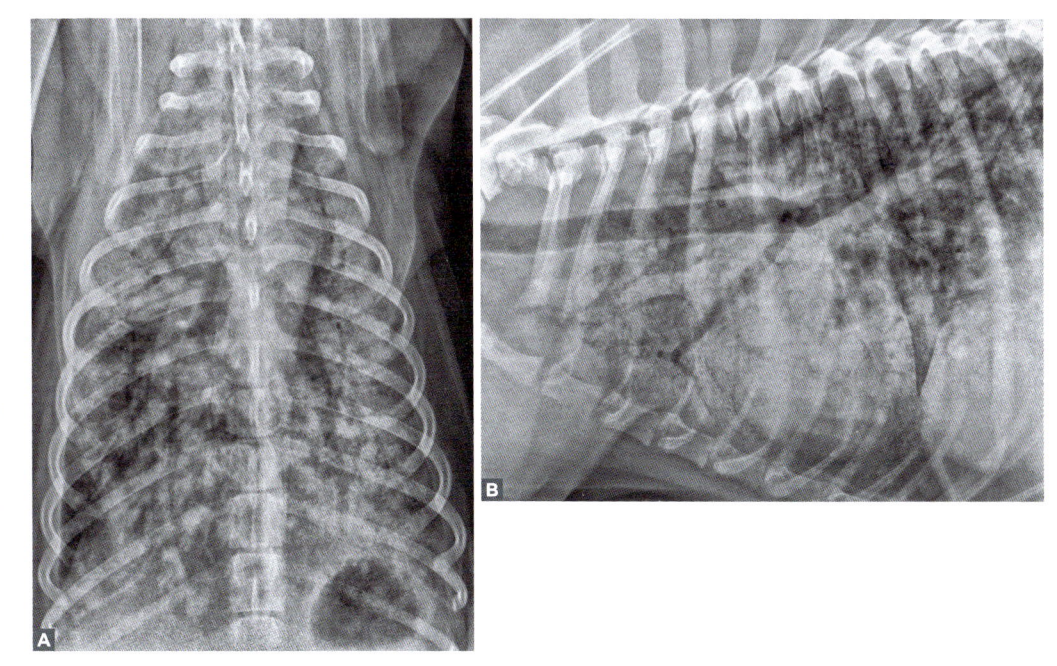

SECTION IV THORAX

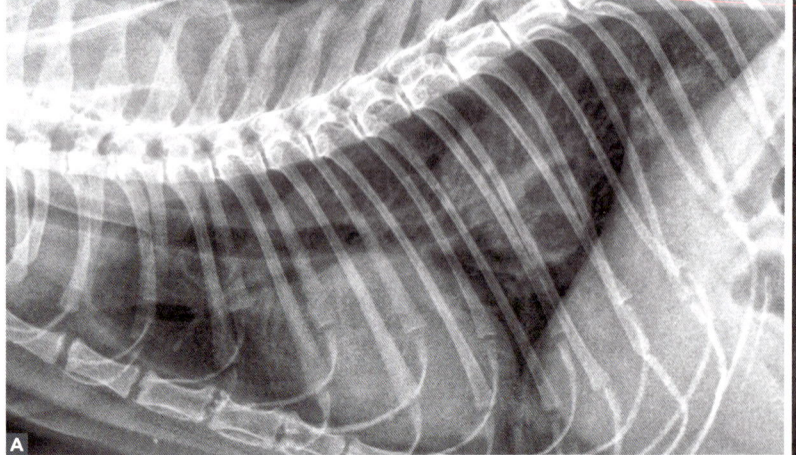

Fig. 23.49 A 14-year-old castrated female Persian cat with a sudden onset of painful left forelimb lameness. Thoracic radiographs, left lateral recumbency (**A**) and ventrodorsal (**B**) projections reveal a large, round soft tissue mass in the central zone of the left caudal lung lobe (outlined by arrows in image **B**). This mass was confirmed to be an adenocarcinoma. An additional 5 mm in diameter adenocarcinoma nodule was found in the right cranial lung lobe on necropsy. This nodule is not visible in the radiographs. It is known that nodules up to 5 mm or slightly larger may not be radiographically visible. The cat's lameness and pain in the left forelimb were caused by ischemia from a tumor embolus in the radial artery.

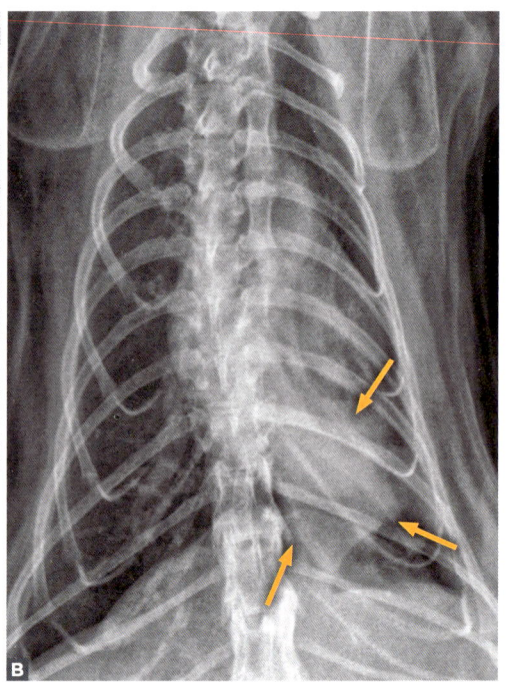

Fig. 23.50 A 12-year-old Persian female cat with moderate pleural effusion. (**A**, **B**) Left lateral recumbency and dorsoventral projections of the thorax before pleural drainage. All lung lobes are retracted from the thoracic wall and surrounded by a homogeneous soft tissue opacity. Therapeutic centesis with follow-up radiography after drainage can help identify lesions crucial for diagnosis. In this case, a poorly defined cavitated mass lesion in the caudododorsal periphery of the right caudal lung lobe is more clearly visualized in both the left lateral recumbency (**C**) and dorsoventral (**D**) projections after drainage.

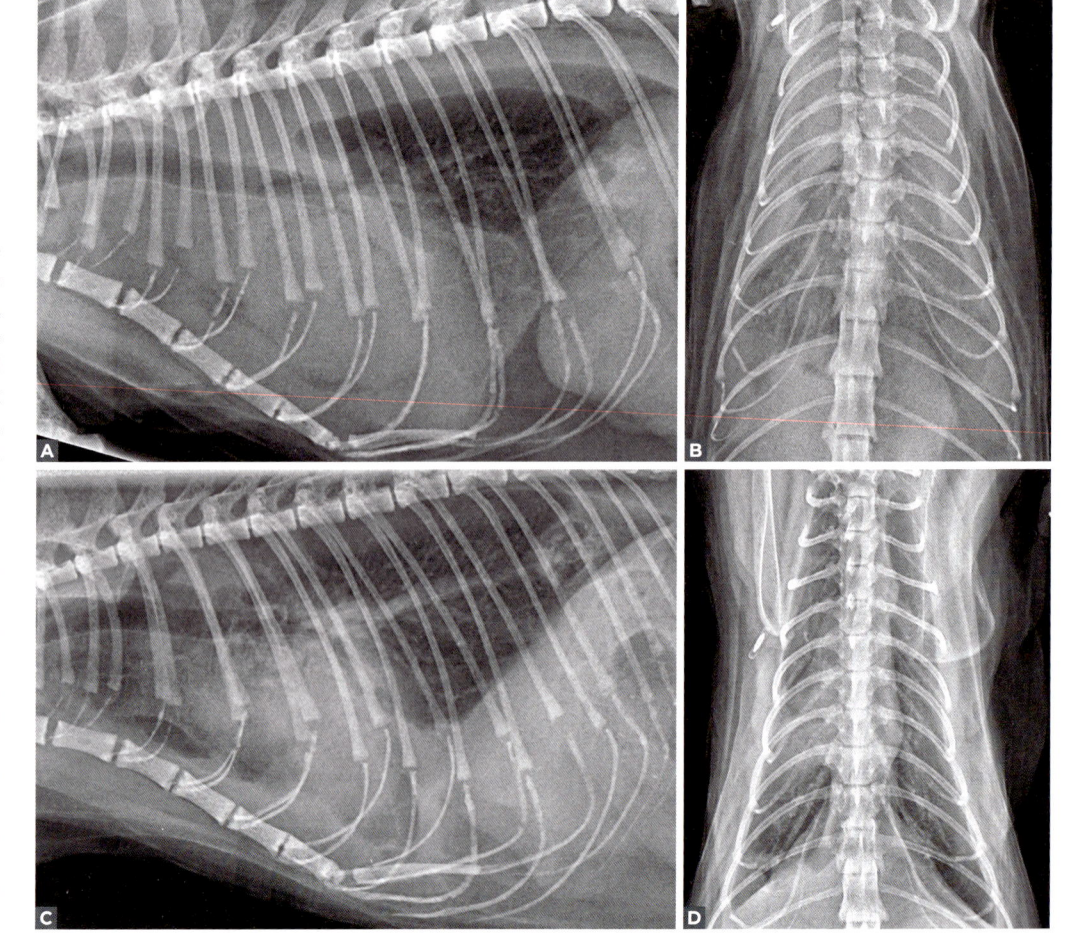

392

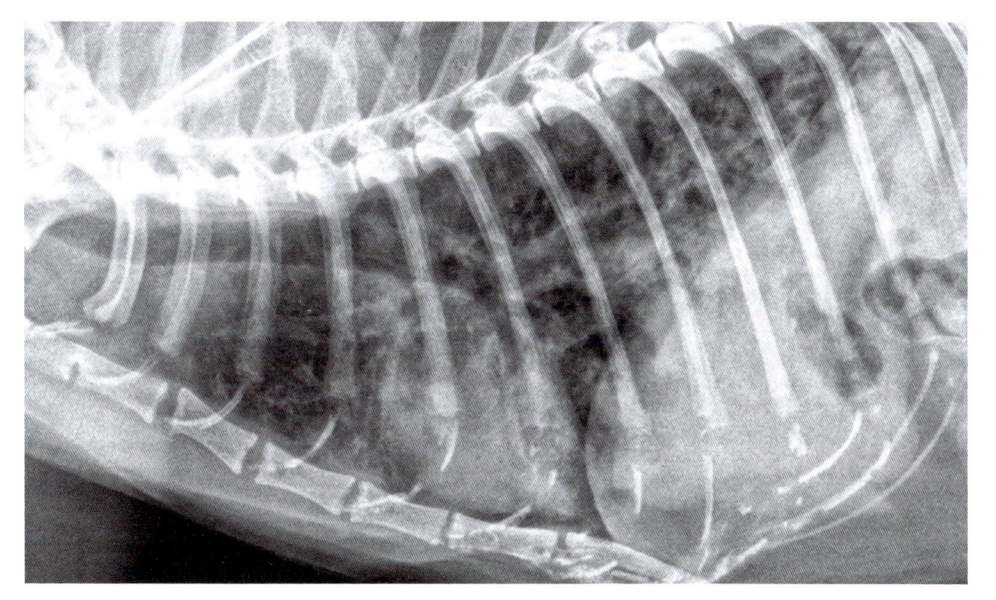

Fig. 23.51 A 13-year-old Domestic shorthair cat with confirmed diffuse spread of adenocarcinoma in all lung lobes. Right lateral recumbency thoracic radiograph shows patches of severe unstructured interstitial opacity interposed between areas of bronchointerstitial pattern. Necropsy also showed metastases to mediastinal and tracheobronchial lymph nodes, not apparent on the radiograph.

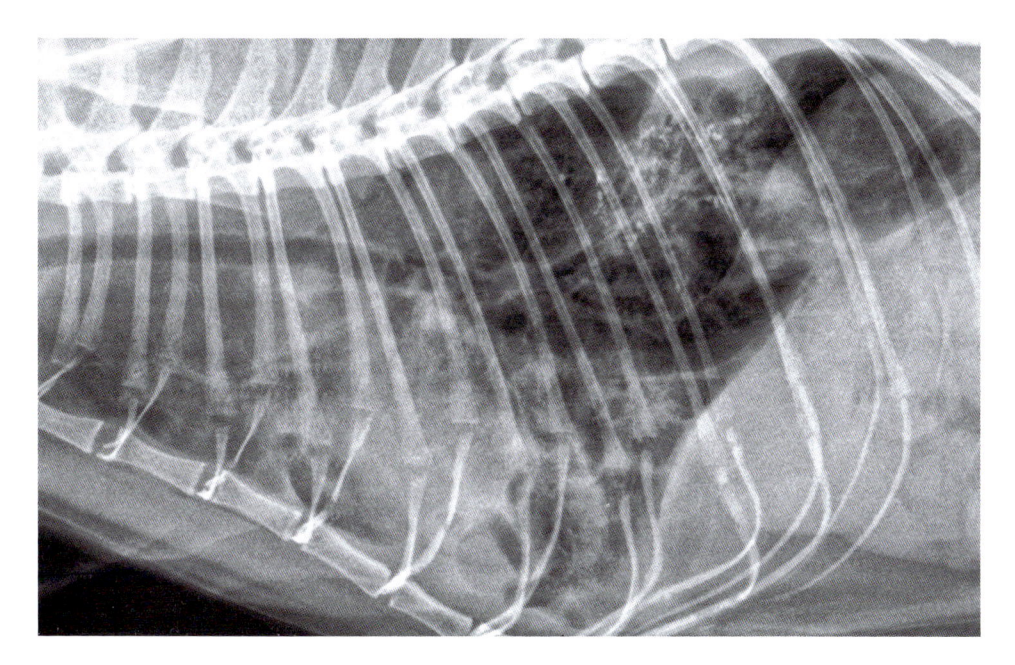

Fig. 23.52 A nine-year-old Domestic shorthair cat with confirmed multifocal adenocarcinoma in several lung lobes. A lateral projection of the thorax. Most of the pulmonary parenchyma is abnormal, with multiple foci of poorly defined heterogenous soft tissue opacity, a combination of mass lesions and severe interstitial opacity. Multiple small amorphous mineral opacities are present within a lesion in the caudal lung lobes.

Histiocytic sarcoma

Histiocytic sarcoma is a neoplasia of dendritic cell origin that can affect the lungs and many other organs. It has previously also been called malignant histiocytosis and disseminated histiocytic sarcoma. The tumor type appears in dogs and cats but is quite rare in cats. Two forms are described, a localized histiocytic sarcoma and a disseminated histiocytic sarcoma, depending on if one or multiple organs are affected. Both localized and disseminated forms can affect the lungs. Breed predisposition is reported mainly for the Bernese Mountain dog, but also for Flat Coated Retrievers, Rottweilers, and Miniature Schnauzers.[25]

As with many lung neoplasias, the appearance of histiocytic sarcoma may vary. However, histiocytic sarcoma is a likely diagnosis in patients with pulmonary masses and sternal and tracheobronchial lymphadenopathy.[22] (**figs. 23.53** and **23.54**). Other reported findings include pleural effusion, generalized interstitial pattern, patchy consolidations, and concurrent skeletal and abdominal lesions[25] (**figs. 23.55** and **23.56**).

SECTION IV THORAX

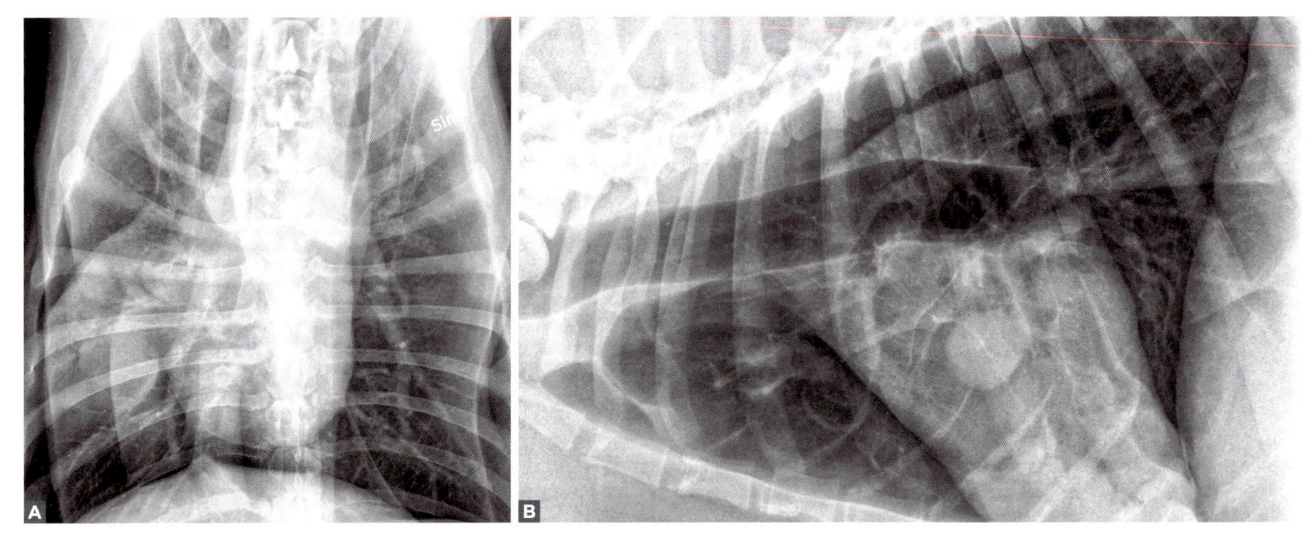

Fig. 23.53 A seven-year-old male Bernese Mountain dog. Thoracic radiographs, ventrodorsal and left lateral recumbency projections. In the ventrodorsal projection (**A**) there is an ovoid well defined mass within the right middle lung lobe. A second mass is partly visible in the hilar part of the lobe. An alveolar pattern with air bronchograms, creating a lobar sign between the aerated right cranial lung lobe and the opaque part of the right middle lung lobe is present. In the left lateral recumbency projection (**B**), one of the round mass lesions is located in the mid zone of the lobe, and the alveolar opacity is in the ventral periphery of the right middle lung lobe. These lesions were histiocytic sarcoma, and this breed has a known predisposition.

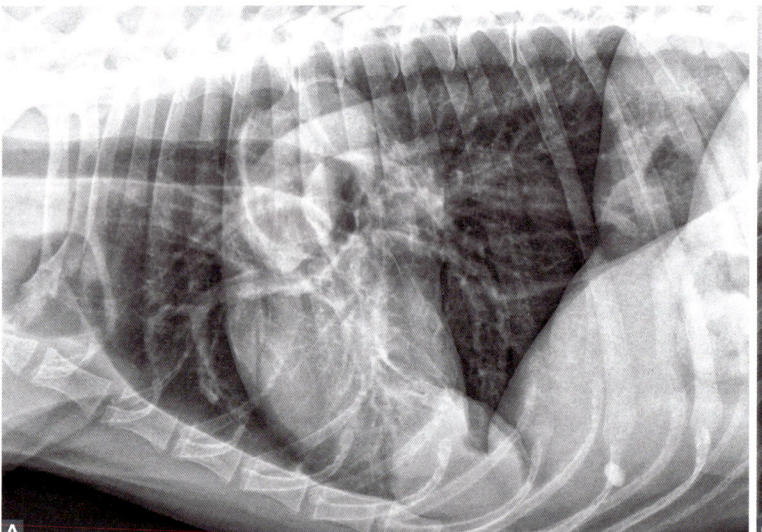

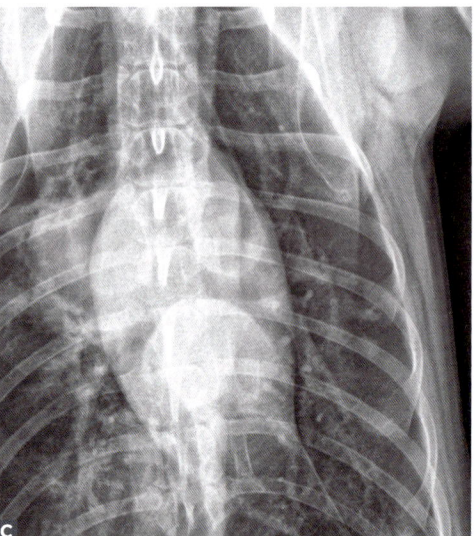

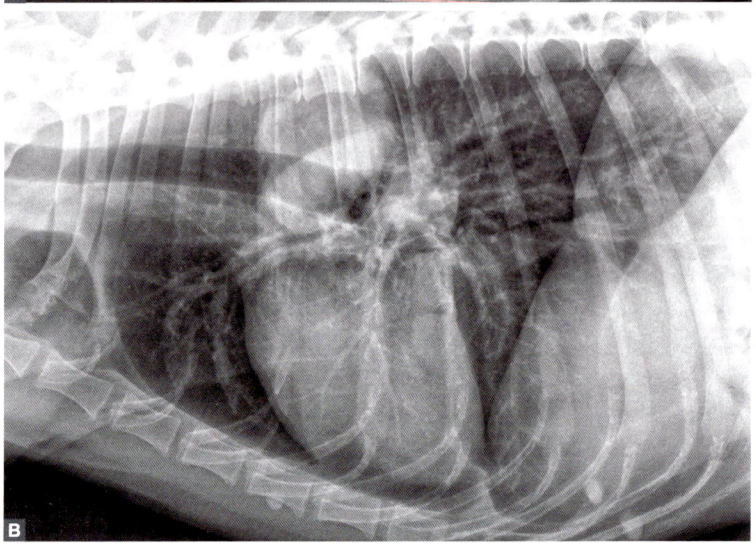

Fig. 23.54 (**A**) Left lateral recumbency, (**B**) right lateral recumbency and (**C**) ventrodorsal thoracic radiographs of an eight-year-old female Pharaoh Hound. A mass is located in the ventral periphery of the right middle lung lobe and is seen clearly in the left lateral recumbency projection. It is faintly visible in the right lateral recumbency projection (**B**) due to dependent atelectasis. A lobulated soft tissue mass lesion is present in the hilar zone of the right lung and surrounds both the tracheal bifurcation and the hilar portion of the right cranial lobar bronchus (**C**). The mass causes a ventral deviation of the bronchus to the right cranial lung lobe (seen in image **A**) and lateral displacement of the caudal lobar bronchi in the ventrodorsal projection (**C**). The changes indicate severe enlargement of the tracheobronchial lymph nodes. Necropsy confirmed histiocytic sarcoma in the right cranial and middle lung lobes and severely enlarged tracheobronchial and mediastinal lymph nodes.

CHAPTER 23 Pulmonary infiltrations

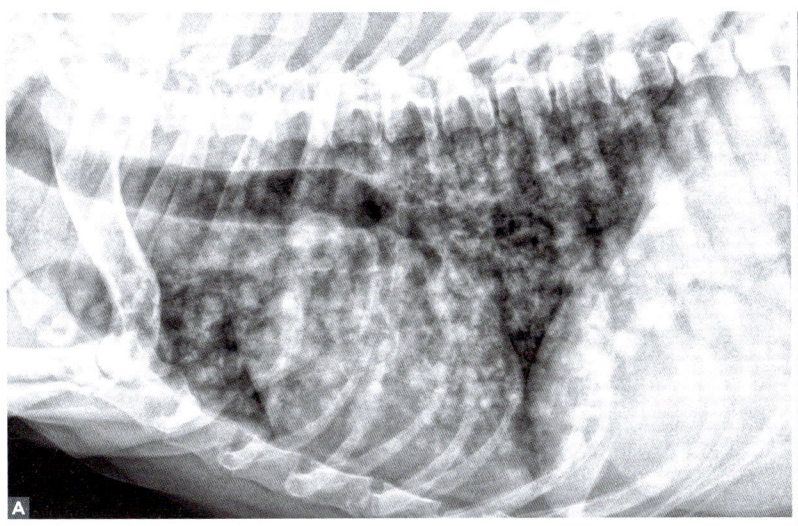

Fig. 23.55 A 14-year-old female Glen of Imaal Terrier. Left lateral recumbency (A) and ventrodorsal (B) projections of the thorax. A generalized nodular interstitial pattern is present in all lung lobes with varying sized nodules. The dog had several skin nodules diagnosed as histiocytic sarcomas, and the pulmonary nodules very likely represent the same neoplasm. There are so many overlapping nodular lesions that individual lesions are hard to discern. Discrete nodules are more readily seen in thin parts of the lung, such as the ventral thorax overlying the heart.

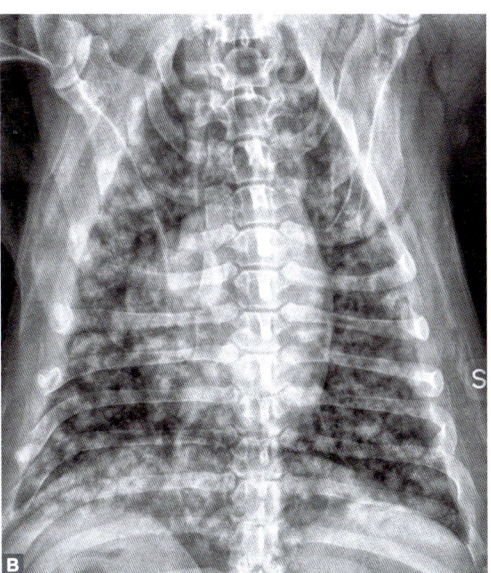

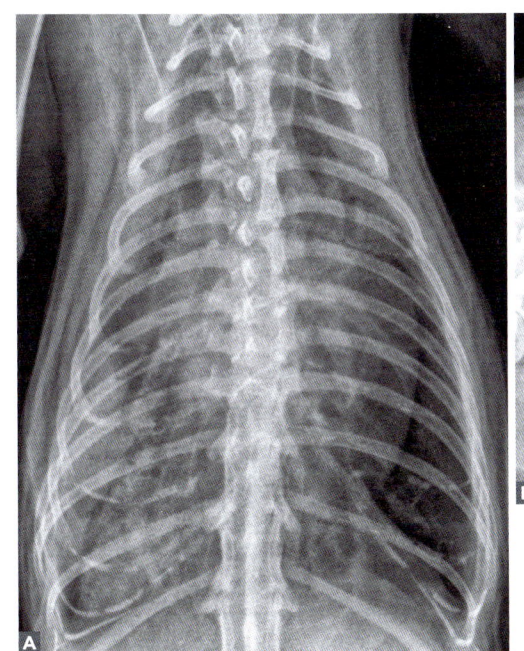

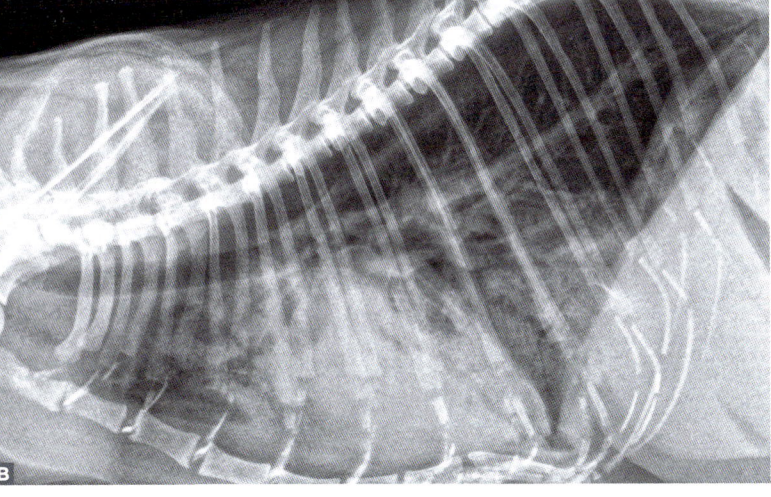

Fig. 23.56 A nine-year-old Domestic shorthair cat. In the dorsoventral projection (A) there is an alveolar pattern in the right lung and left cranial lung lobe, with air bronchograms and border effacement of the right hemidiaphragm and cardiac silhouette. In the left lateral recumbency projection (B), the alveolar opacity partly effaces the entire cardiac silhouette, and effaces the vasculature to the cranial and middle lung lobes, the caudal vena cava and cupola of the diaphragm. There is a compensatory hyperinflation of the caudal lung lobes. This cat had a round cell neoplasia, likely histiocytic sarcoma in the pulmonary parenchyma.

Granulomas

Granulomas and abscesses can cause focal or multifocal nodular and mass lesions in the pulmonary parenchyma depending on their origin. With a systemic hematogenous spread, the distribution is more likely to be generalized or affecting multiple lung lobes. Granulomas can have parasitic or fungal origins. Granulomas and abscesses can also be caused by inhaled foreign bodies and such lesions have a caudodorsal distribution in the lungs. Small migrating foreign bodies can cause a low-grade chronic cough, with subtle localized radiographic findings or normal radiographs. In contrast, larger foreign bodies can create considerable mass lesions, radiographically mimicking primary lung neoplasia (**fig. 23.57**).

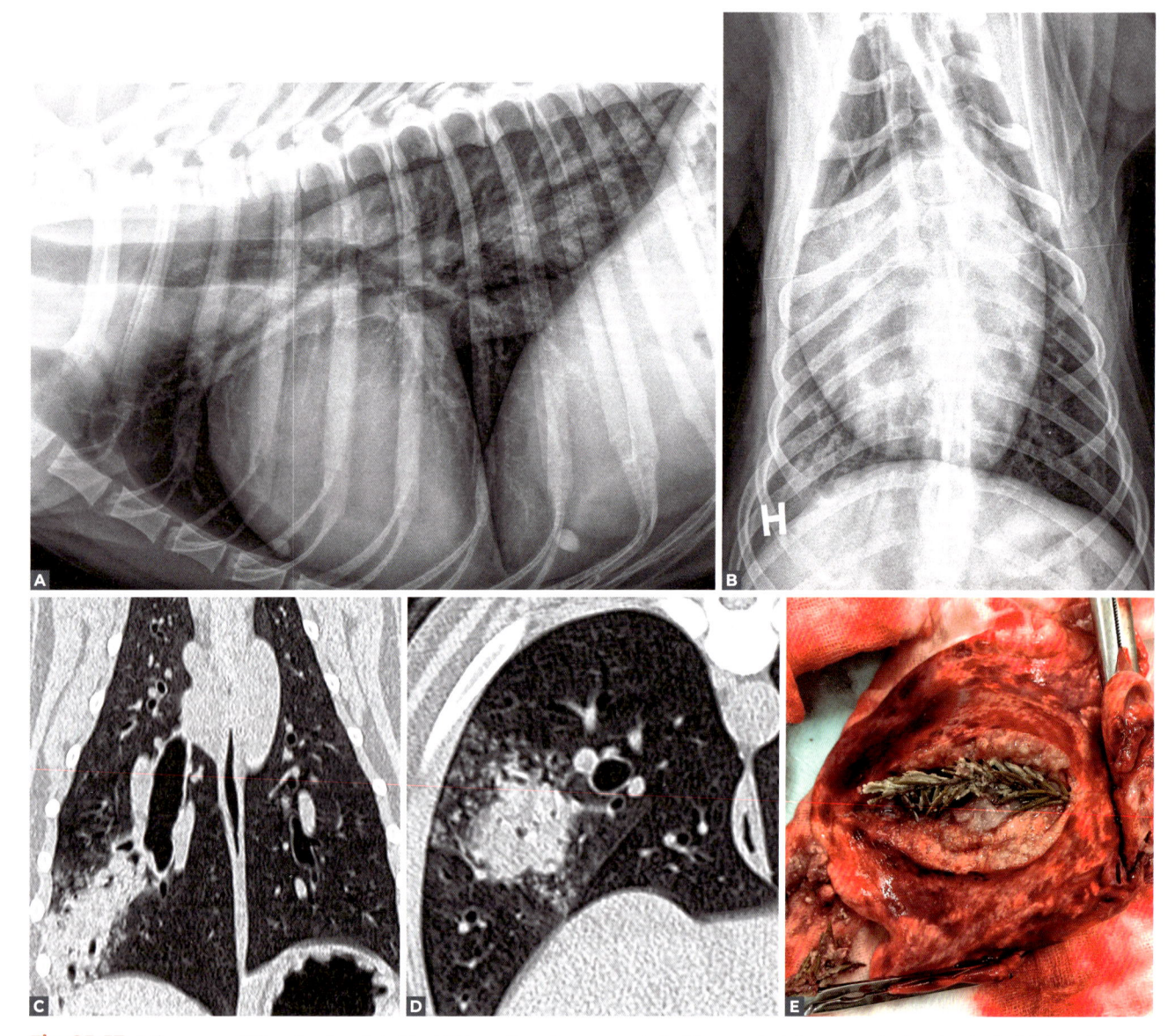

Fig. 23.57 A three-year-old hunting dog of the Finnish Hound breed was presented with a cough of three-months duration. In the left lateral recumbency (**A**) radiograph, focal poorly defined, heterogenous alveolar opacity is seen in the caudodorsal lung field between the caudal vena cava and aorta. The same lesion is seen in the right caudal lung field in the ventrodorsal projection (**B**). To further characterize the lesion, a CT was performed. (**C**) Dorsal plane reconstruction of the thorax at the level of the caudal lung lobes, windowed for lungs. An elongated area of consolidated lung tissue containing multiple small gas pockets is seen in the right caudal lung lobe conforming to a secondary bronchus. The bronchus is obliterated. (**D**) Transverse plane reconstruction of the right caudal lung lobe, showing the consolidated area in cross-section. A discrete foreign body cannot be seen but there is a significant relatively circumscribed lesion associated with the airway. The location in the mid zone of the right caudal lung lobe closely associated with the airways is a frequent site for an inhaled foreign body and this is the most likely diagnosis. The right caudal lung lobe was removed. (**E**) Cut through the lung lesion that reveals a 5 cm long branch from the European spruce tree (*Picea abies*), still with most of the needles in place. The lesion is a foreign body granuloma.

Lung lobe torsion

Lung lobe torsion occurs in both dogs and cats. The most common localization is the right middle lung lobe in large breed dogs, while the left cranial lung lobe is more commonly affected in small breed dogs. The affected lobe has diffusely increased soft tissue opacity, which may be uniform. In some cases, there is lobar soft tissue opacity with numerous interspersed small gas bubbles, resembling a sponge or foam, referred to as a vesicular pattern. The affected lobe is usually enlarged from congestion, causing a mediastinal shift away from the affected lobe. In some cases, the hilar segment of the lobar bronchus remains visible but is abruptly truncated. The bronchus may also have an abnormal orientation or a visible twist, resembling a pigtail. Pleural effusion may be present either adjacent to the affected lobe or throughout the pleural space and can obscure the abnormal lobe. With ultrasound, the affected lobe appears hypoechoic in the periphery, with hyperechoic foci in the central portion from residual air. The sonographic changes are not specific, and it is not possible to obtain a confirmed diagnosis with this technique. Computed tomography is the preferred imaging modality to diagnose lung lobe torsion. Findings are an abruptly ending bronchus and pleural effusion with enlargement, consolidation, emphysema of the affected lung lobe, and a mediastinal shift. Interestingly, the rotated lung lobes do not enhance, whereas adjacent collapsed and aerated lung lobes do, and this is another useful feature to differentiate to other diagnoses such as neoplasia.

References

1. Lee EA, Johnson LR, Johnson EG, Vernau W. Clinical features and radiographic findings in cats with eosinophilic, neutrophilic, and mixed airway inflammation (2011-2018). J Vet Intern Med 34:1291-1299, 2020.
2. Hahn H, Specchi S, Masseau I, Reinero C, Benchekroun G, Rechy J, et al. The computed tomographic "tree-in-bud" pattern: Characterization and comparison with radiographic and clinical findings in 36 cats. Vet Radiol Ultrasound 59:32-42, 2018.
3. Suter PF, Lord PF. Thoracic radiography: a text atlas of thoracic disease in the dog and cat. Wettswil, Switzerland, 1984.
4. Masseau I, Reinero CR. Thoracic computed tomographic interpretation for clinicians to aid in the diagnosis of dogs and cats with respiratory disease. Vet J 253:105388, 2019.
5. Rozanski E. Canine chronic bronchitis: an update. Vet Clin North Am Small Anim Pract 50:393-404, 2020.
6. Johnson LR, Johnson EG, Hulsebosch SE, Dear JD, Vernau W. Eosinophilic bronchitis, eosinophilic granuloma, and eosinophilic bronchopneumopathy in 75 dogs (2006-2016). J Vet Intern Med 33:2217-2226, 2019.
7. Fina C, Vignoli M, Terragni R, Rossi F, Wisner E, Saunders JH. Computed tomography characteristics of eosinophilic pulmonary granulomatosis in five dogs. Vet Radiol Ultrasound 55:16-22, 2014.
8. Johnson LR, Johnson EG, Vernau W, Kass PH, Byrne BA. Bronchoscopy, imaging, and concurrent diseases in dogs with bronchiectasis: (2003-2014). J Vet Intern Med 30:247-254, 2016.
9. Norris CR, Samii VF. Clinical, radiographic, and pathologic features of bronchiectasis in cats: 12 cases (1987-1999). J Am Vet Med Assoc 216:530-534, 2000.
10. Hawkins EC, Basseches J, Berry CR, Stebbins ME, Ferris KK. Demographic, clinical, and radiographic features of bronchiectasis in dogs: 316 cases (1988-2000). J Am Vet Med Assoc 223:1628-1635, 2003.
11. Cannon MS, Johnson LR, Pesavento PA, Kass PH, Wisner ER. Quantitative and qualitative computed tomographic characteristics of bronchiectasis in 12 dogs. Vet Radiol Ultrasound 54:351-357, 2013.
12. Laurila HP, Rajamaki MM. Update on canine idiopathic pulmonary fibrosis in West Highland White Terriers. Vet Clin North Am Small Anim Pract 50:431-446, 2020.
13. Evola MG, Edmondson EF, Reichle JK, Biller DS, Mitchell CW, Valdés-Martínez A. Radiographic and histopathologic characteristics of pulmonary fibrosis in nine cats. Vet Radiol Ultrasound 55:133-140, 2014.
14. Han HJ, Kim JH. Concurrent pulmonary hypoplasia and congenital lobar emphysema in a young dog with tension pneumothorax: a rare congenital pulmonary anomaly. Acta Vet Scand 61:37, 2019.
15. Reetz JA, Caceres AV, Suran JN, Oura TJ, Zwingenberger AL, Mai W. Sensitivity, positive predictive value, and interobserver variability of computed tomography in the diagnosis of bullae associated with spontaneous pneumothorax in dogs: 19 cases (2003-2012). J Am Vet Med Assoc 243:244-251, 2013.
16. Berry CR, Gallaway A, Thrall DE, Carlisle C. Thoracic radiographic features of anticoagulant rodenticide toxicity in fourteen dogs. Vet Radiol Ultrasound 34:391-396, 1993.
17. Dicker SA, Lisciandro GR, Newell SM, Johnson JA. Diagnosis of pulmonary contusions with point-of-care lung ultrasonography and thoracic radiography compared to thoracic computed tomography in dogs with motor vehicle trauma: 29 cases (2017-2018). J Vet Emerg Crit Care (San Antonio) 30:638-646, 2020.
18. Bouyssou S, Specchi S, Desquilbet L, Pey P. Radiographic appearance of presumed noncardiogenic pulmonary edema and correlation with the underlying cause in dogs and cats. Vet Radiol Ultrasound 58:259-265, 2017.

19. Diana A, Guglielmini C, Pivetta M, Sanacore A, Di Tommaso M, Lord PF, et al. Radiographic features of cardiogenic pulmonary edema in dogs with mitral regurgitation: 61 cases (1998-2007). *J Am Vet Med Assoc* 235:1058-1063, 2009.
20. Egenvall A, Hansson K, Sateri H, Lord PF, Jonsson L. Pulmonary oedema in Swedish hunting dogs. *J Small Anim Pract* 44:209-217, 2003.
21. Geyer NE, Reichle JK, Valdes-Martinez A, Williams J, Goggin JM, Leach L, et al. Radiographic appearance of confirmed pulmonary lymphoma in cats and dogs. *Vet Radiol Ultrasound* 51:386-390, 2010.
22. Barrett LE, Pollard RE, Zwingenberger A, Zierenberg-Ripoll A, Skorupski KA. Radiographic characterization of primary lung tumors in 74 dogs. *Vet Radiol Ultrasound* 55:480-487, 2014.
23. Aarsvold S, Reetz JA, Reichle JK, Jones ID, Lamb CR, Evola MG, et al. Computed tomographic findings in 57 cats with primary pulmonary neoplasia. *Vet Radiol Ultrasound* 56:272-277, 2015.
24. Marolf AJ, Gibbons DS, Podell BK, Park RD. Computed tomographic appearance of primary lung tumors in dogs. *Vet Radiol Ultrasound* 52:168-172, 2011.
25. Mullin C, Clifford CA. Histiocytic sarcoma and hemangiosarcoma update. *Vet Clin North Am Small Anim Pract* 49:855-879, 2019.

SECTION V
ABDOMEN

CHAPTER 24

Abdominal cavity and retroperitoneal space

Christopher R. Tollefson

> **KEY POINTS**
>
> - Orthogonal projections of the abdomen should always be performed when doing survey radiographs.
> - Multiple radiographic projections may be required to evaluate the body wall, but ultrasound and CT are more sensitive and specific at detecting lesions.
> - Decreased peritoneal detail occurs from numerous etiologies, and additional investigation such as abdominal ultrasound and cytology is usually needed.
> - Free gas within the abdomen may be easiest to identify with a horizontal beam projection.
> - Abdominal masses have several possible organs of origin, and differentials, ultrasound, CT, and cytology/histopathology are usually needed to refine the differential list.
> - Abdominal lymph nodes are usually visible on radiographs only when severely enlarged and are better assessed with US and CT.
> - Ultrasound or computed tomography are helpful for evaluating the adrenal glands, deciphering the origin of most abdominal masses, or evaluating patients with large volumes of peritoneal effusion.

An integral part of the interpretation of abdominal imaging is a sound knowledge of the anatomical location of the abdominal organs. Radiographs are a great survey imaging modality and are available for many practitioners, but this modality has limitations. CT or ultrasound can also provide a more specific assessment of the abdomen in many cases. With radiographs, taking several projections will help locate an abnormality (**figs. 24.1** and **24.2**).

Due to superimposition, the entire border of an organ is not always outlined on radiographs. For example, the stomach and the liver are in contact, and portions of the outline of both the liver and stomach are obscured. Thus, orthogonal projections help provide a more complete evaluation. Similarly, the right kidney can be challenging to outline due to the close association with the renal fossa of the caudate lobe of the liver and the overlying small intestines on the ventrodorsal projection.

There are a lot of similarities between the dog and cat abdomen, but there are several differences (**figs. 24.3** and **24.4**). In the cat, the left limb of the normal pancreas can occasionally be seen on radiographs in obese patients. In most cats, the tail of the spleen is not visible in the ventral abdomen on lateral projections but is visible in some normal individuals. On a ventrodorsal projection, the normal feline stomach is "J-shaped," and the pylorus is located slightly to the right of the midline.

SECTION **V** ABDOMEN

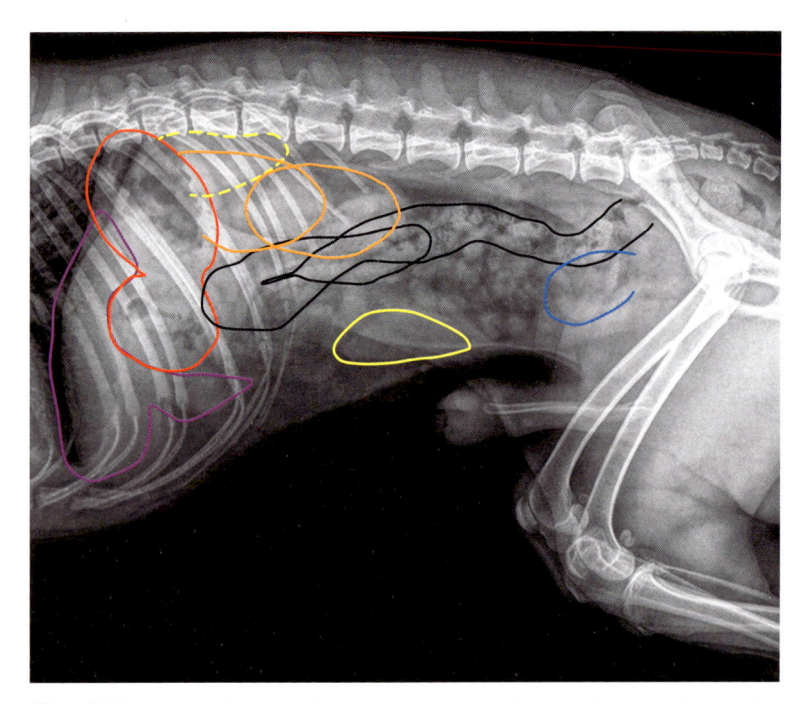

Fig. 24.1 Lateral radiograph of a normal abdomen of a young intact male dog. The liver is outlined in purple. The stomach is outlined in red and silhouettes with the dorsal portion of the liver, head of the spleen, and renal silhouette. The tail of the spleen is solid yellow, with the head of the spleen in yellow. The head of the spleen is not always visible and depends on the body condition of the patient. Care must also be taken when interpreting this area as other organs, such as the adrenal glands, which are not typically visible, may become visible if pathology is present. Orange outlines the renal silhouettes. The colon is outlined in black. Blue is the urinary bladder. The small intestines are between the organs and are not outlined in this figure.

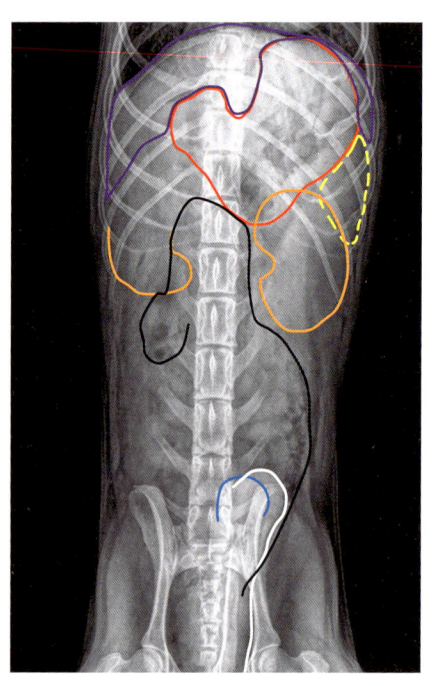

Fig. 24.2 Ventrodorsal radiograph of a normal abdomen of a young intact male dog. The liver is outlined in purple. The stomach is red and silhouettes with the liver, head of the spleen, and renal silhouette. The head of the spleen is yellow. Orange outlines the renal silhouettes. The cranial pole of the right kidney is not definitively identified. The colon is outlined in black. Blue is the visible portion of the urinary bladder. The small intestines are between the organs and are not outlined in this figure. The prepuce is outlined in white and should not be mistaken for a mass.

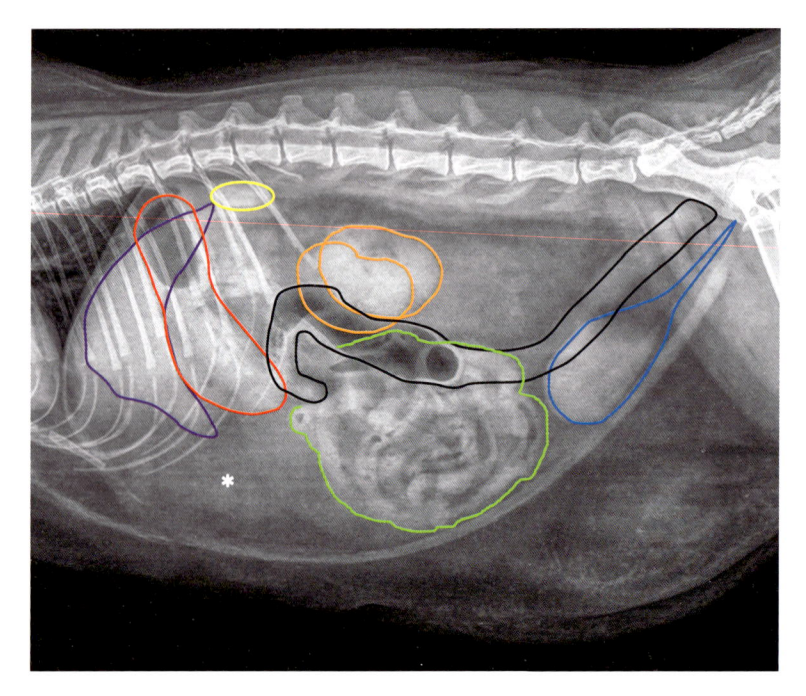

Fig. 24.3 Lateral radiograph of a normal female spayed cat. Purple outlines the hepatic silhouette. The ventral portion includes the gallbladder, which is occasionally seen ventrally as a convex, soft tissue opaque bulge. The stomach is red and is variable in size depending on the degree of filling. The small intestines are bundled together and are outlined in green. Orange outlines the renal silhouettes. Yellow is the head of the spleen. This is not always visible and depends on the patient's body condition. Black is the colon. Blue is the urinary bladder and urethra. Notice the abundant falciform fat that is ventral to the liver (asterisk).

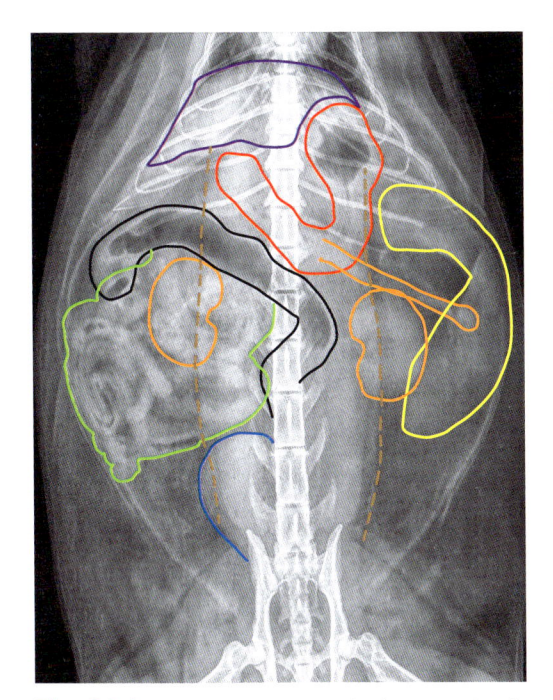

Fig. 24.4 Ventrodorsal radiograph of a young female spayed cat. The liver is outlined in purple and is partially superimposed over the stomach. The stomach (red) is J-shaped with the pylorus slightly right to the midline, unlike dogs. The left limb of the pancreas is outlined in white. This is a normal finding in a well-conditioned cat. Yellow outlines the spleen, with the head of the spleen cranial and the tail caudal. Black is the colon. The colon is partially superimposed with the spine and pelvis, impeding complete evaluation distally in this case. Blue outlines the urinary bladder, which, like the colon, is partially superimposed with the spine and pelvis. The dashed tan line outlines the hypaxial muscles.

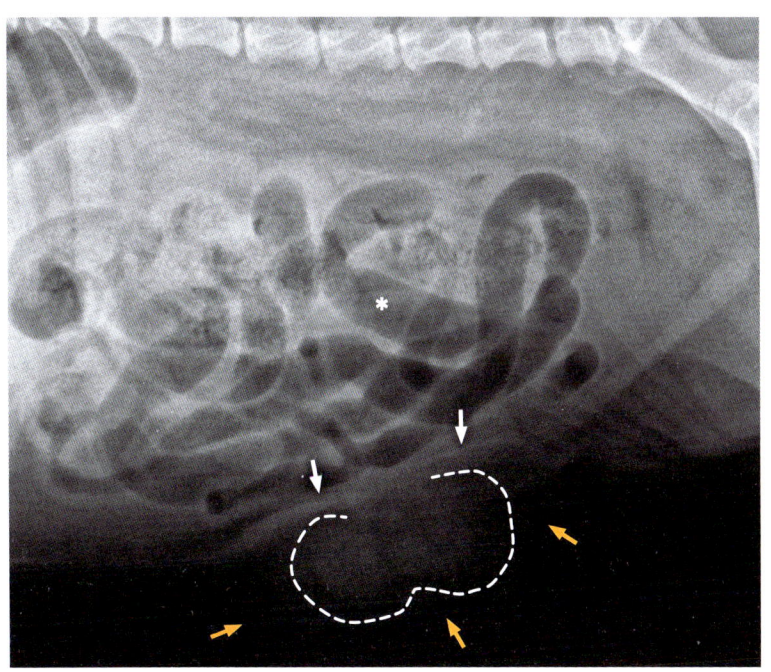

Fig. 24.5 Collimated left lateral radiograph of a ten-year-old dog that presented for vomiting. Several loops of small intestine are dilated with gas (white asterisk). There is broad-based superficial swelling of the ventral abdominal wall (orange arrows). Within this region, there is a lobulated soft tissue opaque structure (within the dashed white line). The body wall at this site is dorsally deviated (white arrows). This dog has a loop of small intestine herniated through a rent in the body wall that is entrapped, causing small intestinal obstruction.

Body wall

The body wall is the lateral and ventral confines of the abdominal cavity. The body wall is composed of the rectus abdominis, transversus abdominis, external abdominal obliques, and internal abdominal obliques.[1] Because of this, it is possible to see discontinuity of the muscle bellies, particularly on the ventrodorsal projection in well-conditioned patients when fat is deposited within the fascial planes. The body wall is challenging to evaluate as it is a curved structure and small rents or defects are usually not visible on radiographs. On **fig. 24.5**, there is a body wall hernia, but the exact location is not determined due to the superimposition of the intact parts of the body. As in this case, detection of a body wall hernia on radiographs almost always depends on visible herniation of abdominal viscera. Occasionally, obliqued projections are helpful in identifying a defect (**fig. 24.6**).

When trauma is an inciting cause, secondary signs may be easier to detect, such as thickening of the body wall, edema, peritoneal effusion, or herniated abdominal organs (**fig. 24.7**). Computed tomography is the best imaging modality to identify body wall ruptures if radiographs are inconclusive (**fig. 24.8**).

Survey radiographs can also be used to assess dehiscence of surgical wounds. However, radiographs are unlikely to detect a defect in the muscle of the body wall unless there is herniation of the intestine. Ultrasound is more sensitive for assessment of dehiscence of laparotomy incision, as the two

SECTION V ABDOMEN

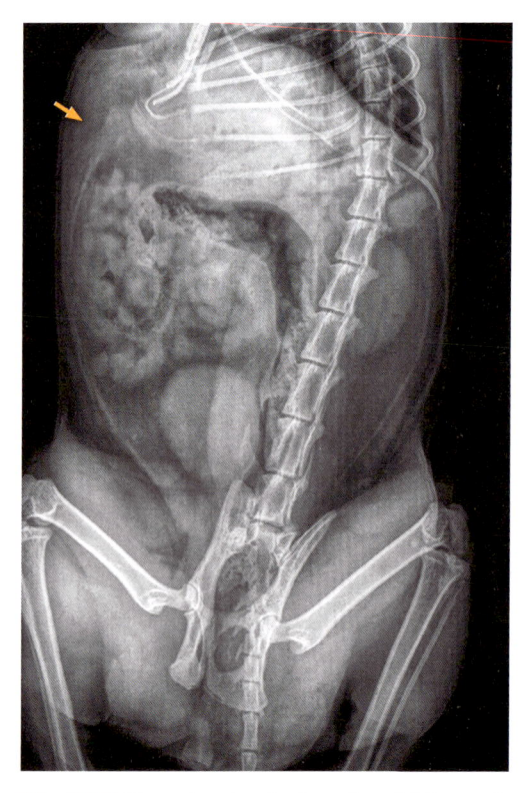

Fig. 24.6 Ventrodorsal projections of an adult Domestic shorthair cat with an abdominal wall rupture. The defect was not visible on the standard ventrodorsal positioning. When the patient was obliqued, the defect became easier to visualize. Notice the discontinuity of the abdominal wall muscles at the arrow.

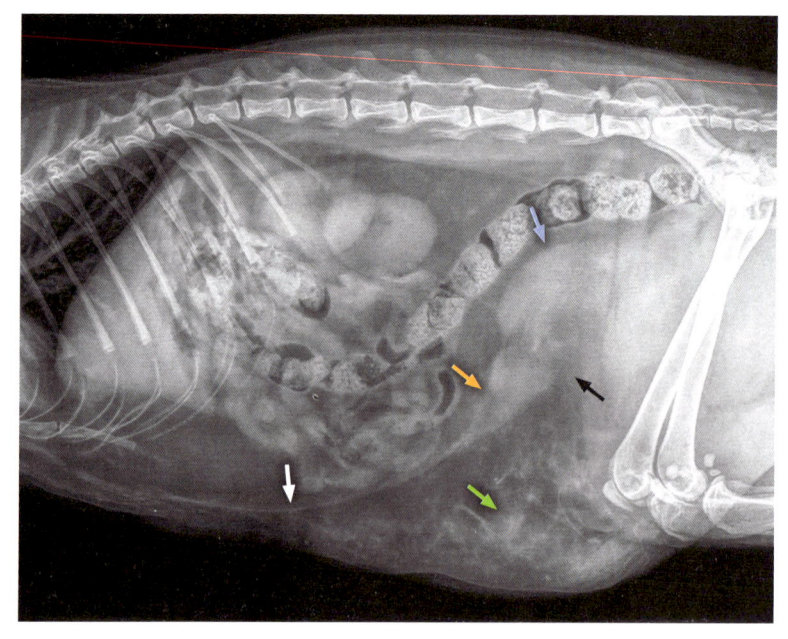

Fig. 24.7 Left lateral projection of a cat with traumatic body wall rupture. Notice the normal thin abdominal body wall (white arrow) cranially. Caudally the body wall becomes thickened (orange arrow) and indistinct from hemorrhage and edema (black arrow). These changes are suspicious for a rupture of the abdominal body wall, but a discrete defect is not visible. There is focal loss of abdominal serosal detail within the caudal abdomen, obscuring some of the borders of the urinary bladder (blue arrow). There is wispy soft tissue opaque material in the superficial ventral abdominal soft tissues (green arrow) from hemorrhage and/or edema.

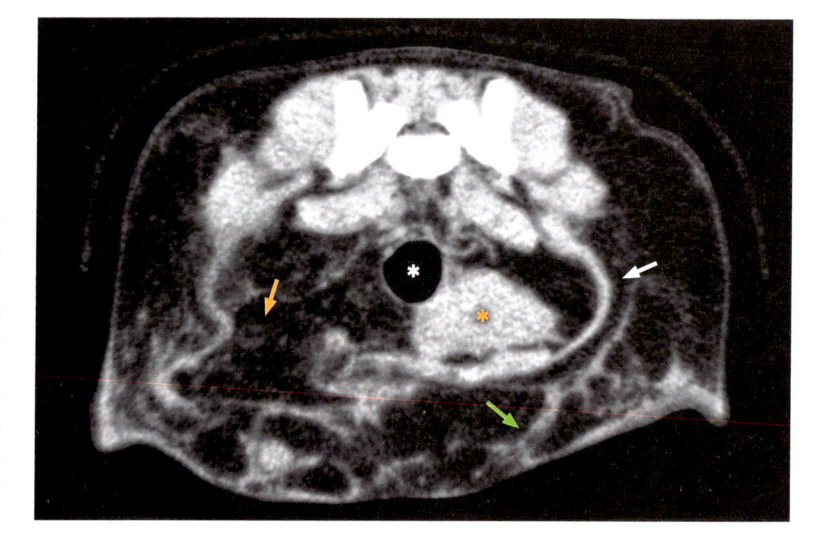

Fig. 24.8 A transverse computed tomographic image in a soft tissue window of the same cat as in fig. 24.7. The patient's right is towards the left of the image, and the dorsum is towards the top of the image. The colon is denoted with a white asterisk. A normal, smooth, and thin portion of the abdominal wall is depicted (white arrow). The urinary bladder is denoted with a orange asterisk. Notice the disruption of the body wall along the right ventral aspect (orange arrow). The hemorrhage and or edema are again seen within the superficial ventral abdominal soft tissues (green arrow).

rectus abdominis muscles on either side of the linea alba are easily recognized. The suture material may also be visible as hyperechoic foci causing acoustic shadowing. Dehiscence of the linea alba is seen as the separation of the two rectus abdominis muscle bellies. Ultrasound may also demonstrate herniation of mesentery, omentum, or intestine with greater sensitivity than radiographs. CT can also be used to assess wound dehiscence, as the excellent contrast between fat and muscle tissue and lack of superimposition will clearly show a defect if one is present. The diaphragm is the cranial border of the abdomen and is discussed in a separate chapter.

Serosal detail

The abdominal organs, connective tissues, and inner margins of the body wall are lined by the peritoneum, which is a thin serous membrane.[1] Between two layers of peritoneum, there is a space (peritoneal space) that contains a minimal amount of fluid that allows the organs to move without friction. Normal peritoneal serosal margin detail in the abdomen is dependent upon the presence of fat. In patients with normal or obese body condition, intra-abdominal fat deposited in the mesentery, omentum, and retroperitoneal fascia, highlights the serosal or outer margin of the viscera within the peritoneal space, that is, the liver, spleen, stomach, small intestine, colon, and urinary bladder. At least part of the outer margin of these organs should be visible on good-quality abdominal radiographs. The inner margin of the muscle layer of the body wall should also be visible.

Before determining if peritoneal serosal margin detail is normal or abnormal, the overall body condition of the patient should be assessed, as this determines how good or poor peritoneal serosal margin detail will be. In juvenile patients, there is limited intra-abdominal brown fat, which has significant water content, and as a result, absent or minimal visible serosal margin detail. Mature cats and dogs in normal body condition will have at least some fat within the abdomen. In obese patients, there is usually a large volume of fat within the abdomen. In dogs, obesity results in greater accumulation of fat in the retroperitoneal space. In cats, fat is selectively deposited in the falciform ligament in individuals with obese body condition. Serosal detail in thin, athletic patients or cachectic patients is limited or even absent. Such patients usually have little or no subcutaneous fat, a helpful extra-abdominal control. The shape of the abdomen is an important clue when deciding if patients without body fat also have peritoneal effusion. In cachectic patients, the abdomen usually has a tucked appearance. A pendulous or distended abdomen with effaced peritoneal serosal margins in a patient without body fat almost certainly indicates the presence of peritoneal fluid contributing to the distention. The detail in the retroperitoneal space, in the dorsal abdomen, is also an important internal control when deciding if serosal detail is normal or reduced from the presence of fluid in the peritoneal space. In both cats and dogs with normal or obese body condition, there is fat deposition in the fascial planes of the retroperitoneal space. This clearly outlines the left kidney and sometimes the right. The ventral margin of the epaxial muscles is also usually visible. In some obese patients, the abdominal aorta and caudal vena cava may also be visible.

Fluid within the peritoneal space will reduce or eliminate serosal detail depending upon a balance between the volume of fluid present and the quantity of fat within the abdomen. Thus, in an obese patient, the presence of a small volume of peritoneal fluid results in a streaky or mottled appearance with indistinct serosal margins. With an increasing volume of intraperitoneal fluid, there is progressive blurring and ultimately complete effacement of peritoneal serosal margin detail. When a large volume of fluid is present, this will result in complete loss of peritoneal serosal margin detail and a pendulous or distended abdomen, even in patients with normal body condition.[2]

The radiographic appearance of peritoneal fluid is the same regardless of the type of fluid present. Decreased serosal detail is a relatively common finding. Because the fat within the abdomen provides the contrast for the visualization of the serosal margins of the abdominal organs, a loss of the fat will cause decreased abdominal serosal detail. For this reason, patients with a decreased body condition and those with a tucked-up abdomen will have poor detail. Other features such as scalloping of the soft tissues along the lumbar spinous processes may help indicate a decreased body condition. Radiographically, abdominal effusion can be identified by wispy soft tissue opaque material superimposed over the abdomen and decreased distinction of the serosal detail of the abdominal organs up to a complete loss of the serosal margins of the abdominal organs, leaving just intestinal gas being visualized. Possible causes of decreased serosal detail include modified transudate, pure transudate, sterile or septic exudate, chyle, bile, urine, hemorrhage, or neoplastic effusion/carcinomatosis (**fig. 24.9**).[2]

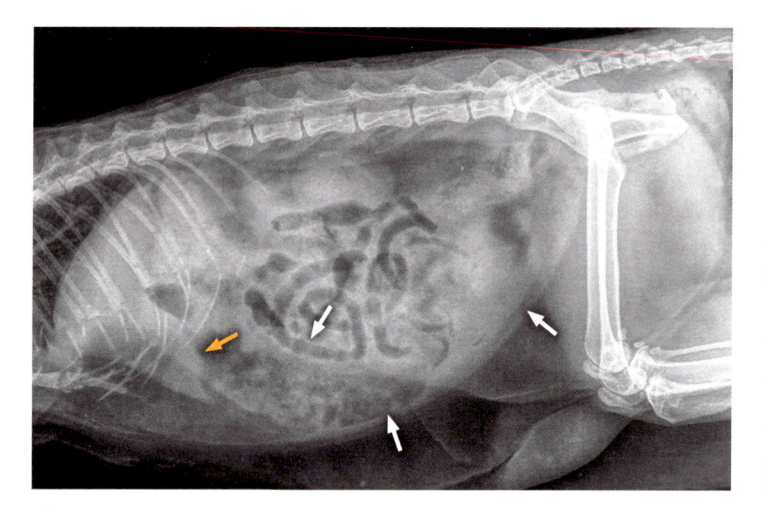

Fig. 24.9 A ten-year-old neutered male Domestic shorthair cat presented for vomiting and diarrhea for 1 month. There is decreased peritoneal detail with loss of the serosal margins of the small intestines and urinary bladder (white arrows). The caudal margin of the hepatic silhouette is mildly undulating. This patient had numerous nodules along the peritoneum, peritoneal effusion, and hepatic nodules on ultrasound. Carcinomatosis was suspected based on cytology.

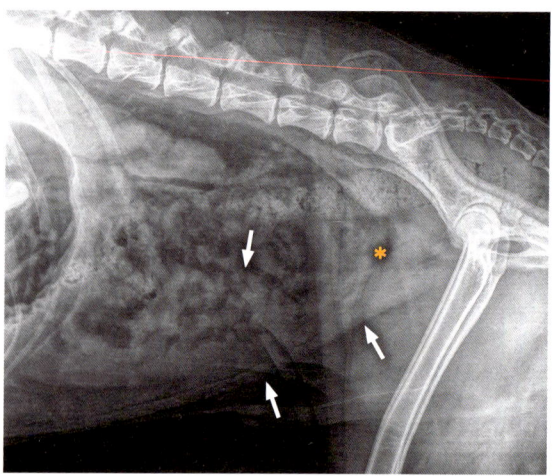

Fig. 24.10 Caudal lateral radiograph of a two-year-old German shepherd. There is decreased serosal detail of the peritoneal space causing border effacement of the small intestines (white arrows). Notice that the outer margin of the urinary bladder is not visible (asterisk). Peritoneal effusion is present. Abdominocentesis was performed, and uroperitoneum was diagnosed, which was found to be from a urinary bladder rupture. A cystogram can confirm the diagnosis.

Reduced peritoneal serosal margin detail can be mimicked by wet hair artifact if the patient was wet or had an ultrasound study prior to radiography. Some peritoneal effusion is normal following laparotomy and may persist for up to 2 weeks.[2] Normal postoperative peritoneal effusion has a radiographic appearance similar to postoperative septic peritonitis, and these cannot be distinguished based on radiographs only. With moderate to large volumes of peritoneal fluid, the abdominal viscera will be partly or completely obscured, significantly limiting radiographic assessment (**fig. 24.10**).

Normal juvenile patients up to a few months of age typically also have absent or limited serosal margin detail within the abdomen as they have intra-abdominal brown fat, which has a higher water content, thus an opacity similar to the soft tissues. The detail gradually increases as white fat replaces the brown fat and, for most patients, is similar to adults by 5 to 6 months of age (**fig. 24.11**). Peritoneal serosal detail in obese patients, especially cats, is typically excellent as the fat also results in some separation of organs.

When peritoneal fluid is identified on abdominal radiographs, the abdomen is assessed for evidence of organ enlargement or a mass lesion. If the serosal margin detail is reduced but not effaced, organ enlargement or a mass lesion may be visible as in a patient without effusion. In patients with complete effacement of serosal margin detail, organ enlargement or the presence of a mass lesion can sometimes be inferred by displacement of organs within the abdomen, particularly the intestine. This is not always reliable, and the suspected abnormality should be confirmed by ultrasound or CT. Patients with peritoneal effusion should have thoracic radiographs to confirm or exclude cardiac disease, metastatic neoplasia, or multicentric neoplasia as the etiology.

Ultrasound is the preferred imaging modality for the evaluation of peritoneal fluid. The sonographic appearance of the fluid may be helpful, but sampling should always be performed for analysis and cytologic assessment. Anechoic fluid is more likely to represent acellular fluid such as transudate or modified transudate. If the fluid in the peritoneal space is echogenic, this likely indicates the presence of cellular debris and/or protein such as hemorrhage or exudate. The liver should be evaluated to confirm or exclude hepatic venous congestion, which would indicate right-sided congestive cardiac failure as the cause of effusion. The liver, spleen, gastrointestinal tract, and lymph nodes should be evaluated for the presence of a mass lesion or enlargement.

The retroperitoneal space is a potential space in the dorsal abdomen. This is bounded dorsally by

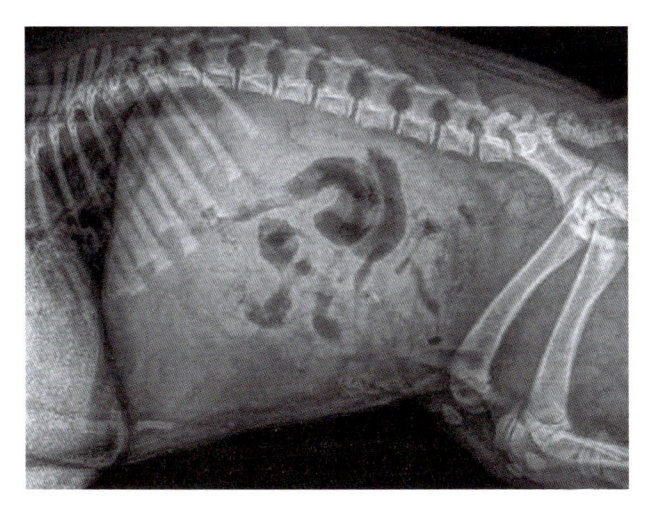

Fig. 24.11 Left lateral projection of a two-month-old intact female French Bulldog presenting for vomiting. Notice the absence of serosal detail. This is a normal appearance for the patient's age. No free fluid was identified on abdominal ultrasound, and no foreign bodies were present. The radiographs and abdominal ultrasound were normal.

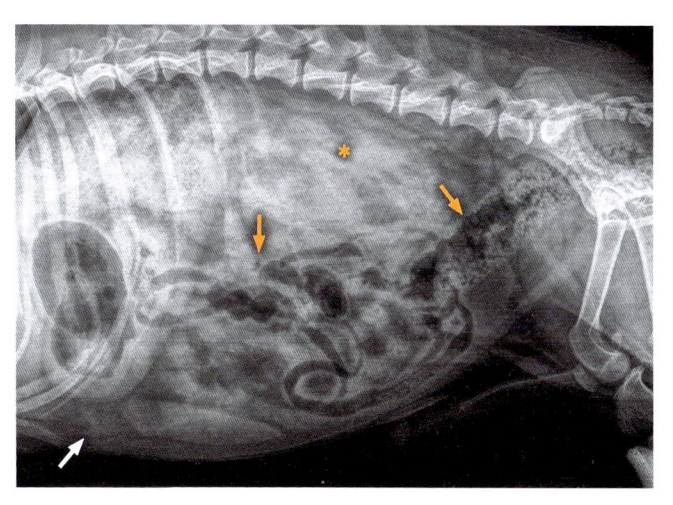

Fig. 24.12 Left lateral abdominal radiograph of a dog with retroperitoneal mass effect and effusion. Notice the effacement of the renal silhouettes and ventral border of the epaxial muscles and diffuse wispy soft tissue opacity (asterisk) compared to normal peritoneal serosal margin detail by the ventral aspect of the stomach and spleen (white arrow). The retroperitoneal space is expanded, causing ventral displacement of the intestines (orange arrows).

the epaxial muscle, cranially by the diaphragm, and ventrally by the peritoneal membrane. The retroperitoneal space communicates with the mediastinum via the openings in the diaphragm for the aorta and esophagus and caudally is contiguous with the fascia of the pelvic canal. The retroperitoneal space contains the aorta, caudal vena cava, kidneys, adrenal glands, and lumbar aortic lymph nodes. Comparison of detail within the peritoneal space and retroperitoneal space is a useful internal control within the abdomen, as pathologic processes do not usually cause accumulation of fluid in both areas. Patients with normal body condition and peritoneal fluid have preserved retroperitoneal detail, and the outline of at least one of the kidneys remains visible. Fluid accumulation within the retroperitoneal space will obscure the renal silhouettes and the ventral margin of the epaxial muscle, well serosal margin detail in the peritoneal space is preserved (**fig. 24.12**).

The presence of a mass and/or fluid in the retroperitoneal space may result in expansion of the space. On lateral radiograph, this is evidenced by ventral displacement of the small and large intestine.[3]

Increased serosal detail is usually a more significant finding. The most common reason for the presence of peritoneal gas is recent abdominal surgery. Gas may persist for up to 4 weeks following laparotomy.[2] Pathologic etiologies of intraperitoneal gas include rupture of the gastrointestinal tract, rupture of an intra-abdominal abscess with gas-forming organisms, and penetrating trauma of the body wall (**fig. 24.13**).

Gas within the peritoneal space may enhance the visibility of serosal margins if there is sufficient volume present. When a relatively large volume of gas is present within the peritoneal space, it will rise to the highest part of the abdomen. On lateral radiographs, this is usually most evident interposed between the crura of the diaphragm, liver, and gastric body/fundus and the cranial dorsal abdomen. On ventrodorsal projections, gas will accumulate

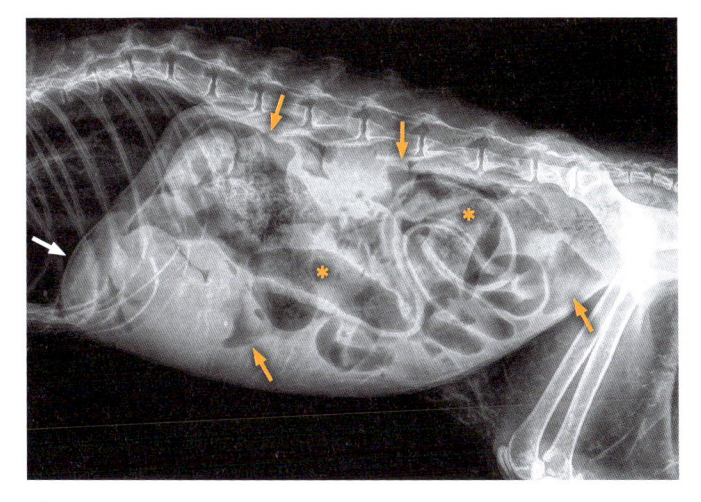

Fig. 24.13 A geriatric Domestic longhair cat with cachexia. The abdominal margin of the diaphragm is outlined by gas (white arrow). A few large, triangular gas bubbles are present throughout the peritoneal space (orange arrows). Notice the gas dilated loops of small intestine (asterisks). A definitive cause of the pneumoperitoneum was not identified, and euthanasia was elected.

in the cranial ventral abdomen and may outline the caudal margin of the cupula of the diaphragm. If the volume of gas present is small, small pockets of gas may be dispersed in the abdomen, usually located in folds of the mesentery and omentum. These small pockets of gas may be difficult to distinguish from normal pockets of intestinal luminal gas. Peritoneal gas may be noted in the periphery of the abdomen beyond the normally expected location of the small intestine. If there is suspicion of peritoneal gas, the patient should be allowed to lie undisturbed for a few minutes on the radiographic table after the first images are obtained. A repeat radiograph is then obtained. Gas within the intestine seldom appears in the same location on radiographs obtained more than a few seconds apart because of peristalsis. Gas pockets that do not change location over several minutes should increase suspicion of peritoneal gas. The shape of the gas bubbles may also be a helpful clue, as these conform to the serosal margin of adjacent segments of the intestine and may have a triangular or comma shape rather than the normal circular or ovoid shape of intestinal luminal gas bubbles. If possible, horizontal plane radiographs are the preferred method to diagnose peritoneal gas. The patient can be positioned in left recumbency to avoid confusion with gas in the body of the stomach, and ventral dorsal or dorsoventral radiographs are obtained with a horizontal beam centered on the upper body wall. This will show a gas pocket below the body wall. Alternatively, the patient can be placed in dorsal recumbency and a horizontal beam laterolateral radiograph obtained, centered on the highest point of the cranial ventral abdomen. Ultrasound is also quite sensitive for the detection of small volumes of gas within the peritoneal space. The sonographic appearance of the gas bubbles is the same as intestinal luminal gas, but ultrasound shows that the gas pockets are located outside the gastrointestinal tract.

Abdominal masses

Organomegaly and masses are a common indication for abdominal radiographs. When organomegaly or masses are present, displacement of adjacent organs can be helpful to determine the origin (**fig. 24.14**). When a mass is identified in the abdomen on radiographs, the adjacent viscera, particularly the gastrointestinal tract, are assessed for displacement. The normal abdominal organs are displaced away from the site of origin of the mass, and structures or organs that are normally located in this region of the abdomen are the most likely origin. For example, a mass lesion in the left mid-abdomen that causes rightward and caudal displacement of the small and large intestines is most likely of splenic origin. The absence of a normal visible splenic shadow would also support this conclusion. Identification of a discrete abdominal mass may not be possible when there is fluid within the peritoneal space. In such patients, the term "mass effect" is used to describe the displacement of viscera such as the small intestine when a discrete mass is not identified, but the organ displacement is suspicious of the presence of such a lesion.

Differentials for abdominal masses include neoplasia, granuloma, hematoma, cyst, and abscess. Abdominal ultrasound is usually more helpful in confirming the origin of abdominal masses. When a mass is identified with ultrasound, the objective is to connect the mass to a specific abdominal organ if possible (**fig. 24.15**).

Nodular fat necrosis or "Bates bodies" are seen more frequently in cats than in dogs. They are usually well-defined spherical, ovoid, or irregular nodules with an eggshell-like rim and inconsistent internal mineralization.[4] These structures are benign, inconsequential findings and should not be mistaken for small intestinal foreign bodies or neoplastic abdominal masses (**fig. 24.16**).

Intra-abdominal lipomas or infiltrative lipomas occasionally occur in dogs and less frequently in cats. These have uniform fatty opacity and cause organ displacement that depends upon the point of origin within the abdomen. In some patients, these can be exceedingly large at the time of diagnosis.

CHAPTER **24** Abdominal cavity and retroperitoneal space

The large lipoma may cause displacement and compression of the viscera into a quadrant of the abdomen resulting in radiographs that show relatively uniform opacity in the abdomen and appear devoid of normal viscera, which could potentially be confused with intraperitoneal effusion by the casual observer. Liposarcomas are relatively rare in canine and feline patients. In most cases, these neoplasms have a soft tissue component in addition to fatty tissue and do not have the uniform fatty opacity of lipomas and infiltrative lipomas (**fig. 24.17**). Ultrasound imaging of these lesions is frequently unhelpful, as fatty tissue appears as amorphous tissue of heterogenous echogenicity without internal features. CT of the abdomen is usually much more helpful to assess the gross extent of the lesion and determine the origin and assist with surgical planning for resection or debulking.

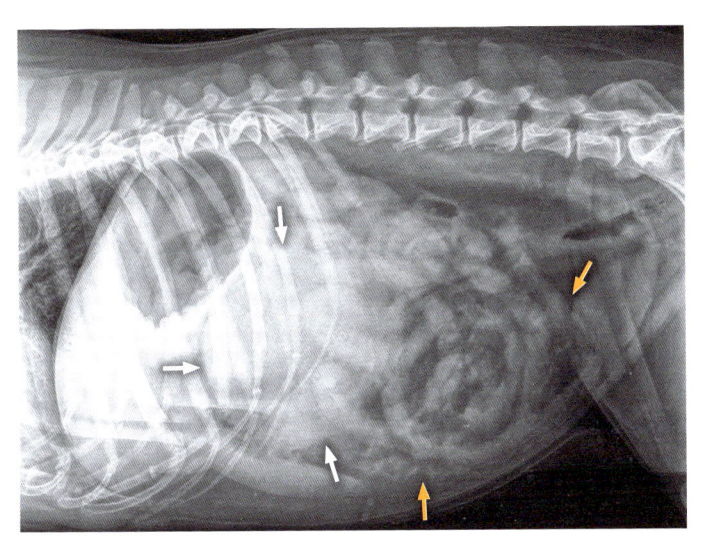

Fig. 24.14 Lateral radiograph of an adult mixed breed dog with a midabdominal mass causing caudal displacement of the small intestines (white arrows). There is wispy soft tissue opaque material throughout the abdomen which is likely due to a moderate volume of peritoneal effusion (orange arrows).

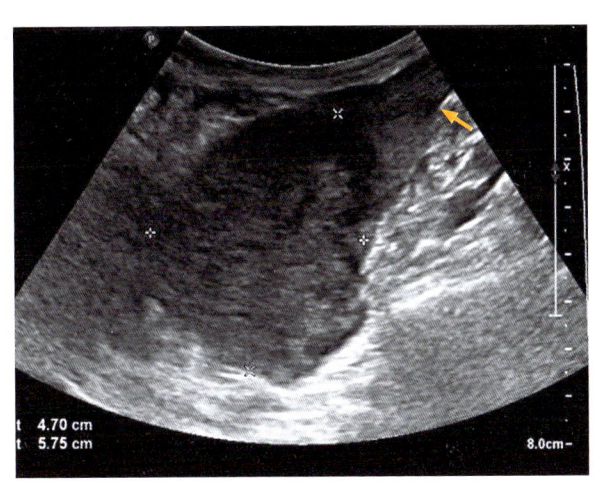

Fig. 24.15 Ultrasound image of an adult dog presenting for an abdominal mass. The mass was identified and outlined with the calipers. The mass is also arising from the spleen (orange arrow).

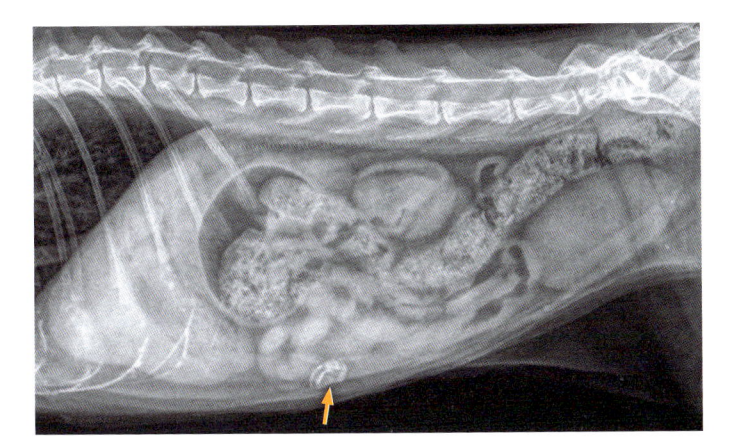

Fig. 24.16 Left lateral abdominal radiograph of an adult Domestic shorthair cat. There is a smoothly marginated, ovoid, fat opaque structure with a thin mineral opaque rim within the ventral aspect of the mid-abdomen (arrow). This structure is not within a loop of the bowel. Notice the small intestines adjacent to the structure are smaller in diameter and normal in size. The opaque mineral structure represents nodular fat necrosis, often referred to as a "Bates body", and should not be confused with a small intestinal foreign body.

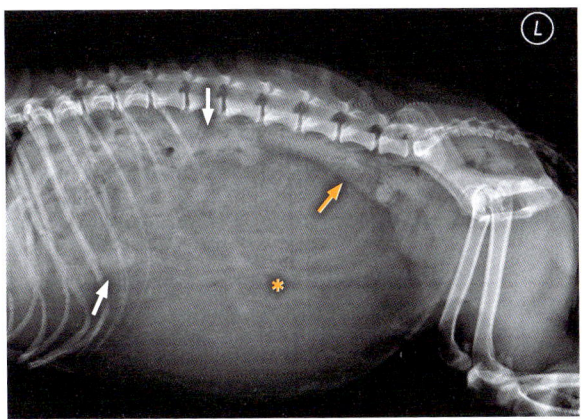

Fig. 24.17. Left lateral radiograph of a dog with a large intra-abdominal lipoma that fills most of the abdomen. Notice the displacement of the small intestines (white arrows) and colon (orange arrow) cranially and dorsally. The serosal margins of these structures are still visible. There are a few thin, curvilinear soft tissue opaque structures superimposed over the mid aspect of the abdomen (asterisk), which likely represent vessels.

Lymph nodes

There are numerous lymph node groups within the abdomen. Normal lymph nodes are not visible with radiography and are only identified if severely enlarged. Ultrasound or cross-sectional imaging is usually necessary to fully evaluate these structures. One consistent set of lymph nodes is in the medial iliac lymph nodes (**fig. 24.18**).

These lymph nodes are situated caudal to the deep circumflex veins, ventral to the L6-L7 vertebrae, and dorsal to the colon. When they are enlarged, a sharp margin can be identified and cause ventral displacement of the colon (**fig. 24.19**).

Differentials of lymphadenomegaly include neoplasia, either metastatic or multicentric, and reactive lymphadenopathy. When enlarged lymph nodes are identified, further investigation and evaluation are recommended to look for a primary lesion (**fig. 24.20**).

On ultrasound, puppies may have similar to slightly larger abdominal lymph nodes than adult dogs. Their lymph nodes may also be homogenously hypoechoic or hyperechoic with a hypoechoic rim.[5]

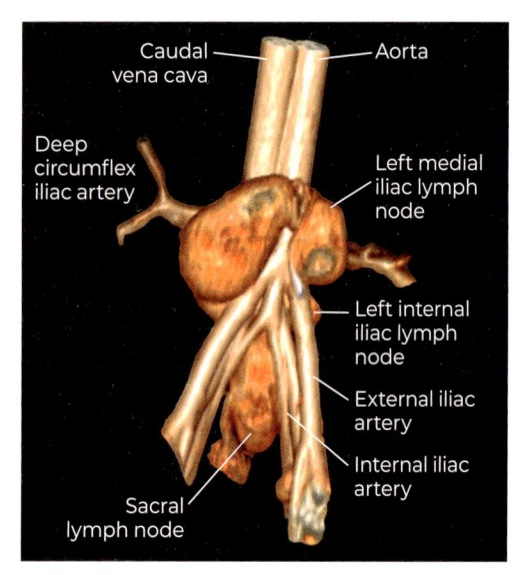

Fig. 24.18 3D reconstruction of the terminal aorta and caudal vena cava in a dog with lymphadenopathy. The patient's right is towards the left of the image, and the ventral aspect is facing the reader. The medial iliac lymph nodes are ventral to the vascular structures. The internal iliac lymph nodes are along the dorsal aspect of the trifurcation and positioned between the external iliac artery and the internal iliac artery. The sacral lymph node is associated with the median sacral artery (not seen).

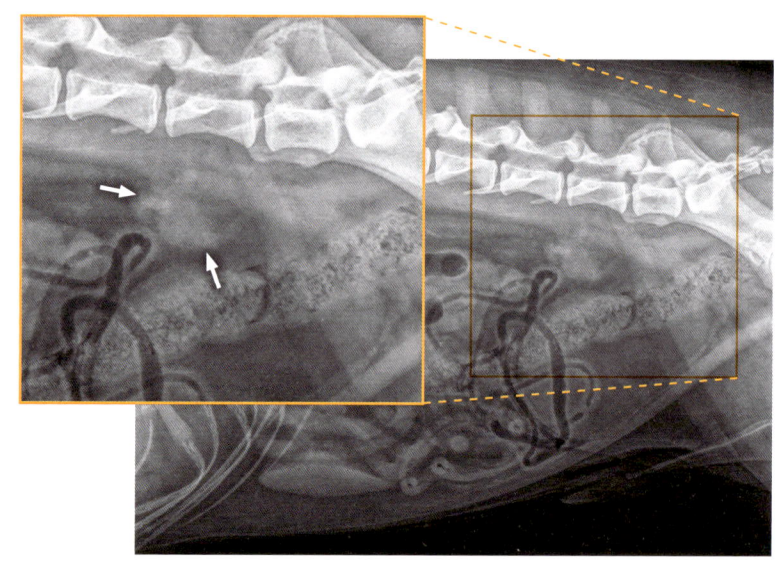

Fig. 24.19 Caudal lateral radiograph of a six-year-old neutered male Golden Retriever mix. The patient presented with exercise intolerance and anorexia. There is a smoothly marginated, ovoid, soft tissue opaque structure ventral to the L6-L7 vertebrae (white arrows). This mass was confirmed on ultrasound to be an enlarged medial iliac lymph node and ultimately diagnosed as lymphoma.

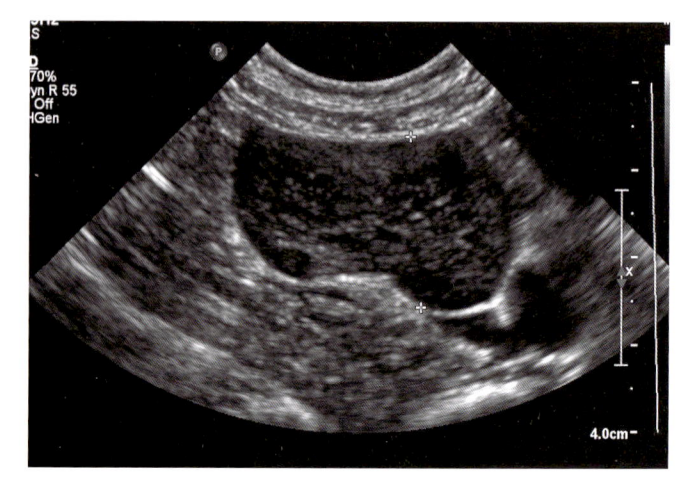

Fig. 24.20 Ultrasound image of the same dog as in fig. 24.19 with an enlarged and heterogeneously hypoechoic right medial iliac lymph node. Lymphoma was diagnosed after fine-needle aspirates were obtained.

Adrenal glands

Normal adrenal glands in both dogs and cats are not visible on survey radiographs. Dystrophic mineralization of the adrenal glands is an occasional incidental finding in geriatric cats and is clinically inconsequential. Larger mass lesions originating from the lymph nodes are rarely of sufficient size to be visible on radiographs. These appear as mass lesions at the cranial medial aspect of the ipsilateral kidney. Smaller adrenal mass lesions may exhibit mineralization, rendering them visible on radiographs, but this is also quite rare. Malignant adrenal neoplasms are locally invasive and may cause acute retroperitoneal hemorrhage from invasion and rupture of one of the renal veins or caudal vena cava. Affected patients presented in hypovolemic shock from hemorrhage. Survey radiographs show diffuse increased opacity in the retroperitoneal space that is also expanded, causing ventral displacement of the intestine (**fig. 24.21**).

Ultrasound is more widely used for the assessment of the adrenal glands and, with practice, the normal adrenal glands can be identified in most canine and feline patients (**fig. 24.22**). Although the adrenal glands are close to the kidneys, the anatomic relationship is relatively variable. The relation to vascular landmarks is much more consistent and reliably allows identification of these glands. The left adrenal gland is located at the lateral border of the aorta, immediately cranial to the origin of the left renal artery. The left renal artery courses cranial and lateral from the aorta at the lateral aspect of the left adrenal gland. The celiac artery and cranial mesenteric artery originate from the ventral aspect of the aorta at the level of the adrenal gland. The left renal vein passes across the caudal pole of the left adrenal gland to the caudal vena cava. The left phrenicoabdominal artery and vein pass across the dorsal and ventral mid-body of the left adrenal gland, respectively. The right adrenal gland is located at the lateral or dorsal lateral aspect of the caudal vena cava, immediately cranial to the origin of the right renal artery. The adrenal gland is usually slightly cranial to the origin of the celiac and cranial mesenteric arteries. Similar to the left adrenal gland, the right phrenicoabdominal artery and vein pass across the dorsal and ventral mid-body of the right adrenal gland.

Normal adrenal glands have hypoechoic parenchyma in comparison to the adjacent fat and fascia. With a high-frequency transducer, the adrenal cortex and medulla can sometimes be resolved in a normal patient. The left adrenal gland in dogs varies from a short, thin ovoid structure to an elongated bilobed structure. In most patients, the right adrenal gland has a similar shape. In some patients, the right adrenal gland may be arrowhead-shaped, pointed cranially. In cats, the adrenal glands are normally discrete short ovoid hypoechoic structures. Adrenal gland size is variable depending on

Fig. 24.21 Lateral and collimated ventral dorsal radiographs of an adult dog with an adrenal adenocarcinoma. On the radiographs, the mass is visualized due to the faint mineralization. Given the location, origin from the adrenal gland is most likely with less likely origins to include lymph node, kidney, mesothelium, vasculature, or retained surgical sponge (sometimes called gossypiboma). Differentials include neoplasia, granuloma, or dystrophic mineralization.

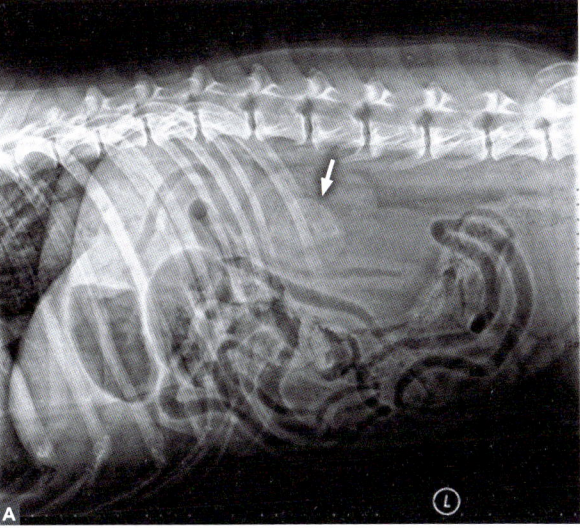

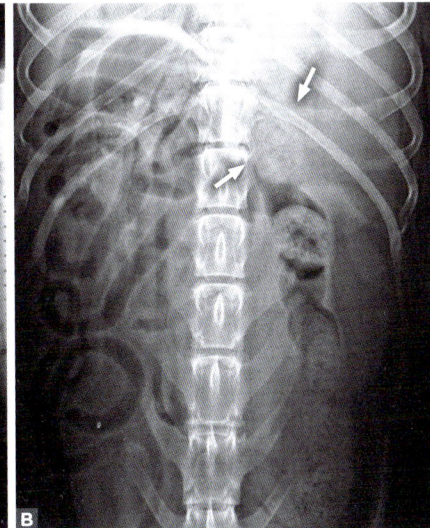

SECTION V ABDOMEN

the dog's size, but on average, a size greater than 0.7 cm in adult large breed dogs is considered the maximum for normal.[2]

Adrenal nodules less than 5 mm in diameter are frequent incidental findings in middle-aged and older dogs (**fig. 24.23**). In many patients, these are benign and non-functional, and there are no associated clinical signs. Endocrine testing and repeat sonographic imaging are usually recommended to monitor these lesions. Mass lesions greater than 2 cm in diameter are significantly more likely to represent malignant adrenal neoplasia. Sonographic evidence of invasion of the renal veins, phrenicoabdominal veins, or caudal vena cava is the most reliable sign of malignant neoplasia such as adrenal adeno-

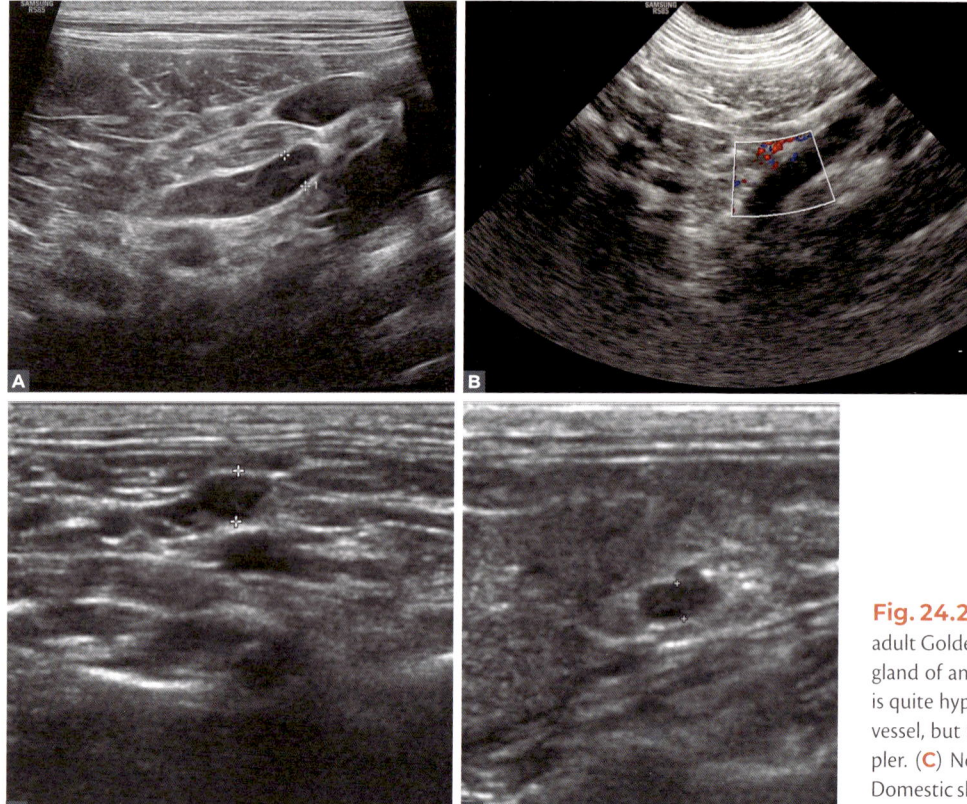

Fig. 24.22 (**A**) Normal left adrenal gland of an adult Golden Retriever. (**B**) Normal right adrenal gland of an adult Golden Retriever. The adrenal is quite hypoechoic and could be mistaken for a vessel, but there is no blood flow on color Doppler. (**C**) Normal left adrenal gland of an adult Domestic shorthair cat. (**D**) Normal right adrenal gland of an adult Domestic shorthair cat.

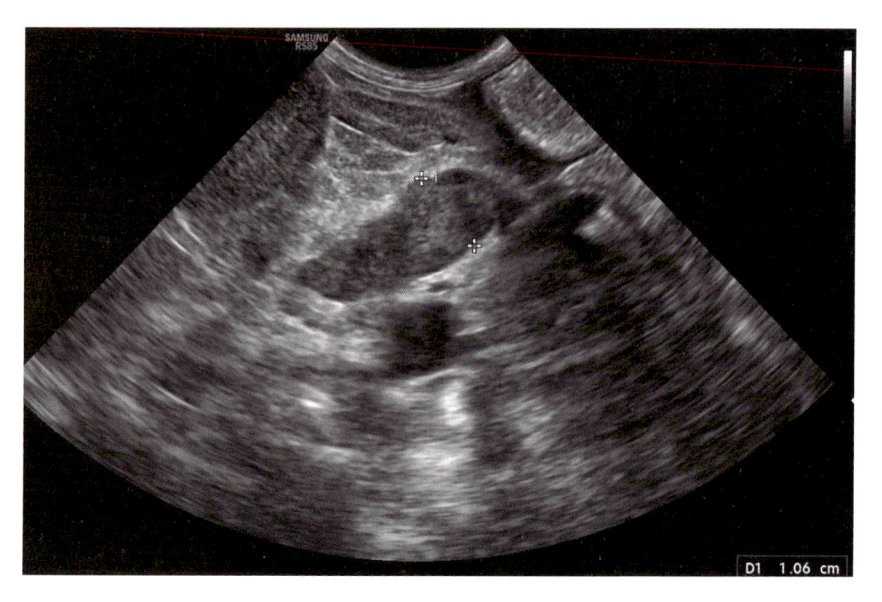

Fig. 24.23 Left adrenal gland of an adult mixed breed dog. The overall size of the caudal pole is enlarged, measuring greater than 1 cm in thickness (between the calipers). Within the caudal pole, there is a round, ill-defined, hyperechoic nodule.

carcinoma or pheochromocytoma. The presence of an echogenic thrombus within the lumen of the renal vein or caudal vena cava adjacent to an adrenal mass should be interpreted as vascular invasion (**figs. 24.24** and **24.25**). In some patients, the thrombus can be quite large, causing almost complete occlusion of the cava or renal vein. In some patients, there may be sonographic evidence of invasion of the kidney or infiltration of the epaxial musculature by a malignant adrenal mass. Although ultrasound can be helpful to evaluate adrenal masses and look for vascular invasion, computed tomography may also be helpful for evaluating the extent of invasion or evaluating difficult to identify masses (**fig. 24.26**).

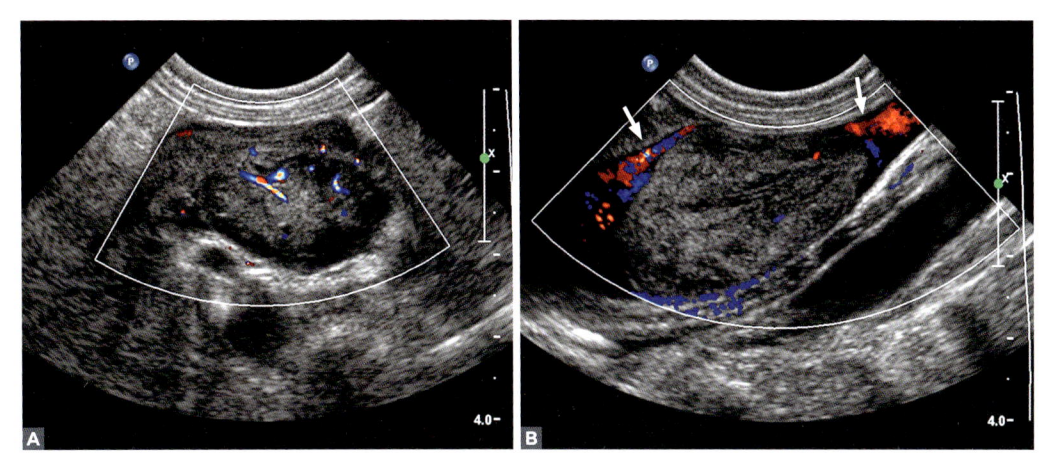

Fig. 24.24 (**A**) Ultrasound image with color Doppler. A mass was identified in the region of the left adrenal gland, and a normal left adrenal gland was not identified. The mass demonstrated blood flow. (**B**) Evaluation of the caudal vena cava showed an extension of the mass into the vessel. The mass caused partial occlusion with turbulent blood flow passing around the mass (arrows). These findings indicate a malignant neoplasm such as adenocarcinoma or pheochromocytoma.

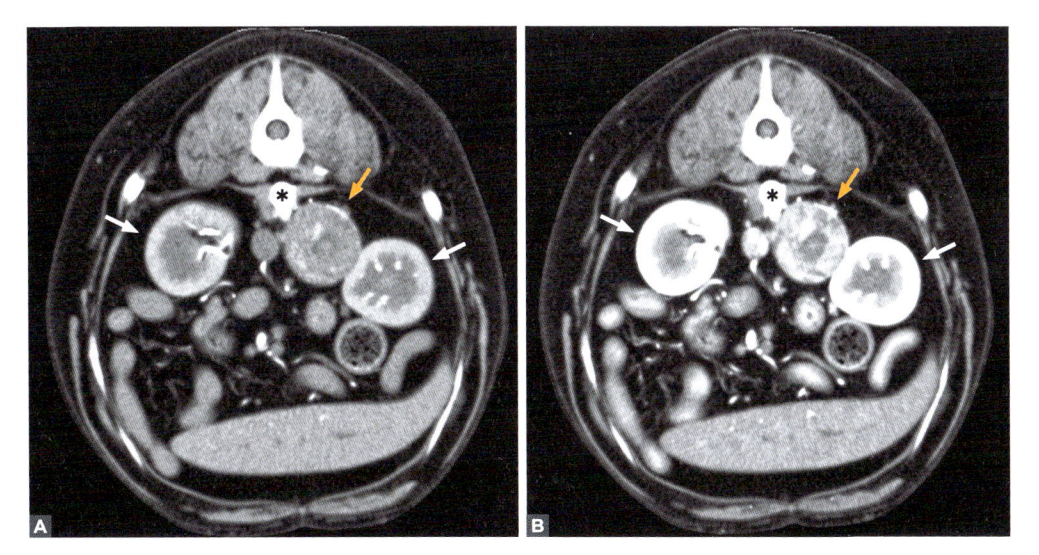

Fig. 24.25 Post-contrast computed tomographic transverse slices in a soft tissue window of a nine-year-old spayed female Labrador Retriever. The patient's right is to the left of the image. (**A**) This image was acquired during the early arterial phase. (**B**) This image was acquired during the late arterial phase. Notice the strong contrast enhancement of the aorta (asterisk) in both phases. The renal cortices are mildly contrast-enhancing in the early phase, then strongly contrast-enhancing in the late arterial phase (white arrows). Medial to the left kidney, there is a heterogeneously contrast-enhancing, soft tissue, and fluid attenuating mass (orange arrows). The mass is of adrenal origin with a central region that does not enhance, likely indicating necrosis. Given the size and contrast enhancement pattern, pheochromocytoma and cortical adenocarcinoma are most likely.

SECTION V ABDOMEN

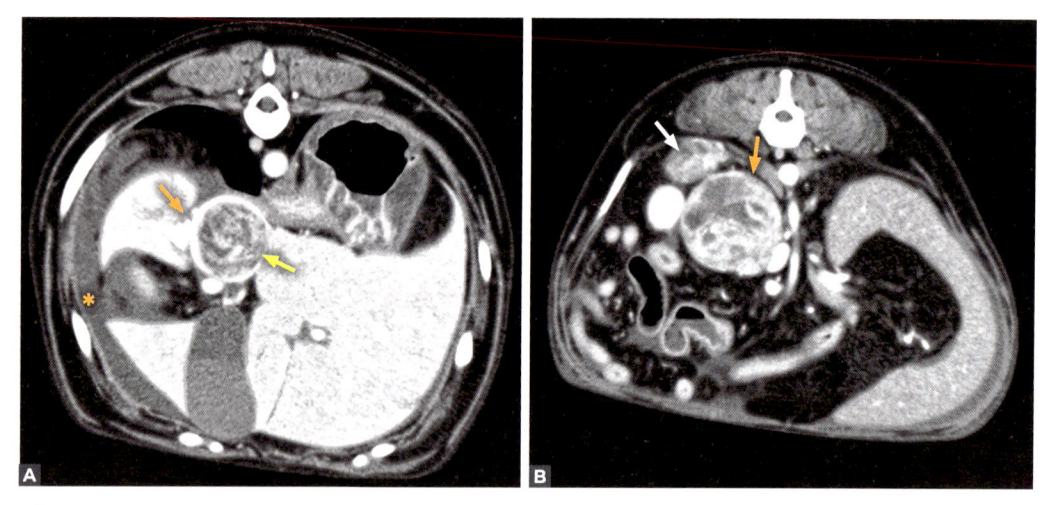

Fig. 24.26 The patient's right is to the left of the image. Transverse computed tomographic images of a dog with a right adrenal mass and invasion into the caudal vena cava. (A) The caudal vena cava is markedly dilated and almost completely filled with a heterogeneously contrast-enhancing mass (yellow arrow) surrounded by a thin, contrast-filled lumen (orange arrow). There is a moderate amount of fluid within the abdomen (asterisk). (B) A more caudal transverse image showing the adrenal mass (orange arrow). A large tumor thrombus dilates the right phrenicoabdominal vein as it courses dorsally to the adrenal mass (white arrow).

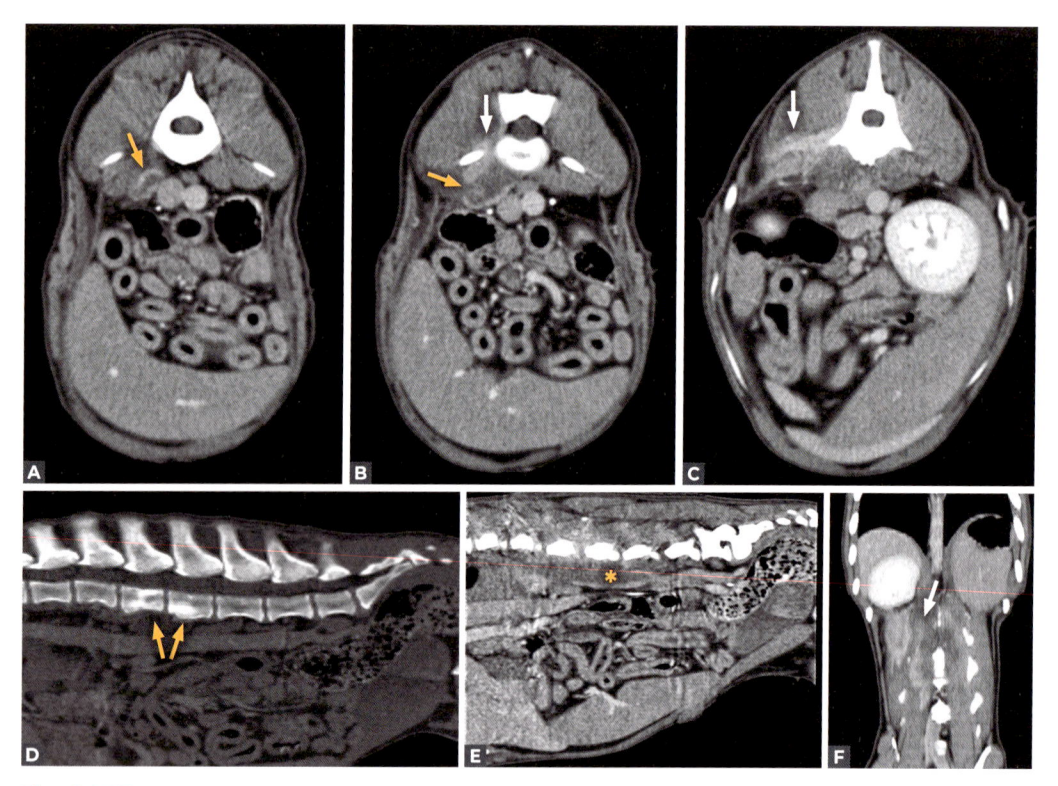

Fig. 24.27 Computed tomography study of a 14-month-old mixed breed dog. (A, B) The post-contrast study shows a fistula with a well visible contrast-enhancing wall containing fluid (orange arrows). (B-F) Contrast enhancement of the psoas and epaxial muscles was also visible, leading to a diagnosis of myositis (white arrows). The sagittal reconstruction in the one window (D) shows bone sclerosis of the body of L3 and L4, which is a sign of spondylitis. In a parasagittal reconstruction in soft tissue window (E), the fluid containing mass is visible (asterisk), consistent with an abscess.

Migrating foreign body

Migrating foreign bodies can have a wide variety of clinical signs, presentations, and signalment depending on where they are, what they are, and what organ systems are involved.

One such foreign body is presumed to be the wire bristles from the grill brushes. These are frequently encountered in canine patients within the peritoneal space and are almost always incidental. They are curvilinear and varying in length, metal opaque structures.

Another common migrating foreign body is aspirated plant material. Hunting dogs and puppies may present with clinical signs of sneezing, coughing, fever, or nasal discharge with foreign bodies that enter the respiratory system. These foreign bodies may have a wide variety of clinical signs depending on the route and extent of migration. Foreign bodies such as fox awns can migrate through the lungs and become implanted in the body wall or retroperitoneal space. This material tends to migrate caudally and dorsally through the bronchi and reach the ventral aspect of the L3-L4 vertebrae as this is the location for the attachment of the crus of the diaphragm. This may cause columnar periosteal proliferation and osteomyelitis along the ventral aspects of the L3-L4 vertebrae (**fig. 24.25**).

In addition to radiographs, computed tomography, magnetic resonance imaging, or ultrasound can be more helpful in locating suspected foreign material and is more sensitive and specific for identification. Typically, the resulting granulomatous reaction and secondary inflammation appear as amorphous, disorganized tissue, but the foreign material appears as a discrete hyperechoic structure, sometimes with acoustic shadowing.

Plant foreign material can be difficult to identify even with advanced imaging. Wood, for example, will have different appearances based on the different water content and chronicity of the foreign material (**figs. 24.27- 24.29**).[6]

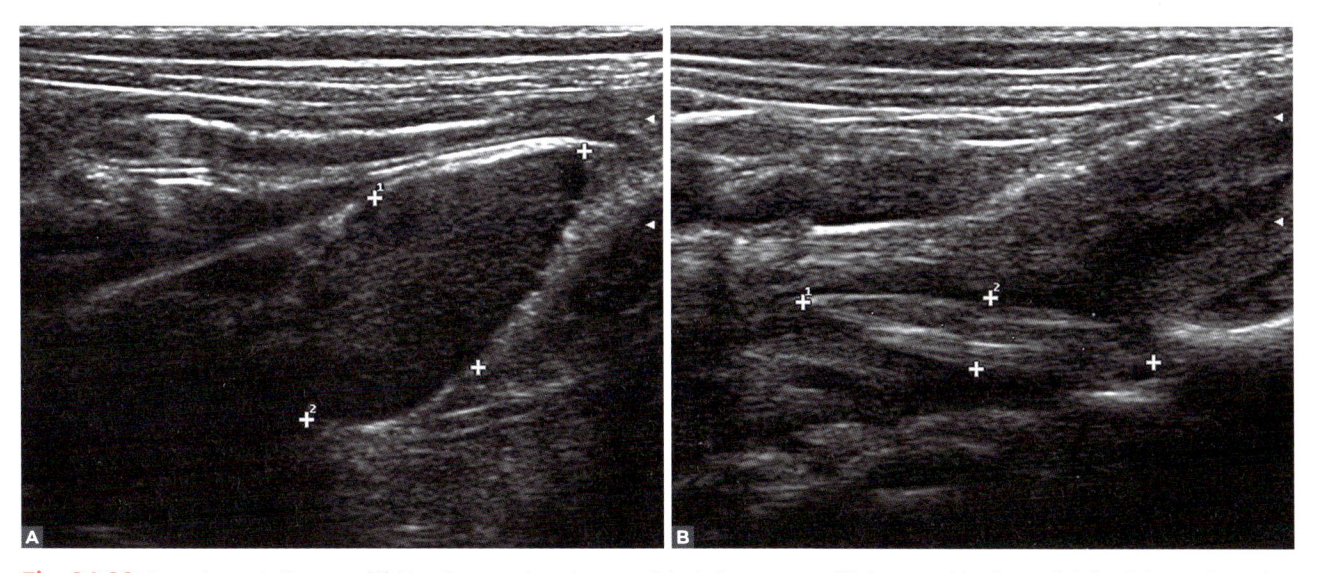

Fig. 24.28 Same dog as in fig. 24.27. (**A**) The ultrasound on the area of the lesions seen on CT shows a sublumbar well-defined abscess formation, (**B**) and adjacent to it a vegetal foreign body. The dog underwent surgery, and the foreign body was removed with ultrasound guidance.

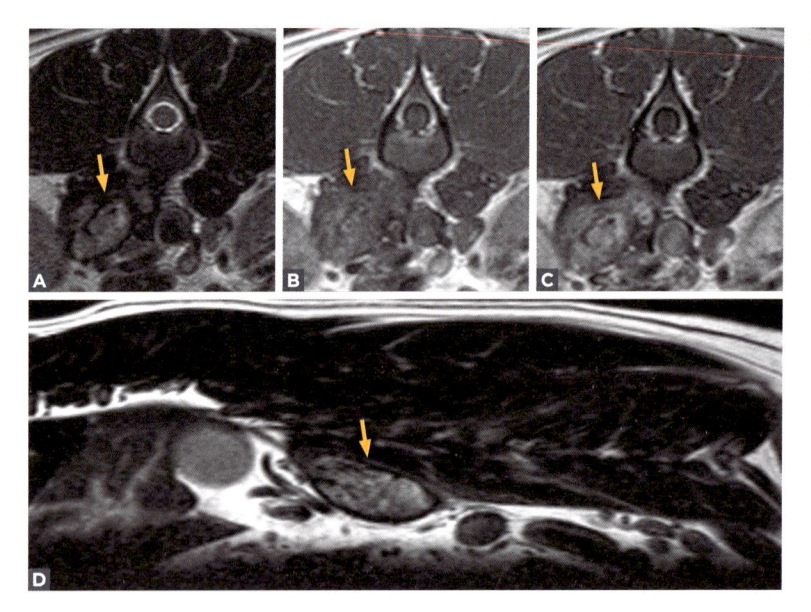

Fig. 24.29 Magnetic resonance imaging study of a four-year-old male Basset in pain when hunting and not comfortable lying down. It showed pain when the lumbar region was palpated. The images weighted in T1 FSE and T2 showed a sublumbar abscess (arrows).

References

1. Hermanson JW, de Lahunta A, Evans HE. The muscular system. In Hermanson J, de Lahunta A (editors). Miller and Evans' Anatomy of the Dog 5th edition. St. Louis, Elsevier, 2020.
2. Thrall DE (editor). Textbook of Veterinary Diagnostic Radiology 6th edition. St. Louis, Elsevier, pp 659-678.
3. Liptak JM, Dernell WS, Ehrhart EJ, Rizzo SA, Rooney MB, Withrow SJ. Retroperitoneal sarcomas in dogs: 14 cases (1992-2002). *J Am Vet Med Assoc* 224:1471-1417, 2004.
4. Schwarz T, Morandi F, Gnudi G, Wisner E, Paterson C, Sullivan M, Johnston P. Nodular fat necrosis in the feline and canine abdomen. *Vet Radiol Ultrasound* 41:335-339, 2000.
5. Krol L, O'Brien R. Ultrasonographic assessment of abdominal lymph nodes in puppies. *Vet Radiol Ultrasound* 53:455-458, 2012.
6. Ober CP, Jones JC, Larson MM, et al. Comparison of ultrasound, computed tomography, and magnetic resonance imaging in detection of acute wood foreign bodies in the canine manus. *Vet Radiol Ultrasound* 49:411-418, 2008.

CHAPTER 25

Gastrointestinal contrast studies

Lorrie Gaschen

KEY POINTS

- Contrast studies are performed when survey radiography is equivocal or functional information is required to make a diagnosis.
- Intraluminal, mural and extramural classifications of obstruction can be diagnosed.
- Static esophagrams aid in the diagnosis of foreign bodies, strictures, paraesophageal masses, diverticuli, and bronchoesophageal fistulae.
- Videofluoroscopy is necessary for diagnosing oral, pharyngeal, cricopharyngeal and esophageal dysfunction.
- Barium contrast studies are contraindicated if there is a suspicion of perforation based on the presence of cavity effusions or free gas in the thorax or abdomen.
- Pneumocolonogram is helpful for differentiating gas dilated small vs. large bowel in dogs and cats with suspected mechanical ileus.
- Negative contrast studies of the stomach and colon can be used for detection of foreign bodies and mural masses.

Contrast studies of the gastrointestinal tract are valuable for ruling out obstructions of the esophagus, stomach, and small and large intestines. Esophagrams, upper gastrointestinal studies and barium enemas are the most common procedures performed. Chapters 18, 26, and 28 cover the radiographic interpretation of esophageal, gastric, and large intestinal disorders while this chapter will focus on performing and making a diagnosis using contrast studies in those regions.

Contrast esophagram

Indications for performing an esophagram are dysphagia or regurgitation without a definitive etiologic lesion on survey radiographs. An esophagram can be used for investigation of diagnoses such as esophageal foreign body, strictures, esophageal and paraesophageal masses, diverticuli, bronchoesophageal fistula, and motility disorders. The main contraindication is the presence of pneumomediastinum or pleural effusion which can be associated with esophageal rupture. Contrast esophagography is best avoided in patients with pneumonia as aspiration of contrast may cause significant worsening of pneumonia. Barium containing contrast media are most commonly used but should be avoided if esophageal rupture is suspected or endoscopy is planned following the study. Non-ionic iodinated contrast media is preferred in these instances. Ionic iodinated contrast media are not used as these are hyperosmolar and will cause potentially lethal pulmonary edema if

BOX 25.1 ESOPHAGEAL CONTRAST STUDY PROCEDURES

Prior to performing the study:
- Survey radiographs of the oropharyneal, laryngeal and cervical region, lateral and ventrodorsal.
- Survey orthogonal views of the thorax.
- Screen for pneumothorax and pleural effusion, which can indicate esophageal perforation.
- Do not perform if esophageal perforation is suspected.
- Screen for radiopaque foreign body, mass, and segmental or generalized megaesophagus which carry an aspiration potential.

Perform a liquid followed by a solid phase static esophagram, with both barium-soaked soft food and kibble:
- Liquid can pass a narrowing that soft food or kibble cannot.

Static liquid barium esophagram:
- Oral administration with syringe.
- 60% weight/volume pre-formulated barium sulfate suspension:
  - Small dog: 15 mL.
  - Large dog: 20-30 mL.
  - Cat: 5-7 mL.
- Lateral radiographs of the neck and thorax immediately after administration, then ventrodorsal of the thorax.
- Perform opposite lateral radiograph of the thorax.
- Repeat thoracic radiographs to monitor passage of any residual contrast in the esophagus.

Static barium meal:
- Used to identify incomplete obstructions.
- If liquid barium esophagram is negative, administer a barium meal.
- If dog or cat can swallow water but not food.
- Soak soft food and kibble separately with barium sulfate suspension liquid:
  - Dog: 1 cup of food and 10 mL of liquid barium.
  - Cat: ½ cup of food and 10 mL of liquid barium.
- Allow dog or cat to eat from the bowl and immediately perform lateral cervical and thoracic images.
- Perform opposite lateral radiograph of the thorax.
- This procedure may be repeated a number of times as necessary.

Iodinated esophagram:
- If esophageal perforation is suspected.
- If endoscopy is going to be performed afterwards.
- Oral administration with syringe.
- Use a 50:50 mixture of non-ionic iodinated contrast medium and tap water:
  - Dog: 10-15 mL.
  - Cat: 5-10 mL.
- Perform radiographs as for liquid barium suspension.

Modified from: Wallack ST. Static barium esophagram. In Wallack ST (editor). The handbook of veterinary contrast radiography, Solana Beach, 2003, Veterinary Imaging, pp 45-53.

aspirated. Static radiographic esophagrams can be performed to diagnose foreign bodies, strictures, and masses, while functional swallowing disorders require dynamic contrast fluoroscopy. **Box 25.1** outlines the procedures for performing static liquid and solid phase esophagrams.[1] Videofluoroscopic contrast swallow studies are indicated for dogs and cats to assess oral, pharyngeal, cricopharyngeal, esophageal, and caudal esophageal sphincter function in real time. Images should be acquired at a minimum of 30 frames per second. Patients that cannot prehend food, drop food, drool, or have repeated attempts to swallow food or water without success require dynamic swallow studies. If videofluoroscopy equipment is not available, patients may need to be referred to a specialty center to diagnose swallowing disorders.

Esophagram diagnosis of obstruction

Segmental dilation of the esophagus on survey radiographs in a patient with esophageal clinical signs is an indication for performing a liquid and solid phase static barium esophagram to identify a potential site of narrowing and its extent. Positive contrast filling the esophagus has three potential variations from normal when an obstruction is present: luminal, mural and extramural (**box 25.2**).[2] Liquid is used to assess the borders of the contrast column while the solid phase study is used to identify a site of incomplete obstruction that allows passage of liquid (**fig. 25.1**).

Intraluminal foreign body obstruction

A foreign body can lead to a complete or partial obstruction (**fig. 25.2**). Acquired strictures can develop at the site of obstruction, especially when obstruction is long standing. The foreign body can have variable opacities and lead to variable degrees of esophageal dilation, both segmental and generalized. If a radiopaque foreign structure is not directly visualized radiographically or a soft tissue mass is identified in the region of the esophagus in a patient with regurgitation, a contrast esophagram is indicated.

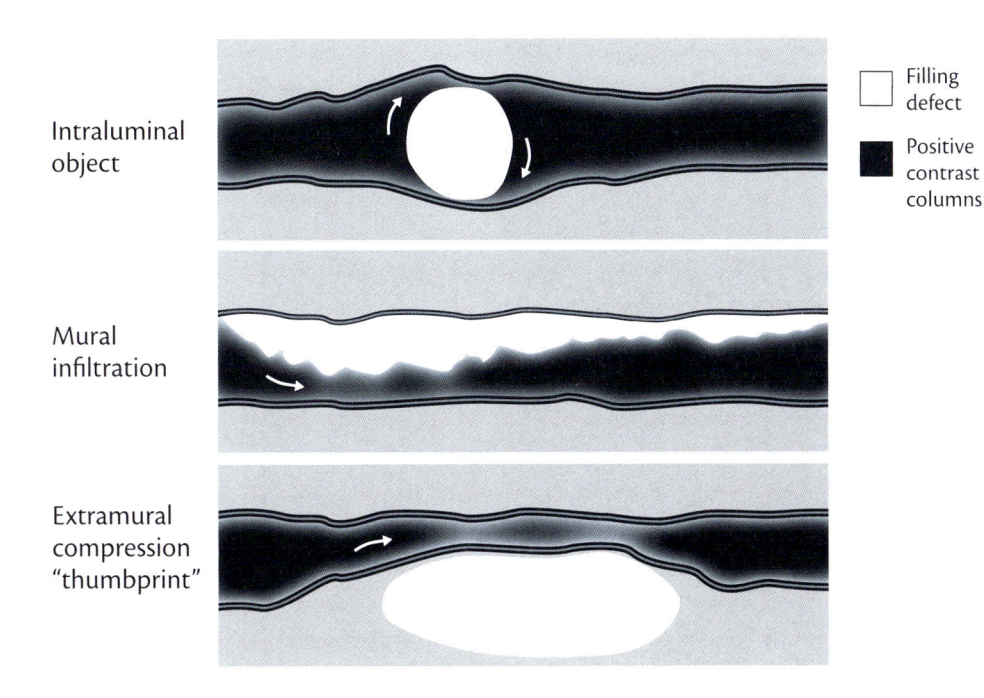

Fig. 25.1 Schematic of the three types of obstructions that can be diagnosed from a positive contrast study of the alimentary tract. Intraluminal lesions such as foreign bodies typically have contrast medium surrounding them. Mural lesions such as tumors, fungal infiltration, ulcers, and strictures are partially surrounded by contrast medium which has irregular margins at the site of the lesion. Extramural compressive lesions are external to the alimentary tract due to a mass effect causing luminal narrowing. The columns of contrast in both intraluminal and extramural compression are typically smoothly marginated.

SECTION V ABDOMEN

BOX 25.2 — PATTERNS OF OBSTRUCTION OF THE GASTROINTESTINAL TRACT

Intraluminal
- Filling defect in the contrast contrast medium.
- Focal dilation common with foreign body obstruction on lateral and ventrodorsal views.
- Contrast column borders remain smooth at mucosal border.
- Gradual transition zone from dilated to normal diameter.
- Incomplete and partial obstructions can have similar abnormalities.
- Complete stop or passage on all sides the intraluminal structure.
- Shape dependent on the type of content:
  - Linear foreign body with plication.
  - Outline shape of the foreign body.

Mural
- Thickening or ulcerations of the bowel wall:
  - Fungal and neoplastic infiltration.
  - Benign ulceration.
- Usually cause incomplete obstruction.
- Narrowing of the lumen.
- Contrast columns have an irregular border with the mucosa.
- Intestinal diameter orad from the lesion may be dilated.
- Thickening can be concentric or eccentric, symmetric or asymmetric.
- Ulcers form a "crater-like" mural filling defect in the contrast column:
  - An outpouching of contrast across the wall.

Extramural
- Narrowing of the intestinal lumen is due to external compression.
- Examples include adhesions from previous surgery and an organ mass such pressing on the intestine.
- A "thumb print" sign is present in the contrast column at the site of narrowing:
  - Smooth contrast columns at the mucosal border.
  - Narrowed lumen in one orthogonal view, widened in the other view.

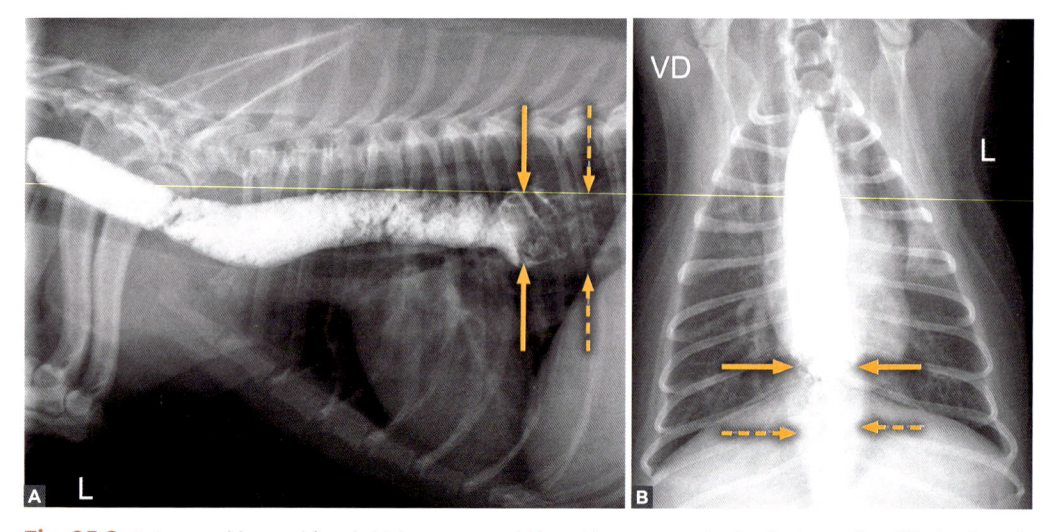

Fig. 25.2 A six-year-old spayed female Maltese ate a rawhide and began regurgitating. Barium sulfate fills the thoracic esophagus which is moderately and uniformly distended. Between the carina and diaphragm there is an abrupt stop of the contrast column which partially surrounds a filling defect in the lumen of the caudal esophagus (solid arrows). The esophagus is focally distended and soft tissue opaque at the site of the rawhide foreign body (dashed arrows).

Mural infiltration

Fungal, parasitic, neoplastic, and ulcerative disease can lead to thickening and irregularity of the wall causing narrowing and obstruction (fig. 25.3). The esophagus is typically dilated cranial to the lesion. Contrast columns at the transition from normal to the site of infiltration will have an irregular border at the site of luminal narrowing, indicating that infiltration of the wall is most likely. Mural lesions may be eccentric or circumferential.

Extramural compression

Extramural compression of the esophageal lumen in juvenile patients is usually from a vascular ring anomaly (VRA), most commonly persistent right aortic arch (PRAA). Masses within the mediastinum or surrounding structures are the most common causes in adult patients. PRAA is a vascular anomaly that leads to extraluminal compression of the esophagus cranial to the carina that typically occurs in puppies and kittens (fig. 25.4). Some patients have adult onset of clinical signs.[3,4] Esophageal dilation from VRA is typically segmental involving the cervical and cranial thoracic segments cranial to the carina. The esophagus can form a large diverticulum located ventral to the trachea at the thoracic inlet. Occasionally, the esophagus can develop generalized dilation in animals with PRAA, and in these cases the prognosis is worse. The contrast column will be concentrically narrowed at the site of obstruction and have smooth borders. Contrast enhanced computed tomography is necessary to characterize the vascular anomaly for confirmation and surgical planning.

Fig. 25.3 An eight-year-old Labrador Retriever with a history of chronic regurgitation and progressive anorexia and ptyalism. An esophagram was performed with a liquid phase contrast (A) and with barium-soaked kibble bolus (B). In both studies there is focal dilation of the mid-cervical esophagus. In the liquid phase, the dorsal margin of the contrast column is irregular, and the ventral border is smooth (solid arrows). Contrast passes the point of dilation with a typical linear pattern of the normal folds of the esophageal mucosa (dashed arrows). (B) The barium-soaked kibble cannot pass beyond the cervical esophagus and there is a broad based hemispherical mucosal mass lesion at the site of mucosal irregularity in the liquid phase (solid arrows). An ultrasound examination was performed and a soft tissue mass in the wall of the esophagus was identified and guided tissue sampling for cytology was diagnostic for esophageal squamous cell carcinoma.

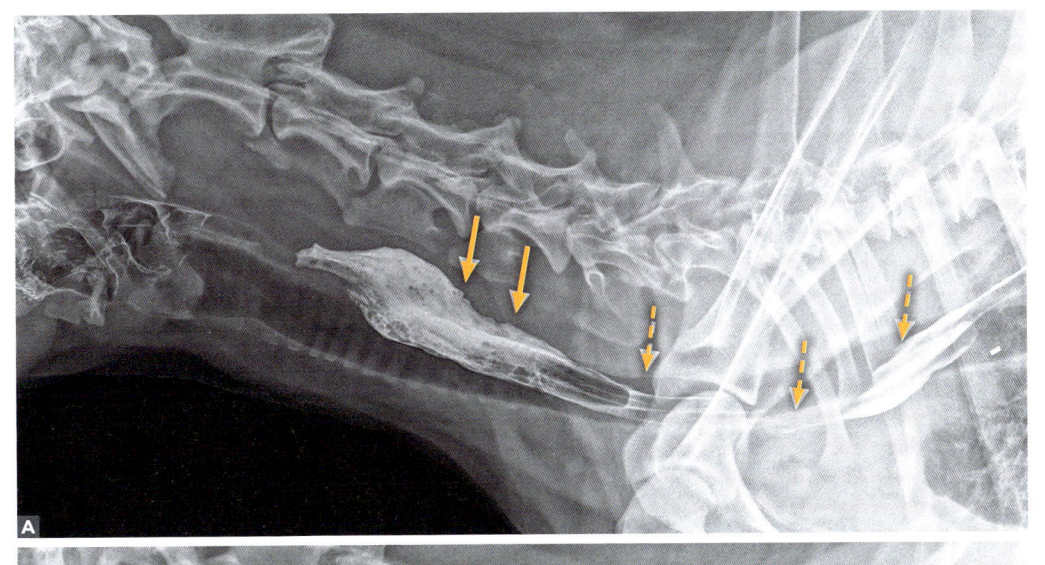

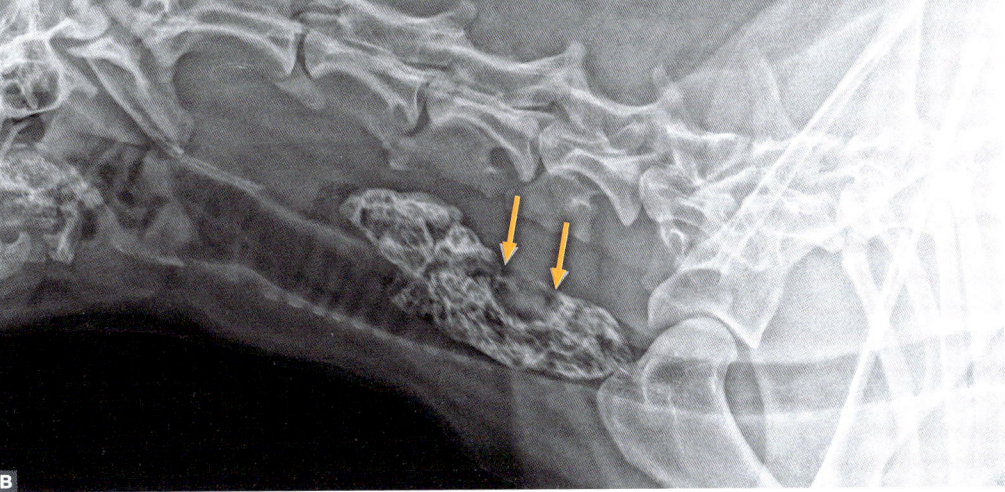

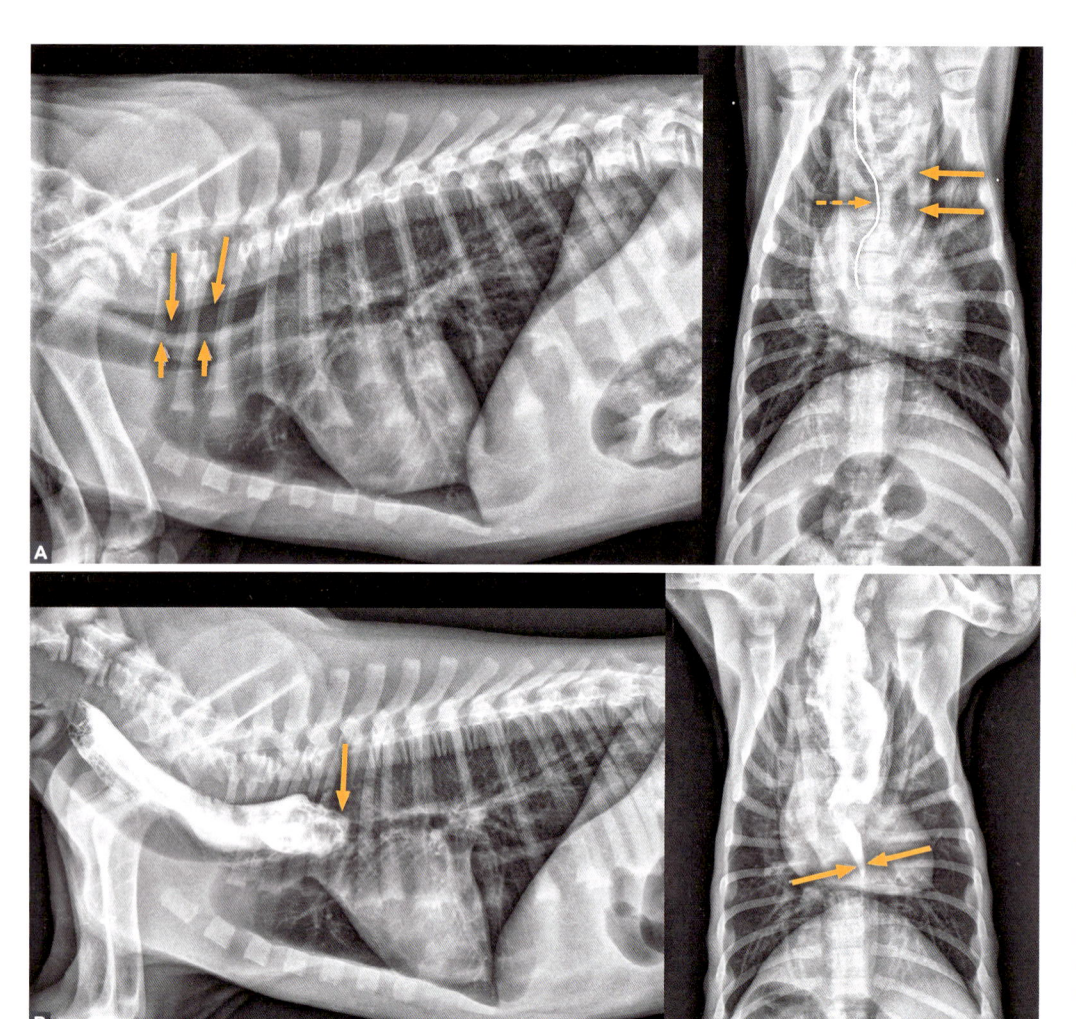

Fig. 25.4 (**A**) An eight-week-old female German Shepherd dog with regurgitation of solid food at four weeks of age and not gaining weight since that time. Survey radiographs of the thorax show gas dilation of the cranial thoracic esophagus and esophageal stripe sign (solid arrows). The trachea is ventrally and leftward displaced from the first to fourth thoracic vertebrae. The caudal esophagus is not distended. (**B**) A barium sulfate esophagram was performed and the esophagus is dilated from the level of the larynx to the fourth thoracic vertebra where the contrast is abruptly truncated and tapers with smooth borders to a point (solid arrows), indicating an extraluminal compression cranial to the heart base. A persistent aortic arch was diagnosed with computed tomography angiography and a ligamentum arteriosum was transected surgically.

Dysphagia

Oral, pharyngeal, cricopharyngeal

Lateral radiographs of the head and neck are important for ruling out structural abnormalities or foreign bodies. Videofluoroscopy recorded at 30 frames per second to observe and quantify the passage of a bolus is required to diagnose functional swallowing disorders.[5-7] Liquid barium sulfate suspensions (5-20 mL of 45-85% weight/volume) and barium soaked soft and hard food should be administered to completely assess swallowing (**figs. 25.5-25.8**). Ideally, the study should be carried out in standing with horizontal beam fluoroscopy but can be performed in lateral recumbency. Eating a food bolus tests normal prehension. Once the food is prehended or liquid contrast medium is administered orally, the bolus is formed by the tongue propelled to the oropharynx, the oropharynx contracts, pushing the bolus to the cranial esophageal sphincter which opens while the epiglottis covers the laryngeal opening. The sphincter closes immediately to prevent retrograde movement or reflux of the bolus into the nasopharynx or oral cavity.

Retention of the bolus in the oral cavity occurs in animals with oral dysphagia. Retention of the bolus in the pharynx or reflux into the nasopharynx indicates pharyngeal dysphagia such as aerodigestive disorders, and pharyngitis. Cricopharyngeal dysphagia is recognized by retention of the bolus in the pharynx, delayed or intermittent opening of the cranial esophageal sphincter, and repeated forceful attempts to swallow while the sphincter remains closed preventing transit of a bolus into the esophagus (**fig. 25.9**). The bolus can also be aspirated into the larynx or trachea in animals with dysphagia.

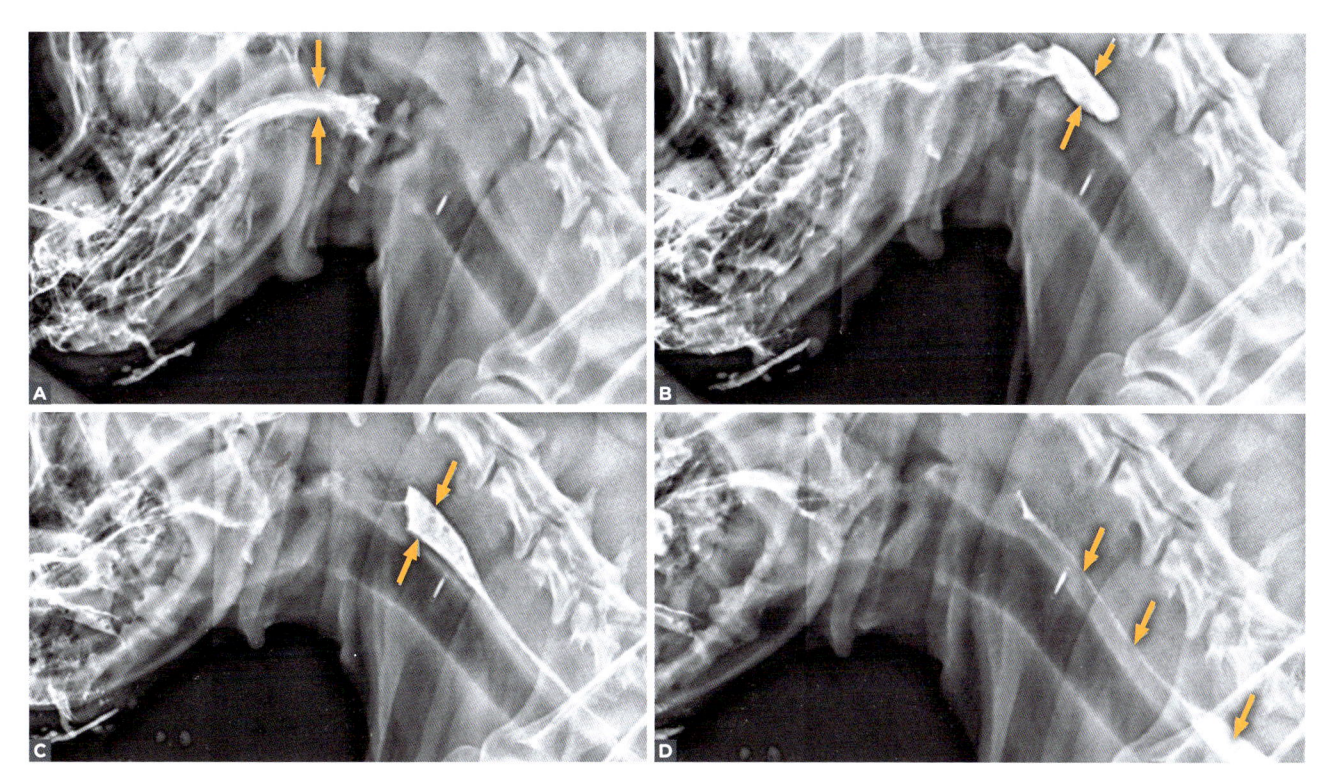

CHAPTER 25 Gastrointestinal contrast studies

Fig. 25.5 Static images from a 30 frame/second videofluoroscopic barium sulfate suspension liquid phase swallow study performed with a horizontal beam in a standing normal dog. There is liquid barium coating the mouth and oral cavity and the bolus is shown with solid arrows. (**A**) Pharyngeal contraction; (**B**) opening of the cranial esophageal sphincter; (**C**) normal shape of the tight bolus passing into the cranial esophagus, and (**D**) normal thin linear remnant of contrast coating the esophageal mucosa after passage of the bolus.

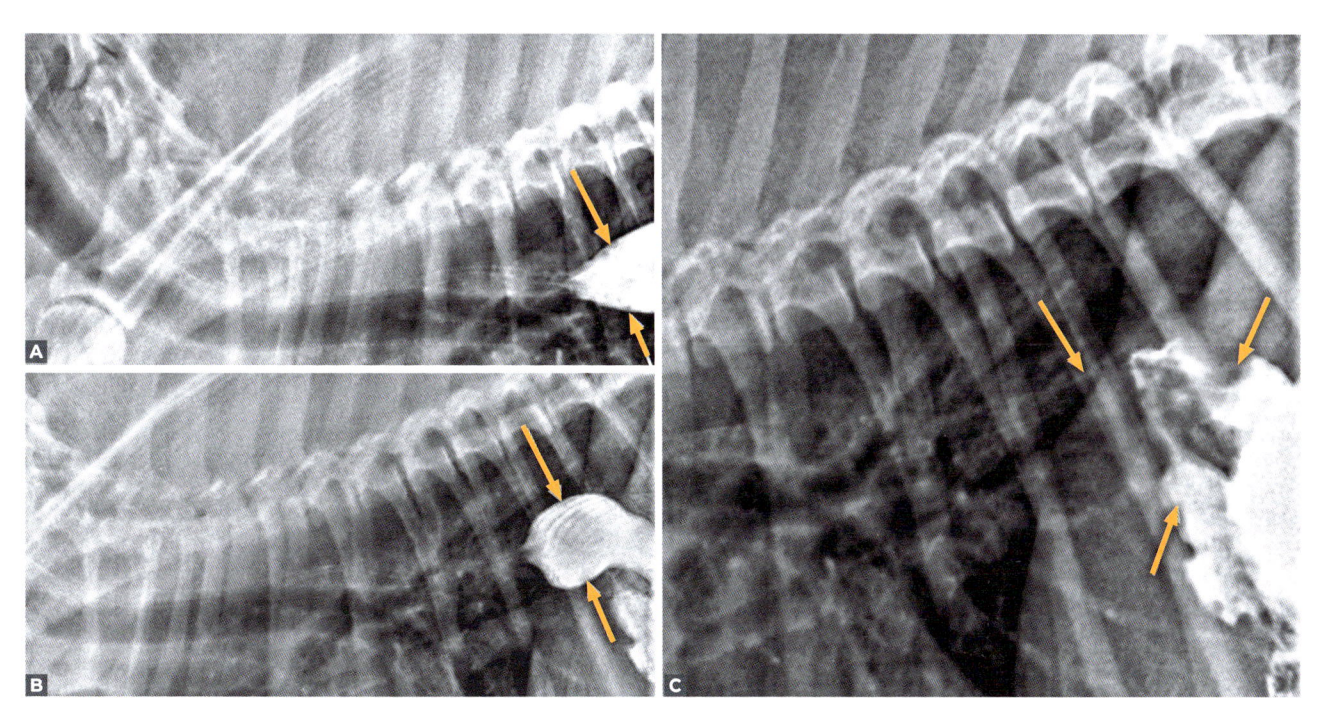

Fig. 25.6 Static images from a 30 frame/second videofluoroscopic barium sulfate suspension liquid phase swallow study performed with a horizontal beam in the same standing normal dog as in fig. 25.5 (**A**). The esophagus is contracted after passage of the bolus and thin layer of contrast coats the esophageal lining. (**B**) The bolus (solid arrows) is tight and passes through the open caudal esophageal sphincter. (**C**) The caudal esophageal sphincter is now closed and barium has entered the stomach.

421

SECTION V ABDOMEN

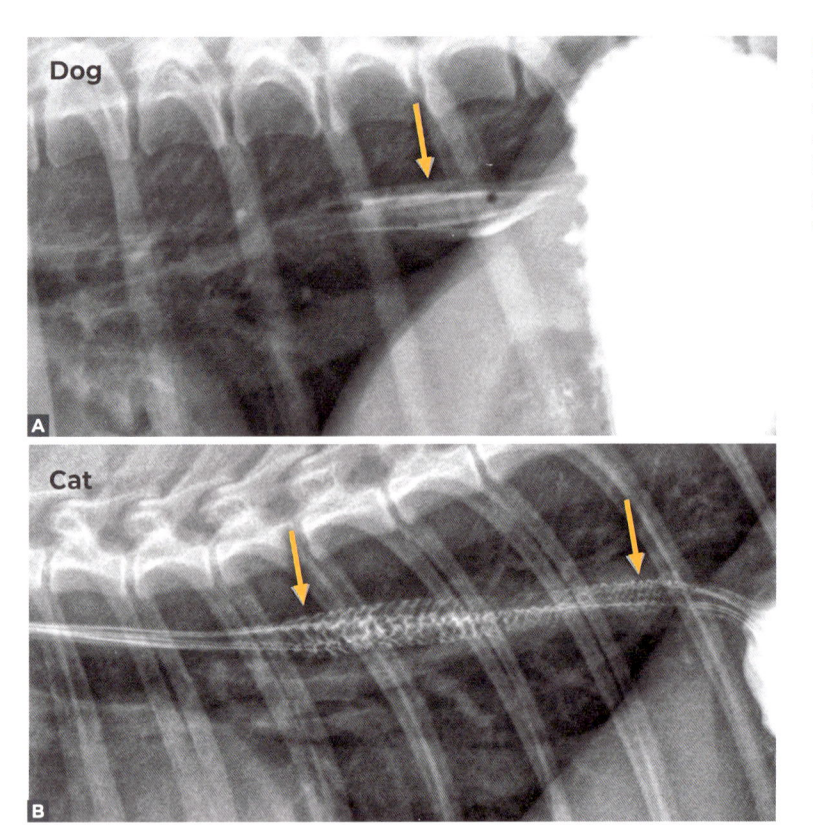

Fig. 25.7 Radiographic images showing the differences in the caudal esophagus in normal dogs and cats. Barium coating the mucosa in dogs shows fine linear folds and has smooth borders (arrows) while in the cat the mucosa has a herringbone pattern (arrows) in the caudal thorax due to the presence of striated muscle in the caudal thoracic esophageal wall in this species.

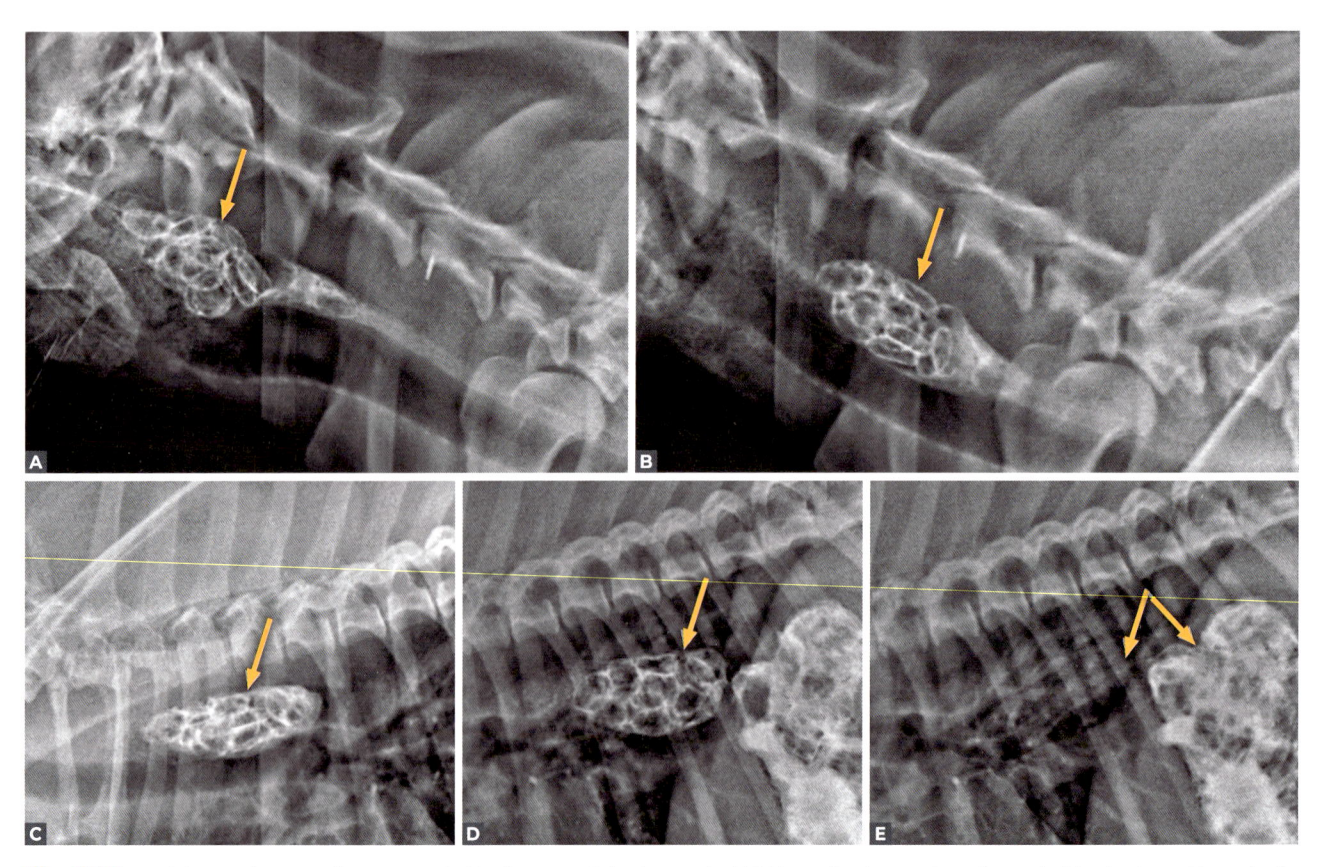

Fig. 25.8 Static images from a 30 frame/second videofluoroscopic barium-soaked kibble swallowing study performed with a horizontal beam in the same standing normal dog as in fig. 25.5 (**A**). The kibble bolus (solid arrow) is in the oropharynx as the cranial esophageal sphincter begins to open. (**B**) The tight kibble bolus enters the cervical esophagus. (**C**) The kibble bolus passes into the thoracic esophagus cranial to the carina and maintains its tight shape. (**D**) The bolus passes to the esophageal hiatus of the diaphragm. (**E**) The bolus is now present in the stomach and there is no residual kibble in the caudal esophagus.

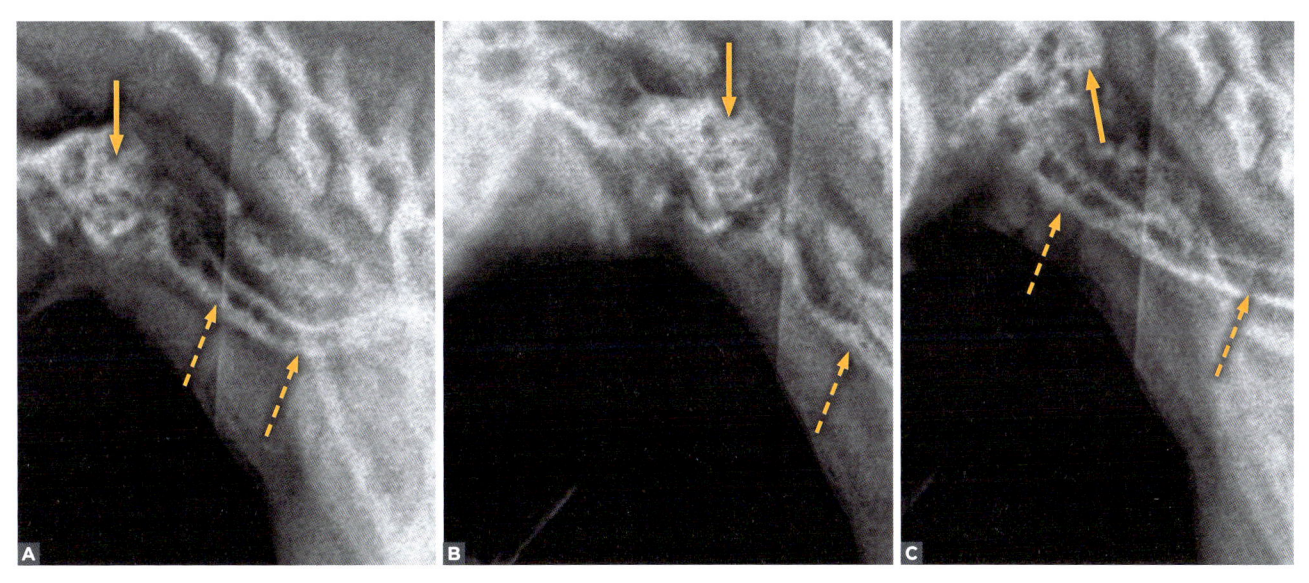

Fig. 25.9 A three-year-old neutered male Cocker Spaniel with chronic idiopathic megaesophagus, regurgitation, inability to swallow and recurrent aspiration pneumonia. Static images from a 30 frame/second videofluoroscopic barium-soaked kibble bolus swallow study performed with a horizontal beam with the patient standing. The liquid phase swallow study performed prior showed multiple attempts to swallow before the cranial esophageal sphincter opened. Liquid barium was aspirated into the trachea (dashed arrows). (**A**) Barium-soaked kibble bolus in the oropharynx and lack of opening of the cranial esophageal sphincter. (**B**) Subsequent attempts do not lead to opening of the sphincter and the bolus remains in the oropharynx. (**C**) The bolus is retropulsed into the nasopharynx and the sphincter does not open. The bolus never passed the sphincter in this dog. The diagnosis was acquired cricopharyngeal achalasia causing inability to swallow solid food boluses and tracheal aspiration.

Esophageal dysmotility and megaesophagus

Generalized megaesophagus can be congenital or acquired. Causes include juvenile idiopathic, adult idiopathic, neuromuscular (myasthenia gravis), myositis, immune-mediated, polyneuropathy, inflammatory, toxic, neoplastic, and obstructive (foreign body or stricture), and caudal esophageal sphincter achalasia. Contrast esophagrams are indicated when diseases causing hypomotility have been ruled out as a cause for generalized esophageal dilation and clinical concern for a caudal stricture or caudal esophageal achalasia is present. Videofluoroscopy is used to assess transport of the bolus via primary and secondary peristaltic waves to the caudal esophageal sphincter (**figs. 25.10-25.13**). Videofluoroscopic swallow studies are indicated for investigation of suspected caudal esophageal achalasia and hiatal disorders which can be intermittent and difficult to diagnose on static esophagrams. Gravity-assisted esophageal transit studies using a Bailey chair in dogs with megaesophagus and lower esophageal sphincter disease, such as achalasia, provides improved diagnostic efficacy and provides better management strategies.[8]

SECTION V ABDOMEN

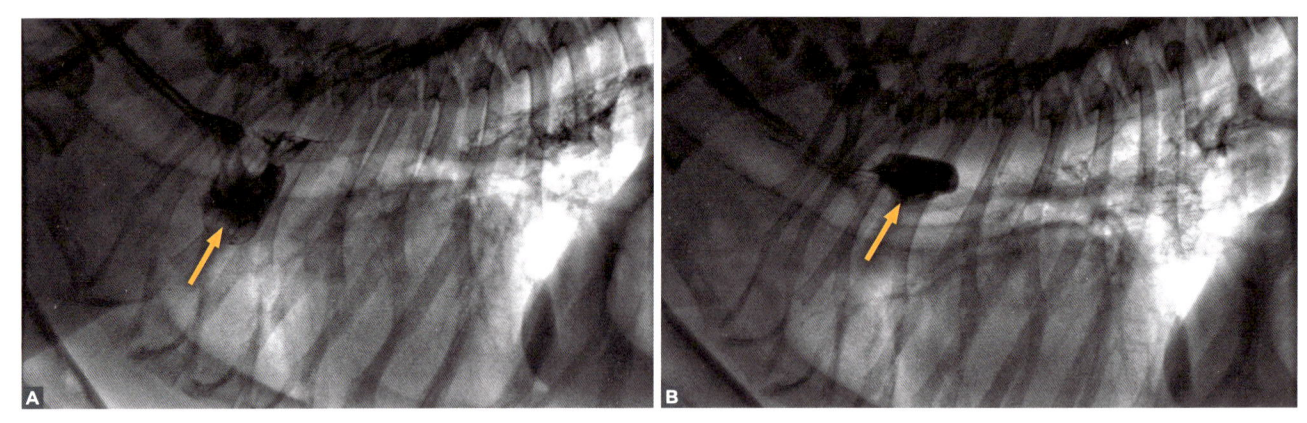

Fig. 25.10 Static images of a liquid phase lateral recumbency videofluoroscopy in a two-year-old neutered male English Bulldog that was regurgitating 3-4 times per week. (A) Sigmoid-shaped ventral deviation of the liquid barium contrast filling the esophagus is present at the thoracic inlet (arrows). (B) A second liquid bolus showed the ventral deviation is transient. A diagnosis of incidental redundant esophagus was made. A redundant loop of the esophagus at the thoracic inlet is a common inconsequential finding in brachycephalic dogs.

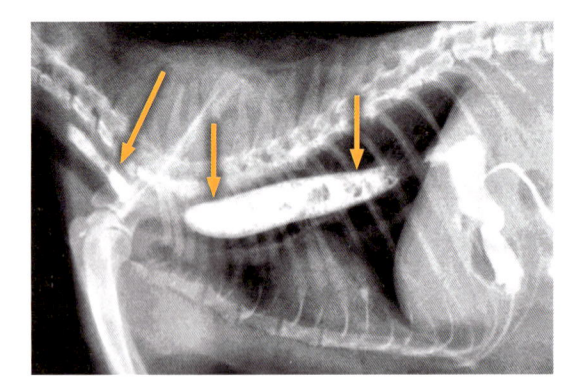

Fig. 25.11 A 14-year-old Domestic longhair spayed female cat with difficulty swallowing and regurgitation had a barium sulfate liquid phase and soft food barium-soaked phase swallow study. The pharyngeal and cricopharyngeal phases were normal. In the esophageal phase, there was mild cervical and severe thoracic esophageal dilation with the soft food material and contrast (arrows). A tight bolus was never formed, and the dilation persisted in the esophagus without evidence of peristalsis. Only liquid passed into the stomach. The cat was diagnosed with acquired megaesophagus and dysmotility. Differentials included idiopathic, inflammatory, and neuromuscular disease.

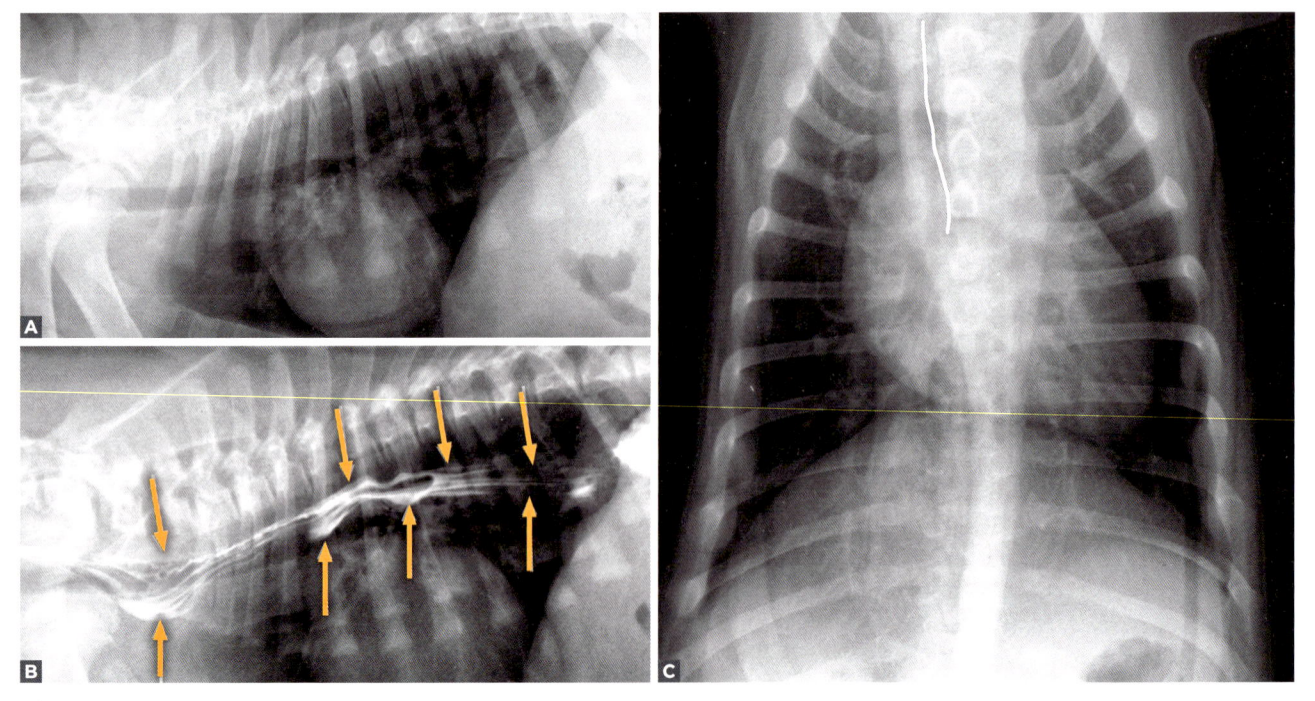

Fig. 25.12 A three-month-old male Mastiff with frequent regurgitation presented for a swallow study. Survey radiographs (A, B) were normal and did not show dilation of the esophagus. (C) Liquid phase barium sulfate administered orally showed retention of contrast in the esophagus with mild dilation (arrows). Peristalsis was not observed with extended real time imaging. The diagnosis of esophageal phase dysphagia due to juvenile idiopathic dysmotility was made. (B) Note the normal position of the trachea in the ventrodorsal view (white line). The lack of segmental esophageal dilation cranial to the carina almost certainly excludes vascular ring anomaly as the etiology of regurgitation in this juvenile patient.

424

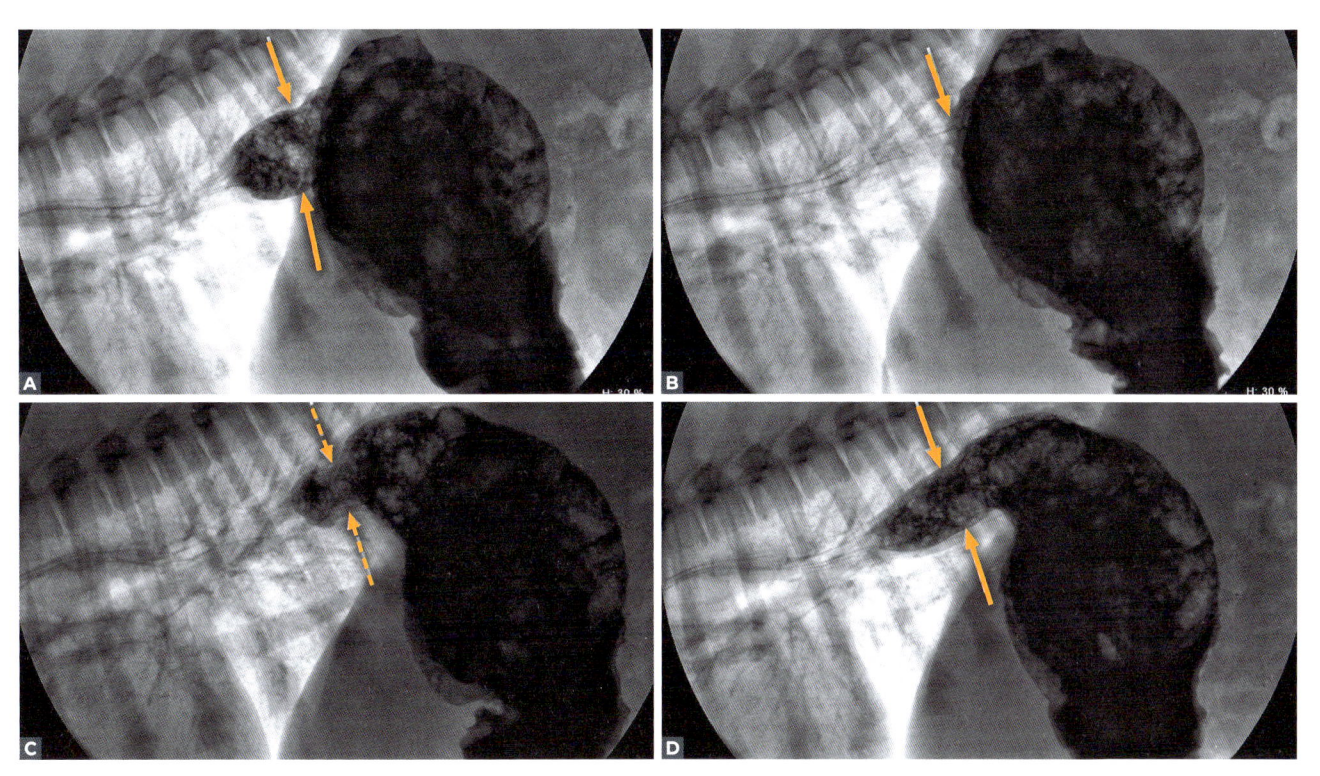

Fig. 25.13 A four-month-old female Belgian Malinois with an eight-week history of regurgitation. A barium-soaked kibble phase swallow study was performed following an unremarkable liquid phase study. (**A**) Opening of the caudal esophageal sphincter (arrow) as the bolus passes through, and (**B**) closing of the sphincter (arrow) immediately after. (**C**) Cranial displacement of the caudal esophageal sphincter (dashed arrows) and cardia into the thorax at the esophageal hiatus, and (**D**) continued cranial displacement of the gastroesophageal junction and cardia (arrow) into the thorax. The dog was diagnosed with a congenital sliding hiatal hernia.

Upper gastrointestinal contrast study

An upper gastrointestinal (GI) study examines the stomach and jejunum for transit time, partial or complete obstructive disease (luminal, mural and extramural types listed in **box 25.2**), and is also used for animals with hematemesis and melena. Main indications include situations where survey radiographs are equivocal for the cause of the gastrointestinal signs in dogs and cats with acute or chronic vomiting, chronic diarrhea, mass effect in the abdomen, and chronic weight loss (**figs. 25.17-25.21**). **Box 25.3** lists the procedures for an upper GI study using barium and iodinated contrast media.[1,9,10] Barium is the preferred contrast medium due to its inert properties and ability to coat the gastrointestinal mucosa (**figs. 25.14-25.16**). Nonionic iodinated contrast medium is reserved for patients with a suspicion of bowel perforation based on the presence of peritoneal effusion or free gas in the abdomen (**fig. 25.17**). Animals that are dehydrated should receive fluid therapy prior to an upper GI study, as even nonionic iodinated agents will cause some sequestration of water in the intestine. Iodinated contrast medium is not ideal for evaluating the mural lesions and barium is preferred if this is suspected. Both barium suspension and iodinated contrast medium can be used to confirm complete obstructions but can pass through a partial obstruction and sufficient images should be obtained to avoid missing such a lesion. Nonionic iodinated contrast medium should be diluted with water to be approximately isotonic to plasma for oral administration which minimize osmotic dilution and still allows adequate assessment of the gastrointestinal tract.[10]

Iodinated contrast medium can also be mixed with carboxymethylcellulose (CMC, carboxymethylcellulose sodium salt, Sigma Chemical Co, St Louis, Mo and Kukjeon Pharm, Seoul, Republic of Korea) which is nontoxic, nonimmunogenic, biodegradable, and bioabsorbable substance with low risk of causing adverse reaction if aspirated into the lungs or abdominal cavity.[9] See **box 25.3** for mixture and dosages.

BOX 25.3 — BARIUM ENEMA AND PNEUMOCOLONOGRAM PROCEDURES

Barium upper GI study
- Evaluate GI transit and emptying times, diagnose luminal foreign bodies, mural infiltrative disease and potential causes of hematemesis or melena.
- Contraindications include suspicion of perforation and presence of peritoneal gas or fluid.
- Iodinated contrast medium can be used instead of barium if perforation is suspected (see below).

Prior to performing the study
- Perform without sedation which affects transit time and emptying.
- 12-24-hour food fast, water can be provided up to 2 hours prior to study.
- Survey abdomen, right and left lateral and ventrodorsal views preferred.
- If gastric ingesta is present, continue fasting and repeat survey radiographs until resolved.
- If feces are present, perform an enema and repeat survey radiographs until resolved.
- Administer barium sulfate suspension orally via syringe or orogastric tube.
- Administer 30-60 % weight/volume solution:
  - Dog: <20 kg, 8-12 mL/kg; >20 kg, 5-7 mL/kg.
  - Cat: 12-20 mL/kg
- Perform right and left lateral, VD and DV radiographs immediately.
- Repeat right and left lateral and VD at 30, 60, and 90 minutes, and every 30 mintues thereafter until barium reaches the colon.

Emptying and transit times for barium upper GI studies
- Normal gastric emptying:
  - Dog: 30-120 minutes.
  - Cat: 15-60 minutes.
- Small intestinal transit:
  - Dog: 30-120 minutes.
  - Cat: 30-60 minutes.
- Small intestinal emptying:
  - Dog: 180-300 minutes.
  - Cat: 30-60 minutes.

Modified from Wallack ST. Static barium esophagram. In Wallack ST (editor). The handbook of veterinary contrast radiography, Solana Beach, 2003, Veterinary Imaging, pp 45-53.

Iodinated upper GI
Prior to performing the study
- The animal must be well hydrated to prevent life-threatening shock due to the hyperosmolarity of the contrast medium.
- Prepare the animal as for the barium upper GI outlined above.

Iodinated contrast media type, preparation and administration
- Non-ionic iodinated contrast medium is preferred due to lower osmolarity.
- Ionic iodinated contrast medium can be used but should be diluted.
- Dilute iodinated contrast medium 1:3 with tap water prior to oral administration.
- Iodinated contrast medium can be mixed with carboxymethylcellulose: 8.5 mL of 0.5% CMC/kg mixed with 1.5 mL iohexol/kg.
- Administer iodine via orogastric tube, as aspiration from oral syringe administration can lead to acute pulmonary edema.
  - Dog: 10 mL/kg. Right, left and VD radiographs at time 0, 15, 30, 60, 90, 120, and 150 minutes until it reaches colon. Normal gastric emptying: 30-120 minutes. Small intestinal transit: 60-90 minutes.
  - Cat: 10 mL/kg. Right, left and VD radiographs at time 0, 15, 45, 60, 75, and 90 minutes until it reaches colon. Normal gastric emptying: 30-90 minutes. Small intestinal transit: 15-75 minutes.

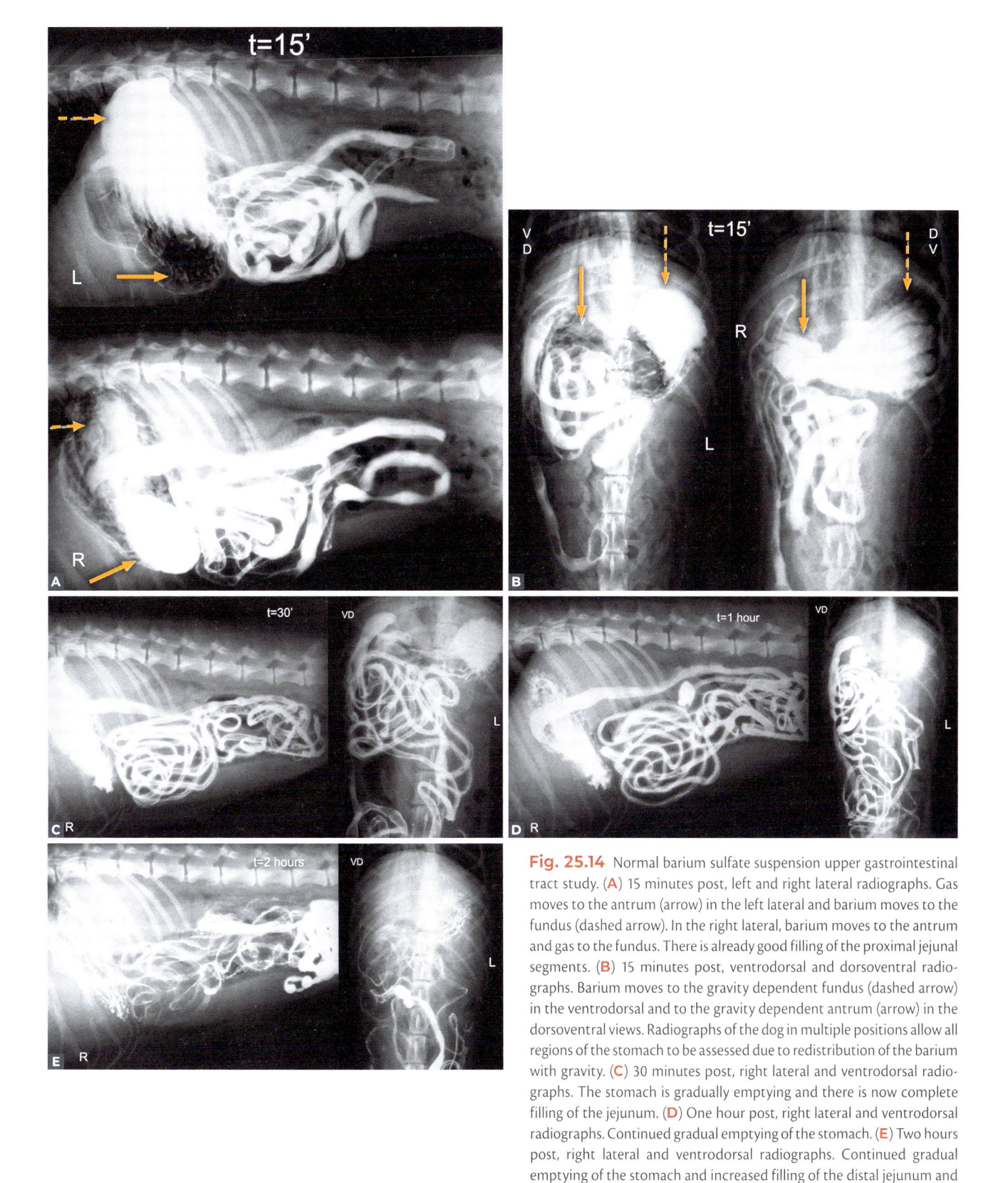

CHAPTER 25 Gastrointestinal contrast studies

Fig. 25.14 Normal barium sulfate suspension upper gastrointestinal tract study. (**A**) 15 minutes post, left and right lateral radiographs. Gas moves to the antrum (arrow) in the left lateral and barium moves to the fundus (dashed arrow). In the right lateral, barium moves to the antrum and gas to the fundus. There is already good filling of the proximal jejunal segments. (**B**) 15 minutes post, ventrodorsal and dorsoventral radiographs. Barium moves to the gravity dependent fundus (dashed arrow) in the ventrodorsal and to the gravity dependent antrum (arrow) in the dorsoventral views. Radiographs of the dog in multiple positions allow all regions of the stomach to be assessed due to redistribution of the barium with gravity. (**C**) 30 minutes post, right lateral and ventrodorsal radiographs. The stomach is gradually emptying and there is now complete filling of the jejunum. (**D**) One hour post, right lateral and ventrodorsal radiographs. Continued gradual emptying of the stomach. (**E**) Two hours post, right lateral and ventrodorsal radiographs. Continued gradual emptying of the stomach and increased filling of the distal jejunum and emptying of the proximal jejunum.

SECTION V ABDOMEN

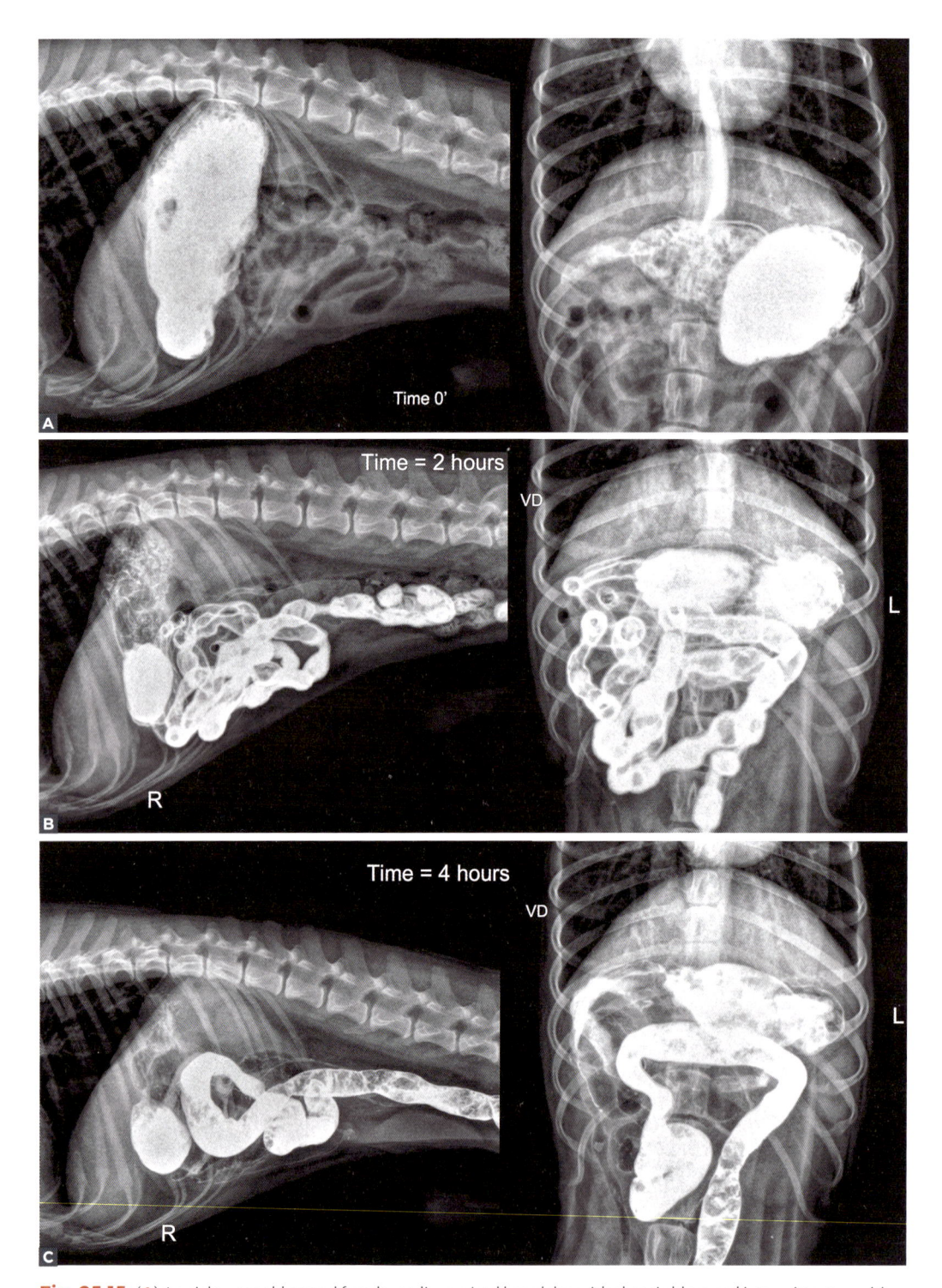

Fig. 25.15 (**A**) An eight-year-old spayed female medium mixed breed dog with chronic bloat and intermittent vomiting. The upper gastrointestinal study with barium sulfate suspension showed normal filling of the stomach at 15 minutes. (**B**) At two hours post, there is progressive emptying of the stomach but with a moderate amount of residual contrast (compared to fig. 25.14E). The jejunum has progressive normal filling. (**C**) At four hours post, the colon has a large amount of contrast filling and there is a moderate amount of residual contrast in the stomach, similar to the two-hour time point. This dog has delayed gastric emptying without evidence of obstruction and has differentials of functional ileus due to gastritis, idiopathic, and pancreatitis causing regional inflammation.

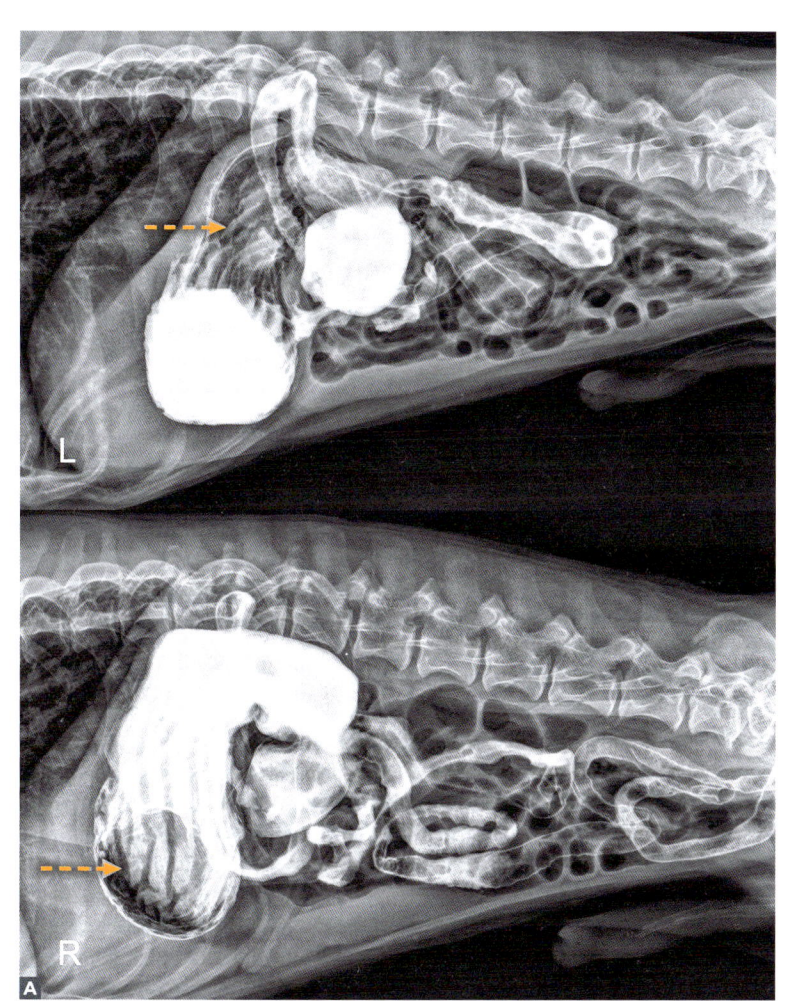

CHAPTER 25 Gastrointestinal contrast studies

Fig. 25.16 (**A**) A six-year-old male Basset Hound with intermittent chronic bloat and regurgitation. The barium sulfate upper gastrointestinal study showed malposition of the stomach. In the left lateral, the antrum should be filled with gas, but is now filled with gravity-dependent barium, indicating it is malpositioned on the left side of the dog. In the right lateral, there are rugal folds in the ventrally positioned part of the stomach indicating this is the fundus and body. The pyloric antrum should be located (dashed arrows) in the cranioventral abdomen. (**B**) In the ventrodorsal and dorsoventral images, the fundus (dashed arrow) and antrum (arrow) are both located on the left. Exploratory laparotomy confirmed gastric malpositioning which was corrected with gastropexy.

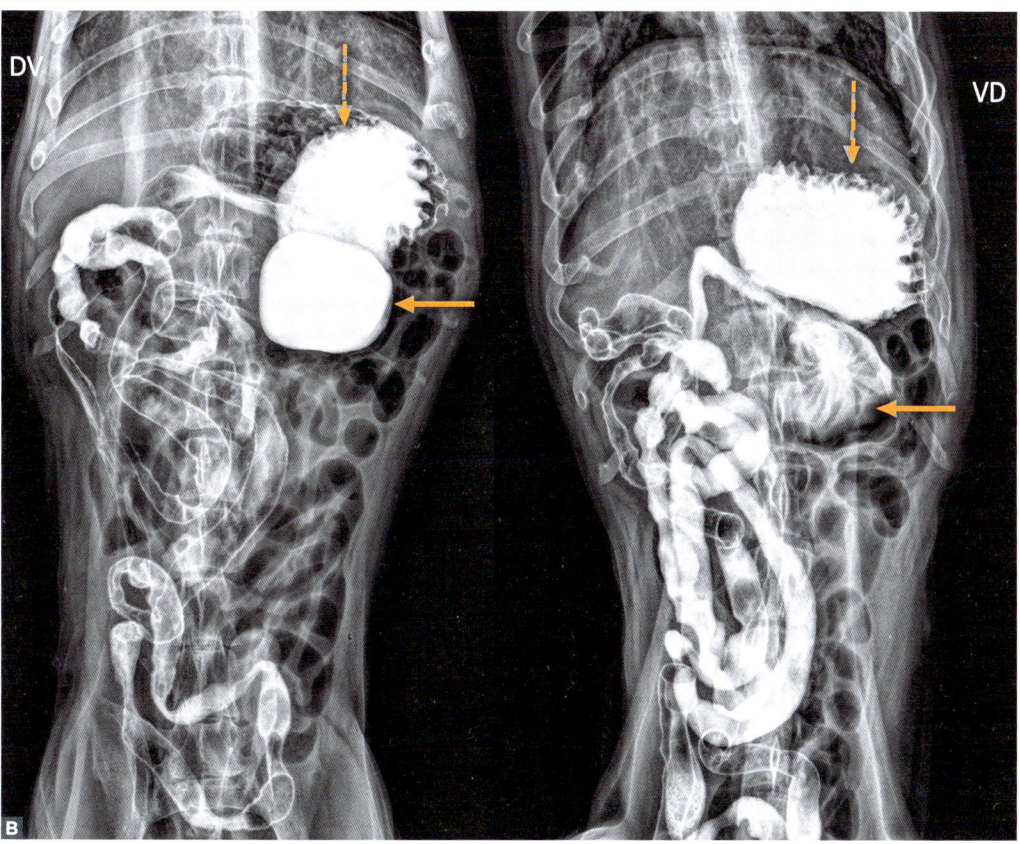

429

SECTION V ABDOMEN

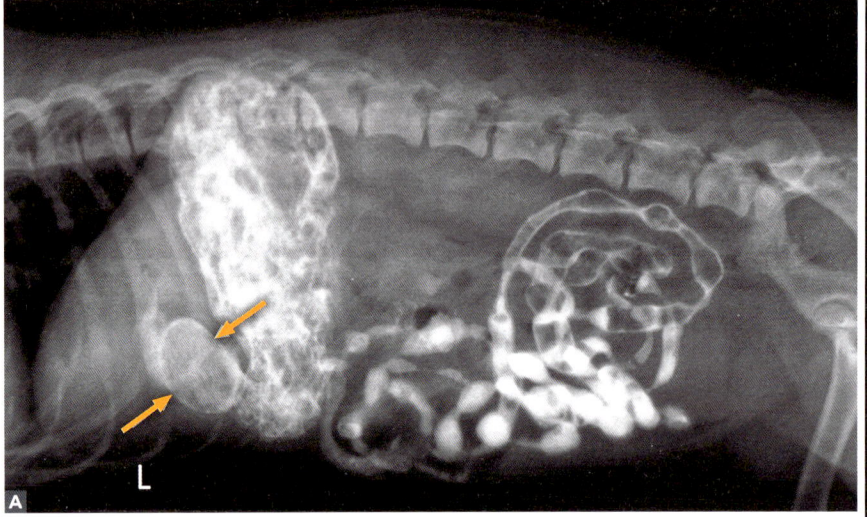

Fig. 25.17 A one-year-old spayed female Lhasa Apso after three days vomiting. The survey radiographs were equivocal. The barium upper gastrointestinal study showed an ovoid luminal filling defect with smooth contrast columns surrounding it (arrows) within the gastric antrum. The outflow obstruction was not complete and liquid barium could pass to the jejunum. Endoscopy was performed and a plastic toy was removed.

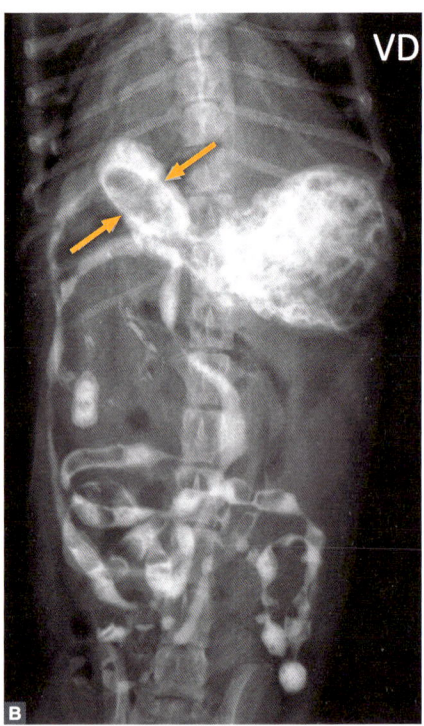

Fig. 25.18 A three-year-old Domestic shorthair neutered male cat with acute vomiting. A negative contrast gastrogram was performed and highlighted a large clump of striated soft tissue content that had a "wavy" pattern (arrows). The material in the stomach has relatively distinct margins highlighted by air which is not usually seen with food. Gastroscopy was performed and a wad of rubber hair bands was removed.

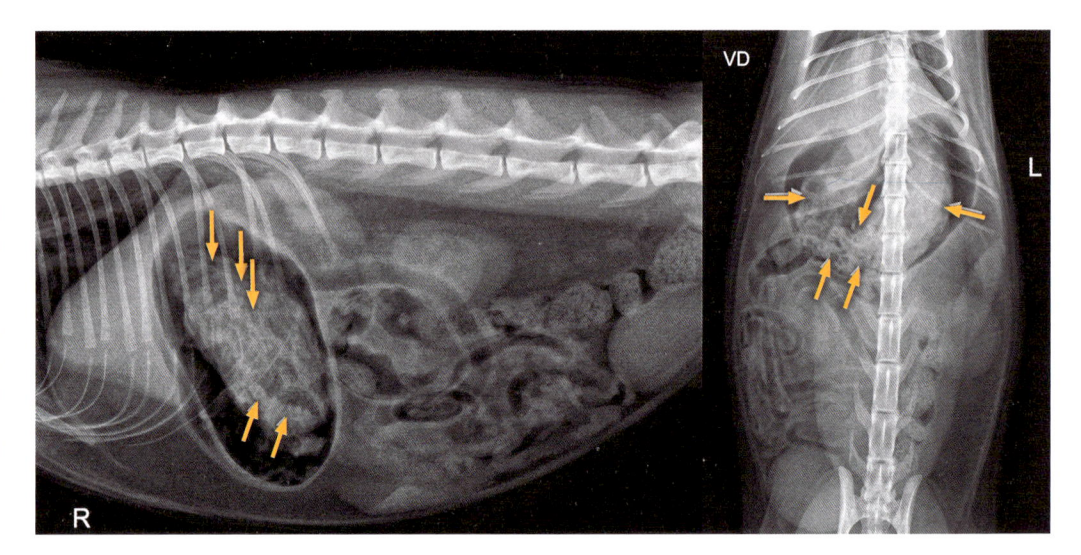

Negative contrast gastrography

Negative contrast gastrogram is performed in order to rule out the presence of a gastric mass or intraluminal structure (**fig. 25.18**). Patients should be fasted, and the stomach must be completely empty in order to perform this procedure and survey radiographs are used to ensure this. If large amounts of feces are present in the ascending or transverse colon, an enema should be given to empty the colon an hour or two prior to the procedure. Room air or 5 mL/kg body weight of carbonated non caffeinated beverages can be introduced via orogastric tube to distend the stomach. A minimum of right and left lateral and ventrodorsal radiographs and, if possible, a dorsoventral radiograph are performed immediately.[1]

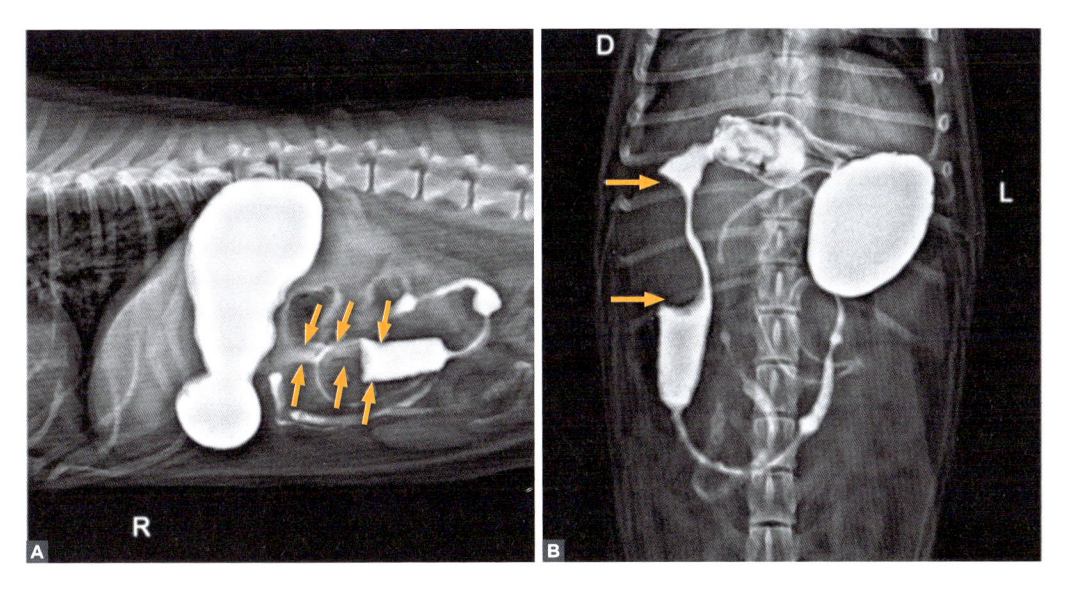

CHAPTER 25 Gastrointestinal contrast studies

Fig. 25.19 A nine-year-old neutered male Dachshund with subacute vomiting and weight loss for six days. The upper gastrointestinal barium study showed a duodenal obstruction (arrows). The narrowed portion of the descending duodenum has smoothly bordered contrast column borders and a "thumbprint" sign indicating that the compression is extramural. Exploratory surgery diagnosed a non-resectable pancreatic carcinoma mass causing compression of the duodenum.

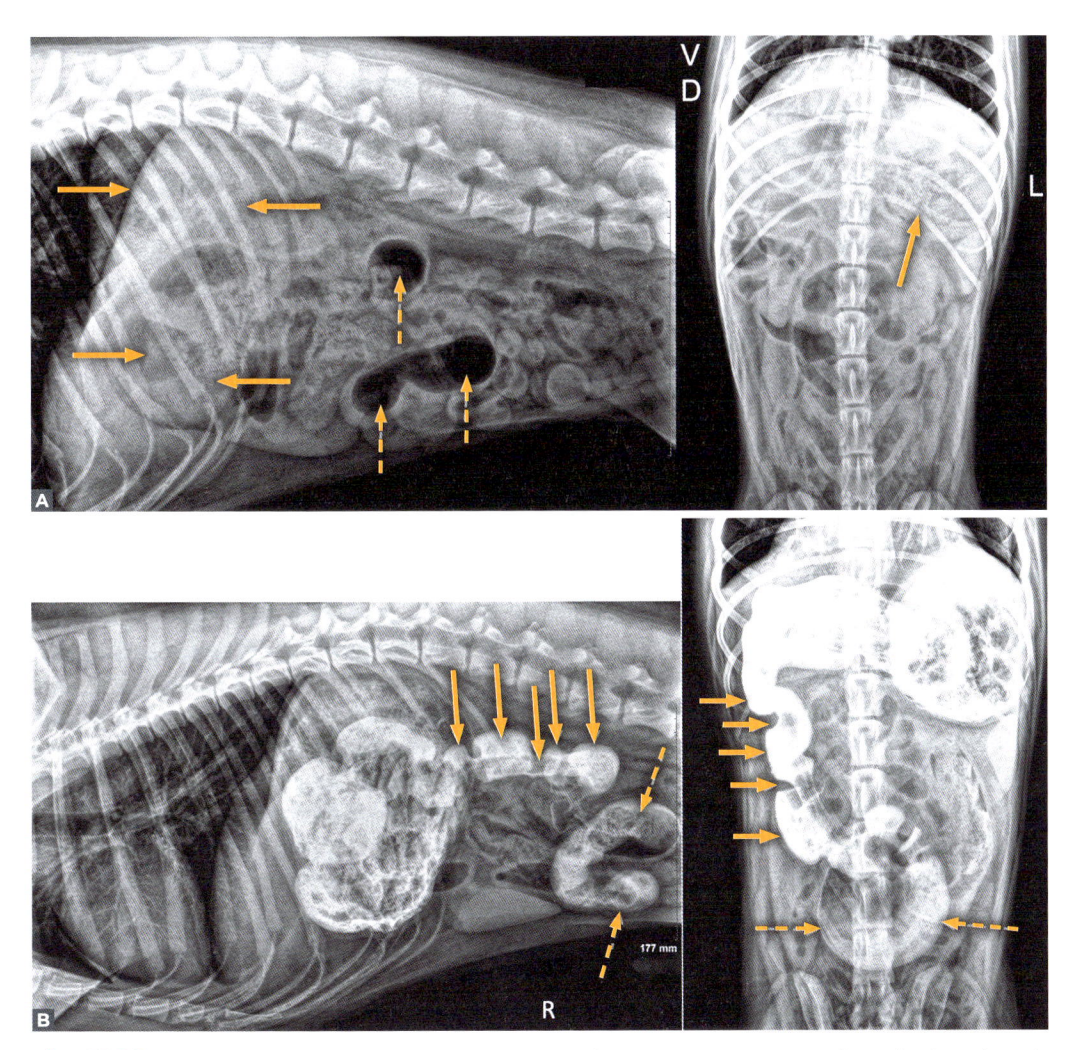

Fig. 25.20 (**A**) A 1.5-year-old neutered male Border Collie with acute vomiting. Survey radiographs showed gastric distention with heterogeneous mixed soft tissue and gas ingesta (arrows) and multiple severely gas dilated mid abdominal jejunal segments (dashed arrows). (**B**) The upper gastrointestinal barium study showed coating of gastric ingesta and plication of the duodenum (arrows). The proximal jejunal segments are partially filled with barium and are severely dilated, matching the same dilated segments in the survey image (dashed arrows). A linear foreign body was diagnosed with extension into the jejunum with mechanical ileus.

431

SECTION V ABDOMEN

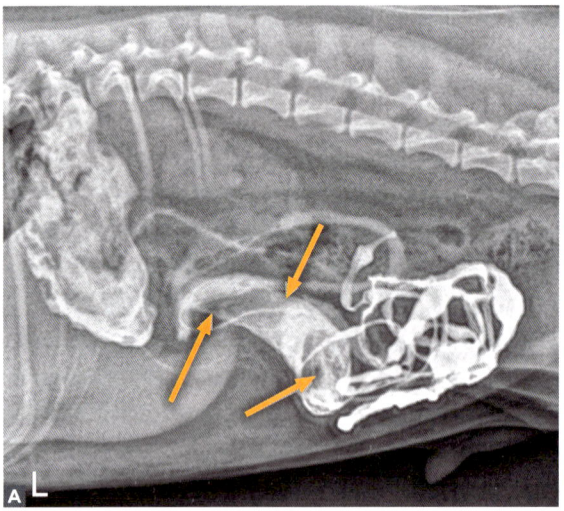

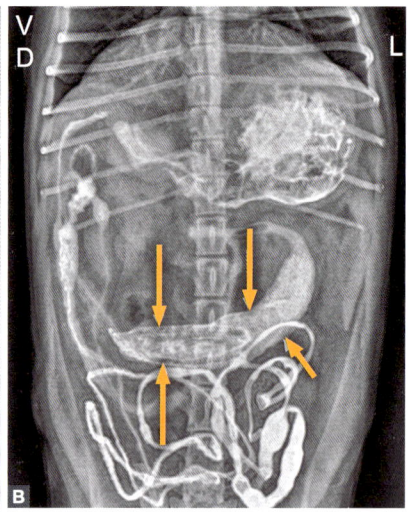

Fig. 25.21 A five-year-old neutered male small mixed breed dog with acute vomiting for two days. Radiographs obtained two hours after contrast administration showed residual contrast in the stomach and a segmental small intestinal dilation, which was localized to the distal duodenum/proximal jejunum (arrows). Within the dilated segment, contrast passes around a luminal structure that creates a filling defect. Liquid barium passes to the distal jejunal segments which are not dilated. A cloth foreign body was surgically removed from the proximal jejunum.

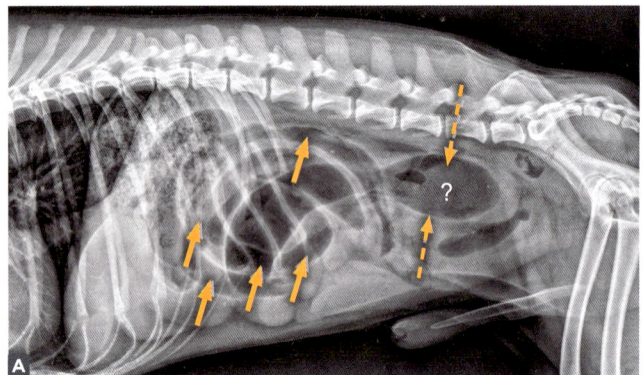

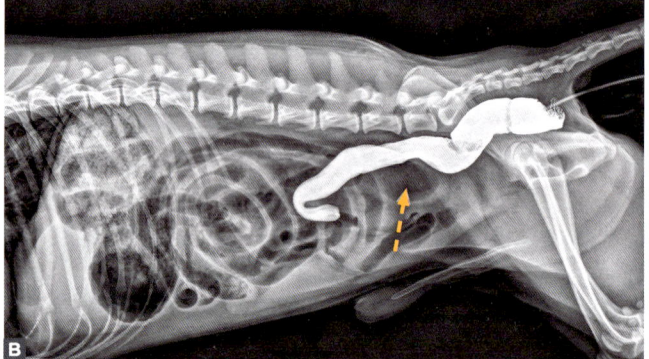

Fig. 25.22 An eight-year-old neutered male King Charles Spaniel after four days vomiting with a painful abdomen. Survey radiography showed multiple gas-dilated bowel segments which are localized to the jejunum (arrows). In the caudal abdomen, there is severe segmental gas dilation of a bowel segment that is difficult to localize to the jejunum vs. the colon (dashed arrows). A barium enema was performed and the barium-filled colon is dorsal to and separate from the severe gas dilated segment, now confirmed to have a jejunal origin and mechanical ileus of the jejunum was diagnosed. A foreign body was surgically removed.

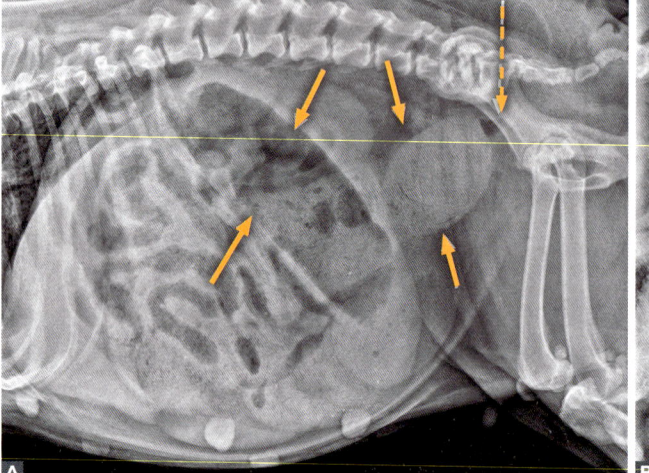

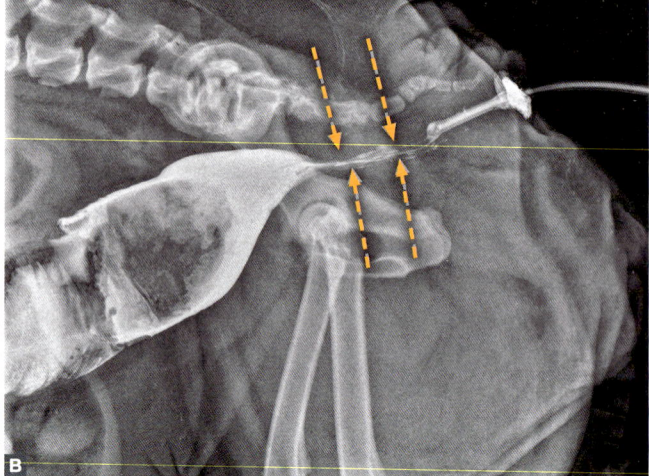

Fig. 25.23 A six-year-old female English Bulldog with vomiting and no defecation for four days. Survey radiographs showed severe colonic dilation with gas and feces (arrows). A barium enema was performed and there is focal narrowing of the colorectal segment with smooth uniform borders (dashed arrows). A stricture was diagnosed with colonoscopy.

Barium enema

Barium enemas are indicated for determining the cause of constipation, hematochezia, and painful defecation causing colonic distention such as stenosis and fungal and neoplastic wall infiltrative disease (**figs. 25.22** and **25.23**). Colonic torsion and volvulus can also be confirmed with a barium enema by identifying a site of narrowing of severely gas-dilated bowel. **Box 25.4** outlines the procedures for performing a barium enema.[1]

Pneumocolonogram

The pneumocolonogram is valuable for differentiating gas dilated jejunum from the colon or determining if feces-like material is in the colon or jejunum in dogs and cats with vomiting (**figs. 25.24** and **25.25**). Gas-filled large intestines and gas-dilated jejunal segments can be difficult

---

BOX 25.4 | BARIUM ENEMA AND PNEUMOCOLONOGRAM PROCEDURES

Barium enema
- Evaluate large bowel for location, volvulus, intussusception, and luminal, mural or extramural obstructions.

Prior to performing the study
- 24-hour food fast, water can be provided.
- Survey abdomen to confirm the colon is devoid of feces.
- Give enema and repeat if feces are present.
- Sedate or anesthetize.
- Place a lubricated Foley catheter in the rectum or descending colon and inflate bulb.
- Administer 20-25% weight/volume barium sulfate suspension.
- Start infusing the lower end of the dosages:
  - Dog: 11-30 mL/kg body weight.
  - Cat: 7-20 mL/kg body weight.
- Repeat right lateral to evaluate filling, repeat if required.
- Perform left lateral and VD once colon is filled.

Pneumocolonogram
- Discriminate between gas-filled large and small intestines and identify strictures or masses.

Prior to performing the study
- If the colon contains feces on survey radiographs, perform and enema and repeat.
- Place animal in right lateral recumbency.
- Sedation may be necessary to alleviate pain and discomfort.
- Place a lubricated rubber catheter in the rectum or descending colon.
- Administer room air using a large syringe.
- Repeat right lateral radiographs.
- Perform VD radiographs once the colon is filled with air.

Modified from Wallack ST. Static barium esophagram. In Wallack ST (editor). The handbook of veterinary contrast radiography, Solana Beach, 2003, Veterinary Imaging, pp 45-53.

to differentiate from one another due to superimposition. Feces-like content can accumulate in the distal jejunum or ileum with subacute and chronic obstruction and must be distinguished from normal feces in the colon. Pneumocolonography can also be used to diagnose a wall-associated colonic wall mass or stricture. Introducing gas into the colon when feces are present will confound interpretation of the pneumocolonogram. A cleansing enema and repeat radiographs should be performed before this procedure and may obviate the contrast study. **Box 25.3** outlines the technique for dogs and cats.[1]

Complications of contrast studies

Aspiration of barium sulfate suspensions can occur especially when administered orally by syringe. Small amounts in the airways are usually expectorated and normally does not lead to lung injury (**fig. 25.26**). Aspirations of large volumes may lead to serious complications. Aspiration of barium

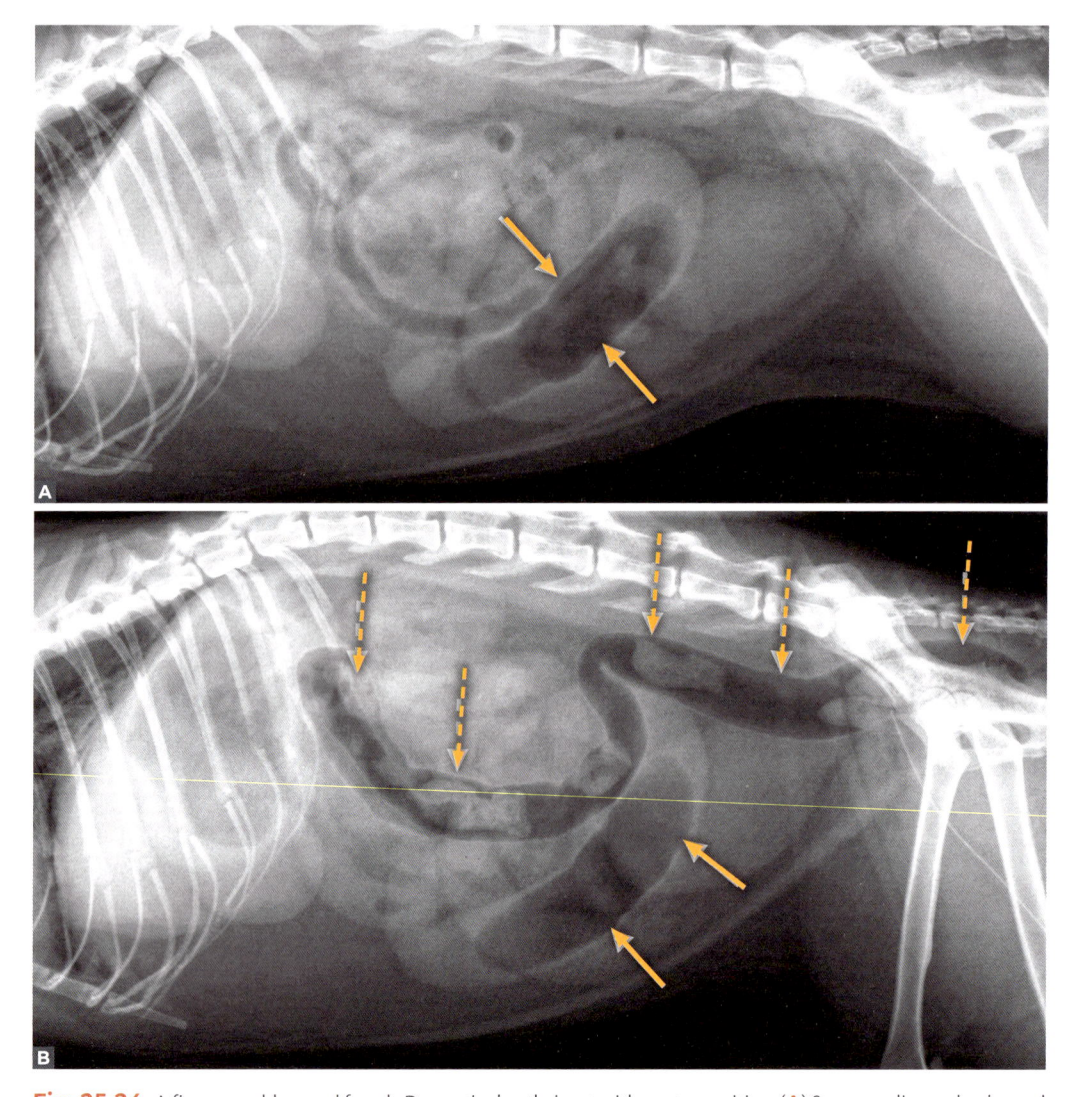

Fig. 25.24 A five-year-old spayed female Domestic shorthair cat with acute vomiting. (**A**) Survey radiographs showed a severe segmental gas and fluid dilation of a bowel segment (arrows). The colon could not be traced to determine if this segment represented a small or large bowel. (**B**) A pneumocolonogram (dashed arrows) was performed and showed that the dilated segment was the jejunum and not the colon. Mechanical ileus was diagnosed and a foreign body removed surgically.

Fig. 25.25 (**A**) Survey radiographs of a four-year-old neutered male Jack Russell Terrier with vomiting for three days showed an accumulation of coarse granular mineral opacity debris in the intestine, referred to as a gravel sign (arrows), in the right mid-abdomen and some punctate mineral content in some of the small intestinal segments. No additional intestinal dilation was present. It could not be determined with certainty if the mineral debris was located in the ascending colon or a jejunal segment. (**B**) A pneumocolonogram was performed and the gravel sign was not located in the colon (dashed arrows). The mineral material was not highlighted or surrounded by gas after the pneumocolonogram and was determined to be present in a jejunal segment, likely due to a partial obstructive foreign body or stenosis. A partially obstructing cloth foreign body was removed from the end jejunum.

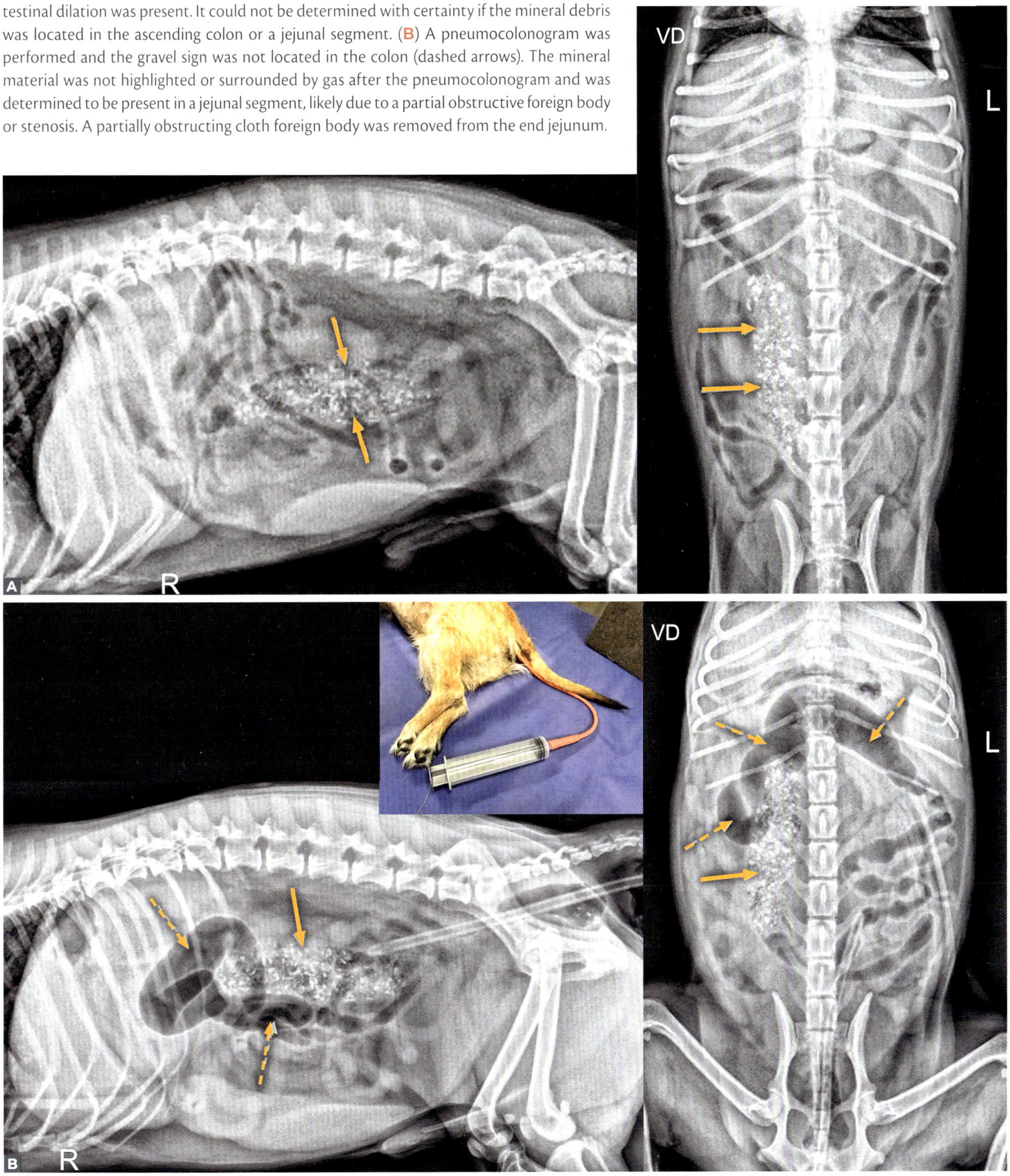

SECTION V ABDOMEN

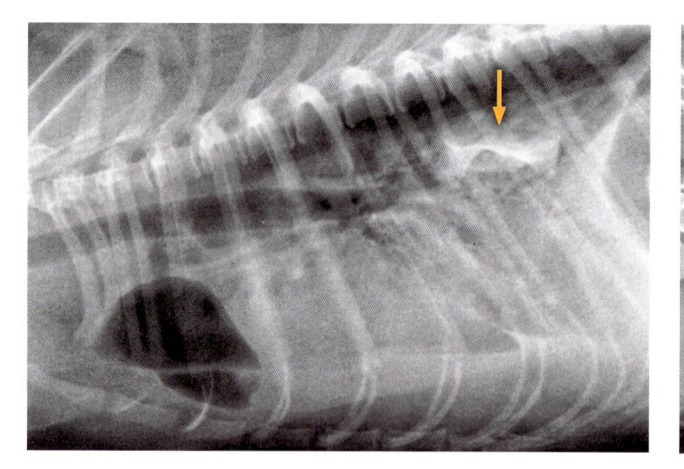

Fig. 25.26 Lateral radiograph of a dog with chronic regurgitation for one week that developed a fever and respiratory distress. Severe pleural effusion is present and a bone opaque foreign body is present in the caudal esophagus (arrow). This is an example of a strict contraindication for administering oral barium. The dog had a ruptured esophagus and resultant pleural effusion due to pyothorax.

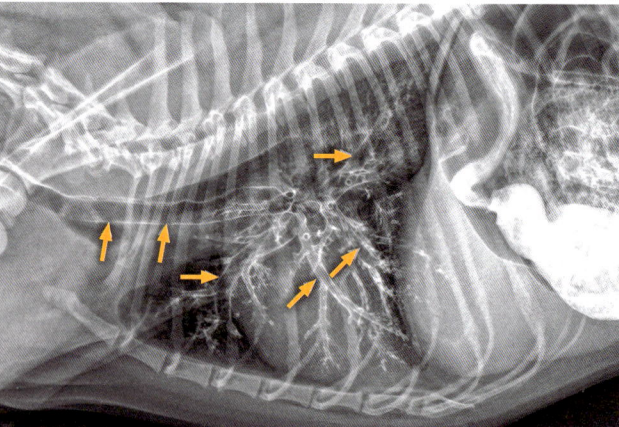

Fig. 25.27 The same dog as in fig. 25.9 with cricopharyngeal achalasia and tracheal aspiration of barium liquid. Barium coats the tracheal and bronchial mucosal surfaces. This is a potential complication of administering barium orally with a syringe in dogs with dysphagia. Small amounts of barium such as this do not usually lead to additional issues and repeat radiographs can be performed to monitor its clearance in the following days.

suspension with preexisting pneumonia may cause significant exacerbation. Barium leakage into the mediastinum, pleural space or peritoneal space secondary to esophageal or gastrointestinal perforation can lead to severe mediastinitis, pleuritis or peritonitis (**fig. 25.27**). Barium granulomas, fibrosis and adhesions can develop in the peritoneal cavity and mediastinum. Iodinated contrast agents have high osmolarity, and chemical toxicity and should be diluted for oral administration to minimize adverse reactions including hypovolemic shock with puppies and kittens and dehydrated patients at greater risk. Aspiration of hyperosmolar iodinated contrast medium can also lead to life-threatening pulmonary edema and for this reason ionic contrast agents should not be used. In addition, the hypertonicity of ionic agents causes water sequestration in the intestine and dilution frequently rendering a study nondiagnostic.[9,10]

References

1. Wallack ST (editor). The handbook of veterinary contrast radiography, Solana Beach, 2003, Veterinary Imaging.
2. Burk R, Ackerman, IN. The Abdomen 2nd edition. Philadelphia, 1996, WB Saunders.
3. Shannon D, Husnik R, Fletcher JM, Middleton G, Gaschen L. Persistent right aortic arch with an aberrant left subclavian artery, Kommerell's diverticulum and bicarotid trunk in a 3-year-old cat. *JFMS Open Rep* 1:2055116915614590, 2015.
4. Blank C, Ahuja R, McGovern D, Gaschen F, Gaschen L. Adult-onset regurgitation in two dogs with partial esophageal constriction caused by vascular ring anomaly. *J Small Anim Pract* 61:717, 2020.
5. Pollard RE: Imaging evaluation of dogs and cats with Dysphagia. *ISRN Vet Sci* 2012:238505, 2012.
6. Pollard RE. Videofluoroscopic evaluation of the pharynx and upper esophageal sphincter in the dog: a systematic review of the literature. *Front Vet Sci* 6:117, 2019.
7. Pollard RE, Marks SL, Cheney DM, Bonadio CM. Diagnostic outcome of contrast videofluoroscopic swallowing studies in 216 dysphagic dogs. *Vet Radiol Ultrasound* 58:373-80, 2017.
8. Haines JM, Khoo A, Brinkman E, Thomason JM, Mackin AJ. Technique for evaluation of gravity-assisted esophageal transit characteristics in dogs with megaesophagus. *J Am Anim Hosp Assoc* 55:167-77, 2019.
9. Kang J, Oh D, Choi J, Kim K, Yoon J, Choi M. Evaluation of a dual-purpose contrast medium for radiography and ultrasonography of the small intestine in dogs. *Am J Vet Res* 81:950-957, 2020.
10. Williams J, Biller DS, Myer CW, Miyabayashi T, Leveille R. Use of iohexol as a gastrointestinal contrast agent in three dogs, five cats, and one bird. *J Am Vet Med Assoc* 202:624-627, 1993.

CHAPTER 26

The stomach

Lorrie Gaschen

KEY POINTS

▮ Right lateral, left lateral and ventrodorsal radiographs of the abdomen in vomiting dogs are necessary to assess the stomach for obstructive foreign material in the gastric outflow tract.
▮ Repeat radiographs with fasting and fluid therapy are useful for monitoring the passage of gastric content to differentiate food from foreign material which appears similar radiographically.
▮ Gastric ultrasound is important for identifying infiltrative stomach disease, which is difficult to diagnose radiographically.
▮ Computed tomography can aid in diagnosing gastric wall ulceration which is more difficult with ultrasonography.
▮ Lesions at the porta hepatis can originate from the stomach, liver, lymph node, and pancreas and are difficult to differentiate without the use of computed tomography.

Acute or chronic vomiting are the most common indications for radiographic investigation of the stomach. Other potential indications are acute onset of severe abdominal distention and large and giant breed dogs and evaluation of cranial abdominal mass lesions, particularly in cats.

In dogs, a three-view radiographic study of the abdomen is the current standard for assessing the stomach and, in particular, the gastric outflow tract which includes the antrum, pylorus, and duodenum (**figs. 26.1-26.4**).[1] This has not been shown to be necessary for cats unless the stomach is very dilated.[2]

Normal anatomy and appearance

In a normal adult dog, the gastric fundus and body are located in the left cranial abdomen, and the junction of the gastric body and the pyloric antrum is approximately on the midline or slightly to the right of the midline. The pyloric antrum is located in the right cranial abdomen. On lateral projections, the stomach appears as an elongated ovoid or bilobed structure, immediately caudal to the liver and oriented in a dorsal to ventral direction. On ventrodorsal projections, the stomach lies transversely across the abdomen. The appearance of the normal feline stomach on a lateral projection is similar to that of the canine patient. On the ventrodorsal projection, the normal feline stomach has a "J" shape on the ventrodorsal projection, with the gastric body oriented in a slightly caudal direction and the pyloroduodenal junction on or slightly to the right of the midline.

In canine patients who have been completely fasted, the stomach usually contains a small to moderate volume of air and a small volume of fluid from normal secretions. The volume of luminal air is variable and may be increased in dogs and cats that are dyspneic or tachypneic, or stressed. The

SECTION V ABDOMEN

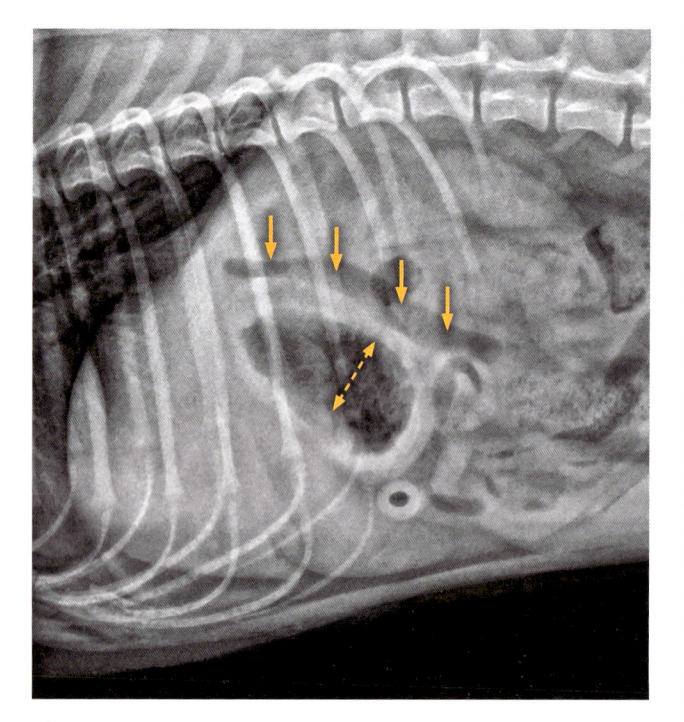

Fig. 26.1 Normal left lateral radiograph of the dog's stomach. In left lateral recumbency, the antrum, pylorus, and duodenum, which are right-sided anatomic structures, are non-dependent and gas distributes into those regions. Any fixed soft tissue opaque foreign material could potentially be highlighted by gas surrounding it in the gastric outflow tract, making the identification of an obstruction more likely. *Orange arrows:* duodenum filled with gas; *double-headed arrow:* antrum filled with gas.

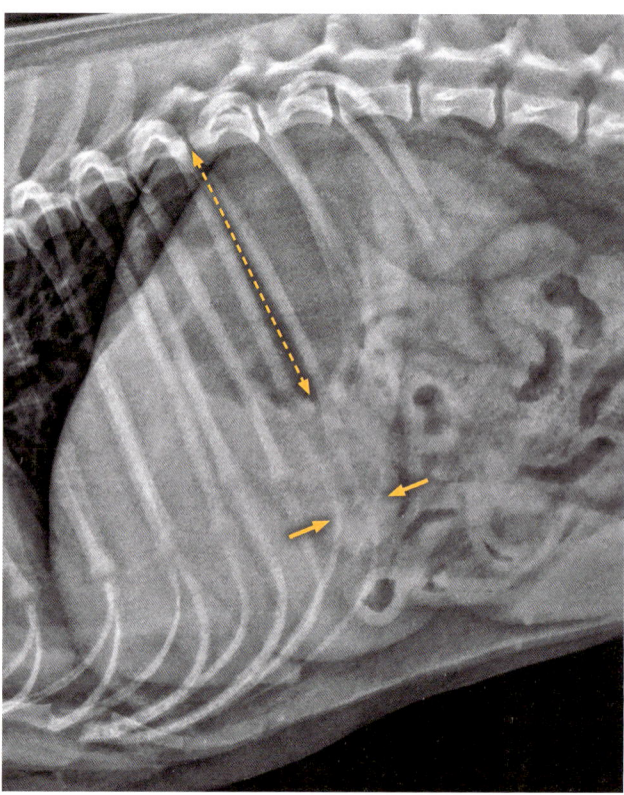

Fig. 26.2 Normal right lateral radiograph of the dog's stomach. In right lateral recumbency, the antrum, pylorus, and duodenum, which are ventral right-sided structures, are dependent and not filled with gas. The antrum in this dog is soft tissue opaque (arrows). Gas fills the nondependent fundus and body (double-headed arrow).

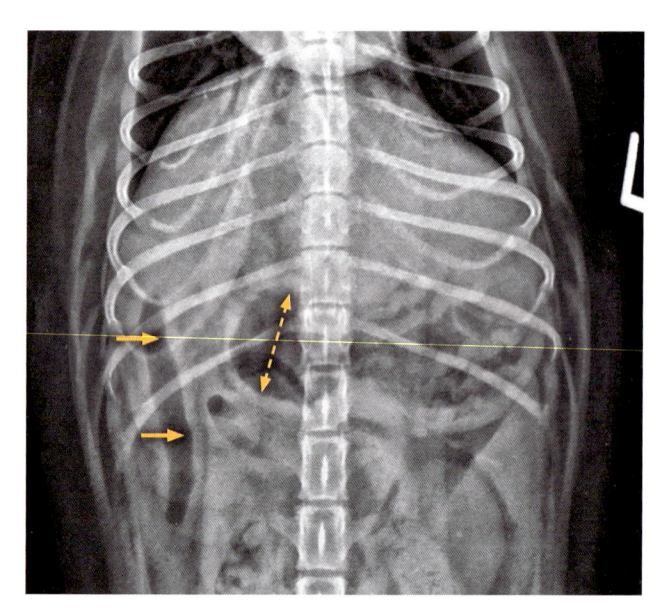

Fig. 26.3 Ventrodorsal radiographic images of the dog's stomach. The antrum (double-headed arrow) and gastric body are filled with gas in the ventrodorsal position. Normal rugal folds are present in the gastric body. The duodenum (arrows) is also filled with gas.

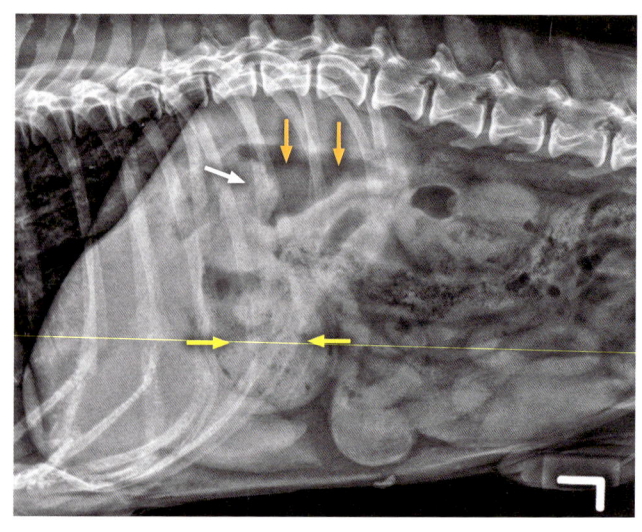

Fig. 26.4 Left lateral radiograph of the cranial abdomen in a neutered male Dachshund that presented after 4 days of vomiting and lethargy. Left lateral abdominal radiograph. Gas redistributes to the right-sided duodenum (orange arrows) and highlights a soft tissue foreign body (white arrow) at the pyloroduodenal junction. The antrum (yellow arrows) is also filled with similar soft tissue content. Fabric was surgically removed from the stomach.

rate of gastric emptying in normal dogs is extremely variable, depending upon the type and volume of food ingested. This can also be slowed by extraneous factors such as stress or pain. The presence of residual food material in the stomach 12 to 16 hours after ingestion of a large meal is not unusual in dogs. Gastric emptying in cats is somewhat quicker.

The normal radiographic appearance of the stomach varies depending upon the patient's positioning and the luminal content. When the patient is in right recumbency, gas in the stomach will rise to the upper part of the stomach, the fundus, and the body. Any fluid in the stomach will migrate toward the dependent part of the gastric lumen, in this case, the pyloric antrum. The fluid-filled pyloric antrum frequently appears as an almost circular discrete uniform soft tissue opacity structure in the cranial ventral abdomen on right lateral projections and normal dogs and should not be mistaken for a gastric foreign body. On a left lateral projection, gas will rise to the uppermost part of the stomach, the pyloric antrum. The gastric fundus and body may be filled with gas, fluid, or a combination of both. On a ventrodorsal projection, fluid will tend to fill both the gastric fundus. Gas will fill the distal part of the gastric body and pyloric antrum. On a dorsoventral projection, gas will fill the gastric fundus. The pyloric antrum is usually fluid-filled unless a relatively large volume of gas is present in the stomach.

The significance of radiopaque material in the stomach must be correlated to the timing of the last meal or suspected ingestion of foreign material. Repeat radiographs in vomiting dogs and cats with a distended stomach containing heterogeneous soft tissue opaque ingesta are often necessary after 12-24 hours (or less if the animal's clinical status deteriorates) to monitor the passage of the content (**fig. 26.5**).[3] Food and foreign content can appear very similar radiographically, and repeat radiographs after confirmed fasting and fluid therapy provide an important diagnostic method to differentiate them. The stomach should empty, at least in part, either from continued vomiting or normal peristalsis. The persistence of content without changes increases suspicion of foreign material, but additional testing is needed for confirmation. In cats, the stomach wall has alternating bands of soft tissue and fat that can appear as a "wagon wheel" radiographically due to fat in the submucosal layer, which is a feature particular to cats (**fig. 26.6**).

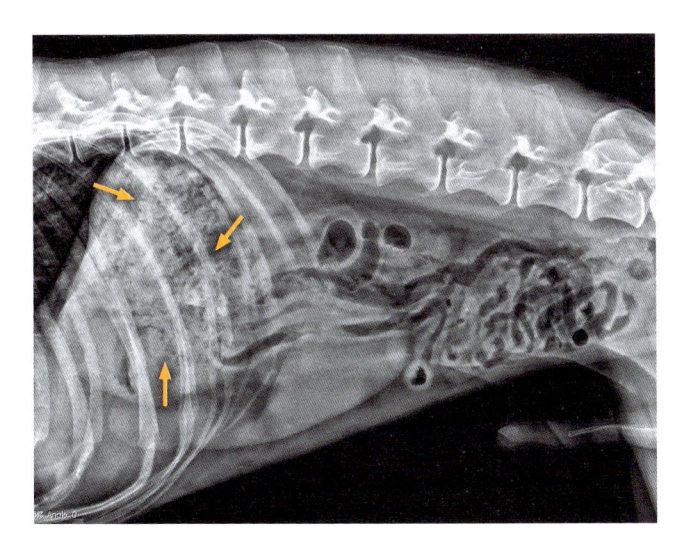

Fig. 26.5 Right lateral abdominal radiograph performed after a 24-hour fast and fluid therapy in a dog with acute vomiting. There is a large volume of heterogeneous soft tissue content filling the stomach (arrows). The jejunal segments are normal in size and contain a normal small volume of gas. The colon is almost empty and practically devoid of feces. Tampons were removed from the stomach with gastroscopy. This finding underscores the principle that food and foreign content, especially fabric, appear similar radiographically. Fasting with repeat radiographs is a good method of differentiating food from foreign material.

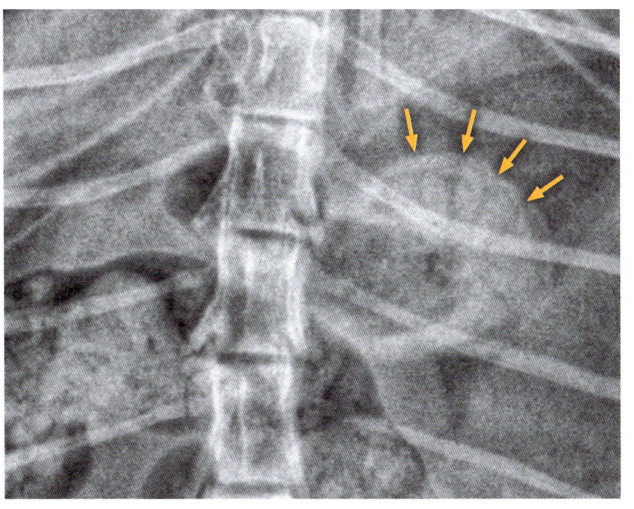

Fig. 26.6 Ventrodorsal image of the normal cat stomach. An empty stomach with a wagon wheel-like appearance due to the alternating soft tissue opaque rugal folds with the fat of the submucosa between them (arrows).

Ultrasonography is routinely employed as a complementary imaging modality to survey radiographs for evaluation of the stomach. Ultrasound can be used to assess the gastric wall for abnormalities such as alteration or effacement of the layering and thickening. Ultrasound also provides some information about the gastric content, but imaging is often significantly limited by the presence of luminal gas and resulting artifacts. The normal gastric wall should have five alternating hyperechoic and hypoechoic layers as in the small intestine. The luminal border of the mucosa appears as a bright echogenic line. The mucosal layer is hypoechoic, which overlies the more echogenic submucosal layer. The muscularis layer is hypoechoic, while the serosal margin appears as a thin hyperechoic line. The gastric body and pyloric antrum have numerous rugal folds. Measuring the gastric wall to confirm or exclude thickening should only be performed when the stomach is at least moderately distended. Peristaltic waves are usually observed in real-time in normal patients, averaging approximately 4-5 per minute.

Ultrasonography should be performed prior to endoscopy or barium studies if possible. For the ultrasonographic evaluation of the stomach, high-frequency curved array transducers are recommended. Linear transducers can be used in smaller dogs or cats but are less useful for imaging medium or larger dogs due to their large contact area, limited field of view, and subcostal location of the stomach to use to assess the stomach in larger animals. A 7.5 MHz transducer is adequate for large dogs, whereas frequencies >7.5 MHz are best for smaller dogs and cats. The ultrasound examination of the stomach should include an assessment of the peritoneum, mesentery, and regional lymph nodes. Even under ideal conditions, it is usually not possible to examine the entire stomach during abdominal ultrasound.

Ultrasonographic evaluation of the stomach should include an assessment of wall thickness, layering, and symmetry, localization and distribution of thickening, motility, and luminal content.

Contrast-enhanced computed tomography of the stomach is an excellent modality to examine the stomach and regional structures. CT allows assessment of wall layering and thickness, mechanical outflow obstructions, luminal foreign bodies, acute hemorrhage such as associated with mucosal ulcers, gastric wall perforation, and infiltrative disease such as neoplasia.

Gastric foreign bodies and foreign material

A gastric foreign body or foreign material is a common etiology of acute onset vomiting, particularly in canine patients. Some gastric foreign objects such as stones, rocks, or metallic objects are straightforward to identify on radiographs. In some patients, gastric foreign objects may pass through the small intestine and be eliminated through the colon, but unfortunately, it is not possible to reliably predict the size of foreign objects likely to cause small intestinal obstruction. Soft tissue opacity foreign objects in the gastric lumen are often significantly more difficult to diagnose, as these may be obscured by luminal fluid. Obtaining three views of the abdomen increases the likelihood that the foreign object will be outlined by luminal air, particularly if the foreign object is fixed in the pyloric antrum.

A limited gastric contrast study can be used when there is significant suspicion of ingestion of a soft tissue opacity foreign object, but this is not identified on survey radiographs. A small volume of diluted barium suspension is administered (approximately 5 to 25 mL of 30% weight/volume, depending upon the patient's size). Left lateral, right lateral and ventrodorsal, and dorsoventral radiographs of the abdomen are obtained. The small volume of contrast may outline a discrete foreign object such as a plastic or rubber ball (**fig. 26.7**). If these radiographs do not yield a diagnosis, additional barium can be administered to perform a complete upper gastrointestinal contrast study.

The presence of heterogeneous soft tissue material in the gastric lumen is a frequent finding in canine patients presented with acute onset vomiting. The radiographic appearance of such content is

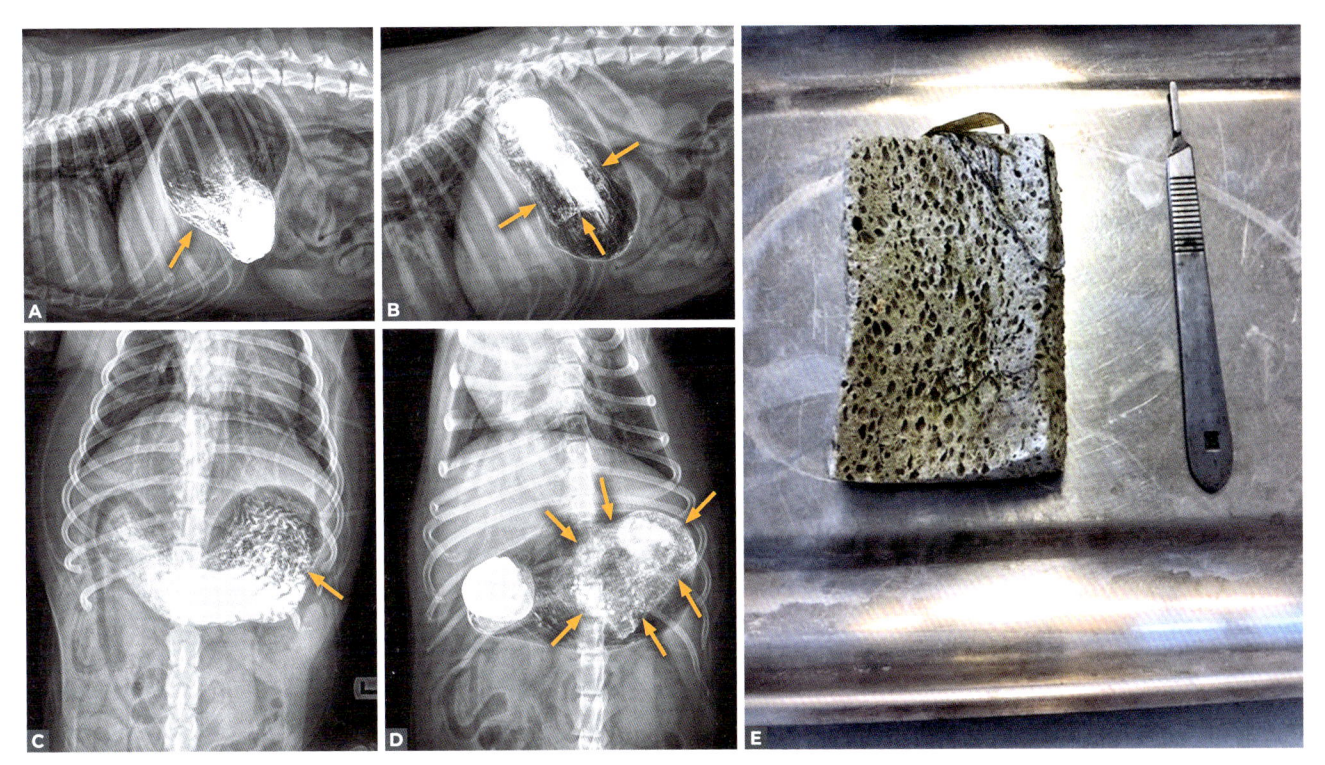

Fig. 26.7 Small volume contrast study in a dog with a gastric foreign body. The study shows a foreign body impregnated with barium resembling a sponge in the left lateral and ventrodorsal views (**B, D**). In the right lateral and dorsoventral views, the foreign body is not or barely visible due to the superimposition of the rugal folds.

nonspecific and residual food or foreign material such as fabric or clothing, plastic, trichobezoars, or phytobezoars can all appear relatively similar on radiographs. Fabric or clothing foreign material and phytobezoars may have a striated appearance from gas pockets entrapped within the structure of the material. The presence of radiopaque material in the stomach must be correlated to the timing of the last meal or clinical suspicion of ingestion of foreign material. Repeat radiographs after confirmed fasting and fluid therapy provide an important diagnostic method to differentiate between food and foreign material. Repeat radiographs should be obtained after fasting for 12-24 hours (or less if the animal's clinical status deteriorates) to monitor the passage of the content (**fig. 26.5**).[3] The stomach should empty, at least in part, from peristalsis, although this may be slower than expected in stressed patients. Persistence of content without change increases suspicion of foreign material, but endoscopy, a contrast upper gastrointestinal study, or laparotomy may be needed for confirmation.

Gastric dilation disorders

Gastric distension may be caused by excess quantities of gas, food, and/or fluid in the stomach and is one of the most common findings in vomiting dogs and cats on survey radiographs. Causes include gastric bloat, atony, gastritis, gastric dilation volvulus, mechanical outflow obstruction, and infiltrative disease of the gastric wall such as neoplasia.

Gastric bloat and atony

When the stomach is dilated and food-filled but positioned normally, "food bloat" is one of the most likely diagnoses (**fig. 26.8**). Delayed gastric emptying and gastritis are occasional causes of this finding (**figs. 26.9-26.11**). Repeat radiographs can be used in these instances to monitor the passage of the ingesta after medical management since food, and foreign material can appear similar radiographically.

SECTION V ABDOMEN

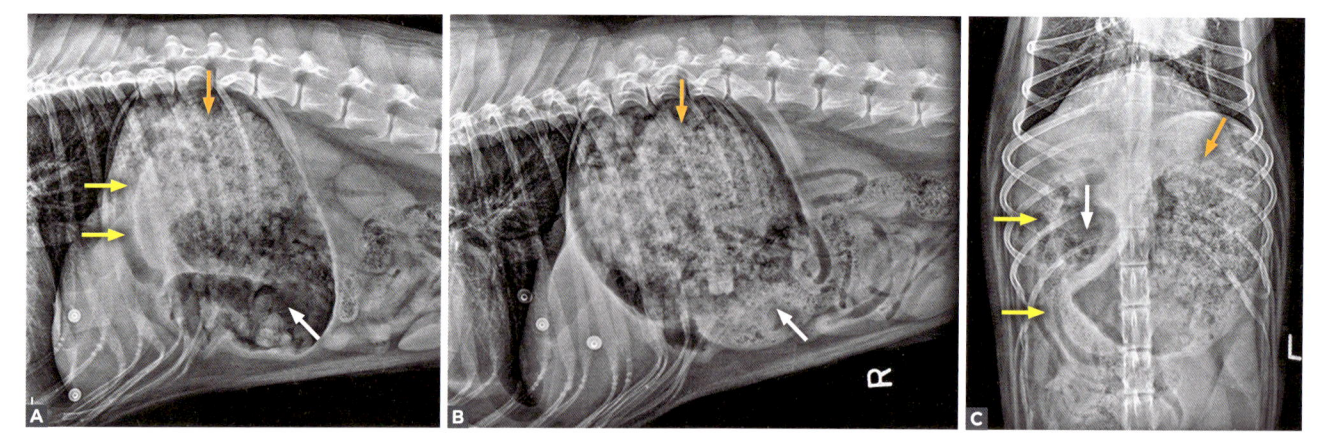

Fig. 26.8 Left and right lateral and ventrodorsal radiographs of the cranial abdomen of a Great Dane mixed breed dog that presented with acute vomiting. The stomach has a normal position with the fundus (orange arrow) and antrum (white arrow) in their normal positions. The stomach is markedly distended with a heterogeneous soft tissue and gas mixed ingesta that has a granular appearance. The duodenum is visible in the left lateral and ventrodorsal views and contains gas (yellow arrows). The granular appearing content could represent food, foreign material, or a combination of food mixed with foreign material, and these cannot be differentiated radiographically. The content in this dog was food, and the diagnosis was food bloat.

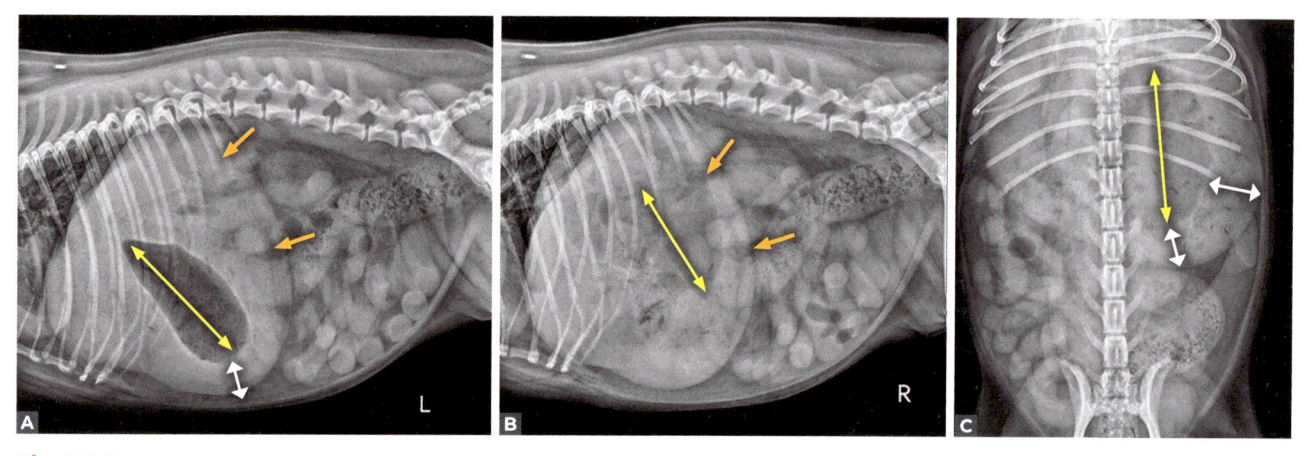

Fig. 26.9 Right and left lateral and ventrodorsal radiographs of the abdomen of a Pug dog that presented with retching, vomiting, and a distended abdomen. The stomach is markedly dilated due to a large amount of fluid and gas content. This presence of fluid (orange arrows) with a superimposed large gas bubble (yellow arrows) is often mistaken for a thickened gastric wall (white arrows). The margin of the gas bubble is only showing the border with fluid in the stomach, not the gastric mucosa, so a determination of wall thickness cannot be made and requires ultrasound. In the right lateral and the ventrodorsal images, the gas bubble has heterogeneous opacity, which is due to the superimposition of fluid and the gas bubble. This opacity is diagnostic for the presence of fluid and gas in the stomach. Differentials for the fluid and gas distended stomach include functional ileus (gastritis and pancreatitis), a gastric outflow obstruction (pyloric stenosis, foreign body), and gastric wall infiltration with neoplasia (less common).

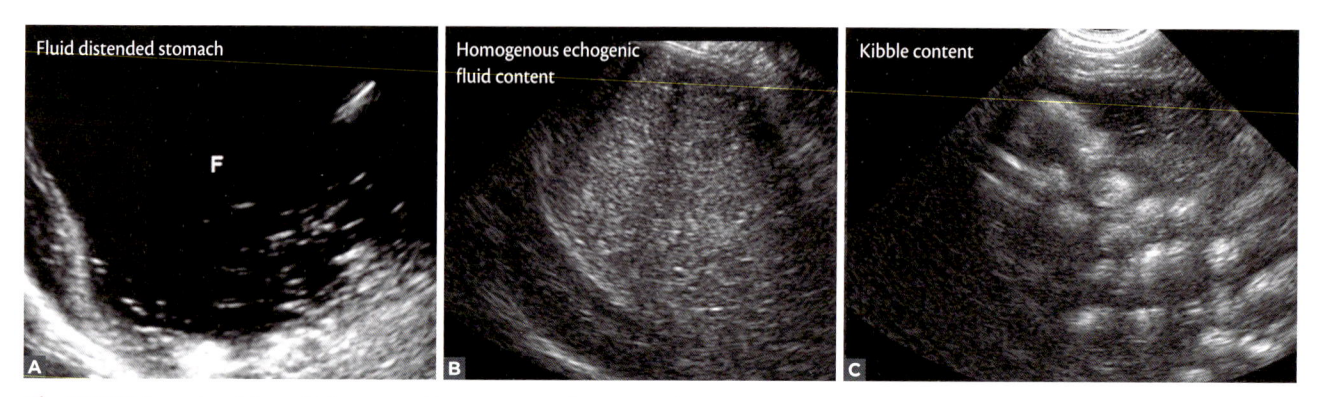

Fig. 26.10 Examples of the variable sonographic appearance of content in the stomach. Ultrasound images of the stomach of three different dogs. All three dogs have a dilated stomach. (A) The stomach is fluid distended. Hyperechoic stipples within the fluid are due to small gas bubbles. (B) Distention of the stomach filled with a homogenous echogenic fluid ingesta that represented soft food mixed with fluid. (C) Multiple round hyperechoic nodular structures surrounded by fluid in the distended stomach due to recent ingestion of kibble.

Fig. 26.11 Ultrasound image of the stomach of a dog that had recently eaten a meal consisting of soft chunks of food. Compared to kibble in fig. 26.10, soft food such as meat and potatoes have a hypoechoic appearance (arrows) and are often partly outlined by gas (labeled gas in the stomach) surrounding them in the lumen of the stomach.

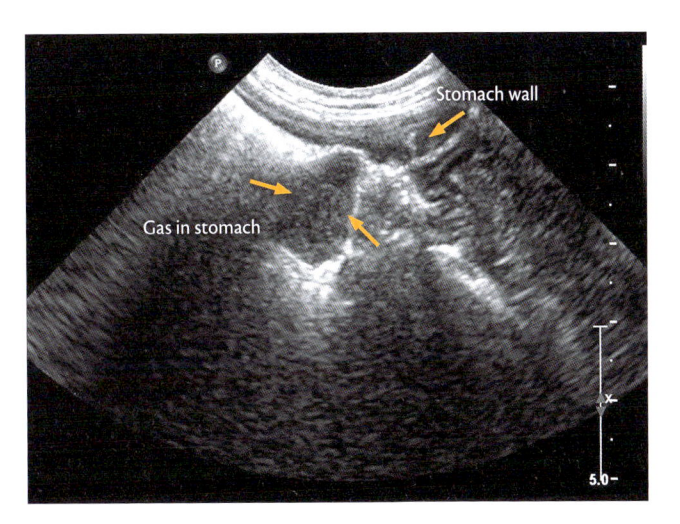

Fig. 26.12 An eight-year-old spayed female small mixed breed dog presented with chronic vomiting and weight loss. (**A**) A left lateral radiograph and (**B**) transverse ultrasound image of the gastric antrum are shown. The left lateral radiograph shows the stomach wall to have a thickened, undulant shape (arrows), but this could be an artifact from adherent content. In the corresponding transverse ultrasound image of the antrum, the thickened, undulant shape of the stomach wall is confirmed. In the ultrasound image, the thickened wall has a transmural hypoechoic loss of wall layering. Gastric biopsy diagnosed a lymphoma.

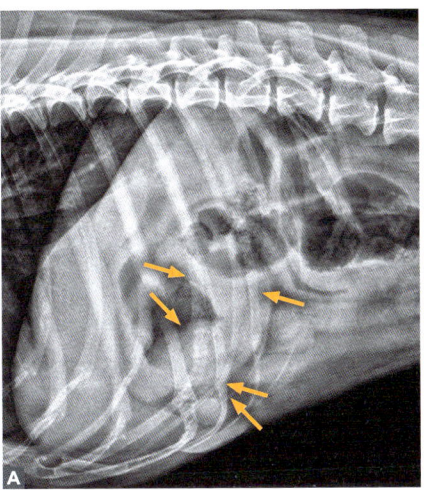

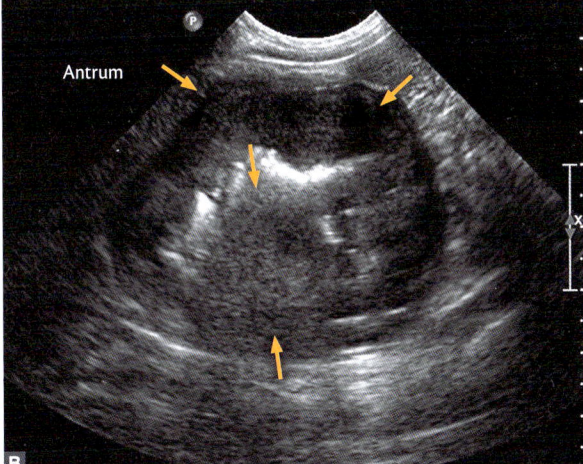

Gastritis and ulcers

Gastritis and ulceration can lead to thickening of the gastric wall. Gastric wall thickness cannot be accurately assessed on survey radiographs, and thickening of the stomach wall is commonly over-interpreted. Silhouetting of luminal fluid with the stomach wall adjacent to a gas bubble in the lumen can give the false appearance of wall thickening (**fig. 26.9**). Confirmation of wall thickening requires either an upper gastrointestinal contrast study (chapter 25), ultrasonography, or contrast-enhanced computed tomography for diagnosis (**fig. 26.12**).

Ultrasonographically, thickening of the stomach wall can be characterized as focal or diffuse, concentric, or asymmetric (**fig. 26.13**). Focal thickening with disrupted wall layering may be caused by neoplasia with or without ulceration, granulomas, and benign ulcers. Generalized thickening is more commonly seen with inflammatory disease but can also occur with diffuse neoplastic infiltration. Thickening of the gastric wall is considered to be present when the wall thickness is greater than 5 mm in dogs or 3 mm in cats. Gastric wall measurements should not be obtained when the stomach is empty and collapsed, as folding of the gastric wall renders it difficult to identify the wall layers, and thickness is usually grossly overestimated. When measuring the thickness of the gastric wall, the wall should be measured between rugal folds to avoid overestimating wall thickness.

Gastric wall edema can occur in dogs with vomiting secondary to pancreatitis and in dogs with hypoalbuminemia.[4,5] Edema of the gastric wall can lead to wall thickening >5mm. Ultrasonographic features of gastric wall edema include some or all of the following: a thickened wall, complete loss of wall layering, thickening of the submucosa, and muscularis thickening.[4] In dogs with hypoalbumine-

SECTION V ABDOMEN

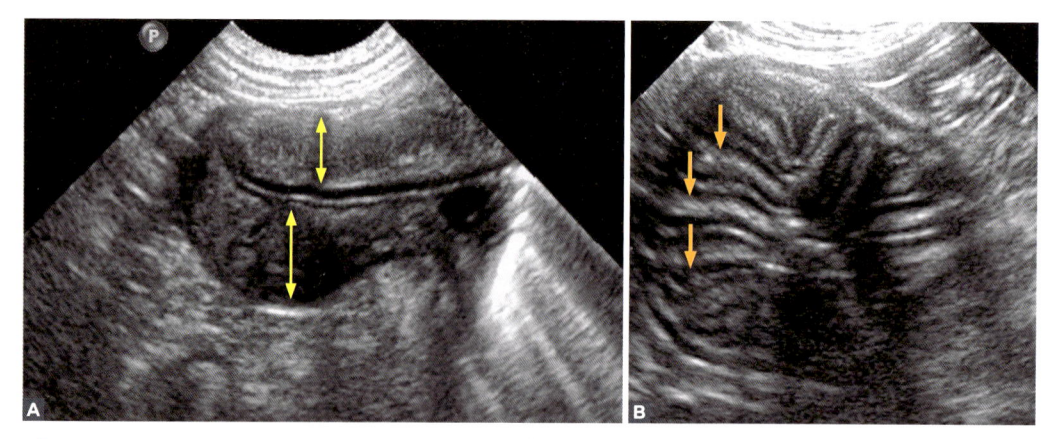

Fig. 26.13 A six-year-old neutered male Bassett Hound presented with acute vomiting and hematemesis. (**A**) Ultrasound examination of the gastric fundus showed a diffusely thickened submucosal layer of the wall with preserved mucosal layering (yellow arrows). (**B**) Three days later, following medical management, the gastric wall thickness and layering of the fundus resolved to normal with normal radiating rugal folds (orange arrows). The diagnosis was non-specific gastritis and gastric wall edema. The thickened gastric wall in a vomiting dog can appear like infiltrative infectious or neoplastic causes, and repeat sonography of the stomach following medical management and when vomiting is resolved is worthwhile to determine if the findings are static or not.

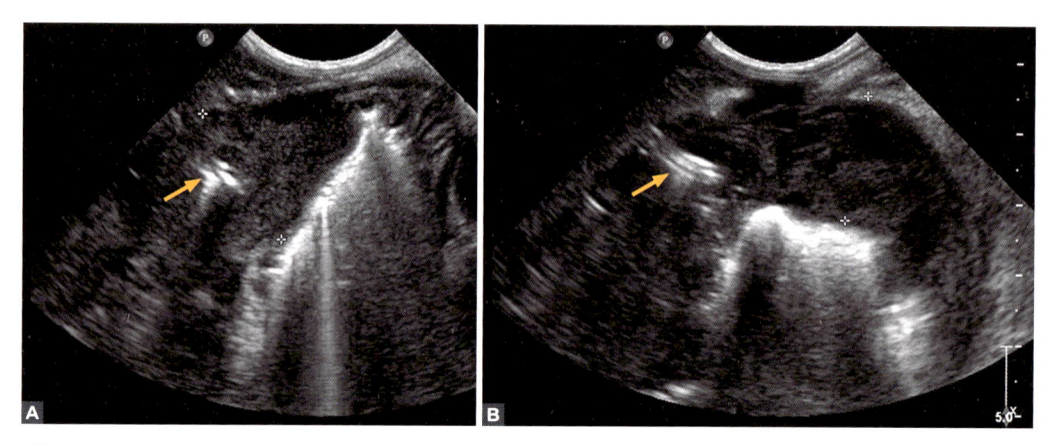

Fig. 26.14 Ultrasound images of the stomach in a six-year-old neutered male medium mixed breed dog that presented with chronic vomiting and melena. The dog had been receiving non-steroidal anti-inflammatory drugs for orthopedic pain. The gastric antral wall shows focal severe thickening (calipers) up to 2.12 cm. The thickened regions have transmural hypoechoic loss of wall layering. Within the thickened regions, there are multiple hyperechoic stipples with reverberation artifacts (arrows) that represent necrosis and gas filling an ulcer crater. The dog was diagnosed with benign ulcers.

mia, 21.4% showed gastric wall thickening with a mean of 10.0 mm ± 2.0 mm, preserved mucosal layering, thickening of the submucosa, and alterations in the regular wall layering.[5] Gastric wall thickening in dogs with vomiting, pancreatitis, or hypoalbuminemia should be monitored for sonographic resolution of wall thickening once clinical signs have ceased in order to rule out neoplastic infiltration. Gastric ulcers lead to disruption of the mucosa and cannot be diagnosed using survey radiography. Diagnosis requires a barium contrast study, ultrasound, contrast-enhanced computed tomography, or endoscopy. Endoscopy is the preferred method for diagnosis of small mucosal ulcerations, which are difficult or impossible to detect with all other modalities due to their small size and lack of secondary wall thickening. Wall thickening in combination with a surface defect or crater is necessary to detect ulcerations using most imaging modalities. Ultrasonographically, benign ulcers appear as a localized wall thickening (**fig. 26.14**).[6] Mucosal craters with an irregular surface and the adherence of gas bubbles may also be seen. The presence of luminal gas and food creates artifacts that make the ultrasonographic detection of gastric ulcers difficult. Benign ulcers lead to focal gastric wall thickening and loss of wall layering that may appear similar to malignant ulcers. CT is the best

CHAPTER **26** The stomach

imaging modality for the assessment of the gastric wall as neither superimposition nor luminal gas interfere with imaging. Distension of the stomach with water or gas reduces artifacts from folding of the gastric wall and allows assessment of all of the gastric wall. At the same time, assessment of the lymph nodes and liver for local and regional metastasis.

The presence of focal wall thickening and loss of layering requires tissue sampling to differentiate benign from malignant gastric wall infiltrative disease.

Gastric dilation and volvulus

Severe dilation together with displacement of the stomach is a sign of gastric volvulus, most often diagnosed and large and giant breeds dogs and rarely in smaller dogs. The stomach rotates approximately 180 degrees around the long axis of the abdomen, resulting in the location of the pyloric antrum and the left cranial dorsal abdomen and the location of the fundus and gastric body in the right and midline ventral abdomen. In dogs with gastric volvulus, the stomach may appear compartmentalized or segmented with band-like soft tissue opacities apparent between the gas-filled segments (**fig. 26.15**). As the pylorus is usually displaced dorsally and to the left, a right lateral radiograph results in gas filling of this abnormally positioned segment of the stomach and is usually sufficient to make the diagnosis. The esophagus is often dilated and gas-filled, secondary to occlusion of the gastroesophageal junction. In many patients, there is also generalized gaseous dilation of the small intestine from paralytic ileus caused by ischemia and pain. Gastric dilation and volvulus is extremely rare in cats.[7] Partial volvulus is also possible in dogs, and the stomach has an atypical location but is not consistent with a complete volvulus (**fig. 26.16**). Intermittent volvulus and

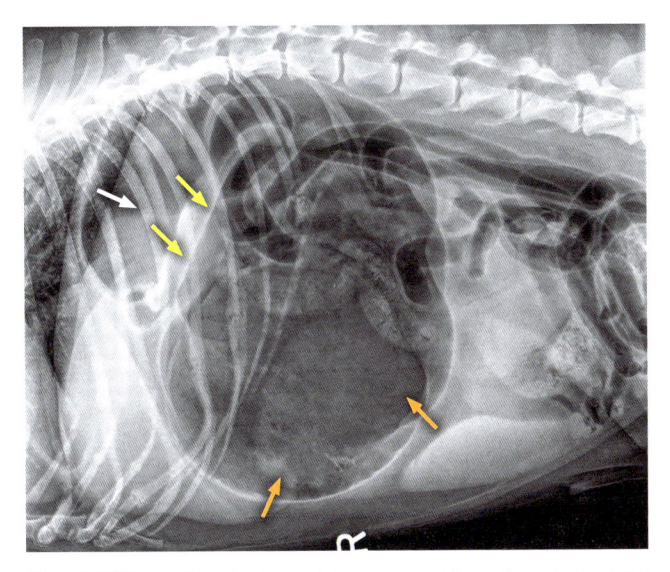

Fig. 26.15 A Collie-mixed breed dog presented for a distended, painful abdomen and retching. A right lateral radiograph was performed and showed the fundus and body to be displaced caudoventrally (orange arrows) and the antrum craniodorsally (white arrow). Compartmentalization is present, denoted by a soft tissue band between the antrum and fundus (yellow arrows). This is a gastric dilation and volvulus requiring surgical intervention.

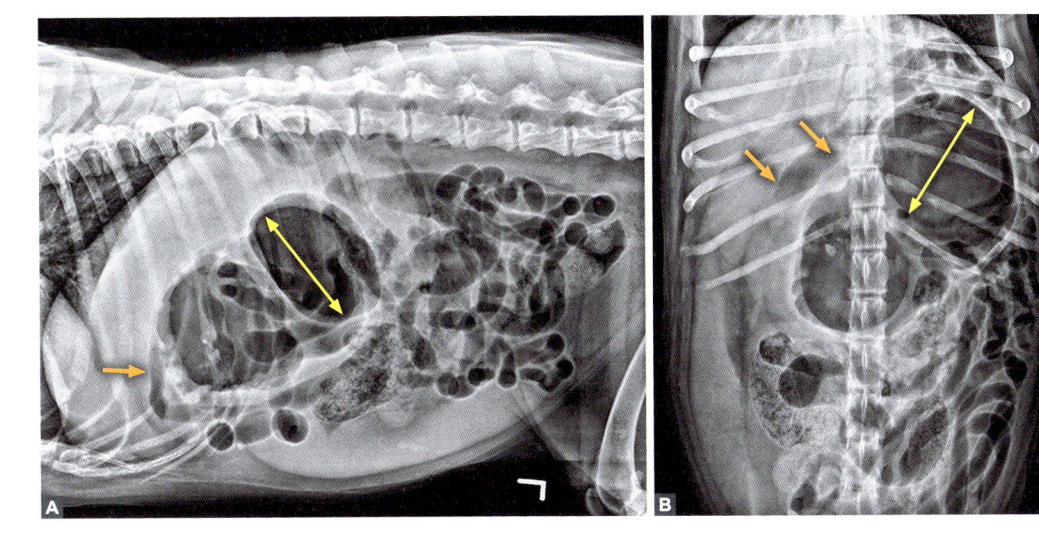

Fig. 26.16 Left lateral and ventrodorsal radiographs of the abdomen in a Cane Corso dog presenting for chronic intermittent vomiting for 2 months. The gastric positioning is abnormal. The gas-filled gastric body (yellow arrows) is located to the left mid-dorsal abdomen. The gastric fundus is positioned on the midline caudal to the gastric body on the ventrodorsal view. The duodenum is shifted medially (orange arrows), and the spleen is enlarged and displaced to the right. The entire jejunum is displaced into the left mid-abdomen. A partial volvulus of the stomach was confirmed surgically, and the spleen was displaced to the right and congested.

SECTION V ABDOMEN

Fig. 26.17 Right lateral abdominal radiograph of a dog with gastric dilation and volvulus that ruptured. The fundus and body are malpositioned in the caudoventral abdomen (white arrow), and there is free gas throughout the peritoneal space highlighting the serosal margins of multiple intestinal segments (orange arrows) and the caudal margin of the diaphragm.

Fig. 26.18 Right and left lateral abdominal radiographs of a ten-month-old cat with acute vomiting. The stomach is dilated with fluid and gas that redistributes based on the recumbency of the cat. (**A**) Gas fills the outflow tract of the antrum and duodenum (orange arrows). A foreign body is highlighted in the dilated proximal duodenum (yellow arrow). (**B**) Fluid fills the pyloric antrum and duodenum (orange arrows). This study is a good example of gastric outflow obstruction, which is characterized by a dilated stomach and empty jejunal segments. Once the obstruction occurs, the intestine distal to the obstruction empties, and the stomach becomes more dilated with time.

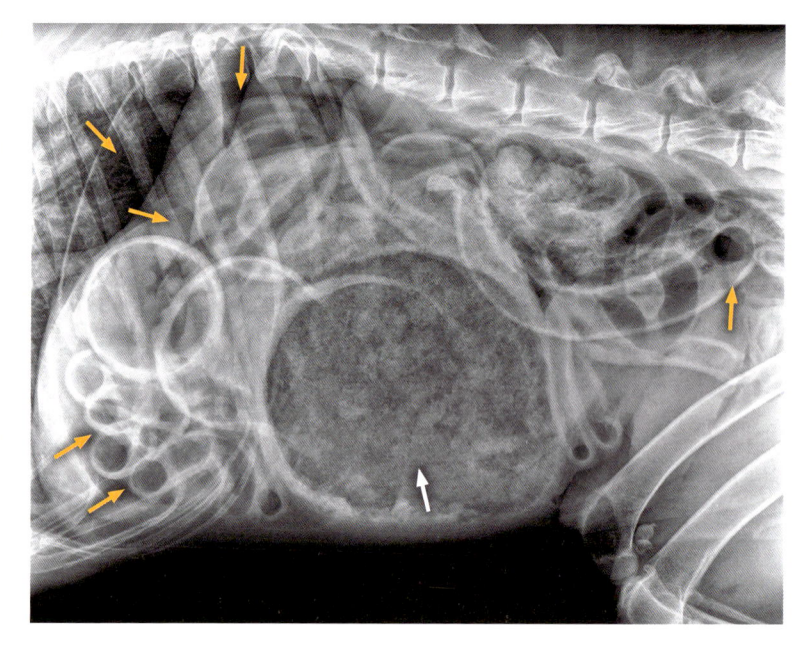

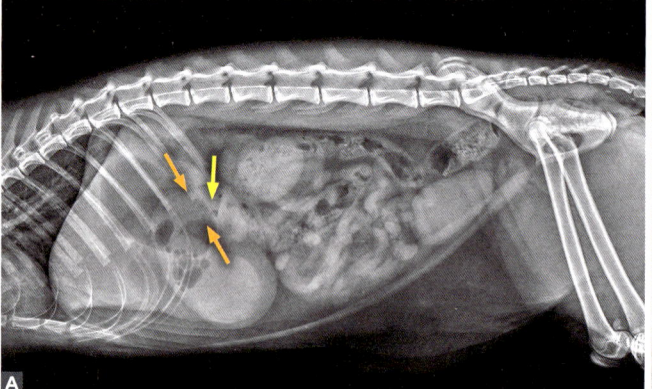

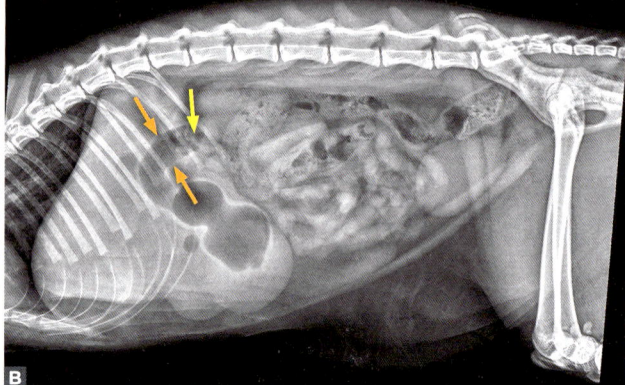

volvulus without dilation can also occur in dogs. An uncommon complication of gastric dilatation and volvulus is rupture which results in the release of a large volume of gas into the peritoneal cavity (**fig. 26.17**). Gas may also be seen within the gastric wall and portal veins with necrosis of the stomach from dilation and volvulus. Computed tomography can be helpful for diagnosing gastric malposition in dogs, and the location of the pyloric canal in the left cranial abdomen near the gastric cardia and the antrum to the left or ventral of the fundus are typical features.[8]

Gastric outflow obstruction

Gastric outflow obstruction can occur from narrowing of the lumen of the antrum and pylorus because of wall thickening or mechanical blockage of the orifice. Survey radiographs usually show some degree of gastric distension. In a left lateral recumbent position, gas in the stomach rises up to the non-dependent side (right side), and soft tissue opacity foreign bodies in the outflow tract are easier to detect when highlighted by luminal gas. In right lateral recumbency, fluid fills the right-sided outflow tract making luminal foreign material more difficult to detect (**figs. 26.18** and **26.19**). In cats, however, obtaining both right and left lateral images is not helpful for assessing the gastric outflow tract unless there is moderate to severe gastric dilation present.[2] Gastric foreign bodies may not cause a complete outflow obstruction when they are freely mobile within the gastric lumen but can

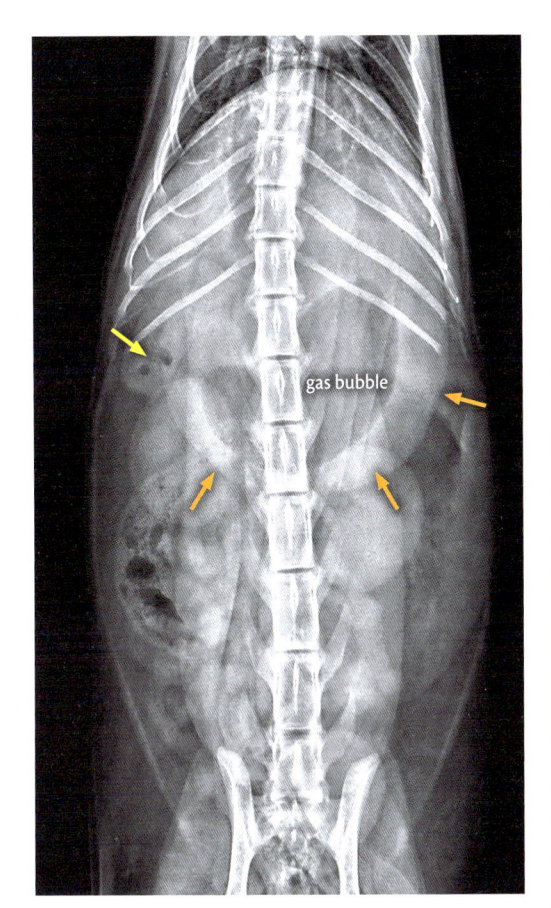

Fig. 26.19 Ventrodorsal radiograph of the same cat as in fig. 26.18. The stomach is severely distended with fluid and gas (orange arrows identify caudal serosal margins of the stomach). A gas bubble is superimposed on the fluid opacity in the stomach and should not be misinterpreted as gastric wall thickening. A proximal duodenal foreign body (yellow arrow) is present.

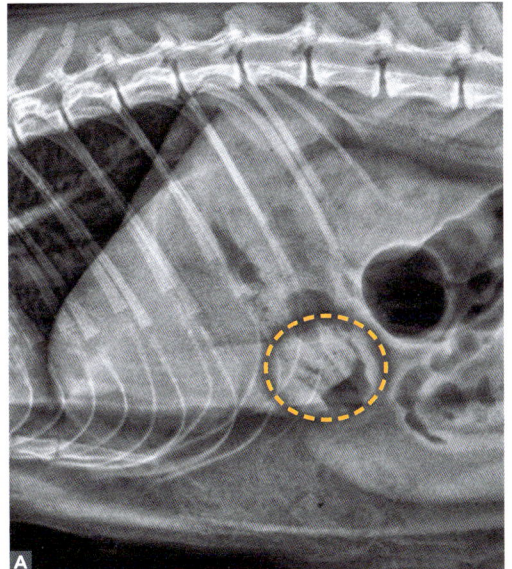

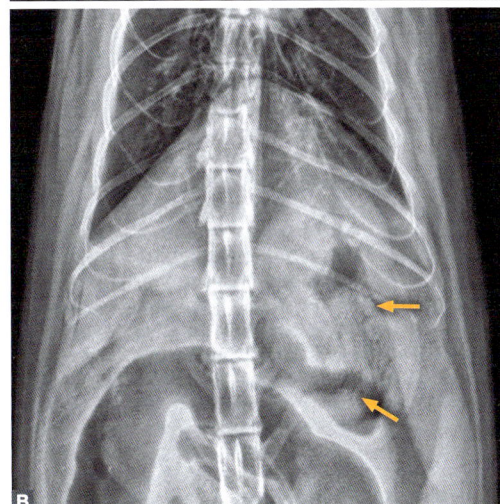

Fig. 26.20 A four-year-old neutered male cat with retching and vomiting for 24 hours. There is a soft tissue opaque structure with a striated appearance (orange arrows) surrounded by gas in the stomach that is mobile and moves from the fundus in the ventrodorsal view to the body in the left lateral image (circle). A hairball was removed from the stomach with gastroscopy. The stomach was not distended as the hairball was not causing complete gastric outflow obstruction.

cause intermittent obstruction and vomiting (**fig. 26.20**). Positive contrast upper gastrointestinal tract studies (chapter 25) and ultrasonography are very helpful for identifying outflow tract disorders causing gastric obstruction when radiographs are equivocal. These may be due to foreign bodies, polyps, or severe inflammatory infiltrates or neoplasms.

Differentiating hypertrophic pyloric stenosis from inflammatory infiltrates or neoplasia is often not possible with diagnostic imaging since all lead to a narrowing of the pyloric orifice due to annular thickening and have a similar appearance radiographically and sonographically (**figs. 26.21** and **26.22**). Congenital hypertrophic pyloric stenosis shows circumferential thickening (>3 mm) of the muscularis layer on ultrasound and can be recognized by a hypoechoic layer that appears like a ring in cross-section (**fig. 26.23**). Strong peristaltic contractions due to the stenotic lumen of the outflow tract can also be observed. Reflux of the gastric ingesta can be observed sonographically, and little to no content passes to the duodenum on repeated contractions. Chronic hypertrophic gastritis can appear like hypertrophic pyloric stenosis, but the mucosa is usually also thickened. Polypoid thickening can be identified at the pyloric antrum and is eccentric, not concentric, as with pyloric hypertrophy. These structures can be sessile or pedunculated and cause intermittent obstruction of the gastric outflow tract (**fig. 26.24**). Concentric thickening of the pylorus can also occur with neoplastic and fungal infiltration, and a definitive diagnosis requires histopathology (**fig. 26.25**).

SECTION V ABDOMEN

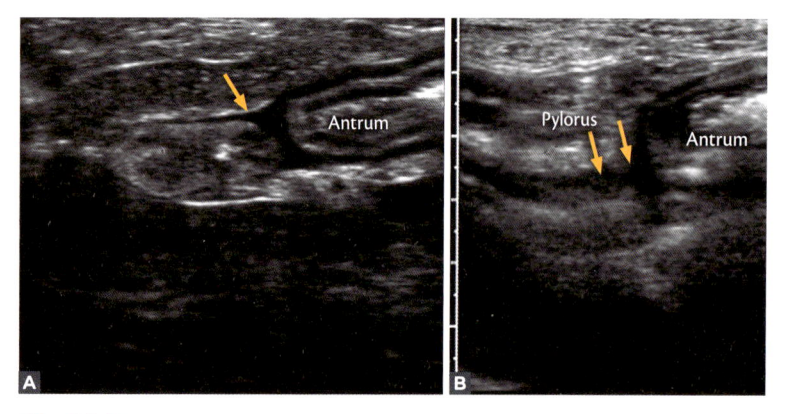

Fig. 26.21 Normal cat (**A**) and dog (**B**) ultrasound images of the pylorus. In the cat, there is a hypoechoic region of the pyloric wall that should not be mistaken for thickening and is normal for this species.

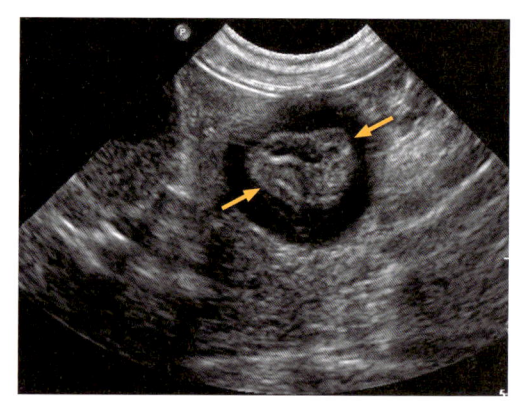

Fig. 26.22 Transverse image of the pylorus of an 11-year-old neutered male Dachshund with chronic vomiting. The muscularis layer (arrows) of the pylorus is circumferentially thickened due to idiopathic pyloric hypertrophy.

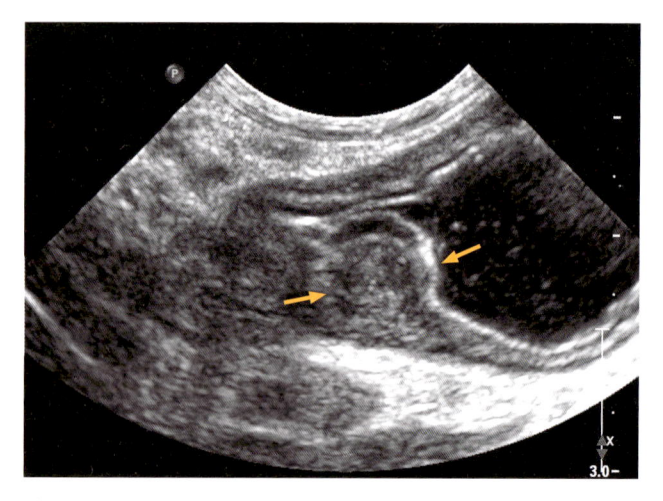

Fig. 26.23 A 12-year-old neutered male Dachshund presented with chronic vomiting for 3 weeks. Ultrasound of the stomach showed a discrete round mural nodule at the pylorus protruding into the lumen (arrows). The nodule was diagnosed as a polyp. Polyps in this location can cause intermittent gastric outflow obstructions.

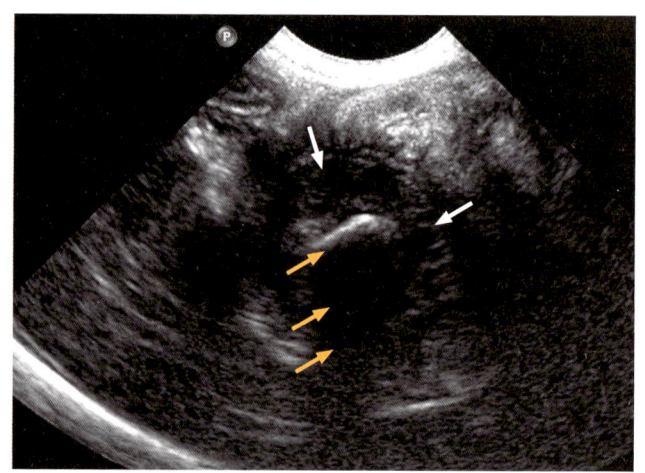

Fig. 26.24 Transverse ultrasound image of a dog with chronic vomiting. There is circumferential hypoechoic transmural thickening of the antral wall (white arrows). In the lumen, there is a hyperechoic linear interface with strong acoustic shadowing (orange arrows). The dog had a foreign body lodged in the pyloric antrum with secondary wall thickening causing outflow obstruction.

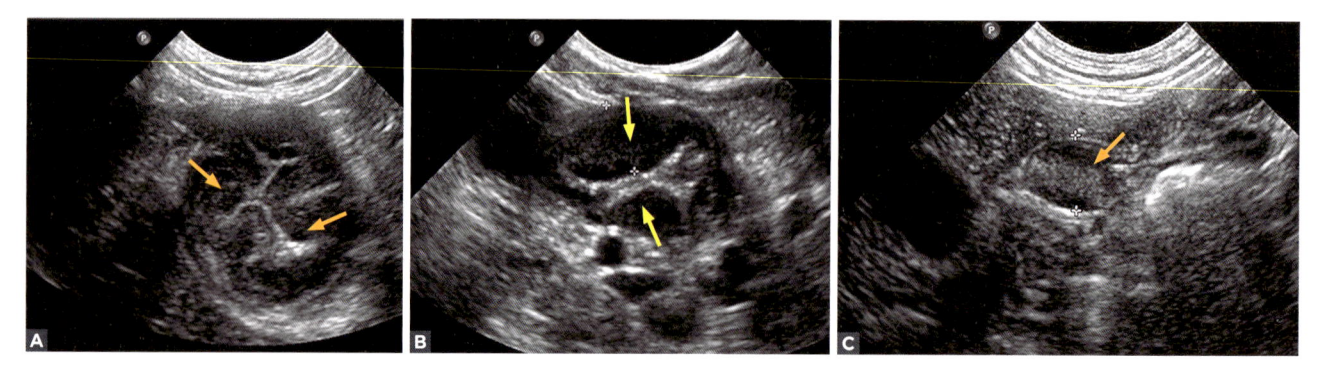

Fig. 26.25 Gastric ultrasound images of a four-year-old male Jack Russell Terrier dog that presented for 2 weeks of hematochezia and generalized lymphadenopathy. (**A**) The stomach has diffuse, transmural hypoechoic wall thickening with disrupted wall layering (orange arrows). (**B**) There is also multifocal transmural hypoechoic wall thickening along the wall of the descending colon (yellow arrows). This is a transverse image of the mid descending colon. (**C**) The gastric lymph node is enlarged (orange arrows). Differentials for these findings are neoplastic and fungal infiltrative disease such as histoplasmosis, and requires tissue sampling to differentiate. This dog was diagnosed with lymphoma.

Infiltrative disease of the gastric wall

Gastric neoplasia is relatively uncommon, and carcinoma is the most common type of gastric neoplasia in dogs with lymphoma being the most common in cats. Gastric neoplasia is difficult to diagnose on survey radiographs unless there is a large mass highlighted by luminal gas. Diffuse stomach wall infiltrations are even more difficult and often impossible to diagnose radiographically. Focal gastric wall masses are typical with carcinoma, leiomyoma, and leiomyosarcoma, while generalized wall thickening may be seen with several other conditions, including chronic hypertrophic gastritis, gastric wall edema, eosinophilic gastritis, fungal infiltrations, and neoplasms, such as lymphoma or histiocytic sarcoma. Diffuse and localized gastric wall infiltrations and masses are better imaged with ultrasound, which often eliminates the need for gastrointestinal contrast studies. Neoplasms can be recognized during abdominal ultrasound by observing thickening of the wall and a disruption of the normal wall layering (fig. 26.24). The neoplastic lesion usually shows a decreased echogenicity and may create the appearance of pseudolayering.[9] Regional lymph nodes are often enlarged. Gastric lymphoma occurs in both dogs and cats and causes a generalized, hypoechoic thickening of the gastric wall with loss of wall layering.[10]

Ultrasound-guided percutaneous fine-needle aspiration or biopsy of the gastric wall can be performed to differentiate neoplastic, and inflammatory infiltrates. Fine-needle aspiration can be performed with a 20-gauge needle, or biopsies can be taken with an automated 18-gauge biopsy device when the gastric wall is thicker than 2 cm.

Contrast-enhanced computed tomography has been shown to be helpful in staging canine gastric tumors.[11] CT features of lymphoma, carcinoma, leiomyoma and inflammatory polyps overlap. However, CT is advantageous for diagnosing local invasion and distant metastasis for staging purposes in addition to characterization of the origin and extent of the lesion (fig. 26.26).[11] Helical hydro CT (HHCT) has been found easy to perform and is useful for diagnosing gastric tumors in dogs and cats (fig. 26.27). For this technique, the stomach is intubated and filled with water at a dose of 30 mL/kg. The abdomen is scanned before and after intravenous injection of water-soluble iodinated contrast. This technique allows complete assessment of the gastric wall without interference from luminal gas such as ultrasound and allows accurate assessment of the size and extent of mural gastric lesions for treatment planning. The technique is also useful for the evaluation of the local and regional lymph nodes.[12]

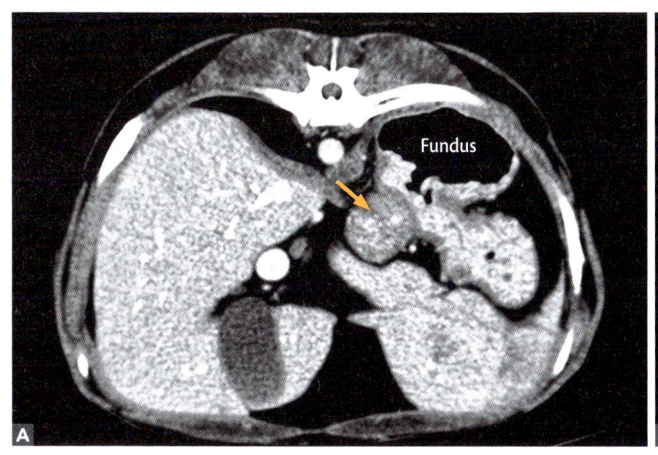

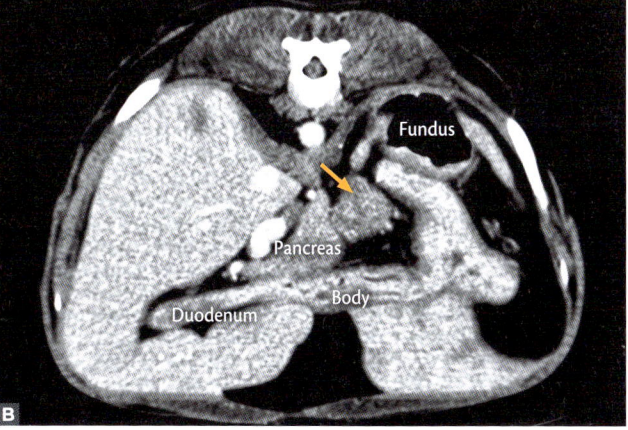

Fig. 26.26 CT images of a 13-year-old spayed female Terrier mixed dog with vomiting and a mass near the porta hepatis identified on ultrasound. Post-contrast CT scan soft tissue window showed a mass in the wall at the lesser curvature of the stomach close to the cardia. The esophagus is not affected. The mass effaces the muscular layer of the stomach and extends beyond the serosal border, protruding into the surrounding fat near the porta hepatis. The proximity of the mass to the porta hepatis can make it difficult to distinguish from a lesion originating from the pancreas or hepatic lymph node using ultrasonography. The rest of the stomach is unremarkable. Differentials of leiomyoma and leiomyosarcoma were given based on their predilection for the muscularis layer. Other gastric neoplasms such as carcinoma are possible. This mass would require either ultrasound-guided sampling or laparotomy to obtain tissue for diagnosis since it does not extend through the wall into the mucosa/lumen, precluding endoscopic sampling.

SECTION V ABDOMEN

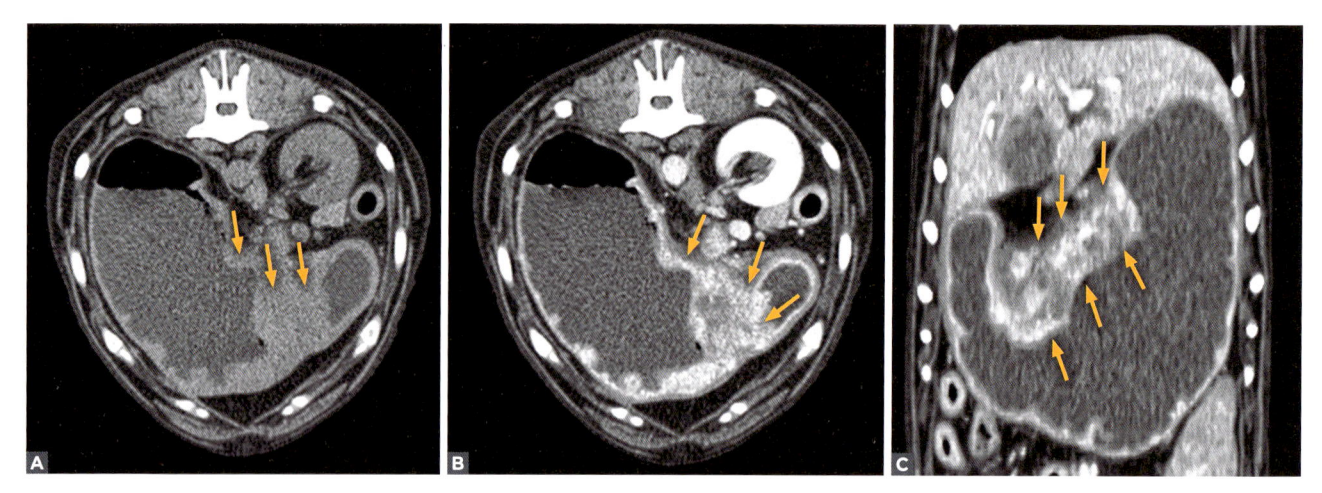

Fig. 26.27 HHCT of a nine-year-old female mixed breed dog with gastric neoplasia. Pre- (**A**) and post- (**B**) contrast transverse views of a dog with severe thickening of the smaller curvature (arrows), well visible after the stomach distension. The dorsal MPR reconstruction (**C**) clearly shows the involvement of the less curvature of the stomach. Final diagnosis was gastric carcinoma.

References

1. Vander Hart D, Berry CR. Initial influence of right versus left lateral recumbency on the radiographic finding of duodenal gas on subsequent survey ventrodorsal projections of the canine abdomen. *Vet Radiol Ultrasound* 56: 12-17, 2015.
2. Paradise, H, Gaschen L, Wanderer M, Liu C, Granger LA. Performing both lateral abdominal radiographs may not improve the visualization of gas in the gastric outflow tract of cats. *Vet Radiol Ultrasound* 60:633-639, 2019.
3. Miles S, Gaschen L, Presley T, Liu C, Granger LA. Influence of repeat abdominal radiographs on the resolution of mechanical obstruction and gastrointestinal foreign material in dogs and cats. *Vet Radiol Ultrasound* 62:282-288, 2021.
4. Murakami M, Heng HG, Lim CK, Parnell NK, et al. Ultrasonographic features of presumed gastric wall edema in 14 dogs with pancreatitis. *J Vet Intern Med* 33:1260-1265, 2019.
5. Murakami M, Heng HG, Lim CK, Parnell NK, Sola M. Ultrasonographic features and prevalence of presumed gastric wall edema in dogs with hypoalbuminemia. *J Vet Intern Med* 34:1867-1871, 2020.
6. Penninck D, Matz M, Tidwell A. Ultrasonography of gastric ulceration in the dog. *Vet Radiol Ultrasound* 38:308-312, 1997.
7. Leary ML, Sinnott-Stutzman V. Spontaneous gastric dilatation-volvulus in two cats. *J Vet Emerg Crit Care (San Antonio)* 28:346-355, 2018.
8. White C, Dirrig H, Fitzgerald E. CT findings in dogs with gastric malposition: 6 cases (2016-2019). *J Small Anim Pract* 61:766-771, 2020.
9. Penninck DG, Moore AS, Gliatto J. Ultrasonography of canine gastric epithelial neoplasia. *Vet Radiol Ultrasound* 39:342-348, 1998.
10. Richter KP. Feline gastrointestinal lymphoma. *Vet Clin North Am Small Anim Pract* 33:1083-1098, 2003.
11. Tanaka T, Akiyoshi H, Mie K, Okamoto M, et al. Contrast-enhanced computed tomography may be helpful for characterizing and staging canine gastric tumors. *Vet Radiol Ultrasound* 60:7-18, 2019.
12. Terragni R, Vignoli M, Rossi F, Laganga P, et al. Stomach wall evaluation using helical hydro-computed tomography. *Vet Radiol Ultrasound* 53:402-405, 2012.

CHAPTER 27

The small intestine

Lorrie Gaschen

> ### KEY POINTS
>
> - It is not possible to assess intestinal wall thickness on survey radiographs, which requires either an upper gastrointestinal contrast study or ultrasonography.
> - Fluid-distended intestines can be misinterpreted as being thickened due to the summation of fluid within the intestinal wall.
> - Repeat radiographs can be used to monitor intestinal diameter and content over time when the patient is clinically stable and radiographs are equivocal.
> - Mechanical obstruction is recognized by a mixed population of dilated and non-dilated intestinal segments both radiographically and sonographically.
> - Spoon compression can aid in better visualizing individual intestinal segments by eliminating superimposition.
> - Ultrasonography is useful when radiographs are equivocal in vomiting and diarrheic animals to assess luminal content, wall layering, and thickness.
> - Ultrasonography can be used to assess peristalsis when functional ileus is suspected clinically.
> - Causes of transmural loss of intestinal wall layering cannot be differentiated sonographically and requires tissue sampling to diagnose the cause.
> - Muscularis thickening in cats can be due to either inflammatory bowel disease or lymphoma.
> - Computed tomography of the small intestines is typically reserved for patients with equivocal radiographic findings or more complex intestinal masses as a means of pre-surgical planning and is not used as a first-line diagnostic test.

Indications for survey radiographs to assess the small intestine include vomiting, acute abdomen, diarrhea, weight loss, anorexia, or a palpable mass. In dogs and cats with clinical disease suspected of the small intestines, a three-view radiographic study consisting of right and left lateral and ventrodorsal radiographs should be performed as a minimum database and prior to performing abdominal ultrasound. Survey radiographs allow an overall assessment of the small intestinal diameter, distribution, and content, which is important for diagnosing functional vs. mechanical ileus. Radiopaque small intestinal foreign material can also be identified and monitored in repeat studies. Ultrasonography is typically performed when survey radiographs of the small intestines are equivocal and is important for diagnosing intussusceptions, pancreatitis, intestinal wall thickening, presence of peristalsis, luminal content, and infiltrative disease.

SECTION V ABDOMEN

As a rule, anorectic animals or animals held off food (>12 hours) should not have small bowel segments containing soft tissue opaque or granular material resembling food. Granular or more opaque small bowel contents may be detected in patients with a partial or complete obstruction.

Normal small intestinal diameter in healthy dogs should be less than 1.6 times the height of the mid lumbar vertebral body of L5. In cats, the maximum intestinal diameter is 12 mm, or twice the height of the L2 vertebral body.

The normal duodenum in dogs has a specific location in the mid-right lateral abdomen spanning from cranial to caudal along the right abdominal wall. In cats, the duodenum has a cranial and midline location. The jejunal segments in dogs and cats are localized to the mid to caudal abdomen between the caudal margin of the stomach, cranial margin of the urinary bladder, and ventral and superimposed with the colon in dogs and cats (**figs. 27.1** and **27.2**). In cats with large deposits of intra-abdominal fat, the jejunum often migrates into the right mid-abdomen and can even collect into a "clump" of intestines that can be confused with a linear foreign body (**fig. 27.2B**).

Compression views of the abdomen can be very useful for assessing the small intestine. Because the jejunal segments and colon are often superimposed with one another and have variable gas and soft tissue content, it can be challenging to differentiate small from large bowel and to assess the shape of the intestines (**fig. 27.3**). In cats, this is important to differentiate bunching as with a linear foreign body. A radiolucent spoon such as a wooden cooking spoon can be used to apply gentle pressure to the abdomen and serves to separate the jejunal segments from one another.

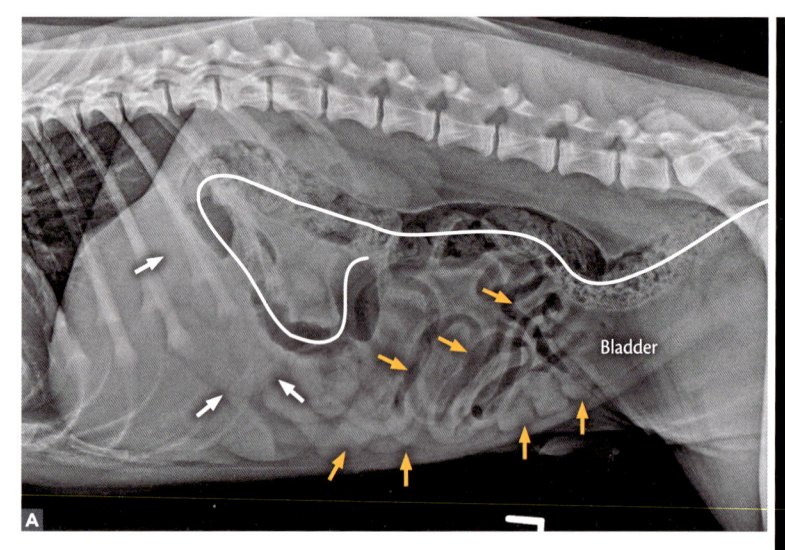

Fig. 27.1 (**A**) Left lateral abdominal radiograph of a normal dog showing the appearance of normal small intestines. The dog is fasted, and the stomach is devoid of content (white arrows). The jejunum is a uniform population of normal diameter and has variable soft tissue opacity and gas content (orange arrows). The gas content has low volume, and the intestines are not distended. The jejunal segments are distributed in the mid-ventral abdomen between the stomach and aspect of the urinary bladder and approximately ventral to the colon. There is gas in the ascending and transverse colon, with feces filling the length of the descending colon (the white line traces the path of the colon). Important to note is the excellent serosal detail at the margins of the jejunal segments outlined by peritoneal fat even though they are superimposed with one another. (**B**) Ventrodorsal abdominal radiograph of a normal dog. The stomach is devoid of content (white arrow). The jejunum is a uniform population of diameter and has a normal distribution in the mid-abdomen and more accumulated on the right, which is normal. The jejunum is variably opaque soft tissue, and some segments contain gas and have a continuous tubular shape. The cecum has some granular soft tissue content and can be mistaken for a dilated jejunal segment but its location in the right mid-abdomen and sigmoid shape is typical for this segment (dotted line). The transverse colon contains gas, and the descending colon is filled with feces (traced by the white line).

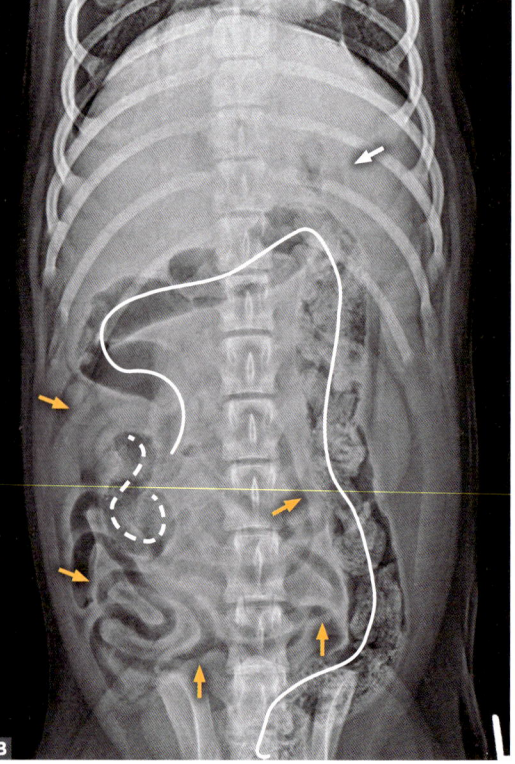

CHAPTER **27** The small intestine

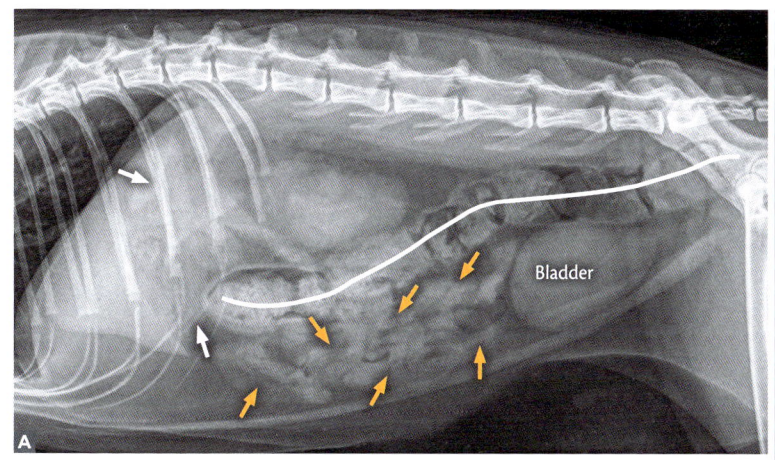

Fig. 27.2 (**A**) Right lateral abdominal radiograph of a normal cat. The stomach is devoid of content (white arrows). The jejunum (orange arrows) is a uniform population of normal diameter and has a normal distribution and tubular shape in the mid-ventral abdomen between the stomach and bladder and ventral to the colon (the white line traces the colon path). (**B**) Ventrodorsal abdomen of a normal cat. The stomach is devoid of content (white arrows). The jejunum (orange arrows) is a uniform population of normal diameter and distributed into the right mid-abdomen, which is very typical in cats. The colon is traced with a white line to show its location.

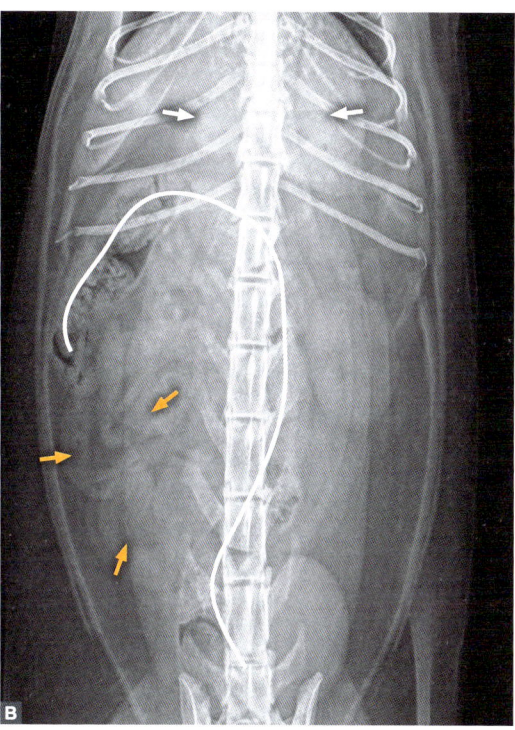

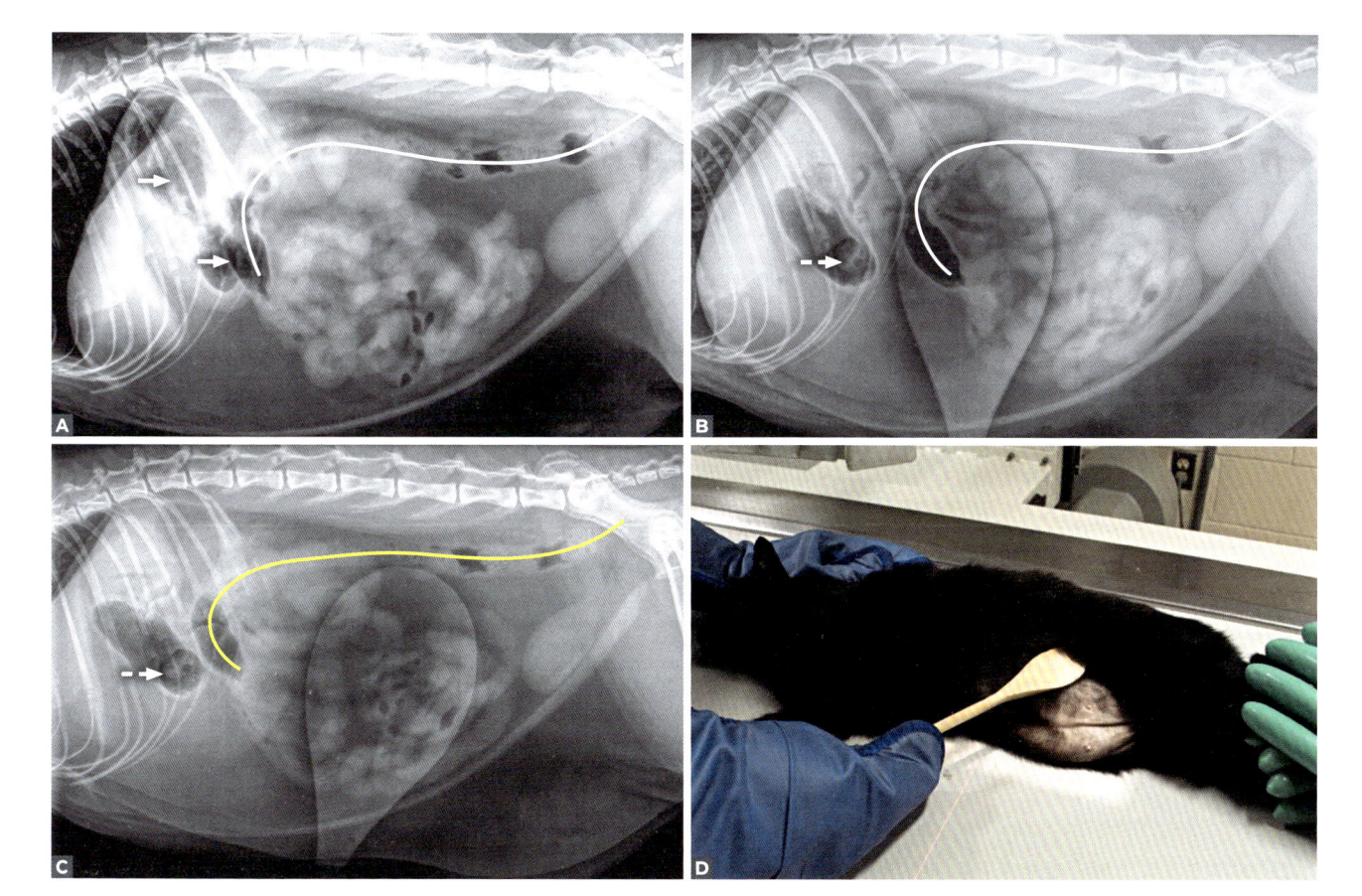

Fig. 27.3 (**A**) Lateral radiographs in a cat that presented with vomiting. The stomach contains gas (white arrows), and a small foreign body was identified in the stomach (dashed arrows) and was the ultimate cause of the vomiting. (**B, C**) A wooden cooking spoon was used to do a compression view to assess the jejunal segments better. Pressing down with the spoon in the cranial (**B**) and mid (**C**) abdomen allows the small intestines to be separated away from one another and individually assessed for size and content. This also helps to rule out a linear foreign body where the intestines are bunched together and will not spread out under spoon compression. The jejunal segments in this cat are normal. (**D**) Demonstrating the use of spoon compression for assessment of the small intestines in a cat. The wooden spoon is slowly pressed down on the abdomen to separate the small intestinal superimposition.

Ileus

Ileus is a failure of the intestinal contents to be transported and is recognized radiographically by the presence of dilated bowel segments. The radiographic appearance of ileus is dependent on its duration, location, and type. Ileus can be either functional or mechanical. In mechanical ileus, acute or proximal obstructions may be associated with little intestinal dilation radiographically, whereas chronic or more distally located obstructions will be associated with more severely dilated intestinal segments. Mechanical ileus may be partial or complete and has a luminal, mural, or extramural location. Examples of diseases causing mechanical obstruction include foreign bodies, herniation of small intestinal segments, intussusception, adhesions, granulomas, or infiltrative disease due to fungal or neoplastic causes. Small intestines are considered mildly dilated when they are >1.6 times the mid height of the fifth lumbar vertebral body L5 in dogs. When generalized mild small intestinal dilation is present, it is known as functional or paralytic ileus (**figs. 27.4-27.6**). Functional ileus results in obstruction since the intestinal contents pool in the gastrointestinal tract due to lack of motility. It may also affect the

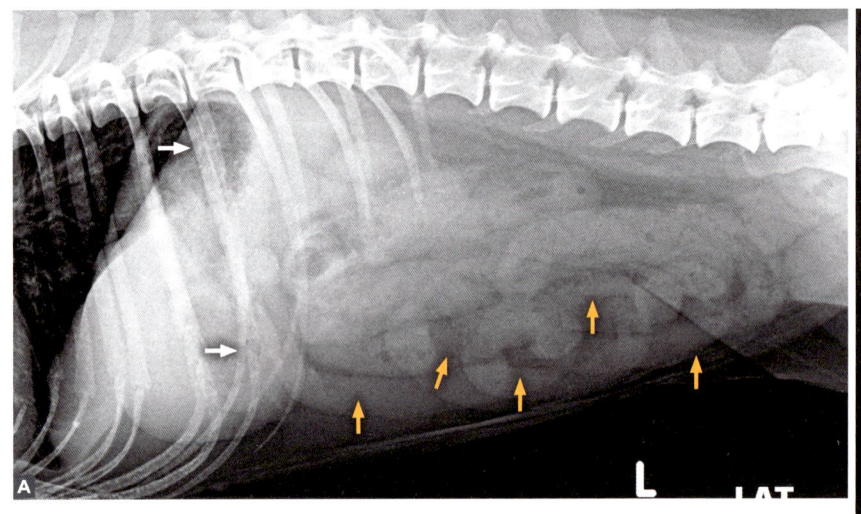

Fig. 27.4 (**A**) Lateral abdomen in a dog with vomiting and diarrhea. The stomach contains a frothy gas and fluid mixture but is not overly distended (white arrows). The jejunum is mildly dilated, and the segments are uniform in diameter. The jejunum also contains frothy fragmented gas bubbles and fluid (orange arrows). The colon is devoid of feces and contains fluid and gas. The radiographic diagnosis was functional ileus, and the dog had non-specific gastroenteritis. (**B**) Ventrodorsal view. The stomach contains a frothy gas and fluid mixture but is not overly distended (white arrows). The jejunum is mildly dilated, and the segments are uniform in diameter. The jejunum also contains frothy fragmented gas bubbles and fluid (orange arrows). The colon is devoid of feces and contains fluid and gas. The radiographic diagnosis was functional ileus, and the dog had non-specific gastroenteritis.

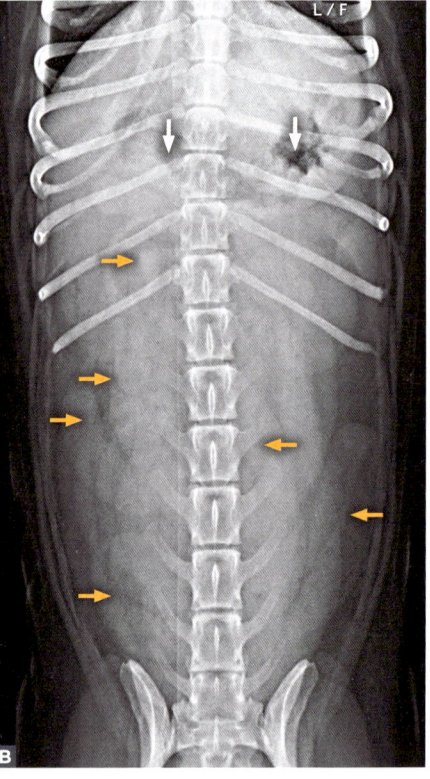

Fig. 27.5 Lateral abdominal radiograph of a cat with vomiting and diarrhea. There is gas and fluid mildly distending the stomach (white arrows). The jejunum is mildly distended and predominantly fluid opaque with mild gas in a few loops (orange arrows). The transverse colon contains gas, and the descending colon is fluid opaque (white line outlines large bowel). The cat was diagnosed with non-specific gastroenteritis. Fluid and gas in the colon had passed from the upper gastrointestinal tract resulting in diarrhea.

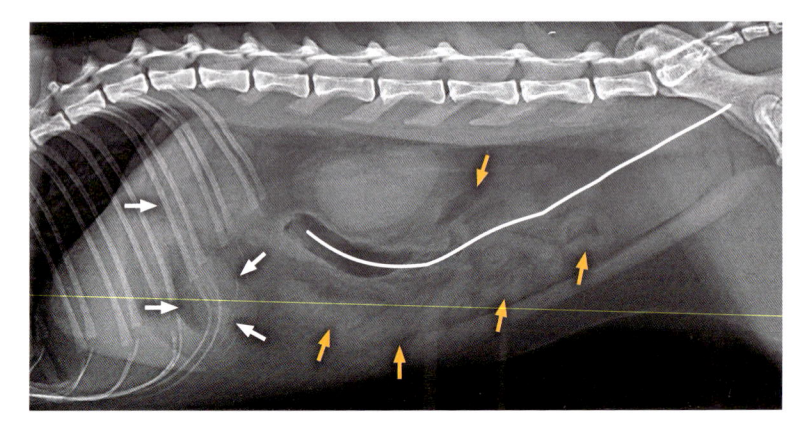

CHAPTER 27 The small intestine

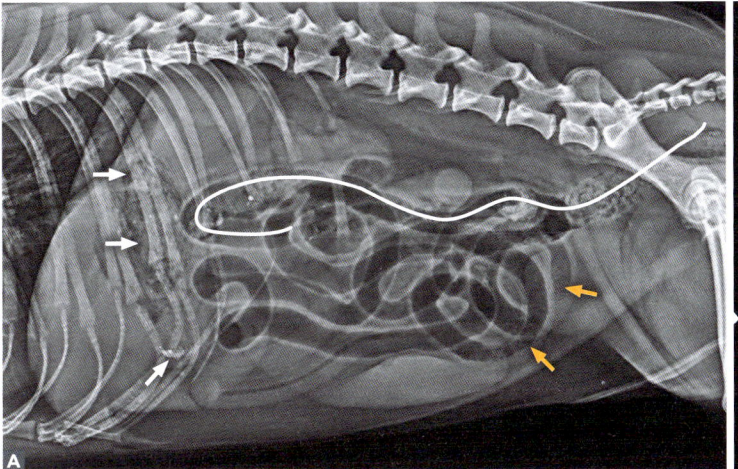

Fig. 27.6 (A) A two-year-old neutered male small breed dog presented with acute vomiting and diarrhea. There is a small volume of heterogenous gastric content, including some mineral opacities that form a conglomerate (white arrows). The jejunum is mildly dilated and has a normal tubular course and location in the abdomen. The jejunal content is predominately gas, and some segments have a frothy appearance (orange arrows). There is a mild amount of feces in the colon that also contains some mineral content similar to the stomach. The diagnosis is functional ileus due to non-specific gastroenteritis following indiscriminate ingestion. The path of the colon is traced with a white line. (B) Ventrodorsal image. There is a small volume of heterogenous gastric content that includes some mineral opacities that form a conglomerate (white arrow). The jejunum is mildly dilated and has a normal tubular course and location in the abdomen. The jejunal content is predominately gas, and some segments have a frothy appearance (orange arrows). There is a mild amount of feces in the colon that also contains some mineral content similar to the stomach. The diagnosis is functional ileus due to non-specific gastroenteritis following indiscriminate ingestion. The path of the colon is traced with a white line.

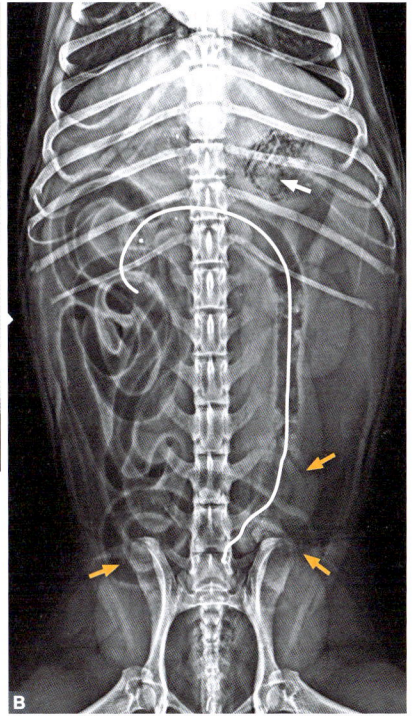

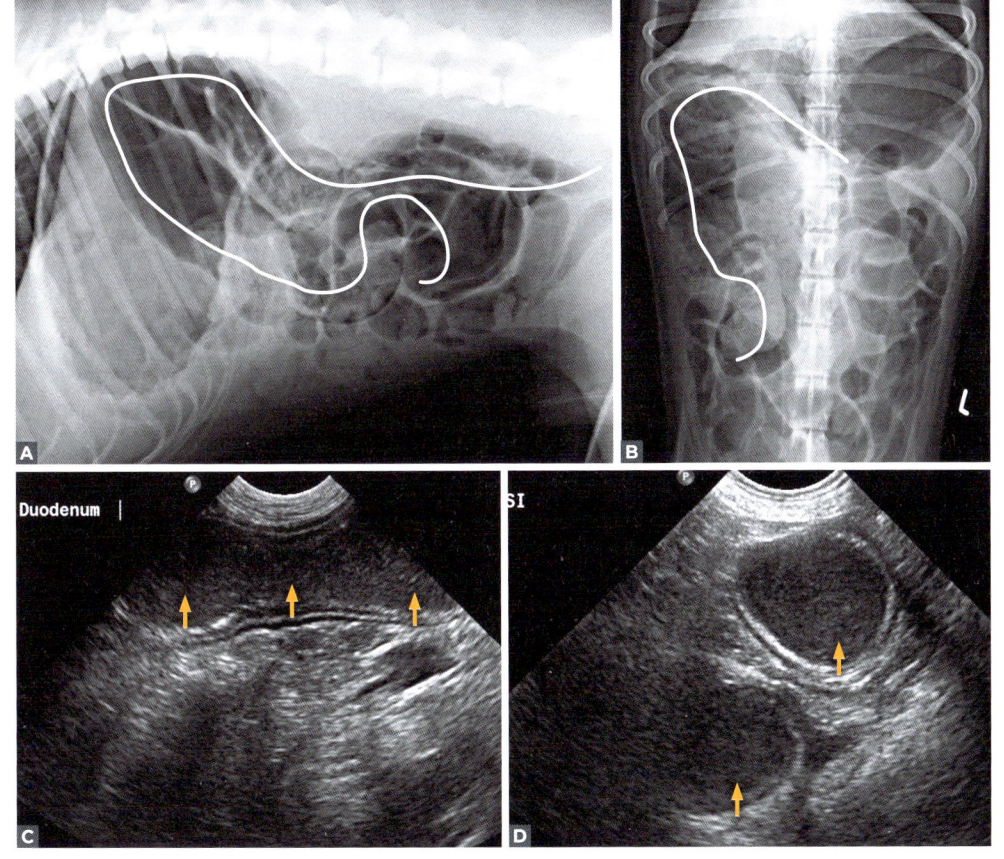

Fig. 27.7 (A) Lateral and (B) ventrodorsal radiographs of a dog with vomiting and hemorrhagic diarrhea. There is generalized moderate to severe gas dilation of the entire gastrointestinal tract, which poses a challenge in trying to rule out mechanical ileus. There are some formed feces in the cecum and ascending colon (white line traces the path of this region). The combination of generalized gas dilation and the clinical signs prioritizes a radiographic diagnosis of functional ileus even though the small intestines are more than mildly dilated. There is also some soft tissue content in the dilated jejunal segments. The next steps for this dog may include continued fasting, fluid therapy, and repeat radiographs to assess the size and content of the gastrointestinal segments with time, depending on its clinical status. Ultrasound images of the (C) duodenum and (D) jejunal segments in a dog with vomiting and diarrhea diagnosed with functional ileus due to non-specific gastroenteritis. The duodenum and all jejunal segments did not have peristalsis and were moderately dilated with fluid (orange arrows).

455

stomach, small intestines, or large intestines simultaneously and, when severe, makes the radiographic pattern challenging to interpret and differentiate large from small intestine (**fig. 27.7**). Radiographically, the small intestinal segments with functional ileus may have a homogeneous soft tissue opacity when they are fluid-filled, or a mixed pattern of gas and fluid may also be present. Small volume soft tissue luminal content can also be present. It is not possible to assess intestinal wall thickness on survey radiographs. A segment of intestine with gas and fluid content can have the appearance of a thickened wall due to the silhouetting effect between the fluid and intestinal wall.

The most common cause of the gastrointestinal pattern consistent with functional ileus is acute non-specific enteritis or acute hemorrhagic diarrhea syndrome (AHDS), and dogs have clinical signs of both vomiting and diarrhea. This intestinal pattern can be also due to the administration of pharmaceutical agents such as parasympatholytics or sedatives. Other causes are peritonitis, blunt abdominal trauma, electrolyte imbalance, or enteritis of various causes. Dysautonomia is a disorder of the autonomic nervous system that can also lead to generalized dilation of the gastrointestinal tract in both dogs and cats. A complete obstruction in the distal jejunum or at the ileocecal level may also lead to the same radiographic appearance. Decreased peristalsis may be limited to the duodenum in patients with pancreatitis.

In partial obstructions, because fluid passes through the narrowed lumen, the contents remaining proximal to the partial obstruction become physically denser and, therefore, radiographically opaquer and lead to a gravel sign (**fig. 27.8**).

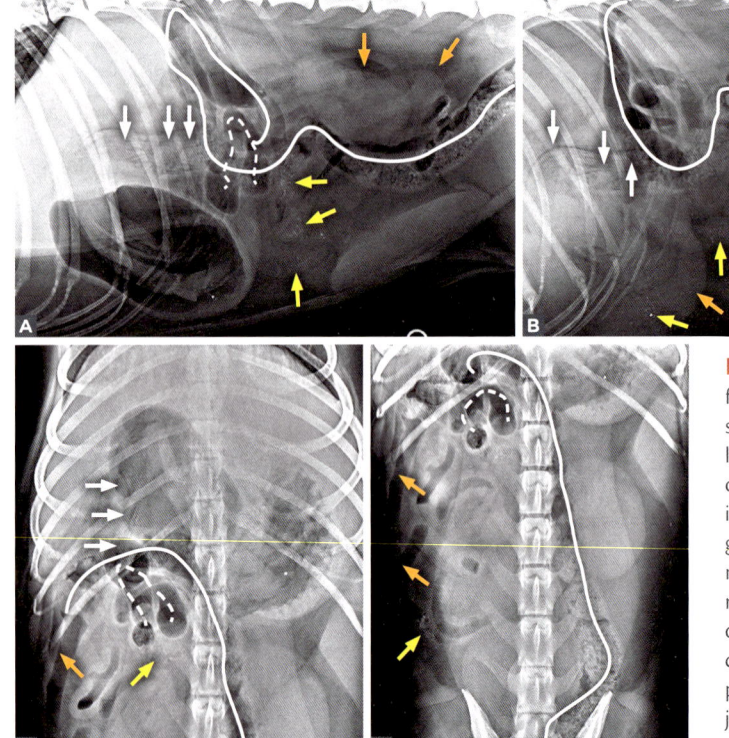

Fig. 27.8 (**A**) Left lateral radiograph of a dog with acute vomiting for 24 hours and a history of eating foreign objects at home. The stomach is dilated, and gas fills the antrum highlighting a large tubular foreign body that extends through the pylorus and into the duodenum (white arrows). There are a few segments of small intestine in the cranial and mid-abdomen that are mildly dilated and have a gravel sign: focal mineral opaque structures within the lumen of the mildly dilated segments (yellow arrows). The rest of the jejunum has mild variable dilation with fluid and gas (orange arrows). The path of the colon is traced with a white line. The cecum is traced with a dotted white line. This dog had a duodenal fabric foreign body and partially obstructive small intestinal foreign bodies in the proximal jejunum. (**B**) Right lateral radiograph. The stomach is dilated, and a striated soft tissue tubular foreign body is in the duodenum (white arrows). There are a few segments of small intestine in the cranial and mid-abdomen that are moderately dilated and have a gravel sign: focal mineral opaque structures within the lumen of the mildly dilated segments (yellow arrows). The rest of the jejunum has mild variable dilation with fluid and gas (orange arrows). This dog had a duodenal fabric foreign body and partially obstructive small intestinal foreign bodies in the proximal jejunum. (**C**) Cranial and caudal ventrodorsal radiographs. The stomach is dilated, and a striated soft tissue tubular foreign body is in the duodenum (white arrows). The distal descending duodenum contains gas (orange arrow). There are a few segments of small intestine in the cranial and mid-abdomen that are moderately dilated and have a gravel sign: focal mineral opaque structures within the lumen of the mildly dilated segments (yellow arrows). The rest of the jejunum has mild variable dilation with fluid and gas (orange arrows). This dog had a duodenal fabric foreign body and partially obstructive small intestinal foreign bodies in the proximal jejunum.

More severe dilations, usually with gas, are seen in animals with complete obstructions, which are termed mechanical ileus (**fig. 27.9**). Dilation (1.5-2 times the height of the body of L5 in dogs) is seen proximal to the site of obstruction, and the segments distal to it usually appear empty and contracted. Due to this, the jejunal segments appear to have highly variable diameters and are described as having a mixed population. Feces may still be present in the colon, depending on the duration of the obstruction. Distal jejunal obstructions may cause generalized dilation and resemble a functional ileus radiographically or a mesenteric volvulus, and the clinical status of the dog plays an important role in differentiating these. Using a small intestine to L5 ratio of 1.7, the diagnosis of intestinal obstruction has a 66% sensitivity and specificity.[1] The low sensitivity and specificity of comparing the small intestinal diameter to vertebral body height underscores that this method should be used as an initial indicator and that other methods, such as continued fasting with fluid therapy and repeat radiographs or ultrasonographic examination are required when the initial radiographs are equivocal or for the purposes of monitoring for passage of intestinal content (**fig. 27.10**).[2]

Ultrasonography has the advantage that it can be used to inspect the small intestines for wall layering, thickness, dilation, and peristalsis, as well as for intraluminal, intramural, and extraluminal causes of obstruction. Lack of peristalsis occurring together with generalized dilation of the small intestines can be seen with functional ileus. Small intestinal contractions can be observed, and approximately 1-3 per minute is considered normal, and ultrasound can be used to monitor peristalsis.[3]

Radiolucent intestinal foreign bodies may be detected by ultrasound, especially when they cause mechanical obstruction at the junction of dilated and empty jejunal segments (**figs. 27.11** and **27.12**). The finding of severe dilation of one or more segments of the jejunum and the stomach together with empty, contracted bowel segments distally may indicate a complete or partial obstruction (**fig. 27.13**). Solid luminal material generally appears as a hyperechoic interface, which creates an acoustic shadow. Care should be taken not to misinterpret a gas-liquid interface in a dilated bowel segment as an obstruction. Balls and pieces of balls will have a round or curvilinear

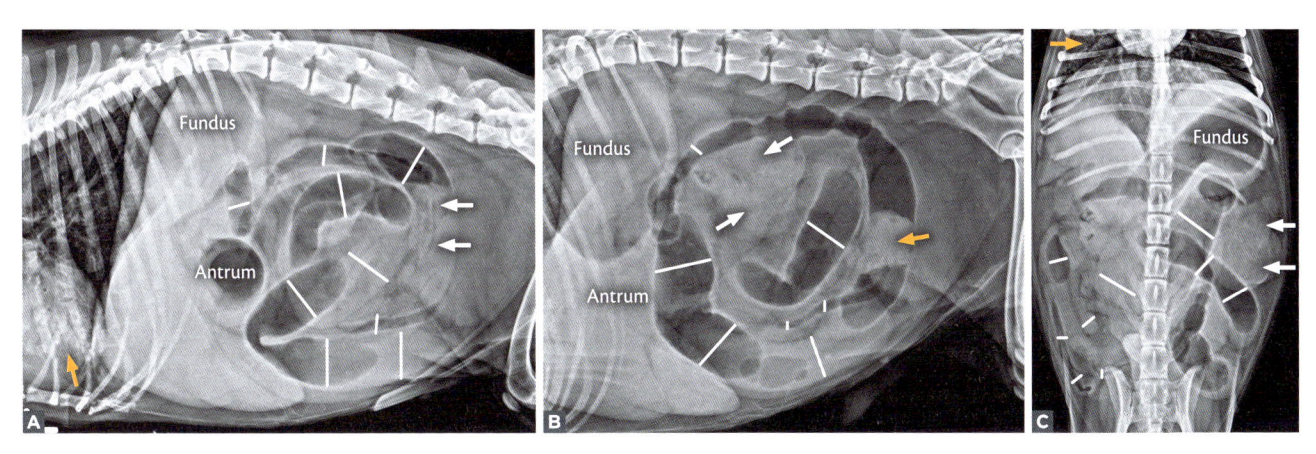

Fig. 27.9 (**A**) Left lateral radiograph of a ten-year-old neutered male Cocker Spaniel presented with acute vomiting. The dog historically had a splenic mass (white arrows). The gastrointestinal pattern is mechanical ileus: there is a mixed population of severely dilated jejunal segments together with normal to mildly dilated ones (bars show variable diameters). There is heterogenous luminal content in some of the dilated segments as well (white arrows). The colon is devoid of content. In the left lateral image, gas has migrated to the gastric antrum (labeled). The diagnosis was a fabric intestinal foreign body causing complete obstruction. The dog also developed aspiration pneumonia (orange arrow) in the right middle lung lobe due to vomiting. (**B**) Right lateral radiograph. The gastrointestinal pattern is mechanical ileus: there is a mixed population of severely dilated jejunal segments together with normal to mildly dilated ones (bars show variable diameters). There is heterogenous luminal content in some of the dilated segments as well (orange arrow). In the right lateral image, fluid in the stomach migrates to the antrum compared to gas content in left lateral view (fig. 27.9A). The diagnosis was a fabric intestinal foreign body causing complete obstruction. (**C**) Ventrodorsal radiograph of a ten-year-old neutered male Cocker Spaniel that presented with acute vomiting. The dog historically had a splenic mass (white arrows). The gastrointestinal pattern is mechanical ileus: there is a mixed population of severely dilated jejunal segments together with normal to mildly dilated ones (bars show variable diameters). There is heterogenous luminal content in some of the dilated segments as well. The diagnosis was a fabric intestinal foreign body causing complete obstruction. The dog also developed aspiration pneumonia (orange arrow) in the right middle lung lobe due to vomiting.

SECTION V ABDOMEN

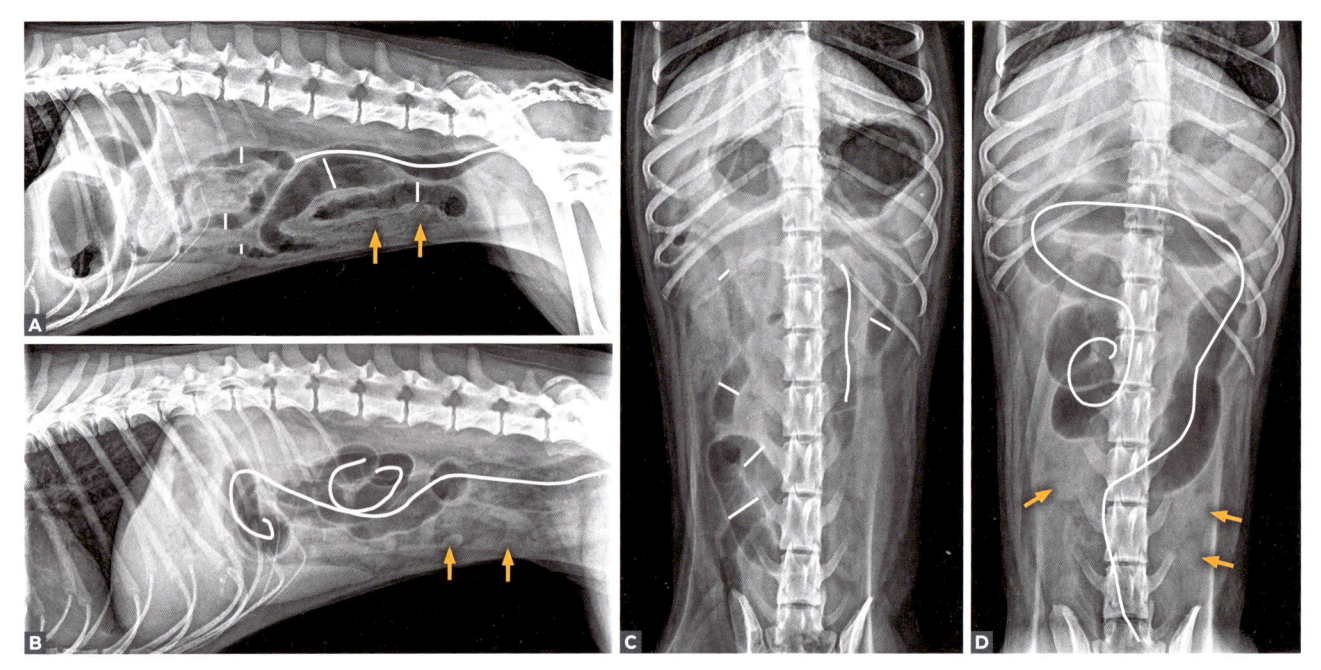

Fig. 27.10 A seven-year-old spayed female medium-sized mixed breed dog presented with acute vomiting for 24 hours. (A) In the initial radiographs, the stomach is dilated with gas, and mechanical ileus is present with a mixed population of small intestinal diameter ranging from normal to severely dilated with gas. In the mid-ventral abdomen, a single jejunal segment has heterogeneous soft tissue content (arrows). Based on the stable condition of the dog, a decision was made to continue fasting and fluid therapy and repeat the radiographs. (B) This radiograph was performed 8 hours later, the abnormal content had passed and the mechanical ileus had resolved. The colon is now distended with gas, and the jejunum is devoid of content and normal in size. (C) In the initial radiographs, the stomach is dilated with gas, and mechanical ileus is present with a mixed population of small intestinal diameter ranging from normal to severely dilated with gas (white bars). In the mid-ventral abdomen, a single jejunal segment has heterogeneous soft tissue content. Based on the stable condition of the dog, a decision was made to continue fasting and fluid therapy and repeat the radiographs. (D) This radiograph was performed 8 hours later, and the abnormal content had passed, and the mechanical ileus had resolved. There is considerably less gas dilation of the stomach. The cecum and colon are now distended with gas (traced with white line), and the jejunum is devoid of content and normal in size (arrows).

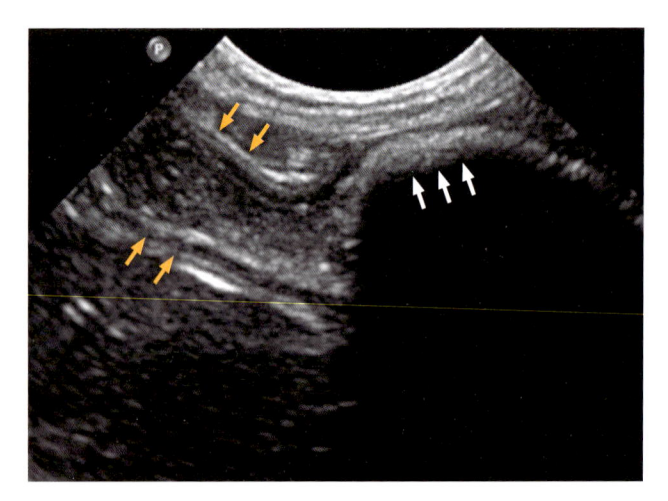

Fig. 27.11 A single segment of jejunum is moderately dilated with fluid (orange arrows) and there is a focal expansion of the segment due to an intraluminal object. The object is curvilinear with a strong distal acoustic shadow (white arrows). An intestinal foreign body was removed surgically that was causing mechanical ileus.

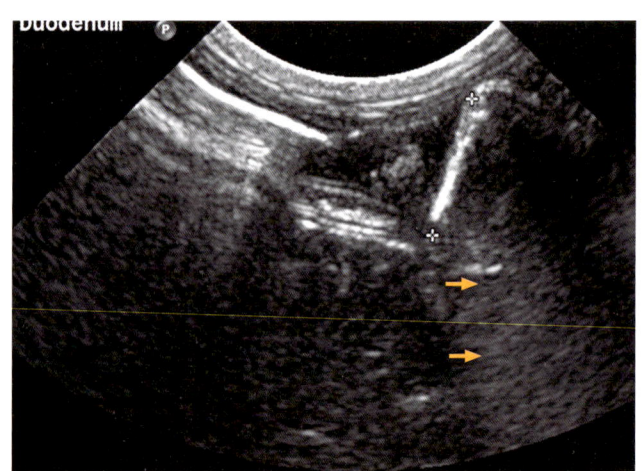

Fig. 27.12 An intraluminal structure is present in the duodenum that has a straight border (between calipers), and a distal acoustic artifact is present. The acoustic artifact is not as hypoechoic as in fig. 27.11 as the material is not as solid to create a clean hypoechoic shadow. The foreign body was causing mechanical ileus and gastric outflow obstruction. A piece of foam was removed surgically.

CHAPTER **27** The small intestine

surface, peach pits are irregular, and bones generally have a smooth regular surface. Linear foreign bodies can sometimes be identified in plicated segments of small bowel as a thin hyperechoic structure with the small intestines bunched along it (**figs. 27.14-27.17**). Much like radiography, unclear or equivocal findings regarding hyperechoic luminal content can be re-examined on a follow-up ultrasound examination.

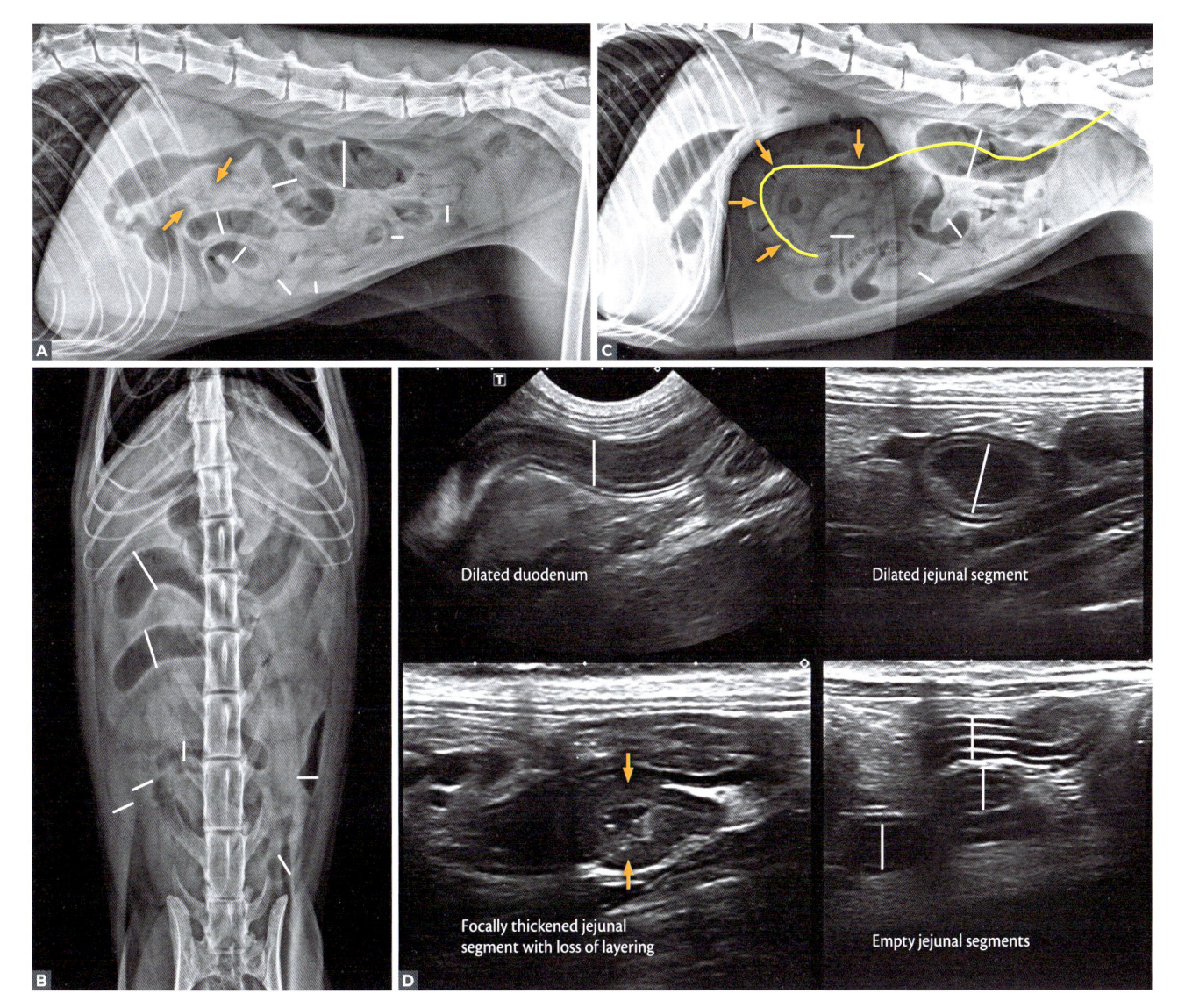

Fig. 27.13 (**A**) Lateral abdominal radiograph of a ten-year-old female spayed cat that presented with acute vomiting and collapse. There is a mixed population of small intestinal diameter present (white bars), with the proximal jejunal segments moderately gas dilated and the more caudal segments mildly dilated with gas or fluid opacity. There is a segment of bowel with a soft tissue granular content (orange arrows) in the mid-abdomen that cannot be differentiated from feces in the large intestine. (**B**) Ventrodorsal abdominal radiograph of a ten-year-old female spayed cat presented with acute vomiting and collapse. There is a mixed population of small intestinal diameter present (white bars), with the proximal jejunal segments moderately gas dilated and the more caudal segments mildly dilated with gas or fluid opacity. (**C**) Spoon compression was performed. The granular content is now identified as fecal balls in the transverse colon (orange arrows), and the path of the colon can be traced (yellow line). The mixed population of jejunal segment diameter remains, and the diagnosis is mechanical ileus. An ultrasound examination was performed. (**D**) Ultrasound examination of the same cat showed a mixed population of dilated fluid-filled duodenum and proximal jejunal segments and many empty caudal segments (white bars). A focal narrowing of the lumen was present and associated with concentric wall thickening and loss of layering (orange arrows). Exploratory laparotomy was performed, and a stricture was identified, causing mechanical obstruction.

SECTION V ABDOMEN

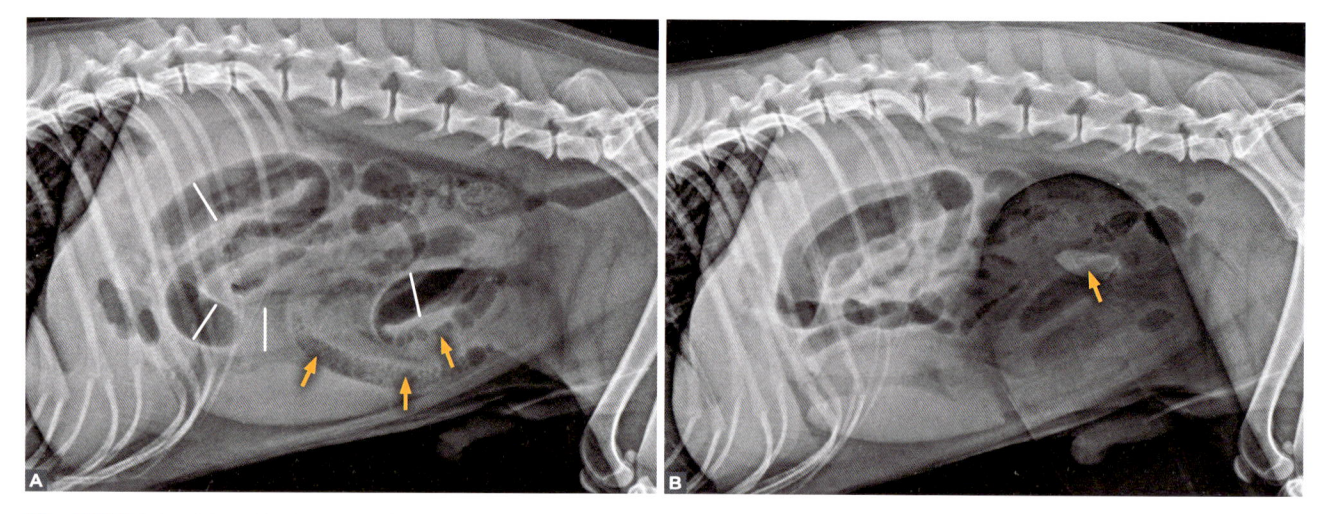

Fig. 27.14 (**A**) Left lateral radiographs of an eight-year-old Jack Russel Terrier presented with four days of vomiting and 24 hours of anorexia. A mechanical ileus pattern is present with a mixed population of jejunal dilation ranging from severe to normal diameters (white bars). There is frothy gas and fluid in a few of the mid-ventral abdominal segments (arrows). (**B**) Spoon compression was applied, and a mineral opaque intestinal foreign body (arrow) was identified in the small intestines, which was subsequently removed surgically and was found to be a hard rubber object.

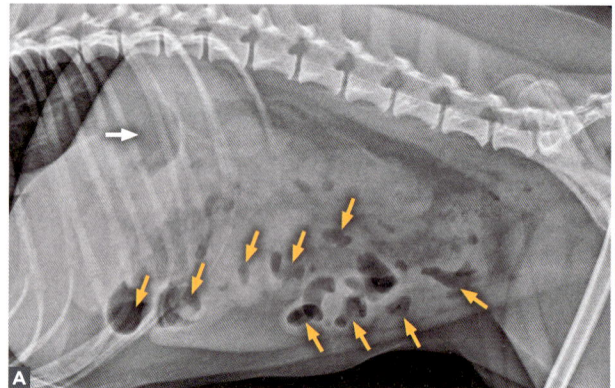

Fig. 27.15 (**A**) Left lateral radiograph of a small breed dog with acute and persistent vomiting for three days. The stomach contains some gas (white arrow). The jejunum has an abnormal shape with bunching and fragmented irregularly shaped gas content (orange arrows). This is a linear foreign body. (**B**) Ventrodorsal radiograph. The stomach contains some gas (white arrow). The jejunum has an abnormal shape with bunching and fragmented irregularly shaped gas content (orange arrows). This is a linear foreign body.

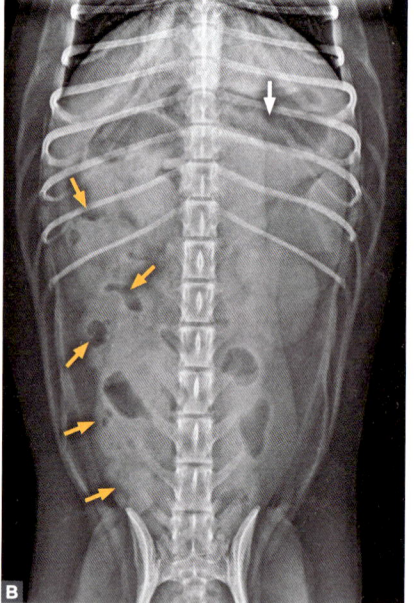

Complicated forms of ileus

Complicated types of ileus include bowel perforation with peritonitis, free gas in the abdominal cavity, and bowel ischemia due to thromboembolism, intussusception, or volvulus at the root of the mesentery. Linear foreign bodies can also lead to a complicated form of ileus that can lead to ischemia and perforation. The presence of pneumoperitoneum together with abdominal effusion on an abdominal radiograph should alert the clinician to the fact that bowel perforation has occurred. The detection of free intra-abdominal gas may require the use of ventrodorsal horizontal beam radiography with the patient in left lateral recumbency. Free air can be detected just under the right abdominal wall and lateral to the duodenum. Linear foreign bodies produce characteristic changes on abdominal radiographs in both dogs and cats (**figs. 27.15-27.17**). The small intestinal segments appear convoluted and gathered or clumped together at one site (usually in the mid-right abdomen), and intraluminal fragmented gas bubbles appear asymmetrical and irregularly shaped. It is important to recognize the difference between hyperperistalsis and linear foreign body as the two can be confusing. Hyperperistalsis due to spasms, such as with enteritis, can create a corrugated or string of pearls appearance (fig. 27.16). A string of pearls pattern has no bunching, and the gas patterns are continuous rather than irregular and fragmented. Ultrasonographically, the small intestinal segments will appear gathered up with the linear foreign material binding them together (figs. 27.18 and 27.19). The surrounding

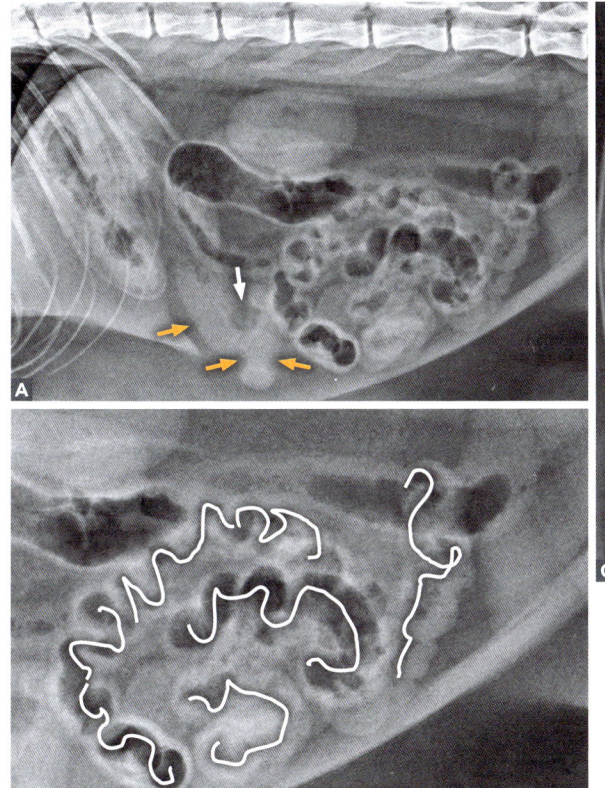

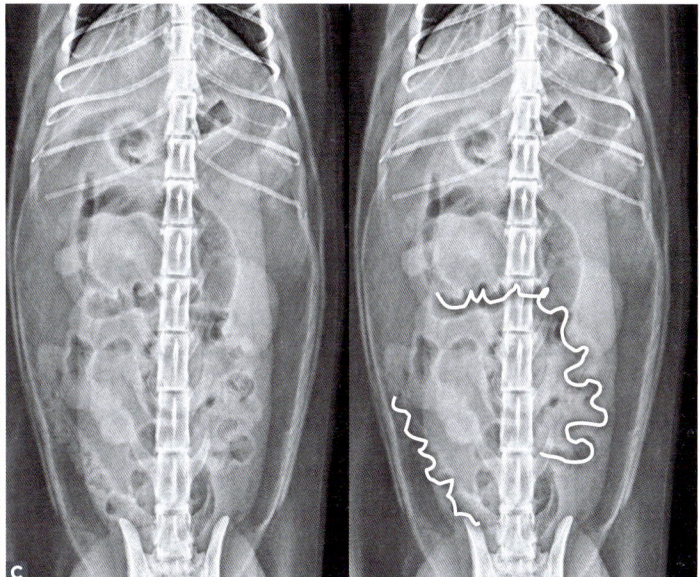

Fig. 27.16 (A) Right lateral abdominal radiograph of a three-year-old cat with acute vomiting for 48 hours and now anorexia. The stomach contains mild gas, and the duodenum is dilated and has an irregular undulant shape and fragmented gas bubbles (orange arrows). (B) Magnified image of the jejunum. The jejunum has generalized plication recognized by bunching and fragmented gas content (white line drawing). Fragmented gas appears as irregularly shaped luminal gas that does not have a tubular course typical of normal jejunum. (C) Ventrodorsal radiograph. The stomach contains mild gas, and the duodenum is dilated and has an irregular shape and gas content. The jejunum has generalized plication recognized by bunching and fragmented gas content. Fragmented gas appears as irregularly shaped luminal gas that does not have a tubular course typical of normal jejunum (white line drawing).

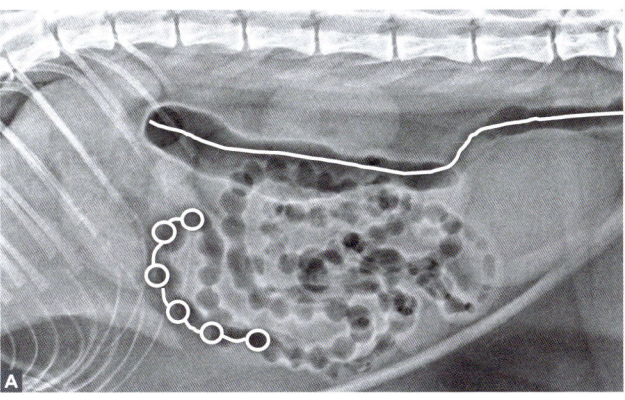

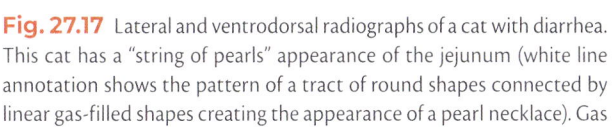

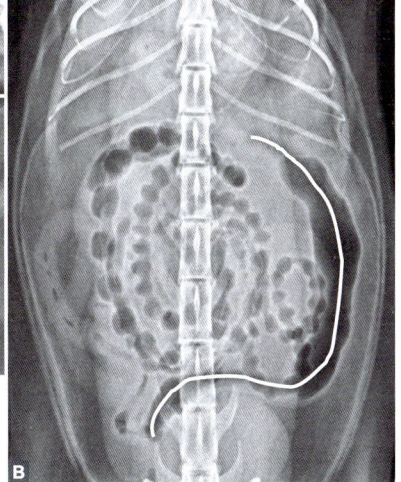

Fig. 27.17 Lateral and ventrodorsal radiographs of a cat with diarrhea. This cat has a "string of pearls" appearance of the jejunum (white line annotation shows the pattern of a tract of round shapes connected by linear gas-filled shapes creating the appearance of a pearl necklace). Gas fills the colon, which is devoid of feces. Hyperperistalsis can create this appearance of the jejunum that can be misinterpreted as plication. The jejunum is not bunched, and the gas in the lumen is continuous, not fragmented as with a linear foreign body. The path of the gas-filled colon is shown with a white line.

SECTION V ABDOMEN

mesentery should be examined for increased echogenicity and free fluid, which could be indicative of rupture. Figure **27.20** shows the use of spoon compression to aid in the diagnosis of linear foreign material in the jejunum that is anchored in the gastric antrum.

Volvulus or mesenteric thromboembolism can be recognized by the presence of generalized, severely dilated, and gas-filled jejunal segments (**fig. 27.21**). Generalized dilation due to severe functional ileus or end jejunal/ileal obstruction can be difficult to differentiate radiographically, and the dog's clinical signs play an important role in therapeutic decision-making. The dogs in **fig. 27.7** and **27.21** look similar radiographically but have different clinical status. The dog in **fig. 27.21** has more severe generalized dilation due to mesenteric volvulus, while the dog in **fig. 27.7** had functional ileus and was clinically stable.

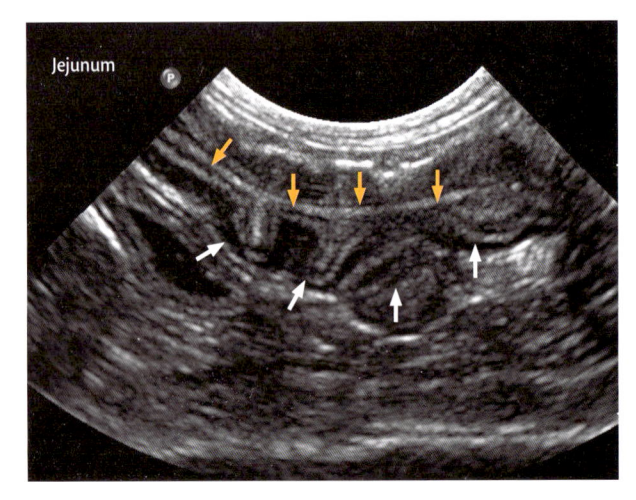

Fig. 27.18 Ultrasound image of a linear foreign body. A thin hyperechoic structure (white arrows) is centrally located within a section of jejunum that is bunched and plicated over it (orange arrows).

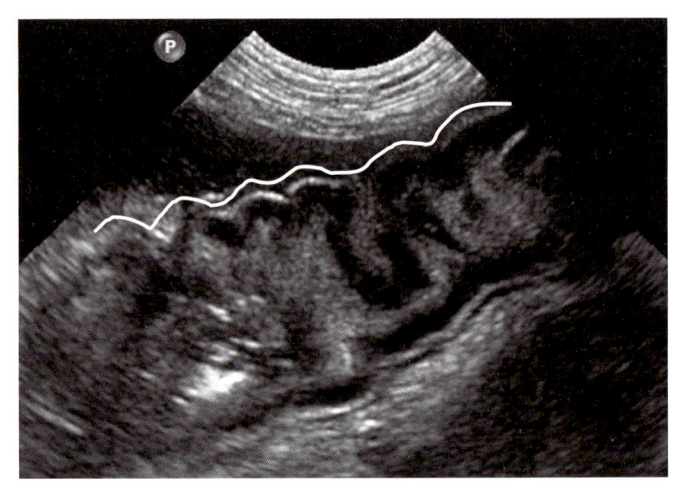

Fig. 27.19 Ultrasound image of a dog with duodenitis secondary to non-specific gastroenteritis. The intestinal segment is corrugated: it has a tubular course that is undulating, but there is no plication of string in the lumen (the undulating white line shows this shape). This pattern can be confused with a linear foreign body. The corrugation is often secondary to spams that come and go. Observing the segment over time can help differentiate the shape change as dynamic vs. static. Pancreatitis is another cause of spasms of the duodenum that can cause corrugation.

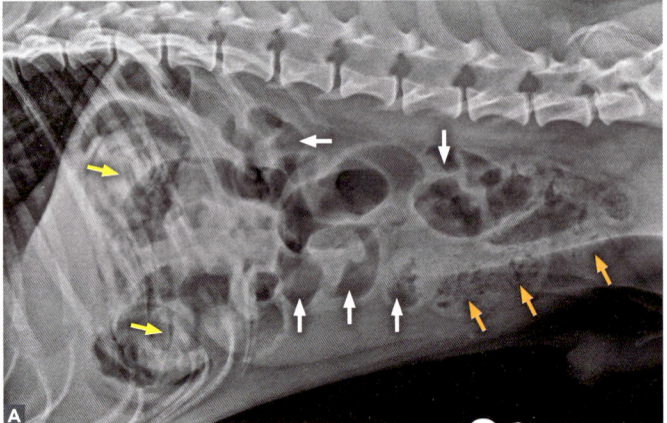

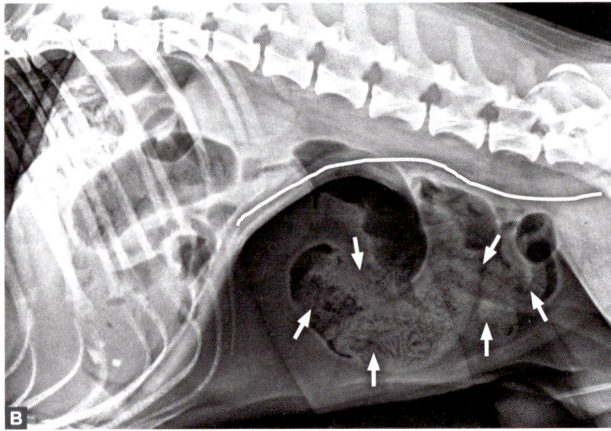

Fig. 27.20 (**A**) A four-year-old neutered male Boston Terrier dog after vomiting for two days. The dog was fasted, and radiographs were performed. There are heterogeneous soft tissue conglomerates in the stomach (yellow arrows); the gas-filled jejunal segments are dilated, and some are plicated (white arrows). In the mid-ventral abdomen, there is a large volume of heterogeneous soft tissue content in the intestine that is difficult to assign to a specific small vs. large bowel (orange arrows). (**B**) Spoon compression showed the abnormal content to be isolated to multiple small intestinal segments (white arrows) and aided in differentiating this content from the large bowel. The colon is dorsal to this region and devoid of content (white line). The diagnosis was a linear foreign body anchored in the pylorus at surgery.

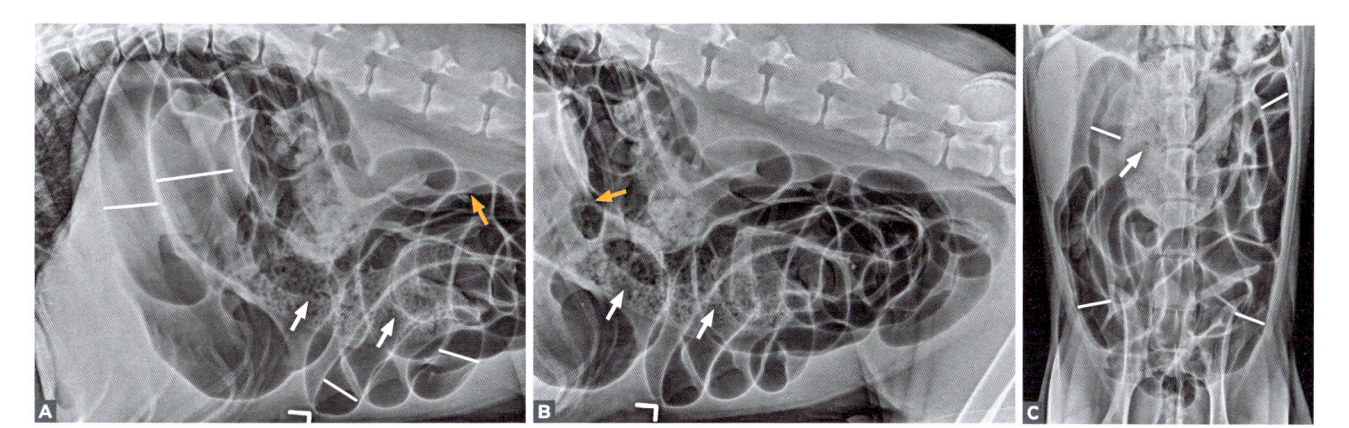

Fig. 27.21 Left lateral radiographs of the cranial (**A**) and caudal (**B**) abdomen of a four-year-old Great Dane presented with bloating, collapse, and hypovolemia. The entire small intestinal tract is severely dilated with gas (white bars show some of the intestines as an example, and the pattern is generalized). The colon cannot be discerned from the small intestines, and there is a mid-cranial segment with granular content (white arrows). This pattern has differentials of end jejunal or ileal obstruction and mesenteric volvulus. Due to the dog's clinical status, exploratory surgery was performed, and a mesenteric volvulus was diagnosed. (**C**) Ventrodorsal radiographs of the caudal abdomen show the entire small intestinal tract severely dilated with gas as in the lateral images. The colon cannot be discerned from the small intestines, and there is a mid-abdominal segment of intestine with granular content (white arrows). This pattern has differentials of end jejunal or ileal obstruction and mesenteric volvulus. Due to the dog's clinical status, exploratory surgery was performed, and a mesenteric volvulus was diagnosed.

Infiltrative small intestinal disease

Localized mural infiltrations due to inflammation, infection, or neoplasia can narrow the intestinal lumen and lead to partial or complete obstructions. Clinical signs tend to be more chronic compared with foreign body obstruction. Some degree of intestinal dilation is often resent, and solid foreign material such as small stones can collect proximal to the stricture. Ultrasonographically, neoplastic infiltrates produce intestinal wall thickening, often with a loss of wall layering. Lymphoma is the most common intestinal tumor in cats but also occurs frequently in dogs. It commonly leads to either a symmetrical or asymmetrical, transmural, circumferential thickening. The wall layers are difficult to identify, and the entire wall appears hypo- to anechoic. The infiltration of the intestinal wall may be solitary, diffuse, or multifocal, and regional lymph nodes may be enlarged. However, complete intestinal obstruction often does not occur. Intestinal carcinoma often produces a solitary intestinal mass, as can polyps, leiomyomas, or leiomyosarcomas. Carcinomas tend to be annular, irregular infiltrations that invade the lumen and cause obstructions and have more heterogeneous or complex echogenicity of the infiltrated wall. Granulomatous infiltrations due to fungal infections may also cause diffuse or focal infiltrations of the bowel wall and are difficult to distinguish from neoplasia ultrasonographically. Histoplasmosis, for example, can produce localized and severe wall infiltrations that resemble lymphoma. Feline gastrointestinal eosinophilic sclerosing fibroplasia is an inflammatory disease that causes wall thickening and loss of layering in the stomach, duodenum, jejunum, and colon and has been described as having similar sonographic features to neoplasia or fungal infiltration.[4] Because the ultrasonographic appearance of the intestinal wall alone is not sufficient for a definitive diagnosis, either full-thickness biopsies, ultrasound-guided percutaneous biopsies, or fine-needle aspirates of the bowel wall are required for a definitive diagnosis of wall infiltrative diseases that thicken the wall or disrupt wall layering. Figures **27.22** through **22.29** show normal and abnormal ultrasound examples of jejunal abnormalities.

SECTION V ABDOMEN

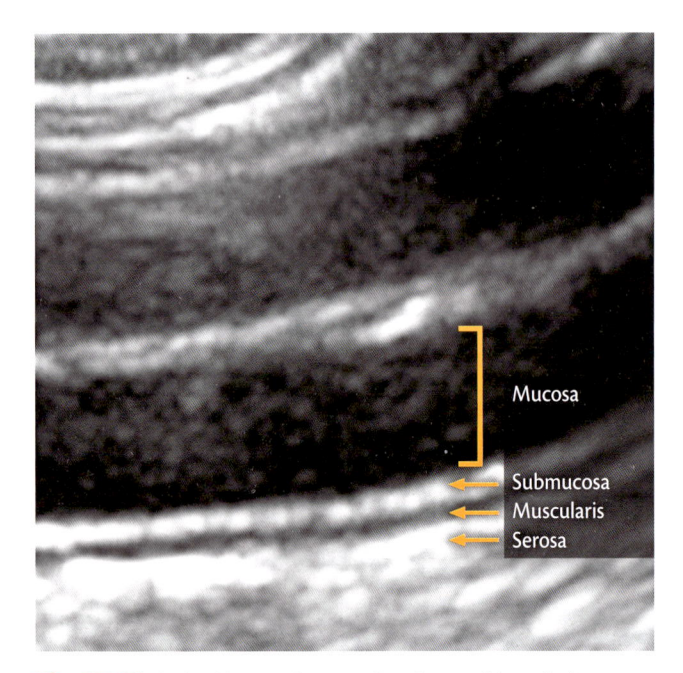

Fig. 27.22 Sagittal image of a normal canine small intestinal segment using a 7.5 MHz curved array probe. The muscularis is hypoechoic, shown with a bracket. The outer three layers are alternating hyperechoic (submucosa), hypoechoic (muscularis), and the hyperechoic serosa. The outer three layers are thin and approximately the same size. The mucosa is the thickest layer. The lumen is empty and appears as a thin hyperechoic interface.

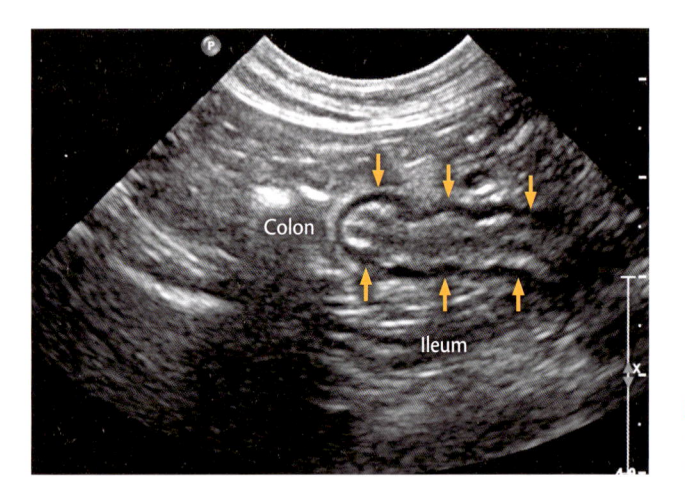

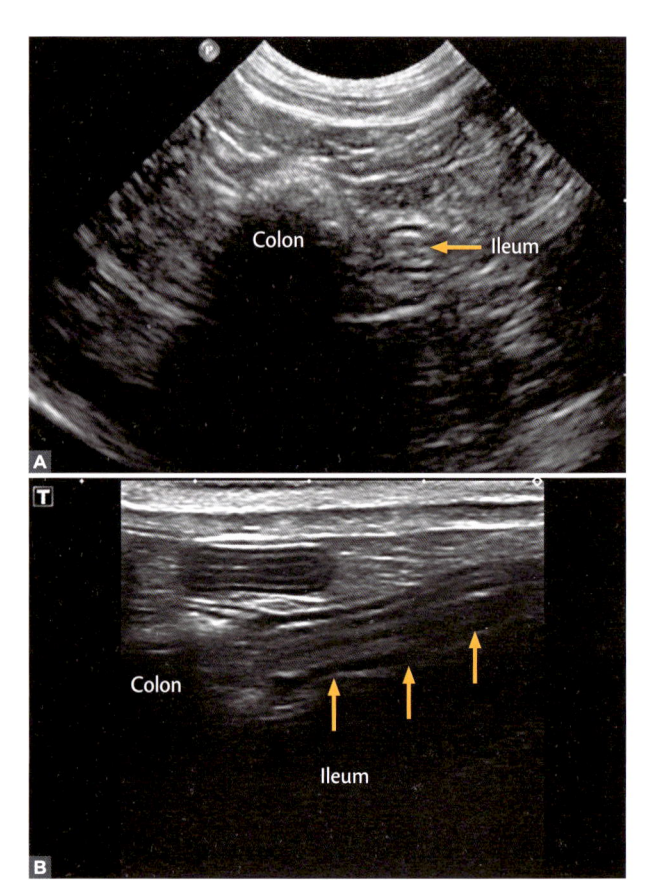

Fig. 27.23 Transverse (**A**) and sagittal plane (**B**) images of the ileocecocolic junction showing the appearance of the normal canine ileum. The ileum has the same wall layering as the jejunum, but the muscularis layer is more prominent. In transverse, the ileum has a rosette appearance (**A**).

Fig. 27.24 Sagittal image of the normal cat ileum. The ileum is shorter in cats compared to dogs but has a similar sonographic appearance with a more prominent muscularis compared to the jejunal layering.

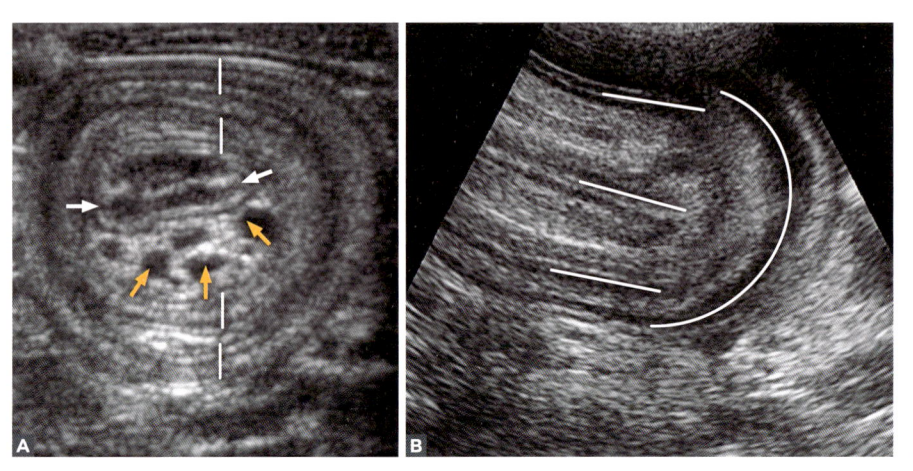

Fig. 27.25 A four-month-old Boxer dog with chronic diarrhea presented with acute vomiting. A soft mass was palpated in the mid-abdomen. The transverse (**A**) and sagittal (**B**) ultrasound images were diagnostic for jejunal intussusception. (**A**) There are concentric rings of intestine (white bars show stacked intestinal walls in a concentric pattern) with a central contracted segment of intestine (dotted arrow) together with many mesenteric vessels (white arrows). (**B**) The sagittal image appears like a pitchfork or trident with a blunted or curvilinear shape (white line) at one end and the stacked intestinal segments aligned at the other (white bars).

CHAPTER **27** The small intestine

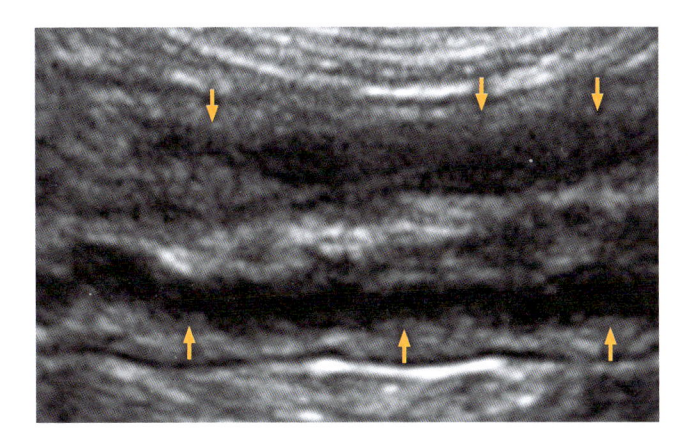

Fig. 27.26 Sagittal ultrasound image of a small intestinal segment in a dog with *Heterobilharzia americana* infection. This infection causes pathology at the submucosa, and in this dog, the submucosa has a common finding of thickening and irregularity (arrows).

Fig. 27.27 Examples of focal transmural hypoechoic loss of wall layering (arrows) of the jejunum in some examples in cats that had histological samples taken from the lesions. (**A**) Sagittal image of a cat with mast cell tumor with a hypoechoic infiltrative mass of the jejunal wall disrupting the wall layering. (**B**) Transmural hypoechoic loss of layering in a cat with histoplasmosis. (**C**) Focal transmural hypoechoic severe thickening with loss of wall layering in a cat with feline idiopathic eosinophilic sclerosing fibroplasia. (**D**) Focal transmural thickening that is hypoechoic and no wall layering, which was diagnosed as lymphoma. Transmural loss of layering is not specific for a specific etiology, and the diagnosis requires tissue sampling.

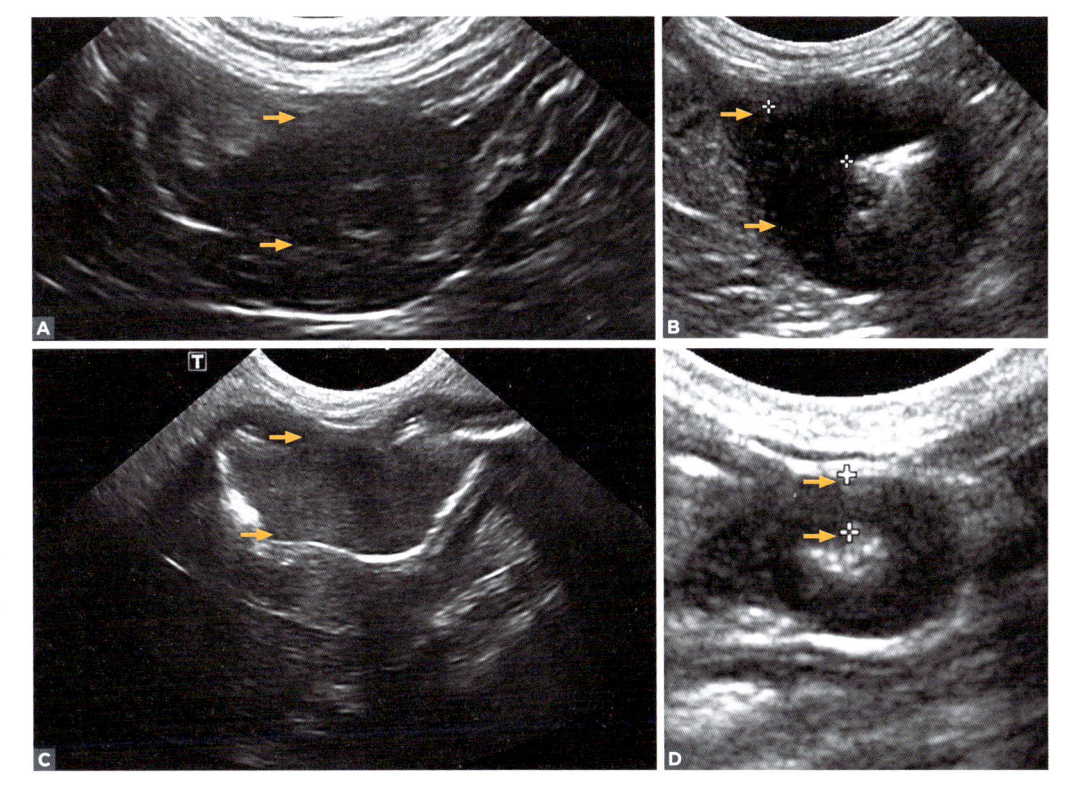

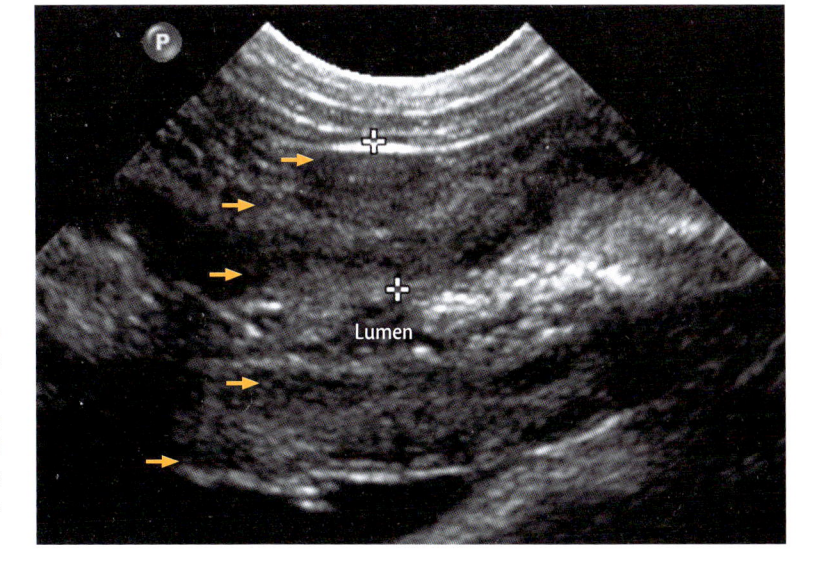

Fig. 27.28 A two-year-old Labrador Retriever dog with chronic diarrhea and muscle wasting. The sagittal plane ultrasound image of a small intestinal segment with transmural disrupted layering and thickening (6 mm between calipers) was diagnosed with pythiosis. This is a transmural pyogranulomatous infection by *P. insidiosum* that creates alternating bands and random arrangement of the echogenicity of the intestinal wall (arrows).

465

SECTION V ABDOMEN

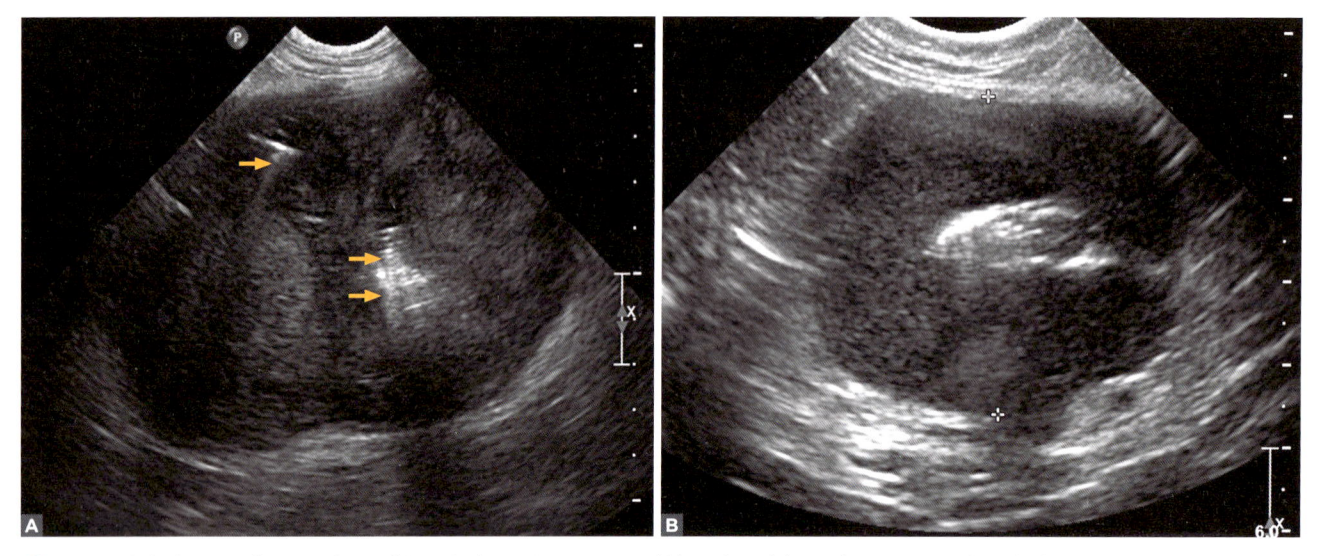

Fig. 27.29 (**A**) Ultrasound image of a small intestinal mass in a ten-year-old large breed dog with vomiting and weight loss. A large 5 cm mass is present in the jejunum that has a heterogenous echostructure with multiple central gas reverberations. This was an emphysematous intestinal carcinoma. (**B**) A similar large jejunal mass in a cat due to B-cell lymphoma. Large intestinal masses can appear similar regardless of their etiology and require tissue sampling to confirm the cause.

Chronic diarrhea and small intestinal disease

Survey radiographs are often nonspecific, and gastrointestinal contrast studies are often unrewarding in patients with chronic diarrhea without vomiting. For detecting intestinal wall infiltrates, ultrasound is superior to survey and contrast radiography but has its own limitations in that it does often not help to identify the underlying cause of diarrhea. However, ultrasound remains a screening tool to assess weight loss and detect gastrointestinal masses as potential causes for gastrointestinal signs. The assessment of the intestinal wall for diffuse disease in dogs and cats with chronic diarrhea rests on the evaluation of wall thickness and layering and evidence of comorbidities (hepatobiliary, pancreatic, and lymphadenopathy). Recently, investigators have tried correlating intestinal wall thickness in healthy dogs with body weight. In that report, the authors suggested normal duodenal wall thickness to be <5.1 mm for dogs up to 20 kg, <5.3 mm for dogs between 20 and 29.9 kg, and <6.0 mm for dogs over 30 kg, and normal values for jejunal wall thickness of <4.1 mm for dogs up to 20 kg, <4.4 mm for dogs between 20 and 39.9 kg, and <4.7 mm for dogs over 40 kg.[5]

Several gastrointestinal diseases can lead to diffuse infiltration of the small intestinal wall. There are no known specific sonographic features that allow differentiation of various infiltrative diseases. The mucosal, submucosal, and muscularis layers are most commonly affected. Figures **27.30** through **27.34** show examples of intestinal abnormalities in dogs and cats. The mucosa may also exhibit alterations in echogenicity varying in severity from diffuse pinpoint hyperechogenic foci to generalized hyperechogenicity. Severe mucosal thickening with increased echogenicity may be seen in animals with protein-losing enteropathy and

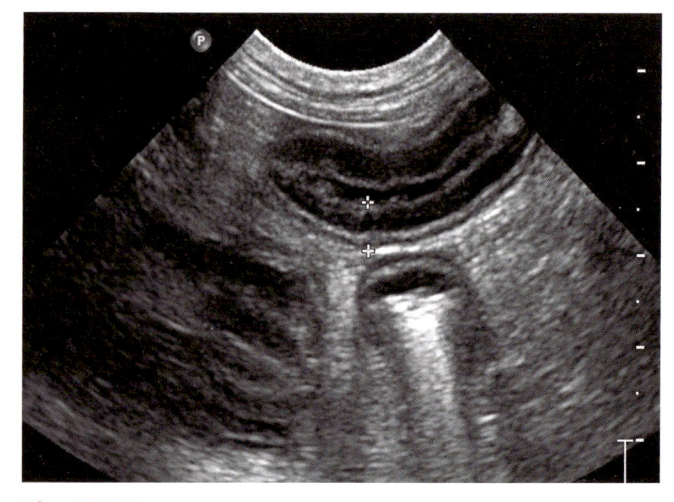

Fig. 27.30 A four-year-old large breed dog with chronic diarrhea and weight loss. Ultrasound images of the jejunum show generalized mild wall thickened (4.8 mm) with normal wall layering and variable low volume fluid and gas content. The dog had intestinal biopsies taken and was diagnosed with severe, chronic lymphocytic plasmacytic enteritis.

CHAPTER 27 The small intestine

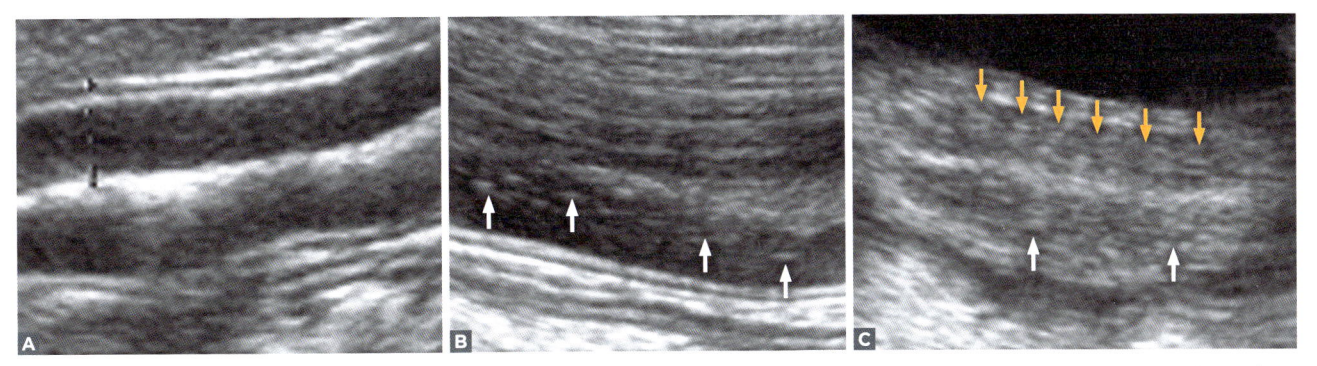

Fig. 27.31 Ultrasound images of the variable appearance of the small intestinal mucosa in dogs. (**A**) A normal mucosa that is homogenous hypoechoic. (**B**) Multiple small hyperechoic speckles (white arrows) in the mucosa. (**C**) Perpendicular hyperechoic striations in the mucosa (orange arrows). All three dogs have histologically diagnosed inflammatory infiltrates. The dog in (**C**) also had lymphangiectasia.

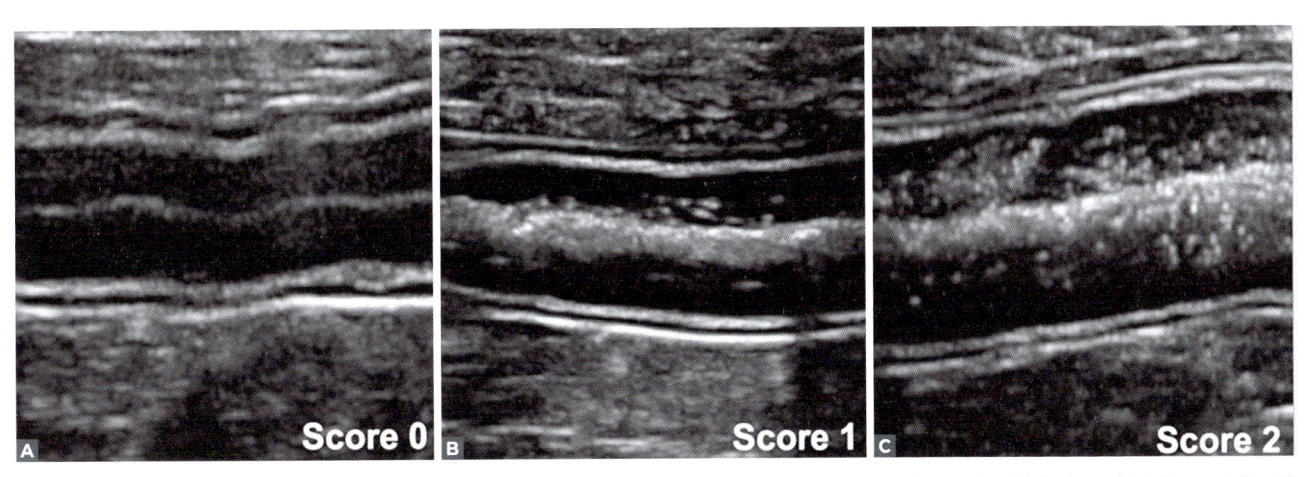

Fig. 27.32 The three ultrasound images are of the same healthy dog that is (**A**) fasted, (**B**) after a low-fat meal, and (**C**) after a high-fat meal. (**B, C**) Variable amounts of mucosal speckles appear after eating, which can be confused with pathologies such as inflammatory bowel disease or lymphangiectasia. Mucosal echogenicity is best interpreted when dogs are fasted.

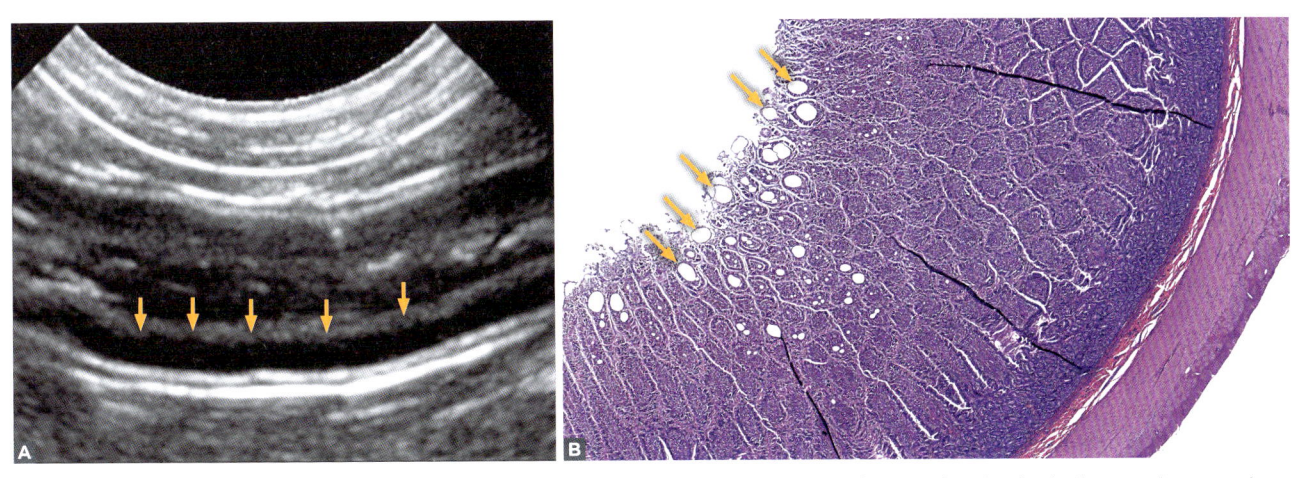

Fig. 27.33 (**A**) Sagittal ultrasound image of a dog that has recently eaten. (**B**) A histology section from another dog that had eaten prior to specimen collection shows that there are fat vacuoles in the tips of the villi (orange arrows) that correspond to the hyperechoic rim at the mucosa-lumen interface. This is a normal feature in dogs that have recently eaten a meal prior to the ultrasound examination.

467

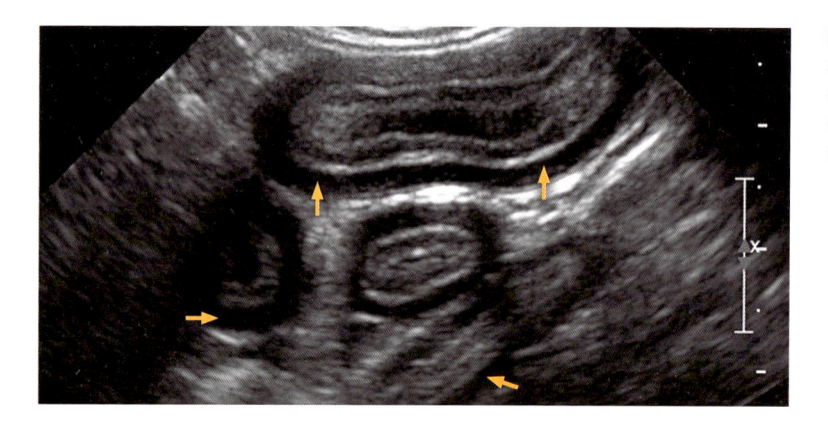

Fig. 27.34 Jejunal ultrasound image of a five-year-old cat with chronic vomiting and weight loss. The muscularis layer was severely thickened in all jejunal segments (arrows), and the total intestinal wall thickened at 3.5 mm. The cat was diagnosed with intestinal T-cell lymphoma.

lymphangiectasia. In addition, the small intestine generally shows some dilation with fluid and gas and may have a decreased motility or a rigid appearance.

Thickening of the intestinal wall or a single layer due to inflammatory disease is difficult to differentiate between fungal or neoplastic infiltration.[6] For example, a thickened muscularis layer alone can occur with either inflammatory or neoplastic infiltration or can be due to smooth muscle hypertrophy.[7] Lymph nodes may appear rounded, heterogeneous, and possibly show target lesions in patients with either disease. Mycotic diseases, such as histoplasmosis, pythiosis, or cryptococcosis, can produce localized infiltrative disease that is sonographically similar to that of neoplasia. However, neoplasia is considered to produce more disruption of wall layering compared to inflammatory disease. Sonographic abnormalities in animals with alimentary lymphoma may include thickening of the gastric or intestinal wall, loss of normal layering, a hypoechoic mass associated with the intestinal wall diffuse muscularis thickening, and abdominal lymphadenomegaly.[8]

Cats with clinical signs of small bowel disease that have diffuse small intestinal wall thickening >3 mm have been shown to correspond to histopathological diseases such as inflammatory infiltrates, lymphoma, or a combination. In these two diseases, thickening of the muscularis contributes to most of the total wall thickness.[9]

References

1. Ciasca TC, David FH, Lamb CR. Does measurement of small intestinal diameter increase diagnostic accuracy of radiography in dogs with suspected intestinal obstruction? *Vet Radiol Ultrasound* 54:207-211, 2013.
2. Miles S, Gaschen L, Presley T, Liu CC, Granger LA. Influence of repeat abdominal radiographs on the resolution of mechanical obstruction and gastrointestinal foreign material in dogs and cats. *Vet Radiol Ultrasound* 62:282-288, 2021.
3. Husnik R, Gaschen FP, Fletcher JM, Gaschen L. Ultrasonographic assessment of the effect of metoclopramide, erythromycin, and exenatide on solid-phase gastric emptying in healthy cats. *J Vet Intern Med* 34:1440-1446, 2020.
4. Weissman A, Pennick D, Webster C, Hecht S, Keating J, et al. Ultrasonographic and clinicopathological features of feline gastrointestinal eosinophilic sclerosing fibroplasia in four cats. *J Feline Med Surg* 15:148-154, 2013.
5. Delaney F, O'Brien RT, Waller K. Ultrasound evaluation of small bowel thickness compared to weight in normal dogs. *Vet Radiol Ultrasound* 44:577-580, 2003.
6. Graham JP, Newell SM, Roberts GD, Lester NV. Ultrasonographic features of canine gastrointestinal pythiosis. *Vet Radiol Ultrasound* 41:273-277, 2000.
7. Daniaux LA, Laurenson MP, Marks SL, Moore PF, Taylor SL. Ultrasonographic thickening of the muscularis propria in feline small intestinal small cell T-cell lymphoma and inflammatory bowel disease. *J Feline Med Surg* 16:89-98, 2014.
8. Grooters AM, Biller DS, Ward H, Miyabayashi T. Ultrasonographic appearance of feline alimentary lymphoma. *Vet Radiol Ultrasound* 35:468-472, 1994.
9. Norsworthy GD, Estep JS, Hollinger C, Steiner JM, et al. Prevalence and underlying causes of histologic abnormalities in cats suspected to have chronic small bowel disease: 300 cases (2008-2013). *J Am Vet Med Assoc* 247:629-635, 2015.

CHAPTER 28

The large intestine

Lorrie Gaschen

> **KEY POINTS**
>
> - Radiography is important to rule out mechanical obstruction of the colon due to abdominal or intrapelvic masses and pelvic canal narrowing.
> - Computed tomography or magnetic resonance imaging are often necessary to investigate mechanical obstruction of the colorectoanal region within the pelvis.
> - Radiography screens for masses associated with the large bowel and associated stenosis and obstipation.
> - Ultrasound is best for assessing loss of wall layering and thickening of the large bowel seen with infiltrative infectious and neoplastic diseases.
> - Colonic torsion and severe colitis can both cause severe gas dilation of the large bowel and look similar.
> - A focal point of narrowing of the severely distended colon is a sign of colonic torsion.
> - Computed tomography and barium enema can be used to diagnose colonic torsion.
> - Congenital anomalies of the rectoanal region usually require contrast studies to diagnose and identify fistulas between the genitourinary tract and large bowel.

Lateral and ventrodorsal radiographs of the pelvic region are an important part of the diagnostic workup in dogs and cats with constipation, hematochezia, and/or painful defecation. Abnormalities of the colon, such as obstruction, megacolon, and constipation can usually be recognized radiographically. Inflammatory disease, parasitic infestation, and dietary hypersensitivity are difficult to diagnose radiographically or sonographically when they affect the colon. Ultrasound is used to trace and examine the colon from the ileocecocolic junction to the pelvic inlet. The rectoanal region can also be examined via a perianal perineal window at the tail base. CT can be used to examine the full extent of the large bowel and to investigate more complex pathology such as colonic torsion or for presurgical planning of masses. CT and MRI are especially useful in diagnosing intrapelvic pathology at the colorectal junction and rectum either due to infiltrative disease, trauma, or a mass effect causing obstruction due to prostatomegaly, lymphadenopathy, or invasive neoplasia from the anal sacs.

Normal large intestine

The normal canine large intestine begins at the ileocecocolic junction in the right mid-abdomen, continues as the ascending colon along a short path in the right cranial abdomen, and curves leftward caudal to the stomach as the transverse colon. The descending colon courses from cranial

SECTION V ABDOMEN

to caudal in the left abdomen (**fig. 28.1**). At the pelvic inlet, the colorectal junction and rectum continue into the pelvic canal, and the rectoanal junction is caudal to the pelvic canal, then finishes as the colorectal junction. The anatomy of the colon forms a "shepherd's hook" or question mark shape on ventrodorsal radiographs. Cats have similar large bowel anatomy, although the cecum is not a radiographically visible structure in cats (**fig. 28.2**). The descending colon location is also variable. It can be shifted into the right side of the abdomen and have a sigmoid course, especially when filled with feces.

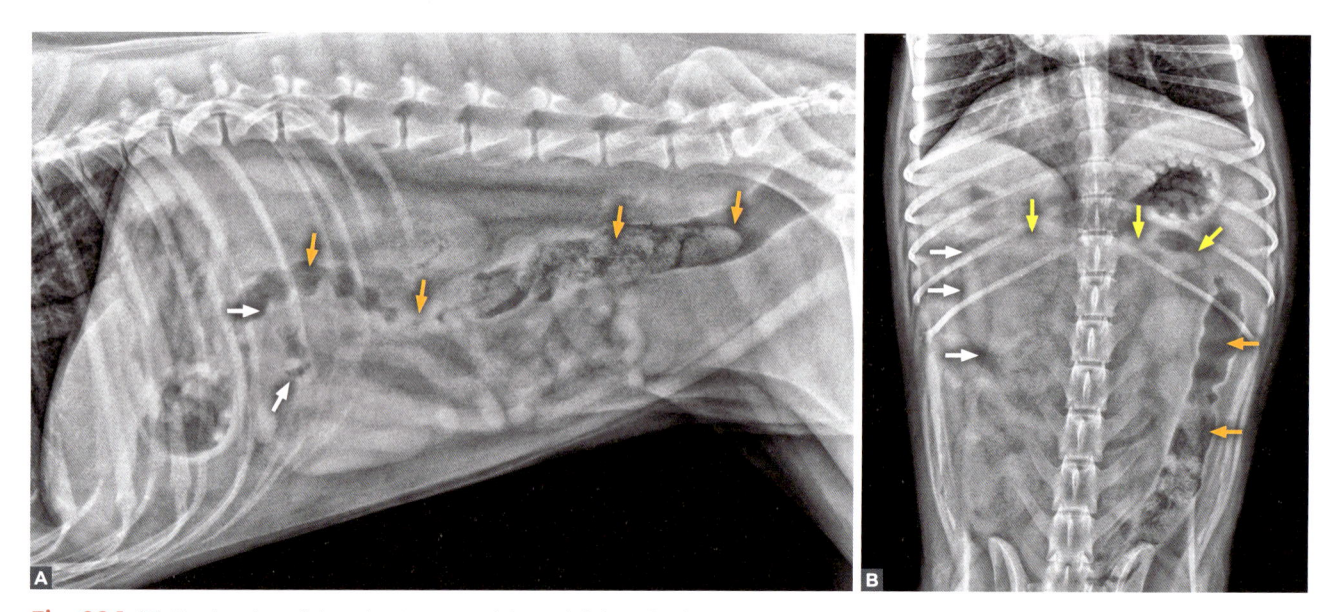

Fig. 28.1 (**A**) The location of the colon in a normal dog. A left lateral radiograph shows the transverse colon (white arrows) and the descending colon (orange arrows) coursing from cranial to caudal in the mid-abdomen. The transverse colon is immediately caudal to the greater curvature of the stomach. (**B**) Normal colon. The ascending colon (white arrows) courses from the mid-abdomen cranially, where it turns toward the midline caudal to the stomach to become the transverse colon (yellow arrows). The descending colon courses from cranial to caudal in the left abdomen (orange arrows).

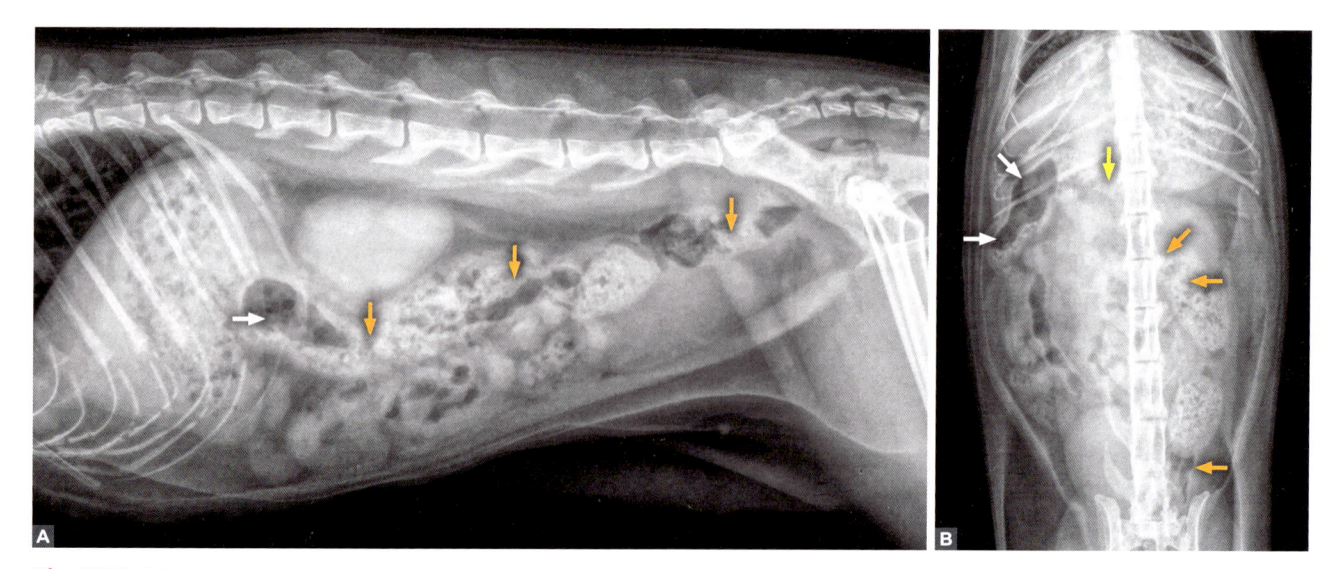

Fig. 28.2 (**A**) Lateral radiograph of the cat's abdomen showing the normal location of the colon. The ascending colon is superimposed with the descending colon in the mid-abdomen, and the two cannot be distinctly differentiated due to superimposition. The transverse colon is located immediately caudal to the stomach (white arrow) and continues from cranial to caudal in the mid-abdomen as the descending segment (orange arrows). The cat is not fasted, and there is soft tissue content in the stomach and some throughout the jejunum. (**B**) Ventrodorsal radiograph of the cat's abdomen showing the normal location of the colon. The ascending colon is located in the cranial right abdomen (white arrows), where it curves to the midline and courses caudal to the stomach (yellow arrow), and continues into the left colon as the descending segment (orange arrows).

CHAPTER **28** The large intestine

On ultrasound, the layering of the colonic wall is seen as alternating bands of hyperattenuating and hypoattenuating thin and equally thick layers consisting of the outer serosa and moving inward the muscularis, submucosa, and the mucosa, the same as the small intestine (**figs. 28.3** and **28.4**). When distended, the wall of the large bowel should have a three-layered appearance and a thickness of 1-2 mm. The empty colon can create a confusing ultrasound image as the folds of the wall are collapsed and can be mistaken for wall thickening (**fig. 28.5**). The ileocecocolic junction is identified by locating the ileum in the transverse and sagittal plane and tracing it back to the large bowel usually recognized by its thin layering and gas content (**fig. 28.6**). The cecum will contain gas in dogs in most instances and be difficult to differentiate

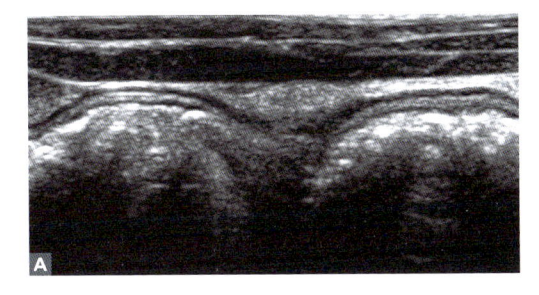

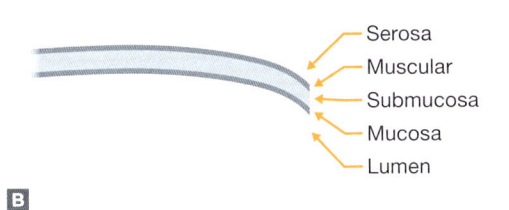

Fig. 28.3 Normal ultrasound image of the colon wall with a schematic showing the wall layering.

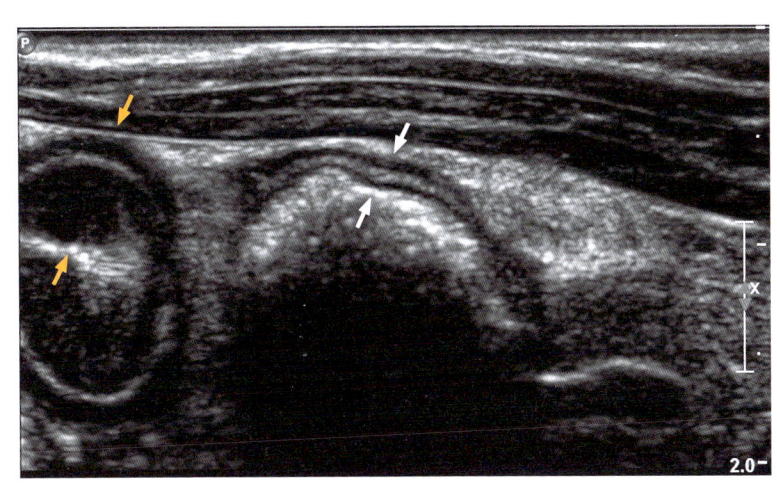

Fig. 28.4 Ultrasound image showing the normal layering of the small intestine (orange arrows) compared to the colonic wall (white arrows).

Fig. 28.5 (**A**) Transverse and (**B**) sagittal ultrasound images of the normal empty colon. The empty colon can be misinterpreted as a thickened wall as the mucosal folds are contracted together (arrows).

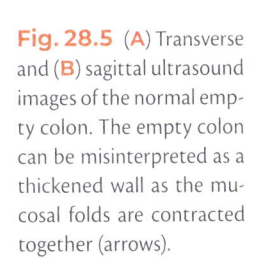

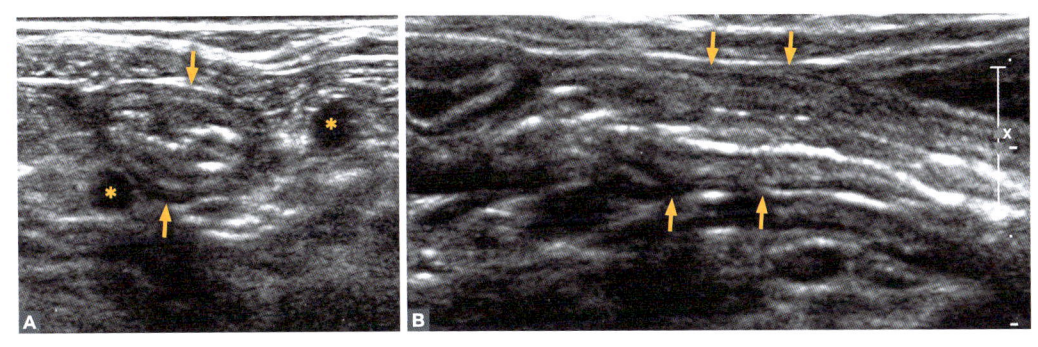

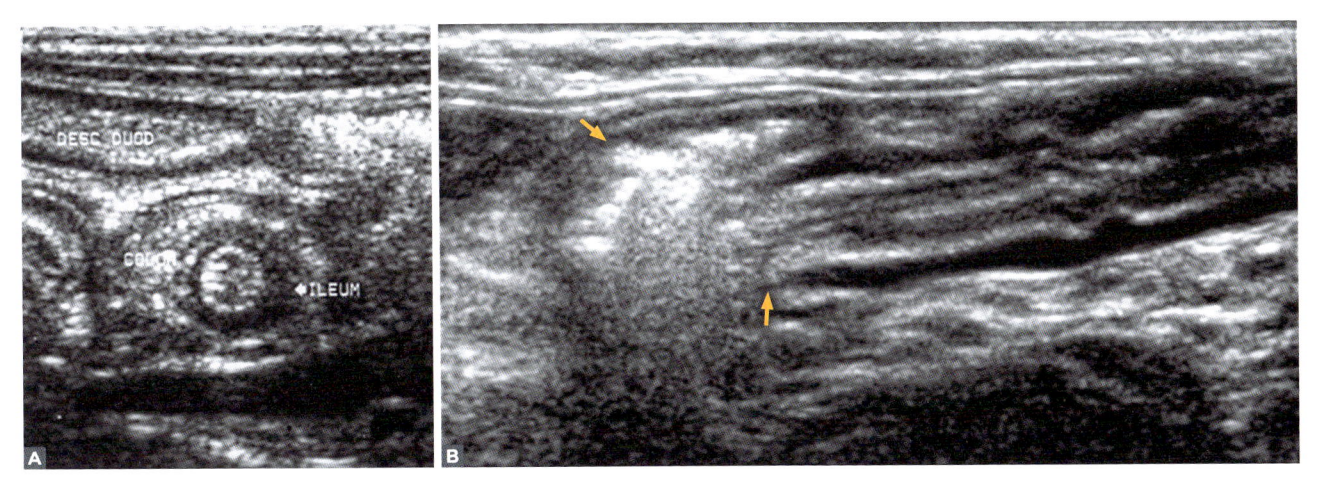

Fig. 28.6 (**A**) Transverse and (**B**) sagittal ultrasound images of the ileocolic junction in a normal dog.

471

from the ascending colon. In cats, the cecum does not typically contain gas (**fig. 28.7**).

The distal rectum and anus can be examined via a perineal approach. Examination of the entire colorectal segment within the pelvis is best performed with CT and MRI. Negative and positive contrast studies of the colon may be performed and are described in chapter 25. Barium enemas can be useful in the diagnosis of ileocolic intussusceptions, cecal inversions, strictures, torsions, or wall infiltrations.

Constipation

Since a large quantity of feces may be present in the colon prior to defecation due to conscious retention in a normal dog or cat, the finding of a radiographically distended colon must be evaluated relative to the patient's clinical signs. The normal colon should not be greater than the length of the seventh lumbar vertebral body in dogs and 1.3 times the length of the fifth lumbar vertebral body in cats, but these values are only meant as general guidelines. Retained feces can also be due to diseases such as idiopathic megacolon causing functional obstruction or mechanical obstruction due to extramural compression, stenosis, foreign body, congenital anomalies, neurologic disorders, neoplasia, and intussusception. Constipation, obstipation, impaction, and megacolon can be difficult to differentiate radiographically and are clinical terms that relate to the chronicity and reversibility of the disorder rather than the radiographic changes. Key features of long-standing feces in the colon include a large volume of feces that have mineral opacity. A large quantity of mineral opaque feces is found with chronic disease, which can be a functional or mechanical obstruction. Functional causes include chronic constipation/obstipation, neuromuscular, and metabolic disorders (**fig. 28.8**). Mechanical causes include foreign body, infiltrative disease-causing wall thickening or a mass, extramural compression, and stenosis (**figs. 28.9-28.12**).

Mechanical obstruction due to previous pelvic canal stenosis from trauma or space-occupying le-

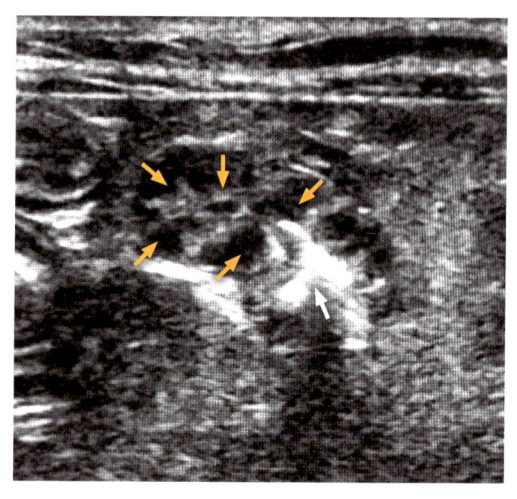

Fig. 28.7 Ultrasound image of the normal feline cecum. The cecum is a small structure with a lobulated appearance with a thick mucosa (orange arrows). Gas from the colon is seen at the junction between both (white arrow).

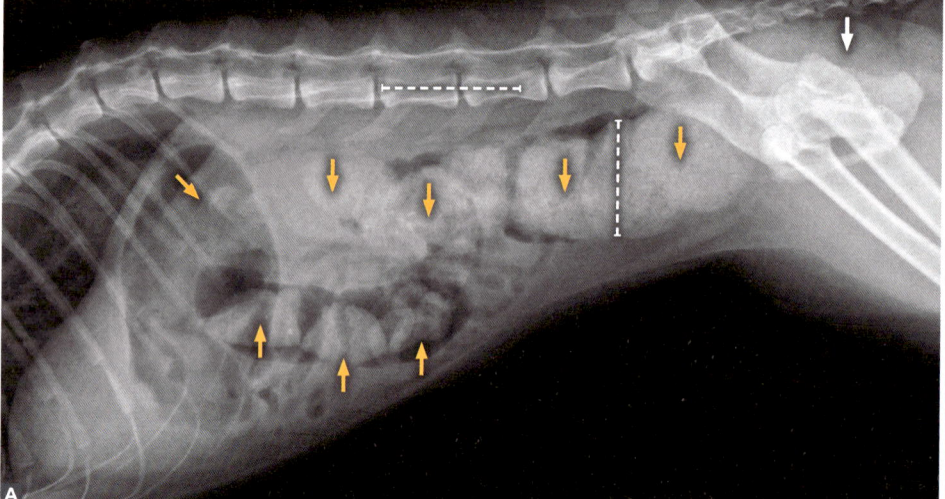

Fig. 28.8 (**A**) Lateral and (**B**) ventrodorsal radiographs of a nine-year-old cat that had idiopathic megacolon for 2.5 years and only had bowel movements on its own up to months at a time. The colon is severely distended with very radiopaque large fecal balls (orange arrows) that are also located in the rectum (white arrow). It is important to examine the entire pelvis radiographically for narrowing or a mass effect. This cat did not have mechanical obstruction and was diagnosed with functional obstruction due to idiopathic megacolon. A measurement of the height of the colon in comparison to the length of the fifth lumbar vertebra showed a ratio >1.3 above the normal upper limit. This is a nonspecific guideline for measuring the colonic diameter.

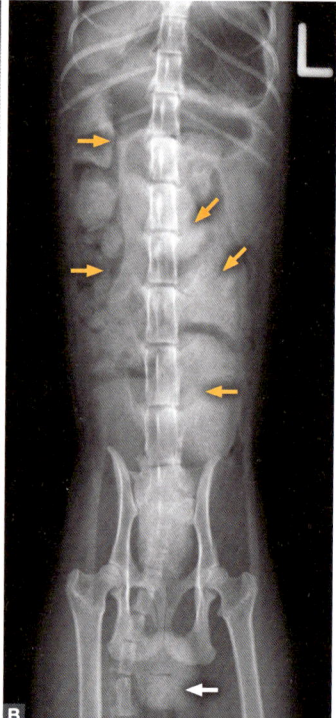

CHAPTER 28 The large intestine

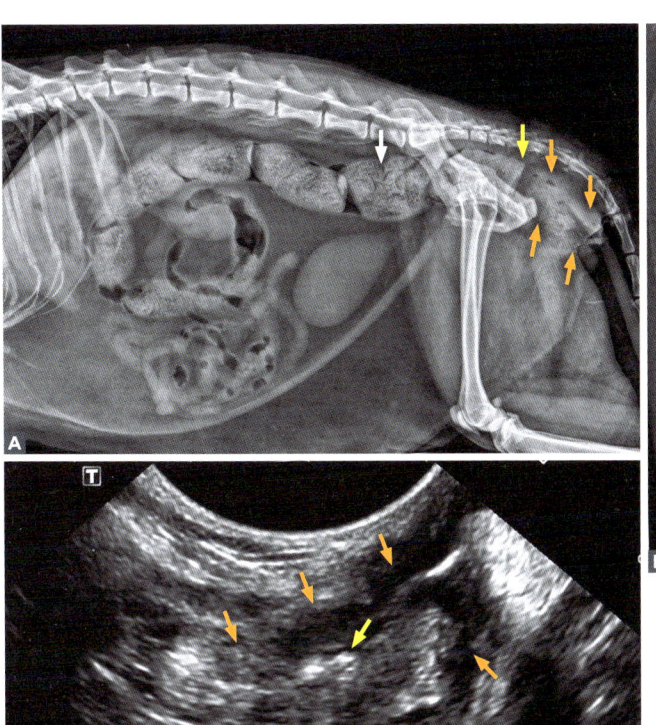

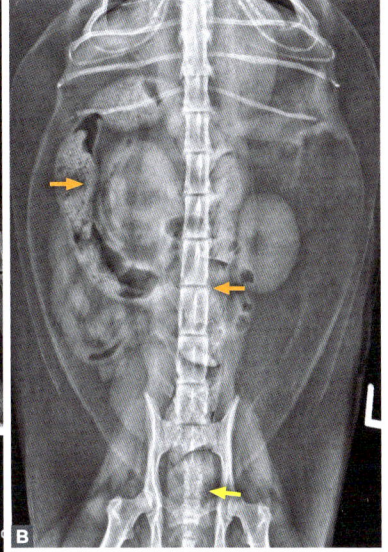

Fig. 28.9 (A) Lateral radiograph of a 12-year-old cat that presented for straining to defecate. The colon is moderately distended with very radiopaque fecal balls. The fecal balls end abruptly (yellow arrow) at a 5 cm length soft tissue opaque mass with multifocal multiple gas foci at the location of the rectoanal junction (orange arrows). (B) Ventrodorsal radiograph of a 12-year-old cat that presented for straining to defecate. The colon is moderately distended with very radiopaque fecal balls. The fecal balls end abruptly (yellow arrow) within the pelvic canal. The rectoanal region is not included in this image. The pelvis is normal. (C) Perineal ultrasound examination of the same cat showing a rectal mass causing obstruction of the colon that resulted in constipation. The curved array probe is placed lateral to the tail head in a sagittal orientation to examine the anorectal structures caudal to the pelvis. A lobulated mass (orange arrows) was detected and was concentric, surrounding the rectum and anus, and had heterogeneous echogenicity. Gas in the rectum (yellow arrow) was helpful for localizing the mass to the anorectal wall. Infiltrative lesions in this region can be due to neoplasms such as adenocarcinoma and lymphoma. A chronic granuloma could also be considered as a differential diagnosis.

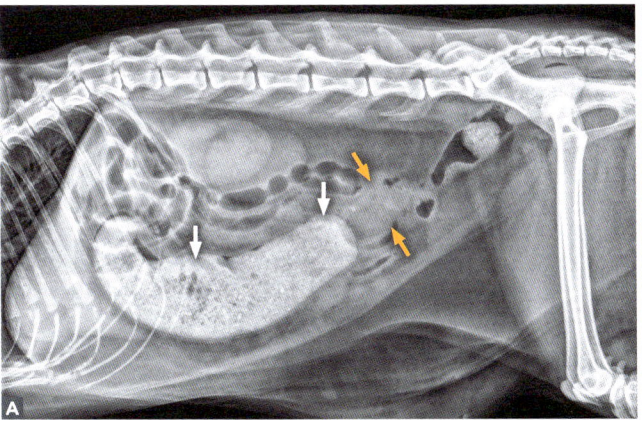

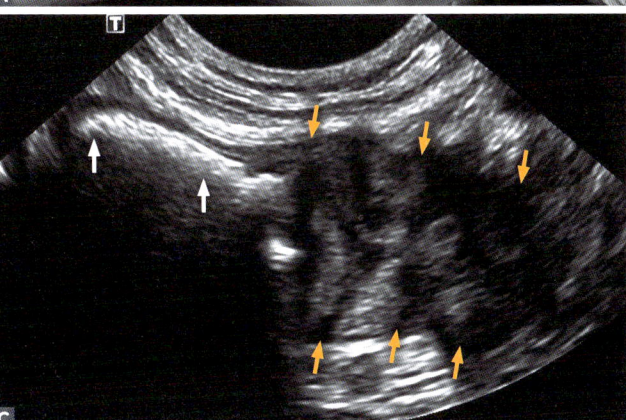

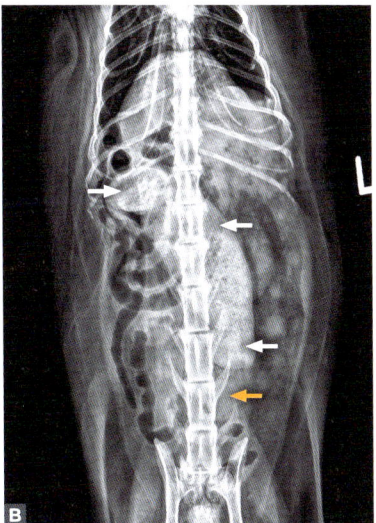

Fig. 28.10 (A) A ten-year-old cat presented with straining to defecate; it had not defecated for 2 weeks. The lateral radiograph shows severe distention of the proximal colon with very radiopaque feces that includes punctate mineralization (white arrows). The feces end abruptly where there is a focal ill-defined soft tissue opaque mass (between orange arrows). The colon and rectum distal to this point have smaller fecal balls present. (B) The ventrodorsal radiograph shows severe distention of the proximal colon with very radiopaque feces that includes punctate mineralization (white arrows). The feces end abruptly where there is a focal ill-defined soft tissue opaque mass (between orange arrows). The colon and rectum distal to this point have smaller fecal balls present. (C) The sagittal ultrasound image of the colon shows fecal material (white arrows) ending abruptly at a large heterogeneous wall infiltrative mural mass (orange arrows) of the distal colon. The lumen of the colon is severely narrowed and causing obstruction of the fecal material seen radiographically. The primary differential for this mass is adenocarcinoma. Tissue sampling is necessary to confirm and rule out other non-malignant causes.

SECTION V ABDOMEN

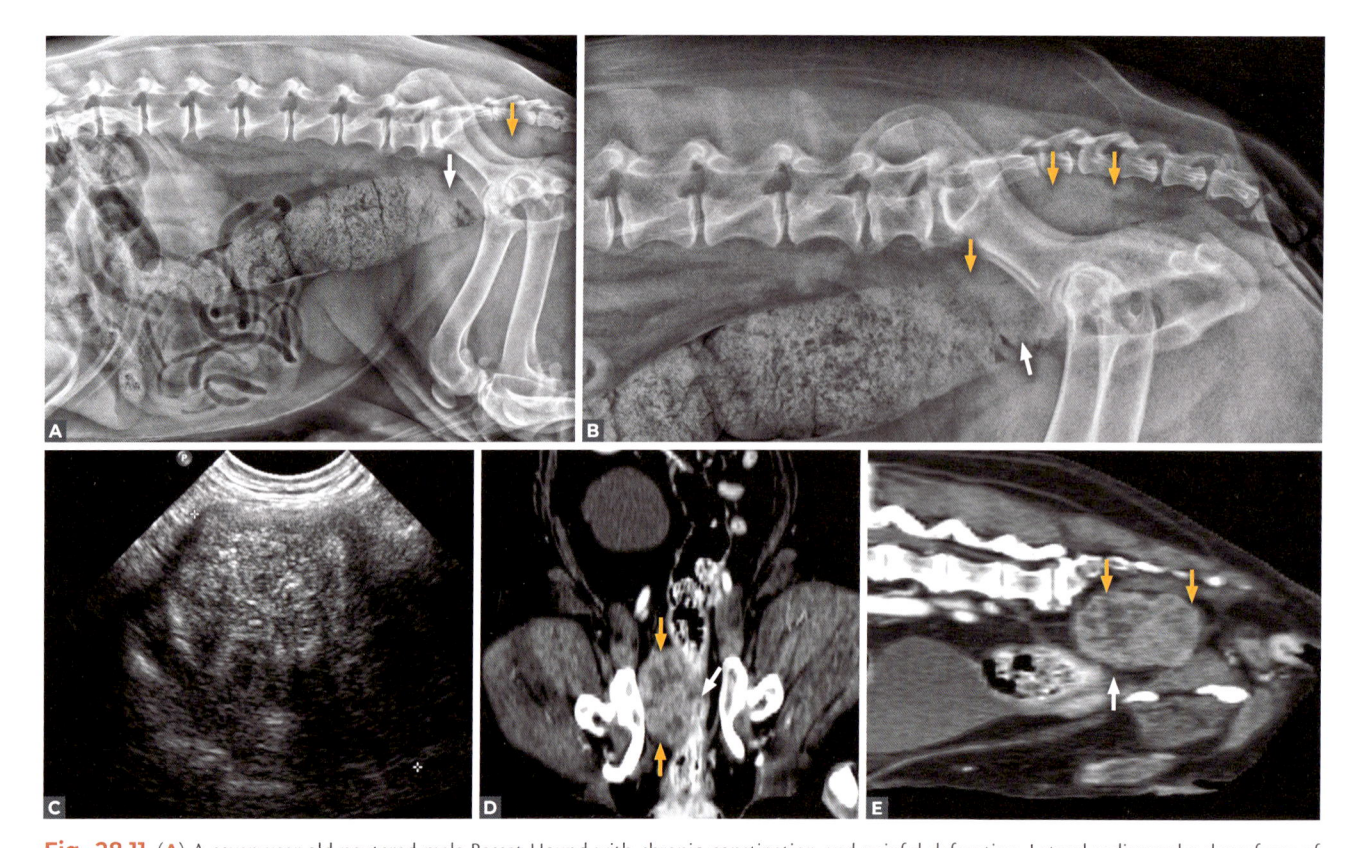

Fig. 28.11 (**A**) A seven-year-old neutered male Basset Hound with chronic constipation and painful defecation. Lateral radiographs show feces of increased opacity present within the descending colon causing some distention. Caudally the descending colon tapers in diameter towards the pelvic canal with ventral (white arrow) deviation and mild compression of the colon. A soft tissue mass is noted within the pelvic canal (orange arrow) dorsal to the rectum and is 8 cm in length. No osseous abnormalities are present. The intrapelvic mass was further examined with ultrasound and computed tomography to determine its origin. Possible causes include constipation secondary to an intrapelvic neoplastic mass such as soft tissue sarcoma, anal sac carcinoma, rectal carcinoma, and a perianal abscess or fistula. (**B**) A lateral focused radiograph of the caudal abdomen and pelvis. Caudally the descending colon tapers in diameter towards the pelvic canal with ventral (white arrow) deviation and mild compression of the colon. A soft tissue mass is noted within the pelvic canal (orange arrow) dorsal to the rectum and is 8 cm in length. No osseous abnormalities are present. The intrapelvic mass was further examined with ultrasound and computed tomography to determine its origin. Possible causes include constipation secondary to an intrapelvic neoplastic mass such as soft tissue sarcoma, anal sac carcinoma, rectal carcinoma, and a perianal abscess or fistula. (**C**) Caudal abdominal sagittal ultrasound image with the probe angled into the pelvic canal. At right dorsolateral position there is a large heterogeneous echogenic mass (between calipers) present that was localized dorsal to the colon and presumed to be retroperitoneal. A retroperitoneal mass was suspected, and the cause for the obstructive constipation noted radiographically. (**D**) Dorsal plane two-dimensional reconstruction CT image post-contrast of the caudal abdomen and pelvis showing a large right-sided heterogenous enhancing mass within the pelvic canal (orange arrows) displacing the rectum to the left and compressing it. (**E**) Sagittal plane two-dimensional reconstruction CT image post-contrast of the caudal abdomen and pelvis showing a large dorsal heterogenous enhancing mass within the pelvic canal (orange arrows) displacing the rectum ventrally and compressing it. The mass could not be definitively localized to any specific organ but was considered to be originating from the lymph nodes in that region. A carcinoma was diagnosed with cytology of the mass.

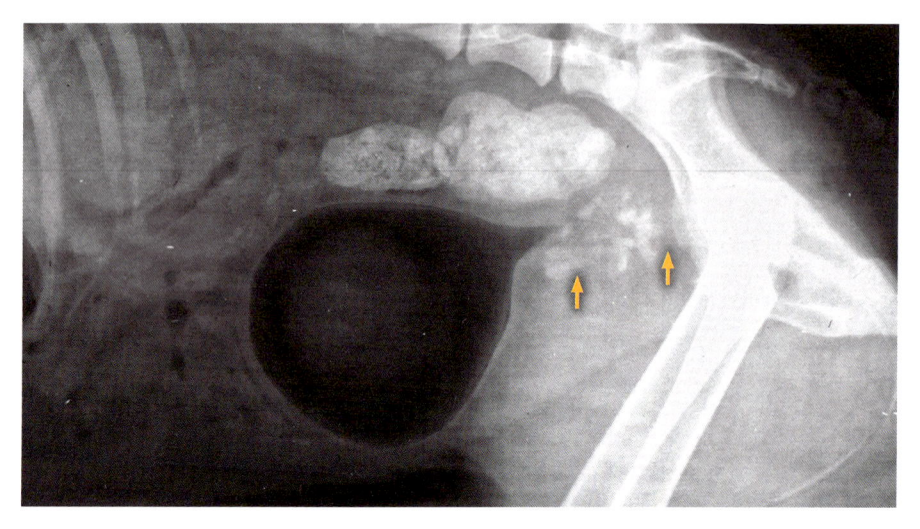

Fig. 28.12 A lateral radiograph of an 11-year-old neutered male dog that was straining to defecate. A negative contrast cystogram was performed as part of the diagnostic workup in this patient for the purposed of localizing the bladder. There are mineral opaque fecal balls in the distal colon. At the bladder neck there is a region of amorphous mineralization present which was diagnosed as prostatic mineralization (arrows). The enlarged mineralized prostate was diagnosed as carcinoma and was causing chronic obstruction of the colorectal junction.

sions as a cause of obstruction of the colon can be screened for radiographically. Sublumbar lymph node enlargement, extension of retroperitoneal masses, prostatomegaly in male dogs and uterine masses in female dogs, and the presence of perineal herniation can also be detected radiographically. Increased soft tissue opacities or displacement or compression of the colon within the pelvic canal indicate the need for further imaging procedures such as ultrasonography, computed tomography, or magnetic resonance imaging.

Intussusception

A soft tissue opaque mass with a curved convex distal interface with gas in the colon is a sign of intussusception. Intussusceptions are more commonly located at the ileocecocolic junction or at any regions along the length of the colon. Radiography is a good screening method to detect a soft tissue mass, but ultrasonography provides a definitive diagnosis of the intussusception (**fig. 28.13**). Intussusception can occur in young dogs and cats with severe enteritis, such as parvovirus infection in dog diarrhea, but can also occur in older animals due to the presence of neoplasia.

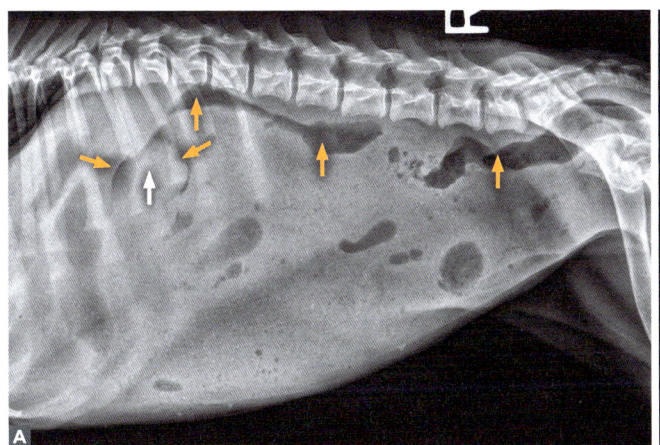

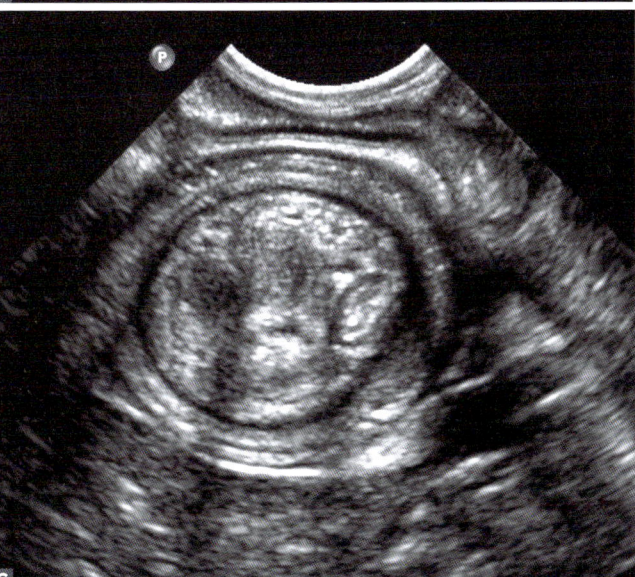

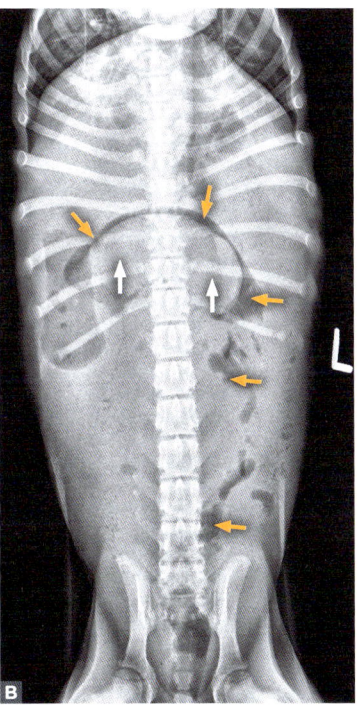

Fig. 28.13 (**A**) A six-month-old female Boxer dog with a 4-month history of diarrhea and weight loss. A lateral radiograph of the abdomen shows generalized loss of detail due to the emaciated body condition. It is difficult to differentiate the origin location of most of the gas opacities to small vs. large intestine. The gas in the distal colon can be traced cranially (orange arrows) to a soft tissue opacity highlighted by gas (white arrow). (**B**) Ventrodorsal radiograph of the abdomen shows generalized loss of detail due to the emaciated body condition. It is difficult to differentiate the origin of most of the gas opacities to small vs. large intestine. The gas in the distal colon can be traced cranially (orange arrows) to a soft tissue opacity highlighted by gas (white arrows), and the gas has a curvilinear shape outlining the mass. (**C**) Abdominal ultrasound was performed. The ultrasound image of the ileocecocolic junction showed the radiopaque mass on the radiographs to be an intussusception with concentric intestinal wall rings and central intestinal segments, vessels, and mesenteric fat.

Colonic torsion

Although not common, colonic torsion is life-threatening and causes severe dilation and displacement of the colon from its normal location (**fig. 28.14**). Radiographic features of colonic torsion include segmental distention, focal narrowing at the site of torsion (torsion sign), displacement of the cecum, and descending colon with mild to no small intestinal distention. CT can be used to confirm colonic torsion, with the main CT feature being the "whirl sign" in addition to displacement and distension of the cecum and colon, focal narrowing of the colon, and distention of the mesenteric vasculature. The whirl sign is created by the spiral path of the twisted tissue and associated blood vessels. Additional CT features may include scant peritoneal effusion, pneumatosis coli, small intestinal distention, portal vein thrombosis, and reduced colonic wall contrast enhancement.

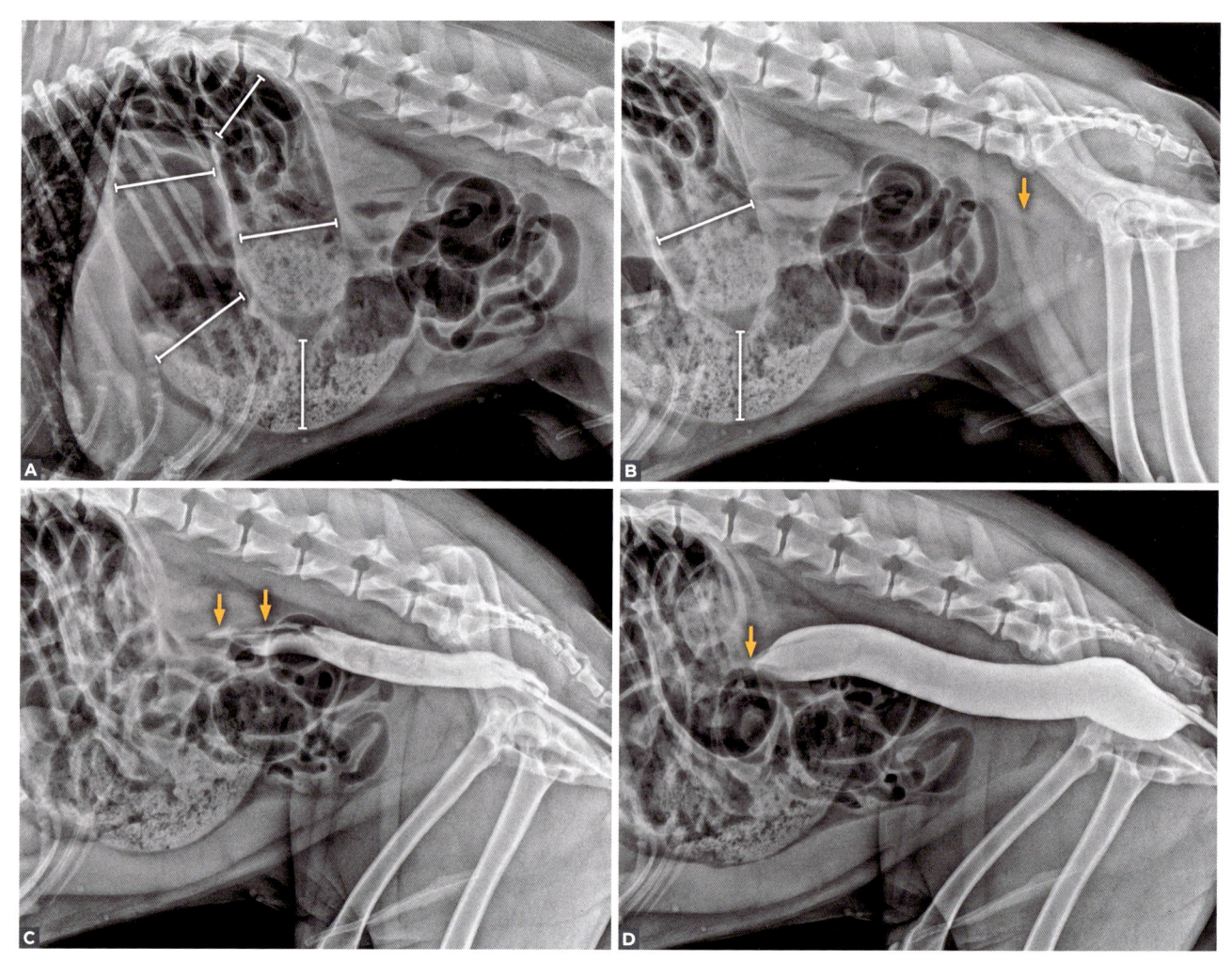

Fig. 28.14 (**A**) Cranial (**B**) and caudal abdomen in a four-year-old neutered male Boxer dog with acute abdomen and no defecation for 5 days. The ascending and transverse colon (white lines) are severely distended with gas and soft tissue opaque granular fecal material. The distal colon cranial to the pelvis is not visible (orange arrow) even though most of the colon is severely distended. (**C, D**) Given the findings of the survey radiographs and suspicion of a colonic torsion, a barium enema using a total of 210 mL barium diluted 1:1 with tap water was performed. (**C**) A rubber catheter is present in the colon with the tip in the proximal rectum. After the instillation of 180 mL of barium, contrast material is present in the descending colon that extends to the level of the L2, where longitudinal striations that twist in a helical pattern (torsion sign, orange arrows) are noted. (**D**) An additional 30 mL of barium was introduced, and the colon is progressively distended, but barium does not extend further cranially. Complete colonic torsion of the proximal descending colon with secondary small intestinal ileus and obstipation was diagnosed.

Infiltrative disease of the large intestine

Soft tissue opaque masses associated with the colon can be recognized radiographically but are not common and can be masked by the presence of feces. Sonographically, focal infiltrations or intramural masses of the colonic wall may be detected and are associated with either neoplasms or fungal granulomas such as pythiosis and histoplasmosis in dogs and cats. Neoplastic causes include carcinoma and lymphoma (**fig. 28.15**). Common sonographic features include a focal mass or diffuse thickening with a loss of wall layering. In cats, feline idiopathic eosinophilic sclerosing fibroplasia is a non-neoplastic cause of wall thickening with loss of layering in the colon.

Colitis

In dogs with diarrhea due to colitis, the colon may appear smoothly bordered or irregularly shaped due to peristalsis, and the colon can be fluid- and/or gas-filled (**fig. 28.16**). Colitis due to diffuse, mild to moderate inflammatory infiltration will often show no radiographic or ultrasonographic changes, and colonoscopy is the diagnostic modality of choice in both dogs and cats. Micronodular lesions in the colonic submucosa can be identified in dogs and cats with inflammatory disease, and these lesions likely represent reactive lymphoid follicles within the wall that resolve with resolution of clinical signs. Transient peristalsis in dogs with colitis can be observed as a corrugated wall shape and variably observed between sequential images (**fig. 28.17**).

Pneumatosis coli is the presence of gas within the colonic wall and is a radiographic sign of infectious colitis but can also be incidental in healthy dogs. Pneumoretroperitoneum and pneumoperitoneum can also occur secondary to pneumatosis coli due to translocation of gas or gas-producing bacteria from the colonic wall (**fig. 28.18**).

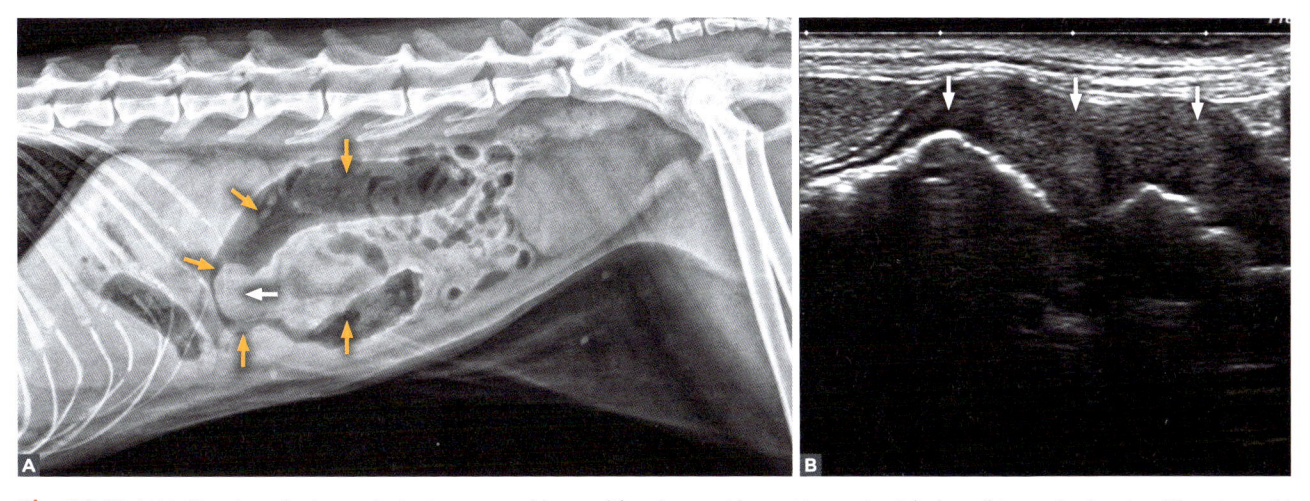

Fig. 28.15 (**A**) Infiltrative colonic neoplasia. A ten-year-old spayed female cat with vomiting and weight loss of 2 months duration. There is a mild small amount of gas and fluid within the stomach and small intestines but no evidence of mechanical ileus. The descending and transverse colon are moderately dilated with gas (orange arrows) and there is a sharply demarcated broad-based soft tissue to gas interface having a homogenous soft tissue opaque rounded interface with the gas at the level of the transverse colon that extends to the ascending colon (white arrow). A colonic mass was diagnosed, and ultrasound was performed to further assess. Possible causes for this radiographic finding include a broad-based wall neoplasm, polypoid benign mass, or granuloma. (**B**) Infiltrative mass of the ascending colon wall. There is marked thickening of the colonic wall with transmural hypoechoic loss of wall layering. The thickened wall measured up to 8.6 mm in diameter and extended from the level of the ileocecocolic junction to the junction with the descending colon. Fine-needle aspiration was performed for cytology. Lymphoma was diagnosed.

SECTION V ABDOMEN

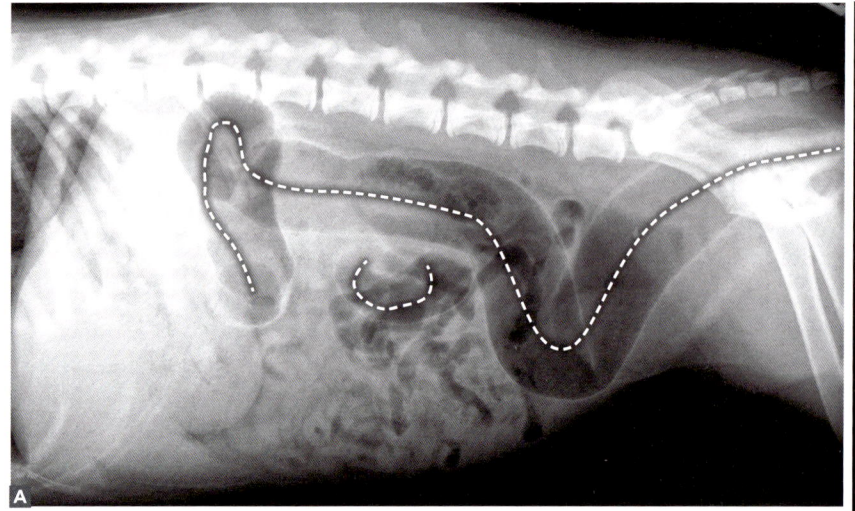

Fig. 28.16 A ten-year-old male mixed breed dog with acute vomiting and diarrhea that was diagnosed with nonspecific gastroenteritis and colitis. (**A**) Lateral and (**B**) ventrodorsal radiographs show the colon is markedly distended with gas and can be traced along its length. The path of the cecum and colon is shown with a white line.

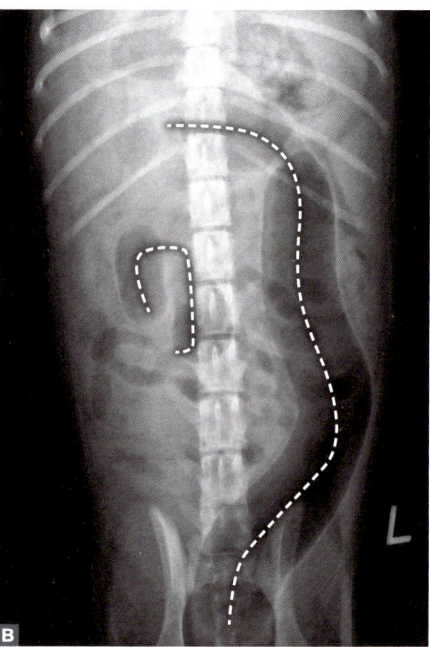

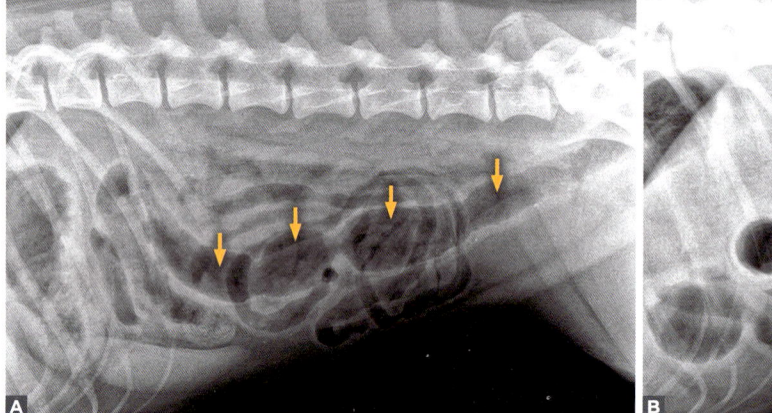

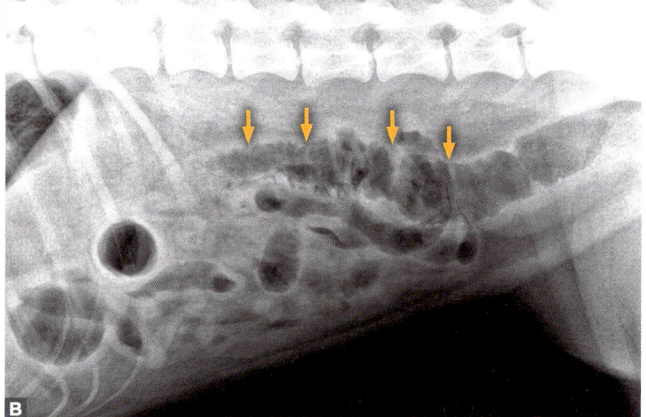

Fig. 28.17 This is an example of the variability of the shape of the colon in a dog with colitis and hematochezia. (**A**) The colon has a smooth border, and there is a focal narrowing at the site of peristalsis/contraction (arrows). (**B**) The descending colon has a corrugated shape due to spasms in radiographs taken within a minute after the first.

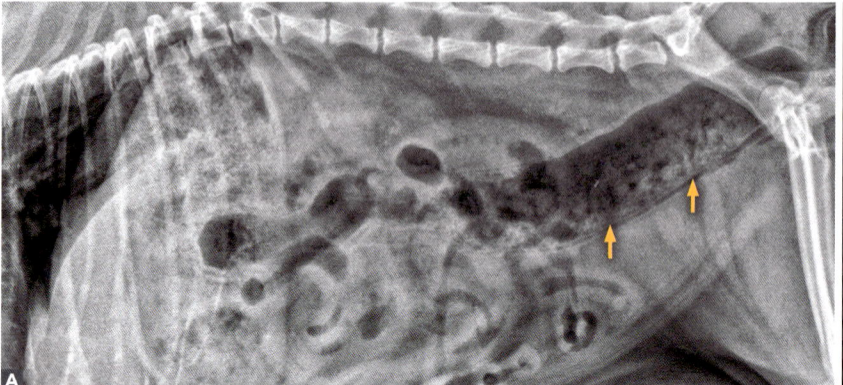

Fig. 28.18 A five-year-old Pomeranian dog with chronic diarrhea and hematochezia. The lateral (**A**) and ventrodorsal (**B**) radiographs of the abdomen show a linear gas opacity within the wall of the distal descending colon (arrows), which is distended with gas and a small amount of soft tissue opaque feces. The diagnosis is pneumatosis coli due to colitis.

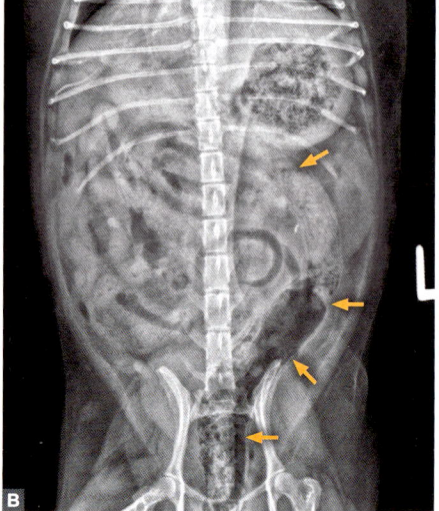

478

CHAPTER 28 The large intestine

Congenital anomalies of the colon

Congenital anomalies of the colon are uncommon and include imperforate anus, atresia coli, and atresia recti, fistulas, diverticulae, duplication, and short colon (**figs. 28.19** and **28.20**). The colon is typically progressively distended with feces, and on physical exam an anal orifice is not present. Radiographically, the distended rectum will end within or caudal to the pelvis and cranial to the location of the anus. Congenital or acquired fistulas can also develop between the vagina, urethra, and rectum. Urine can sometimes be seen to leak from the rectum in patients with a rectourethral fistula and feces may exit the vagina in an animal with fistula formation between the two, which is typically congenital. Positive contrast studies such as a retrograde vaginourethrogram in females or in males a urethrogram can be used to identify fistulas between the urogenital tract and the rectoanal structures. Contrast radiography or CT angiography are methods for examining rectourethral fistulas.

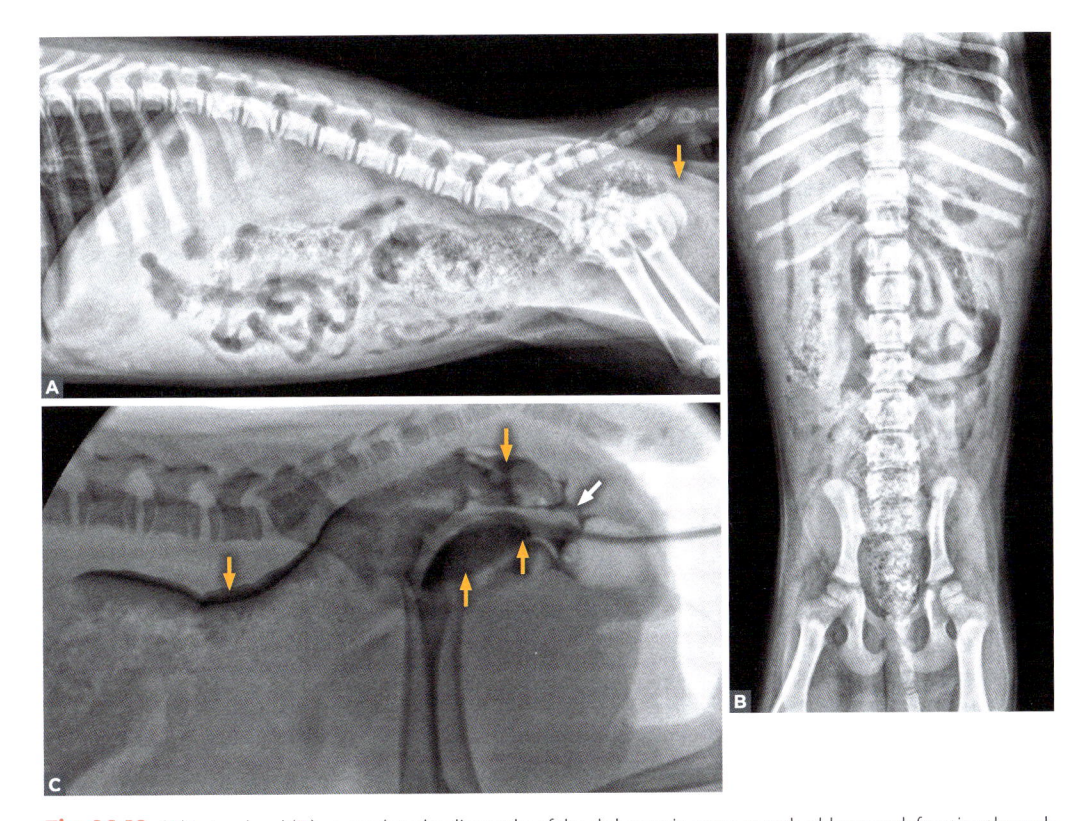

Fig. 28.19 (**A**) Lateral and (**B**) ventrodorsal radiographs of the abdomen in a two-month-old puppy defecating through the vagina. There is an increased amount of fecal material within the colon and abdominal distention. The fecal material ends abruptly cranial to the anus (orange arrow). (**C**) Fluoroscopic vaginourethrogram was performed with iodinated contrast medium. The image is inverted black/white. Contrast medium is visible filling the vagina and the colon (orange arrows) due to a communication between the two (white arrow). There is no evidence of filling contrast of the caudal portion of the rectum or anus. The study is diagnostic for a congenital rectovaginal fistula with atresia ani.

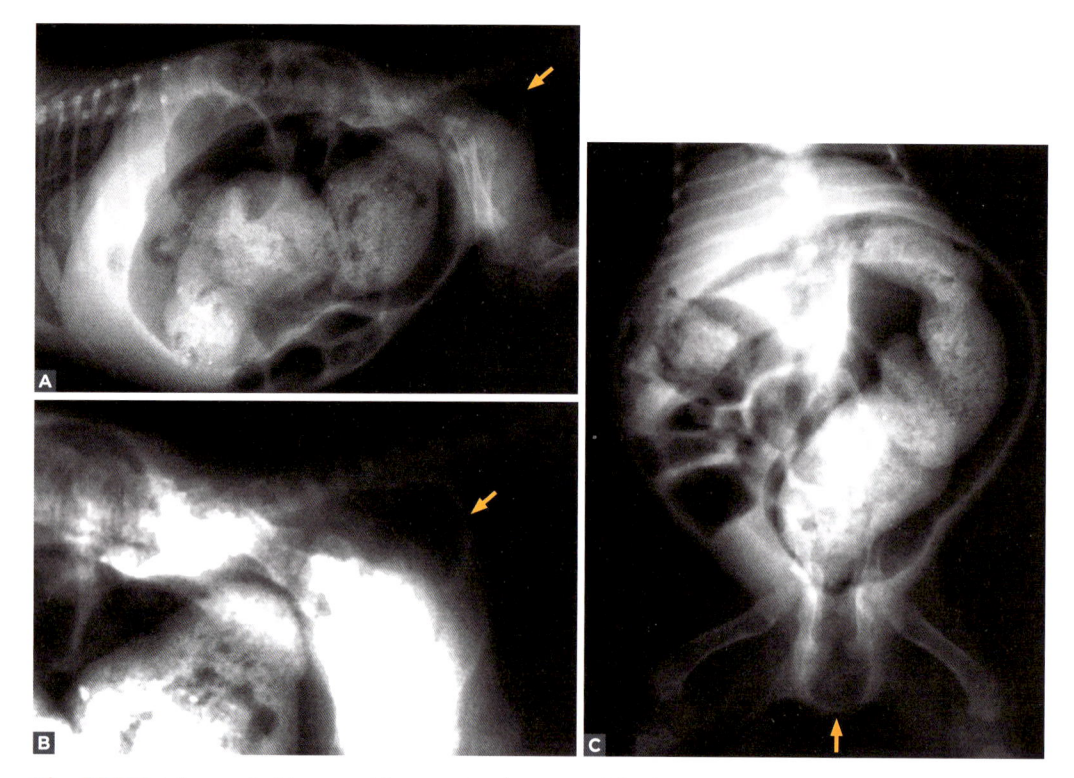

Fig. 28.20 A four-week-old puppy with progressive distention of the abdomen. The lateral (**A**) and ventrodorsal (**B**) radiographs of the abdomen show severe abdominal distention due to severe dilation of the entire colon filled with a large quantity of gas and feces. (**C**) A magnified region of the anus showing the abruptly ending rectum at its junction with the anus, which is also visible in the ventrodorsal image (arrow). The puppy was diagnosed with atresia ani.

References

1. Trevail T, Gunn-Moore D, Carrera I, Courcier E, Sullivan M. Radiographic diameter of the colon in normal and constipated cats and in cats with megacolon. *Vet Radiol Ultrasound* 52:516-520, 2011.
2. Yoon S, Lee SK, Lee J, Baek YB, Cho KO, Choi J. Dual-phase computed tomography angiography of intestinal carcinoid tumor as a lead point for cecocolic intussusception in a dog. *J Vet Med Sci* 81:928-932, 2019.
3. Gremillion CL, Savage M, Cohen EB. Radiographic findings and clinical factors in dogs with surgically confirmed or presumed colonic torsion. *Vet Radiol Ultrasound* 59:272-278, 2018.
4. Barge P, Fina CJ, Mortier JR, Jones ID. CT findings in five dogs with surgically confirmed colonic torsion. *Vet Radiol Ultrasound* 61:190-196, 2020.
5. Chavez-Peon Berle E, KuKanich K, Biller D. Ultrasonographic findings of gastrointestinal histoplasmosis in dogs. *Vet Radiol Ultrasound* 62:108-115, 2021.
6. Slawienski MJ, Mauldin GE, Mauldin GN, Patnaik AK. Malignant colonic neoplasia in cats: 46 cases (1990-1996). *J Am Vet Med Assoc* 211:878-881, 1997.
7. Weissman A, Pennick D, Webster C, Hecht S, Keating J, Craig LE. Ultrasonographic and clinicopathological features of feline gastrointestinal eosinophilic sclerosing fibroplasia in four cats. *J Feline Med Surg* 15:148-154, 2013.
8. Citi S, Chimenti T, Marchetti V, Millanta F, Mannucci T. Micronodular ultrasound lesions in the colonic submucosa of 42 dogs and 14 cats. *Vet Radiol Ultrasound* 54:646-651, 2013.
9. Fisk A, Allen-Durrance A. Pneumatosis coli in a dog. *J Am Anim Hosp Assoc* 55:e55401, 2019.
10. Vianna ML, Tobias KM. Atresia ani in the dog: a retrospective study. *J Am Anim Hosp Assoc* 41:317-322, 2005.
11. Rahal SC, Vicente CS, Mortari AC, Mamprim MJ, Caporalli EHG. Rectovaginal fistula with anal atresia in 5 dogs. *Can Vet J* 48:827-830, 2007.
12. Silverstone AM, Adams WM. Radiographic diagnosis of a rectourethral fistula in a dog. *J Am Anim Hosp Assoc* 37:573-576, 2001.
13. Cruse AM, Vaden SL, Mathews KG, Hill TL, Robertson ID. Use of computed tomography (CT) scanning and colorectal new methylene blue infusion in evaluation of an English Bulldog with a rectourethral fistula. *J Vet Intern Med* 23:931-934, 2009.

CHAPTER 29

Normal liver and hepatic parenchymal disease

Mylène Auger

> **KEY POINTS**
>
> ▍ Radiographs are useful for evaluation of alterations in liver size and opacity.
> ▍ Abdominal ultrasound can detect changes in liver echogenicity, echotexture, margination, identify focal or multifocal lesions, and can help establish a list of differential diagnoses, but seldom provides a specific diagnosis.
> ▍ Spectral Doppler evaluation of the hepatic vasculature, and in particular of the portal vein, can be helpful when portal hypertension and multiple acquired shunts are suspected.
> ▍ CT is often complementary to ultrasound, and is particularly useful when vascular anomalies are suspected, or when evaluating the origin and extent of a hepatic mass.
> ▍ Given the overlap in pre- and post-contrast CT features of hepatic masses, CT cannot accurately predict whether a mass is benign or malignant, or the tumor type, and histopathology remains the gold standard for diagnosis.

Normal hepatic imaging features

Radiographs

The liver has uniform soft tissue opacity and is usually contained within the costal arch, although its caudal extension can vary with patient conformation and breed, inspiratory or expiratory status, and the patient's age, and therefore evaluation of size is somewhat subjective[1,2] (**fig. 29.1**). The ventral liver border may be outlined by falciform fat and is curved and smooth. The lobar borders, such as the junction of the ventral and caudal liver margins on the lateral radiograph, form an acute angle. The position of the stomach can give a more objective assessment of liver size (**fig. 29.2**).

Ultrasound

Several approaches, including subxyphoid and intercostal windows, may be necessary to image the liver.[3,4] In deep-chested dogs and in patients with microhepatia, intercostal windows are particularly useful given that most of the liver is contained within the costal arch. Selection of transducer and frequency depends on the patient and liver size but will usually vary between 5 and 10 MHz.[3,4] The liver should be imaged in sagittal/parasagittal and transverse planes. Complete assessment includes evaluation of size, echogenicity, echotexture, margins, as well as presence and distribution of abnormalities, which can be focal, multifocal or generalized.[5]

Liver size can be difficult to assess with ultrasound; however, the costal arch, the position of the stomach, and liver margins can be used as a reference.[3] Hepatic echogenicity is characterized by com-

SECTION V ABDOMEN

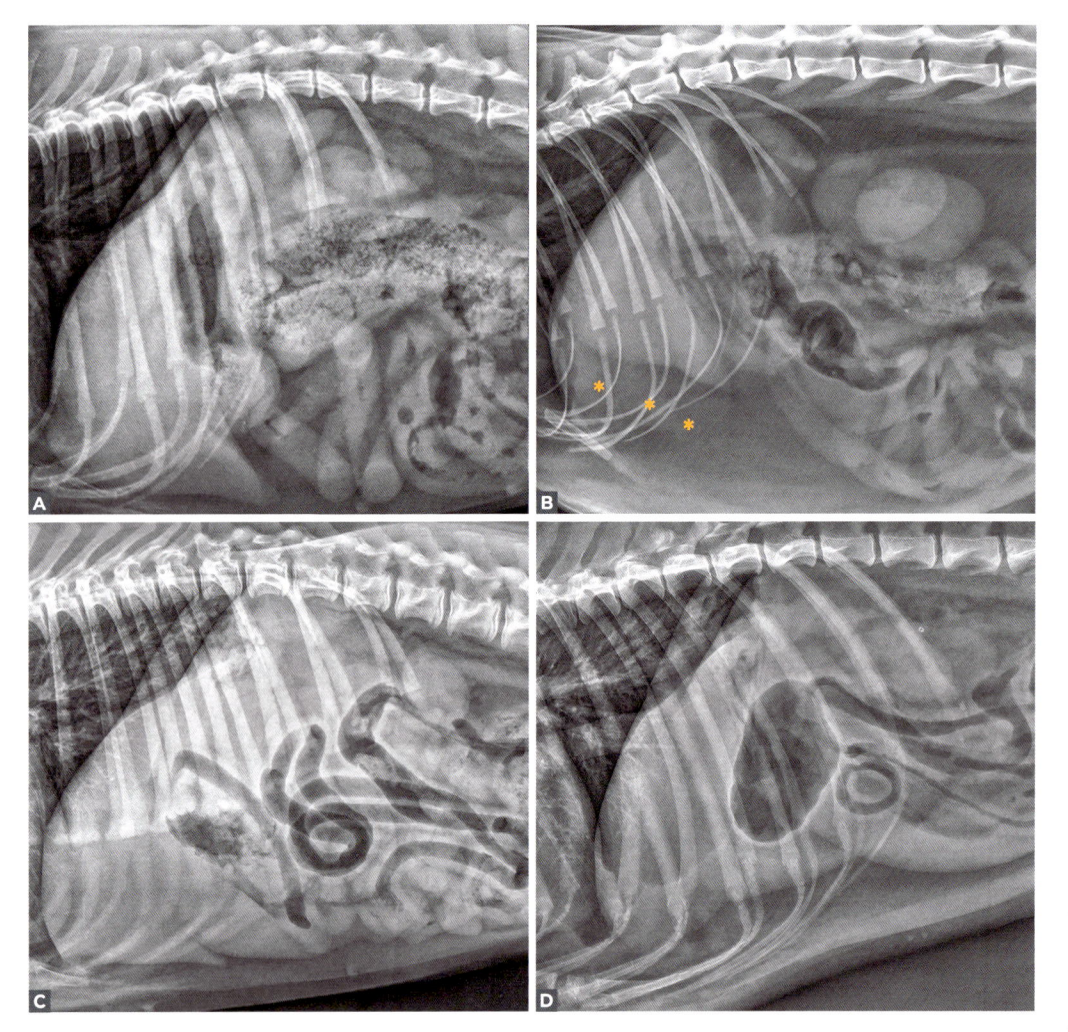

Fig. 29.1 Examples of variations of normal liver size on radiographs. (A) A nine-year-old Chihuahua. The liver extends slightly beyond the costal arch, but has sharp, well-defined margins. This is commonly seen in small breed dogs without evidence of liver disease. (B) Left lateral projection in an obese two-year-old Domestic longhair cat. In obese cats, fat deposition in the falciform ligament (asterisk) is common and should not be mistaken for microhepatia. (C) Left lateral projection in a three-month-old Doberman Pinscher with no evidence of liver disease. The liver extends beyond the costal arch but has sharp well-defined margins. The liver usually appears relatively large in normal juvenile cats and dogs. (D) Left lateral projection in a four-year-old Great Pyrenees. In deep-chested dogs, the liver is often entirely contained within the costal arch which should not be confused with microhepatia.

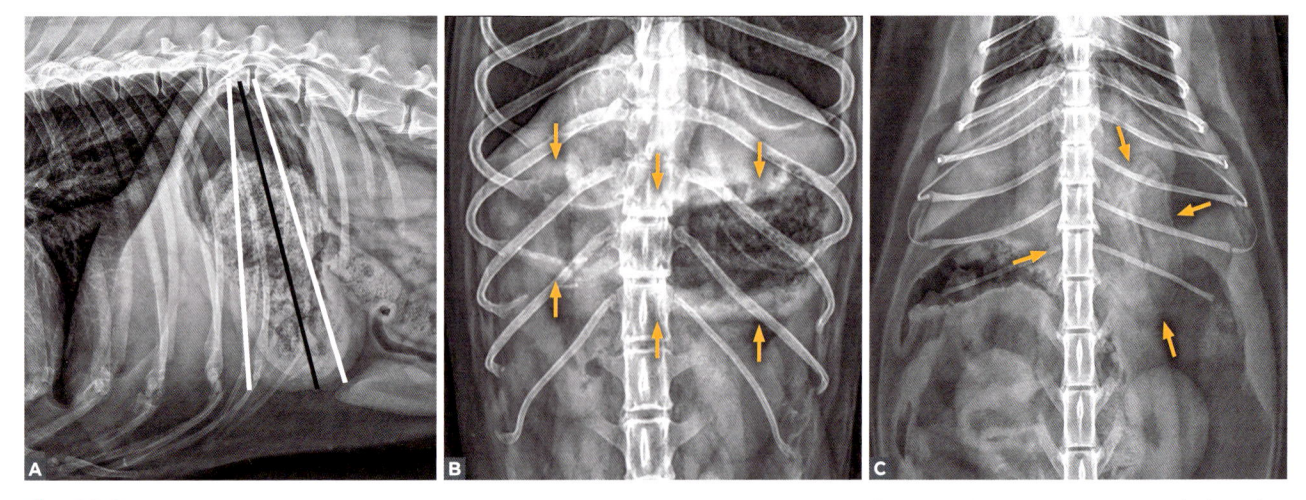

Fig. 29.2 Normal gastric axis. (A) Right lateral radiograph in a nine-year-old Labrador Retriever illustrating the normal gastric axis, which is a line joining the fundus to the antrum on lateral radiographs (black line), and which should range between parallel to the ribs and perpendicular to the spine (white lines). (B) Ventrodorsal radiograph in a nine-year-old Chihuahua. On ventrodorsal radiographs in dogs, the stomach is usually perpendicular to the long axis of the body (arrows). (C) Ventrodorsal view of the abdomen in a two-year-old Domestic longhair cat. In cats, the pylorus is positioned more medially than in dogs, slightly right of midline. The arrows are outlining the stomach.

paring the liver to the spleen and/or kidneys and the visibility of intrahepatic portal veins (**fig. 29.3**). In cats, the liver is often compared to the adjacent falciform fat (**fig. 29.4**).

The intrahepatic portal veins have hyperechoic borders and should taper smoothly.[1] Portal blood flow should be hepatopetal and portal velocity can be measured using spectral Doppler, with an insonation angle correction of less than 60°.[3] Mean portal flow velocity can be calculated by measuring maximal portal velocity, in the center of the portal vein lumen, and then multiplying the maximal velocity by a factor of 0.57.[3] Mean portal flow velocities have been reported to be between 15 ± 3 and 18 ± 8 cm/s in normal dogs, and 10-18 cm/s in normal cats.[3] Hepatic veins are anechoic tubular structures extending through the parenchyma converging on the caudal vena cava. The venous walls are isoechoic to the liver and not visible, although they may be hyperechoic at the confluence with the caudal vena cava[1] (**fig. 29.5**).

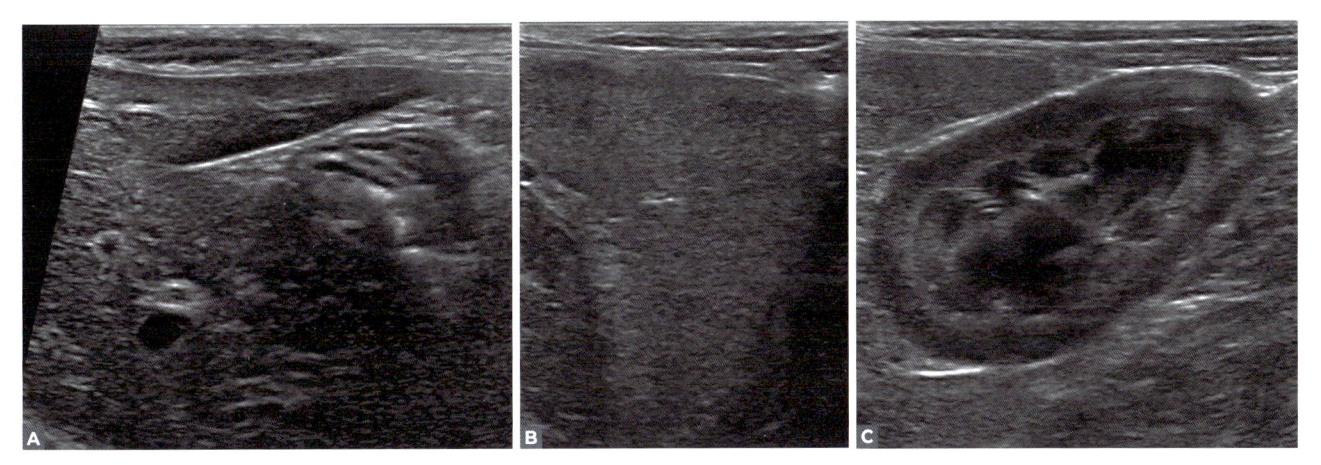

Fig. 29.3 Examples of relative echogenicity between the liver (**A**), spleen (**B**) and kidney (**C**) in a two-year-old mixed breed dog. The liver usually has moderately coarse echotexture and is usually hypoechoic to the spleen and isoechoic to hyperechoic to the renal cortices when compared using the same depth and gain settings.

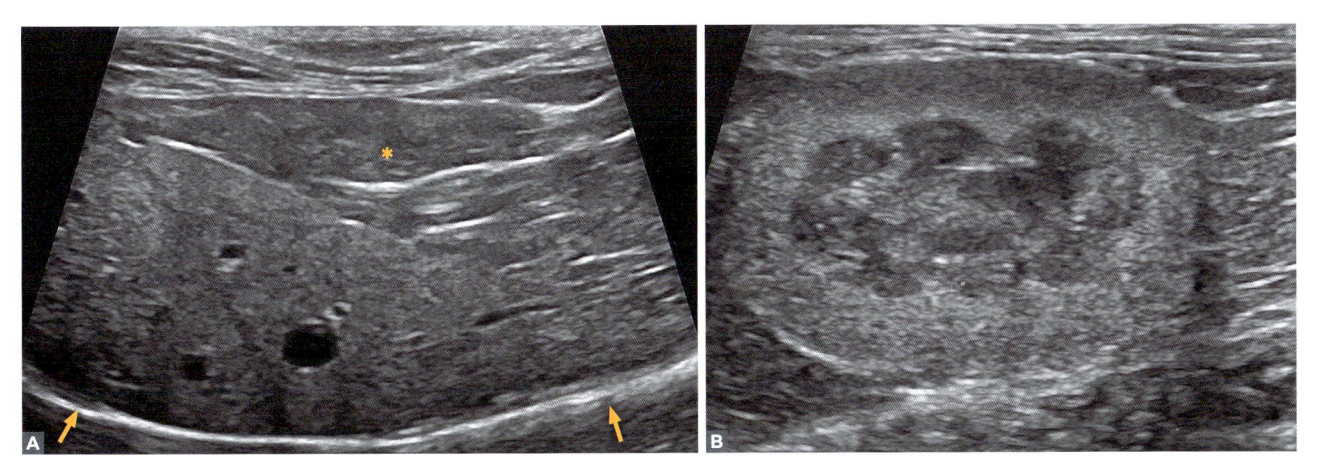

Fig. 29.4 Normal ultrasound variations in cats. (**A**) Transverse sonographic image of the liver in a ten-year-old Somali cat. The falciform ligament is usually isoechoic to slightly hyperechoic to the liver, but in some obese, healthy cats, the liver can be hyperechoic to the falciform ligament (asterisk), as was the case in this cat, who had no clinical or bloodwork evidence of liver disease. A curved hyperechoic line borders the liver cranially and dorsally (arrows), representing the interface between the diaphragm and the lungs/pleura. (**B**) Sagittal sonographic image of the left kidney in the same cat as in (A), demonstrating hyperechogenicity of the renal cortex, likely due to fat deposition, as this cat had no clinical evidence of renal disease. In cats, the renal cortices can occasionally be hyperechoic to the liver.

SECTION V ABDOMEN

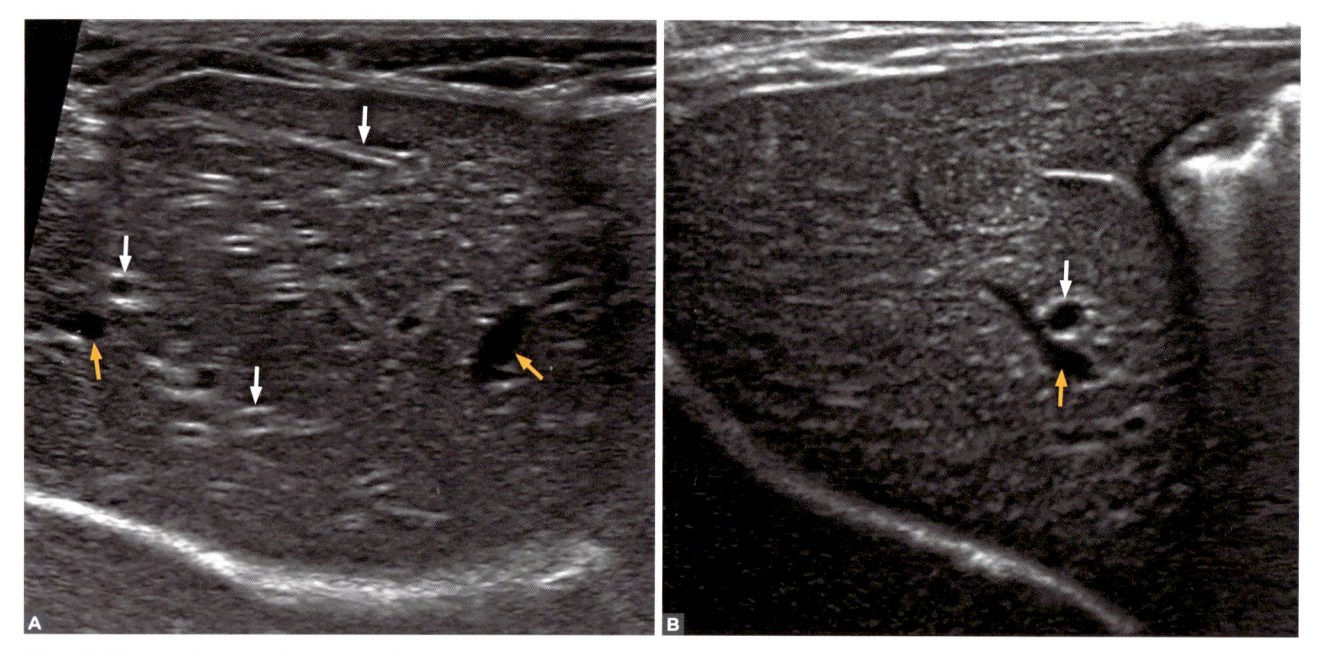

Fig. 29.5 Normal hepatic ultrasound. (**A**) Transverse sonographic image of the liver of a two-year-old mixed breed dog and (**B**) sagittal sonographic image of the liver of a five-month-old mixed breed dog. The intrahepatic portal veins (white arrows) have hyperechoic borders while hepatic veins are anechoic tubular structures extending through the parenchyma (orange arrows). When measured at the same depth, portal veins and hepatic veins should be similar in diameter.

Computed tomography

The liver is normally isoattenuating to the spleen with uniform contrast enhancement. To evaluate the hepatic vasculature, a triple-phase angiogram is recommended, where several post-contrast image acquisitions are precisely timed to highlight the hepatic arterial, hepatic venous and portal venous vasculature (**fig. 29.6**).[6-8]

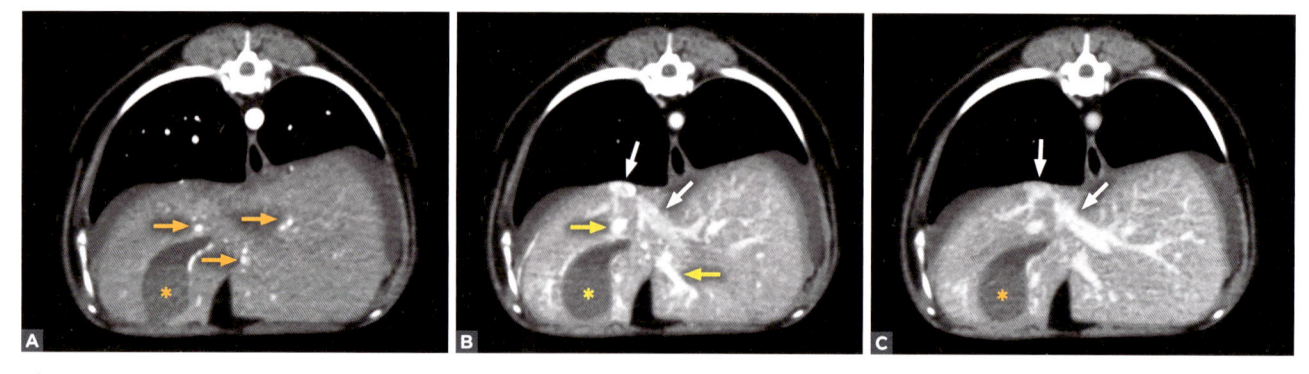

Fig. 29.6 Transverse computed tomographic angiographic study of the normal liver in a three-year-old spayed female mixed breed dog. The gallbladder (asterisk) is hypoattenuating to the liver due to the presence of bile. (**A**) The arterial phase is usually initiated around 13 to 20 seconds post-contrast administration and highlights the hepatic arteries (orange arrows). (**B**) The portal phase is usually initiated around 30 to 40 seconds post-contrast administration and highlights the portal venous system (yellow arrows). In this patient, the caudal vena cava and hepatic veins are partially contrast-enhanced (white arrows) in the portal phase. (**C**) The hepatic parenchymal phase is usually initiated approximately 120 seconds post-contrast administration. The caudal vena cava and hepatic veins are homogeneously contrast-enhanced (white arrows).

Diffuse hepatopathies

Hepatomegaly can be generalized or focal/asymmetric. Increased or decreased liver size can be an indicator of liver disease.[9]

On radiographs, a diffusely enlarged liver extends caudally beyond the costal arch. Rounding or blunting of the liver margins can be a sign of diffuse hepatic parenchymal disease or congestion on radiographs. There may be caudal displacement of the stomach, with craniodorsal to caudoventral orientation of the gastric axis (**fig. 29.7A, B**). In cases of microhepatia, the stomach will be displaced cranially, and the pylorus may be displaced cranially relative to the fundus (**fig. 29.7C, D**).

On ultrasound, alterations in size, changes in echogenicity, an irregular capsular contour or rounded lobar margins suggest a diffuse hepatopathy.[1] Decreased visualization of hyperechoic walls of intrahepatic portal veins, and increased attenuation of the ultrasound beam as it traverses the liver are indicative of liver hyperechogenicity. Hepatic hypoechogenicity usually causes increased conspicuity of intrahepatic portal vein walls. It is important to note that in cases of diffuse, even severe disease, the liver may appear normal sonographically.[5] In cases of suspected hepatopathies, clinical signs and laboratory data need to be taken into consideration, and cytology or histology are usually required for a definitive diagnosis.[1,5]

CT can be complementary to ultrasound in cases of diffuse disease and is preferred if vascular anomalies are suspected. CT angiography (CTA) is superior to abdominal ultrasound for detection and characterization of congenital and multiple acquired portosystemic shunts in dogs and has been

Fig. 29.7 Hepatomegaly and microhepatia. (**A**) Left lateral and (**B**) ventrodorsal radiographs of a 14-year-old Dachshund with steroid hepatopathy, demonstrating hepatomegaly. The liver extends caudally beyond the costal arch with rounded caudoventral margins (white arrows). Note the caudodorsal displacement of the gastric axis (orange arrows) and caudal and medial displacement of the pylorus on the ventrodorsal view (orange arrow). (**C**) Right lateral and (**D**) ventrodorsal radiographs of a four-year-old spayed female mixed breed dog with chronic hepatitis demonstrating microhepatia. The stomach is displaced cranially, reducing the distance between the diaphragm and the stomach (orange arrows). On the ventrodorsal projection, there is cranial displacement of the pyloric antrum. Note the cranial position of the splenic tail (asterisk).

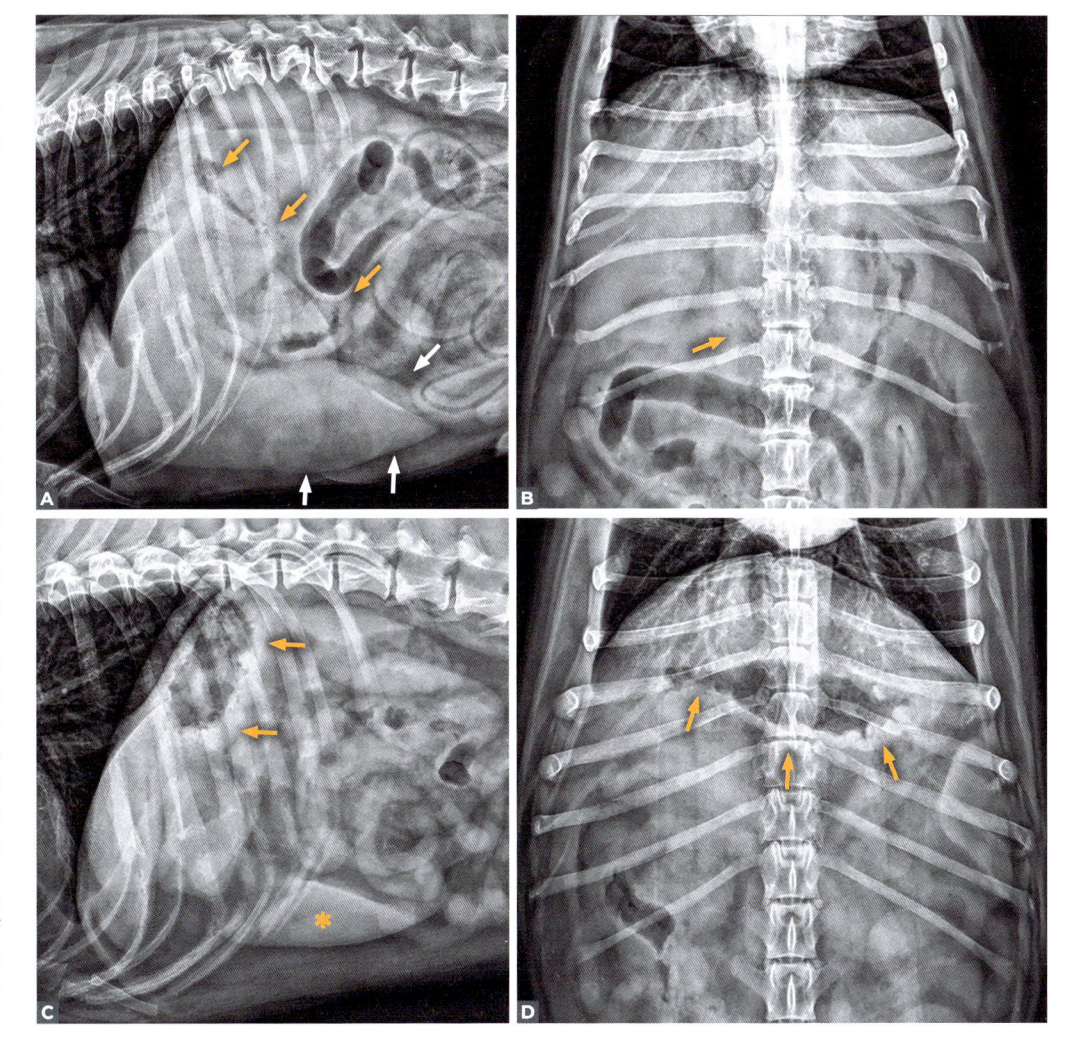

reported to be 5.5 times more likely to correctly ascertain the presence or absence of a portosystemic shunt compared to abdominal ultrasound.[10]

Causes of generalized hepatomegaly include hepatic venous congestion, inflammatory and infiltrative disease, steroid hepatopathy, hepatic lipidosis, and neoplasia.[9] Causes of microhepatia include congenital anomalies of the portal vein, chronic hepatitis, and cirrhosis.[1,9]

Passive hepatic congestion

Passive hepatic congestion (**fig. 29.8**) can occur secondary to obstruction of the hepatic veins or the caudal vena cava, right-sided heart failure, or pericardial disease. It will usually cause hypoechoic hepatomegaly with dilation of the caudal vena cava and hepatic veins, and ascites.

Acute hepatitis

Causes of acute hepatitis (**fig. 29.9**) include infectious agents, toxins, and adverse drug reactions, but may also be idiopathic.[11] Acute hepatitis usually causes diffusely hypoechoic hepatomegaly. Leptospirosis is the most common cause of infectious hepatitis in dogs.[11] In cases of leptospirosis, additional ultrasound findings may include renal abnormalities, biliary abnormalities, perirenal and peritoneal effusion.[12]

Cholangitis/cholangiohepatitis

Cholangitis, which is common in cats, refers to inflammation of the intrahepatic bile ducts while cholangiohepatitis refers to inflammation of the bile ducts that has extended into the hepatic parenchyma[13] (**fig. 29.10**). In cats with cholangitis/cholangiohepatitis, the liver is often diffusely hypoechoic, although it may be normal, hyperechoic or heterogeneous.[3] Biliary abnormalities, such as biliary sludge, cholelithiasis or gallbladder wall thickening (indicative of cholecystitis), and pancreatitis are often seen concurrently.[3]

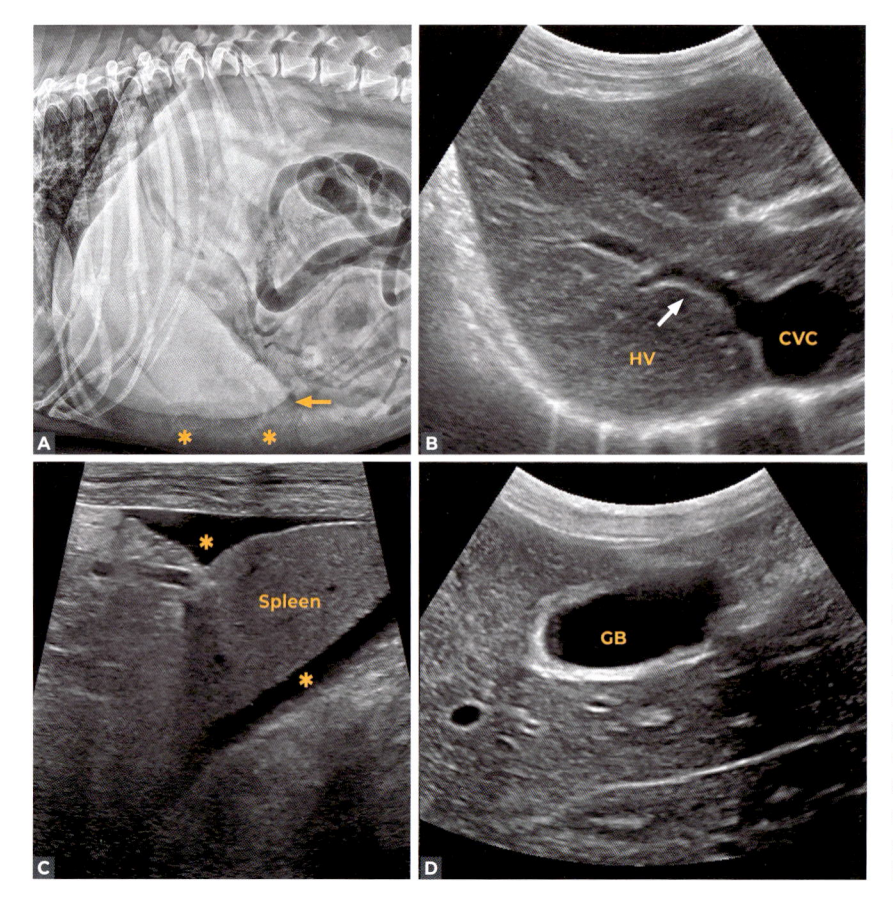

Fig. 29.8 Passive hepatic congestion in an eight-year-old Staffordshire Terrier with right-sided congestive heart failure secondary to tricuspid dysplasia. (**A**) Right lateral radiograph. The liver is moderately enlarged, extending beyond the costal arch with a slightly rounded caudoventral margin (orange arrow). The peritoneal serosal detail is decreased, with fluid-streaking of the peritoneal fat (asterisk), consistent with peritoneal effusion. (**B**) Sagittal ultrasound image of the liver. The hepatic parenchyma is diffusely hypoechoic and the caudal vena cava (CVC), and hepatic veins (HV) are distended. (**C**) Sagittal ultrasound image of the left abdomen. Adjacent to the spleen there is anechoic peritoneal effusion (asterisk). (**D**) Ultrasound image of the gallbladder (GB) displaying gallbladder wall thickening, with triple layering, consisting of thin inner and outer hyperechoic layers and a central hypoechoic layer. This is consistent with gallbladder wall edema, and in this patient, was likely a consequence of right-sided congestive heart failure. The combined findings of hypoechoic hepatomegaly, caudal vena cava and hepatic venous distension, gallbladder wall edema and ascites are consistent with passive hepatic congestion.

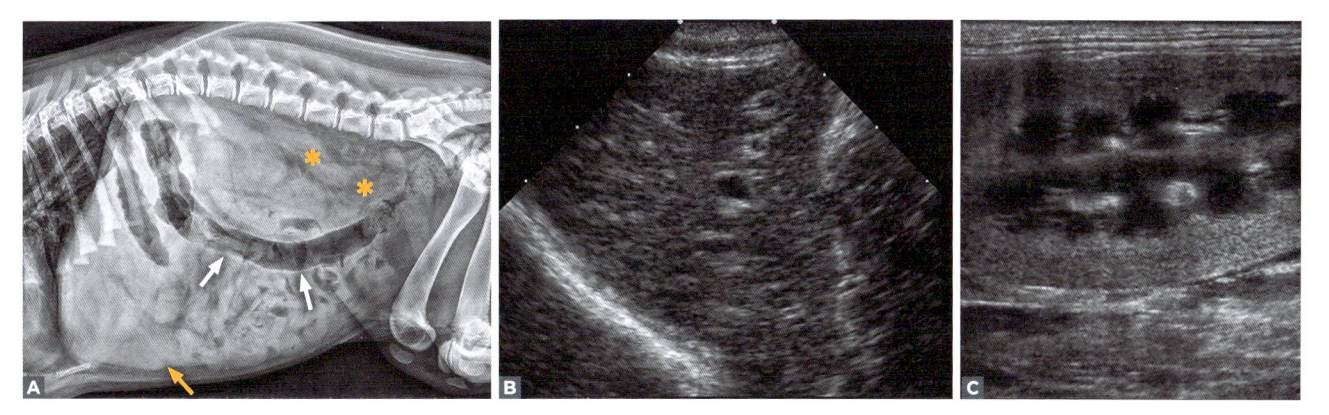

CHAPTER **29** Normal liver and hepatic parenchymal disease

Fig. 29.9 Leptospirosis in a three-month-old Labrador Retriever presenting with acute renal failure and elevated liver enzymes. (**A**) Right lateral radiograph. The liver extends slightly beyond the costal arch (orange arrow). Although overall liver size may be considered normal given the patient's young age, rounding of the liver margins may be an indicator of mild hepatomegaly in this patient. A mass effect is noted in the retroperitoneal space, with fluid streaking of the retroperitoneal fat (asterisk), consistent with retroperitoneal effusion, causing ventral displacement of the descending colon (white arrows). (**B**) Sagittal ultrasound image of the liver. The liver is diffusely hypoechoic, increasing the conspicuity of the portal veins. (**C**) Sagittal ultrasound image of the left kidney. The renal cortex is markedly hyperechoic, accentuating the corticomedullary differentiation. The right kidney had a similar appearance and there was moderate anechoic retroperitoneal effusion. Hepatic hypoechogenicity in this patient is suggestive of acute hepatitis, and in association with renal cortical hyperechogenicity and retroperitoneal effusion, is most consistent with leptospirosis infection. This was confirmed on necropsy.

Fig. 29.10 Feline cholangitis/cholangiohepatitis. (**A**) A three-year-old Domestic shorthair cat with cholangiohepatitis. The liver is normal in echogenicity. There is mild thickening of the gallbladder (GB) wall, suggestive of cholecystitis, and the gallbladder contains a small amount of echogenic debris. (**B**) Same cat as in (**A**) at the level of the duodenal papilla. There is mild thickening of the wall of the distal common bile duct (between cursors) just proximal to the duodenal papilla. (**C**) 14-year-old Domestic shorthair cat with cholangiohepatitis. The liver is normal in overall echogenicity, but is mildly heterogeneous in echotexture. (**D**) Same cat as in (**C**). The gallbladder wall is mildly thickened, indicative of cholecystitis, and the gallbladder (GB) contains echogenic debris. The periportal spaces are thickened and irregular (orange arrows).

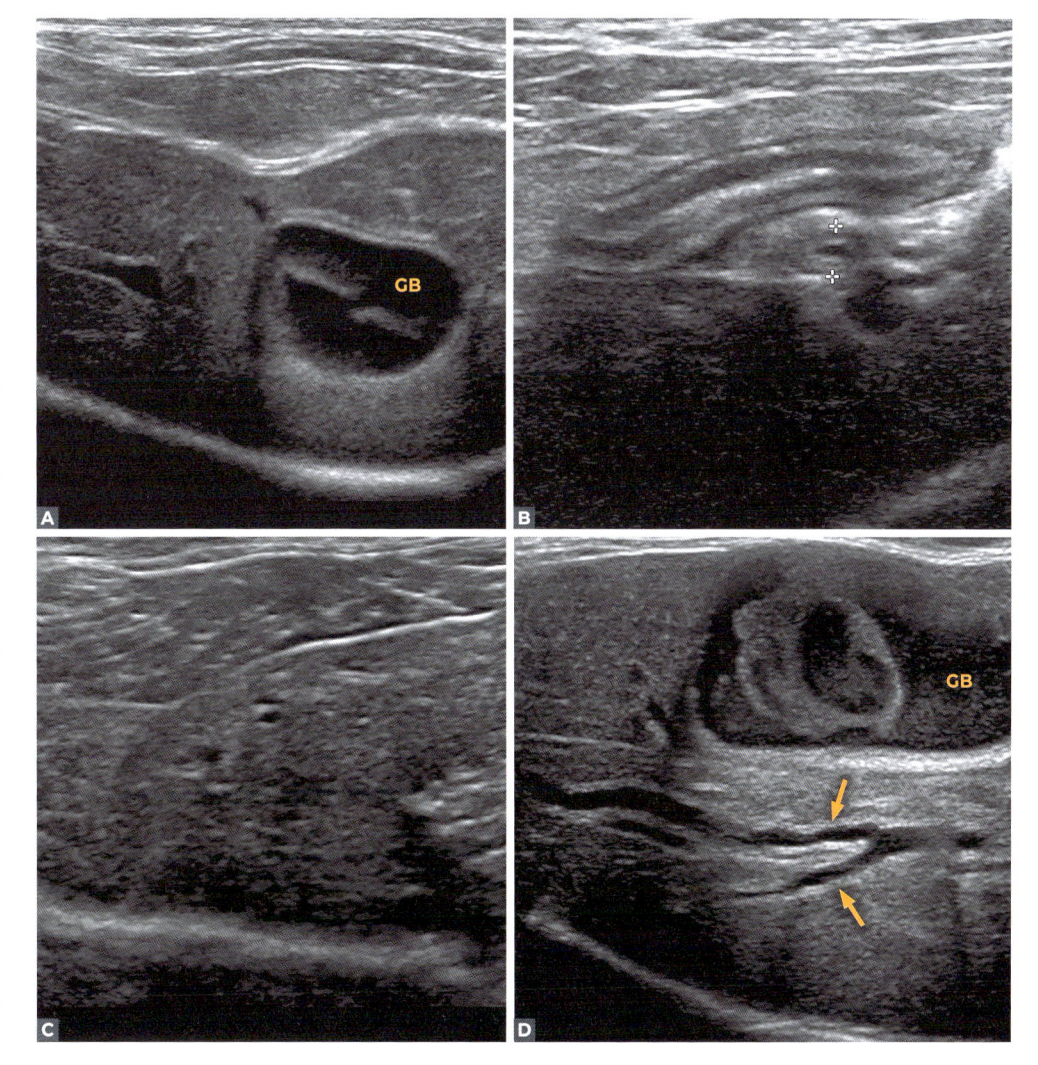

487

SECTION V ABDOMEN

Vacuolar hepatopathy/steroid hepatopathy

In dogs, steroid hepatopathy and other vacuolar hepatopathies such as diabetic hepatopathy, are among the most common diffuse hepatic parenchymal disorders[3] (**fig. 29.11 A, B**). The liver will usually be enlarged and diffusely hyperechoic, and on occasion, may be hyperattenuating.[3] In some cases, ill-defined hypoechoic and/or hyperechoic nodules may be present (consistent with nodular hyperplasia or regenerative nodules).[3]

Hepatic lipidosis

In cats, hepatic lipidosis (**fig. 29.11C, D**) is one of the most common diffuse hepatic parenchymal disorders. With hepatic lipidosis, the liver is sometimes enlarged, and is diffusely hyperechoic, and diffusely hyperattenuating due to fat accumulation within hepatocytes.[1,3]

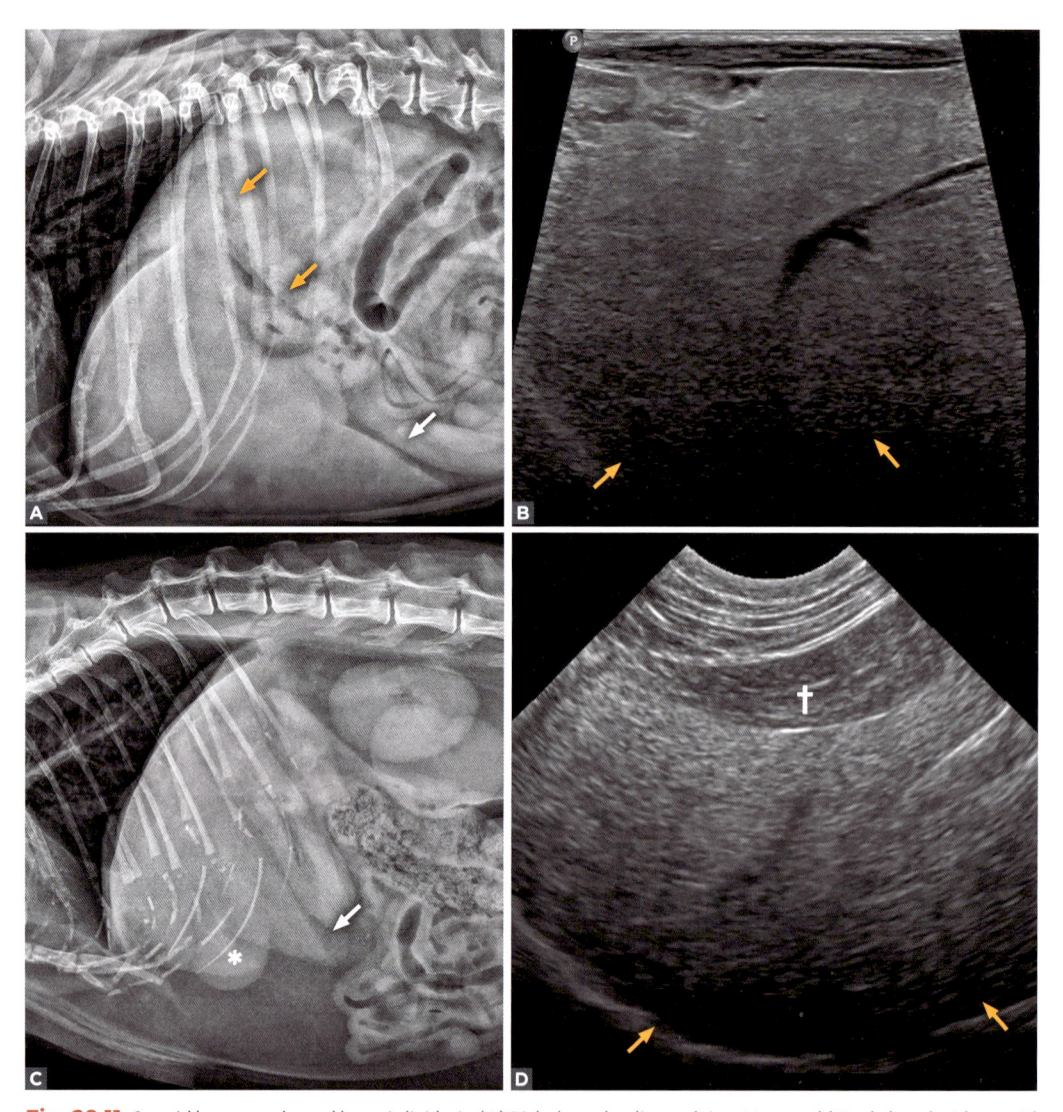

Fig. 29.11 Steroid hepatopathy and hepatic lipidosis. (**A**) Right lateral radiograph in a 14-year-old Dachshund with steroid hepatopathy. The liver is moderately enlarged, extending beyond the costal arch (white arrow) with caudodorsal displacement of the gastric axis (orange arrows). (**B**) Sagittal ultrasound image of the liver of the same dog as in (**A**). The liver is diffusely hyperechoic and hyperattenuating, displaying beam attenuation in the far-field (orange arrows). (**C**) Left lateral radiograph in an 11-year-old Domestic shorthair cat with diabetes mellitus and hepatic lipidosis. The liver is mildly enlarged with sharp caudoventral margins (white arrow). A soft tissue opacity structure with a convex margin extends ventrally beyond the hepatic margin, consistent with distension of the gallbladder (asterisk). (**D**) Sagittal ultrasound image of the liver of the same cat as in (**C**). The liver is diffusely hyperechoic to the falciform fat (†) and is hyperattenuating (orange arrows).

CHAPTER 29 Normal liver and hepatic parenchymal disease

Round cell neoplasia

The ultrasound features of hepatic round cell infiltration can be highly variable (**figs. 29.12-29.14**). Lymphoma may not alter the appearance of the liver or may cause a spectrum of changes including diffuse increased or decreased echogenicity, and focal changes such as hypoechoic nodules or masses.[1,3] Histiocytic sarcoma has been reported to cause hypoechoic nodules and masses but can also cause diffuse hepatic hypoechogenicity.[14]

Mast cell infiltration has been associated with diffuse hyperechoic hepatomegaly, hepatomegaly with normal echogenicity, diffuse hypoechogenicity, and hepatic nodules. Mast cell neoplasia has also been identified in livers with a normal sonographic appearance.[15,16]

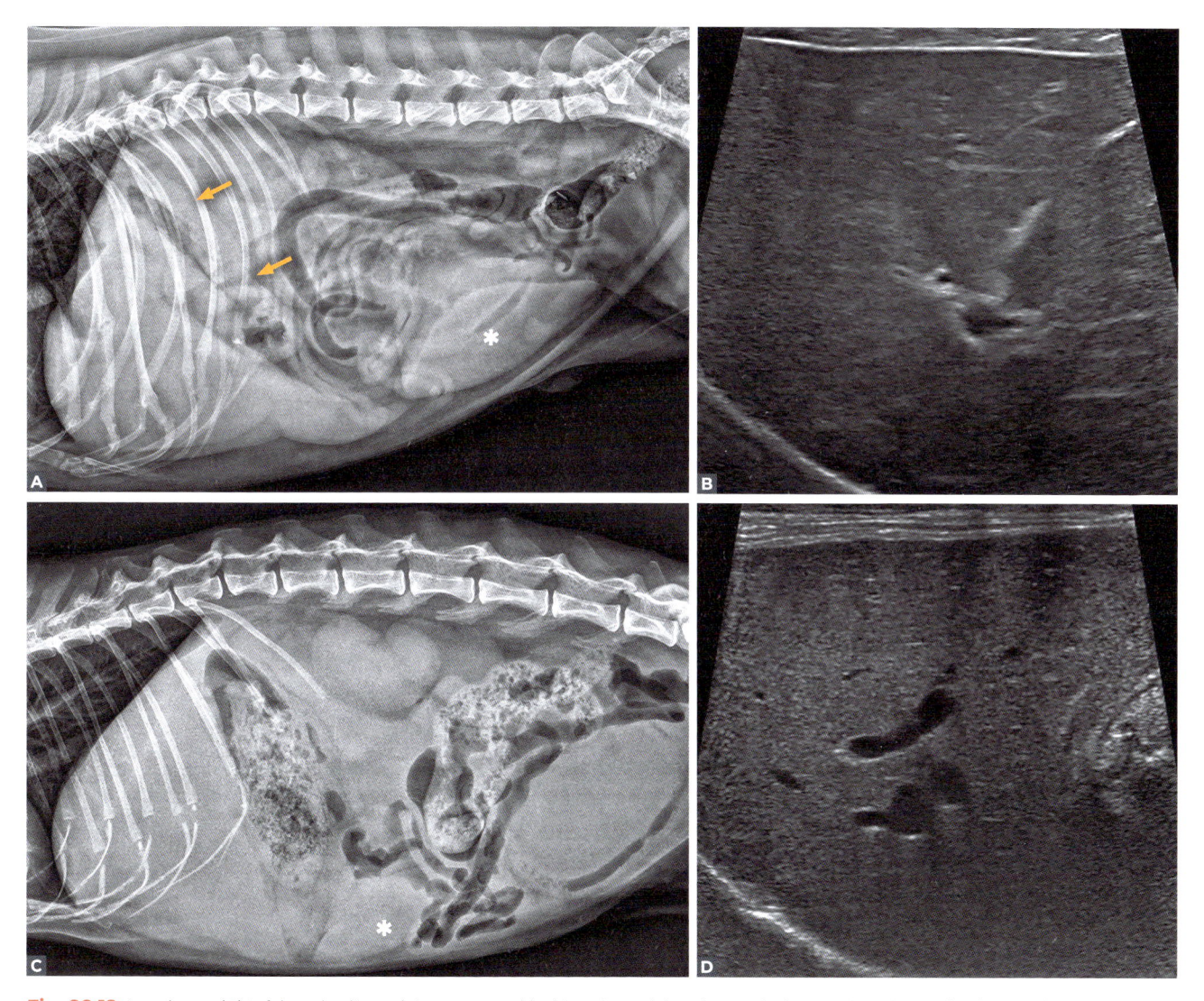

Fig. 29.12 Lymphoma. (**A**) Left lateral radiograph in a ten-year-old Eskimo dog with lymphoma. The liver is enlarged, extending beyond the costal arch, and causing caudodorsal displacement of the gastric axis (arrows). The spleen is also diffusely, smoothly enlarged (asterisk). Hepatosplenomegaly is a common finding with lymphoma. (**B**) Sagittal ultrasound image of the liver, which is enlarged and diffusely hyperechoic, reducing the conspicuity of the intrahepatic portal vessels. Lymphoma was confirmed by cytological analysis of liver and splenic ultrasound-guided fine-needle aspirates. (**C**) Left lateral radiograph in a 12-year-old Domestic shorthair cat with lymphoma. The abdomen is distended, and serosal detail is diffusely decreased, attributed to a combination of visceral crowding due to organomegaly and peritoneal effusion, as retroperitoneal detail is preserved. The liver is moderately enlarged with slightly rounded caudal margins. The spleen is also enlarged (asterisk). (**D**) Sagittal ultrasound image of the liver, which is enlarged and diffusely hyperechoic, reducing the conspicuity of the intrahepatic portal vessels. Lymphoma was confirmed by cytological analysis of liver and splenic ultrasound-guided fine-needle aspirates.

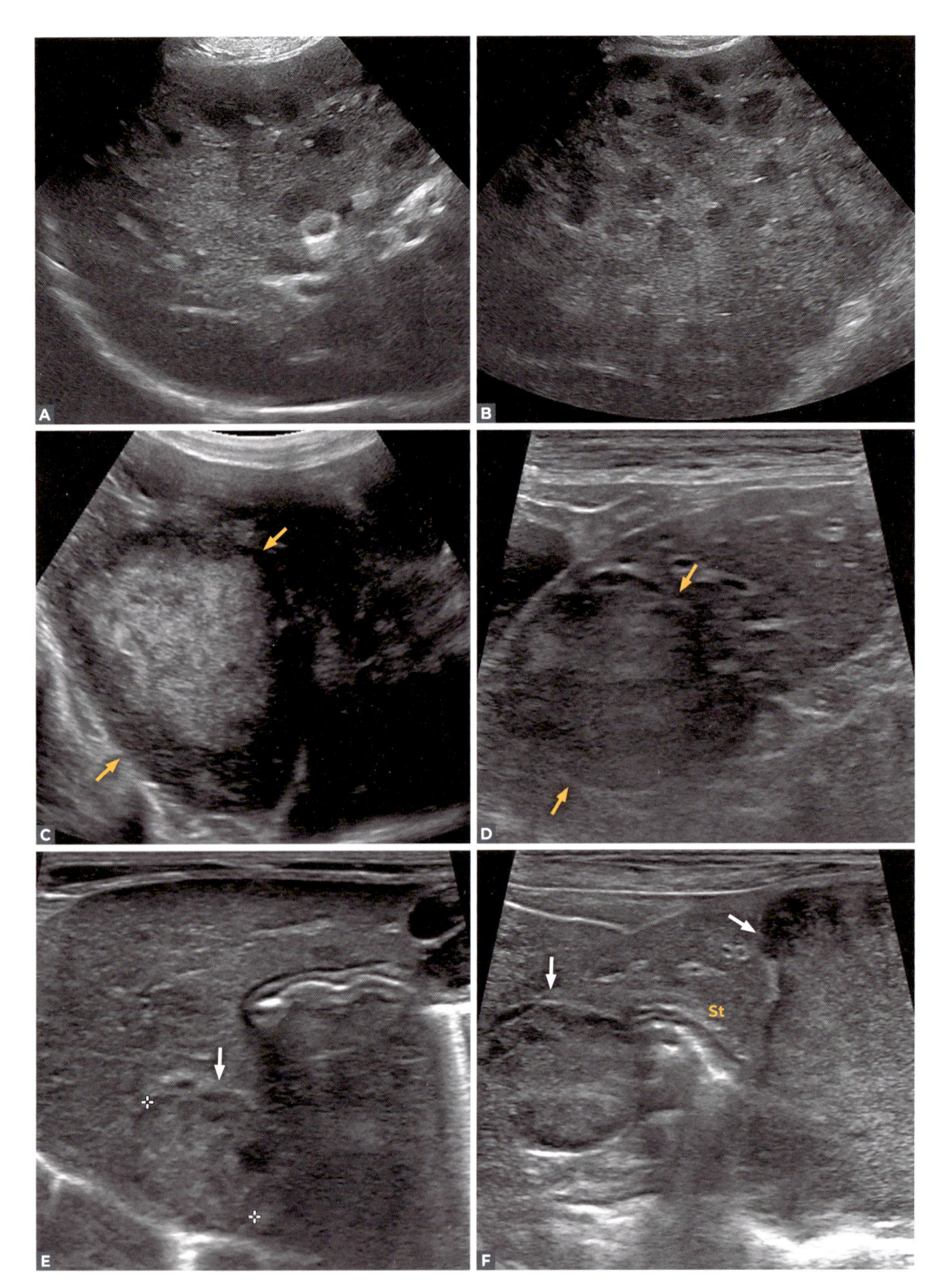

Fig. 29.13 Histiocytic sarcoma. (**A-B**) Ultrasound images of the liver in an eight-year-old Bernese Mountain dog. The liver is diffusely hyperechoic, with numerous variably shaped and sized ill-defined hypoechoic nodules throughout its parenchyma. (**C-D**) Ultrasound images of the liver in an 11-year-old mixed breed dog. A target-like mass is present (**C**), with a hypoechoic periphery and a hyperechoic central portion (orange arrows). There is also an additional ill-defined hypoechoic mass (**D**) (orange arrows). Sagittal (**E**) and transverse (**F**) ultrasound images of the liver in an 11-year-old Maltese. Several large heterogeneous masses are present within the liver (white arrows), adjacent to the diaphragm (**E**) and to the stomach (St) (**F**).

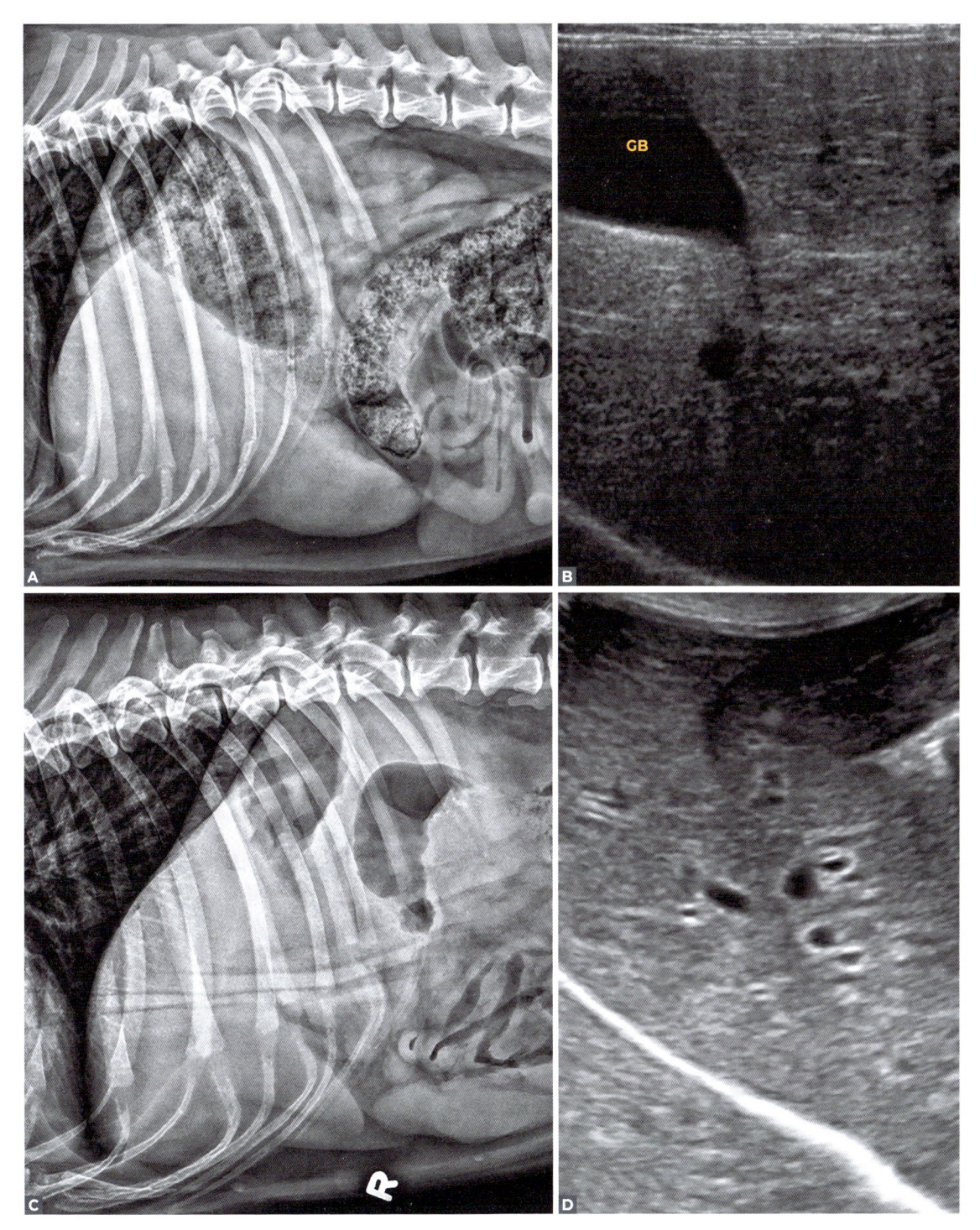

CHAPTER **29** Normal liver and hepatic parenchymal disease

Fig. 29.14 Mast cell tumor (**A-B**) in a ten-year-old mixed breed dog with metastatic mast cell infiltration of the liver. (**A**) Right lateral radiograph. The liver is enlarged, extending beyond the costal arch. (**B**) Sagittal ultrasound image of the liver. The liver is mildly diffusely hyperechoic, reducing the conspicuity of the intrahepatic portal vessels. The gallbladder (GB) is visible in the near field. (**C-D**) An eight-year-old neutered male Staffordshire Terrier with metastatic mast cell infiltration of the liver. (**C**) Right lateral radiograph. The liver is within normal limits for size with a sharp caudoventral margin. (**D**) Sagittal ultrasound image of the liver. The liver is normal in size and echogenicity with sharp margins and without focal lesions. Mast cell infiltration was confirmed by cytological analysis of ultrasound-guided fine-needle aspirates and can be present despite a normal radiographic and sonographic appearance of the liver.

Hepatocutaneous syndrome

Hepatocutaneous syndrome (**fig. 29.15**) causes diffuse hepatic parenchymal lesions, a consequence of marked vacuolar hepatopathy surrounding collapsed areas of relatively normal hepatic parenchyma.[1,3,17] Normal hepatic parenchyma is effaced by hypoechoic foci with surrounding septa of hyperechoic tissue, resembling "Swiss cheese" or "crazy paving". Affected dogs also have dermal lesions in footpads and at mucocutaneous junctions.[1]

Chronic hepatitis/hepatic fibrosis/cirrhosis

Chronic hepatitis in dogs (**fig. 29.16**) is often idiopathic, although infection, toxins, drugs, metabolic causes, and immune-mediated processes are possible etiologies.[11] A commonly identified cause or contributor is excessive copper accumulation in the liver.[11] Chronic hepatitis and cirrhosis tend to be associated with fibrosis, and therefore often cause diffuse heterogenous hyperechogenicity.[1,4] The liver can be normal to small in size, but should not be enlarged.[4] In dogs with cirrhosis, the liver usually has irregular margins, due to the presence of regenerative nodules.[4] Hepatic inflammation, regeneration and fibrosis can eventually cause portal hypertension, seen as reduced velocity of flow within the main portal vein when evaluated with spectral Doppler, and eventually, multiple acquired portosystemic shunts and ascites.[3,4]

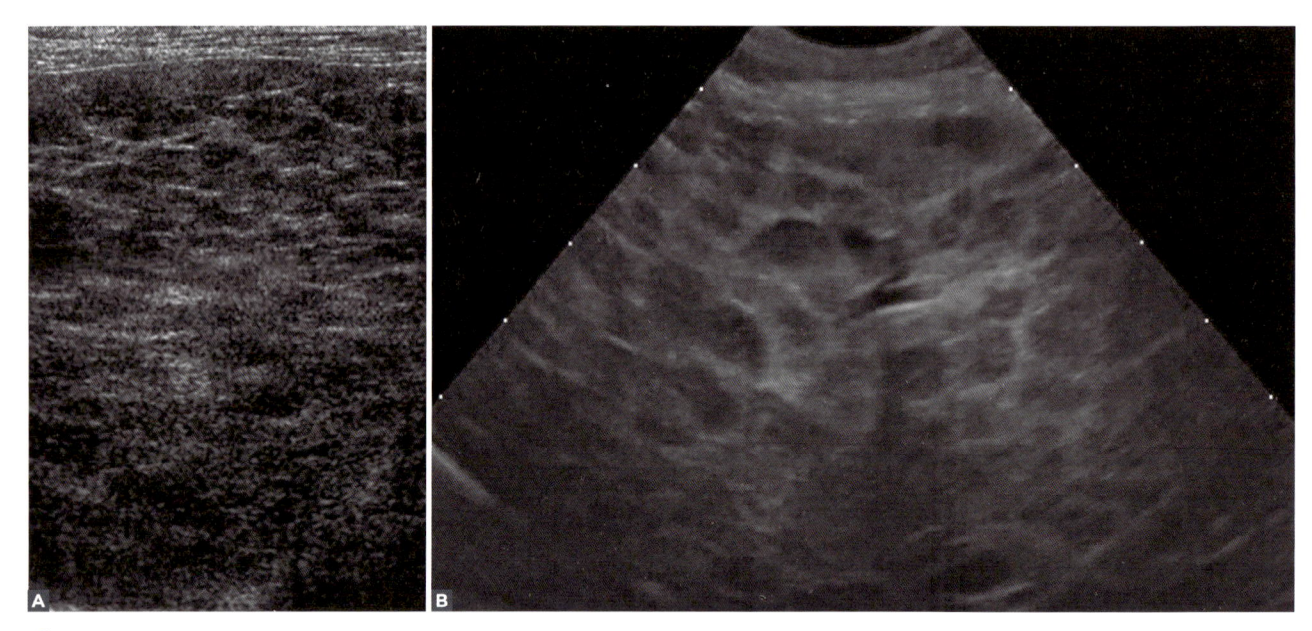

Fig. 29.15 Hepatocutaneous syndrome (superficial necrolytic dermatitis). (**A**) A 12-year-old West Highland White Terrier with hepatocutaneous syndrome. There is a diffuse honeycomb pattern of the liver, with numerous coalescing hypoechoic nodules with surrounding septa of hyperechoic liver parenchyma. (**B**) A ten-year-old Yorkshire Terrier with hepatocutaneous syndrome. Numerous hypoechoic hepatic nodules surrounded by hyperechoic hepatic parenchyma are seen throughout the liver, resulting in a diffuse honeycomb pattern.

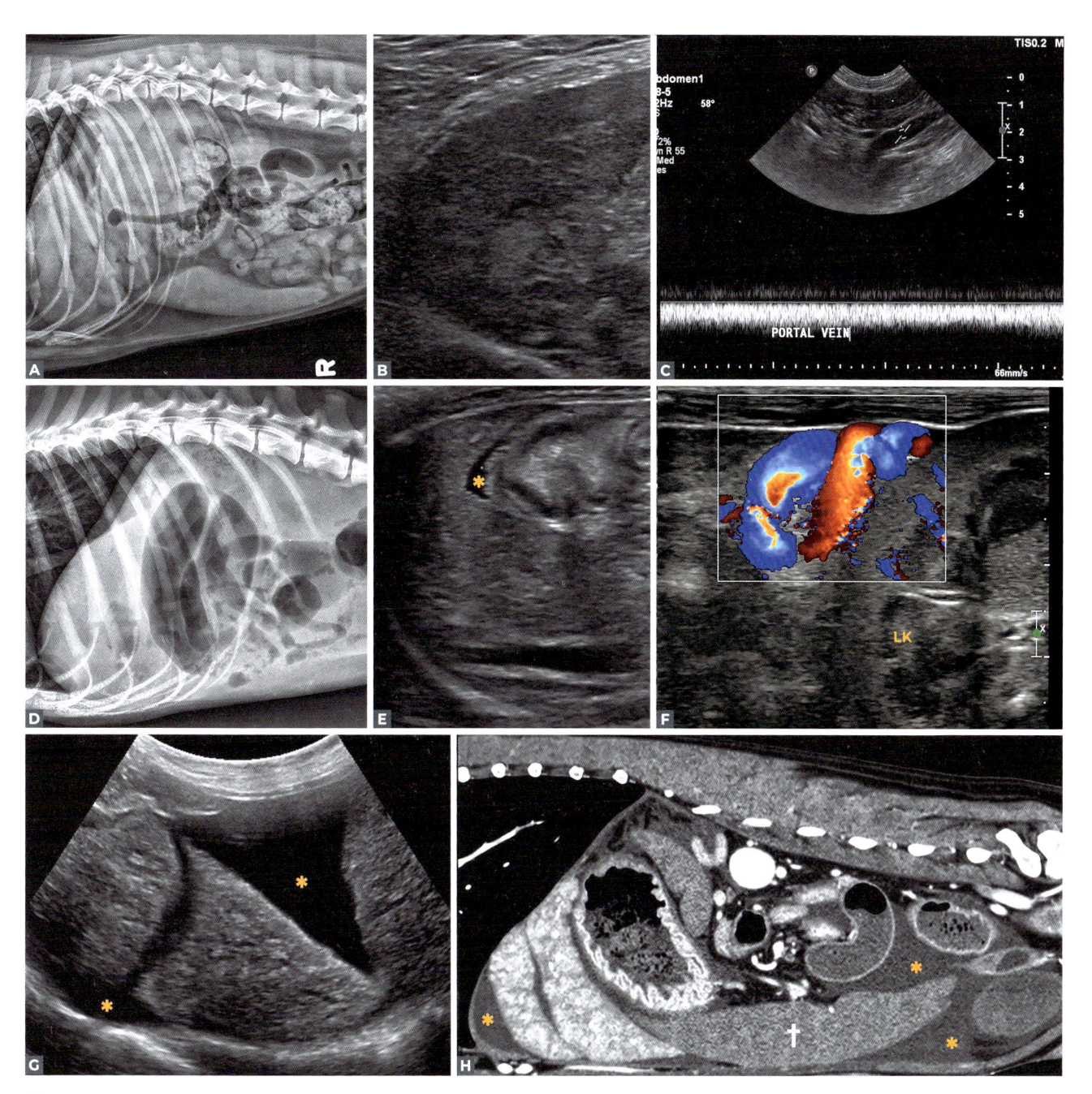

CHAPTER **29** Normal liver and hepatic parenchymal disease

Fig. 29.16 Chronic hepatitis, fibrosis, cirrhosis. (**A-C**) Copper storage hepatopathy and chronic hepatitis in a three-year-old Cavalier King Charles Spaniel. (**A**) Right lateral radiograph. Serosal margin detail is normal, and the liver is slightly small. (**B**) Ultrasound image of the liver. The liver margins are mildly irregular, and the parenchyma is heterogeneous, with coarse echotexture. (**C**) Measurement of portal velocity with spectral Doppler and an angle of insonation of approximately 58°. The blood flow is hepatopetal with a maximal velocity of 20 cm/s. Mean calculated velocity is approximately 11.4 cm/s, lower than the reported normal mean values. No other signs of portal hypertension were present in this patient. (**D-F**) Hepatic fibrosis, portal hypertension, ascites and multiple acquired portosystemic shunts in a one-year-old mixed breed dog. (**D**) Right lateral radiograph. There is decreased serosal detail, consistent with ascites. The liver margins are obscured precluding accurate assessment of size. (**E**) Sagittal ultrasound image of the liver. The liver has a sharp, well-defined caudoventral margin and is slightly heterogeneous. Anechoic fluid is seen between liver lobes (asterisk). (**F**) A plexus of tortuous aberrant blood vessels is seen adjacent to the left kidney (LK) with color Doppler interrogation, consistent with multiple acquired shunts. (**G-H**) Cirrhosis and ascites in a six-year-old mixed breed dog. (**G**) Ultrasound image of the liver, which is mildly heterogeneous with a slightly irregular capsular contour. There is a large volume of anechoic peritoneal effusion (asterisk). (**H**) Post-contrast sagittal multiplanar reconstruction CT image. There is a large volume of peritoneal effusion (asterisk), attributed to portal hypertension. The spleen is enlarged (†), possibly secondary to portal hypertension or general anesthesia. The liver is small, diffusely nodular, and heterogeneous, with a nodular and irregular capsule. The severity of the hepatic changes was underestimated with ultrasound.

Focal and multifocal abnormalities

Focal hepatomegaly

A hepatic nodule or mass can cause enlargement of an individual liver lobe, resulting in displacement of the adjacent viscera depending on the lobe involved.[1] Ultrasound can be used to differentiate cystic or cavitary masses from solid masses as well to evaluate the relationship of a hepatic mass to adjacent structures, in particular large blood vessels, the gallbladder, and the diaphragm. There is significant overlap in the appearance of benign and malignant nodules and masses and ultrasound cannot usually provide a specific diagnosis.

Computed tomography for hepatic masses

CT is complementary to ultrasound for evaluation of hepatic masses, to determine involved lobe or lobes, vascular involvement, and extent of disease. In fact, post-contrast CT has been reported to be more accurate than ultrasound in determining the anatomical origin of hepatic masses.[18] Studies using multiphase contrast-enhanced CT protocols have also attempted to differentiate benign from malignant processes.[19] Despite some features being seen more commonly with primary or metastatic neoplasia in some studies, other studies failed to correlate specific features with benign or malignant lesions.[6-8,19] Histopathology remains the gold standard for diagnosis.

Primary hepatic neoplasia

Hepatocellular carcinoma (**fig. 29.17**) is the most common primary tumor in dogs and can be a focal large mass in a single liver lobe, but can also be invasive, involving several liver lobes, or multifocal and/or coalescing nodules in all liver lobes. On ultrasound, hepatocellular carcinoma can be hypoechoic, hyperechoic or of mixed echogenicity.[1] In cats, biliary cystadenoma, a benign liver tumor, is the most common primary hepatic tumor. These lesions are usually well defined and hyperechoic with numerous small internal cysts.[4]

Metastatic neoplasia

Metastatic neoplasia (**fig. 29.18**) often consists of multifocal nodular or mass-like lesions, which may be hyperechoic or hypoechoic. Target lesions, which can be seen in the liver or spleen, are nodules or masses with a hypoechoic periphery and a hyperechoic to isoechoic center.[20] The finding of one or more target lesions in the liver or spleen has a 74% positive predictive value for malignancy, although the appearance also occurs with benign lesions.[20] A study evaluating triple-phase contrast enhanced CT described metastatic lesions as often being homogeneously hypoattenuating to the liver parenchyma in all post-contrast phases.[6]

Nodular hyperplasia

Hepatic nodular hyperplasia (**fig. 29.19**) is a common benign lesion in older dogs and is usually clinically silent, although affected dogs can have ALP elevations. Lesions can vary in size and echogenicity, although hypoechoic nodules measuring less than 15 mm in diameter with well-defined or poorly defined margins are most common.

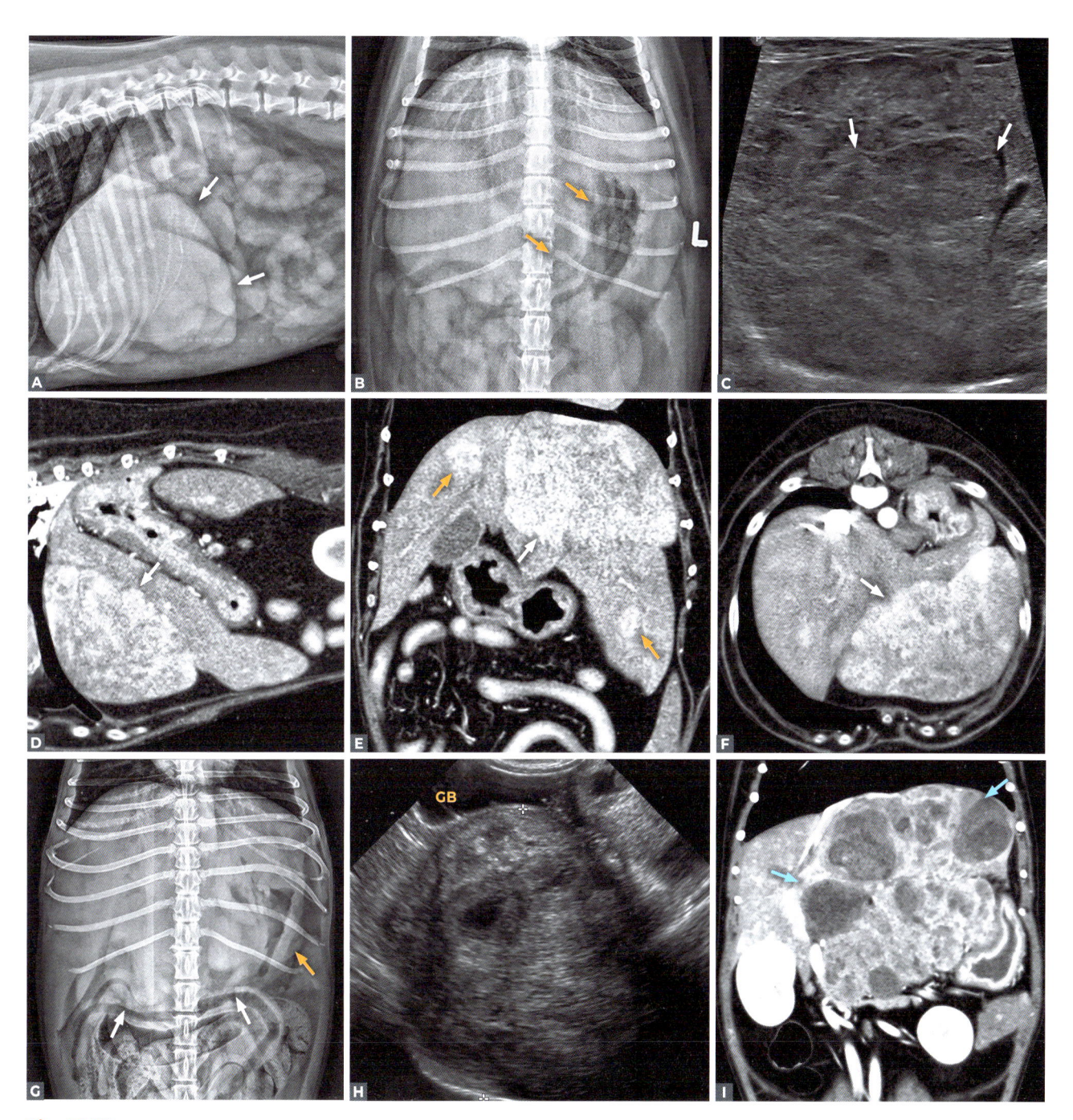

CHAPTER **29** Normal liver and hepatic parenchymal disease

Fig. 29.17 Hepatocellular carcinoma. (**A-B**) Left lateral and ventrodorsal radiographs in a seven-year-old mixed breed dog with hepatocellular carcinoma. There is focal right-sided hepatomegaly (white arrows), displacing the stomach leftward and caudally (orange arrows). (**C**) Ultrasound image in the same patient as (**A**) and (**B**). A large, ill-defined, mildly hypoechoic, and heterogeneous mass is noted in the craniodorsal aspect of the liver. Sagittal (**D**), dorsal (**E**), and transverse (**F**) post-contrast CT images in a ten-year-old mixed breed dog with hepatocellular carcinoma. There is a heterogeneously contrast-enhancing soft tissue attenuating liver mass arising from the left medial liver lobe (white arrows) causing caudal and dorsal displacement of the stomach. Two smaller nodules with similar contrast enhancement features are present within the liver, suggestive of metastases (orange arrows). (**G-I**) Hepatocellular carcinoma in a 12-year-old Pekingese. (**G**) Ventrodorsal radiograph displaying focal central hepatomegaly (white arrows), displacing the stomach leftward and caudal (orange arrow). (**H**) Ultrasound image showing a large, heterogeneously hypoechoic mass in the liver (between cursors) displacing the gallbladder (GB) ventrally. (**I**) Post-contrast dorsal multiplanar reconstruction CT image displaying a large, markedly heterogeneously contrast-enhancing, cavitary liver mass (blue arrows) with leftward displacement of the stomach (asterisk).

SECTION V ABDOMEN

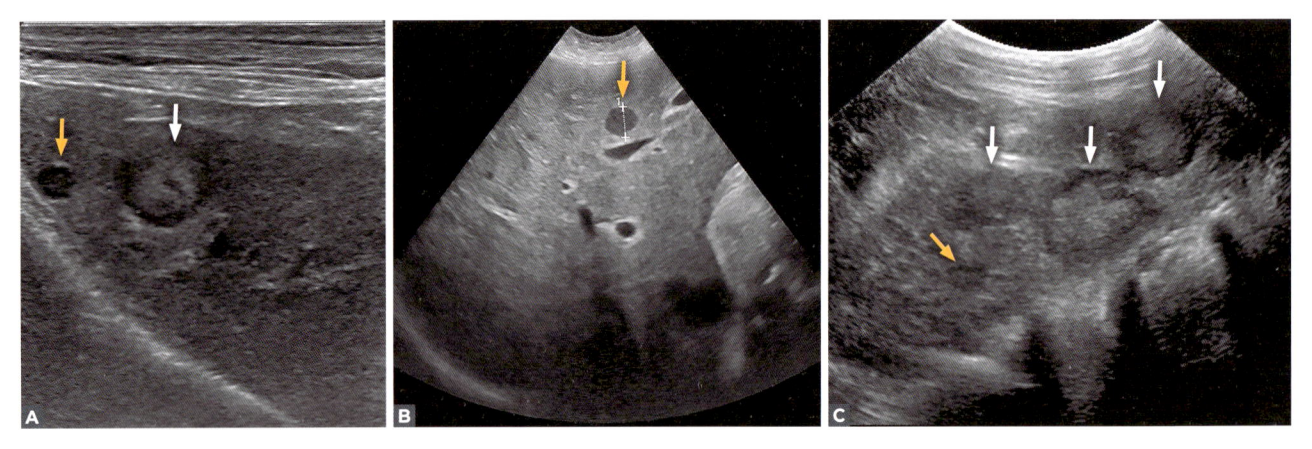

Fig. 29.18 Metastatic neoplasia. (A) Metastatic thyroid carcinoma in a six-year-old mixed breed dog. A target-like nodule, consisting of a hypoechoic periphery and a hyperechoic central portion is noted within the liver (white arrow). A second smaller hypoechoic nodule is also present within the liver. Target nodules are suspicious for metastases, particularly when multiple, and in patients with a known malignant neoplasm. Some benign processes, such as nodular hyperplasia, may have a similar appearance. (B) Metastatic extramedullary plasmacytoma in a ten-year-old Golden Retriever. The liver is diffusely hyperechoic. A well-defined hypoechoic nodule is also present within the liver (orange arrow). (C) Metastatic pancreatic carcinoma in a seven-year-old Golden Retriever. Multiple target-like nodules (white arrows) and an ill-defined hypoechoic nodule (orange arrow) are noted within the liver.

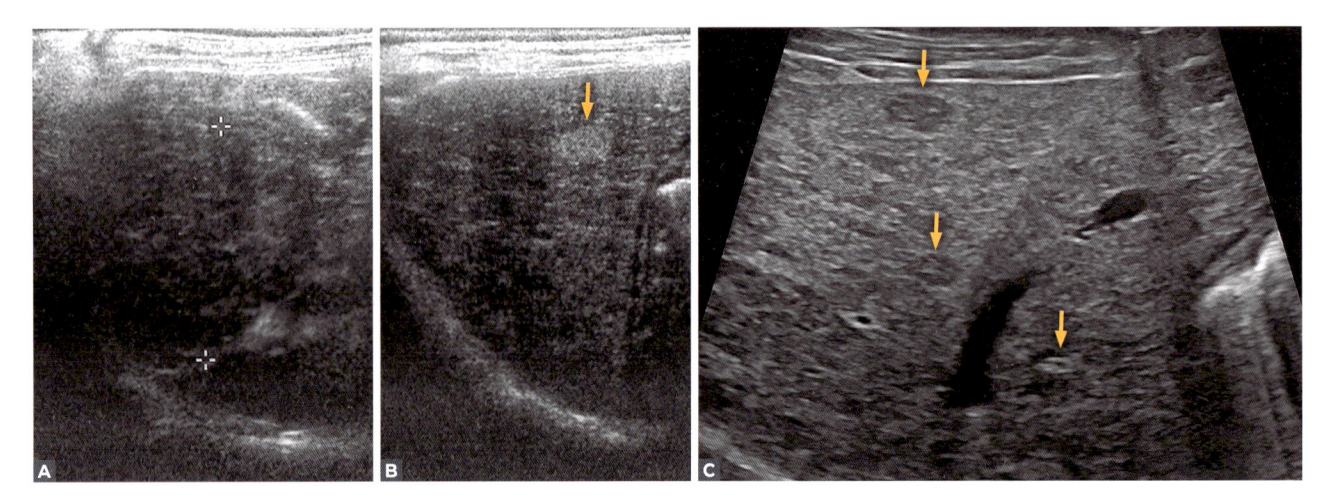

Fig. 29.19 Nodular hyperplasia. (A-B) Nodular hyperplasia in a 13-year-old Cairn Terrier. (A) A large hypoechoic mass (between cursors) and (B) a small hyperechoic nodule (arrow) are noted within the liver, illustrating the variable appearance of benign nodular hyperplasia. (C) A 13-year-old Yorkshire Terrier with hyperadrenocorticism. The liver is diffusely hyperechoic with a coarse echotexture. Several small hypoechoic nodules are noted within the liver (arrows). These findings were consistent with vacuolar hepatopathy and nodular hyperplasia.

References

1. Thrall DE, Larson MM. Liver and Spleen. In Thrall DE (editor). Textbook of veterinary diagnostic radiology 7th edition, St Louis, 2018, Elsevier, pp 792-822.
2. Thrall DE, Robertson ID (editors). Atlas of normal radiographic anatomy and anatomic variants in the dog and cat 2nd edition, St Louis, 2015, Elsevier.
3. Penninck D, d'Anjou MA. Liver. In Penninck D, d'Anjou MA (editors). Atlas of small animal ultrasonography 2nd edition, Hoboken, Wiley Blackwell, 2015, pp 183-238.
4. Nyland TG, Larson MM, Thrall DE. Liver. In Mattoon JS, Nyland TG (editors). Small animal diagnostic ultrasound 3rd edition, St Louis, 2015, Elsevier, pp 332-399.
5. Kemp SD, Panciera DL, Larson MM, Saunders GK, Werre SR. A comparison of hepatic sonographic features and histopathologic diagnosis in canine liver disease: 138 Cases. *J Vet Intern Med* 27:806-813, 2013.
6. Kutara K, Seki M, Ishikawa C, Sakai M, Kagawa Y, Iida G, et al. Triple-phase helical computed tomography in dogs with hepatic masses. *Vet Radiol Ultrasound* 55:7-15, 2014.
7. Fukushima K, Kanemoto H, Ohno K, Takahashi M, Nakashima K, Fujino Y, et al. CT characteristics of primary hepatic mass lesions in dogs. *Vet Radiol Ultrasound* 53:252-257, 2012.
8. Jones ID, Lamb CR, Drees R, Priestnall SL, Mantis P. Associations between dual-phase computed tomography features and histopathologic diagnoses in 52 dogs with hepatic or splenic masses. *Vet Radiol Ultrasound* 57:144-153, 2016.
9. An G, Kwon D, Yoon H, Yu J, Bang S, Lee Y, et al. Evaluation of the radiographic liver length/11th thoracic vertebral length ratio as a method for quantifying liver size in cats. *Vet Radiol Ultrasound* 60:640-647, 2019.
10. Kim SE, Giglio RF, Reese DJ, Reese SL, Bacon NJ, Ellison GW. Comparison of computed tomographic angiography and ultrasonography for the detection and characterization of portosystemic shunts in dogs. *Vet Radiol Ultrasound* 54:569-574, 2013.
11. Ettinger SJ, Feldman EC. Section XIX: Hepatobiliary disease. In Ettinger SJ, Feldman EC, Cote E (editors). Textbook of veterinary internal medicine 8th edition, Saint Louis, 2016, Elsevier, pp 3933-4088.
12. Sonet J, Barthélemy A, Goy-Thollot I, Pouzot-Nevoret C. Prospective evaluation of abdominal ultrasonographic findings in 35 dogs with leptospirosis. *Vet Radiol Ultrasound* 59:98-106, 2018.
13. Boland L, Beatty J. Feline cholangitis. *Vet Clin North Am Small Anim Pract* 47:703-724, 2017.
14. Cruz-Arámbulo R, Wrigley R, Powers B. Sonographic features of histiocytic neoplasms in the canine abdomen. *Vet Radiol Ultrasound* 45:554-558, 2004.
15. Sato AF, Solano M. Ultrasonographic findings in abdominal mast cell disease: a retrospective study of 19 patients. *Vet Radiol Ultrasound* 45:51-57, 2004.
16. Book AP, Fidel J, Wills T, Bryan J, Sellon R, Mattoon J. Correlation of ultrasound findings, liver and spleen cytology, and prognosis in the clinical staging of high metastatic risk canine mast cell tumors. *Vet Radiol Ultrasound* 52:548-554, 2011.
17. Jacobson LS, Kirberger RM, Nesbit JW. Hepatic ultrasonography and pathological findings in dogs with hepatocutaneous syndrome: new concepts. *J Vet Intern Med* 9:399-404, 1995.
18. Lamb CR, Steel R, Lipscomb VJ. Determining the anatomical origin of canine hepatic masses by CT. *J Small Anim Pract* 59:752-757, 2018.
19. Stehlík L, Di Tommaso M, Del Signore F, et al. Triple-phase multidetector computed tomography in distinguishing canine hepatic lesions. *Animals (Basel)* 11:11, 2020.
20. Cuccovillo A, Lamb CR. Cellular features of sonographic target lesions of the liver and spleen in 21 dogs and a cat. *Vet Radiol Ultrasound* 43:275-278, 2002.

CHAPTER 30

Biliary system

Pamela Di Donato and Swan Specchi

KEY POINTS

- Biliary disease is more common in cats than in dogs.
- Cholangitis/cholangiohepatitis may appear with thickened biliary wall, biliary sludge, cholelithiasis and common bile duct (CBD) dilation.
- Gallbladder mucocele (GBM) is common in dogs and rare in cats. Consequences of GBM include biliary obstruction or gallbladder rupture. A typical "stellate" or "kiwi pattern" can be found on ultrasound. Variable appearance in CT, the combination of a hyperattenuating gallbladder material with centrally distributed mineral may be indicative of mucocele.
- Choleliths may be mineral or not. They are generally incidental, or may represent a cause or consequence of biliary stasis, cholangitis, or obstruction.
- Hepatic cysts are often linked to polycystic kidney disease.
- Histology, cytology, and bile culture are valuable diagnostic tools in biliary disease.

The biliary system consists of intrahepatic and extrahepatic structures and include biliary ducts (intra- and extrahepatic component), common bile duct (CBD), cystic duct and gallbladder. The gallbladder is located to the right of the midline within the cranioventral portion of the liver between the right medial and quadrate hepatic lobes in dogs, and between the two parts of the right medial lobe in cats. Sometimes it can protrude as a curved structure from the ventral liver margins on radiographs, especially in cats. Congenital gallbladder anomalies include duplication and agenesis. Gallbladder duplication can be characterized by a septum (partially divided and typically bilobed) (**figs. 30.1** and **30.2**), duplex (double) or multiplex (multiple). Absence of the gallbladder (agenesis) is a rare congenital disease, mostly reported in Chihuahuas with or without associated additional congenital hepatic malformations and ductal plate anomalies.[1]

The gallbladder serves as a reservoir of bile where the bile is stored and concentrated during fasting.[2,3] The cystic duct extends from the gallbladder neck and receives the hepatic biliary ducts forming the CBD, which reaches the duodenum at the major duodenal papilla. The CBD is the extrahepatic pathway that directs the bile towards the duodenum. There is anatomic variation of the communication of the CBD and the duodenum between dogs and cats. In dogs, the CBD empties into the major duodenal papilla a few centimeters beyond the pylorus near the smaller (minor) pancreatic duct while the larger (accessory) pancreatic duct at the minor papilla a little more distally. In cats, the major pancreatic duct joins the CBD prior to its entry into the major duodenal papilla. This anatomical feature predisposes cats to "triaditis", an inflammatory process involving the liver/biliary

SECTION V ABDOMEN

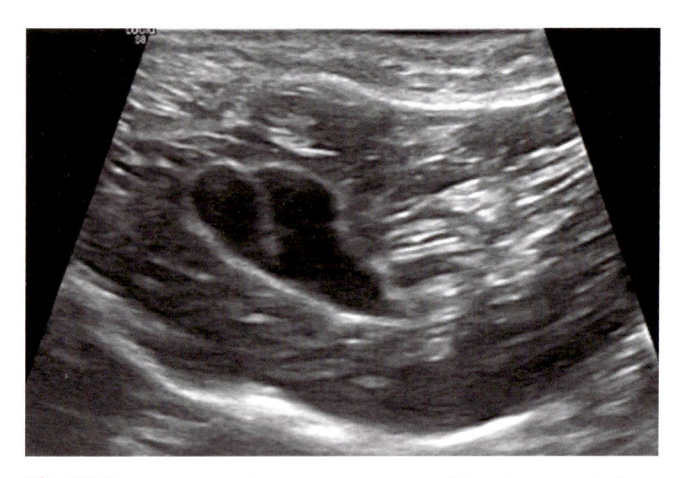

Fig. 30.1 Ultrasonographic image of an 11-year-old female Domestic shorthair cat. The gallbladder lumen is partially divided by an internal echogenic septum resulting in a valentine heart shape (bilobed gallbladder).

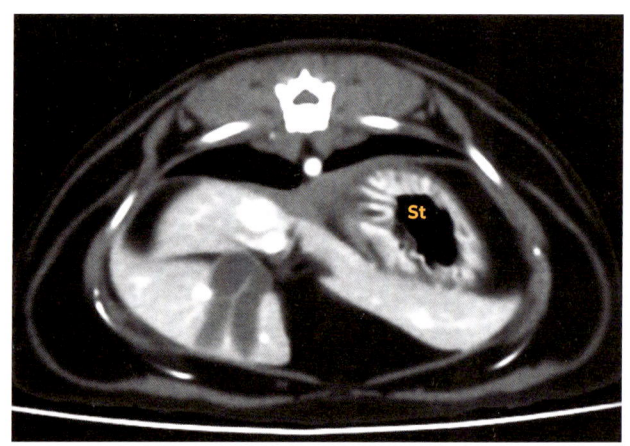

Fig. 30.2 Computed tomographic angiography, transverse image of the abdomen in an 11-year-old Domestic shorthair cat with bilobed gallbladder. *St*, stomach.

system, the intestine and the pancreas. Inflammation of the biliary system is more common in cats than dogs and this may be related to this unique anatomy of cats which may predispose to ascending bacterial infection from the small intestinal tract.[4,5]

The normal wall of the gallbladder and CBD is thin and smooth measuring 1 mm or less.[6] The common bile duct is more visible and routinely visualized in cats than in dogs. It is considered normal up to 3 mm in dogs and 4 mm in cats.[7] The intrahepatic biliary tree is made by variable sized biliary ducts and it is not normally seen in dogs and cats with both ultrasonography and computed tomography (CT) unless dilated.[7,8] A wide spectrum of diseases could affect the biliary system including congenital, inflammatory/infectious, choleliths, mucocele and neoplasia. In cats, diseases of the biliary system are more common than diseases of the liver parenchyma.[2] Diagnostic imaging (radiography, ultrasonography, CT, or MRI), cholecystocentesis and cytology/histology are essential in diagnosis and in guiding therapeutic decisions. Radiography is widely available and can be useful for screening for hepatomegaly, large hepatic masses, to detect radiopaque choleliths, emphysematous cholecystitis, and decreased serosal detail in case of ruptured gallbladder.

Ultrasound is complementary to radiographs and provides detailed information about the hepatobiliary system and surrounding organs. CT and MRI may be indicated in case of liver masses for characterization of the behavior, staging, and surgical planning. Advanced imaging such as CT or MRI are becoming more commonly used for the diagnosis of hepatobiliary disease in dogs and cats. They offer several advantages as the ability to image the patient without superimposition of other organs or gastrointestinal gas, assess vascularization of organs/lesions, possibility to perform 3D/multiplanar reconstructions allowing a more complete assessment of the hepatobiliary system in particular in large and deep-chested dogs. Disadvantages are the need for general anesthesia, increased costs and lack of availability and use of ionizing radiation in case of CT.[9] This chapter focuses on ultrasound, which is the most commonly used and available imaging modality to assess the biliary system. It is a non-invasive diagnostic modality that may help in identifying several hepatobiliary diseases, e.g., dilated bile ducts, liver cysts, choleliths, gallbladder mucocele (GBM), gallbladder wall and parenchymal changes.[2] Ultrasound is sensitive for detecting focal or multifocal disease, while is limited for detecting diffuse infiltrative parenchymal diseases. The absence of ultrasonographic changes does not rule out the possibility of disease. Ultrasound often lacks specificity and cytology, histology and bile culture are required to reach a definitive diagnosis.

Cystic abnormalities and segmental dilatation of the biliary system

Hepatic cystic disease arises from the biliary tract and is considered biliary disease. Biliary cysts can be single or multiple, and they have been correlated with congenital polycystic disease involving the kidneys, liver, and pancreas in cats (Persian) and dogs (Cairn Terriers, West Highland White Terriers, Golden Retriever).[8,10,11] They can be congenital or acquired with or without communication with the biliary tree. Ultrasonographic appearance of hepatic cysts consists of round, thin-walled, anechoic fluid-filled structures with associated distal acoustic enhancement. In CT, they appear as a well-circumscribed, fluid-attenuating lesions with no contrast enhancement within or protruding from the hepatic parenchyma (**fig. 30.3**). Cysts can be difficult to differentiate from cystadenoma. A true hepatic cyst is usually a thin-walled structure generally without septation and contains bile. Aspiration may help differentiate between true cysts and other conditions such as hematomas, abscesses, parasitic cysts, malignant tumours,[12] and bacteriologic culture are advisable as well as serial examinations.[13]

Choledochal cysts (CC) have been recognized in cats as congenital marked segmental cystic dilatation of the CBD without evidence of an obstructive component. In a recent article on four cats with suspected CC, the segmental dilatation of the CBD exceeded 5 mm (sign generally highly supportive of biliary obstruction). Additional ultrasonographic changes include hepatomegaly, tubular/saccular dilatation of the extra and/or intrahepatic biliary ducts, thickening of the biliary walls and biliary echogenic debris accumulation (**figs. 30.4** and **30.5**). Cats with CC may have mild clinical and biochemical changes despite the marked biliary duct dilatation; however, the biliary dilatation may predispose to complications such as biliary stasis, choleliths/debris formation and recurrent biliary infection/cholangitis or cholangiopathies.[14]

Segmental dilatation of the CBD should not prompt immediate emergency surgery, but rather the need for further investigation. Depending on the morphology of the CC some cats may benefit from surgical cyst resection. Long-term medical management is generally required.[14] Caroli's disease has been reported in few dogs (in particular in Boxer and Skye Terrier) and is a congenital dilation of the large and segmental bile ducts communicating with the biliary tree and associated hepatic portal fibrosis and/or bilateral polycystic kidney disease.[15] Calcification of malformed ducts may be observed secondary to bile stagnation and cholangitis.[3] Non-obstructive dilation can be difficult to differentiate from obstructive biliary disease and CT or MRI may help in further characterization of these lesions.

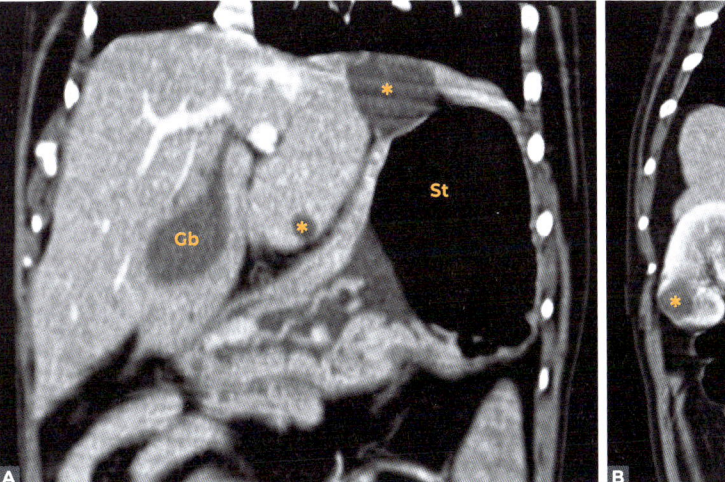

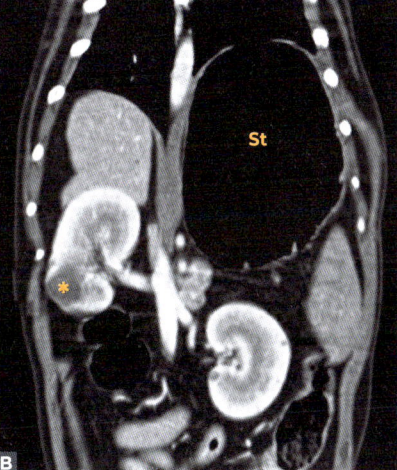

Fig. 30.3 Computed tomographic angiography 2D dorsal reconstruction image, in an 11-year-old crossbred dog with multiple hepatic and renal cysts (asterisk). *GB*, gallbladder; *St*, stomach.

SECTION V ABDOMEN

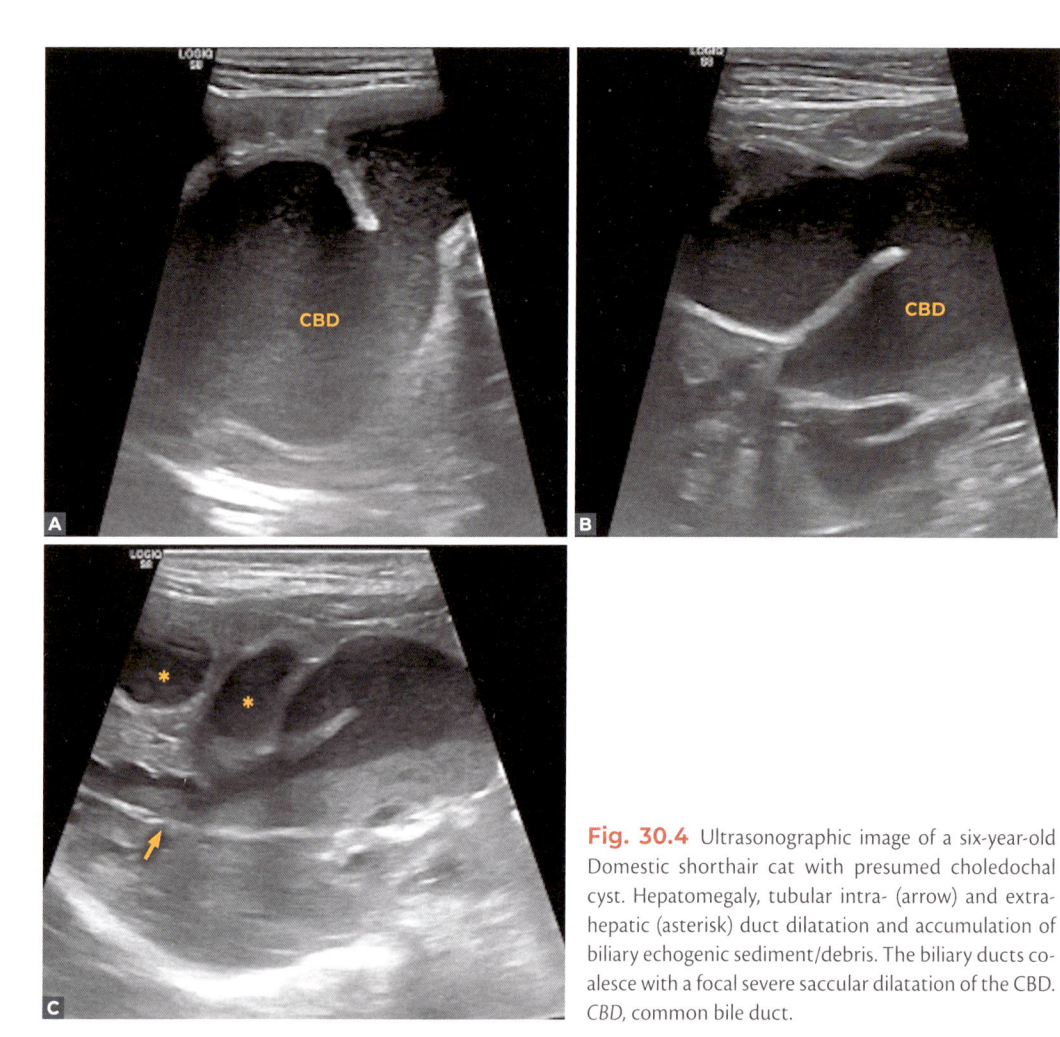

Fig. 30.4 Ultrasonographic image of a six-year-old Domestic shorthair cat with presumed choledochal cyst. Hepatomegaly, tubular intra- (arrow) and extrahepatic (asterisk) duct dilatation and accumulation of biliary echogenic sediment/debris. The biliary ducts coalesce with a focal severe saccular dilatation of the CBD. *CBD*, common bile duct.

Fig. 30.5 Computed tomographic angiography transverse image in a five-year-old Domestic shorthair cat with a presumed choledochal cyst. There is moderate segmental dilatation of the common bile duct (CBD) with moderate thickening and enhancing wall indicative of choledochitis/cholangitis. Multiple dilated bile ducts are visible, including extrahepatic and intrahepatic ducts (arrow).

Biliary sludge

Luminal material within the gallbladder has been described as gravity dependent (mobile) and non-gravity dependent biliary sludge (NDBS) and visible as echogenic material without distal acoustic shadow in ultrasound. The mobility of the sludge is determined by repositioning the animal during the exam.[21] The presence of gravity dependent biliary sludge is a common finding in dogs while in cats biliary sludge can be predictive of increased liver enzymes and total bilirubin.[16] In contrast to this, a recent article found higher prevalence of gallbladder sludge in cats undergoing an abdominal ultrasound and it appears to be non specific.[17] In dogs, gravity-dependent biliary sludge is often seen incidentally, however, it has recently been hypothesized to indicate cholestasis secondary to delayed gallbladder emptying/contractility and possibly represents a risk factor in developing biliary disease (gallbladder mucocele or cholecystitis).[18,19,20] Gravity-dependent biliary sludge may progress to NDBS[20] and gallbladder dysmotility/cholestasis, cholecystitis[21] and cystic mucosal hyperplasia may play a role in dogs. NDBS may indicate changes in viscosity of the bile and potentially increase in mucin content. It has been hypothesized that formation of NDBS precedes the formation of GBM.[18,19,20] Biliary sludge in CT is moderately hyperattenuating relative to normal bile (34-35.8 HU) and generally located in the dependent aspect of the gallbladder/biliary system lumen. Inspissated bile within the gallbladder or CBD may form "sludge balls" and they potentially can lead to biliary obstruction.[22] Gallbladder sludge balls are generally mobile; however, they can firmly adhere to the gallbladder wall and may mimic intraluminal gallbladder echogenic masses (tumors or polypoid form of cystic mucosal hyperplasia). Contrast-enhanced ultrasound (CEUS) may be useful in these cases (if CT is not available) to make distinction between a vascularized structure and non-vascularized biliary sludge ball.[23]

Gallbladder mucocele

Gallbladder mucocele (GBM) is characterized by cystic mucinous hyperplasia resulting in excessive mucin secretion (increase bile viscosity), accumulation of intraluminal inspissated bile/mucus and consequently distension of the gallbladder. The progressive gallbladder distension can lead to pressure wall necrosis that predisposes to rupture with bile peritonitis. Concomitant infection from enteric positive bacteria is possible (14.2%).[24] In case of leakage the bile peritonitis could be septic or aseptic depending on the gallbladder content.[18] GBM can be asymptomatic, or become an emergency/life-threatening condition leading to necrotizing cholecystitis, gallbladder rupture and bile peritonitis. Mucinous plug associated with the mucocele can occlude the gallbladder neck or CBD leading to biliary obstruction. The etiopathogenesis of GBM is unclear and suspected multifactorial. Recognized risk factors for GBM formation include increased age, bile stasis, decreased gallbladder motility, endocrinopathies (such as hyperadrenocorticism, hypothyroidism), and hyperlipidemia. These conditions could predispose to GBM formation by altering the bile composition, impairment of protective mechanism of the epithelium against bile acids and promoting cholestasis/gallbladder dysmotility. Concentrated bile acid may result in wall irritation of the gallbladder, promoting mucinous hyperplasia and eventually gallbladder mucocele.[11,18,19,20] Multiple canine breeds are predisposed, like Shetland Sheepdogs, Cocker Spaniels, Miniature Schnauzers and Border Terriers. GBM is rare in cats, and this may be due to the fact that cats have fewer mucus-secreting glands in the gallbladder wall compared to dogs.[25] Cholecystectomy is generally indicated for GBM causing biliary tract outflow obstruction. Medical management with patient monitoring including follow-up ultrasound exams is a reasonable alternative in stable cases with absence of clinical and biochemical abnormalities.[22] Non-surgical resolution of gallbladder mucocele has been described in two dogs with medical management and treatment of hypothyroidism.[26] Recent studies promote elective cholecystectomy for treatment of GBM as result in best long-term survival and lower mortality compared to medical management.[27,28] In a recent study, dogs undergoing elective cholecystectomy showed lower mortality (2%) compared to those undergoing emergency cholecystectomy (22-40%).[28] On ultrasound, mucocele has a distinctive appearance which makes ultrasound a highly specific and the gold standard modality for diagnosis of this disease. Classic characteristics include an enlarged gallbladder with organized centralized non-dependent hyperechoic sludge distributed in a "stellate" or "kiwi-like" pattern (**fig. 30.6**). This material is immobile with changes in the patient's position. The hypoechoic mucus collected along the gallbladder wall displaces the echogenic bile in the center. The gallbladder wall may be thickened due to edema, inflammation, or necrosis.

Gallbladder rupture may be diagnosed by direct evidence of wall discontinuity or based on indirect signs as pericholecystic hyperechoic fat or fluid accumulation[22] (**fig. 30.7**). The appearance of biliary mucocele has been recently reported in CT. The computed tomographic GBM appearance is variable, and probably depends on the stage of maturity of the mucocele. The presence of hyperattenuating gallbladder material on pre-contrast CT images and centrally distributed mineral can be indicative of mucocele. This distribution was found in ⅔ of the dogs with mucocele with occasionally a radiating or stellate pattern.[29] A cutoff of 48.6 HU (normal bile 34-35.8 HU) has been proposed for diagnosis of mucocele with high specificity (96%) and low sensitivity (52%). Few cases of ruptured gallbladder and migration of the mucocele into the peritoneal cavity have been described[3,30] (**figs. 30.8** and **30.9**).

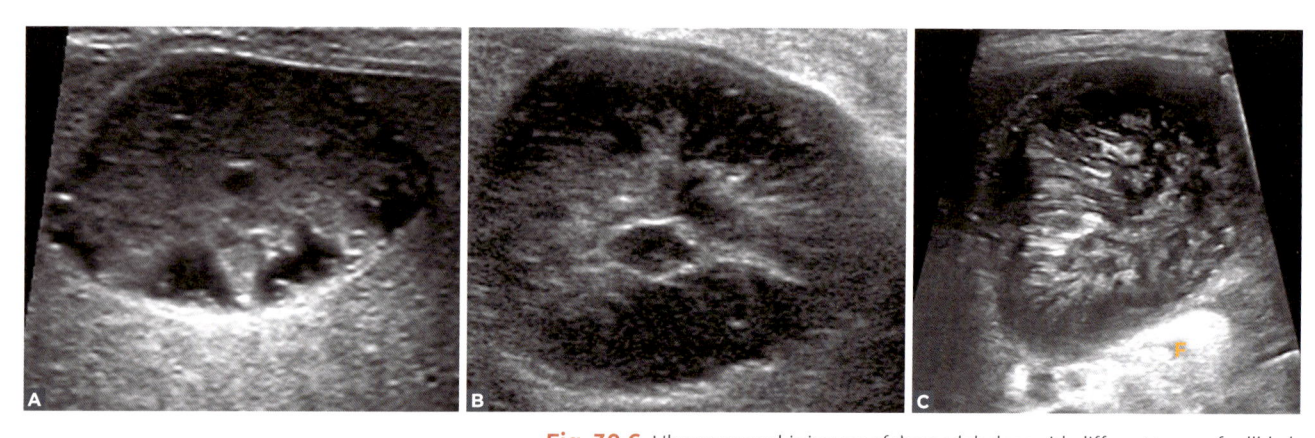

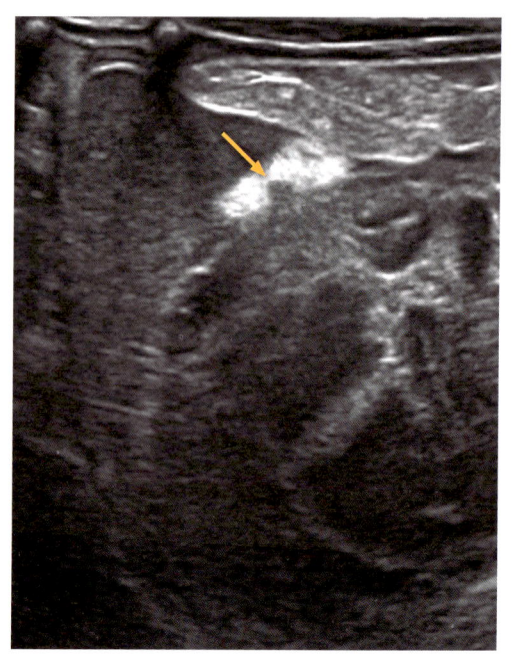

Fig. 30.6 Ultrasonographic images of three adult dogs with different types of gallbladder mucocele. Stellate pattern. (**A**) Multiple hypoechoic bile casts are present along the gallbladder wall with central echogenic bile sludge. (**B**) Kiwi-like pattern (finely striated pattern) and stellate combination. Mobile and poorly echogenic fluidly bile is still present centrally in the lumen. Kiwi fruit-like pattern. F, the fat that surrounds the gallbladder is hyperechoic and suggestive of necrosis/perforation (**C**).

Fig. 30.7 Ultrasonographic image of a 13-year-old Shetland Sheepdog with a ruptured gallbladder mucocele. The mucocele is extruded beyond the wall into the peritoneal cavity through a gallbladder wall defect (arrow). The regional mesenteric fat is hyperechoic. Image courtesy of Dr. Mauro Pivetta.

CHAPTER 30 Biliary system

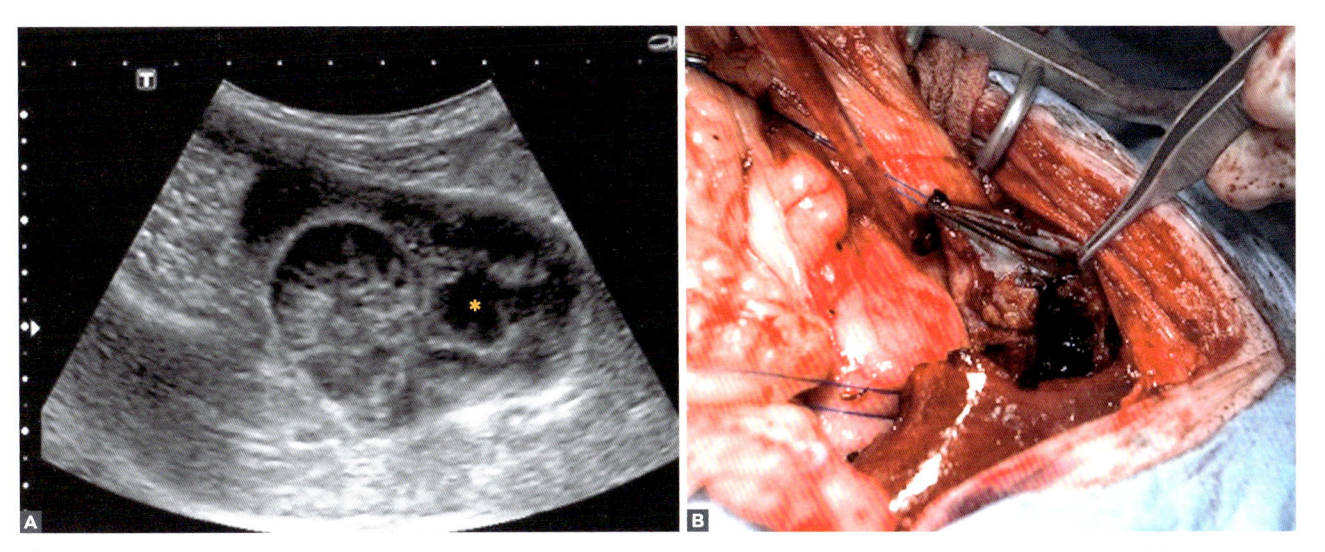

Fig. 30.8 Ultrasonographic image of a 13-year-old Cocker Spaniel with a ruptured gallbladder mucocele. Gallbladder mucocele with kiwi-like patten. (**A**) The gallbladder content extrudes beyond the wall into the peritoneal cavity (asterisk) through a gallbladder wall defect. (**B**) Surgical image of the same dog with confirmation of the gallbladder rupture. Image courtesy of Justus Liebig University Giessen, Germany.

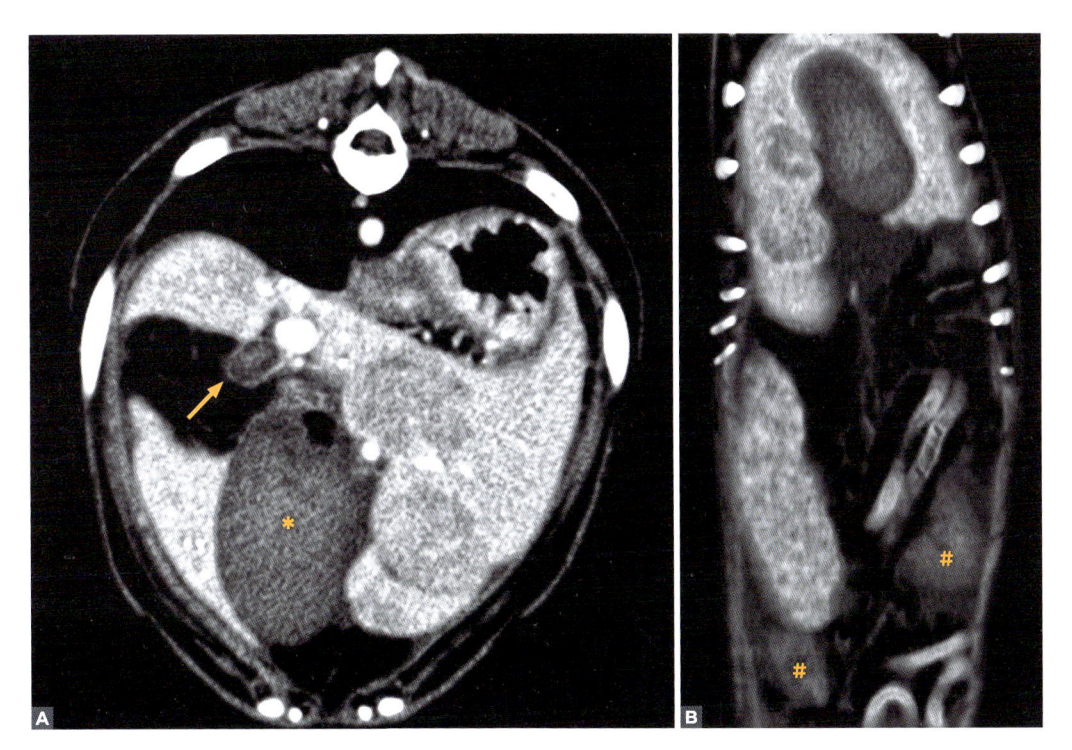

Fig. 30.9 Computed tomographic angiography transverse image (**A**) and 2D dorsal reconstruction (**B**) in a dog with ruptured gallbladder mucocele with multiple foci of extruded/migrating material. The gallbladder is enlarged and filled with a large amount of hyperattenuating centrally located material (pre and post contrast). Similar material (mucinous plug) is filling the common bile duct (arrow). Two organized hyperattenuating structures with a similar pattern to the gallbladder content are present within the peritoneal cavity and representing an extruded gallbladder mucocele (#).

Galbladder rupture

Gallbladder rupture can be secondary to wall ischemia/necrosis/necrotizing cholecystitis as a complication of mucocele, septic cholecystitis, bile sludge, biliary obstruction/choledochitis, neoplasia, impaired vascular supply, or blunt abdominal trauma. Mucocele or bacterial gallbladder infection are reported as the most common concurrent finding in dogs with gallbladder rupture.[31] Necrosis may be secondary to altered perfusion from the cystic artery by gallbladder overdistension, thromboembolism, blunt trauma, or inflammation. Having only a single source of perfusion makes the gallbladder and CBD uniquely susceptible to ischemic necrosis following blunt abdominal trauma. On ultrasound, severely thickened and/or discontinuous appearance of the gallbladder wall ("hole sign") associated with adjacent fluid and regional hyperechoic pericholecystic fat (omental adhesions, peritonitis) suggests necrosis and rupture.[3] Ultrasound has low sensitivity (56.1-81%) and high specificity (81-91.7%) for identification gallbladder rupture.[24,32] The presence of bile pigments in the peritoneal effusion and serum hyperbilirubinemia should lead to the suspicion of biliary rupture. However, lack of these findings should not exclude this diagnosis. Contrast-enhanced ultrasound can be a useful technique to diagnose gallbladder wall necrosis/rupture in dogs with sensitivity and specificity of 100%, higher than conventional ultrasound. Necrosis/rupture presents as a non-vascularized area characterized by a complete absence of contrast enhancement during all contrast phases[32] (**fig. 30.10**).

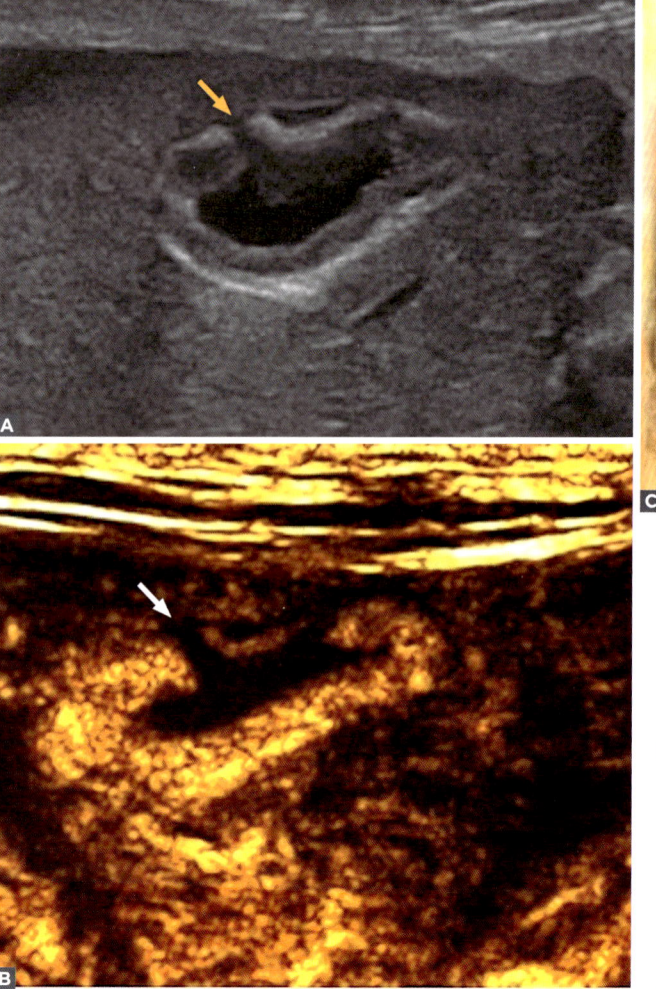

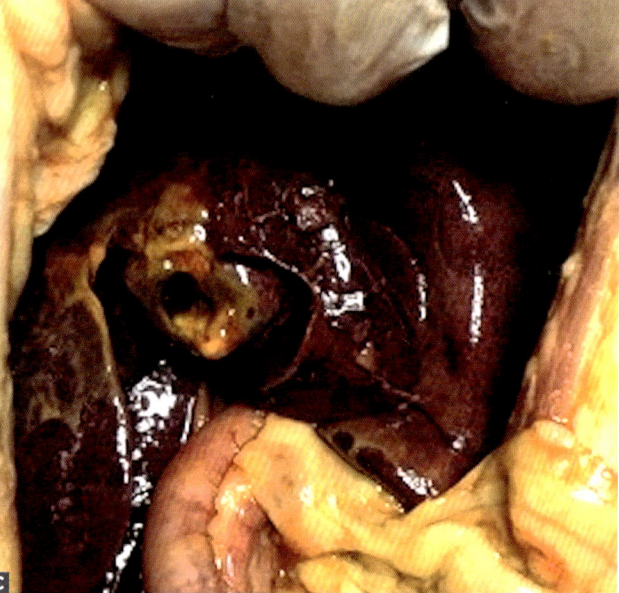

Fig. 30.10 Ultrasonographic B-mode images of an adult dog with gallbladder rupture/necrosis following blunt abdominal trauma. (**A**) The gallbladder wall is diffusely thickened, and there is discontinuity/defect of the wall "hole sign" (arrow). (**B**) CEUS image, showing homogeneous contrast enhancement of the gallbladder wall and the focal, non-vascularized area (arrow) characterized by a complete absence of contrast enhancement corresponding to the area of necrosis/rupture. (**C**) Surgical image of the same dog with confirmation of gallbladder rupture. Image courtesy of Clinica Veterinaria Malpensa, Samarate (VA), Italy.

Cholecystitis, cholangitis and cholangiohepatitis complex

Cholecystitis

Cholecystitis is an inflammatory condition of the gallbladder. It can be acute or chronic with or without bacterial infection. It may be associated with infectious agents, bile stasis, irritation from choleliths, systemic disease, neoplasia, biliary obstruction, or abdominal trauma.[3] Bacterial cholecystitits/cholangitis is a relatively common cause of hepatobiliary disease in dogs and cats, with higher prevalence in cats[33] diagnosed by the combination of ultrasound findings and bile culture. They may be caused by ascending bacterial infection from the intestine or from hematogenous (hepatic portal venous blood) dissemination.[2] The most common isolated pathogens are enteric bacteria. Chronic cholecystitis/cholangitis associated with severe cholestatic liver disease has been reported also caused by liver flukes such as *Platynosomum*[34] (**fig. 30.11**).

Cholecystitis imaging findings include wall thickening (>1 mm) with hyperechoic or doubled-rim appearance, irregular luminal interface, presence of biliary sludge or choleliths.[3,6,22,33,35] Gallbladder wall thickening can be the result of inflammation, edema, or mucosal gland hyperplasia. A double rim appearance results from a central hypoechoic layer between two echogenic layers. It often re-

Fig. 30.11 Ultrasonographic image of a five-year-old Siamese cat with progressive jaundice and anorexia, chronic cholecystitis and cholangitis with cholestasis and suspected EHBDO caused by liver flukes. *Platynosomum* ova were found in the bile from the gallbladder aspirate. (**A**) There is gallbladder (GB) distention, hyperechoic and thickened wall, and moderate luminal echogenic material. The CBD and the bile ducts (asterisk) are moderately distended and tortuous. (**B-C**) The bile duct walls are hyperechoic and thickened. Image courtesy of Antech Imaging Services, Fountain Valley, CA, USA.

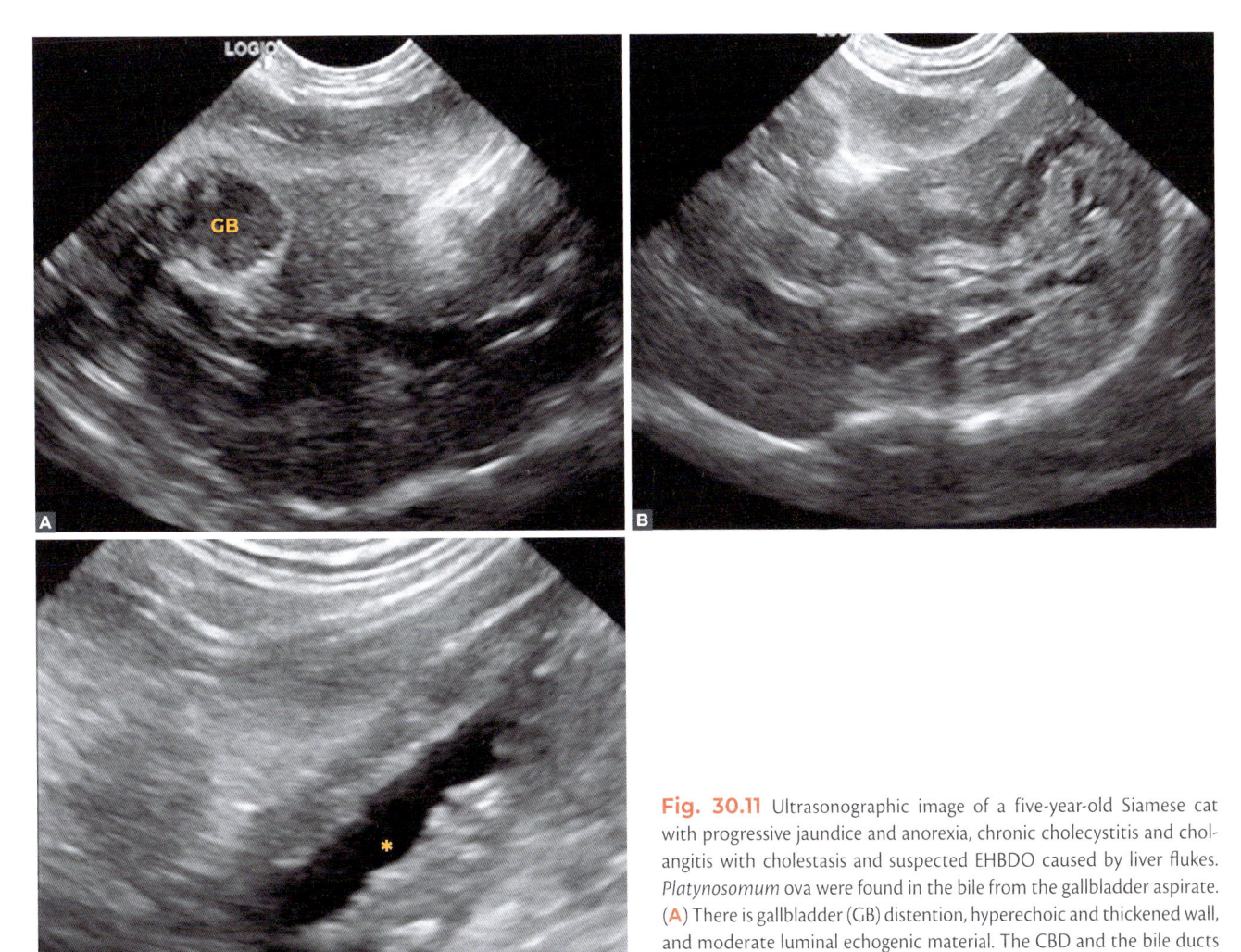

SECTION V ABDOMEN

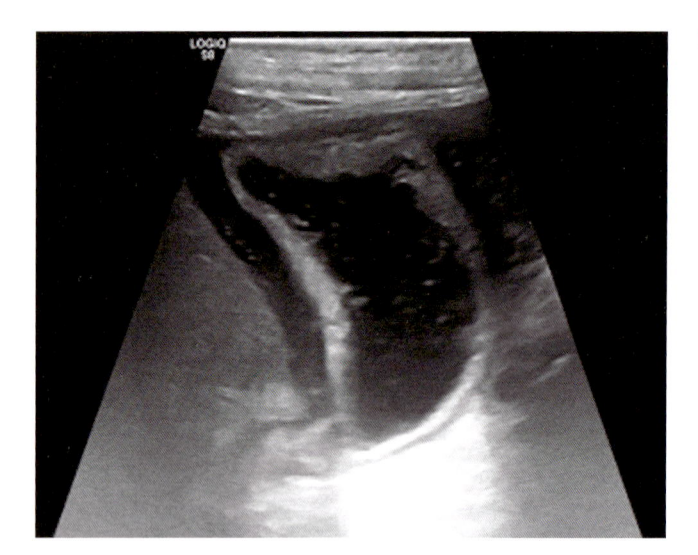

Fig. 30.12 Ultrasonographic image of an eight-year-old crossbred dog with gallbladder wall edema secondary to posthepatic hypertension, pericardial effusion, and suspected cardiac lymphoma. The gallbladder wall is thickened with a double rim appearance.

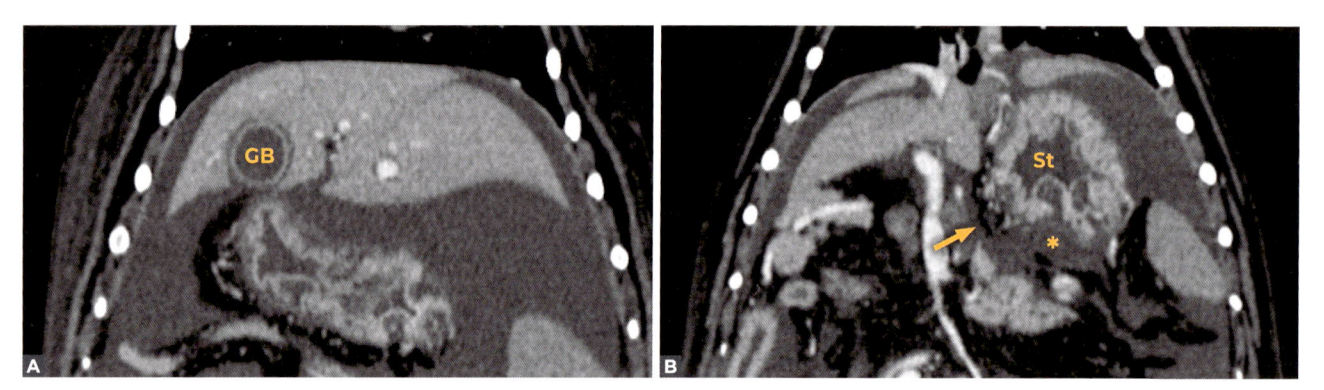

Fig. 30.13 Computed tomographic angiography transverse image in a five-year-old Australian Shepherd dog with gallbladder wall edema secondary to portal hypertension and hepatic fibrosis. The gallbladder wall is thickened with a double rim appearance. (**A**) There is a moderate amount of hypoattenuating peritoneal effusion. Gastric wall edema (asterisk). (**B**) Small tortuous gastroesophageal varices (arrow) are noted within the gastric wall. *GB*, gallbladder; *St*, stomach.

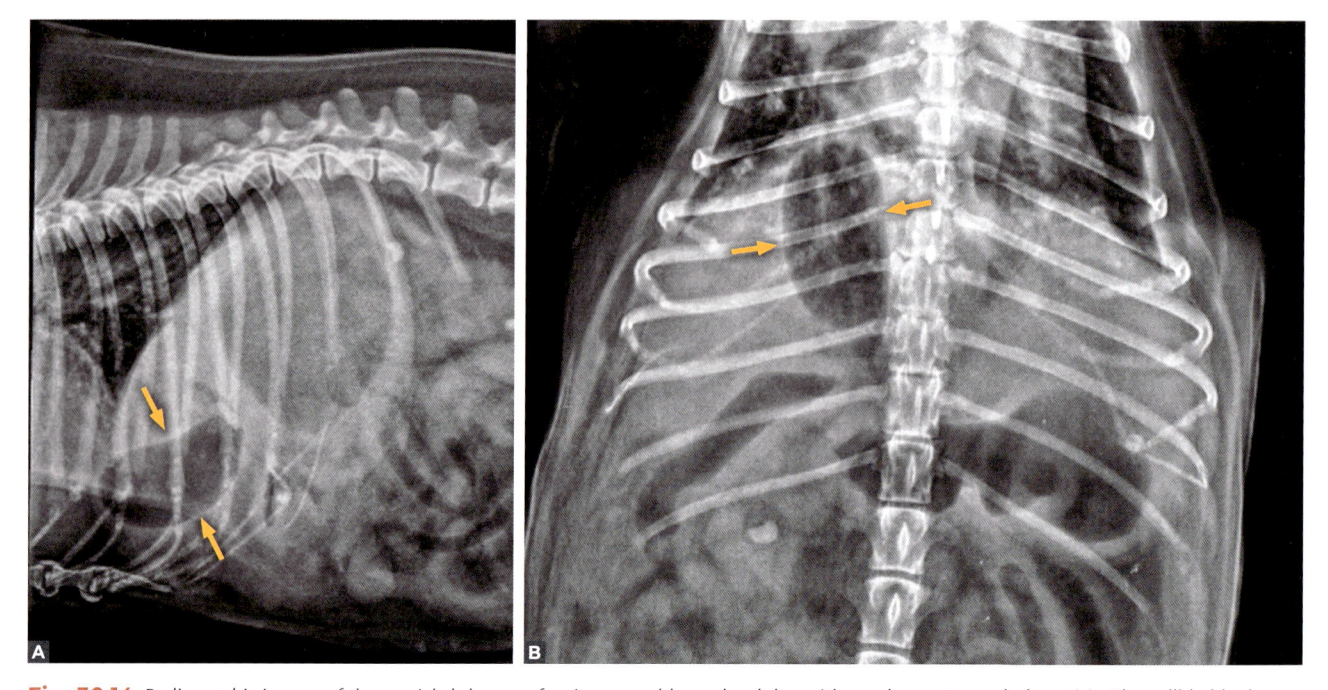

Fig. 30.14 Radiographic images of the cranial abdomen of a nine-year-old crossbred dog with emphysematous cholecystitis. The gallbladder lumen is distended with gas opacity (arrows).

flects edema and may associated with acute cholecystitis, portal hypertension, hypoalbuminemia, anaphylaxis, sepsis, biliary obstruction or artificial due to surrounding peritoneal fluid (**figs. 30.12** and **30.13**). Dystrophic wall mineralization may be present in chronic biliary inflammation. Gallbladder wall thickening is reported to be an accurate finding to predict gallbladder disease in cats, although normal thickness does not rule out mild or chronic inflammation.[6] In dogs with evidence of hepatobiliary disease large amount of biliary a sediment and the presence of immobile biliary sludge is significantly associated with bactibilia and bacterial cholecystitis, however, not pathognomonic.[36] Cholelithiasis may or not be associated with cholecystitis. In another study, abnormal sonographic appearance of the gallbladder (thickened gallbladder wall or presence of bile sludge) had high sensitivity (96%) but low specificity (49%) in cats with positive and negative results of bile bacterial culture, respectively. Cats with normal gallbladder ultrasound were unlikely to have positive bile bacterial culture (negative predictive value of 96%). Gallbladder ultrasound had lower sensitivity (81%), specificity (31%), positive predictive value (20%), and negative predictive value (88%) in dogs. This modality was less predictive of infection in dogs.[33]

Emphysematous cholecystitis

Emphysematous cholecystitis/cholangitis is an infectious disease inducing the formation of gas within the wall and/or the lumen of the gallbladder and usually associated with gas-producing bacteria (*E. coli* and *Clostridium* spp.) and associated with diabetes mellitus, traumatic ischemia, mucocele formation and neoplasia.[13] Aerobic and anaerobic microorganisms may enter the gallbladder by means of reflux from the intestines or via the hepatic circulation. On ultrasound, the presence of gas can be seen intramural or intraluminal as dirty shadow with reverberation and confirmed radiographically or with CT (**fig. 30.14**).[8]

Necrotizing cholecystitis

Gangrenous or necrotizing cholecystitis is characterized by marked wall irregularity, thickening or a discontinuous wall with pericholecystic fluid accumulation. It is due to ischemia, ulceration, hemorrhage, or necrosis of the gallbladder wall.[13]

Cholangitis

Cholangitis is an inflammation of the biliary tree and often seen in conjunction with cholecystitis. It can be acute or chronic, and sterile or secondary to bacterial infection. In cats, cholangitis is commonly associated with concurrent hepatitis (hence the term cholangiohepatitis). Cholangitis/cholangiohepatitis complex is commonly reported in cats and, in many cases, no hepatic and biliary abnormalities are detected on ultrasound.[4,6] When present, ultrasound changes include biliary wall thickening, hyperechoic biliary walls, presence of biliary sludge, cholelithiasis and dilatation of the bile ducts (**fig. 30.15**). The adjacent hepatic parenchyma may be normal, with increased, decreased, or heterogeneous echogenicity.[4,33] Acute cases commonly show decreased parenchymal echogenicity and increased visibility of the portal vasculature. Due to the wide overlap of sonographic changes, histology and cholecystocentesis are recommended for definitive diagnosis. Cholangitis can lead to biliary dilatation as result of inflammation-induced biliary stasis and at times difficult to distinguish from obstructive disease by biliary sludge or choledocholiths. Feline cholangitis is commonly associated with pancreatitis, inflammatory bowel disease and cholecystitis.[4,5] In CT, thickening of the gallbladder and bile duct walls with contrast enhancement can indicate presence of cholangitis.[8]

Cholecystocentesis

Percutaneous US-guided cholecystocentesis can be performed to obtain bile samples for cytologic and culture evaluation in patients with suspected bacterial cholangitis. A transhepatic approach is preferred and ideally the gallbladder should be emptied completely to limit the possibility of bile

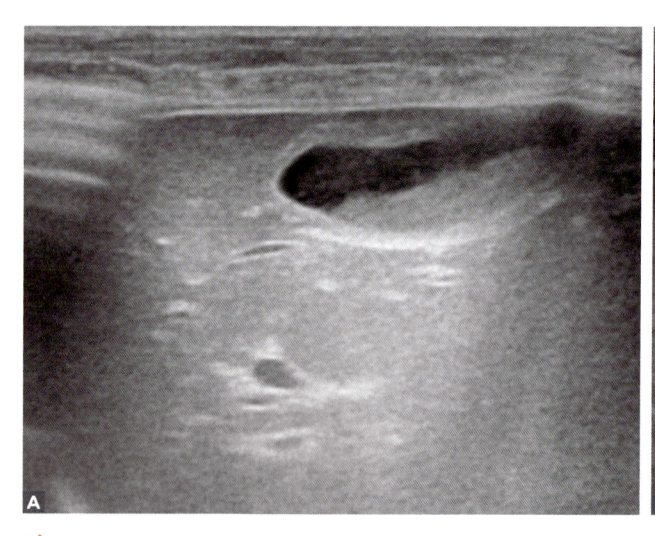

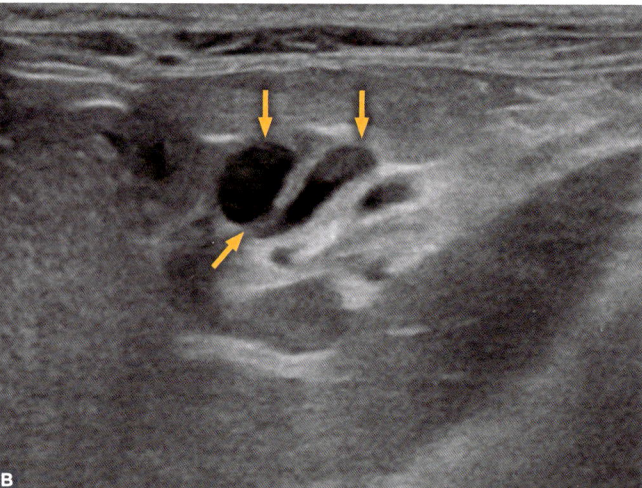

Fig. 30.15 Ultrasonographic image of an adult cat with cholecystitis and cholangitis diagnosed (bactibilia on aspiration, cultured as *Salmonella*). (**A**) The gallbladder has a thickened and hyperechoic wall, dependent echogenic material and some echoes suspended in the bile. (**B**) Tortuous cystic duct with luminal echogenic material and slightly thickened duct walls (arrows). Image courtesy of Royal Veterinary College, Hertfordshire, UK.

leakage into the abdominal cavity. Percutaneous ultrasound cholecystocentesis is a safe technique with low complication rates (0-3.4%).[33,37] Complications include bile leakage/peritonitis, and hemorrhage. There was no predictable relationship between the severity of gallbladder wall changes and risk of complication. This technique should be avoided in cases of EHBDO, obvious gallbladder wall abnormalities or mucocele. Percutaneous ultrasound-guided cholecystocentesis may facilitate the gallbladder rupture in case of wall necrosis.[37]

Choleliths

Choleliths commonly contain mixtures of calcium (calcium carbonate, calcium bilirubinate), bilirubin, mucin, and cholesterol. Radiographs, ultrasound, and CT can be used to visualize choleliths. Visibility on survey abdominal radiographs depends on size and percentage of calcium (**fig. 30.16**). They can be found in the gallbladder, intra and extrahepatic biliary ducts and common bile duct. Choleliths are infrequent and commonly clinically silent. In a recent study, only few dogs with incidental cholelithiasis went on to become symptomatic within the follow-up period.[38] Less commonly, choleliths have been reported to be associated with biliary stasis, altered bile composition and cholecystitis/cholangiohepatitis, the latter being more common in cats.[39] They can form as a consequence of cholangitis, and other way they can damage the bile duct leading to stasis and inflammation.[11] They can also be caused by or as a consequence of biliary obstruction.[40] On ultrasound, mineralized choleliths and choledocholiths present as single or multiple round hyperechoic luminal structures associated with distal acoustic shadowing.

Distal acoustic shadowing becomes more apparent as the size and percentage of calcium content of the calculus increase.[7,11] (**figs. 30.17** and **30.19**). They are usually mobile and located in the dependent portion of the biliary lumen. In the biliary hepatic ducts, they cluster in close proximity and tend to form linear tracts. In CT, the detection of biliary cholelithiasis depends on the chemical composition and calcium-containing concretions present as structures of mineral density (**fig. 30.18**). Non-contrast images should be used to diagnose biliary stone that could be hidden on contrast enhanced series.[8]

CHAPTER 30 Biliary system

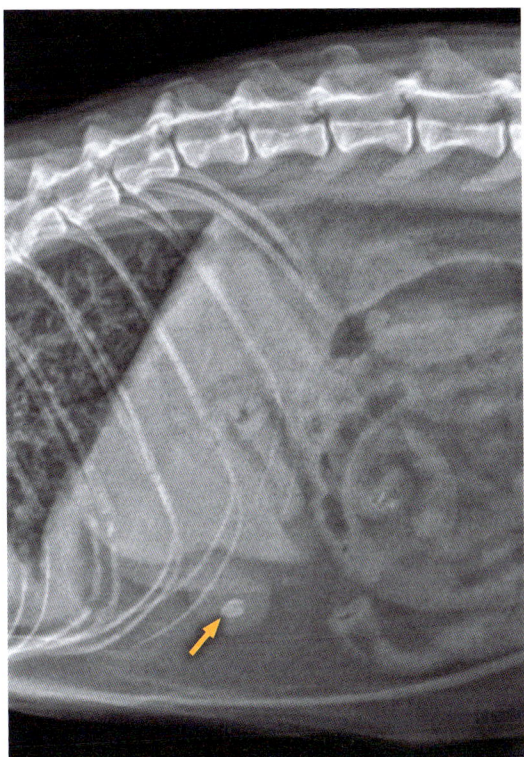

Fig. 30.16 Right lateral radiograph of the cranial abdomen of an eight-year-old Domestic shorthair cat. The gallbladder can be seen as a round soft tissue structure protruding from the ventral liver margin with presence of a single radiopaque cholelith (arrow). Image courtesy of Dr. Mauro Pivetta.

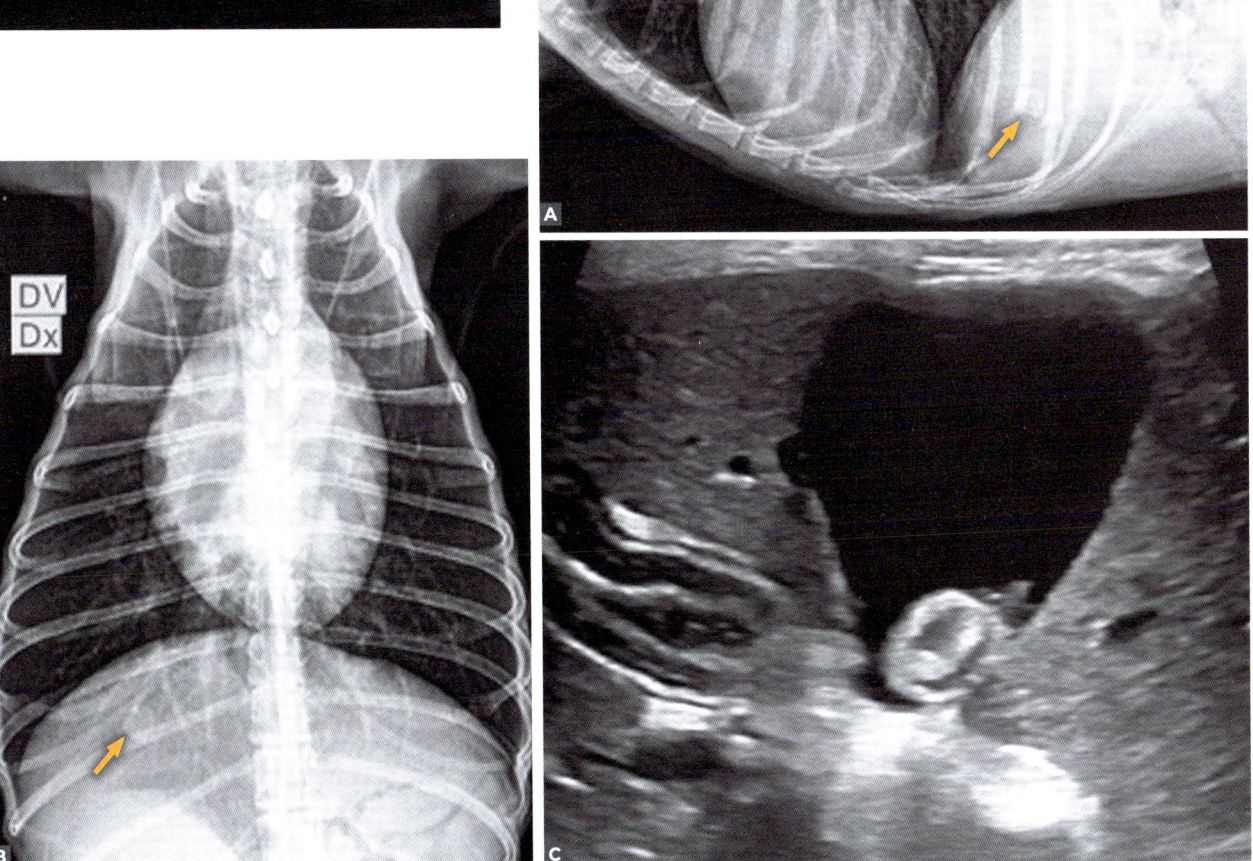

Fig. 30.17 Radiographic images of the thorax and cranial abdomen of a 12-year-old crossbred dog with a single partially mineralized cholelith. There is a well-defined, irregular round, radiopaque structure in the region of the gallbladder (arrow). (A-B) There is a mineral opaque rim present and a less radiopaque center. (C) Corresponding ultrasonographic image of the same dog. The round layered cholelith is associated with weak distal acoustic shadow located in the dependent portion of the gallbladder lumen. *CBD*, common bile duct.

511

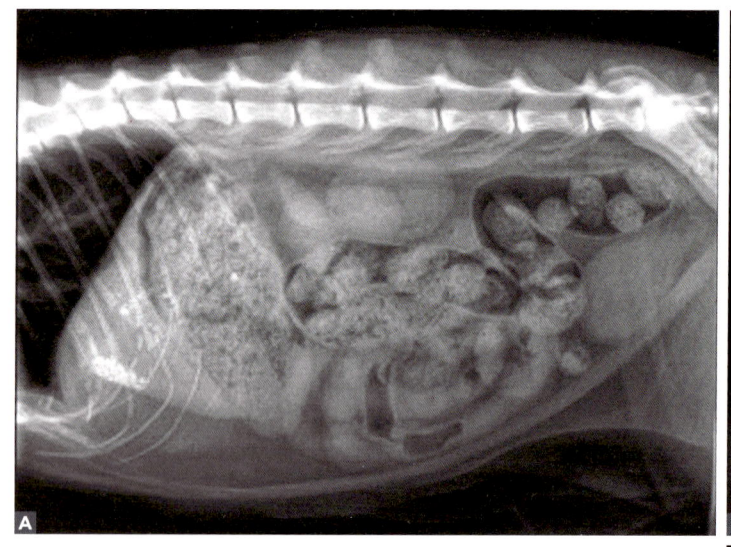

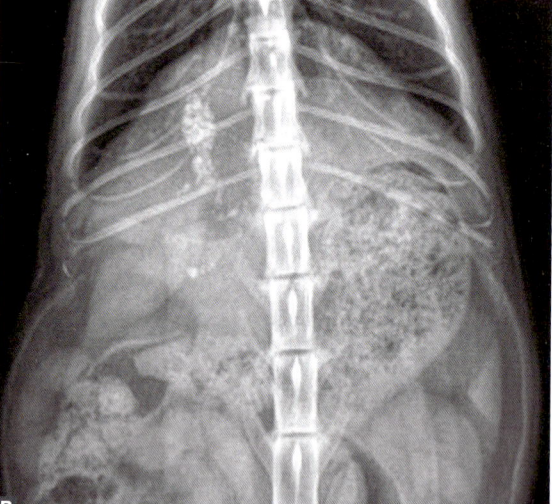

Fig. 30.18 Radiographic images (lateral and ventrodorsal views) of a Domestic shorthair cat with multiple mineral opaque choleliths in the region of the gallbladder and common bile duct (**A-B**). (**C**) Corresponding ultrasonographic image of the same cat with choledocholith in the common bile duct (CBD). Strong acoustic shadowing is present confirming the mineral component. Image courtesy of Antech Imaging Services, Fountain Valley, CA, USA. *CBD*, common bile duct.

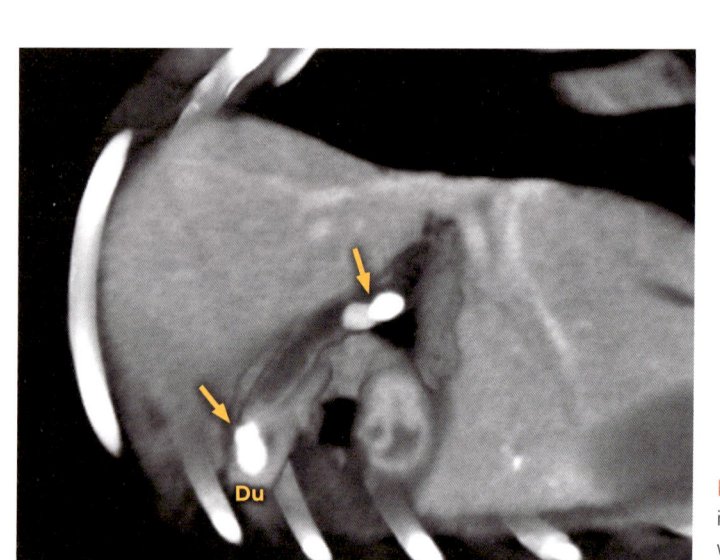

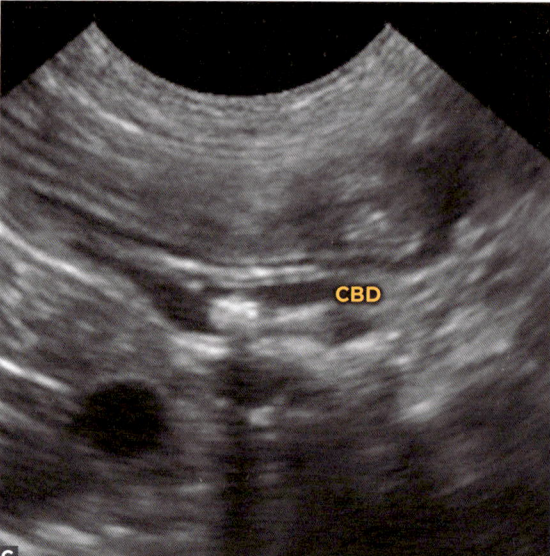

Fig. 30.19 Computed tomographic angiography volume rendered image in an adult dog with multiple hyperattenuating choleliths within the common bile duct (arrows), one at the distal-most aspect adjacent to the major duodenal papilla. *Du*, duodenum.

Extrahepatic biliary obstruction

Causes of extrahepatic biliary duct obstruction (EHBDO) include mucinous plug (e.g., migrating from mucocele), sludge or sludge ball (**fig. 30.20**), choleliths, bile duct stricture, hyperplasia, inflammation/infection (**fig. 30.21**), liver fluke infestation or neoplasia involving liver/biliary system or adjacent organs with intra- or extraluminal compression.[4,7]

Inflammatory/infectious disease of the pancreas or intestine extending to the duodenal papilla and/or CBD can result in stenosis and biliary obstruction.[40] EHBDO secondary to migrating foreign body into the CBD from the duodenum through the major duodenal papilla[41] (**fig. 30.22**) has occasionally been reported. Imaging findings related to EHBDO depend on the duration and severity of the obstruction. After complete obstruction of the CBD, retrograde dilatation is expected that initially affects the

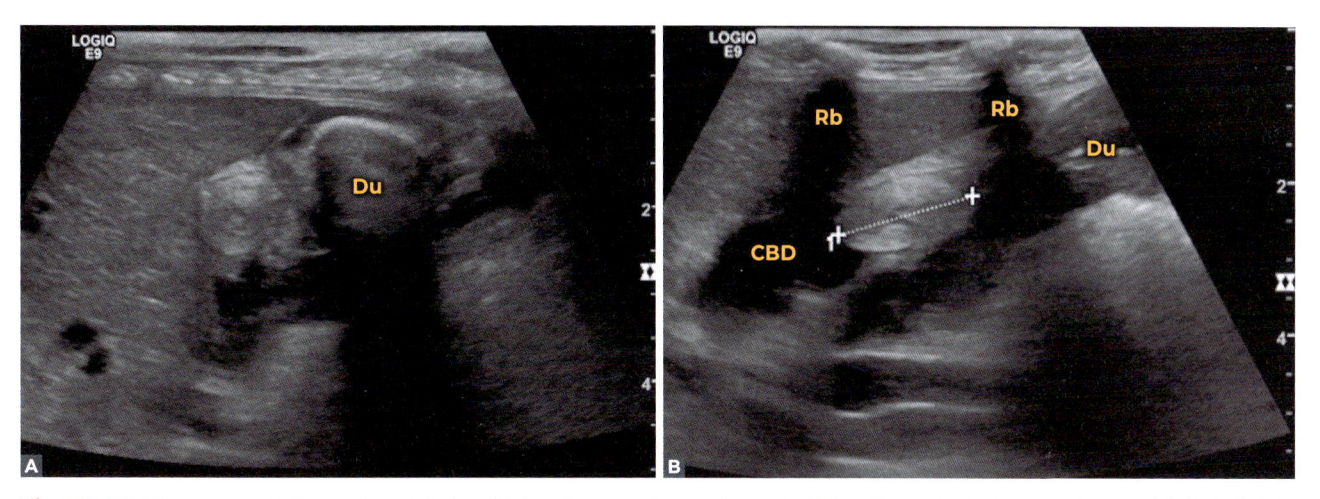

Fig. 30.20 Ultrasonographic image of an adult dog with jaundice secondary to obstructive biliary disease that had a non-mineralized choledocholith/sludge ball in the common bile duct. Note the moderately echogenic well-defined structure without acoustic shadow filling the lumen of the CBD at the duodenal papilla. There is moderate dilatation (>5 mm) of the CBD cranial to the intraluminal structure indicative of obstruction. *CBD*, common bile duct; *Du*, duodenum; *Rb*, ribs. Image courtesy of Justus Liebig University Giessen, Germany.

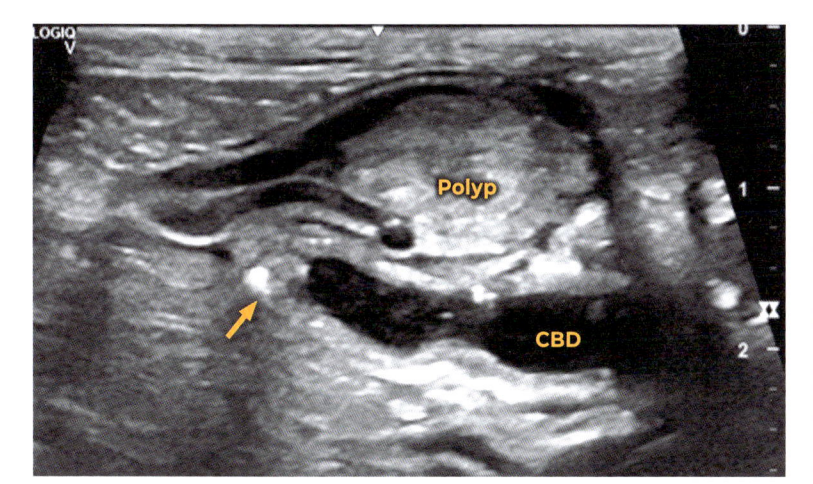

Fig. 30.21 Ultrasonographic images of a Domestic shorthair cat with cholangiohepatitis and partial obstruction of the common bile duct (CBD) presumed to be due to biliary sludge and/or wall thickening at the duodenal papilla (arrow). The dilated common bile duct has moderate thickening and a hyperechoic wall. There is a focal amount of echogenic material at the duodenal papilla. Note also the echogenic nodular lesion filling the lumen of the duodenum diagnosed as duodenal polyp.

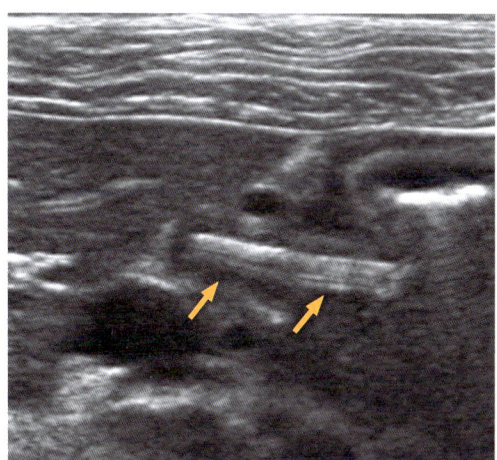

Fig. 30.22 Ultrasonographic images of an adult Domestic shorthair cat with extrahepatic biliary obstruction secondary to a migrating foreign body. A hyperechoic, long, multi-layered spindle shape structure (arrows) is within the lumen of the common bile duct. Image courtesy of Dr. Mauro Pivetta.

CBD, cystic duct and gallbladder within 48h. Within 5-7 days the intrahepatic and extrahepatic ducts become also dilated.[42] Marked distension of the gallbladder is one of the first indicators of complete obstruction in dogs. Differently from dogs, in more than 50% of cats with EHBDO the gallbladder is not distended and, therefore, cannot be used as a reliable indicator of EHBDO alone. This could be due to low gallbladder wall compliance (inflammation with fibrosis) or reduced elasticity of the surrounding hepatic parenchyma. The CBD larger than 5 mm is a more useful indicator of biliary obstruction in cats.[7] Biliary obstruction commonly involves the extrahepatic part of the CBD and particularly the segment in proximity of the duodenal papilla.

Chronic dilatation may predispose to ascending bacterial infection from the intestines. Biliary dilatation may persist to some degree after an obstruction has resolved and, therefore, dilatation of the biliary system is not pathognomonic for the presence of EHBDO.[3] Ultrasound of the gallbladder and bile duct is an accurate method to determine extrahepatic biliary obstruction. If dilated, biliary ducts become visible as anechoic tortuous tubular structures adjacent to the portal vessels also called "shotgun" or "too many tubes" signs. Presence of distal acoustic enhancement (which is not expected for a vessel), intraluminal sludge and color Doppler may help to distinguish them from hepatic vessels.[41] CT and MRI are also reliably diagnostic methodologies. In CT, dilated ducts are non-enhancing vessels adjacent to the portal veins and hypodense compared to the hepatic parenchyma, more clearly visible in portal venous phase as hypoattenuating relative to the surrounding hepatic parenchyma.[8]

Biliary neoplasia

Biliary neoplasia is uncommon in dogs and cats and is a primary hepatic tumor arising from the biliary epithelial cells lining the intra- or extrahepatic bile ducts or gallbladder. Biliary neoplasia may present as cystic or solid form and as focal, multifocal, or diffuse form. They include biliary adenoma/cystadenoma, cholangiocarcinoma/cystadenocarcinoma, and gallbladder tumors (rare). Less commonly, hepatobiliary neuroendocrine carcinoma (carcinoid) has been reported originating from the biliary system.[43] In cats, the most common primary hepatobiliary neoplasms are biliary in origin and benign with cystadenoma up to 65%.[2] In dogs, the most common primary liver neoplasia is from the hepatic parenchyma with malignant hepatocellular carcinoma as most common. Cholangiocarcinoma is the most common malignant hepatobiliary tumor in cats and the second in dogs after hepatocellular carcinoma.[43] Abdominal radiography, ultrasonography and advanced imaging modalities can be used to help identify an abdominal mass. Radiography is not very sensitive and specific for detecting liver neoplasia (depends on the lesion size). Ultrasonography has become the diagnostic tool of choice for screening for abdominal neoplasia. Size, number, and location of hepatobiliary masses can be determined by ultrasound. Sonography, however, is nonspecific and cannot differentiate between benign and malignant disease. Fine-needle aspiration or biopsy remain the accurate way to obtain a diagnosis. CT may help in providing additional preoperative information about the feasibility of surgical resection and presence of distant metastasis. On ultrasound, biliary cystadenoma is typically a moderately echogenic multiloculated mass containing several thin-walled anechoic cysts with distal acoustic enhancement (**fig. 30.23**). They usually are incidental findings unless they become large enough to impinge upon adjacent structures (e.g., stomach) resulting in clinical signs. The hyperechoic portion of the cystadenoma likely represents a combination of fibrous tissue stroma and multiple acoustic interfaces associated with numerous small cysts, resulting in increased sound reflection.[44] On CT, biliary cystadenoma is seen as multiloculated, fluid-attenuating mass with little or no peripheral contrast enhancement. Diagnosis of biliary cystadenoma is challenging, because other cystic lesions such as hepatic cyst, hematoma, abscess, and parasitic cyst can have similar characteristics. Simple cyst contains bile, and it is uncommonly septate. In contrast, biliary cystadenoma or cystadenocarcinoma contain clear or mucinous fluid rather than bile and often present complex structure with septation.[44] Cholangiocarcinoma has a high metastatic rate, and it spreads often to the regional lymph nodes, lungs, and peritoneum (carcinomatosis). It can present as a solid or cystic mass (cystadenocarcinoma). On ultrasound, cystadenocarcinoma presents as a poorly defined multiloculated mass with distal acoustic enhancement due to the presence of multiple hypoattenuating fluid-filled cavities. They can be difficult to differentiate from the benign form without histopathological exam.[43] On CT, they present as poorly encapsulated masses with relative hypoattenuation on both unenhanced and contrast-enhanced images[8] (**fig. 30.24**). Gallbladder masses are rare, benign, or malignant and include polyp due to cystic mucosal hyperplasia, adenomas/adenocarcinomas, and carcinoid tumors. CEUS may help discriminated between vascularized (polypoid lesion and tumor) and non-vascularized intraluminal echogenic masses (sludge and mucocele).[23]

CHAPTER 30 Biliary system

Fig. 30.23 Ultrasonographic images of an adult cat with presumed biliary cystadenoma. A solitary, poorly demarcated and moderately echogenic multiloculated mass (arrows) containing several thin-walled anechoic cysts with distal acoustic enhancement is present in the liver (asterisk). Both solid and characteristic cystic components are present within this mass.

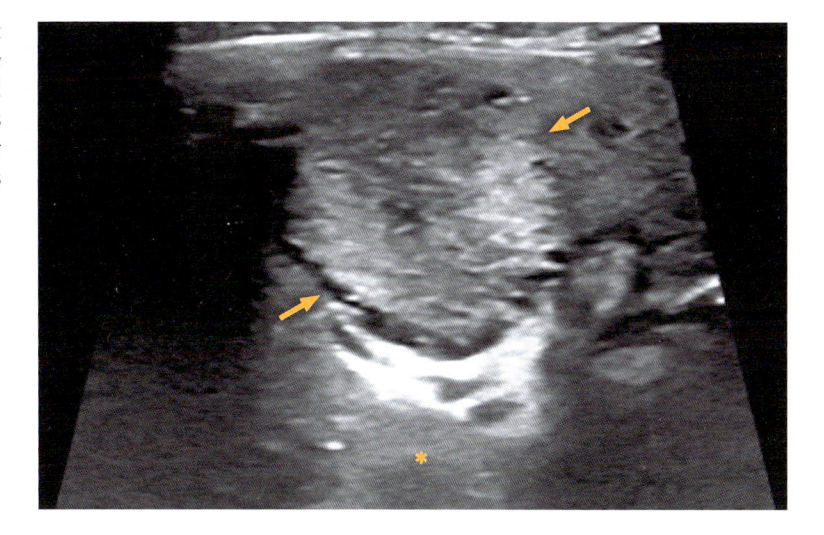

Fig. 30.24 Computed tomographic angiography volume rendered image in a cat with a diagnosis of cholangiocarcinoma. A multilobulated complex mass in the caudate hepatic lobe is present with relative hypoattenuation on both unenhanced and contrast-enhanced images and multiple cystic lesions.

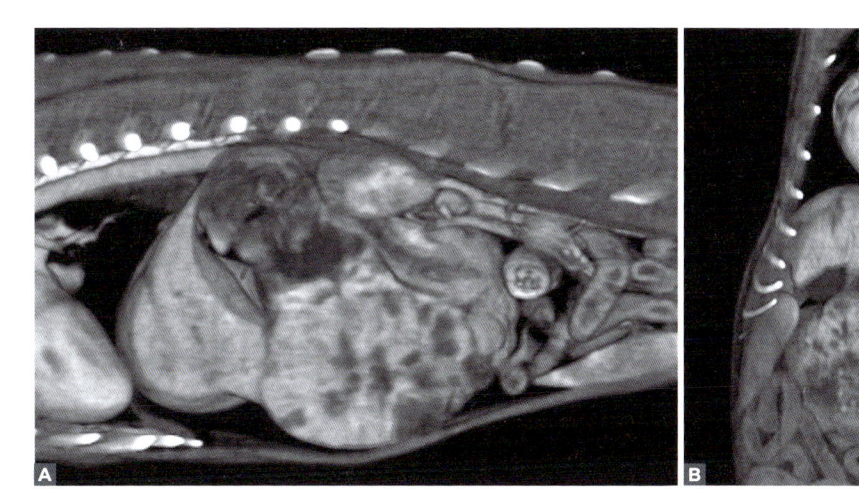

References

1. Sato K, Sakai M, Hayakawa S, Sakamoto Y, Kagawa K, Kutara K, Teshima K, Asano K, Watari T. Gallbladder agenesis in 17 dogs: 2006-2016. *J Vet Intern Med* 32:188-194, 2018.
2. Otte CMA, Penning LC, Rothuizen J. Feline biliary tree and gallbladder disease. Aetiology, diagnosis and treatment. *J Feline Med Surg* 19:514-528, 2017.
3. Center SA. Diseases of the gallbladder and biliary tree. *Vet Clin North Am Small Anim Pract* 39:543-598, 2009.
4. Marolf AJ, Leach L, Gibbons DS, Bachand A, Twedt D. Ultrasonographic findings of feline cholangitis. *J Am Anim Hosp Assoc* 48:36-42, 2012.
5. Callahan Clark JE, Haddad JL, Brown DC, Morgan MJ, Winkle TJV, Rondeau MP. Feline cholangitis: a necropsy study of 44 cats (1986-2008). *J Feline Med Surg* 13: 570-576, 2011.
6. Hittmair KM, Vielgrader HD, Loupal G. Ultrasonographic evaluation of gallbladder wall thickness in cats. *Vet Radiol Ultrasound* 42:149-155, 2001.
7. Gaillot HA, Penninck DG, Webster CR, Crawford S. Ultrasonographic features of extrahepatic biliary obstruction in 30 cats. *Vet Radiol Ultrasound* 48:439-447, 2007.
8. Bertolini G. Gallbladder and biliary system. In Bertolini G (editor). Body MDCT in Small Animals, 2017, Springer International Publishing, pp 127-141.
9. Marolf AJ. Diagnostic imaging of the hepatobiliary system. *Vet Clin North Am Small Anim Pract* 555-568, 2017.
10. Best EJ, Bush DJ, Dye C. Suspected choledochal cyst in a Domestic shorthair cat. *J Feline Med Surg* 12:814-817, 2010.
11. Center SA. Diseases of the gallbladder and biliary tree. *Vet Clin North Am Small Anim Pract* 39:543-598, 2009.
12. Nyland TG, Koblik PD, Tellyer SE. Ultrasonographic evaluation of biliary cystadenomas in cats. *Vet Radiol Ultrasound* 40:300-306, 1999.
13. Larson MM, Mattoon JS, Lawrence Y, Sellon RK. Gallbladder and biliary tract. In Mattoon J, Sellon R, Berry C (editors). Small Animal Diagnostic Ultrasound 4th edition. Saunders, 2021, pp 389-405.
14. Spain HN, Penninck DG, Webster CR, Daure E, Jennings SH. Ultrasonographic and clinicopathologic features of segmental dilatations of the common bile duct in four cats. *J Feline Med* Surg 1-9, 2017.
15. Last RD, Hill JM, Roach M, Kaldenberg T. Congenital dilatation of the large and segmental intrahepatic bile ducts (Caroli's disease) in two Golden retriever littermates. *Tydskr S Afr Vet Ver* 77:210-214, 2006.

16. Harran N, d'Anjou MA, Dunn M, Beauchamp G. Gallbladder sludge on ultrasound is predictive of increased liver enzymes and total bilirubin in cats. *Can Vet J* 52:999-1003, 2011.
17. Villm J, DeMonaco S, Larson M. Prevalence of gallbladder sludge and associated abnormalities in cats undergoing abdominal ultrasound. *Vet Radiol Ultrasound* 1:8, 2022.
18. Cook AK, Jambhekar AV, Dylewski AM. Gallbladder sludge in dogs: ultrasonographic and clinical findings in 200 patients. *J Am Anim Hosp Assoc* 52:125-131, 2016.
19. Tsukagoshi T, Ohno K, Tsukamoto A, Fukushima K, Takahashi M, Nakashima KO, Fujino Y, Tsujimoto H. Decreased gallbladder emptying in dogs with biliary sludge or gallbladder mucocele. *Vet Radiol Ultrasound* 53:84-91, 2012.
20. DeMonaco SM, Grant DC, Larson MM, Panciera DL, Leib MS. Spontaneous course of biliary sludge over 12 months in dogs with ultrasonographically identified biliary sludge. *J Vet Intern Med* 30:771-778, 2016.
21. Besso JD, Wrigley RH, Gliatto JM, Webster CRL. Ultrasound appearance and clinical findings in 14 dogs with gallbladder mucocele. *Vet Radiol Ultrasound* 41:261-271, 2000.
22. Gaschen L. Update on hepatobiliary imaging. *Vet Clin Small Anim* 39:439-467, 2009.
23. Bargellini P, Orlandi R, Paloni C, Rubini G, Fonti P, Righi C, Peterson ME, Rishniw M, Boiti C. Contrast-enhanced ultrasound complements two-dimensional ultrasonography in diagnosing gallbladder diseases in dogs. *Vet Radiol Ultrasound* 59:345-356, 2018.
24. Jaffey JA, Graham A, VanEerde E, Hostnik E, Alvarez W, Arango J, Jacobs C, DeClue AE. Gallbladder mucocele: variables associated with outcome and the utility of ultrasonography to identify gallbladder rupture in 219 dogs (2007-2016). *J Vet Intern Med* 32:195-200, 2018.
25. Griffin S. Feline abdominal ultrasonography: what's normal? What's abnormal? The biliary tree. *J Feline Med Surg* 21:429-441, 2019.
26. Walter R, Dunn ME, d'Anjou MA, Lecuyer M. Nonsurgical resolution of gallbladder mucocele in two dogs. *J Am Vet Med Assoc* 232:1688-1693, 2008.
27. Parkanzky M, Grimes J, Schmiedt C, Secrest S, Bugbee A. Long-term survival of dogs treated for gallbladder mucocele by cholecystectomy, medical management, or both. *J Vet Intern Med* 33:2057-2066, 2019.
28. Youn G, Waschak MJ, Kunkel KAR, Gerard PD. Outcome of elective cholecystectomy for the treatment of gallbladder disease in dogs. *J Am Vet Med Assoc* 252:970-975, 2018.
29. Fuerst JA, Hostnik ET. CT attenuation values and mineral distribution can be used to differentiate dogs with and without gallbladder mucoceles. *Vet Radiol Ultrasound* 60:689-695, 2019.
30. Soppet J, Young BD, Griffin JF, Gilmour LJ, Heffelman V, Tucker-Mohl K, Biller DS, Wolff CA, Spaulding KA. Extruded gallbladder mucoceles have characteristic ultrasonographic features and extensive migratory capacity in dogs. *Vet Radiol Ultrasound* 59:744-748, 2017.
31. Crews LJ, Feeney DA, Jessen CR, Rose ND, Matise I. Clinical, ultrasonographic, and laboratory findings associated with gallbladder disease and rupture in dogs: 45 cases (1997-2007). *J Am Vet Med Assoc* 234:359-366, 2009.
32. Bargellini P, Orlandi R, Paloni C, Rubini G, Fonti P, Peterson ME, Rishniw M, Boiti C. Evaluation of contrast-enhanced ultrasonography as a method for detecting gallbladder necrosis or rupture in dogs. *Vet Radiol Ultrasound* 57:611-620, 2016.
33. Smith RP, Gookin JL, Smolski W, Di Cicco MF, Correa M, Seiler GS. Association between gallbladder ultrasound findings and bacterial culture of bile in 70 cats and 202 dogs. *J Vet Intern Med* 31:1451-1458, 2017.
34. Koster L, Shell L, Illanes O, Lathroum C, Neuville K, Ketzis J. Percutaneous ultrasound-guided cholecystocentesis and bile analysis for the detection of *Platynosomum* spp.-induced cholangitis in cats. *J Vet Intern Med* 30:787-793, 2016.
35. Tamborini A, Jahns H, McAllister H, Kent A, Harris B, Procoli F, Allenspach K, Hall EJ, Day MJ, Watson PJ, O'Neill EJ. Bacterial cholangitis, cholecystitis, or both in dogs. *J Vet Intern Med* 30:1046-1055, 2016.
36. Lawrence AY, Ruaux CG, Neminic S, Milovancev M. Characterization, treatment, and outcome of bacterial cholecystitis and bactibilia in dogs. *J Am Vet Med Assoc* 246:982-989, 2015.
37. Schiborra F, McConnell JF, Maddox TW. Percutaneous ultrasound-guided cholecystocentesis: complications and association of ultrasonographic findings with bile culture results. *J Small Anim Pract* 58:389-394, 2017.
38. Ward PM, Brown K, Hammond G, Parkin T, Bouyssou S, Coia M, Nurra G, Ridyard AE. Cholelithiasis in the dog: prevalence, clinical presentation, and outcome. *J Am Anim Hosp Assoc* 1-7, 2020.
39. Eich CS, Ludwig LL. The surgical treatment of cholelithiasis in cats: a study of nine cases. *J Am Anim Hosp Assoc* 38:290-296, 2002.
40. Mayhew PD, Holt DE, McLear RC, Washabau RJ. Pathogenesis and outcome of extrahepatic biliary obstruction in cats. *J Small Anim Pract* 43:247-253, 2002.
41. Brioschi V, Rousset N, Ladlow JF. Imaging diagnosis – extrahepatic biliary tract obstruction secondary to a biliary foreign body in a cat. *Vet Radiol Ultrasound* 6:628-631, 2014.
42. Nyland TG, Gillett NA. Sonographic evaluation of experimental bile duct ligation in the dog. *Vet Radiol* 23:252-260, 1982.
43. Mullin C, Clifford AC. Biliary Neoplasia. In Mott J, Jo Ann Morrison JA (editors). Blackwell's Five-minute Veterinary Consult Clinical Companion: Small Animal Gastrointestinal Diseases. Wiley Blackwell, 2019, pp 1-7.
44. Nyland TG, Koblik PD, Tellyer SE. Ultrasonographic evaluation of biliary cystadenomas in cats. *Vet Radiol Ultrasound* 40:300-306, 1999.

CHAPTER 31

Portosystemic shunts

Lorrie Gaschen

KEY POINTS

- Portosystemic shunts may be congenital or acquired.
- They manifest not only in young animals, and even congenital forms can present later in life.
- Radiography is limiting for a diagnosis.
- Ultrasonographic features include:
  - Small liver.
  - Large kidneys.
  - Urolithiasis.
  - PV/Ao ratio <0.65.
  - Direct visualization of an anomalous intra- or extrahepatic vessel.
  - Increased numbers and size of portal vessels in the abdomen, indicating secondary shunting and portal hypertension.
- Definitive diagnosis and presurgical planning vs. medical management may require advanced imaging techniques such as portograms of CT angiography.

Imaging diagnosis of dogs and cats suspected of having a portosystemic shunt involves identifying indirect signs such as a small liver and urolithiasis as well as directly identifying the anomalous vessel/s either sonographically or with positive contrast studies. Cats and small breed dogs mainly have extrahepatic portosystemic shunts, while large breed dogs typically have intrahepatic anomalies. Extrahepatic congenital portosystemic shunts are mainly found in small breed dogs and include portocaval (splenocaval, splenophrenic, right gastric caval), portoazygous, and portocolonic. Congenital shunts in large breed dogs are often intrahepatic and are either left divisional (ductus venosus), central, or right divisional. It is important to remember that adult animals can also present with clinical signs even though they have a congenital shunt. Acquired shunts can be due to congenital portal vein atresia or hypoplasia, or arterioportal fistulas. They can also form secondarily to chronic portal vein thrombosis, hepatic cirrhosis/fibrosis, pericardial tamponade, and right-sided cardiac failure.

Radiography

In dogs with congenital extrahepatic shunts, the liver is often small but can be of normal size. There is often loss of abdominal detail. Microhepatia is diagnosed on lateral abdominal radiographs by assessing the gastric axis (**fig. 31.1**). A line drawn from the gastric fundus dorsally to the antrum should range from parallel to the ribs to perpendicular to the spine. Cranial deviation of the gastric axis and

SECTION V ABDOMEN

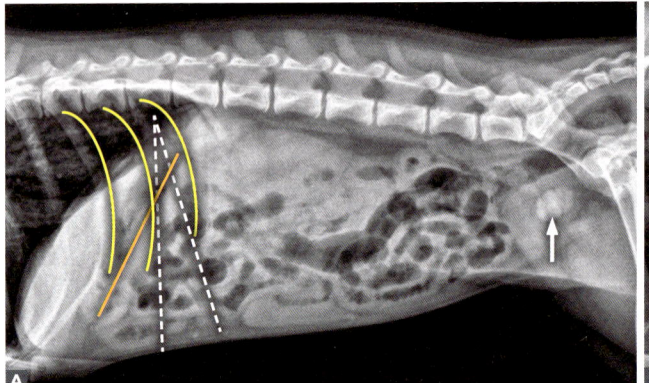

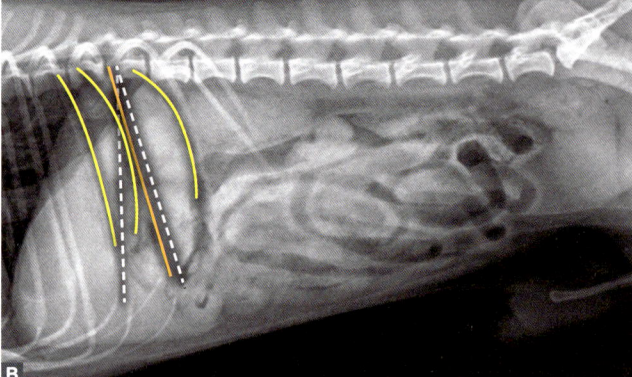

Fig. 31.1 (**A**) A seven-month-old female intact Bichon Frisé presented with hematuria, poor appetite, and failure to thrive. The liver is subjectively small, and the gastric axis (orange line) is cranially deviated. The dotted lines represent the normal range for the gastric axis in association with the spine (perpendicular) and parallel to the ribs (yellow). The white arrow shows a solitary cystolith. (**B**) A one-year-old intact male Yorkshire Terrier with a normal-sized liver. The gastric axis (orange line) is parallel to the ribs (yellow). The dotted lines show the normal range for the gastric axis in association with the spine (perpendicular) and parallel to the ribs (yellow).

subjectively small liver caudal to the diaphragm in a dog or cat with clinical signs or suggestive blood work should be further assessed with either ultrasonography or angiography.

Ultrasonography

The main objectives of the examination are to assess the size of the liver, determine if there are portal vein abnormalities or secondary abnormalities that would suggest a shunt, identify an extra- vs. an intrahepatic shunt, and assess the abdomen for secondary shunts.[1]

In order to answer these questions, the examination should include an assessment of the liver size, kidney size, presence of hyperechoic shadowing structures in the urinary tract, presence of peritoneal effusion, and the presence of too many vessels in the mid-abdomen. Assessment for microhepatia is subjective. The gallbladder and stomach are typically closer to the diaphragm than usual (**fig. 31.2**). In order to search for the anomalous extrahepatic vessel, the main portal vein should be traced from the mid-abdomen from the jejunal and cranial mesenteric veins (**fig. 31.3**) toward the main portal vein in the direction of the liver. The splenic and gastroduodenal veins should be identified near the porta hepatis. The gastroduodenal vein is the final tributary prior to the trifurcation of the portal vein at the porta hepatis. This can be difficult due to small liver size or the presence of gastric ingesta and gas reverberation in that region. As these portal venous structures are traced, an anomalous vessel may be identified in the cranial abdomen. Color Doppler can be used initially to assess flow in the anomalous vessel, at which point pulsed-wave Doppler can be applied to assess the spectral waveform of the vessels. Normal portal veins have a low-velocity monophasic flow (**fig. 31.4**), while anomalous shunting vessels have turbulent, multidirectional flow (**fig. 31.5**). The caudal vena cava can be traced with color Doppler to assess for laminar vs. turbulent flow at the insertion site of a portocaval shunt (**fig. 31.6**).

If an anomalous vessel is not identified on the initial inspection, the dog should be placed in left lateral recumbency with the legs away from the sonographer and head to the left. The probe should be placed dorsally in transverse orientation between the 11th or 12th rib spaces to identify the porta hepatis so that the PV/Ao ratio may be measured (**fig. 31.7**). Angling the probe cranial to caudal is necessary to identify the aorta, the caudal vena cava, and the portal vein in transverse section all in one image so that their diameters can be measured. A PV/Ao value <0.65 is 100% sensitive and 91% specific for the presence of an extrahepatic portosystemic shunt, and proficiency with this technique

CHAPTER **31** Portosystemic shunts

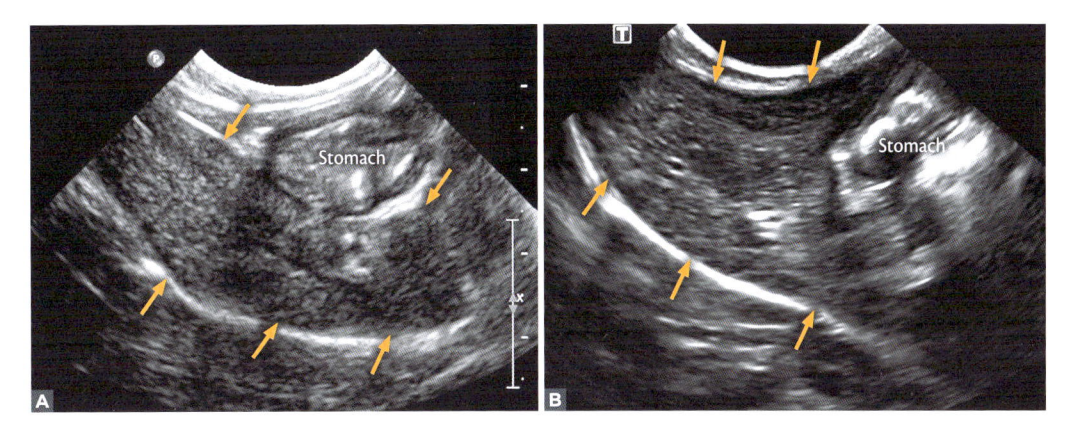

Fig. 31.2 (**A**) Ultrasound images of a ten-month-old female spayed Yorkshire Terrier presented with clinical signs consistent with hepatic encephalopathy and elevated bile acids. Sagittal ultrasound image of the liver. Orange arrows are placed at the ventral (near field) and dorsal (far field) of the liver. The stomach is labeled. The liver is small, and the stomach is located in a more cranial position in close proximity to the diaphragm. (**B**) Sagittal ultrasound image of the liver of a normal Yorkshire Terrier of a similar age as in (**A**). Orange arrows are placed at the ventral (near field) and dorsal (far field) of the liver. The stomach is labeled.

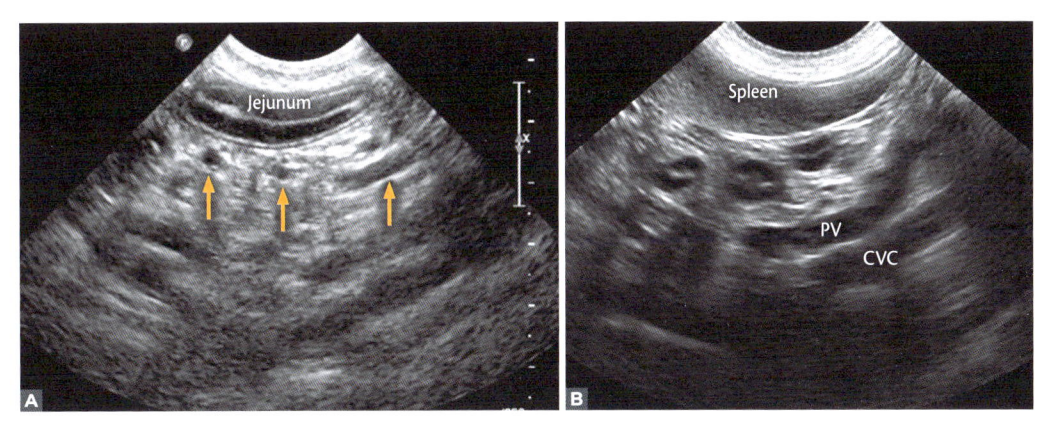

Fig. 31.3 Ultrasound image of the jejunal and mesenteric vein tracing. (**A**) Identification and tracing of the jejunal veins amongst the jejunal intestinal segments. Arrows point out numerous jejunal veins in transverse and longitudinal sections. (**B**) Tracing the jejunal veins cranially to identify the main portal vein in the cranial abdomen and tracing it to the porta hepatis.

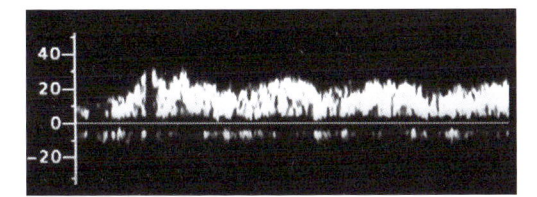

Fig. 31.4 Pulsed wave Doppler showing monophasic, hepatopetal (towards the liver) flow in a normal portal vein. All venous tributaries of the portal vein should have low velocity and monophasic flow, making them easy to identify compared to an artery.

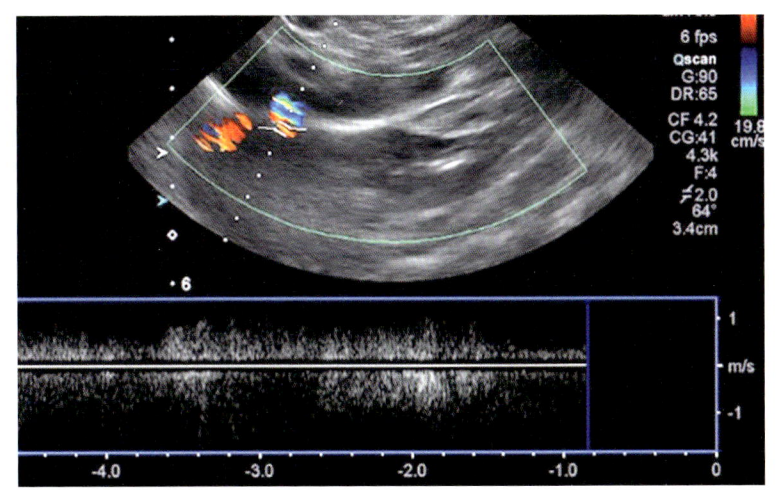

Fig. 31.5 Pulsed wave Doppler showing turbulent flow in a single congenital extrahepatic shunt showing high velocity and bidirectional flow in the region of insertion at the caudal vena cava. The insertion site is seen with color Doppler as a color mosaic representative of turbulent flow.

SECTION V ABDOMEN

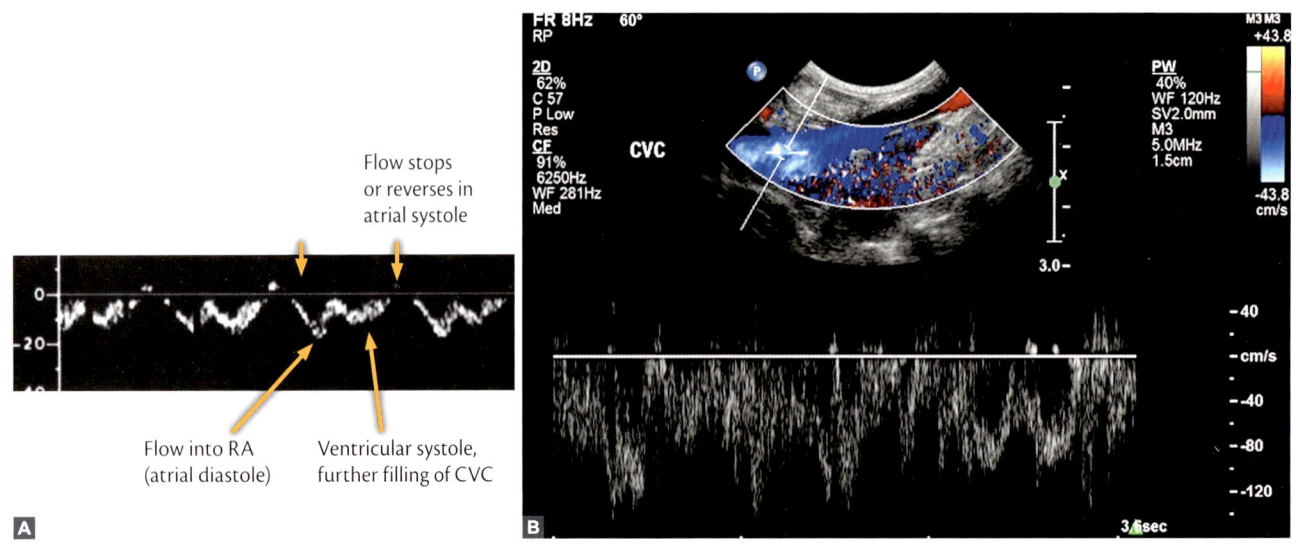

Fig. 31.6 Pulsed wave Doppler of the caudal vena cava. (**A**) Normal pulsed wave Doppler of the caudal vena cava in a normal dog. Caval flow is triphasic in comparison to the monophasic flow of portal veins. (**B**) Dual phased Doppler showing color and pulsed wave imaging of the caudal vena cava (CVC) and its high velocity, nonlaminar flow in the spectral wave form. The caudal vena cava was traced using color Doppler in order to guide the placement of the sample volume of the pulsed wave Doppler beam over the region of turbulence (region of color variance, yellow, etc.) so that its flow characteristics could be analyzed. *RA*, right atrium.

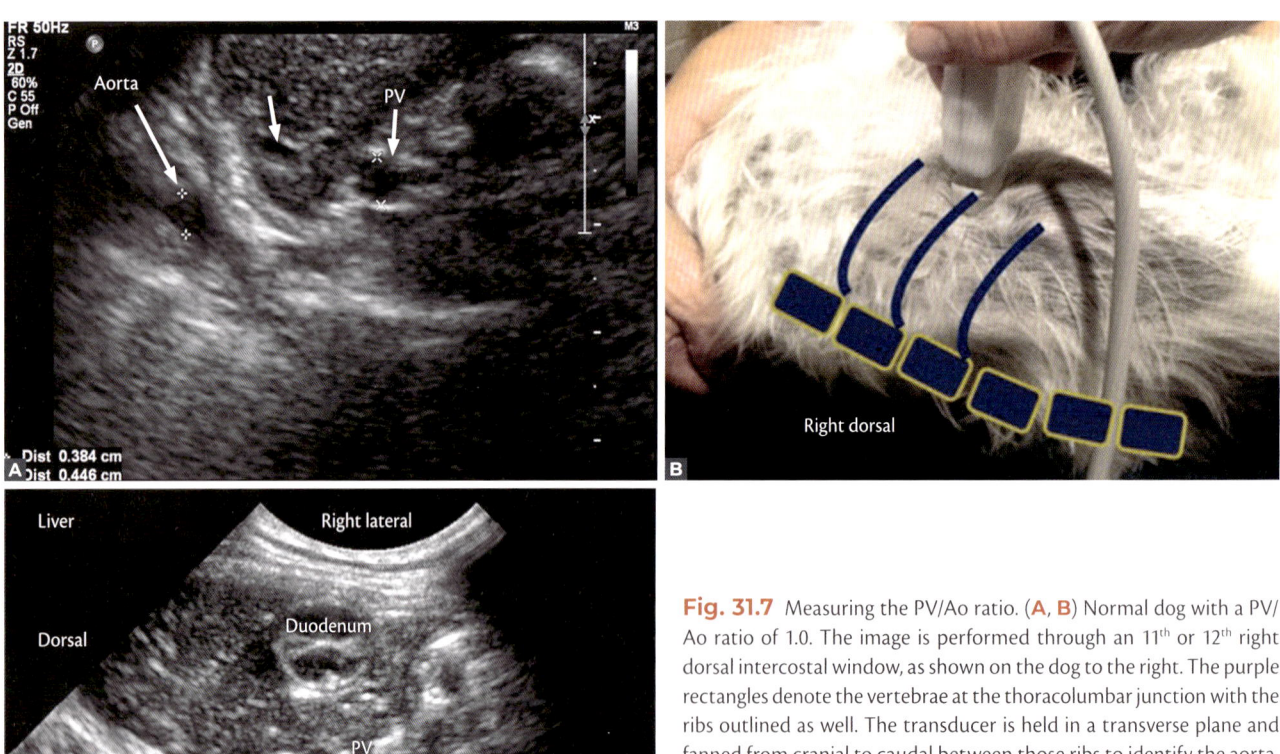

Fig. 31.7 Measuring the PV/Ao ratio. (**A, B**) Normal dog with a PV/Ao ratio of 1.0. The image is performed through an 11th or 12th right dorsal intercostal window, as shown on the dog to the right. The purple rectangles denote the vertebrae at the thoracolumbar junction with the ribs outlined as well. The transducer is held in a transverse plane and fanned from cranial to caudal between those ribs to identify the aorta, the caudal vena cava and the portal vein, marked with white arrows and from left to right, respectively. (**C**) Decreased PV/Ao ratio in a dog with an extrahepatic portocaval shunt. Here the ratio was 0.25, and the portocaval shunting vessel is marked with a orange arrow entering the caudal vena cava. The liver is small, and the duodenum is in the near field in transverse section.

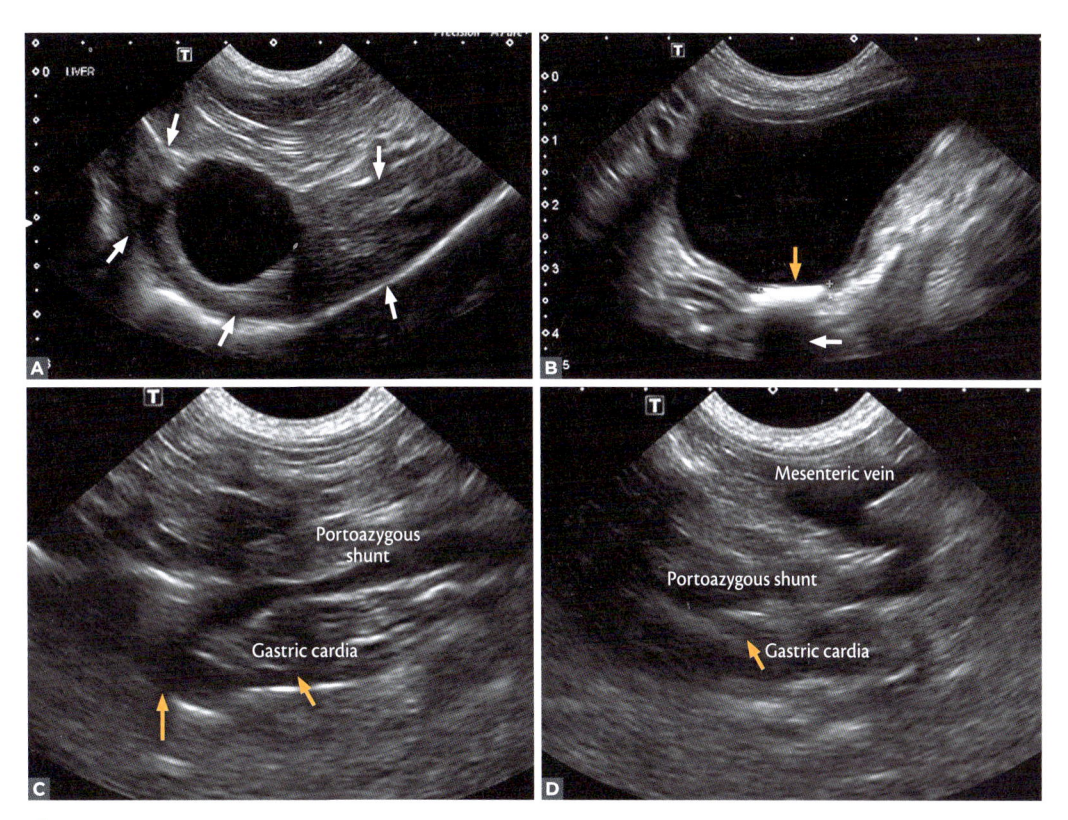

Fig. 31.8 Portoazygous shunt in a six-year-old neutered male Schnauzer detected sonographically. (**A**) Sagittal ultrasound image of the small liver (white arrows). The gallbladder is subjectively the same size as the liver in this frame which is typical of microhepatia. (**B**) The same dog as in fig. 31.10A. Sagittal ultrasound image of the urinary bladder (UB) containing hyperechoic (orange arrow) shadowing (white arrow) cystoliths due to urate stones and crystals. (**C, D**) Portoazygous shunt in the same dog. Tracing the portal vein toward the liver, a large tortuous port.

is achievable with some practice. A PV/Ao ratio >0.8 makes an extrahepatic portosystemic shunt unlikely.[1] Furthermore, the main portal vein will be of normal size or enlarged with an intrahepatic portosystemic shunt.

In the same patient position, the caudal vena cave can be traced in a sagittal plan with color Doppler in order to screen for turbulent flow where an anomalous vessel could terminate in it.

A link between shunt insertion site and clinical signs exists in dogs. Neurologic signs are more common when the shunting vessel enters the caudal vena cava caudal to the liver. This is typical of a splenocaval shunt.[2] Shunts that enter the azygous or phrenic veins, therefore cranial to the liver, for example, have fewer to no clinical signs and may present later in life with a congenital shunt even >5 years of age (**fig. 31.8**).[2,3]

In cats, portosystemic shunts are rare, and the most common is a left gastric vein communicating with the caudal vena cava.[4] Portoazygous, portocaval, and colonic vein shunts have also been described. Ultrasonography has been reported to have a high sensitivity and upwards of 100% in cats.[4] For intrahepatic shunts, the porta hepatis should be examined, and the main portal vein will divide into right, left, and central divisional branches, and this is best identified on a transverse image of the hilus from a ventral window. Large breed dogs <1 year of age are generally affected. The liver will be small, and the intrahepatic shunt appears as a large, anechoic cavity in the center of the liver. It may even look like a second gallbladder. Color Doppler will show a clear connection with the caudal vena cava, and turbulent blood flow will be evident on both color Doppler and pulsed wave Doppler (**fig. 31.9**).

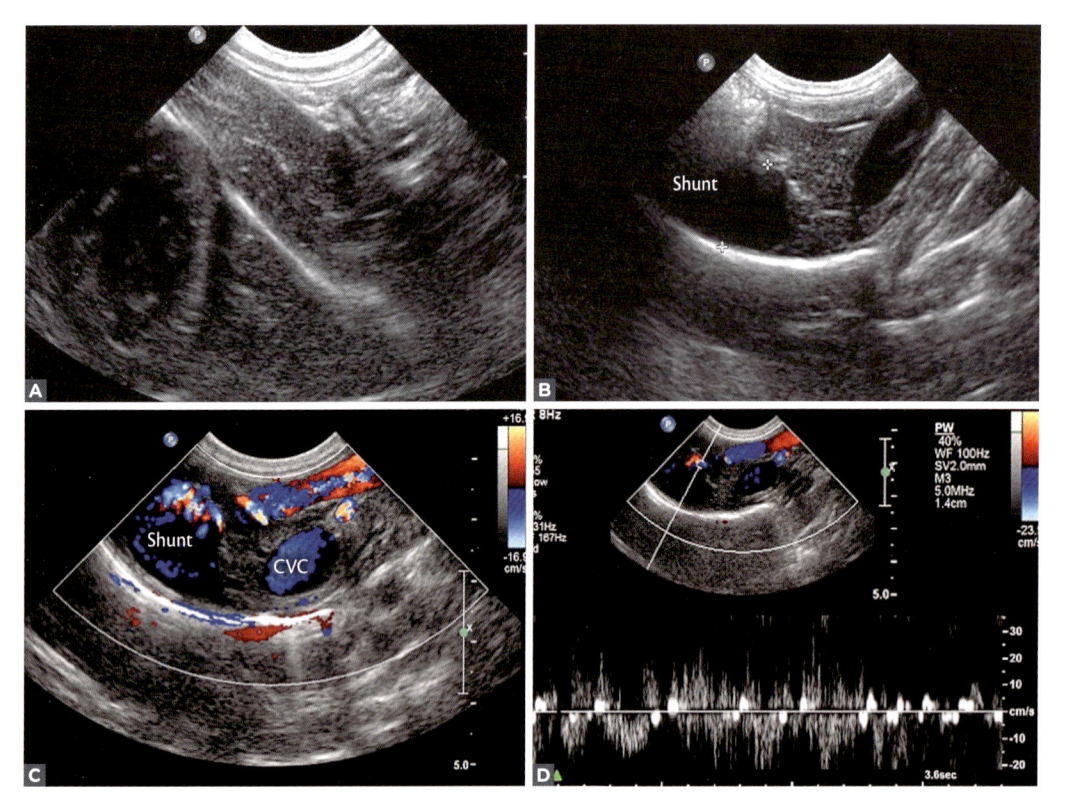

Fig. 31.9 (**A**) A four-month-old intact female Siberian Husky presented with neurologic clinical signs one month before. The dog was blind, circling, and had ptyalism. (**B**) Ultrasound image of the same dog showing a left-sided left divisional intrahepatic shunt. (**C**) Color Doppler ultrasound of the shunt showing a turbulent blood flow within and compared to the caudal vena cava (CVC). (**D**) Pulsed wave Doppler showing bidirectional and high velocity turbulent flow within the intrahepatic shunt.

Contrast studies

Radiographic portography has largely been replaced by computed tomographic angiography for identifying portosystemic shunts. While ultrasound doesn't require anesthesia or intravenous contrast, contrast portography offers a more detailed overview which is most useful for determining if surgical therapy is indicated.

Radiographic portography

Iodinated contrast medium is injected using a surgical approach into an isolated mesenteric vein. Other approaches utilize an intrasplenic injection to create a splenoportogram. Radiographs are performed pre- and immediate post-contrast injection to identify anomalous shunting vessels as well as secondary acquired shunts (**fig. 31.10**).

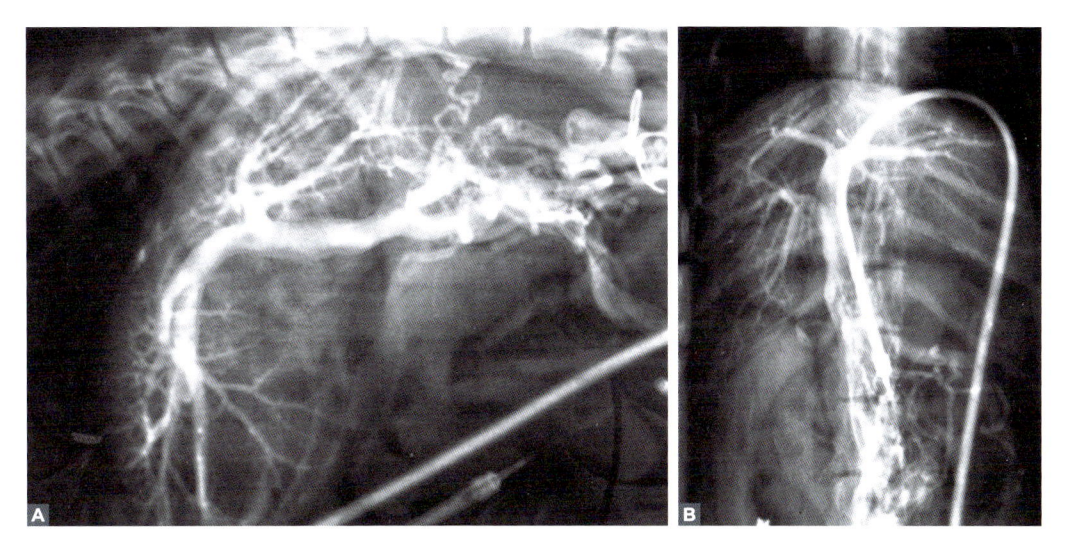

Fig. 31.10 Lateral and ventrodorsal images of an intraoperative mesenteric portogram showing numerous anomalous vessels in the mid-abdomen due to an acquired shunt developed secondary to chronic hepatic fibrosis.

Computed tomographic angiography

This method uses a single peripheral injection of iodinated contrast medium for consistent evaluation of the entire vasculature of the abdomen and can use bolus tracking to assess the arterial and portal phases of contrast distribution for the most accurate detection and description of vascular anomalies.[5] Dual-phase CT allows examination of the hepatic arteries as well as the portal and hepatic veins. This technique allows arteriovenous fistulas as well as venous-venous anomalies to be identified as well.[6] 3D multiplanar reconstructions of the shunts can be performed to assess complex anomalies. In addition, it can help to reduce the risk of inappropriate attenuation site (**fig. 31.11**).

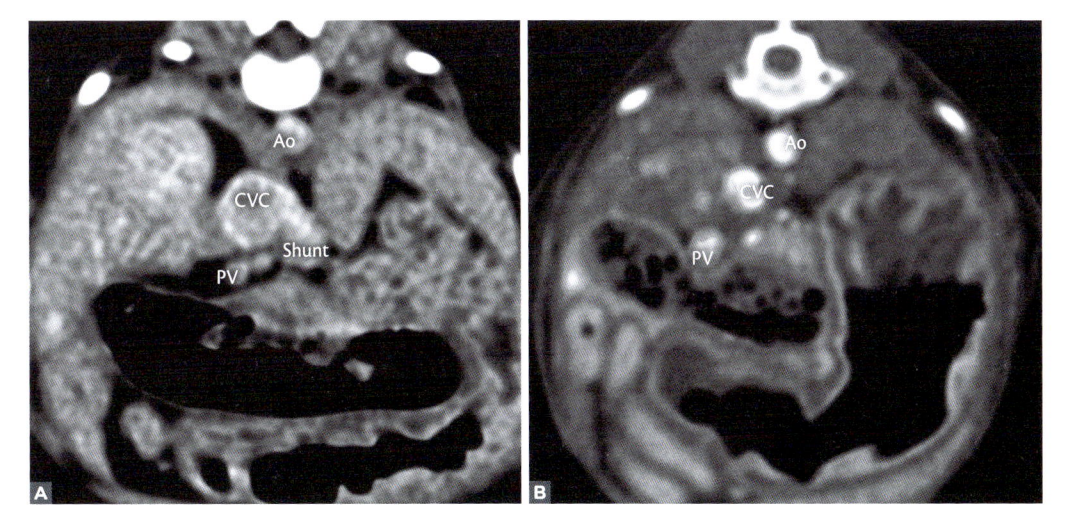

Fig. 31.11 (**A**) Computed tomography angiogram of a seven-month-old male Yorkshire Terrier that presented with chronic vomiting and elevated pre- and postprandial bile acids and after being treated medically for a suspected portosystemic shunt for three weeks without improvement. CT angiography showing a single extrahepatic portosystemic splenocaval shunt. Note the very small diameter portal vein and large size of the caudal vena cava where the shunt inserts. (**B**) CT angiogram of a ten-month-old Yorkshire Terrier showing the normal location and sizes of the portal vein (PV), caudal vena cava (CVC), and aorta (Ao). This dog did not have a portosystemic shunt.

References

1. D'Anjou MA. The sonographic search for portosystemic shunts. *Clin Tech Small Anim Pract* 22:104-114, 2007.
2. Kraun MB, Nelson LL, Hauptman JG, Nelson NC. Analysis of the relationship of extrahepatic portosystemic shunt morphology with clinical variables in dogs: 53 cases (2009-2012). *J Am Vet Med Assoc* 245:540-549, 2014.
3. Worley DR, Holt DE. Clinical outcome of congenital extrahepatic portosystemic shunt attenuation in dogs aged five years and older: 17 cases (1992-2005). *J Am Vet Med Assoc* 232:722-727, 2008.
4. Lamb CR, Forster-van Hijfte MA, White RN, McEvoy FJ, Rutgers HC. Ultrasonographic diagnosis of congenital portosystemic shunt in 14 cats. *J Small Anim Pract* 37:205-209, 1996.
5. Nelson NC, Nelson LL. Anatomy of extrahepatic portosystemic shunts in dogs as determined by computed tomography angiography. *Vet Radiol Ultrasound* 52:498-506, 2011.
6. Zwingenberger AL, McLear RC, Weisse C. Diagnosis of arterioportal fistulae in four dogs using computed tomographic angiography. *Vet Radiol Ultrasound* 46:472-477, 2005.

CHAPTER 32

Pancreas

Angela J. Marolf

> **KEY POINTS**
>
> - The pancreas is a thin V-shaped organ in the cranial abdomen in dogs and cats.
> - Ultrasound imaging of the pancreas can be challenging due to superimposition of overlying stomach and bowel.
> - Computed tomography utilizes intravenous contrast to evaluate the pancreatic parenchyma and eliminates superimposition of adjacent structures.
> - Sonographic changes associated with acute pancreatitis include pancreatic enlargement, changes in pancreatic echogenicity, and peripancreatic inflammation and fluid.
> - Sonographic changes associated with chronic pancreatitis are poorly established. Features may include normal size or enlarged with a heterogenous appearance or have a nodular architecture.
> - CT imaging of pancreatitis includes pancreatic enlargement, changes in pancreatic parenchymal contrast enhancement, peripancreatic inflammation, fluid, and portal vein thrombosis.
> - CT evidence of heterogeneous pancreatic contrast enhancement and portal vein thrombosis indicate a more serious form of pancreatitis.
> - Pancreatic abscesses and pseudocysts are sequelae of pancreatitis.
> - Pancreatic neoplasia may be in the form of primary carcinoma, insulinoma or metastatic. Insulinomas are typically solitary discrete hypoechoic nodules while carcinoma or metastatic disease are more complex with overlapping features with pancreatitis.

The pancreas is located in the cranial and mid-abdomen caudal to the liver. This organ has both exocrine and endocrine functions; the exocrine pancreas produces secretions which aid in digestion. The endocrine pancreas mainly releases insulin which keeps blood sugar levels in a constant range. Imaging of the pancreas can be challenging due to its thin, lobulated shape and proximity to gas and fluid filled structures like the stomach and duodenum. The proximal gastrointestinal tract can become superimposed over the pancreas hindering thorough evaluation.

Inflammation of the pancreas, or pancreatitis, is commonly diagnosed in dogs and cats. Clinical signs associated with pancreatitis can be non-specific and include vomiting, diarrhea, and inappetence. Pancreatitis can range in severity and be accompanied by various sequelae that can affect prognosis. In the past, abdominal radiography was performed in dogs and cats suspected of pancreatitis. Today, ultrasound is the most commonly used modality to diagnose pancreatitis and other pancreatic diseases; however, computed tomography (CT) is becoming more readily utilized in pancreatic imaging.

Normal pancreas

In both dogs and cats, the pancreas is a V-shaped organ with right and left lobes connected by a body. The right lobe lies along the medial side of the duodenum and courses cranially to unite with the body. The body lies near the pylorus and portal vein with the left limb extending laterally near the left kidney and spleen (**figs. 32.1** and **32.2**).

The pancreas has internal ducts to deliver exocrine secretions to the proximal duodenum to aid in digestion. Pancreatic ductal anatomy is different between dogs and cats. The major duct in dogs is the accessory duct which empties onto the minor duodenal papilla. In cats, the major duct is the pancreatic duct which empties onto the major duodenal papilla along with the common bile duct.

Imaging of the normal pancreas

The normal pancreas is not usually identified in the cranial abdominal on standard radiographs. To evaluate the normal pancreas, ultrasound or CT are needed. On ultrasound, the pancreas is typically isoechoic to mildly hypoechoic to the surrounding mesentery and hypoechoic to the adjacent spleen (**figs. 32.3** and **32.4**).[1]

The thickness of the individual right and left lobes and body can vary; however, typically, the pancreas should measure less than 10 mm in thickness in normal dogs[2] and cats.[1] Normal measurements of the pancreatic duct have been obtained for dogs[2] and cats[1] with a general guideline of less than 0.1 mm diameter considered normal. Dilation of the pancreatic duct has been identified as a normal age-related change in cats.[3] Ultrasound imaging of the pancreas can be limited due to overlying gas within the stomach and duodenum or due to operator experience. With CT imaging of the pan-

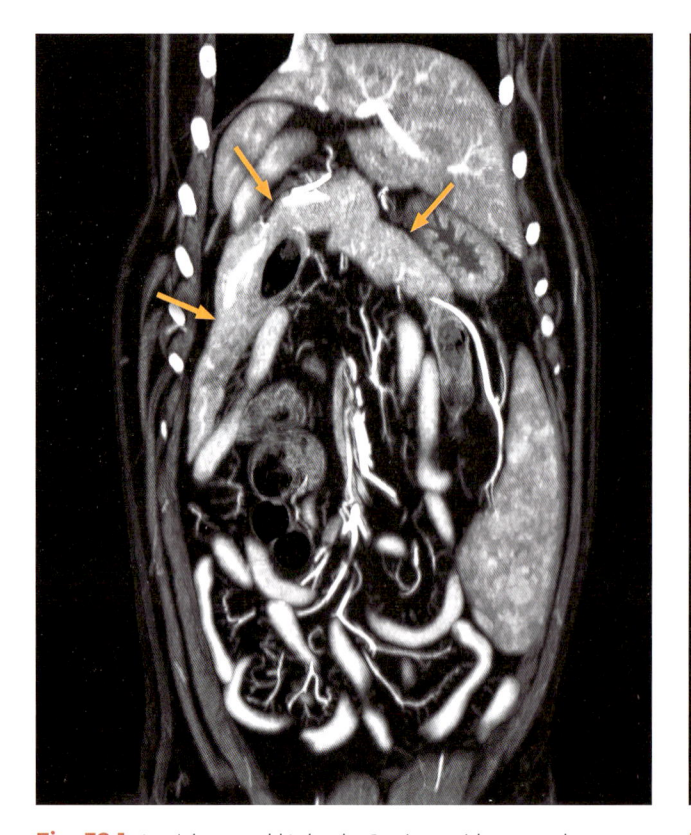

Fig. 32.1 An eight-year-old Labrador Retriever with a normal pancreas. CT dorsal plane reconstruction in venous phase highlighting the normal pancreas location and shape within the cranial abdomen (arrows).

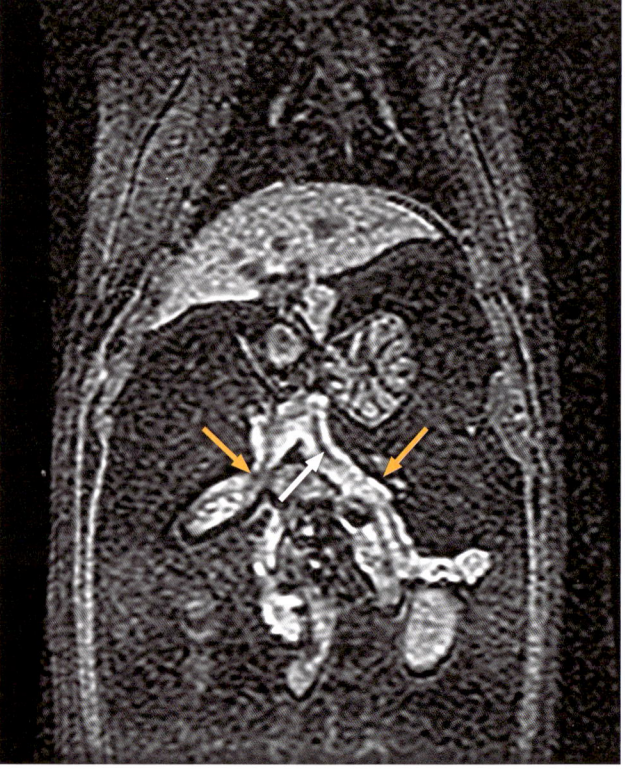

Fig. 32.2 A two-year-old Domestic shorthair cat with a normal pancreas. MRI dorsal plane T1 weighted post-contrast image with fat-saturation highlighting the normal pancreas location and shape within the cranial abdomen (orange arrows). The hypointense tubular structure within the pancreas is the pancreatic duct (white arrow).

creas, intravenous iodinated contrast is needed to evaluate the pancreatic parenchyma. CT imaging of the pancreas demonstrates an iso- to hypoattenuating parenchyma compared to the liver and spleen with homogeneous enhancement of the parenchyma.[4,5] The normal pancreas has smooth margins. Normal size measurements of the right and left limb and body of the pancreas have been established in dogs[4] and cats.[5] Pancreatic duct may be identified on CT imaging in most dogs and cats (**figs. 32.5** and **32.6**).

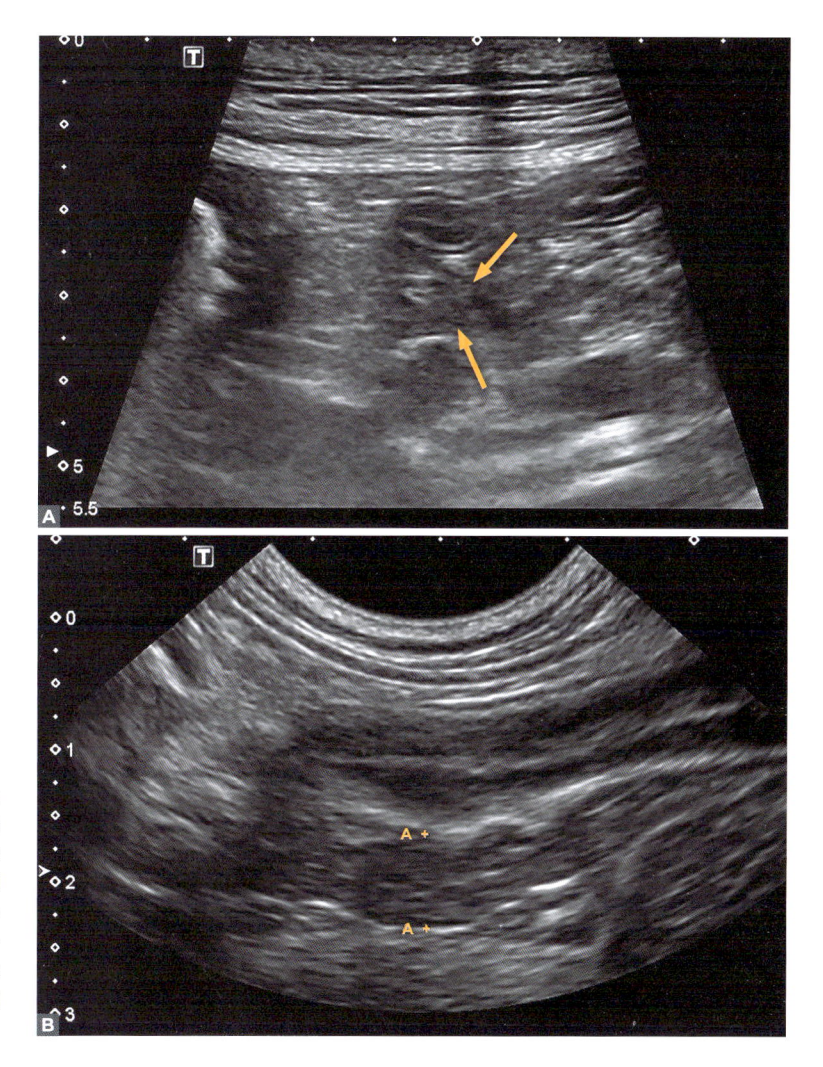

Fig. 32.3 (**A**) A seven-year-old Australian Heeler with a normal left pancreatic lobe. On ultrasound transverse plane imaging, the pancreas is mildly hypoechoic to the surrounding mesentery (arrows). (**B**) A six-year-old mixed breed dog with a normal right pancreatic lobe. On ultrasound sagittal plane imaging, the pancreas is mildy hypoechoic to the surrounding mesentery (calipers). Pancreas measured 7 mm in thickness. The duodenum is located dorsal to the pancreas in the image.

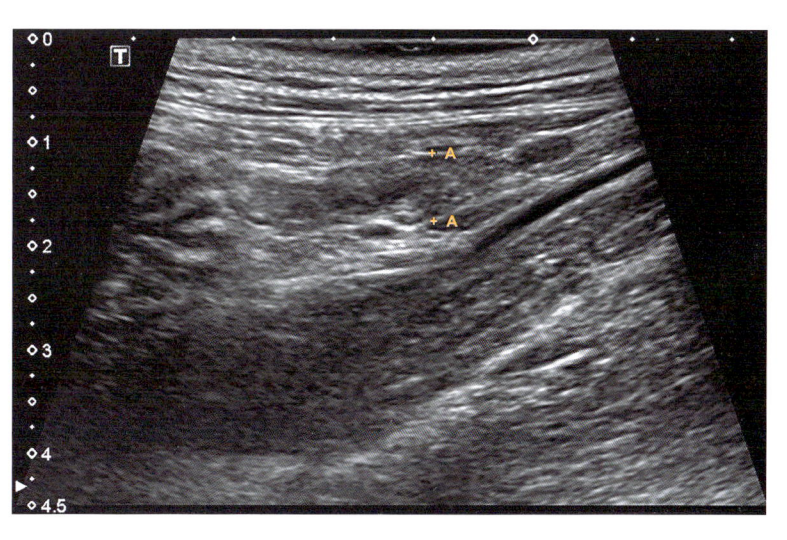

Fig. 32.4 A nine-year-old Domestic shorthair cat with normal left pancreatic lobe. On ultrasound sagittal plane imaging, the pancreas is isoechoic to mildly hypoechoic (calipers). Pancreas measured 6.6 mm in thickness.

SECTION V ABDOMEN

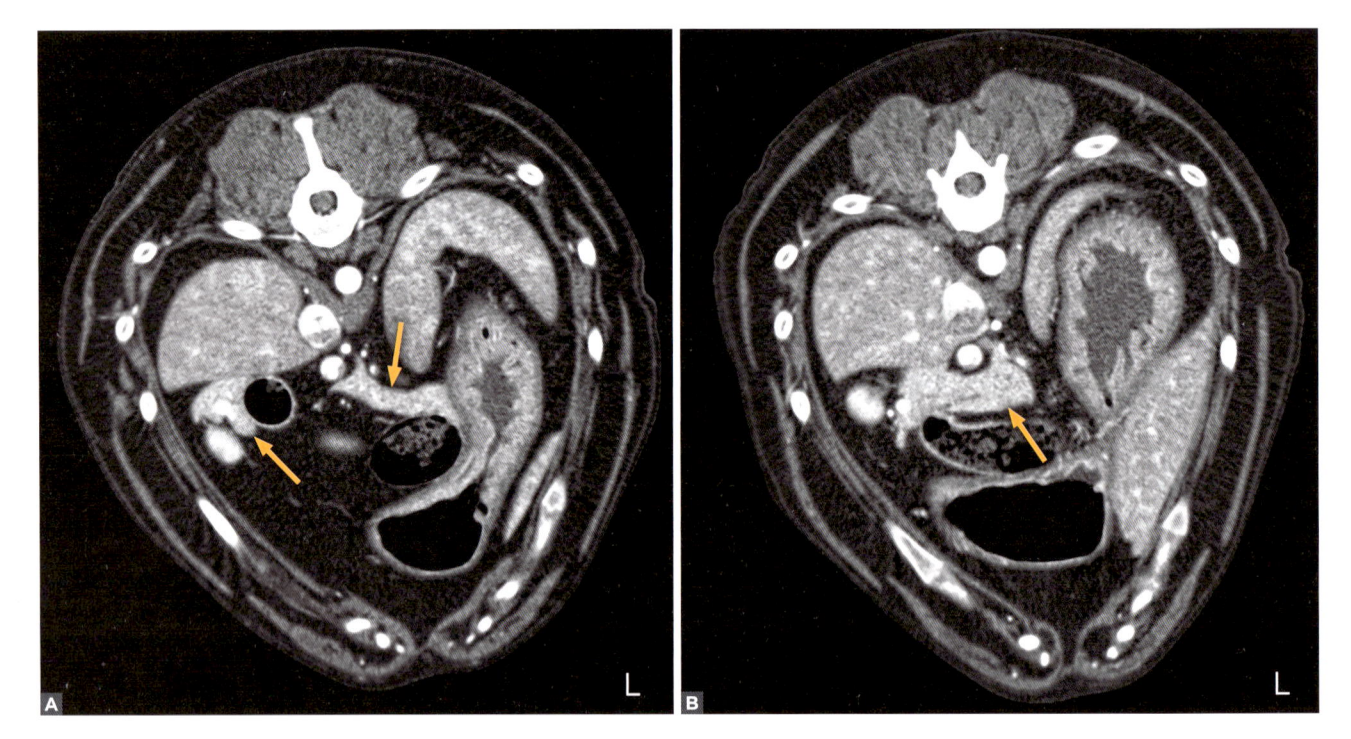

Fig. 32.5 Same dog as in fig. 35.1. CT transverse plane images in venous phase of a normal pancreas. (**A**) Right and left pancreatic lobes (arrows). (**B**) Pancreatic body (arrow). Note the homogeneous contrast enhancement and smooth margins of the pancreas in all images. "L" designated laterality.

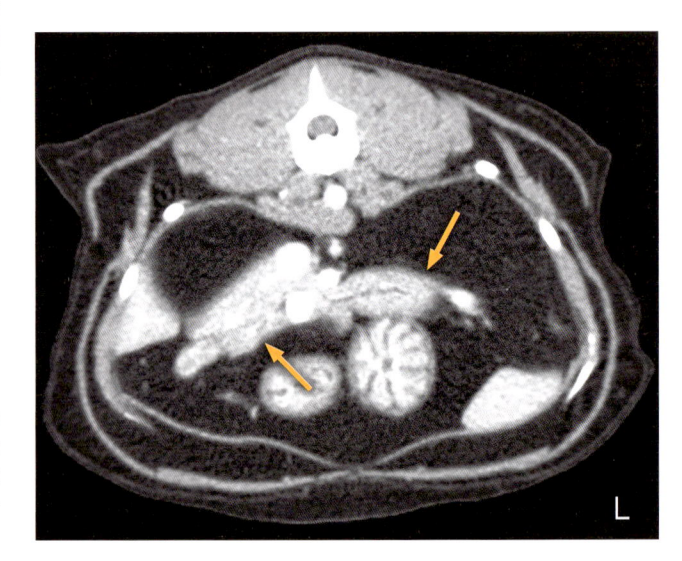

Fig. 32.6 A 16-year-old Domestic shorthair cat. CT transverse plane image in venous phase of a normal pancreas. Portions of the left and right lobes and body are included (arrows). Note the homogeneous contrast enhancement and smooth margins of the pancreas in all images. "L" designates laterality.

Pancreatitis

Pancreatitis is the most common exocrine pancreatic disease in dogs[6] and cats.[7] Acute pancreatitis is more readily apparent on imaging with chronic pancreatitis being more challenging to diagnose. Acute pancreatitis is usually related to release of digestive enzymes that cause inflammation to the pancreatic parenchyma and surrounding tissues, organs, and vasculature. The resulting inflammation within the pancreas results in edema and necrosis.

Imaging of acute pancreatitis

Radiography The radiographic findings associated with acute pancreatitis include decreased serosal detail within the cranial abdomen, a focal mass effect between the pyloroduodenal angle and colon, and mild gas dilation of the duodenum. These changes are not commonly identified on radiographs (**fig. 32.7**).

▎ **Ultrasound** Ultrasound findings in dogs and cats with acute pancreatitis can include pancreatic enlargement, hypoechoic parenchyma, hyperechoic surrounding mesenteric fat, peripancreatic fluid, and common bile duct dilation (**figs. 32.8** and **32.9**).[8]
Pancreatic duct dilation can be seen occasionally. One or more of the above findings may be present, and milder forms of pancreatitis may only show mild enlargement of a portion of the pancreatic parenchyma, i.e., focal increased thickness in one lobe. More severe forms of acute pancreatitis can demonstrate severe thickening of a portion or all of the pancreas with hyperechoic mesentery and free fluid. Extrahepatic biliary duct obstruction due to pancreatic inflammation may occur. Advanced forms of pancreatitis are more easily identified with ultrasound imaging.

▎ **Computed tomography** With CT imaging, the entire pancreas can be evaluated due to lack of superimposition of other organs. This global view of the pancreas and portal vein is advantageous to ensure a thorough evaluation in patients with suspected pancreatitis. CT is becoming more frequently used in the diagnosis of pancreatitis in dogs[9] and cats.[10] Intravenous iodinated contrast allows evaluation of the pancreatic parenchyma for contrast enhancement changes. The common bile duct can be followed as it enters the major duodenal papilla, and extrahepatic biliary duct dilation is readily identified. Additionally, the adjacent vasculature can be reviewed for evidence of thrombosis, particularly in the portal vein. CT imaging of pancreatitis includes pancreatic enlargement, irregular margins, peri-pancreatic changes, and alterations in parenchymal enhancement. Decreases in pancreatic contrast enhancement cause a more heterogeneous enhancement pattern which can be associated with areas of decreased pancreatic perfusion or necrosis. Portal vein thrombosis may be

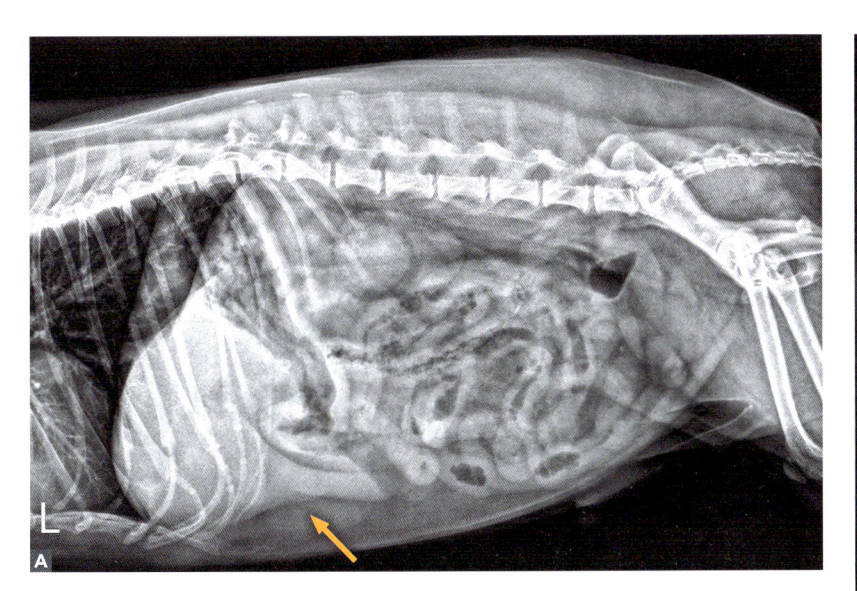

Fig. 32.7 A seven-year-old Bichon Frisé. (**A**) Lateral and (**B**) ventrodorsal abdominal radiographs show decreased detail in the cranial abdomen with mild mass effect caudal to the stomach (arrows). On the VD image, there is mild displacement of the adjacent pylorus and colon. This dog had acute pancreatitis based on ultrasound imaging.

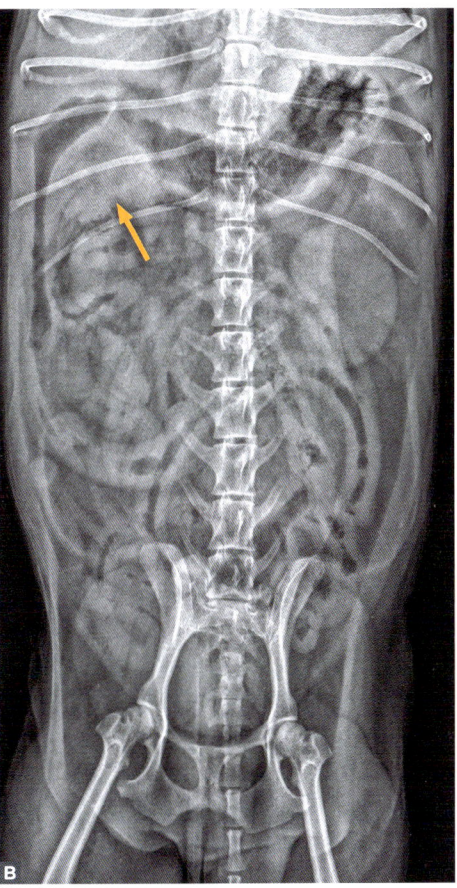

SECTION V ABDOMEN

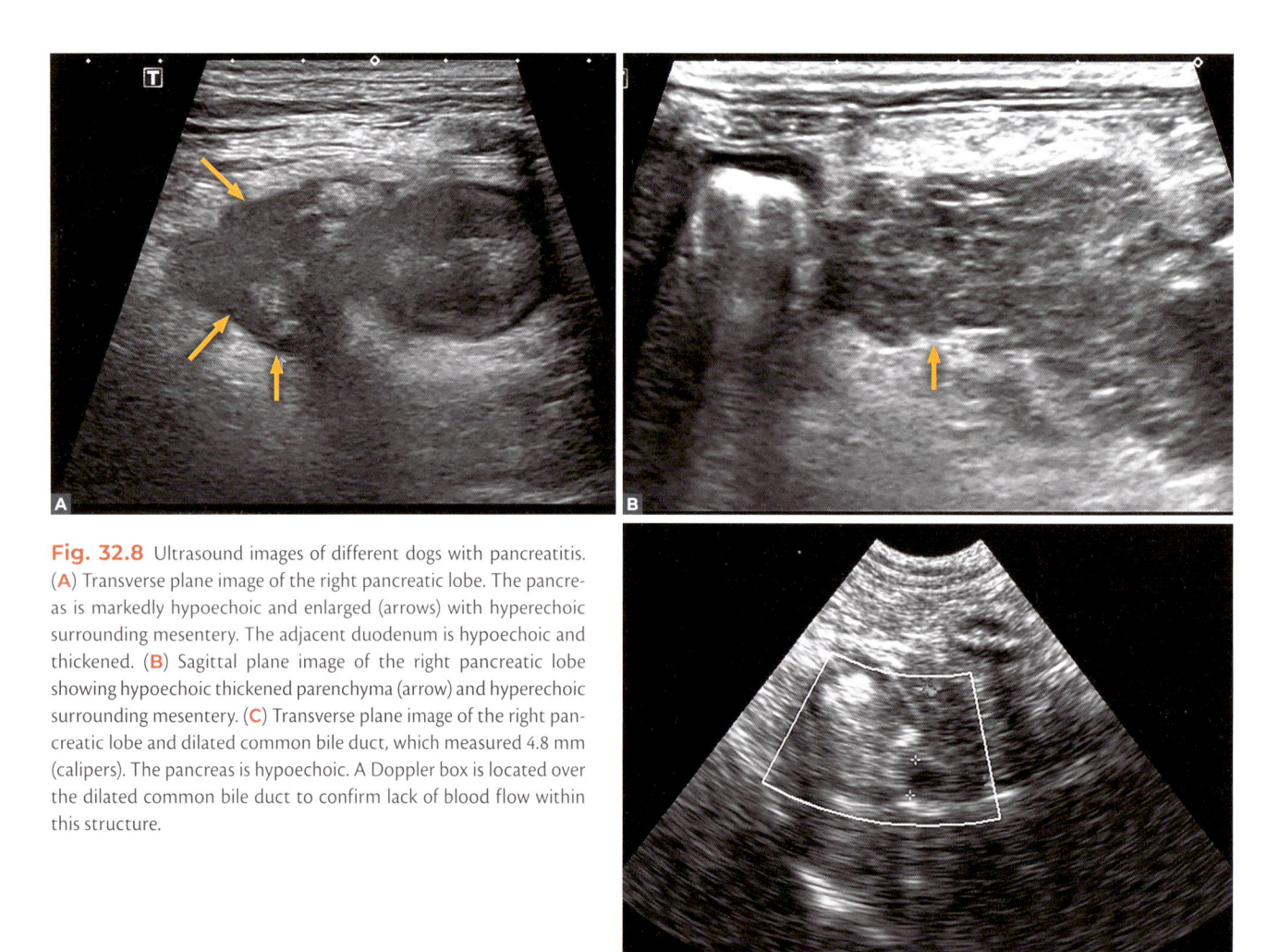

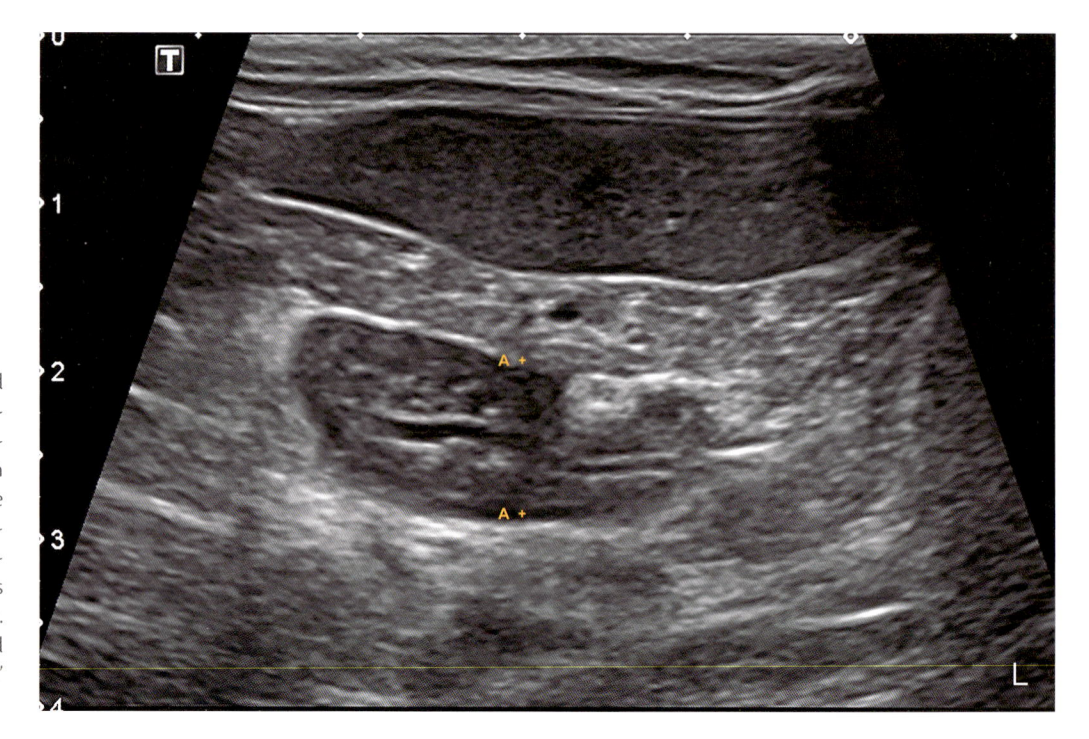

Fig. 32.8 Ultrasound images of different dogs with pancreatitis. (**A**) Transverse plane image of the right pancreatic lobe. The pancreas is markedly hypoechoic and enlarged (arrows) with hyperechoic surrounding mesentery. The adjacent duodenum is hypoechoic and thickened. (**B**) Sagittal plane image of the right pancreatic lobe showing hypoechoic thickened parenchyma (arrow) and hyperechoic surrounding mesentery. (**C**) Transverse plane image of the right pancreatic lobe and dilated common bile duct, which measured 4.8 mm (calipers). The pancreas is hypoechoic. A Doppler box is located over the dilated common bile duct to confirm lack of blood flow within this structure.

Fig. 32.9 A 15-year-old mixed breed dog. CT transverse and dorsal plane reconstruction images in venous phase. Note the mildly thickened pancreatic body and left lobe (arrows) with homogeneous contrast enhancement. This dog was diagnosed with mild pancreatitis. "L" designates laterality.

530

identified with CT imaging in dogs with pancreatitis. Heterogeneous pancreatic contrast enhancement has been associated with portal vein thrombosis and can indicate more severe pancreatitis and a poorer prognosis in dogs.[9] Dogs with milder forms of pancreatitis often have mild thickening of the pancreas with normal homogeneous contrast enhancement. Pancreatic duct enlargement has been noted in cats with CT imaging for suspected pancreatitis (**figs. 32.10** and **32.11**).[10]

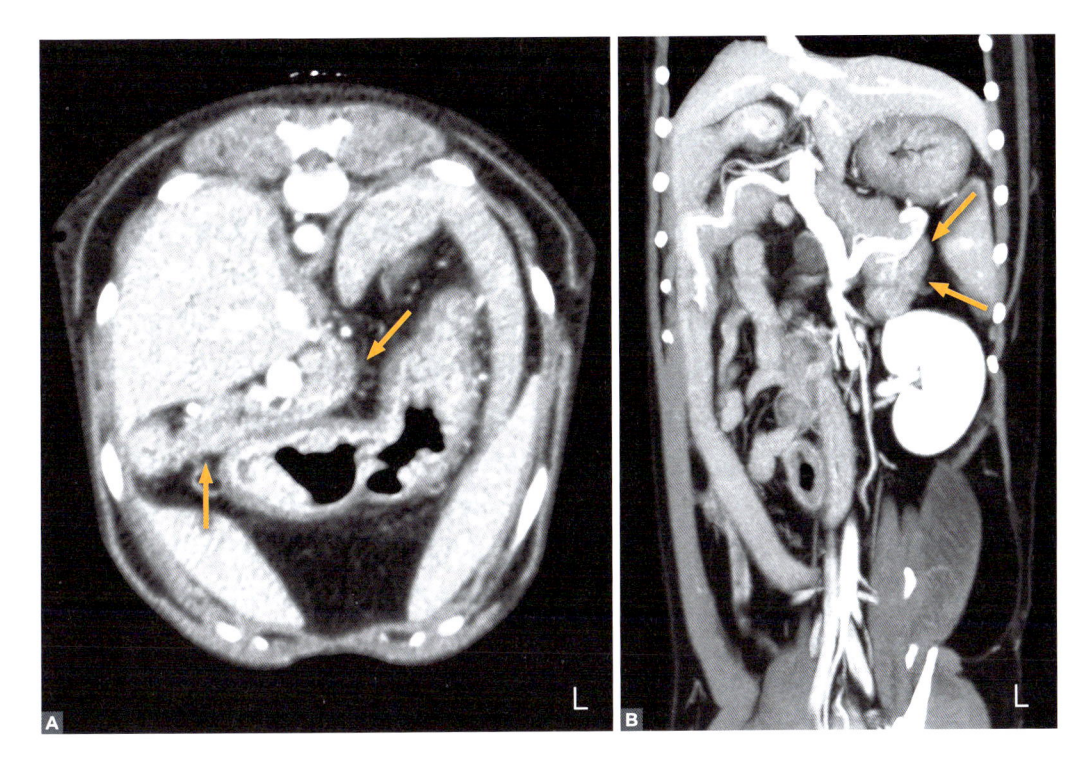

Fig. 32.10 A 15-year-old mixed breed dog. CT transverse and dorsal plane reconstruction images in venous phase. Note the mildly thickened pancreatic body and left lobe (arrows) with homogeneous contrast enhancement. This dog was diagnosed with mild pancreatitis. "L" designates laterality.

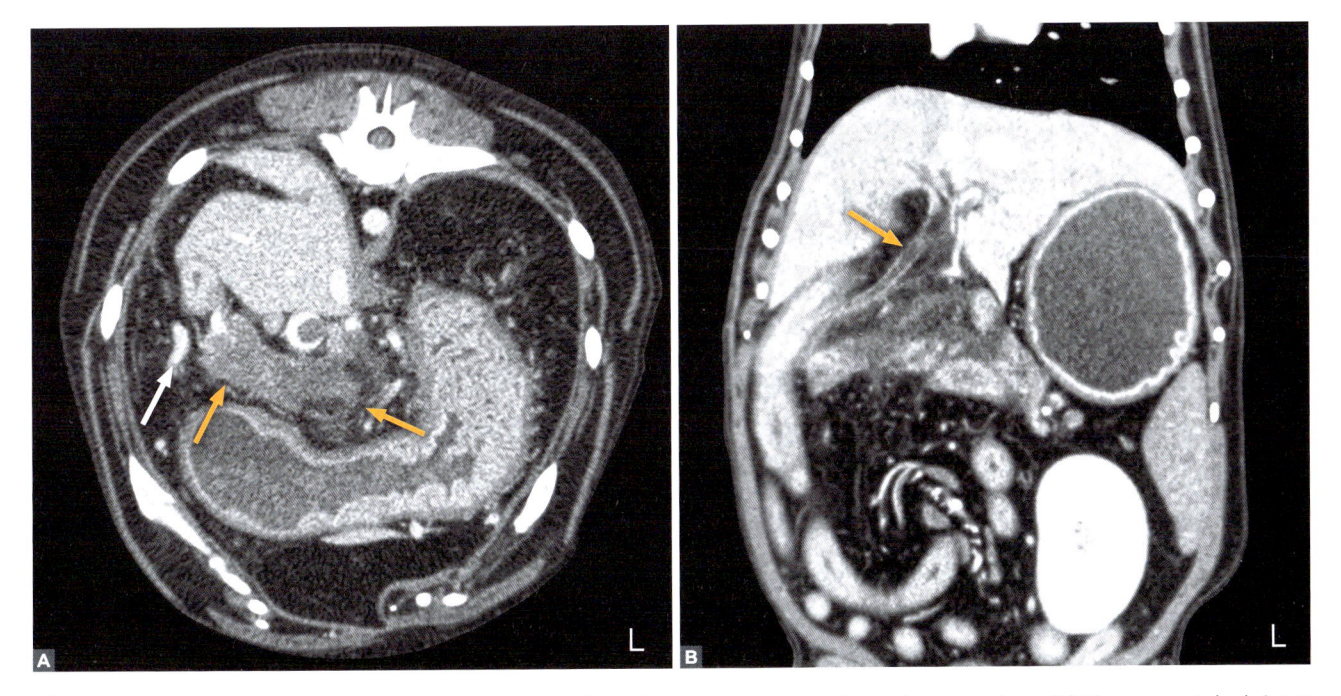

Fig. 32.11 An 11-year-old mixed breed dog. CT transverse and dorsal plane reconstruction images in venous phase. (**A**) The pancreatic body is not minimally contrast enhancing (arrows) with a visible portal vein thrombus (arrowhead). The surrounding mesenteric fat is abnormal and heterogeneous in attenuation. (**B**) Portions of the pancreas show heterogeneous contrast enhancement. The common bile duct is dilated (arrow). This dog was diagnosed with severe pancreatitis. "L" designates laterality.

Pancreatic abscesses/pseudocysts

Abscess and pseudocyst formation can be sequelae of pancreatitis. Pseudocysts are fluid collections that can develop a fibrotic capsule over time that may or may not be infected. Abscess formation is an infected fluid collection within the pancreas. Both of these structures will have hypoechoic (ultrasound) or hypoattenuating (CT) internal fluid with varying degrees of thickened walls. With CT imaging, the walls surrounding pseudocysts and abscesses may contrast enhance. Aspiration and analysis of these structures are necessary for definitive diagnosis and determination of further therapeutic recommendations (**figs. 32.12** and **32.13**).

Chronic pancreatitis

The ultrasonographic appearance of chronic pancreatitis in dogs and cats has not been well described. Recurrent episodes of pancreatitis may lead to chronic changes that can be identified ultrasonographically and mainly consist of fibrosis. The pancreas may be of normal size or enlarged with a heterogenous appearance or have a nodular architecture. Mineralization may be present and may lead to acoustic shadowing (**fig. 32.14**).

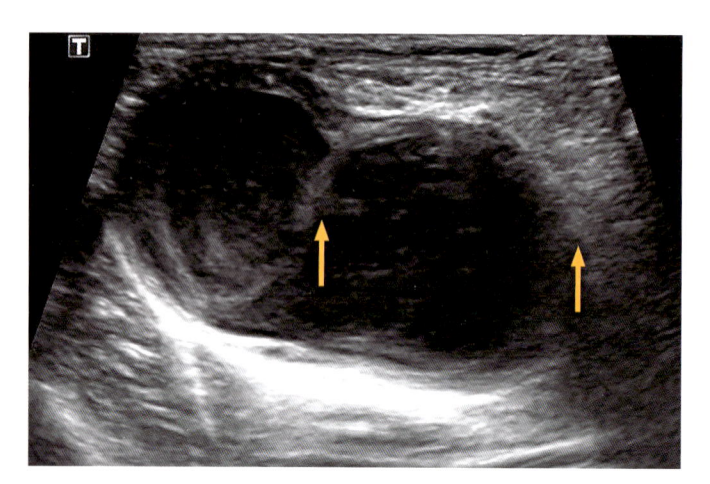

Fig. 32.12 A 15-year-old Domestic shorthair cat. Ultrasound sagittal plane image in the cranial abdomen caudal to the stomach. A large thick wall, fluid-filled structure (arrows) with internal echogenicity was in the region of the pancreas. This cat was diagnosed with a pancreatic abscess.

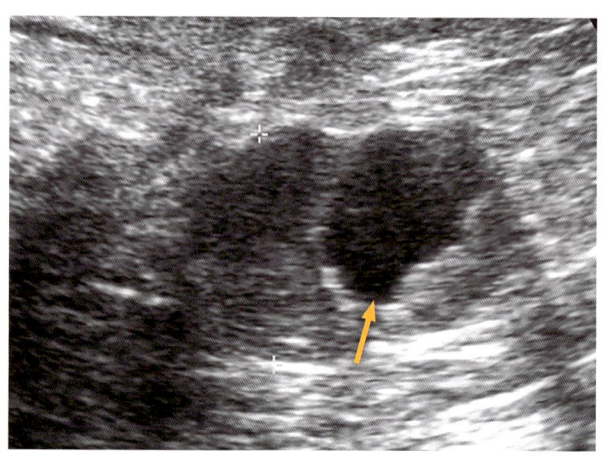

Fig. 32.13 A ten-year-old Domestic shorthair cat. Ultrasound sagittal plane image of the left pancreas. Note the hypoechoic and thickened pancreas, which measured 16 mm (calipers), and internal anechoic thin-walled cyst at the tip (arrow). This cat was diagnosed with a pancreatic cyst.

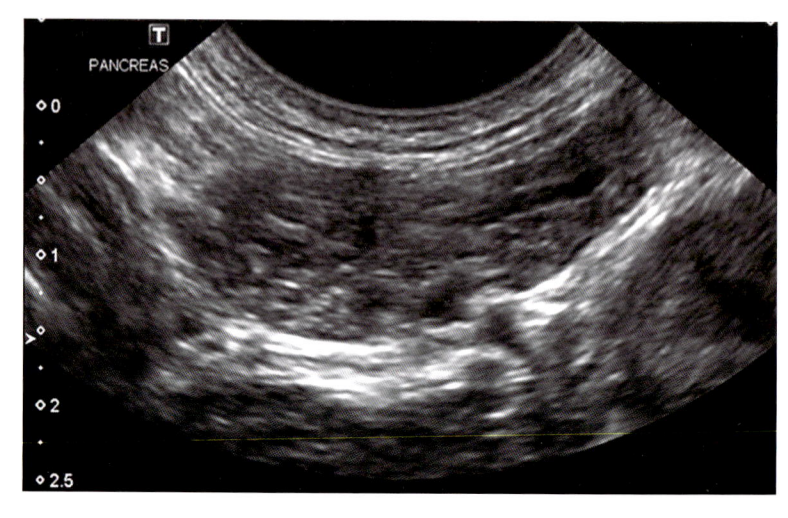

Fig. 32.14 A neutered male 19-year-old Domestic shorthair cat a history of chronic vomiting, diarrhea and lethargy. Ultrasound sagittal plane image of the left pancreas. The pancreas is thickened at 1.9 cm, has a mildly irregular shape and has a heterogenous echotexture with multiple small irregularly shaped hypoechoic nodules. The cat was diagnosed with chronic pancreatitis.

Pancreatic neoplasia

Pancreatic neoplasia is much less common than pancreatitis in both dogs and cats.[11] Neuroendocrine tumors are the most common pancreatic neoplasia, followed by adenocarcinoma and metastatic tumors. Differentiation of pancreatitis and pancreatic neoplasms with ultrasound is not always easy due to the overlapping nature of their appearance. Lymphadenomegaly can occur with either and surrounding tissues are often similarly altered.[11] Fine-needle aspiration or true-cut, laparoscopic, or surgical biopsy is often needed for conclusive differentiation. Involvement of multiple organs can occur in both severe suppurative pancreatitis or primary liver, pancreatic, or bile duct neoplasia.[11] Neoplasia of any one of these structures may invade adjacent organs and simulate inflammatory or granulomatous disease. In such cases, biopsy of both the liver and pancreas is warranted. Diffuse infiltrative disease of the pancreas, liver, and other organs such as the stomach, duodenum, spleen, and lymph nodes may be seen in suppurative, granulomatous, as well as neoplastic disorders. Depending on the size of a pancreatic nodule, the amount of gastrointestinal gas, and thoracic conformation of the patient, pancreatic neoplasms such as insulinomas and adenocarcinomas may be difficult to detect ultrasonographically. CT angiography may improve the diagnosis of insulinomas in dogs and a case report showed a distinctly enhanced mass in the arterial phase (**figs. 32.15- 32.17**).[12]

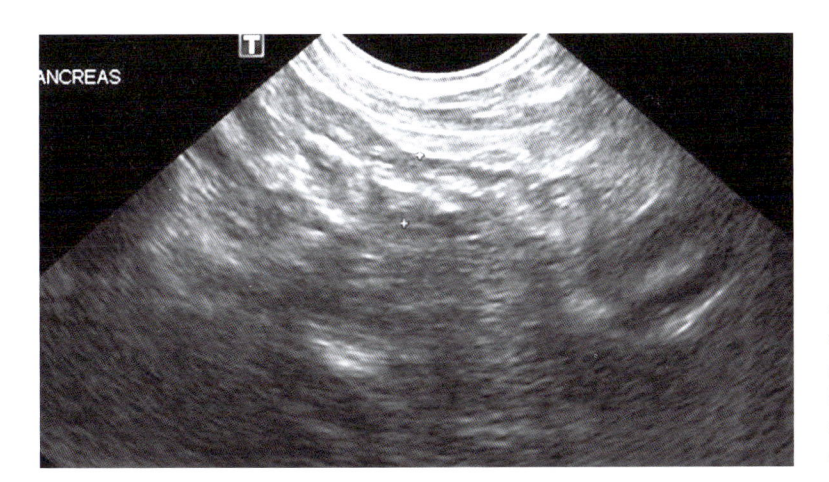

Fig. 32.15 A spayed female ten-year-old Boston Terrier with a previous history of pancreatitis and currently free of clinical signs. Ultrasound sagittal image of the right pancreas. The pancreas is not enlarged (8 mm thick), but is diffusely heterogenous with multifocal ill-defined hyperechoic regions and a mildly irregular shape. The dog was diagnosed with chronic pancreatitis.

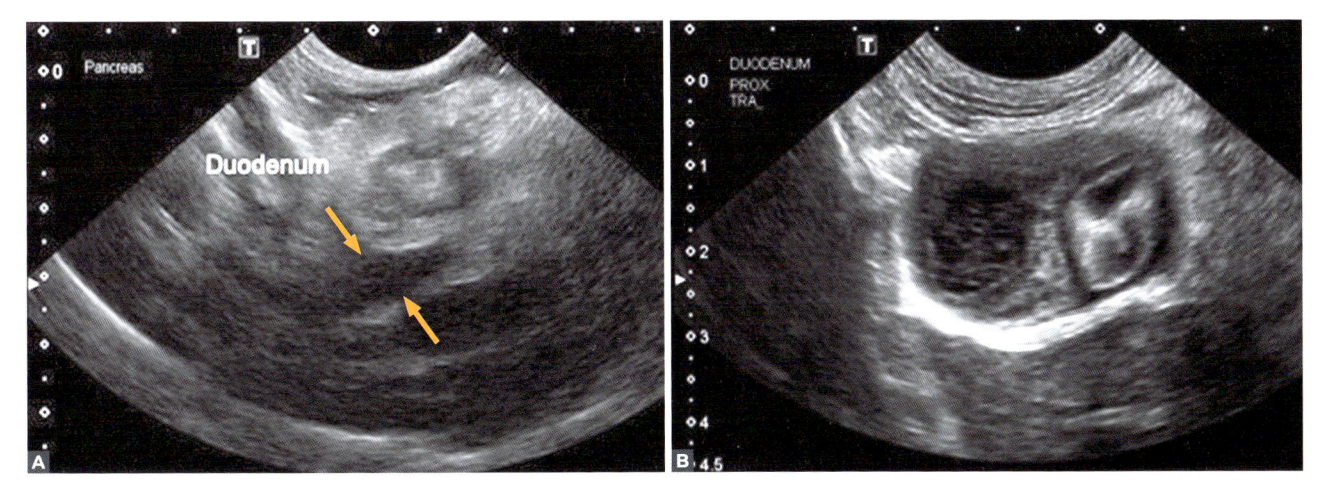

Fig. 32.16 A neutered male nine-year-old Dachshund with a one-week history of vomiting and inappetence. (**A**) Sagittal ultrasound image of the right pancreas where there is a focal, irregularly shaped and heterogenous mass present (between arrows). The pancreas is surrounded by hyperechoic mesentery. (**B**) Transverse image of the proximal duodenum and pancreatic body which is attached to the wall of the duodenum and has a central hypoechoic cavity. The dog had an exploratory laparotomy and the pancreas and mesentery were infiltrated such that resection was not possible. Histopathology diagnosed pancreatic carcinoma. This case illustrates the overlap in ultrasound features between acute pancreatitis, abscesses and pancreatic neoplasia and underscores the need for tissue sampling.

Fig. 32.17 A neutered male eight-year-old Beagle-mixed dog with a history of hypoglycemia and weakness. There is a well-marginated, hypoechoic 9.9 mm diameter nodule in the right pancreas diagnosed as an insulinoma. The duodenum is visible in the near field.

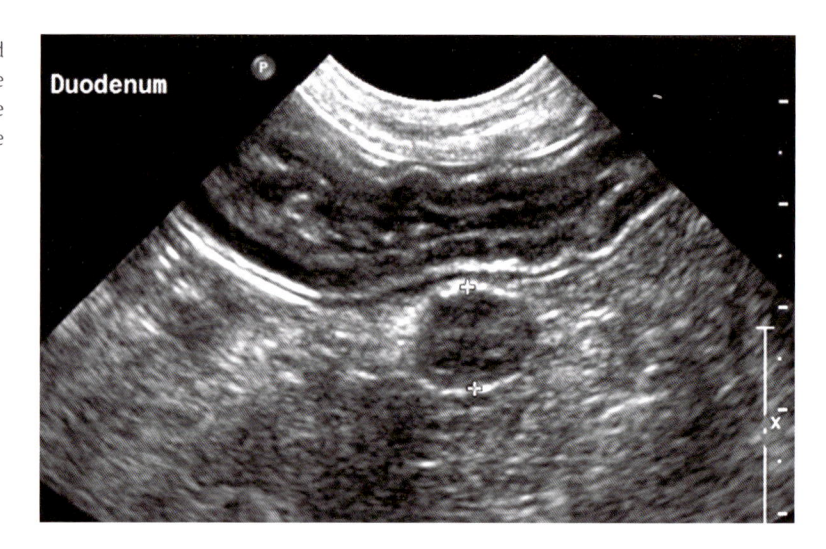

References

1. Etue SM, Penninck DG, Labato MA, Pearson S, Tidwell A. Ultrasonography of the normal feline pancreas and associated anatomic landmarks: a prospective study of 20 cats. *Vet Radiol Ultrasound* 42:330-336, 2001.
2. Penninck DG, Zeyen U, Taeymans ON, Webster CR. Ultrasonographic measurement of the pancreas and pancreatic duct in clinically normal dogs. *Am J Vet Res* 74: 433-437, 2013.
3. Larson M, Panciera DL, Ward DL, Steiner JM, Williams DA. Age-related changes in the ultrasound appearance of the normal feline pancreas. *Vet Radiol Ultrasound* 46: 238-242, 2005.
4. Caceres AV, Zwingenberger AL, Hardam E, Lucena JM, Schwarz T. Helical computed tomographic angiography of the normal canine pancreas. *Vet Radiol Ultrasound* 47:270-278, 2006.
5. Secrest S, Sharma A, Bugbee A. Triple phase computed tomography of the pancreas in healthy cats. *Vet Radiol Ultrasound* 59:163-168, 2018.
6. Newman SJ, Steiner JM, Woosley K, Williams DA, Barton L. Histologic assessment and grading of the exocrine pancreas in the dog. *J Vet Diagn Invest* 18:115-118, 2006.
7. De Cock HE, Forman MA, Farver TB, Marks SL. Prevalence and histopathologic characteristics of pancreatitis in cats. *Vet Pathol* 44:39-49, 2007.
8. Penninck DG. Gastrointestinal tract. In: Penninck DG, d'Anjou MA, editors. Atlas of small animal ultrasonography 2nd edition, Ames, Iowa, 2015, Blackwell Publishing, p 259.
9. French JM, Twedt DC, Rao S, Marolf AJ. Computed tomographic angiography and ultrasonography in the diagnosis and evaluation of acute pancreatitis in dogs. *J Vet Int Med* 33:79-88, 2019.
10. Park JY, Bugbee A, Sharma A, Secrest S. Feline pancreatic ducts are consistently identified on CT and more likely to be dilated in the body of pancreas in cats with elevated feline pancreatic lipase immunoreactivity. *Vet Radiol Ultrasound* 61:255-260, 2020.
11. Bennett PF, Hahn KA, Toal RL, et al. Ultrasonographic and cytopathological diagnosis of exocrine pancreatic carcinoma in the dog and cat. *J Am Anim Hosp Assoc* 37:466-473, 2001.
12. Iseri T, Yamada K, Chijiwa K, et al. Dynamic computed tomography of the pancreas in normal dogs and in a dog with pancreatic insulinoma. *Vet Radiol Ultrasound* 48:328-331, 2007.

CHAPTER 33

Spleen and lymph nodes

Margret S. Thompson

> **KEY POINTS**
>
> - The abdominal lymph nodes and the spleen are complex filtration organs and key components of the body's immune system.
> - Ultrasonography is the most used diagnostic imaging tool in the evaluation of the lymphatic system in the dog and cat, though other cross-sectional modalities (e.g., CT and MRI) provide similar information.
> - Patterns of abnormalities are useful for diagnostic and prognostic prioritization.
> - Familiarity with lymph node drainage patterns is necessary for providing diagnostic and prognostic information in abdominal pathology.
> - Lymph node or splenic size, homogeneity, and margination may help to separate benign from malignant causes, but cytologic and histologic confirmation is usually necessary given the overlap of findings.

Providing complex filtration of body fluids and immune function, the abdominal lymph nodes, and the spleen should be routinely and completely evaluated in relation to other system pathology in small animal abdominal imaging studies.

Lymph nodes

Challenging to identify because of their small size and deep locations, the abdominal lymph nodes require anatomical knowledge of vascular landmarks for localization. Lymphatic drainage patterns must be known to determine the significance of abnormalities. Lymphadenopathy is often marked before being detected on radiographs in cats and dogs. On cross-sectional imaging modalities like ultrasound, CT and MRI, lesions with similar can represent local, regional or systemic disease, and the extent of nodal involvement is important, but size and shape vary with age, species and lymph center. Relatively larger lymph nodes like the jejunal and medial iliac nodes are routinely included in complete abdominal ultrasound scanning protocols. Smaller nodes, like hepatic and renal nodes, are more oval and smaller, and often not identified.[1-3] Identifying abdominal lymph nodes using vascular landmarks can often help with the diagnosis and determination of lesion significance in adjacent organs.

Canine and feline abdominal lymph nodes can be divided into lymph centers of the abdominal and pelvic walls (parietal) including lumbar, iliosacral, and iliofemoral lymph centers and visceral abdominal lymph node subgroups associated with specific organs. The celiac lymph center includes those nodes associated with organs supplied by the celiac artery, including the hepatic, splenic, gastric and pancreaticoduodenal lymph nodes.[4] Often called portal nodes, hepatic nodes lie beside the portal vein just caudal to the hilus of the liver. These nodes drain the liver, stomach, duodenum and pancreas. Gastric lymph nodes, if abnormal, can often be seen in dogs and cats. These lymph nodes are variable in number and lie near the lesser curvature of the stomach draining the esophagus, stomach, diaphragm, and lesser omentum with drainage to the hepatic or splenic lymph nodes. Smaller nodes in the celiac group, including the splenic and pancreaticoduodenal, are less commonly seen if normal.[1-4]

The cranial mesenteric lymph center consists of the jejunal nodes and colic nodes, which should be evaluated as part of a systematic abdominal ultrasound or CT scan. The jejunal lymph nodes, commonly called mesenteric nodes, are the largest lymph nodes of the abdomen and are most often paired along the vascular trunk of the mesentery. Placing a probe slightly to the right of the umbilicus will commonly localize jejunal lymph nodes in the mid-abdomen of most dogs and cats. More commonly multiple than other lymph centers, one to five lymph nodes may be seen on the right and/or left of the mesenteric vasculature, draining the jejunum, ileum, and pancreas. These lymph nodes are normally elongated, measuring up to 0.5 cm thick and up to 3 to 4 cm long in dogs.[1-3] In cats, these nodes are similar in appearance with normal thickness up to 0.3 cm.[1-3] The jejunal lymph nodes are usually reactive and larger in young dogs and cats up to 1 year of age.[4-6] The colic lymph nodes are located in the mesocolon, draining the ileum, cecum and colon, and are often grouped into the mesenteric node evaluation.[4]

The medial iliac lymph nodes are part of the iliosacral lymph center and are routinely evaluated as part of an abdominal ultrasound examination, particularly in the dog. Draining the most caudal aspect of the body, the medial iliac lymph nodes are single, large nodes located lateral to the great vessels just cranial to the origin of the iliac vessels. Placing a probe transversely on the great vessels and tracing caudally to the trifurcation is an easily learned method for localizing and measuring medial iliac lymph nodes (**fig. 33.1**). In many dogs, identification of the lymph nodes is easier using a lateral imaging approach. Size, shape, margination, and echogenicity should be evaluated. Canine medial iliac lymph nodes are typically fusiform to oval in shape and isoechoic to slightly hypoechoic relative to the surrounding fat. Short-axis (transverse) measurements up to 5 mm in thickness and long-axis (sagittal) 2-4 cm in length have been reported in normal adult dogs. In cats, the medial iliac lymph nodes are less commonly identified when normal and enlargement is less common than in dogs. The imaging approach is the same as employed for canine patients. These lymph nodes are often accessible for sampling, which is helpful to obtain a diagnosis and determine local spread from pathology originating in the caudal abdomen, pelvic canal and perineum.[1-3, 8-9]

The large drainage area of these nodes includes the skin of the dorsal abdominal wall caudal to the last rib, the skin of the pelvic region, the tail root, the craniolateral aspect of the thigh and stifle, abdominal muscles, muscles and bones of the pelvic limb, pelvic and lumbar muscles, colon, rectum, anus, vagina, vulva, testis, prostate, ureter, bladder, urethra, aorta, spinal cord meninges with efferent vessels from deep, superficial inguinal, left colic, sacral and internal iliac lymph nodes. The internal iliac lymph nodes, formerly known as the hypogastric lymph nodes, are small, paired nodes located between the internal iliac and median sacral artery.[4] The sacral lymph nodes are not always differentiated from the internal iliac lymph nodes but lie along the dorsal musculature of the pelvic canal. These nodes are not easily imaged by abdominal ultrasound but can be clinically important in urogenital and pelvic neoplasia. Enlargement is more easily identified on CT or MRI examination.[8]

Three abdominal and pelvic parietal lymph centers are present. Up to 17 parietal nodes along the aorta and caudal vena cava drain the lumbar vertebrae, last ribs, abdominal body wall and lumbar musculature, aorta, spinal cord, meninges, parietal pleura and peritoneum, diaphragm, kidneys, adrenal glands, ovaries, testicles, and axillary/inguinal lymph nodes. Limited literature is available describing normal and abnormal imaging of these nodes, but these are rarely visible on ultrasound if normal.[4] The superficial inguinal lymph nodes are normally small and deep in the inguinal fat. If abnormal, these nodes should be sampled in patients with mammary or pelvic limb neoplasia.

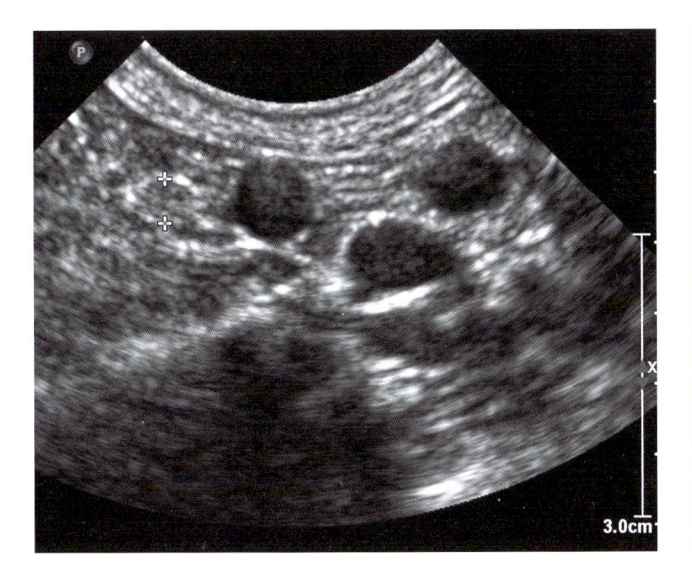

Fig. 33.1 Normal right medial iliac lymph node in a large breed dog. The use of anatomic landmarks, particularly the trifurcation of the aorta scanned in a transverse plane, are useful for localization of these lymph nodes.

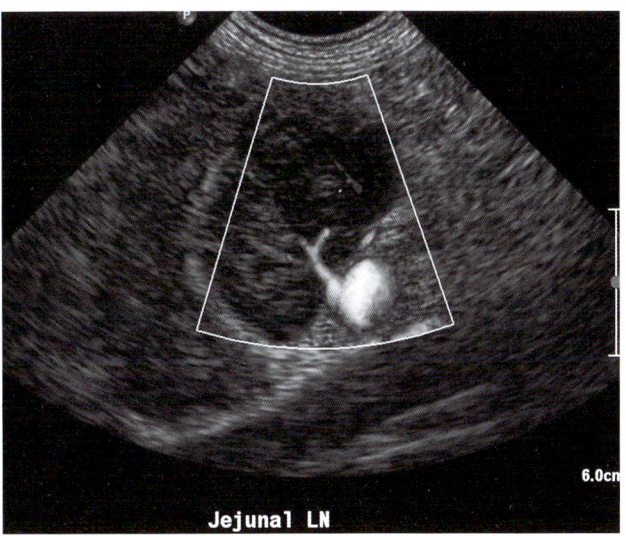

Fig. 33.2 Hilar blood flow in an enlarged, hypoechoic, round abdominal lymph node. Intranodal vascular patterns (hilar flow = benign, absence of hilar flow = more likely malignant) have not been identified as useful in dogs or cats, compared to human cancer patients where particularly in superficial lymph nodes this distinction is useful.[10]

On routine abdominal ultrasound scans, a systematic approach should include evaluation of the region of all described lymph centers and definitive measurement of jejunal and medial iliac lymph nodes. Diseased lymph nodes enlarge, become more hypoechoic and rounded (**fig. 33.2**). Late in disease, variable echogenicity and irregular margins can be noted.[9]

Lymphatic drainage in normal dogs and cats is generally well described, but limited descriptions of draining node patterns in diseased and neoplastic processes, reportedly altered due to neovascularization in people, are available.[10]

Diseases of lymph nodes fall into three primary categories with similarly abnormal nodal characteristics:

- Multifocal or generalized lymphadenopathy.
- Focal lymphadenopathy with local disease (sentinel node).
- Focal or center lymphadenopathy is useful in prognostication.

Abnormal lymph nodes are typically enlarged, hypoechoic with surrounding focal effusion or hyperechoic fat. Degree, distribution, and adjacent pathology determine significance.

Multifocal or generalized lymphadenopathy

Common in dogs, uncommon in cats, round cell, systemic neoplasia may present as multifocal enlarged and hypoechoic lymph nodes with or without organ pathology (**fig. 33.3**). Lymphoma, histiocytic and mast cell appear similarly on cross-sectional imaging. Regionally, systemic infections like *Pythium* and fungal diseases can have a similar cross-sectional appearance. Fine-needle aspiration for cytologic diagnosis is routine.[1-3]

Focal lymphadenopathy with local disease (sentinel node)

Features of metastasis to lymph nodes such as spread to the medial iliac lymph nodes from an anal sac carcinoma include enlargement, rounding, and hypoechogenicity.[1-3,8,10] In addition, focal effusion or hyperechoic fat may surround the abnormal lymph node in dogs.[11] Untreated systemic neoplasia like lymphoma causes greater nodal enlargement and shape change than metastasis in general. Specific evaluation and sampling of lymph nodes draining suspected or known neoplasms is recommended.[1-3]

Table 33.1 Abdominal organ, draining lymph node to be evaluated if significant pathology (e.g., neoplasia) identified and whether this lymph node can commonly be identified with abdominal ultrasound or CT should be considered.[4]

Organ	Draining lymph node	Ease of identification	Prompt pathology evaluation
Liver	Hepatic	Seen with specific effort/disease	Hepatic mass
Gallbladder	Hepatic	Seen with specific effort/disease	Luminal mass
Esophagus	Lumbar aortic	Not normally seen	
Diaphragm	Lumbar aortic, splenic	Not normally seen	
Stomach	Gastric, hepatic, splenic	Seen with specific effort/disease	Gastric mass
Duodenum	Hepatic, splenic, pancreaticoduodenal	Seen with specific effort/disease	Differentiation of inflammatory versus neoplastic processes
Pancreas	Hepatic, splenic, pancreaticoduodenal	Seen with specific effort/disease	Differentiation of inflammatory versus neoplastic processes
Peritoneum/omentum	Splenic, pancreaticoduodenal, sternal	Seen with specific effort/disease	CT may be needed
Spleen	Splenic	Not normally seen	Not commonly used to prognosticate
Adrenal glands	Lumbar aortic	Not normally seen	Vascular invasion of mass is a better prognostic tool
Kidney	Renal	Seen with disease	Not commonly used to prognosticate
Jejunum, ileum, cecum, colon	Jejunal, colic	Part of complete abdominal scan	Differentiation of inflammatory versus neoplastic processes
Rectum	Colic, medial iliac	Part of complete abdominal scan	Differentiation of inflammatory versus neoplastic processes
Anus/anal sac	Medial iliac	Part of complete abdominal scan	Differentiation of inflammatory versus neoplastic processes (may have sacral and internal iliac involvement that is not easily detected on ultrasound)
Ovaries	Lumbar aortic	Seen with disease	CT may be needed
Vagina/vulva	Medial iliac	Part of complete abdominal scan	
Scrotum, prepuce, penis	Superficial inguinal	Seen with disease	
Testis/epididymis	Lumbar aortic	Seen with disease	
Prostate	Medial and internal iliac	Part of complete abdominal scan	Differentiation of inflammatory versus neoplastic processes (may have internal iliac involvement that is not easily detected on ultrasound)
Ureter	Medial iliac	Part of complete abdominal scan	
Urinary bladder	Lumbar and internal iliac	Seen with specific effort/disease	CT may be needed
Urethra	Internal iliac	Seen with specific effort/disease	CT may be needed
Thoracic mammary gland	Axillary	Seen with specific effort/disease	Benign versus neoplastic processes and recurrence
Abdominal mammary gland	Axillary and inguinofemoral	Seen with disease	Benign versus neoplastic processes and recurrence
Inguinal mammary gland	Inguinofemoral and popliteal	Seen with disease	
Lumbar vertebrae	Lumbar aortic	Seen with specific effort/disease	CT may be needed
Pelvic limbs/tail			

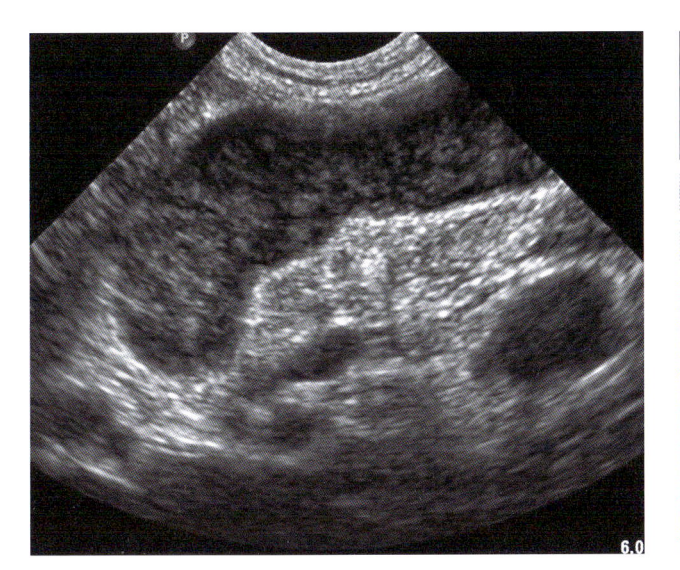

Fig. 33.3 Jejunal lymphadenopathy can be seen in systemic diseases like lymphoma or local disease, like gastrointestinal lymphoma.

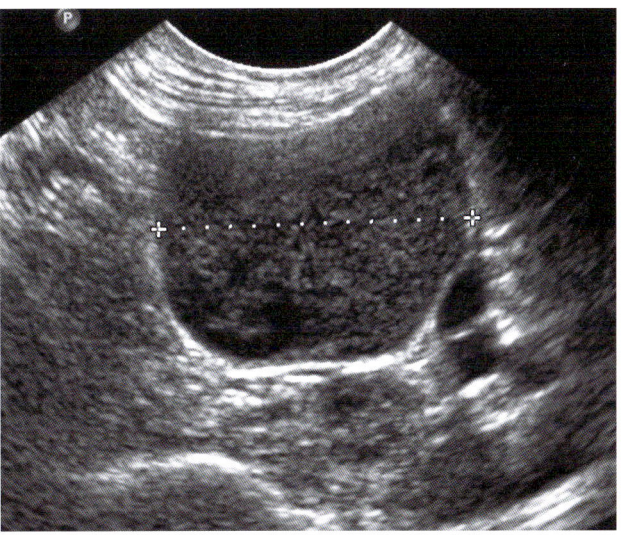

Fig. 33.4 Moderately enlarged, hypoechoic right medial iliac lymph node in a middle-aged Golden Retriever with systemic lymphoma. The use of anatomic landmarks, particularly the trifurcation of the caudal vena cava and aorta scanned in a transverse plane, are useful for the localization of these lymph nodes.

Focal or center lymphadenopathy useful in prognostication

Degree of regional lymphatic abnormality can be helpful in ranking disease. In cats, prioritization of gastrointestinal lymphoma versus inflammatory bowel disease pre-endoscopic sampling or empiric treatment is routine. Similar enlargement, hypoechogenicity, and perinodal hyperechoic fat can be seen in these lymph nodes with both processes. Degree of nodal abnormality, along with signalment and presenting signs be used to rank differentials (**fig. 33.4**). Fine-needle aspiration can sometimes be helpful in confirming gastrointestinal lymphoma versus other inflammatory intestinal pathologies in the cranial mesenteric lymph center, but ultimately biopsy may be needed to obtain a confirmed diagnosis.[1-3]

Spleen

The spleen is the largest secondary lymphatic organ, and has limited, overlapping abnormal imaging appearances with many local or systemic causes. The spleen is located in the left cranial abdomen, approximately parallel to the greater curvature of the stomach, and is elongated tongue-shaped in the normal cat and dog. The position may vary with gastric filling and the spleen may be entirely subcostal if the stomach is empty, especially in deep-chested dogs. The dorsal extremity is relatively fixed in the left dorsal abdomen and requires specific attention during ultrasound evaluation. The dorsal extremity is usually visible as a triangular soft tissue opacity structure in the left cranial abdominal quadrant in both dogs and cats. It is interposed between the body wall, gastric body, left kidney and colon. The tail of the spleen is quite mobile and may be located in the ventral abdomen extending to right of the midline, oriented obliquely across the abdomen, or lie parallel to the inner margin of the left body wall. The tail of the spleen is almost always seen on lateral abdominal radiographs in the dog but is far less commonly identified in the cat. If the spleen is visible on lateral radiographs of a feline patient, this may indicate enlargement and warrants investigation.[1-3] On ultrasound, splenomegaly in dogs is generally recognized as a splenic thickness greater than 3 cm and in cats greater than 1 cm.[1-3]

Blood enters the spleen through the splenic artery, a branch of the celiac artery, which can be identified on ultrasound and contrast-enhanced CT. This supply divides into many branches (up to 25 reported) along the long hilus that course through the capsule dividing into smaller vessels that become surrounded by lymphoid tissue. Similar segmentation exists in the venous system, ending into the gastrosplenic vein at the hilus. The spleen stores red blood cells and removes them from circulation, has an important immune function as a site of lymphocyte and monocyte production, and is responsible for blood platelet formation from megakaryocytes.[4] On imaging studies, the spleen is typically homogenous in appearance, with smooth margins and functional divisions are not identifiable (**fig. 33.5**). These functions can be assumed by other organs if the spleen is removed.[4] Accessory spleens are rare and, in the author's experience lymph nodes are often mistaken for "daughter spleens". Like lymph nodes, changes in size, shape, echogenicity, and texture of the spleen may be a normal response or represent disease. As with most organs, a normal imaging study of the spleen does not equate with absence of pathology.[1-3] Diseases of the spleen fall into seven common categories in dogs and cats:

- Single or few nodules.
- Focal, multifocal infarction or splenic torsion.
- Masses.
- Diffuse micronodular disease.
- Inhomogeneous parenchymal change.
- Normal appearance with increased size.
- Hyperechoic splenic nodules.

Hyperechoic splenic nodules are almost always benign fatty lesions (myelolipomas) or mineralization. Myelolipomas are small, benign, round-to-irregularly shaped, hyperechoic foci of varying sizes (**fig. 33.6**). Typically found at the hilus centered on veins, they are very commonly seen in dogs and less commonly in cats.[13] Dystrophic parenchymal mineralization of varying patterns and distribution can also sometimes be identified as hyperechoic speckles and thin lines throughout the spleen, often thought to be associated with chronic endocrinopathies.[1-3]

Few, small hypoechoic nodules

Hypoechoic splenic nodules, less than one centimeter in diameter, often represent benign processes if another pathology is not identified during the patient's workup (**fig. 33.7**). If unchanged on se-

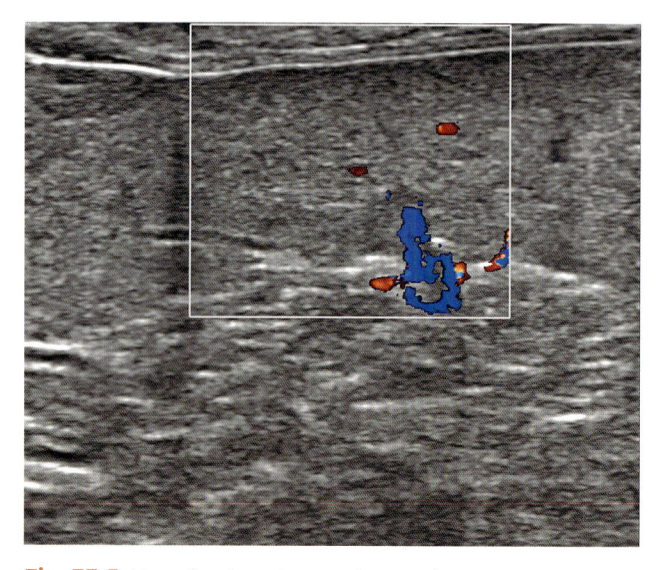

Fig. 33.5 Normal canine spleen on ultrasound.

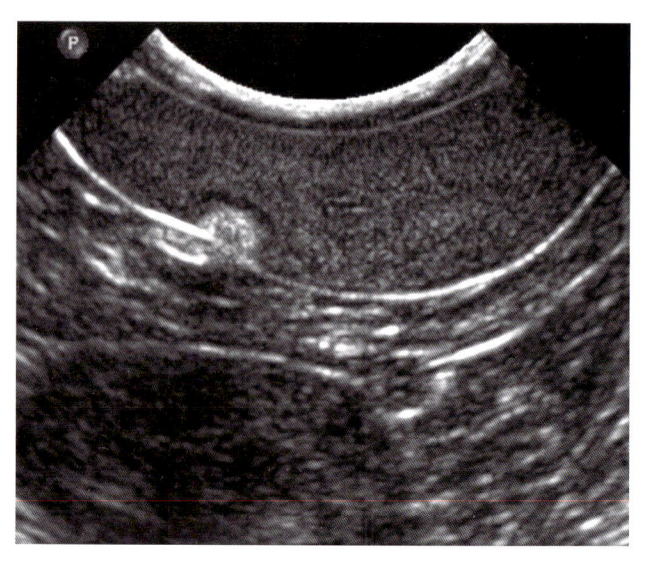

Fig. 33.6 Benign myelolipoma: a small, hyperechoic subcapsular nodule in a normal canine spleen, centered on peripheral, hilar vessels.

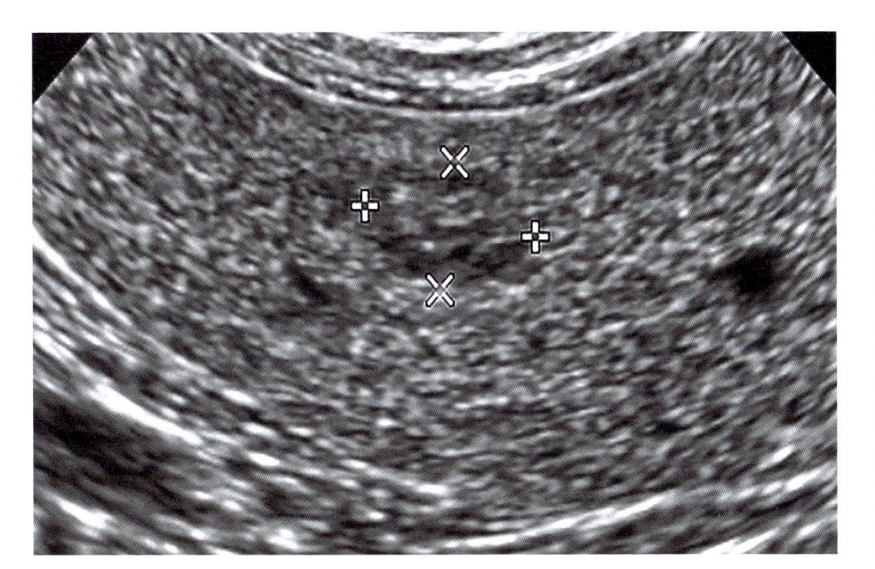

Fig. 33.7 Benign nodular hyperplasia in an older Cocker Spaniel found incidentally during evaluation of urinary tract signs without evidence of neoplastic process. These small, hypoechoic, well-defined nodules (less than 1 cm in diameter) in dogs, in otherwise normal spleens will maintain a similar size on sequential examinations.

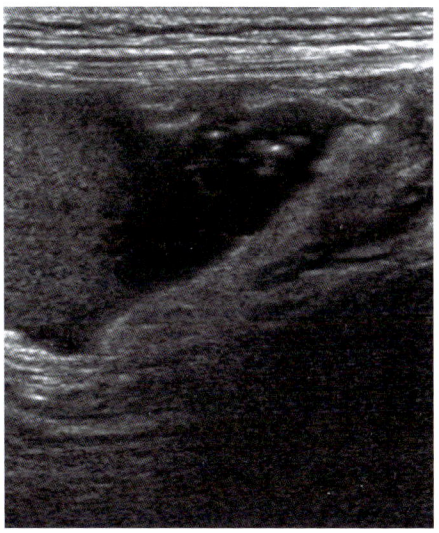

Fig. 33.8 Wedge-shaped, peripheral hypoechoic infarct in a canine spleen. The few hyperechoic foci may represent intra-parenchymal gas. The trace adjacent fluid, hyperechoic mesentery and possible intra-lesional gas (e.g., hyperechoic foci with distal reverberation) should prompt consideration of infectious splenitis or necrosis.[1-3]

quential exams, extramedullary hematopoiesis or lymphoid hyperplasia is most likely in dogs.[1-3] Often identified incidentally on abdominal CT examinations as well, contrast enhancement patterns can further help provide prioritized diagnoses as highly contrast-enhancing nodules (greater than 90 HU) are more likely benign, nodular hyperplasia.[14]

Vascular compromise

Focal splenic infarction occurs secondary to embolism or thrombosis within the arterial system of the spleen moderately common in the dog. Neoplasia, septic processes, hypercoagulable conditions of varied etiology, and thrombosis associated with cardiovascular disease are reported as underlying diseases. Most commonly wedge-shaped at the periphery on cross-sectional imaging, focal infarcts in the spleen vary in appearance, with a degree of infarction and age impacting appearance with poorly marginated, hypoechoic, or complex abnormalities indistinguishable from other focal splenic lesions (**fig. 33.8**). Infarcts and clots within vessels within vary in appearance varying depending on age, initially iso- to hypoechoic becoming progressively hyperechoic over days. As revascularization occurs, local fibrosis may shrink and distort the shape of the spleen.[1-3] Color doppler sampling with detection of venous flow and normal vessels is required to rule out vascular compromise. Fully evaluating the patient for systemic disease when splenic infarcts are identified is key, as these vascular lesions are often secondary.

Whole organ vascular compromise/splenic torsion

Splenic torsion is mostly seen in large breed dogs. Some patients present with acute severe signs including anorexia, lethargy, weakness, and abdominal pain. Patients may also present with similar less severe chronic signs. Splenic torsion can also occur in conjunction with gastric dilatation and volvulus. Splenic torsion can be difficult to diagnose on radiographs with potential changes including diffuse enlargement, sometimes with an abnormal C-shape. Some patients have peritoneal fluid and a mid-abdominal mass effect with caudal and rightward displacement of the intestine suggesting a splenic origin. These changes should prompt a sonographic study. On ultrasound, splenic torsion

SECTION V ABDOMEN

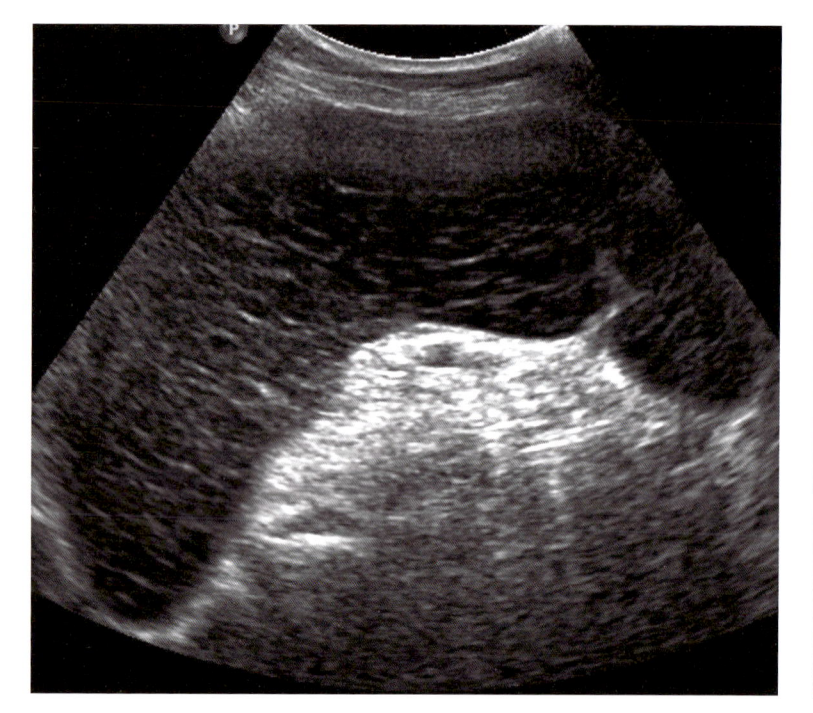

Fig. 33.9 Chronic splenic torsion in an adult female Belgian Malinois with abdominal pain. The spleen is enlarged, rounded, severely hypoechoic with "lacey" echotexture. Doppler interrogation did not identify normal blood flow.

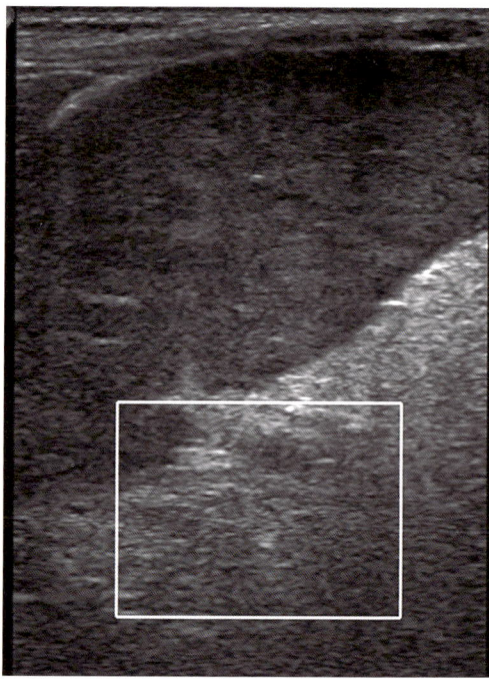

Fig. 33.10 The characteristic triangular hyperechoic hilar lesion reported as a sign for splenic torsions is demonstrated in this presumptively less chronic torsion with more mottled echogenicity.[13]

is characterized by moderate to severe diffuse enlargement of the spleen, rounding of margins with varied echogenicity change from mottled to lacey to severely hypoechoic (**fig. 33.9**). The sonographic appearance of the parenchyma may change within hours or days in patients with an acute presentation. A hyperechoic hilar "triangle" has also been described as suggestive of torsion (**fig. 33.10**). Most vessels in the spleen are not visible on ultrasound but using color-flow Doppler, both arterial and venous flow can be seen in splenic parenchyma. Blood flow in the hilar veins is often visible without color Doppler when normal, but this is needed to show flow in the hilar arteries. In patients with torsion, echogenic thrombi may be seen in larger splenic veins, or color Doppler can confirm lack of flow in the hilar veins and smaller parenchymal veins. Color Doppler interrogation of the splenic parenchyma confirms the absence of flow in smaller vessels. Arterial flow may be partly preserved, depending upon the degree of torsion and chronicity.

Many variably sized nodules or small masses

When many nodules or irregularly shaped margin distorting nodules or masses are detected on ultrasound or CT cross-sectional imaging of the spleen, fine-needle sampling for cytology should be performed as systemic neoplastic processes such as round cell tumors and metastasis are more likely than benign processes (**fig. 33.11**).[3]

Large single mass with peritoneal fluid

Splenic masses are common in canine patients with etiologies including lymphoid hyperplasia, hematoma, and neoplasia such as hemangiosarcoma, histiocytic sarcoma, and lymphoma. The sonographic appearance is variable with significant overlap and cannot be used to make a diagnosis. Some lesions have uniform echogenicity but more often masses have a disorganized heterogeneous appearance, from necrosis and intralesional hemorrhage. When identified in conjunction with hemorrhagic peritoneal fluid, splenic masses are more likely to be malignant neoplasms, but peritoneal hemorrhage can occur with benign lesions. Doppler blood flow pattern, contrast enhancement on ultrasound, contrast enhancement on CT and sonographic features have not proven useful in determining the likelihood of malignant splenic neoplasia (e.g., hemangiosarcoma) versus benign hematoma (**figs. 33.12** and **33.13**). Clinically, the presence of easily detected abdominal hemorrhage with a splenic mass is the most common presentation of primary malignant splenic neoplasia, though also seen in benign hematomas. A limited sonographic examination can be used for confirmation of a splenic mass and fluid sampling. Approximately ⅔ of splenic masses are neoplastic; ⅔ of splenic masses with peritoneal hemorrhage are hemangiosarcomas.[1-3] Splenectomy and histopathology are required to obtain a confirmed diagnosis.

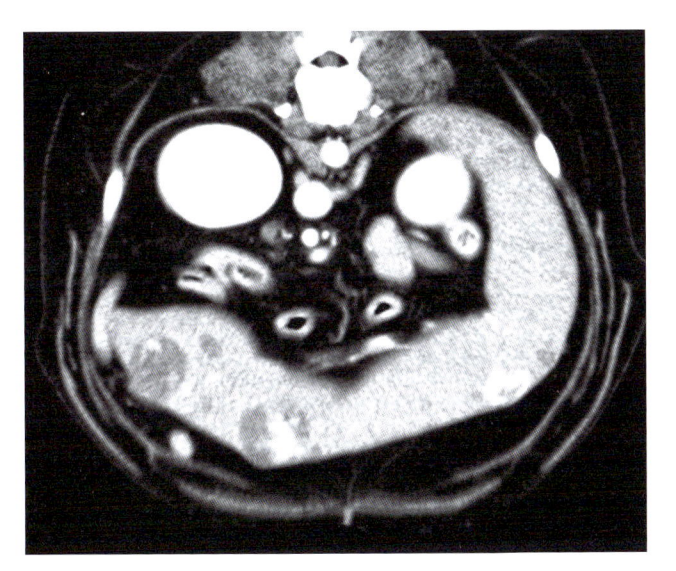

Fig. 33.11 Transverse, post-contrast CT of the mid-abdomen of an adult Flat Coated Retriever with lethargy. Multiple mixed density, variably contrast-enhancing small splenic masses (as well as hepatic masses) were seen. FNA and cytology found malignant histiocytosis.

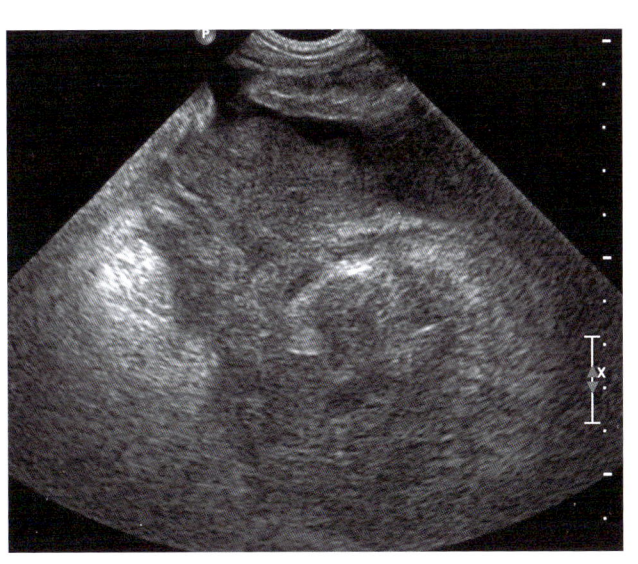

Fig. 33.12 Hemangiosarcoma of the spleen in an adult German Shepherd dog. Limited abdominal ultrasound is often used for diagnosis of hemoabdomen from rupture of a splenic mass in emergency practice.

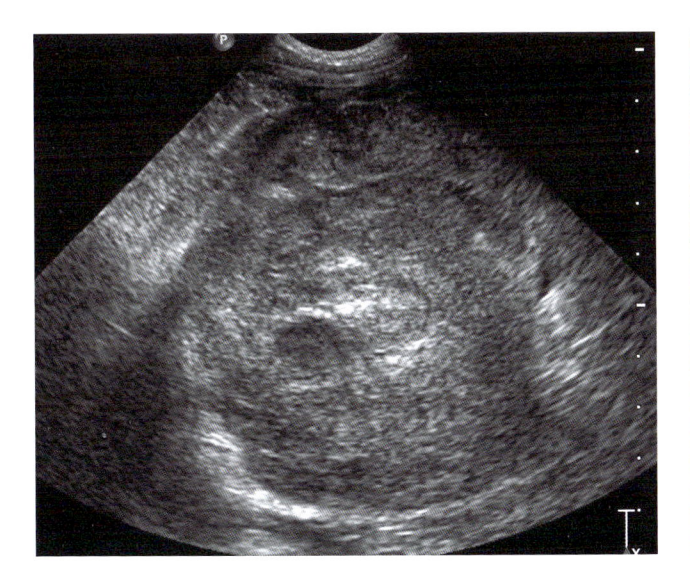

Fig. 33.13 Multiple probe placements/orientations are often needed to confirm peritoneal fluid. It is often easier to scan any visible normal spleen to demonstrate attachment to the mass than vice versa. Additional image of the same dog as in fig. 33.12.

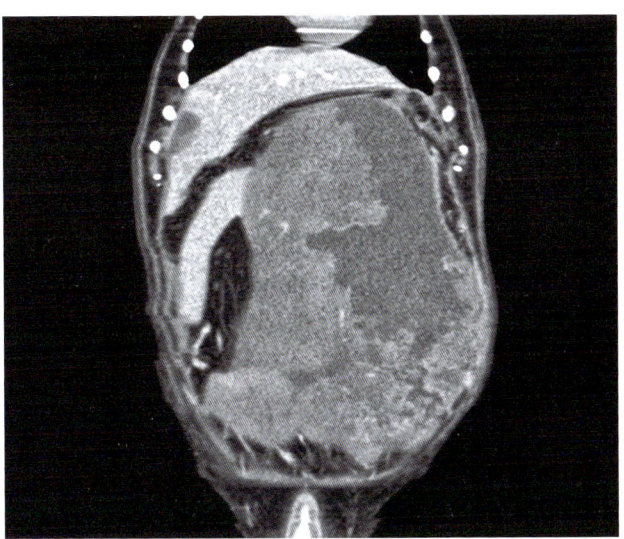

Fig. 33.14 Dorsal plane CT post-contrast in an old neutered male Beagle. The very large, inhomogeneously contrast-enhancing splenic mass was diagnosed as a benign neoplasm. CT is often necessary to identify the organ of origin, as splenic versus hepatic origin can be difficult to determine on abdominal ultrasound. Abdomen filling splenic masses in dogs, without peritoneal hemorrhage, are more likely to be less aggressive disease.[15]

Large single mass without or minimal volume peritoneal fluid

Abdomen-filling splenic masses, so large that determining the organ of origin is sometimes difficult or impossible, have been reported to be more commonly non-neoplastic masses or benign or less aggressive neoplasms in dogs (**fig. 33.14**).[15] Non-cavitated, larger masses (>2 cm in diameter) may be aspirated for cytologic evaluation with accurate diagnosis; however, as with cavitated, large mass lesions, this step is sometimes not performed, as neoplastic disease is more accurately diagnosed with splenectomy and histopathologic diagnosis.[15]

Diffuse micronodular parenchymal change

Diffuse micronodular change in the spleen of dogs and cats is seen frequently and is more likely to be visible when using high-frequency linear transducers (e.g., 10-18 MHz) versus micro-convex transducer use (e.g., 5-8 MHz).[16] Benign and malignant causes are equally common, and splenic size must be evaluated in addition to echotexture. In young dogs and cats, benign extramedullary hematopoiesis is characterized by a normal size spleen with diffuse, poorly defined, tiny hypoechoic nodules (**fig. 33.15**).[1-3]

If splenic enlargement (increased thickness and/or rounding of margins) is present with a diffuse micronodular echotexture, other differentials such as infiltrative round cell neoplasia are more likely, most often lymphoma (**fig. 33. 16**).[1-3]

Inhomogeneous parenchymal change with enlargement

Diffuse, inhomogeneous, or patchy changes in the spleen of a dog or cat should be further investigated. Vascular compromise and malignant neoplasia such as hemangiosarcoma and round cell tumors are possible differential diagnoses (**fig. 33.17**).

Inhomogeneous parenchymal change with normal size

Inhomogeneous echogenicity or patchy-to-nodular contrast enhancement on CT similar to diffuse micronodular change can be normal or extramedullary hematopoiesis in normal-sized organs. Sedation and blood pressure may play a role, causing splenic enlargement in dogs.[1-3,17] A non-specific finding, FNA with cytology should be considered if clinical signs or concurrent disease warrant further characterization versus sequential recheck.

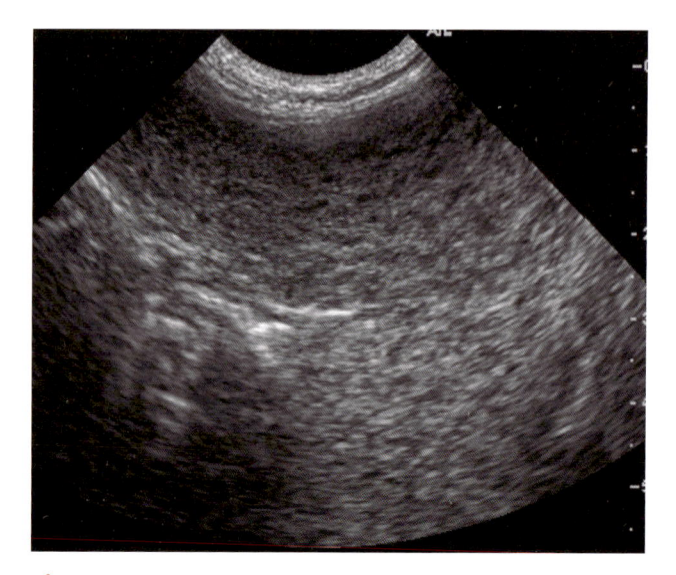

Fig. 33.15 Normal size spleen in a ten-month-old, large mixed breed dog. Extramedullary hematopoiesis was diagnosed on fine-needle aspiration and cytology.

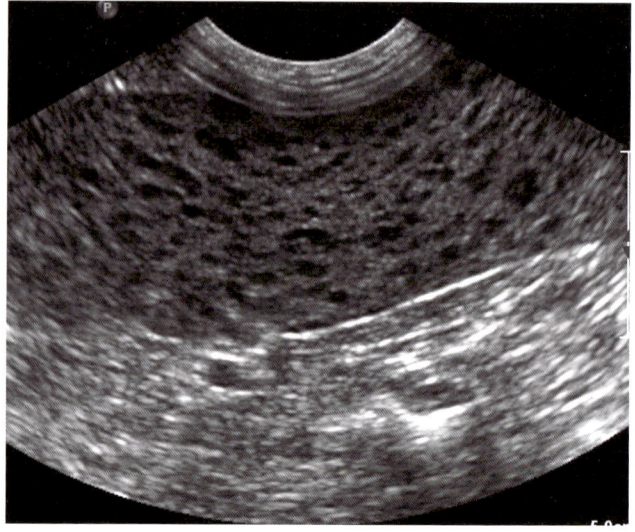

Fig. 33.16 Enlarged, rounded, micro-nodular spleen in a ten-year-old neutered male Golden Retriever. Lymphoma was diagnosed on fine-needle aspiration of the spleen and enlarged peripheral lymph nodes.

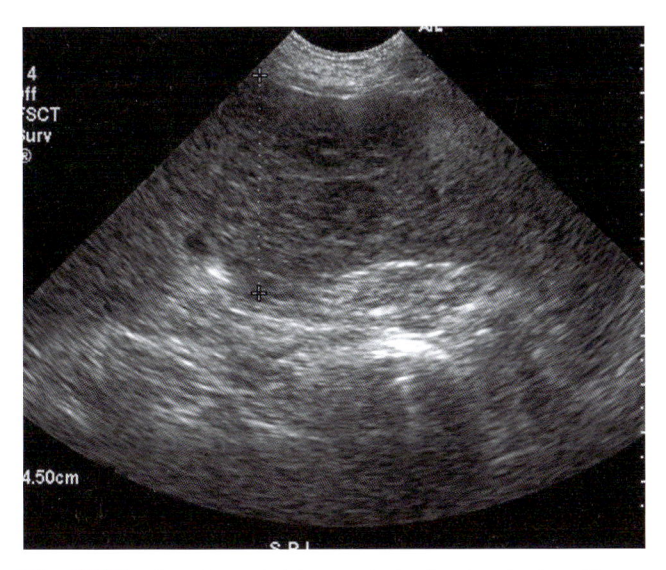

Fig. 33.17 Enlarged, rounded, heteroechoic spleen in a dog (roughly normal thickness is 3 cm); lymphoma was diagnosed on fine-needle aspiration.

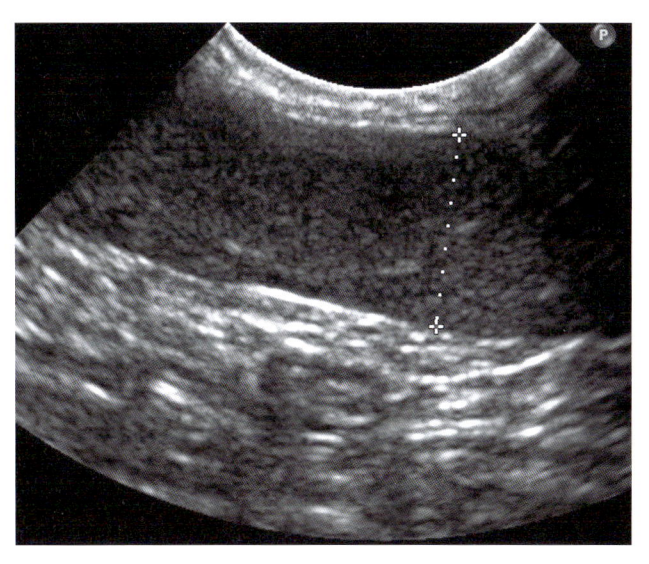

Fig. 33.18 An enlarged (3 cm thickness), rounded, spleen with normal echogenicity in a cat (roughly normal thickness is 1 cm), lymphoma was diagnosed on fine-needle aspiration.[1-3]

Normal appearance with increased size

Splenic size is quite variable in normal dogs and this diagnosis should be made with care. Young, active dogs, especially working breeds, often have a larger spleen than sedentary, older patients. Splenomegaly in dogs is generally recognized as a splenic thickness greater than 3 cm and in cats greater than 1 cm.[1-3] Rounded margins are a somewhat more reliable indicator of enlargement than size. Causes include pharmacological, congestion, immune stimulation/infection, and infiltrative neoplasia. Generalized feline splenomegaly may be neoplastic or infectious, with lymphoma, infectious splenitis (e.g., *Cytauxzoon* infection), and mast cell neoplasia more common diagnoses (**fig. 33.18**).[1-3] Generalized splenomegaly in the dog with otherwise normal findings is more commonly benign, or the result of overzealous interpretation.[1-3] Sedative and anesthetic administration have been shown to cause splenic enlargement in dogs, with a normal appearance on ultrasound and CT. Acepromazine, detomidine, dexmedotomidine, propofol, barbiturates, and alfaxalone have been reported to cause this change. This does not seem to occur in feline patients. Smooth muscle relaxation of the splenic capsule and vascular pooling resulting in increased volume are suspected in this drug-induced change seen in dogs.[17-18]

Conclusions

▌ Learning to identify and evaluate lymph nodes is clinically useful especially in oncology patients but requires practice and systematic scanning.
▌ Review lymphatic drainage of primary lesion using anatomy reference.
▌ Use vascular landmarks to identify lymph nodes, and examination of the lymph system and additionally as a prompt to assess vessels.
▌ Measure thickness and compare to published normal (over 0.3 cm in cats and 0.7 cm in dogs may be abnormal).
▌ Evaluate shape, remembering that some nodes are longer (jejunal) or rounder (hepatic) normally. Irregular margins are abnormal but uncommon; rounding is abnormal and common in pathology.
▌ Evaluate echogenicity: mottling or decreased echogenicity relative to adjacent fat is abnormal.
▌ Perform sampling if feasible and safe.

During ultrasound evaluation of the spleen, a systematic approach can be used to construct and prioritize differentials.

During a complete, routine examination of the abdomen, slide off the left lateral liver to identify the spleen lateral to the left kidney. Use a grid pattern to fully evaluate, including specifically scanning dorsally to evaluate the head of the spleen.

- If possible, compare echogenicity to the left lateral liver, with the spleen normally more echogenic than the liver.
- Look at splenic margins; they should be sharp and pointed. If rounded, enlargement is likely.
- Measure thickness at mid-body. Cats are normally less than 1 cm thick and big dogs, less than 3 cm. If thick, reassess margins and echogenicity/echotexture.
- Look at overall echogenicity in enlarged spleens; if very hypoechoic, vascular interrogation should be performed to rule out splenic torsion in dogs.
- Look for focal echogenicity changes: characterizing nodules, masses, and wedge-shaped (e.g., infarcts) lesions. Use color Doppler to interrogate blood flow in abnormal regions.
- Hyperechoic nodules are usually benign (e.g., myelolipomas, mineralization).
- Small (less than 1 cm and well-defined) hypoechoic nodules are often benign (e.g., extramedullary hematopoiesis or nodular hyperplasia). Serial rechecks may be warranted.
- Moderate to large hypoechoic or mixed echoic nodules, particularly those with irregular margins, should be sampled (FNA) and are more likely malignant neoplasia or uncommon diagnoses like abscessation.
- If a splenic mass is found, also evaluate for peritoneal fluid and sample if present.

References

1. Mattoon J, Sellon R, Berry C, editors. Small Animal Diagnostic Ultrasound 4th edition. St. Louis, Elsevier, 2020.
2. Penninck D, d'Anjou M (editors). Atlas of Small Animal Ultrasonography 2nd edition. Ames, IA, Wiley Blackwell, 2015.
3. Thrall DE, editor. Textbook of Veterinary Diagnostic Radiology 7th edition. St. Louis, MO, Elsevier, 2018.
4. Evans HE, De Lahunta A. Miller's Anatomy of the Dog 4th edition. St. Louis, MO, Elsevier, 2013.
5. Kinns J, Mai W. Association between malignancy and sonographic heterogeneity in canine and feline abdominal lymph nodes. Vet Radiol Ultrasound 48:565-569, 2007.
6. Schreurs E, Vermote K, Barberet V, et al. Ultrasonographic anatomy of abdominal lymph nodes in the normal cat. Vet Radiol Ultrasound 39:68-72, 2008.
7. Agthe P, Caine AR, Posch B, Herrtage ME. Ultrasonographic appearance of jejunal lymph nodes in dogs without clinical signs of gastrointestinal disease. Vet Radiol Ultrasound 50:195-200, 2009.
8. Llabrés-Díaz FJ. Ultrasonography of the medial lymph nodes in the dog. Vet Radiol Ultrasound 45:156-165, 2004.
9. Palladino S, Keyerleber MA, King RG, Burgess KE. Utility of computed tomography versus abdominal ultrasound examination to identify iliosacral lymphadenomegaly in dogs with apocrine gland adenocarcinoma of the anal sac. J Vet Intern Med 30:1858-1863, 2016.
10. Ying M, Bhati, KSS, Lee YP, Yuen HY, Ahuja AT. Review of ultrasonography of malignant neck nodes: greyscale, Doppler, contrast enhancement and elastography. Cancer Imaging 13: 658-669, 2013.
11. De Swarte M, Alexander K, Rannou B, et al. Comparison of sonographic features of benign and neoplastic deep lymph nodes in dogs. Vet Radiol Ultrasound 52:451-456, 2011.
12. Hardie EM, Vaden SL, Spaulding K, et al. Splenic infarction in 16 dogs: a retrospective study. J Vet Intern Med 9:141-148, 1995.
13. Mai W. The hilar perivenous hyperechoic triangle as a sign of acute splenic torsion in dogs. Vet Radiol Ultrasound 47:487-491, 2006.
14. Fife WD, Samii VF, Drost WT, Mattoon JS, Hoshaw-Woodard S. Comparison between malignant and nonmalignant splenic masses in dogs using contrast-enhanced computed tomography. Vet Radiol Ultrasound 45:289-297x, 2004.
15. Mallinckrodt MJ, Gottfried SD. Mass-to-splenic volume ratio and splenic weight as a percentage of body weight in dogs with malignant and benign splenic masses: 65 cases (2007-2008). J Am Vet Med Assoc 239:1325-1327, 2011.
16. Quinci M, Sabattini S, Agnoli C, Bettini G, Diana, A. Ultrasonographic honeycomb pattern of the spleen in cats: correlation with pathological diagnosis in 33 cases. J Fel Med Surg 22:800-804, 2020.
17. O'Brien RT, Waller KR III, Osgood TL. Sonographic features of drug-induced splenic congestion. Vet Radiol Ultrasound 45:225-227, 2004.
18. Masiuk MMM, Garcia-Pereira FL, Berry CR, Ellison GW. Effects of a single intravenous bolus injection of alfaxalone of canine splenic volume as determined by computed tomography. Can J Vet Res 82:203-207, 2018.

CHAPTER 34

Urinary tract contrast studies: technique and normal appearance

Micaela Zarelli and Chiara Bergamino

KEY POINTS

- Urinary tract contrast studies use ionic or non-ionic water-soluble iodinated contrast media to evaluate the urinary tract.
- Patient preparation is a key point to obtain a diagnostic study.
- Excretory intravenous urography is performed to evaluate the upper urinary tract.
- For excretory intravenous urography, use a dose of 600 to 700 mg of iodine per kilogram of body weight.
- Cystography is performed to evaluate the urinary bladder.
- For positive cystography use water-soluble iodinated contrast medium diluted to a 20% solution using sterile saline until the bladder is turgid.
- A retrograde urethrography is performed to assess the urethra.
- For retrograde urethrography in male dogs, use 5 to 20 mL of 15%-20% iodinated contrast agent.
- For retrograde vagino-urethrography in female dogs, use contrast medium at a volume of 1 mL/kg

Excretory intravenous urography

Excretory or intravenous urography (IVU) is a contrast radiographic technique that can be used to evaluate the size, shape, position, and pelvis of the kidneys and size, shape, position, and termination of the ureters using ionic or non-ionic water-soluble iodinated contrast media.[1]

The main clinical indications for excretory urography are trauma, hematuria, ectopic ureter, or suspicion of a mass.[2] The main contraindications include known hypersensitivity to contrast media, dehydration/hypovolemia, and hypotension. Oliguria is considered a contraindication as adequate urine output is necessary for a diagnostic study. Iodinated contrast media can cause acute renal failure in patients with reduced urine output, but can occur in any patient.[1] Contrast-induced hypotension is the most common adverse event. Although excretory urography is relatively safe in azotemic patients after adequate hydration, it is quite unlikely to obtain a diagnostic study if the kidneys cannot concentrate adequately.[3]

Patient preparation is essential for a good quality study. The gastrointestinal tract should be completely emptied as it does not enhance visualization of the urinary tract. Food should be withheld for at least 12 to 24 hours before the study and a cleansing enema should be performed a few hours before the procedure. The patient must be adequately hydrated and be normotensive. An intravenous catheter for sedation or general anesthesia and contrast injection is required. Since the contrast medium can affect some parameters, such as specific gravity, samples for urinalysis should be taken before performing contrast studies.[5]

SECTION V ABDOMEN

Prior to injection of contrast, survey radiographs must be taken to confirm good preparation of the patient (**figs. 34.1A** and **34.2A**).

The excretory urography is performed by injecting an intravenous bolus of contrast medium with a dose of 600 to 700 mg of iodine per kilogram of body weight.

The study is a temporal sequence consisting of four phases: arteriogram, vascular nephrogram, tubular nephrogram, and pyelogram.[3]

The arterial phase allows the assessment of the renal arteries,[3,4] which become opacified approximately 5 to 7 seconds after injection of a bolus of contrast medium.[2] In the vascular nephrogram phase the renal parenchyma[4] starts opacifying 10 seconds from the injection as contrast fills the vessels in the kidney. First, the contrast enhancement becomes greater in the cortex than in the medulla and progresses to uniform opacification of the renal parenchyma as contrast is filtered and collects in the tubules, the tubular nephrogram lasting up to 2 minutes, and then fades gradually (**figs. 34.1B** and **34.2B**).[2]

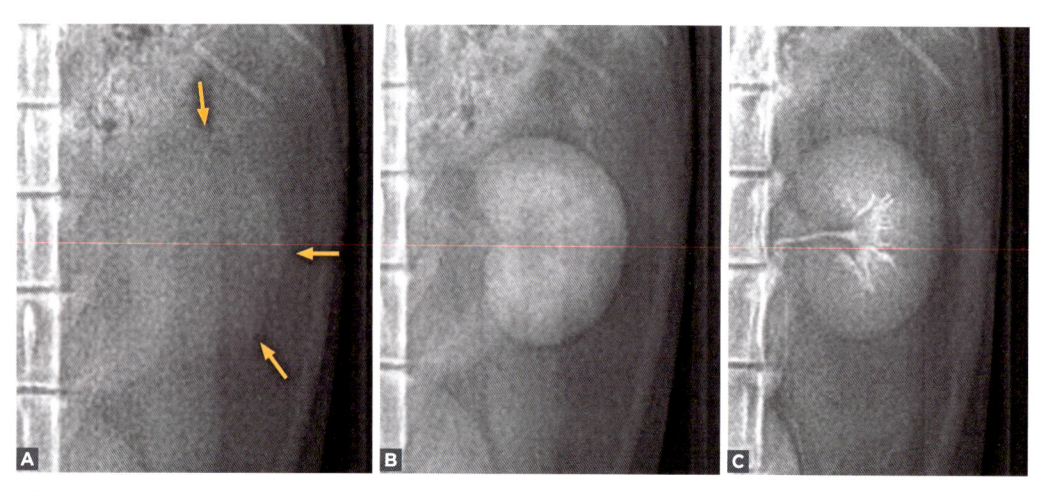

Fig. 34.1 A one-year-old castrated male Domestic shorthair cat. Ventrodorsal projections of the left kidney. (**A**) Survey radiograph showing a normal left kidney (arrows). (**B**) One and half minutes after intravenous iodinated contrast administration. Note the homogenous contrast uptake of the renal parenchyma (tubular nephrogram). (**C**) Three minutes after intravenous iodinated contrast administration. Note the fading of the nephrogram and the contrast accumulation in the left pelvis (pyelogram) and in the proximal left ureter. Normal study.

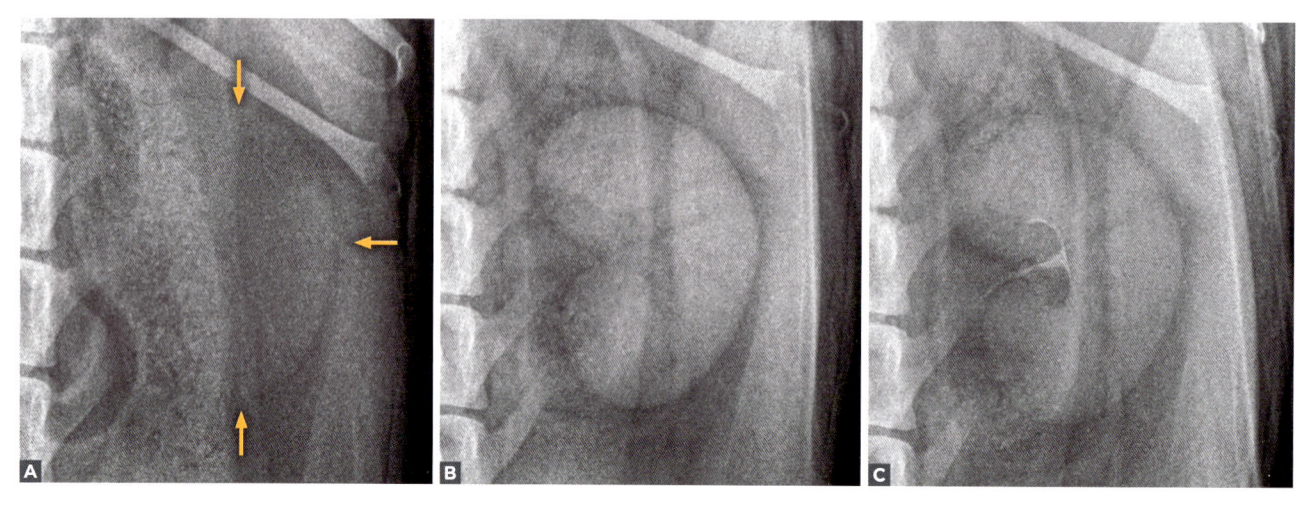

Fig. 34.2 A ten-month-old spayed female Beagle. Ventrodorsal projections of the left kidney. (**A**) Survey radiograph showing normal left kidney (arrows). The abdomen has not been adequately prepared and feces are superimposed on the kidney. (**B**) One minute after intravenous iodinated contrast administration. Note the homogenous contrast uptake of the renal parenchyma (tubular nephrogram). (**C**) Three minutes after intravenous iodinated contrast administration. Note the fading of the nephrogram and the contrast accumulation in the left pelvis (pyelogram) and in the proximal left ureter. Normal study.

As the nephrogram progressively fades, the contrast accumulates in the renal pelvis and ureters, the pyelogram phase (**figs. 34.1C** and **34.2C**).[4]

The patient is positioned in dorsal recumbency before starting the study and 5-10 seconds after contrast injection and a ventrodorsal radiograph is acquired to evaluate the renal arteries in the arteriogram phase. This can only be obtained in smaller patients or when a pressure injector is used in larger patients to ensure rapid injection of a compact bolus of contrast. Following this, a typical study requires ventrodorsal right lateral radiographs to be taken immediately, from 10 seconds to 2 minutes, and then at 5, 20, and 40 minutes. Timing depends upon the area of interest. For example, if the primary goal is to assess one or both kidneys, images should be obtained quickly before contrast washes out. Acquisition times may need to be altered depending on how contrast accumulates in the kidneys and ureters. A dilated ureter may take 20-30 minutes to fill with contrast. For better visualization of the ureters, oblique projections can be added at 5, 20, and 40 minutes. Normal ureters exhibit peristalsis and multiple images are often required at each time point to assess the entire length. The normal renal pelvis does not exceed 3 mm in diameter.[1] The pelvic diverticula may be seen in some dogs and most cats and appear as thin (1 mm) spikes radiating from the pelvis toward the periphery.[2] The ureters measure less than 3 mm in width, have a tubular shape, and show segmentation due to ureteral peristalsis.[1] They terminate at the dorsal aspect of the bladder neck, where they curve cranially for a short distance before entering the wall.[2]

In case of trauma, plain abdominal radiographs are routinely performed as a screening method; however, this technique might be of limited value and complementary imaging modalities are often needed (**fig. 34.3**). Abdominal ultrasound can be used to investigate traumatic injury but cannot confirm a ureteral laceration.[2] In these patients, both excretory urography and retrograde urethrocystography can be useful to examine the entire urinary tract.[6] For trauma patients with suspected ureteral injury, it is essential to ensure adequate hydration and normal blood pressure before performing an IVU. Preparation of the gastrointestinal tract is not needed. The patient is positioned in lateral recumbency, and survey radiographs are obtained. A bolus of contrast is injected, and a lateral radiograph is obtained after 5 minutes. This should show nephrographic enhancement of both kidneys and at least partial

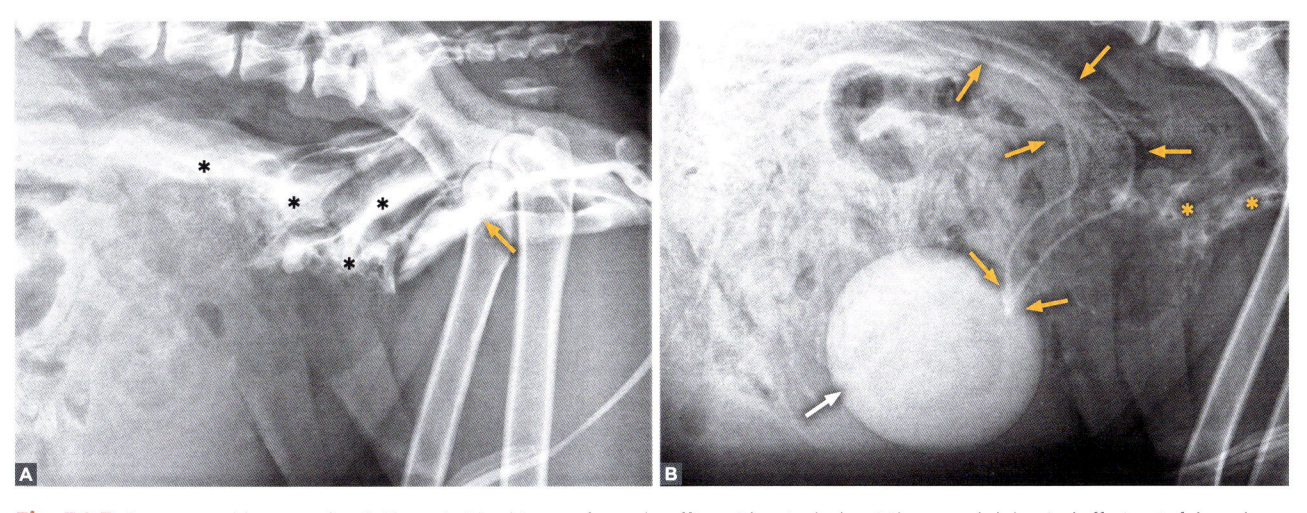

Fig. 34.3 An 11-year-old castrated male Sharpei with a history of a road traffic accident in the last 24 hours and abdominal effusion. Left lateral projections of retrograde urethrogram (**A**) and excretory urogram (**B**). There is decreased serosal detail in the caudal aspect of the peritoneal cavity visible in both projections. (**A**) At the level of the junction between the prostatic urethra and urinary bladder neck the urethra has blunted appearance (orange arrow) and, in this region, the contrast is into the peritoneal cavity (black asterisks). There is no retrograde contrast filling of the urinary bladder. (**B**) After intravenous administration of iodinated contrast medium, both the right and left ureters are identified and normally insert at the level of the trigone (orange arrows). There is residual contrast in the caudal aspect of the peritoneal cavity from the retrograde urethrography (orange asterisks); however, there is no evidence of further contrast leakage in the retroperitoneal space. The urinary bladder is cranially displaced and is filled with contrast and has smooth margins (white arrow); however, the vesicourethral junction is not visible. A traumatic urinary bladder avulsion with secondary uroabdomen was surgically confirmed.

contrast filling of the ureters. Additional lateral radiographs are obtained until both ureters have been filled with contrast and contrast filling of the bladder has been achieved, which confirms the integrity of the upper urinary tract. A renal or ureteral laceration appears as a poorly defined accumulation of contrast in the retroperitoneal space. In case of complete or incomplete renal avulsion, there is no enhancement of the kidney. With renal artery thrombosis, the excretory renal function, and the ability to excrete the contrast may be impaired or completely compromised, thus leading to poor or absent nephrogram depending on the extent of the occlusion.[6,7] Alternatively, contrast could leak in the retroperitoneum or peritoneum suggesting a renal, ureteral laceration.[6,7]

Cystography: pneumocystogram, positive contrast cystogram, double-contrast cystogram

There are three contrast radiographic techniques used to assess the urinary bladder: positive contrast cystography, negative contrast (pneumo-) cystography, and double-contrast cystography, although these have been almost completely supplanted by ultrasound.[3,4,8]

Clinical indications for cystography include trauma, hematuria, dysuria, pollakiuria, nonresponsive bacteriuria, and stranguria. Cystography can also be used to evaluate the integrity of the bladder after trauma.[9] In case of trauma the use of intravenous urography and cystography allows a complete evaluation of the urinary tract.[6]

Contraindications for cystography are few. Fatal air embolism is a rare complication and has been reported in dogs and cats with active mucosal hemorrhage at the time of cystography. Patients should be placed in left lateral recumbency at pneumocystography as this will prevent the circulation of air to the pulmonary arteries from the right heart. The risk of embolization is also reduced by using CO_2 or NO_2 since these gases have higher solubility than room air. Other complications are uncommon; however, trauma and bacterial contamination can result from improper catheterization techniques.[3,8]

Patient preparation is similar to excretory urography. The patient should be sedated or anesthetized before catheterization, and survey radiographs should be taken prior to the contrast study. Catheterization should be performed after filling the catheter with saline or contrast, decreasing air bubbles that may mimic cystic or urethral calculi.[9] Water-soluble iodinated contrast medium diluted to a 20% solution using sterile saline with an approximate dose of 10 mL of contrast medium per kilogram of body weight. The injection should be stopped when the bladder feels turgid on palpation or if back pressure of the syringe plunger occurs (**fig. 34.4**).[9]

Positive contrast cystography is indicated to evaluate urinary bladder position and wall integrity;[3,8] however, this technique is not ideal for assessment of mucosal details.[9]

Pneumocystography is indicated to evaluate the location and shape of the bladder[9], or in combination with an intravenous urography to increase the visibility of the ureterovesical junctions (**fig. 34.5**).[8]

Double-contrast cystography is excellent for demonstrating mural disease and intraluminal filling defects (**fig. 34.6**).[3]

For double cystography, the procedure normally starts with the administration of negative contrast medium (pneumocystography) followed by a few milliliters of undiluted iodinated

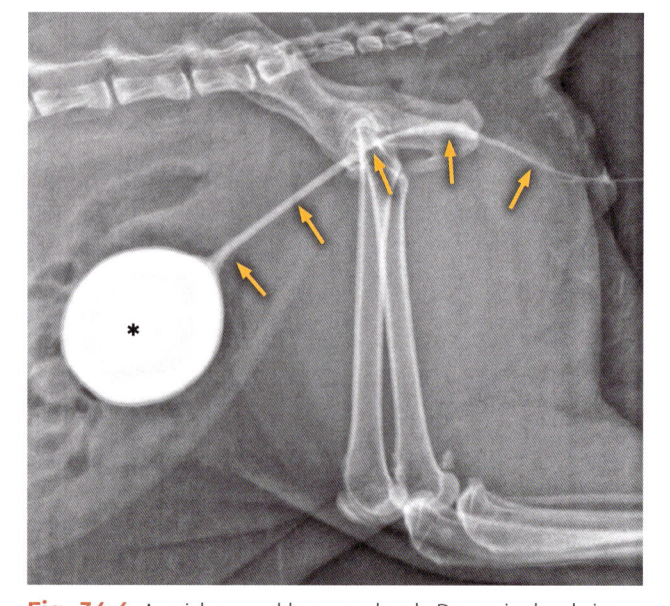

Fig. 34.4 An eight-year-old castrated male Domestic shorthair cat. Right lateral projection of a retrograde cystourethrogram. The study is performed with an iodinated nonionic contrast medium. The urethra (orange arrows) and urinary bladder (black asterisk) have normal positioning and contrast filling. Normal study.

contrast medium (cats 0.5-1 mL; dogs 1-6 mL depending on the size) (**fig. 34.7**).[8] The patient should be gently rolled to distribute the positive contrast along the urinary bladder wall.[8]

For all the contrast techniques, once adequate distension of the urinary bladder is achieved orthogonal projections of the abdomen should be performed. The urinary bladder wall should be smoothly marginated with all contrast media and the content should be homogeneous (radiopaque or radiolucent depending on the technique), without evidence of filling defects.

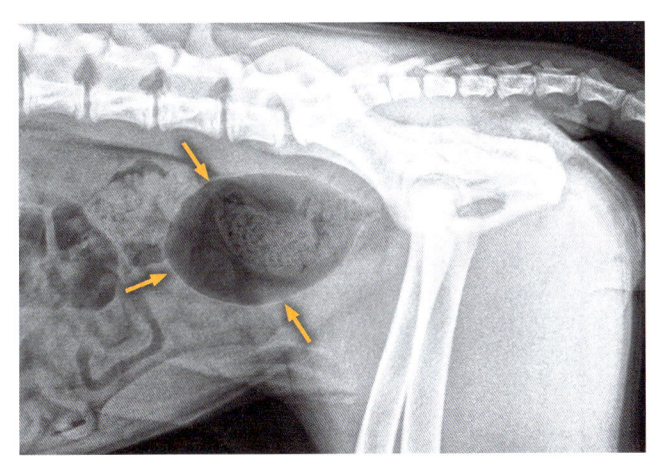

Fig. 34.5 A four-month-old intact female Labrador Retriever. Left lateral projection of a pneumocystography. The study is performed with injection of CO_2 (negative contrast) via a urinary catheter which has been removed. The urinary bladder (arrows) is distended with gas and has normal positioning. The gas allows good visualization of the smooth luminal surface. The colon contains fecal material and is superimposed on the urinary bladder. Normal study.

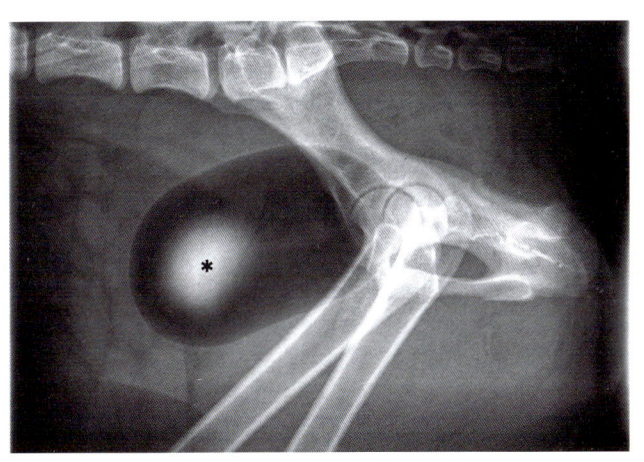

Fig. 34.6 A four-year-old spayed female mixed breed dog. Left lateral projection of a double cystography. The study is performed with the administration of CO_2 (negative contrast) and iodinated nonionic contrast medium (positive contrast). The radiolucent gas fills the urinary bladder, while the iodinated contrast medium forms a radiopaque pool at the dependent (lowest) part of the bladder (black asterisk). The urinary bladder wall is smooth and there are no filling defects in the contrast pool. Normal study.

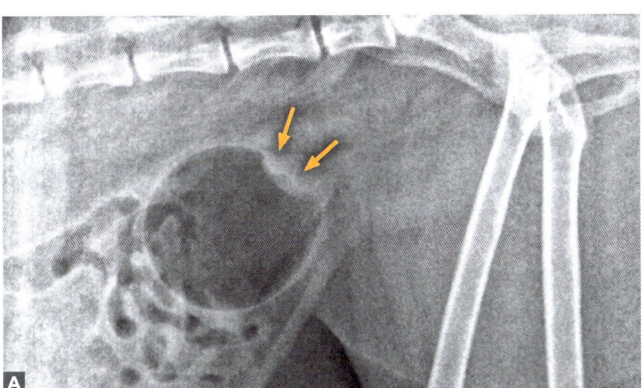

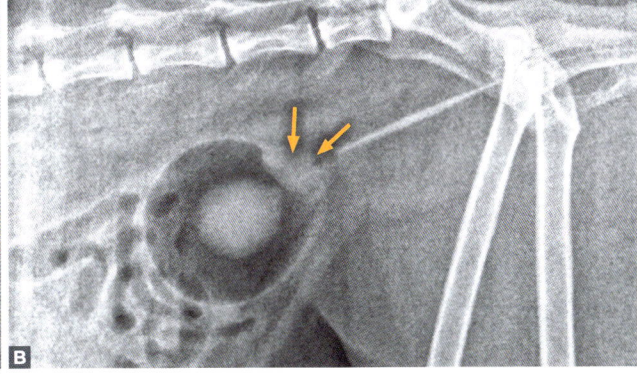

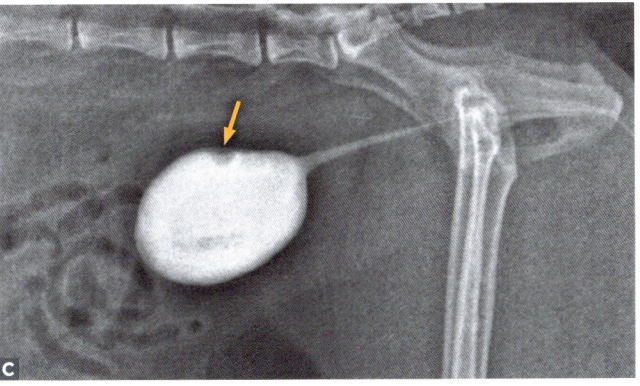

Fig. 34.7 A 12-year-old castrated male Domestic shorthair cat. Left lateral projections of a pneumocystogram (**A**), double-contrast cystogram (**B**), and positive cystogram (**C**). The study is performed with injection of CO_2 and iodinated nonionic contrast medium. There is a lobulated broad-based mural mass in the region of the vesicourethral junction (orange arrows). This mass is much better visualized with the pneumocystography (**A**) and double-contrast cystography (**B**). In the positive cystography (**C**) the contrast filling defect is more subtle and more difficult to visualize, being completely obscured by the contrast. Histopathology confirmed a transitional cell carcinoma.

SECTION **V** ABDOMEN

Contrast urethrogram

A retrograde urethrography is performed to assess the position, integrity, patency, or congenital defect of the urethra.[3,4]

Retrograde urethrogram (males)

Intravenous catheter placement for deep sedation or general anesthesia is required. Survey radiographs should be obtained prior to the contrast study. A urethral catheter with an inflatable balloon is preferred for dogs, as this limits leakage and assists in achieving adequate injection pressure to distend the urethra. A tomcat catheter is used for feline patients. After aseptic preparation, a urinary catheter is introduced with the tip positioned in the distal urethra and 5 to 20 mL of 15%-20% iodinated contrast agent is injected slowly.[3,8] In dogs, at the end of contrast injection, a lateral radiograph is made. Oblique ventrodorsal radiographs are then made at the end of injection of a contrast bolus (**fig. 34.8**).

Normal urethrogram is characterized by smooth margination of the urethra without evidence of contrast leaking or filling defects. The normal canine urethra shows a slight variation in diameter and is usually most narrow within the prostate. The normal feline urethra has a relatively uniform diameter throughout its length.

Normal findings in intact male dogs include contrast reflux into the prostatic ducts.[11]

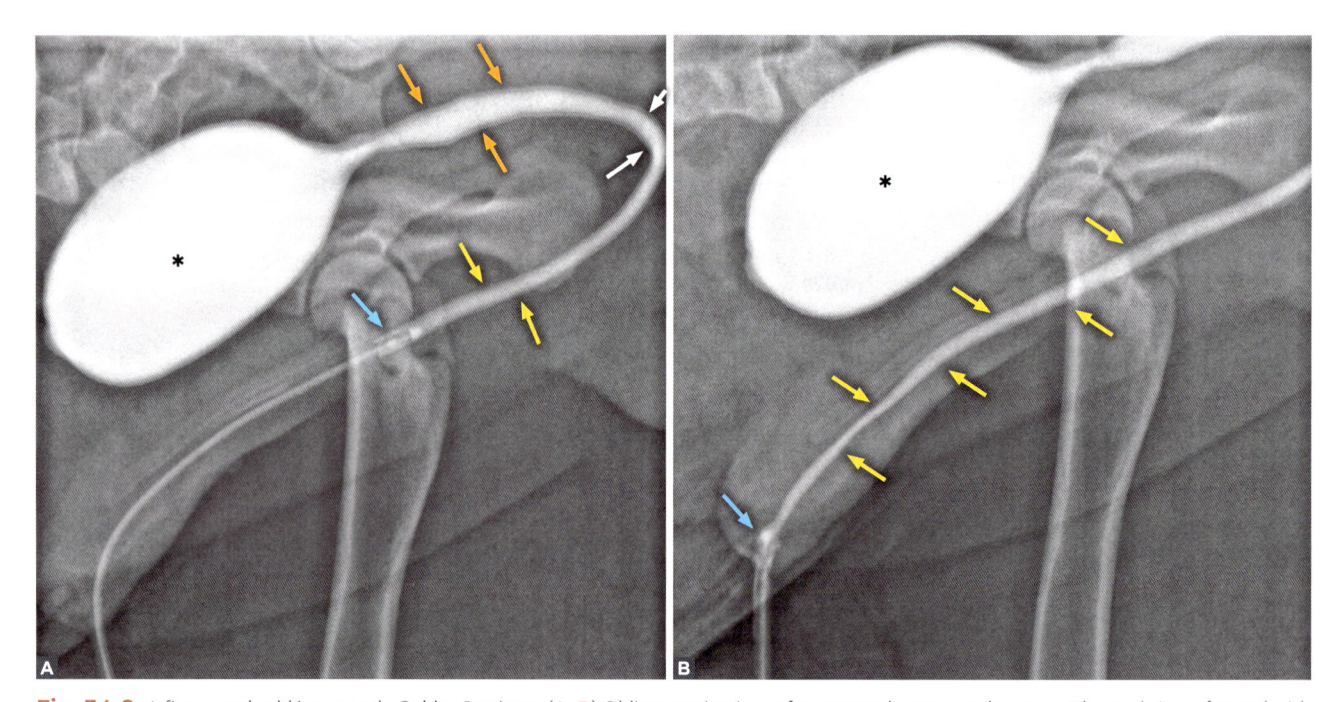

Fig. 34.8 A five-month-old intact male Golden Retriever. (**A**, **B**) Oblique projections of a retrograde cystourethrogram. The study is performed with an iodinated non-ionic contrast medium (positive contrast). The urinary bladder (figs. 34.5A and 34.5B, black asterisk) has normal positioning and contrast filling. To fill the prostatic (fig. 34.5A orange arrows), ischiatic (fig. 34.5A, white arrows) and penile (figs. 34.5A and 34.5B, yellow arrows) segments of the urethra, the tip of the catheter (figs. 34.5A and 34.5B, blue arrows) is repositioned between contrast injections, to ensure good distension of all segments. Normal study.

Retrograde vaginourethrogram (females)

Intravenous catheter placement for general anesthesia is required. Survey radiographs should be obtained prior to the contrast study. After aseptic preparation, a Foley catheter is introduced with the tip in the vaginal vestibule. The balloon should be inflated after the vulvar lips are clamped with atraumatic forceps to avoid leakage. Contrast medium at a volume of 1 mL/kg is injected slowly, avoiding high pressure; opacification of both the vagina and urethra should occur simultaneously.[8] In both dogs and cats, lateral and oblique ventrodorsal radiographs should be taken at the end contrast injection.[4]

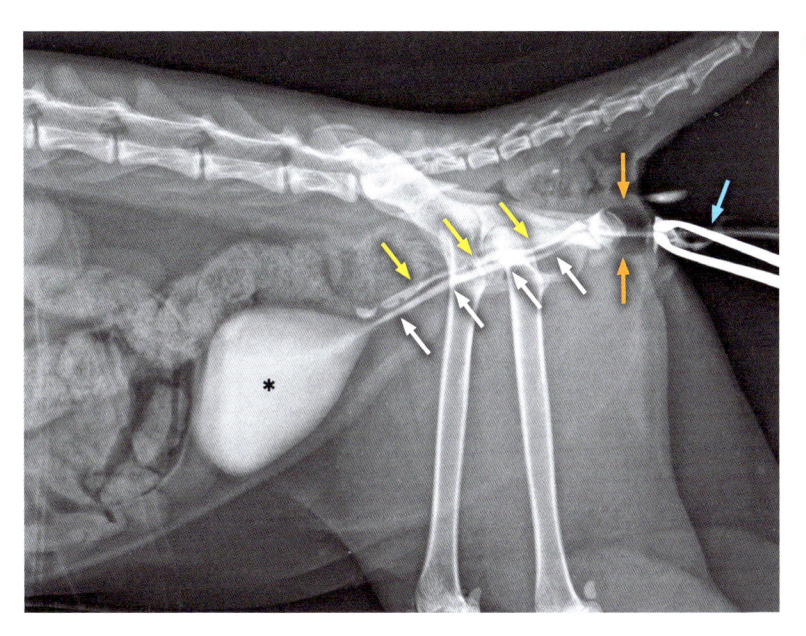

Fig. 34.9 A one-year-old spayed female Domestic shorthair cat. Right lateral projection of a retrograde vaginourethrocystogram. The study is performed with iodinated non-ionic contrast medium (positive contrast). A Foley catheter has a gas-filled balloon (orange arrows), and it is positioned in the vaginal vestibule. A metallic clamp is present to reduce contrast leakage (blue arrow). The urethra (white arrows) and urinary bladder (black asterisk) have normal positioning and contrast filling. The vagina (yellow arrows) is also filled with contrast; however, a few radiolucent defects representing gas bubbles are present in the cranial aspect. Normal study.

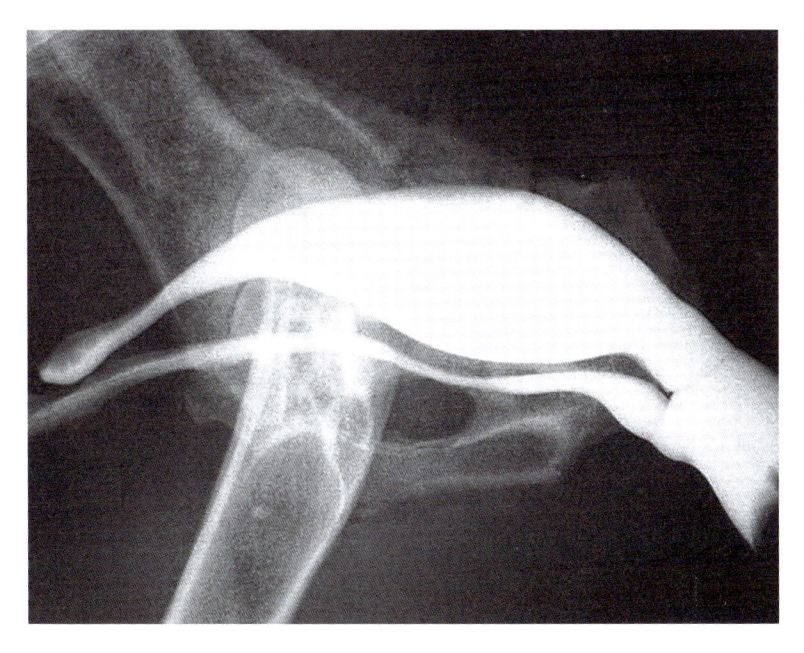

Fig. 34.10 An adult female spayed dog. Right lateral projection of a retrograde vaginourethrocystogram. A study was performed as for fig. 34.9. Courtesy of Prof. Marco Russo.

References

1. Heuter KJ. Excretory urography. Clin Tech Small Anim Pract 20:39-45, 2005.
2. Seiler G. Kidneys and ureters. In Thrall, DE (editor). Textbook of Veterinary Diagnostic Radiology 7th edition. Saunders Elsevier, 2016, pp 823-845
3. Pugh CR, Rhodes WH, Biery DN. Contrast studies of the urogenital system. Vet Clin North Am Small Anim Pract 23:281-306, 1993.
4. Baines E. Practical contrast radiography 3. Urogenital studies. Part III. In Practice 27:466-473, 2005.
5. Feeney DA, Osborne CA, Jessen CR. Effects of radiographic contrast-media on results of urinalysis, with emphasis on alteration in specific gravity. J Am Vet Med Assoc 176:1378-1381, 1980.
6. Morgan JP, Wolvekamp P (editors). Atlas of Radiology of the Traumatized Dog and Cat: The Case-Based Approach 2nd edition. Schlütersche, 2010.
7. Kealy JK, McAllister H, Graham J (editors). Diagnostic Radiology and Ultrasonography of the Dog and Cat 5th edition. Elsevier Saunders, 2010.
8. Hecht S. Diagnostic imaging of lower urinary tract disease. Vet Clin North Am Small Anim Pract 45:639-663, 2015.
9. Essman SC. Contrast cystography. Clin Tech Small Anim Pract 20:46-51, 2005.
10. Johnston GR, Jessen CR, Osborne CA. Effects of bladder distension on canine and feline retrograde urethrography. Vet Radiol:271-277, 1983.
11. Ackerman N. Prostatic reflux during positive contrast retrograde urethrography in the dog. Vet Radiol Ultrasound 24:251-259, 1983.

CHAPTER 35

Kidneys and ureters

Ryan B. Appleby

KEY POINTS

- Renal disease is common in small animals and can present with a variety of signs ranging from localized urinary abnormalities to systemic illness.
- Radiographs are neither sensitive nor specific to underlying etiologies, but they are a valuable screening tool for gross alterations in renal size, shape, and opacity.
- Normal radiographs do not exclude underlying renal disease.
- Ultrasound is the primary diagnostic imaging modality due to its ease of use and accessibility but has limited ability to differentiate specific diagnoses.
- Computed tomography is an excellent diagnostic tool and is valuable in evaluating complex cases and for surgical planning.

Diseases of the upper urinary tract (kidneys and ureters) are common in small animals. Imaging of renal disease often involves several modalities. While radiographs are a frequently used baseline diagnostic tool, they are limited to detecting changes in size, shape, and opacity of the kidneys and ureters and provide no information on function. Radiographic studies are often complemented by or, in some cases, replaced by ultrasound and computed tomography (CT). Regardless of the imaging modality, there is poor correlation between the severity of imaging findings and the severity of azotemia or clinical signs.

Kidneys

Normal kidneys
The normal kidneys in dogs and cats are usually visible as ovoid soft tissue opacity structures in the retroperitoneal space, provided there is sufficient local fatty tissue. In dogs, the left kidney is usually visible, but the right kidney is obscured in about half of patients. In ventrodorsal radiographs, normal kidneys are sometimes obscured by superimposition of the intestine and feces, especially the right kidney (**fig. 35.1**). In cats, both kidneys are usually visible in both lateral and ventrodorsal radiographs but may be obscured by fecal material. Kidneys can be measured in radiographs and are reported to be between 2.5-3.5 times the length of L2 in dogs,[1] though smaller and brachycephalic dogs have relatively larger kidneys compared to larger and dolichocephalic dogs.[2] Normal renal size in cats is reported to be between 1.9 to 3.2 times the length of L2.[3]

SECTION V ABDOMEN

Sonographically, the normal kidney has differentiation between the renal cortex and medulla. The cortex is the outer portion, which is hyperechoic, and the medulla in the inner portion, which is hypoechoic (**fig. 35.2**). In some cases, there is variation in the appearance of the medulla, and a hyperechoic outer medulla is a normal finding, especially in small breed dogs[4] and should not be confused with renal pathology (**fig. 35.2**). Sonographic measurements of the kidneys in dogs have a wide range depending on body size and a renal to aorta ratio between 5.5-9.1 has been described as normal kidney size in dogs.[5] Cats are reported to have a normal renal size on sonography between 3 cm and 4.3 cm.[6]

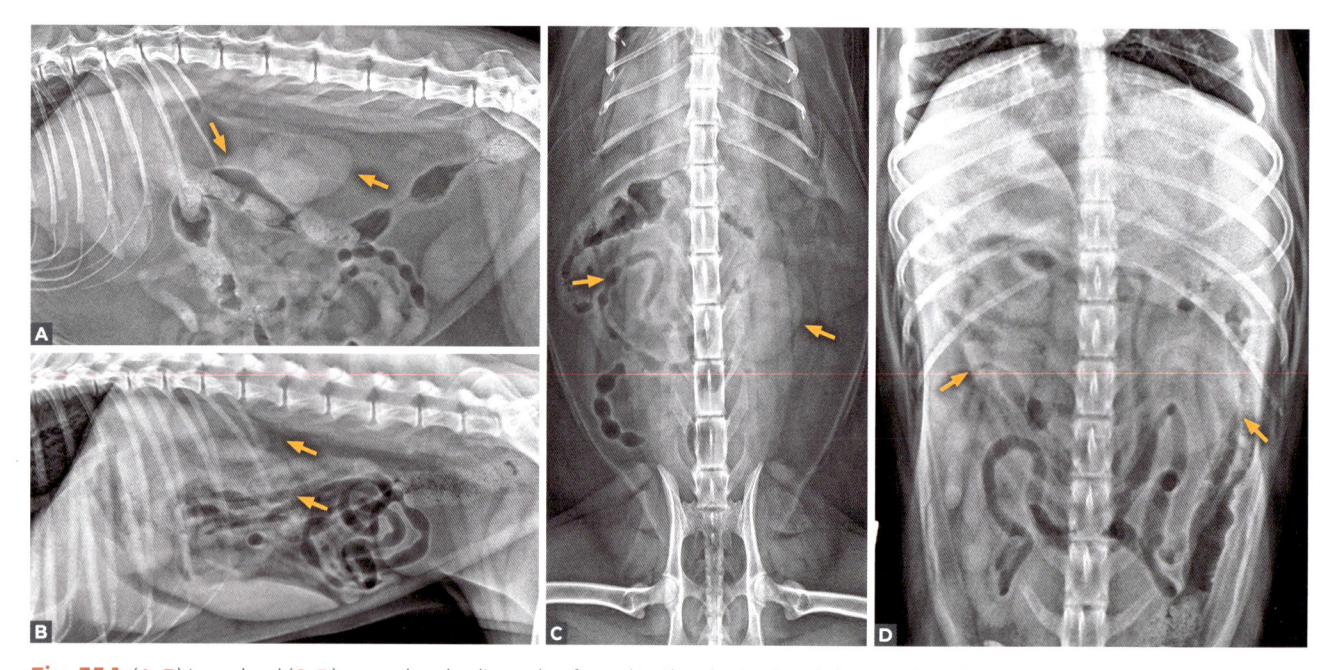

Fig. 35.1 (**A**, **B**) Lateral and (**C**, **D**) ventrodorsal radiographs of a cat (**A**, **C**) and a dog (**B**, **D**) showing the radiographic appearance of normal kidneys (arrows). Notice that the kidneys in the dog are more challenging to delineate due to less fat in the retroperitoneal space and the ventrodorsal projection due to superimposition with other abdominal organs relative to the cat.

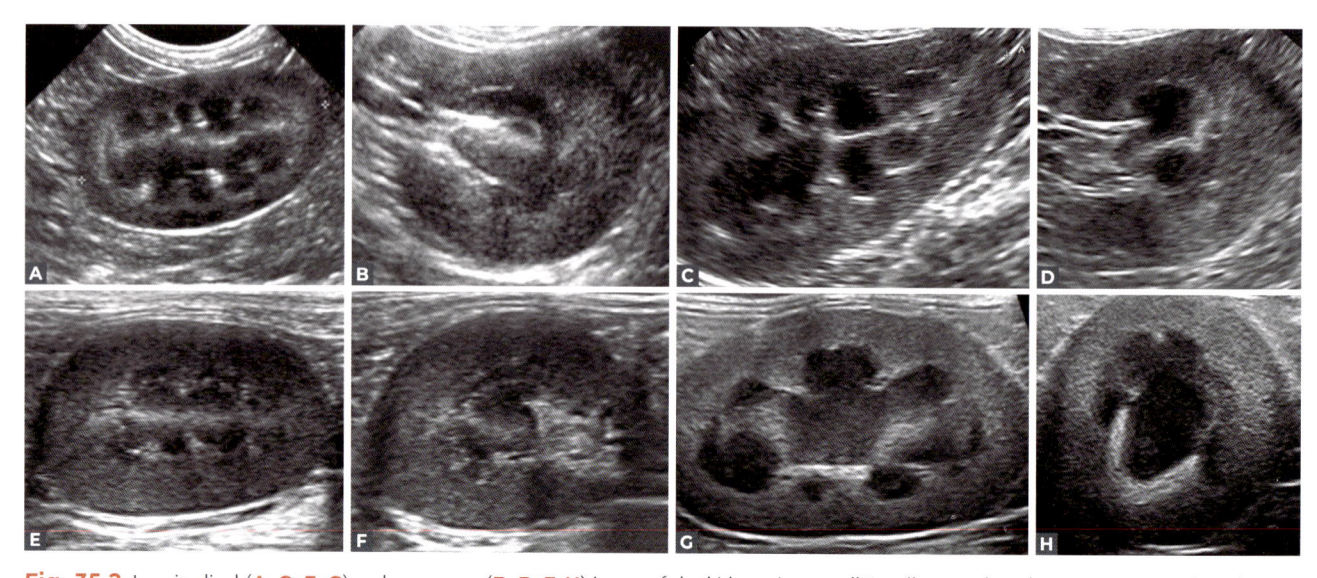

Fig. 35.2 Longitudinal (**A**, **C**, **E**, **G**) and transverse (**B**, **D**, **F**, **H**) image of the kidneys in a small Poodle cross (**A**, **B**), a Boston Terrier (**C**, **D**) and a Domestic shorthair cat (**E**, **F**, **G**, **H**). The outer portion of the kidney is the cortex, typically hyperechoic to the hypoechoic medulla. In some patients, a hyperechoic band is present in the outer medulla (**A**). This finding should not be confused for a medullary band sign, a non-specific indication of disease.

Chronic kidney disease and/or insufficiency

Chronic kidney disease and/or insufficiency is one of the most common renal syndromes affecting at least 1.2% of cats[7] and 0.2% of dogs.[8] Older cats are particularly affected, with over 50% identified as having CKD in some studies.[9] The etiology is poorly understood, and it may arise from a number of different pathways, including renal insult from infection, toxin, or vascular compromise. However, histopathologic findings are commonly and consistently tubulointerstitial fibrosis.[10,11] Renal and ureteral diseases can have non-specific clinical manifestations, including but not limited to weight loss, general malaise, anorexia/hyporexia, vomiting, pain, and polyuria/polydipsia. Laboratory abnormalities often include elevations in serum creatinine, blood urea nitrogen (BUN), symmetric dimethylarginine (SDMA), and hyposthenuria. Imaging findings range from no abnormality to severe morphologic changes. Common imaging findings include infarction (**fig. 35.3**), reduced size (**figs. 35.3** and **35.4A**), and mineralization (**fig. 35.5**).

Sonographically there may be a loss of corticomedullary definition (**fig. 35.4B** and **35.6**) where the normally hypoechoic medulla is increased in echogenicity as well as a reduction in cortical thickness.[12] Hyperechoic bands are sometimes seen in the renal medulla and are a nonspecific finding. A thick hyperechoic band is often associated with CKD when compared to a thin "rim".[13] CKD is best monitored through bloodwork as the severity of imaging abnormalities does not correlate with loss of function and degree of azotemia.

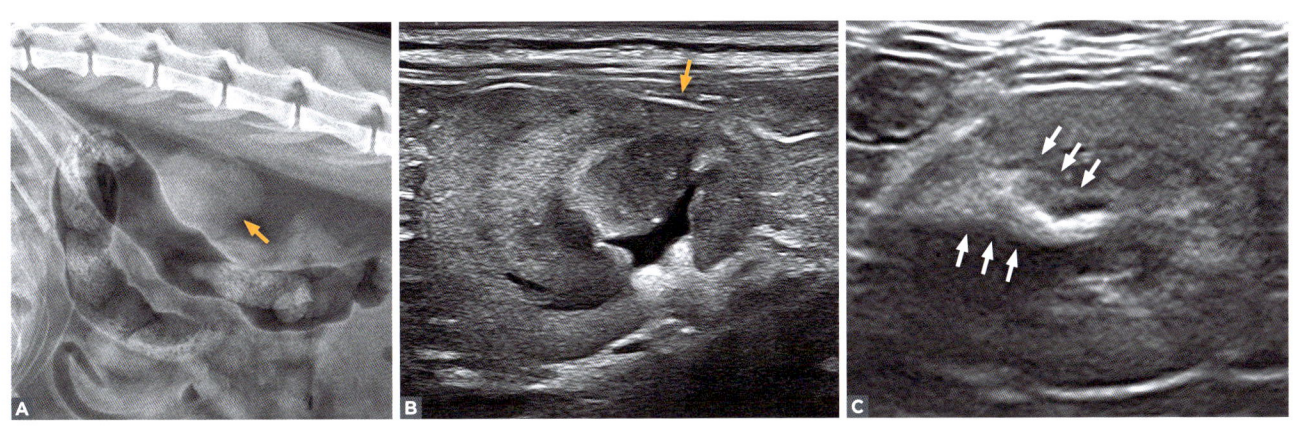

Fig. 35.3 (**A**) Radiograph and (**B**) corresponding longitudinal ultrasound image of a cat with a presumed chronic infarct of the caudal pole of the left kidney. Note the shallow concave defect in the caudal ventral cortical margin of the kidney denoted by the orange arrow in both images. The kidney displays additional evidence of degeneration characterized by a loss of corticomedullary definition and mild dilation of the renal pelvis. (**C**) Some infarcts can be identified on ultrasound as triangular hyperechoic foci with or without concurrent cortical flattening (white arrows).

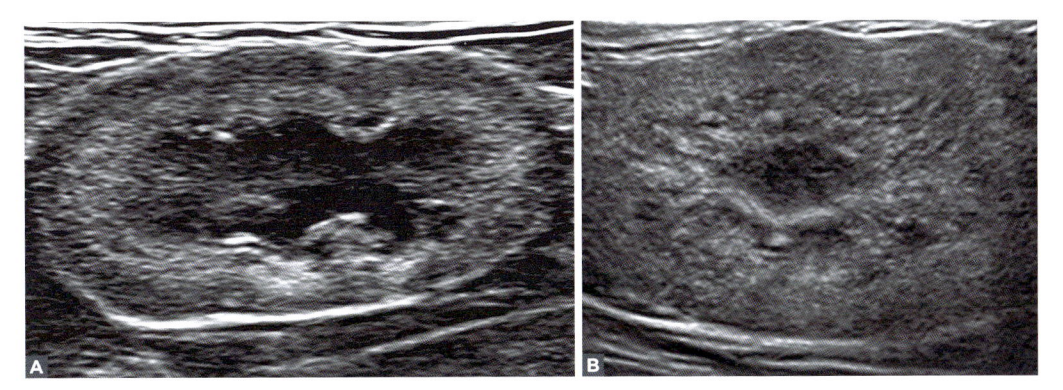

Fig. 35.4 (**A**) Sonographic image of a ten-year-old spayed female Domestic shorthair cat with chronic kidney disease caused by chronic and intermittent ureteral obstruction. The kidney is small in size (~2 cm), with a hyperechoic cortex and hyperechoic speckling in portions of the medulla. (**B**) Longitudinal sonographic image of a ten-year-old old castrated male Domestic shorthair cat with marked loss of corticomedullary definition and relatively hyperechoic medulla.

SECTION V ABDOMEN

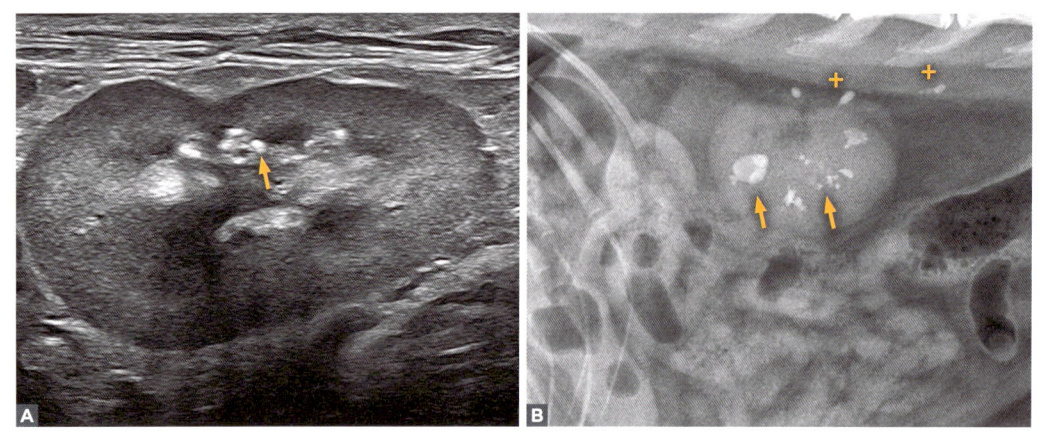

Fig. 35.5 Calculi can be seen either sonographically (**A**) as hyperechoic foci, often in the renal pelvis or peridiverticular tissues (arrows), or radiographically (**B**) as mineral opacity in plane with the kidneys. In this example, calculi are also present in the ureters (+). These images are of a six-year-old castrated male Domestic Shorthair cat (**A**) and a three-year-old Siberian Forest cat (**B**), both presented with acute azotemia.

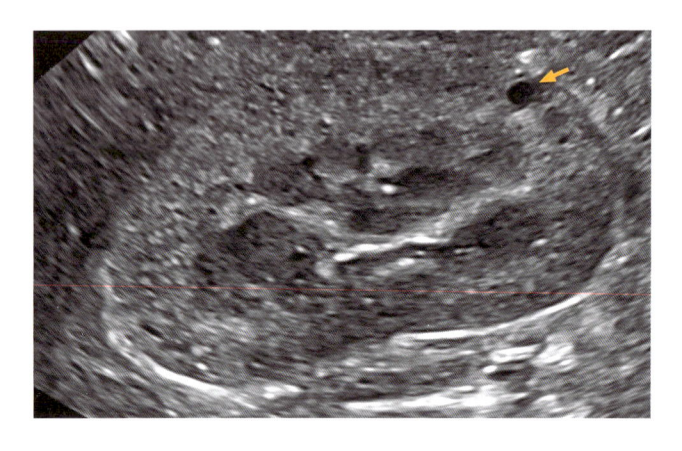

Fig. 35.6 Longitudinal ultrasound image of a feline kidney displaying mild degenerative changes. There is loss of corticomedullary definition, numerous punctate hyperechoic cortical foci, and a caudal pole cyst (arrow).

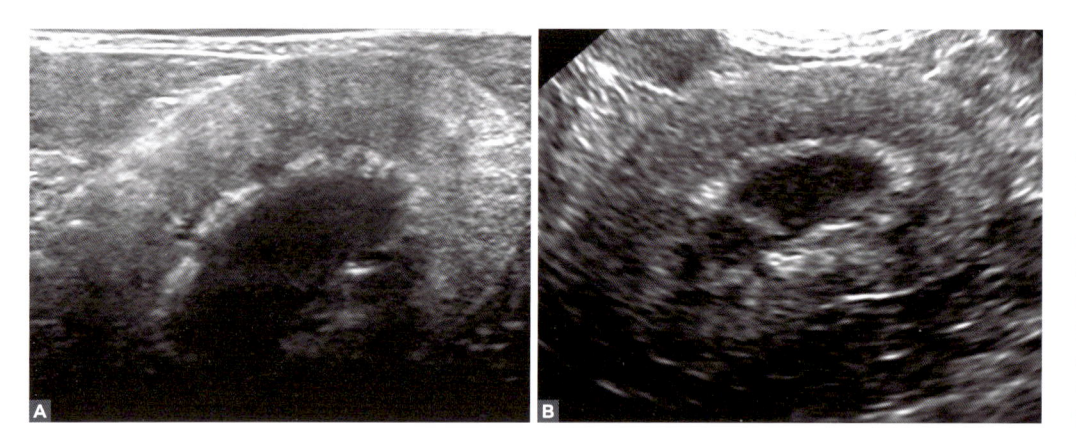

Fig. 35.7 Longitudinal ultrasound images of the left kidney of a ten-year-old female King Charles Cavalier Spaniel with chronic azotemia. A thick medullary band is present, and the cortices are hyperechoic. Detail in the renal cortex is better visualized with a linear probe (**A**) with a higher frequency (18 MHz) when compared to a microconvex probe (**B**) with a lower frequency (9 MHz).

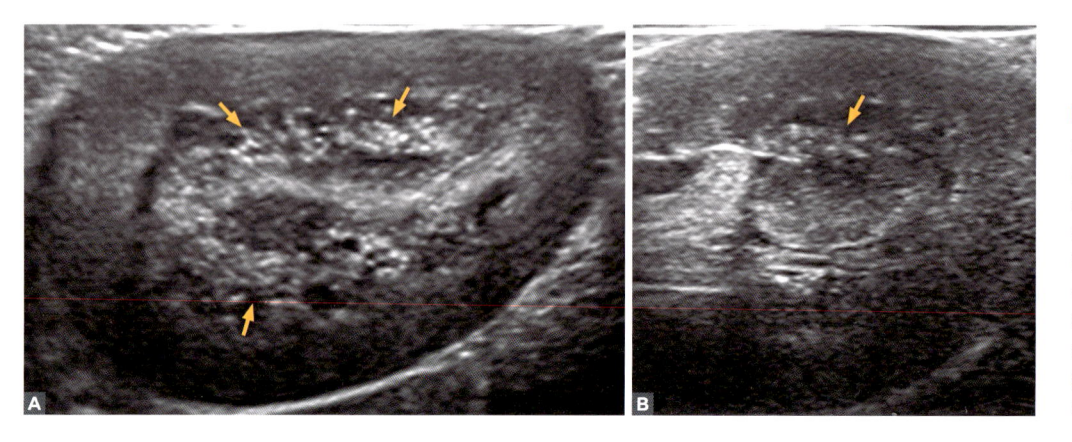

Fig. 35.8 (**A**) Longitudinal and (**B**) transverse images of the left kidney of a nine-month-old female Cairn Terrier presenting for screening for preclinical renal dysplasia. The images identify hyperechoic speckling of the medulla (arrows) compatible with renal dysplasia.

558

Renal dysplasia

Familial renal diseases have been described in a large number of breeds of both dogs and cats with a variety of underlying etiologies, including amyloidosis, polycystic kidney disease, and renal dysplasia.[23] There is significant overlap in the imaging appearance of various diseases, which cannot be distinguished without biopsy or genetic testing. However, the imaging appearance of some disorders has been described.

Renal dysplasia is a hereditary condition where the renal tissue fails to differentiate and develop properly. It has been reported in numerous dog breeds, including Cairn Terriers, Golden Retrievers, Cocker Spaniels, Boxers,[24] Rhodesian Ridgebacks, Shih Tzus, Bull Mastiffs,[25] and Bernese Mountain dogs. While there is significant overlap in the imaging appearance with other causes of chronic kidney disease, the appearance has been described in some groups of dogs (**fig. 35.7**). For example, in Cairn Terriers[26] the sonographic features include decreased corticomedullary definition and either hyperechoic speckling or generalized hyperechogenicity of the renal medulla (**fig. 35.8**). While biopsy is the gold standard for diagnosis, a diagnosis is often made from a combination of signalment (young animal) laboratory data (evidence of renal insufficiency) and imaging appearance (non-specific but marked renal parenchymal changes relative to patient age).

Trauma

Renal trauma occurs relatively uncommonly; however, it can be caused by blunt force trauma (most commonly motor vehicle accidents) or from penetrating injury and ballistic trauma. Trauma can result in either renal avulsion and displacement,[29,30] subcapsular hemorrhage, or perinephric hemorrhage. While subcapsular hemorrhage leads to renal enlargement, perinephric hemorrhage in the retroperitoneal space can obscure the kidneys and appears as a loss of contrast, often with a mass effect expanding the retroperitoneal space. Hemorrhage can also occur secondary to coagulopathy (**fig. 35.9**). Urine leakage into the retroperitoneal space can be caused by ureteral laceration or avulsion. Contrast-enhanced CT can be valuable in cases of trauma. This can allow evaluation of the kidneys to differentiate hematomas neoplastic masses, as neoplasms often have a component of

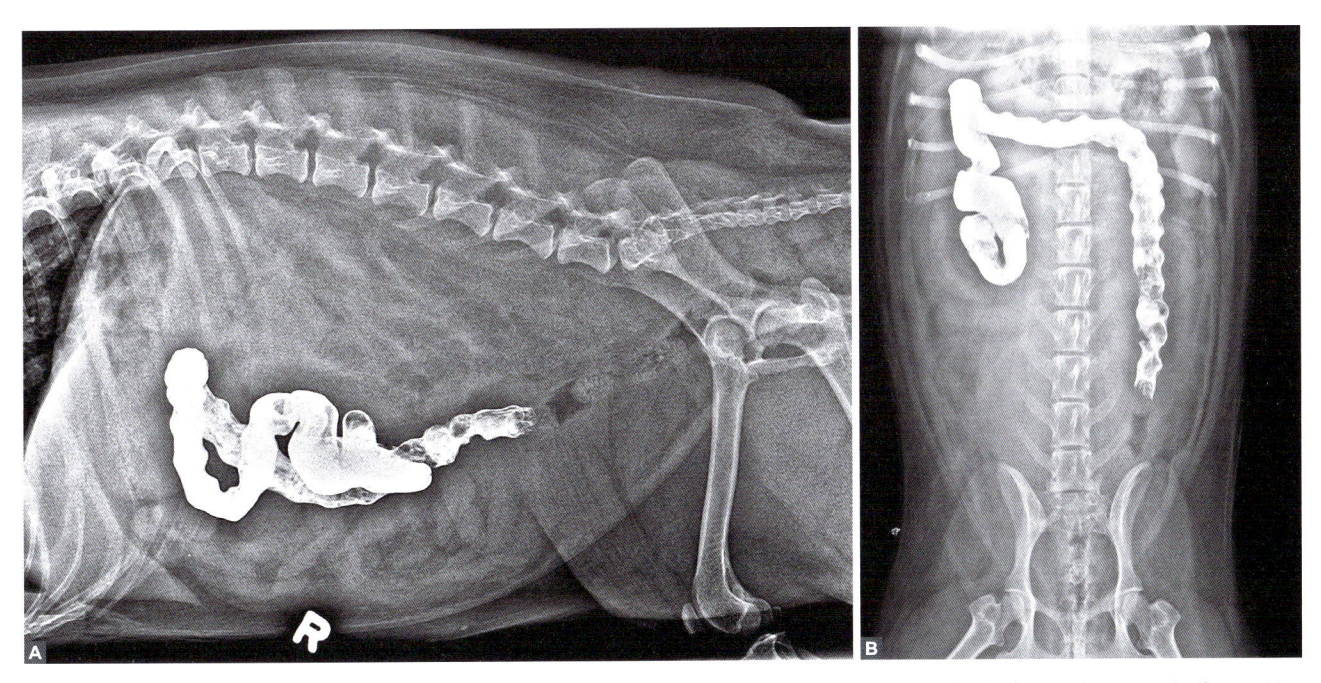

Fig. 35.9 Right lateral and ventrodorsal radiographic projections of a three-year-old spayed female West Highland White Terrier presenting for vomiting and abdominal bruising. There is a moderate volume of fluid expanding the retroperitoneal space, obscuring the kidneys and effacing the ventral margin of the epaxial musculature. This finding is characterized by non-uniform soft tissue opacity and results in ventral displacement of the small intestine and colon, which is barium filled from a previous gastrointestinal contrast study.

SECTION V ABDOMEN

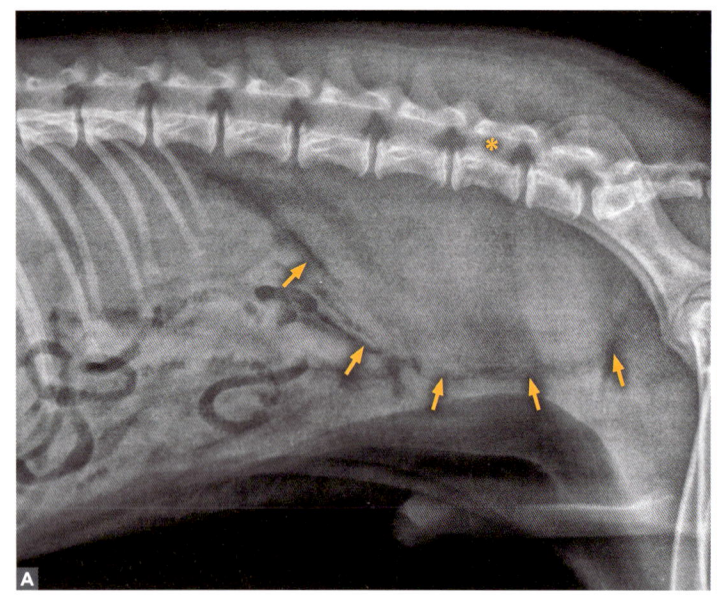

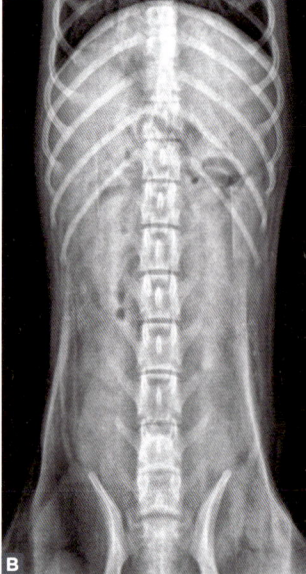

Fig. 35.10 (**A**) Right lateral and (**B**) ventrodorsal projections of the abdomen of a ten-month-old mixed breed dog presenting after a motor vehicle trauma. A caudal abdominal mass effect is present, arising within the retroperitoneal space (arrows) and causing ventral displacement of the distal descending colon. A fracture of the L6 vertebral body (asterisk) is present, characterized by irregularity of the ventral margin.

contrast enhancement. CT can also facilitate the evaluation of the retroperitoneal space in cases of trauma. Hematomas secondary to trauma can also occur in the retroperitoneal space, particularly with pelvic fractures, and can cause a caudodorsal abdominal mass effect. While not arising from the renal system, these patients can present with urinary signs if there is obstruction or compression of the bladder or ureters (**fig. 35.10**).

Trauma can also result in herniation of the kidneys, such as through the body wall to the subcutis. Renal avulsion with displacement into the thorax has been reported in cats.[29,31] Penetrating injuries have been reported to cause local damage to the renal vasculature,[32] and CT may be an important diagnostic tool in surgical planning for these cases.

Neoplasia

While radiography can sometimes identify renal enlargement, it cannot distinguish between causes of renomegaly in most cases. While unilateral renal enlargement or bilateral renal enlargement (**fig. 35.11**) can be identified radiographically, ultrasound and/or CT are required to differentiate between mass lesions and other causes of renomegaly such as hydronephrosis or cysts.

Renal carcinoma is the most common primary renal tumor in dogs and cats.[14,15] Carcinomas can have a heterogeneous appearance and include regions of cysts and solid tissue, with at least partial effacement of normal internal renal architecture. Both ultrasound and CT (**figs. 35.12-35.14**) are valuable in diagnosing renal carcinoma. Ultrasound facilitates fine-needle aspiration to obtain a cytological diagnosis and guide therapy.

Renal lymphoma in cats has a common sonographic appearance where the kidneys are often enlarged (**fig. 35.11**) with a peripheral subcapsular hypoechoic band of tissue (**fig. 35.15**). This appearance can overlap with feline infectious peritonitis (**fig. 35.16**). However, some instances of renal lymphoma do not display the peripheral hypoechoic band. Instead, these cases may display renomegaly alone or evidence of a mass or masses in the kidneys. Renal lymphoma is a large cell lymphoma and affects the kidneys alone[26] 16-48% of the time.[17] The remaining cases have multicentric lymphoma, with a majority of cats having concurrent intestinal masses.[17] When lymphoma occurs in the kidneys of cats, it is always bilateral.[16]

CHAPTER 35 Kidneys and ureters

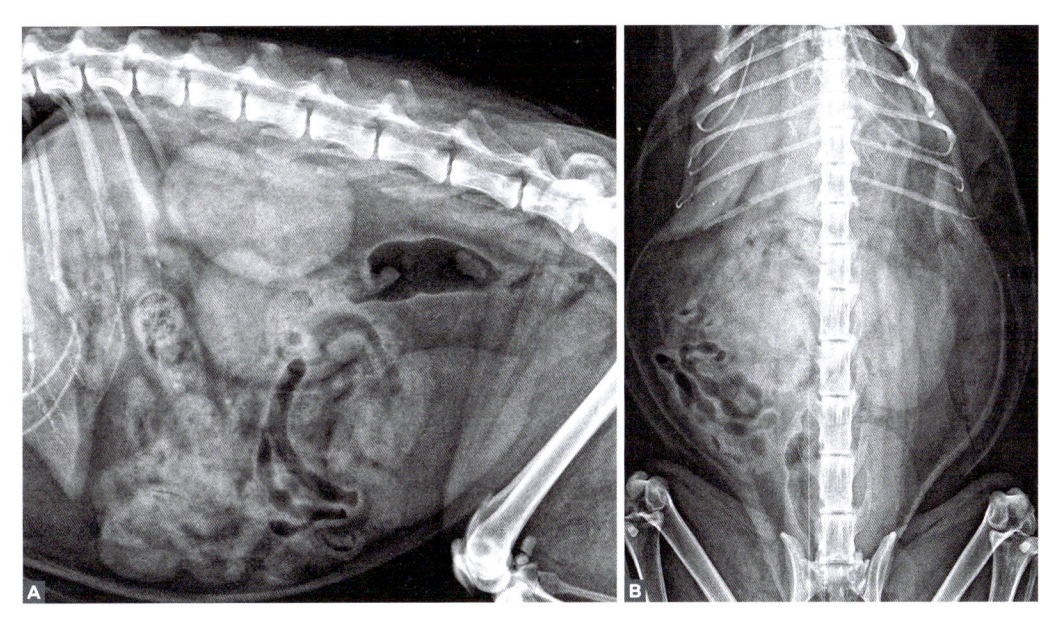

Fig. 35.11 Lateral and ventrodorsal radiographs of a 15-year-old castrated male Domestic shorthair cat with renal lymphoma. There is moderate symmetric enlargement of the kidneys, which are greater than three times the length of the L2 vertebra in the ventrodorsal projection, and are rounded.

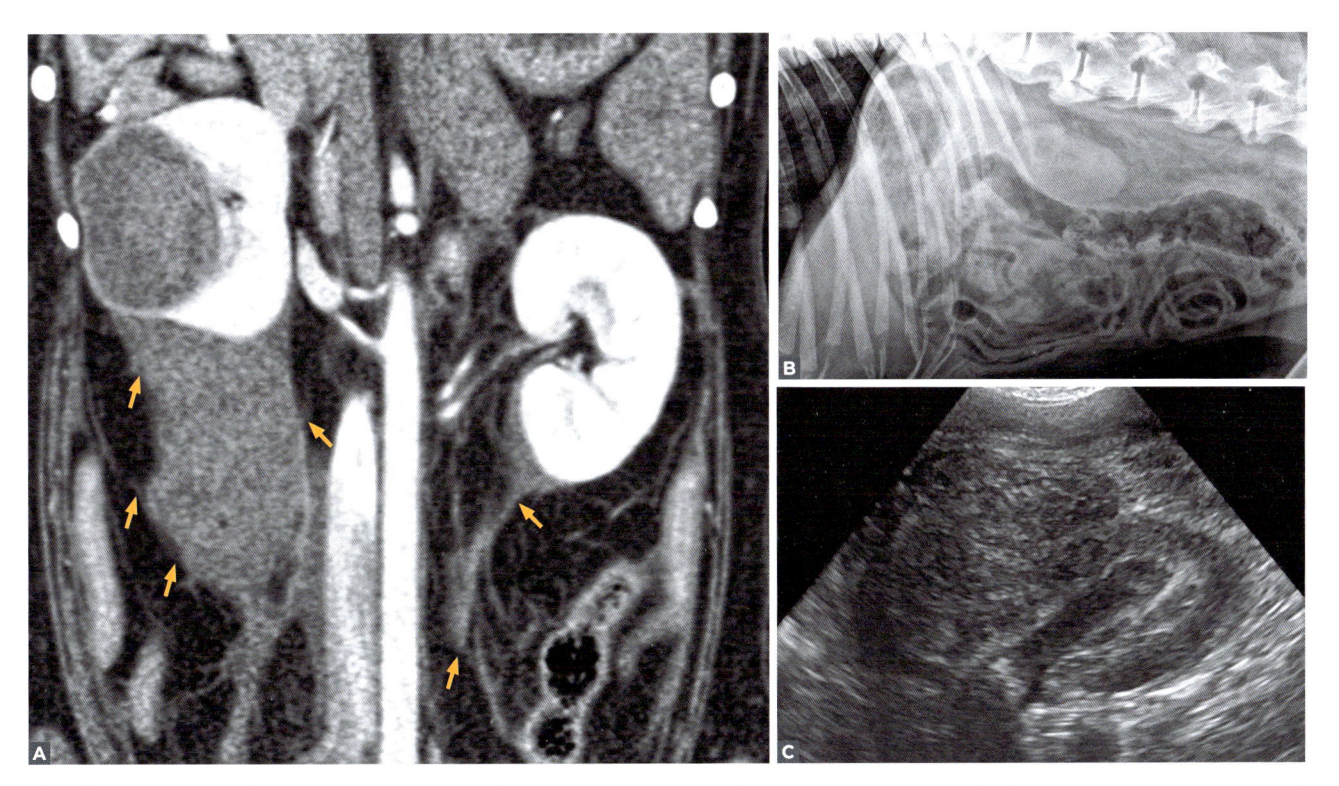

Fig. 35.12 (A) Dorsal plane contrast-enhanced CT, (B) lateral radiograph, and (C) dorsal plane ultrasound of a nine-year-old mixed breed dog with renal carcinoma. Note that the renal mass cannot be seen on radiographs. Wispy soft tissue opacity is present in the retroperitoneal space, indicating fluid in the fascial planes. Ultrasound confirmed the presence of a mass, and CT was used for surgical planning. CT confirms the presence of retroperitoneal fluid, which is non-enhanced material typically between 0-15 HU occupying the retroperitoneal space adjacent to the kidneys (arrows). CT also allows complete staging of the remainder of the abdominal organs. Laparoscopic nephrectomy was performed.

SECTION V ABDOMEN

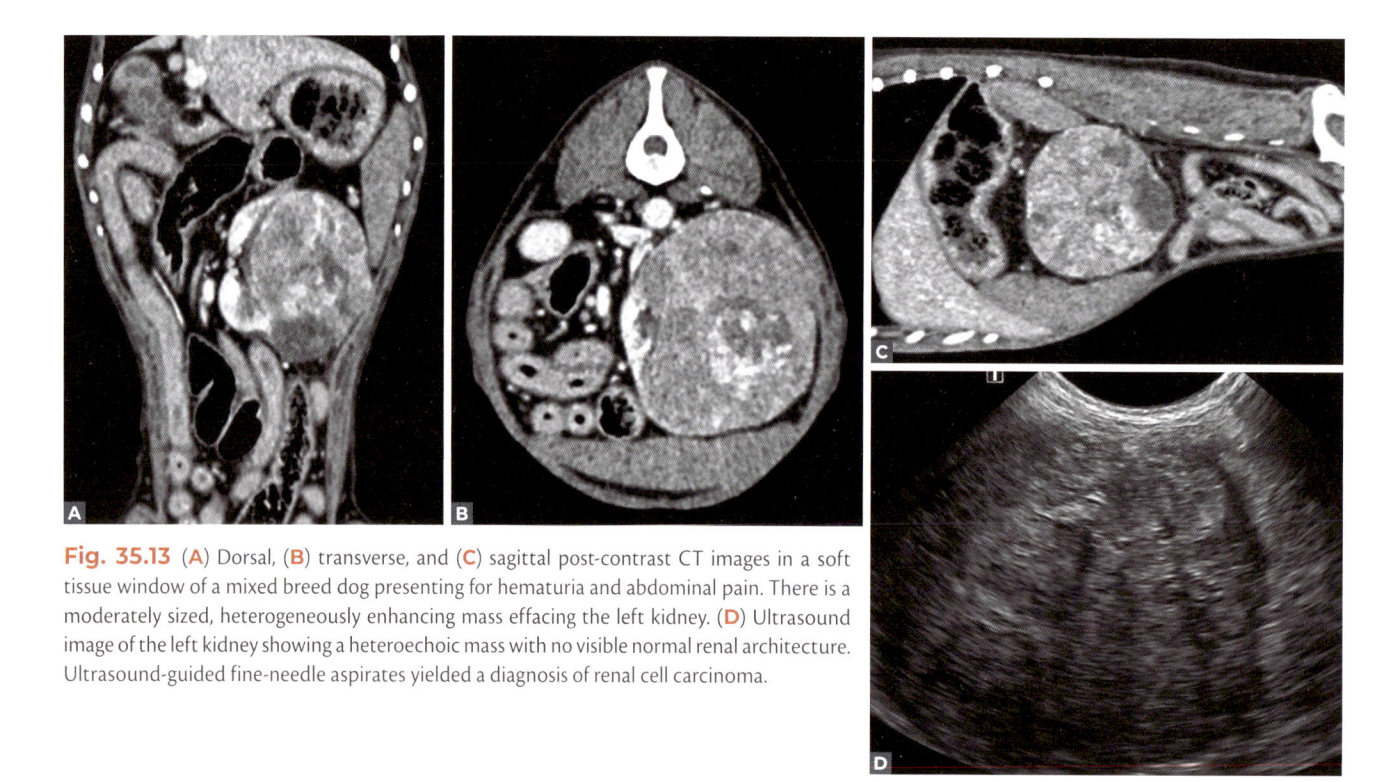

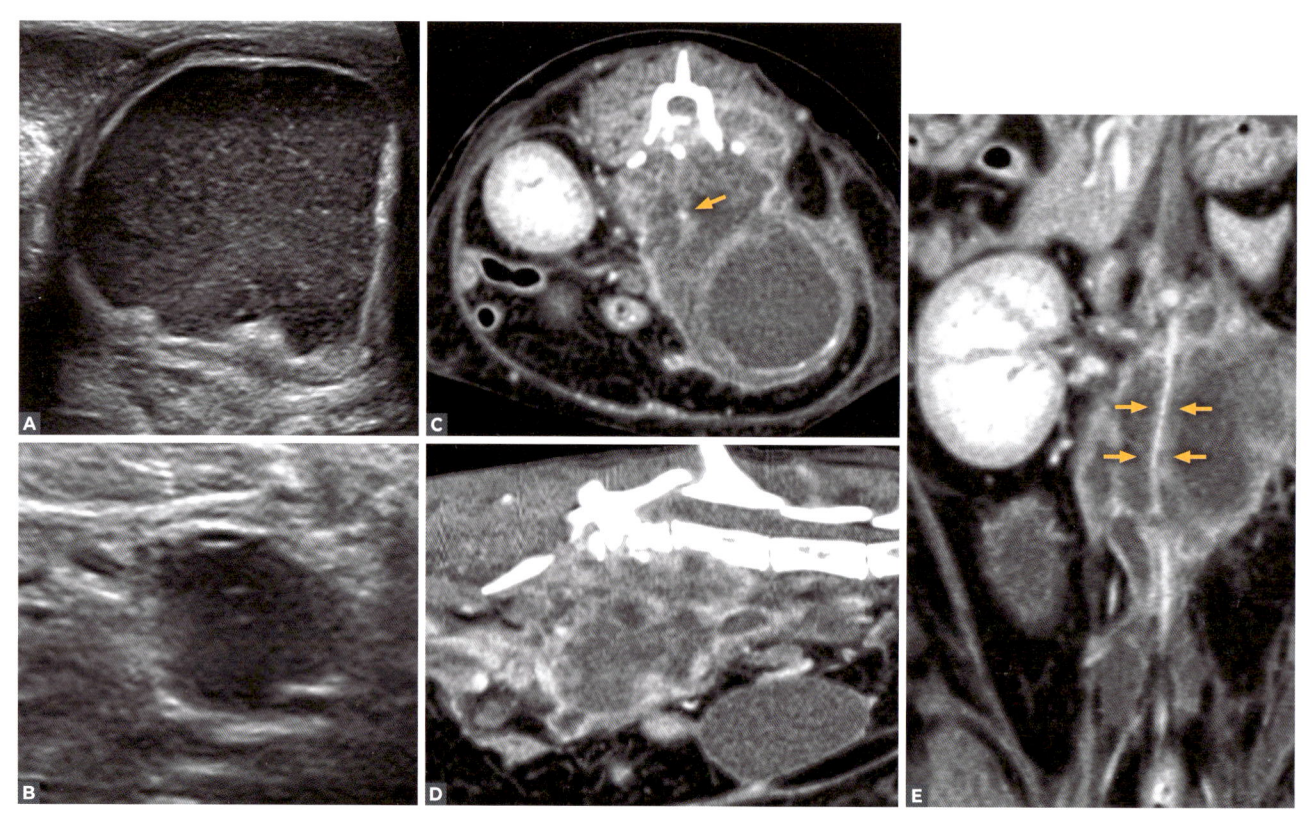

Fig. 35.13 (**A**) Dorsal, (**B**) transverse, and (**C**) sagittal post-contrast CT images in a soft tissue window of a mixed breed dog presenting for hematuria and abdominal pain. There is a moderately sized, heterogeneously enhancing mass effacing the left kidney. (**D**) Ultrasound image of the left kidney showing a heteroechoic mass with no visible normal renal architecture. Ultrasound-guided fine-needle aspirates yielded a diagnosis of renal cell carcinoma.

Fig. 35.14 (**A**, **B**) Ultrasound and (**C**, **D**, **E**) CT images of a two-year-old spayed female Domestic shorthair cat with renal squamous cell carcinoma. The patient presented with back pain and anorexia. Ultrasound identified a large fluid-distended left kidney with echogenic fluid within, what was suspected to be a severely dilated renal pelvis. (**B**) An additional tubular fluid-filled structure was seen extending into the caudal abdomen. The nature of this was unclear, possibly representing a dilated ureter. Inflammation and both peritoneal and retroperitoneal effusion were identified sonographically, and CT was elected to determine if the mass was resectable. (**C**, **D**) CT identified a large, cavitated left renal mass that invaded the vertebrae, and the tubular fluid-filled structure seen on ultrasound was confirmed to be an extension of the mass. (**E**) The mass effaced the caudal vena cava, which was no longer visible and caused marked compression of the aorta seen as a thin contrast medium-filled tubular structure extending through the center of the mass (arrows).

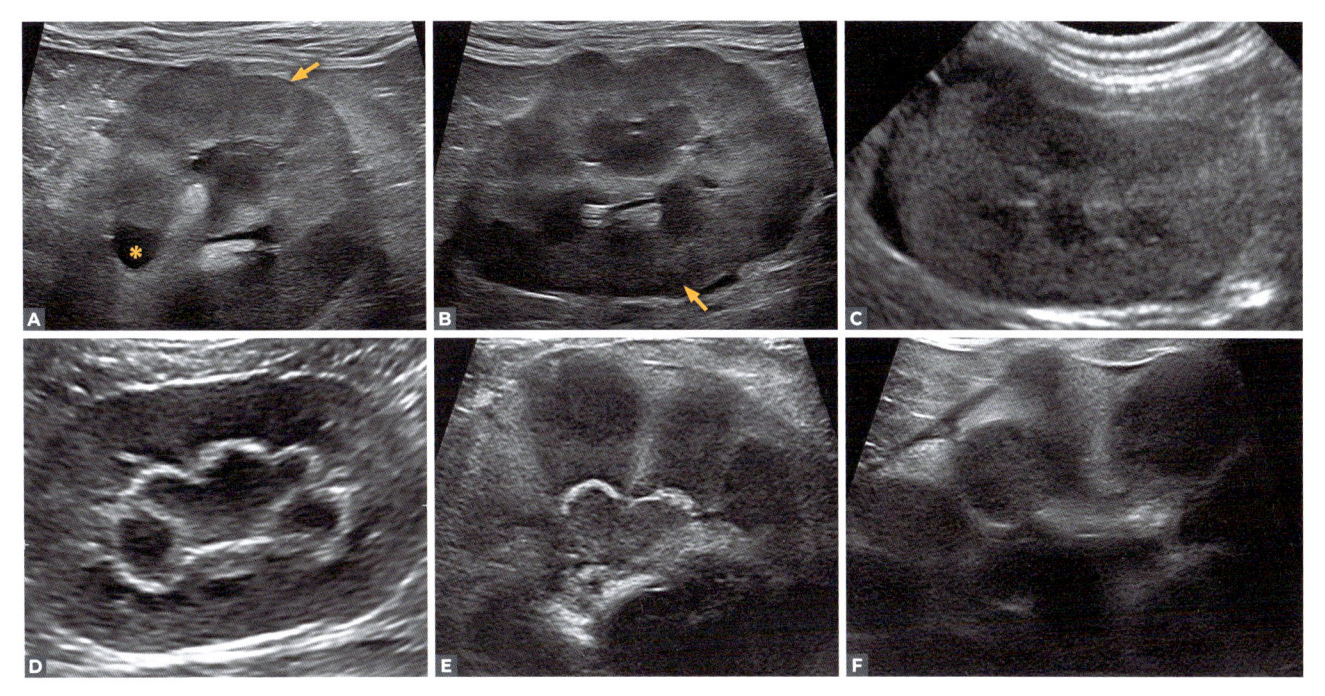

Fig. 35.15 Sonographic images of renal lymphoma in three cats. (**A**) Transverse and (**B**) longitudinal images of a cat with renal lymphoma. Note the thin non-uniform band of hypoechoic tissue around the kidney. This is a common feature of renal lymphoma. There is also a hypoechoic nodule (asterisk) which may reflect a complex cyst or parenchymal change in association with lymphoma. (**C**) Longitudinal ultrasound image that displays a larger volume of hypoechoic subcapsular tissue. (**D-F**) Progression of disease over the course of one month. (**D**) On initial presentation, the patient was diagnosed with gastrointestinal lymphoma, and the kidneys were abnormal with a thick medullary band present; however, they were normal in size (4 cm). (**E, F**) One month later, the patient had marked progression in clinical signs, and the kidneys were enlarged (5.8 to 6 cm). (**D, E**) The left kidney has a change in echogenicity and size with a combination of hypoechoic parenchymal nodules and the previously seen central medullary band. The right kidney shows the common subcapsular hypoechoic tissue and numerous parenchymal nodules.

Fig. 35.16 (**A**) Transverse and (**B**) longitudinal ultrasound images of an 11-year-old castrated male Domestic shorthair cat with FIP. The kidney has a similar appearance to some cases of renal lymphoma, and a thin peripheral subcapsular rim of hypoechoic tissue is present (**A**); there is a non-specific thin medullary band seen.

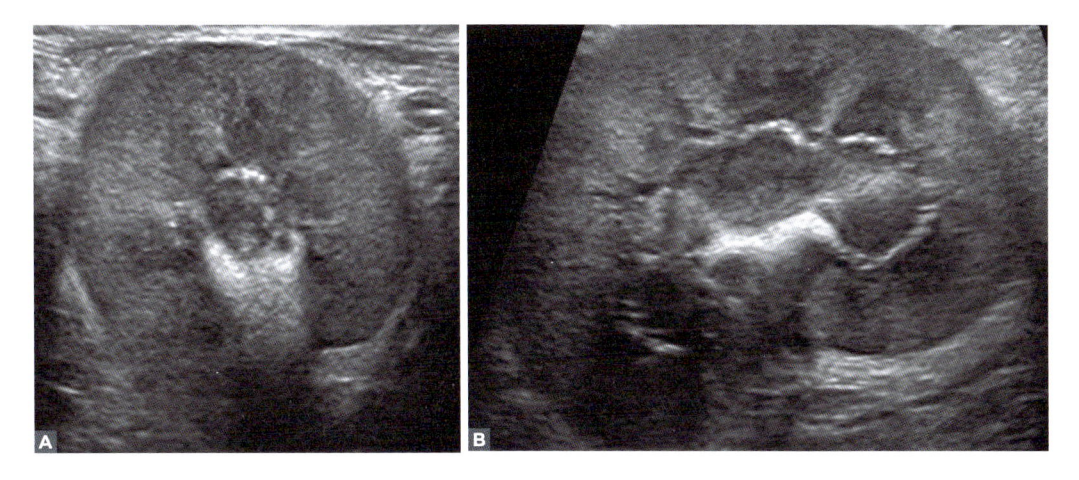

As previously stated, radiography cannot distinguish between causes of renomegaly. For example, radiographically, a nephroblastoma (**fig. 35.17**) cannot be differentiated from a cystadenocarcinoma (**fig. 35.18**). The sonographic and CT appearance is also similar across tumor types, and masses cannot be distinguished based on their sonographic or CT imaging features. However, in some instances, a combination of patient signalment and known tumor features can help differentiate tumors. Nephroblastomas are rare primary tumors of young dogs[18] presenting as large heteroechoic and often solid masses on ultrasound. Cystadenocarcinomas are tumor seen predominantly in German Shepherds and commonly contains numerous small cystic lesions (**fig. 35.18**). These patients can also present with dermatofibrosis.[19]

SECTION V ABDOMEN

Fig. 35.17 (A) Ventrodorsal and (B) lateral radiographs of a 1.5-year-old intact male dog presenting for polycythemia, weight loss, and a palpable abdominal mass. Radiographs identify a large mass that causes ventral displacement of the small intestine and is dorsally confluent with the right renal silhouette in the lateral projections. The mass occupies the right abdomen in the region of the kidney in the ventrodorsal projection (arrows). (C, D) Ultrasound confirms the presence of the mass, which was heterogeneously hyperechoic, expanding the caudal pole of the kidney. Fine-needle aspirates confirmed the mass as a nephroblastoma.

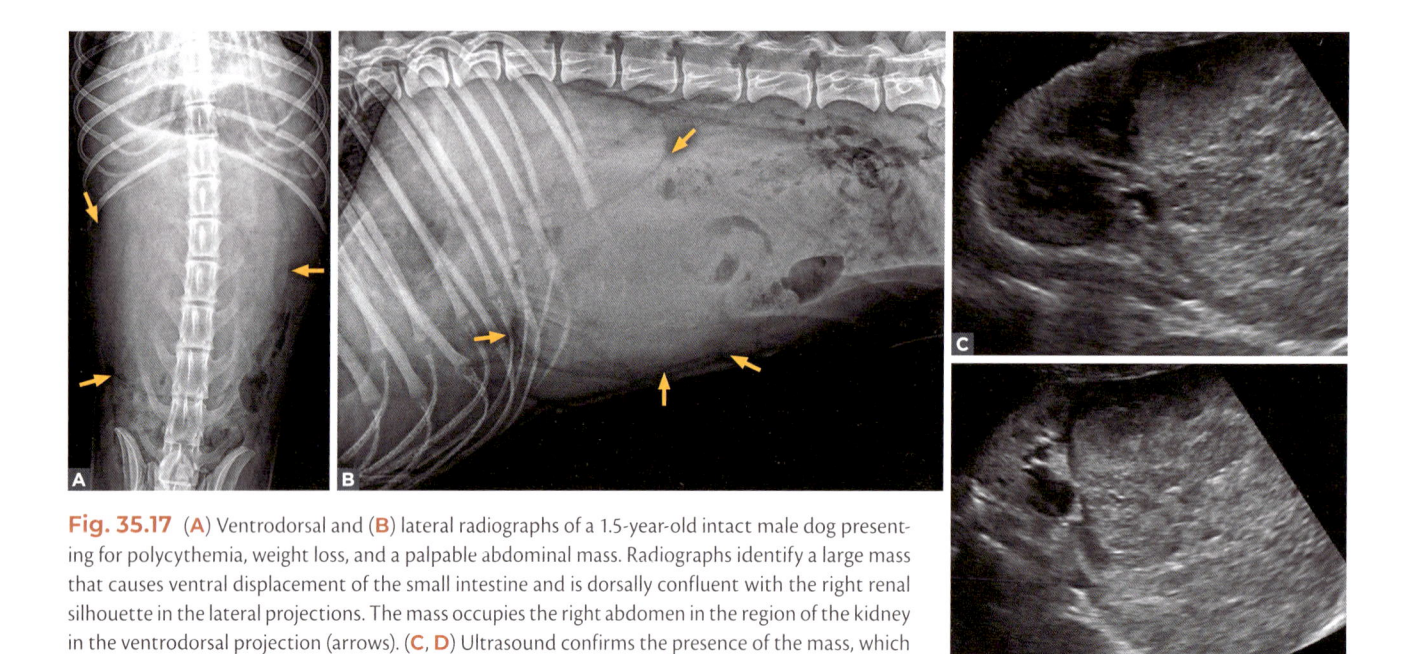

Fig. 35.18 (A) Left lateral, (B) ventrodorsal, and (C) right lateral radiographs of a young male German Shepherd dog presenting for an abdominal mass and nodular cutaneous lesions. The kidneys are enlarged, resulting in ventral and caudal displacement of the intestines. Ultrasound of the right (D, E) and left (F) kidneys confirms multiple cystic lesions throughout the right kidney with partial effacement of normal internal architecture and a large cyst and pyelectasia of the left kidney. Given the breed and presenting complaints, a presumptive diagnosis of renal cystadenocarcinoma and nodular dermatophytosis was made. Images courtesy of Dr. Gabriela Seiler.

CHAPTER 35 Kidneys and ureters

Hydronephrosis

The normal renal pelvis is usually not seen but may be visible as a thin crescent-shaped structure filled with anechoic fluid, measuring up to 2 mm on ultrasound.[20] Mild dilation of the pelvis (up to 2-3 mm) is known as pyelectasia and can often occur secondary to chronic renal disease[17] (fig. 35.19A), IV fluid administration, diuresis, or other causes of polyuria such as hyperadrenocorticism.[20] Partial obstruction of the ureter can also lead to pyelectasia (fig. 25.19B).

Hydronephrosis can be classified as obstructive and non-obstructive. Obstructive hydronephrosis occurs secondary to an impediment to urine flow through the ureters. In cats, this is most commonly calculi. Ultrasound is the primary modality for the identification of obstructive hydronephrosis in small animals. Ultrasound can identify the distended renal pelvis (figs. 35.20 and 35.21) and can

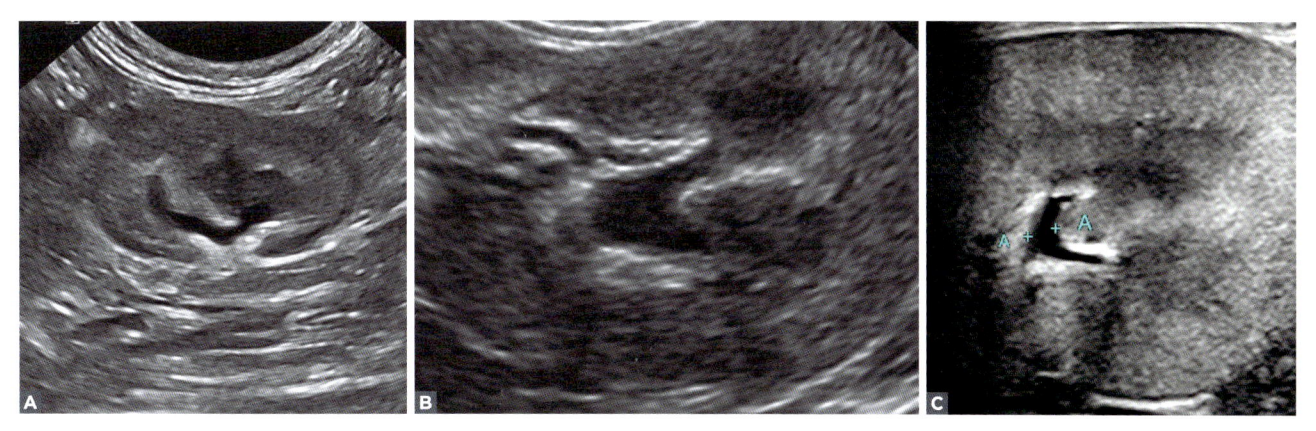

Fig. 35.19 (A) Longitudinal ultrasound of a nine-year-old cat presenting for decreased appetite, mild anemia (HCT 29%), and mild azotemia. The kidney is small (2.48 cm long), with loss of corticomedullary definition, and the renal pelvis is dilated with anechoic fluid. (B) Transverse ultrasound of a seven-year-old Cocker Spaniel with moderate pyelectasia from partial ureteral obstruction secondary to an accumulation of hemorrhage in the urinary bladder resulting in ureteral obstruction. Hemorrhage was due to abnormal platelet function. (C) Transverse ultrasound image of a two-year-old female Maine Coon presenting for pyometra. There is mild pyelectasia (2 mm), loss of corticomedullary definition, and hyperechoic cortical speckling.

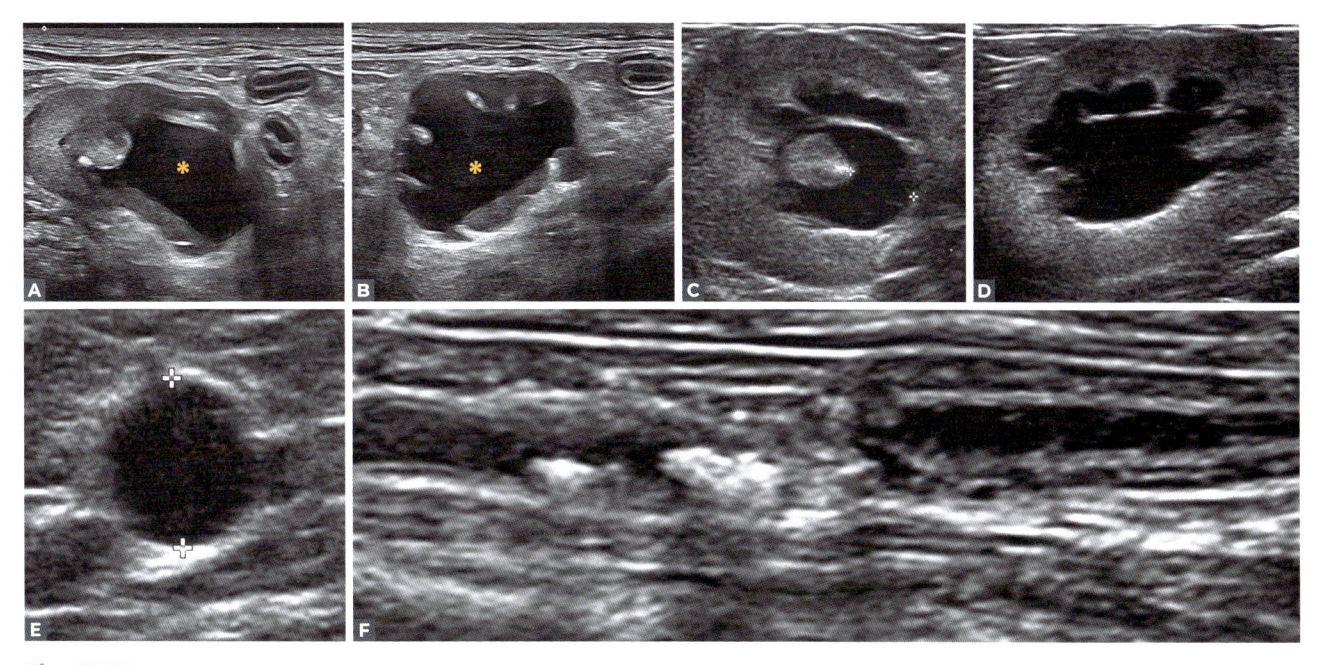

Fig. 35.20 Ultrasound images of two cats with obstructive hydronephrosis. (A) Transverse and (B) dorsal plane ultrasound images of a cat with renal pelvic sediment and calculi resulting in complete obstruction. The renal pelvis (asterisk) is markedly distended. (C-F) A second cat with ureterolithiasis has moderate distention of the renal pelvis up to 8 mm (calipers, C). The renal pelvic dilation is visible in both the transverse (C) and longitudinal planes (D). The proximal ureter is dilated to 9 mm (E), and the ureter tapers to a point where it contains numerous hyperechoic foci compatible with ureteral calculi (F).

SECTION V ABDOMEN

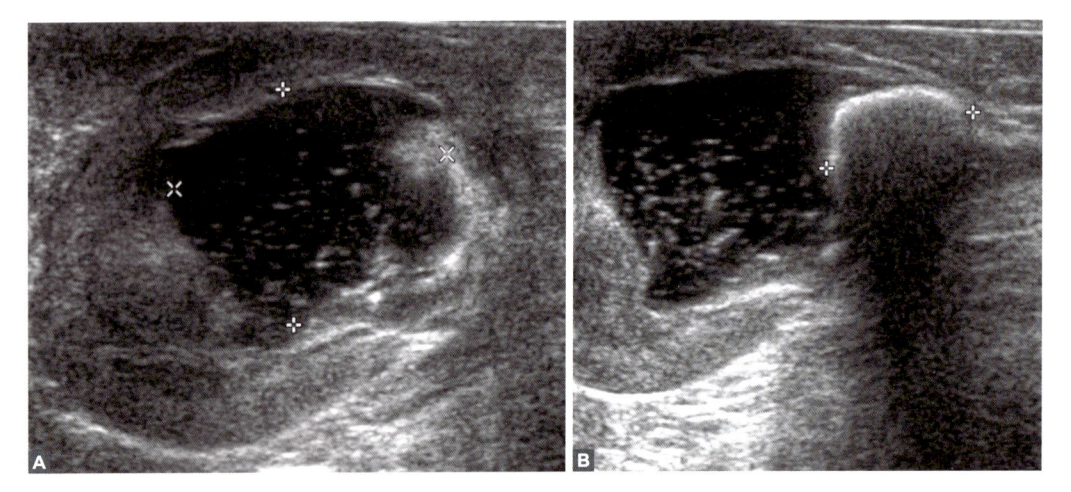

Fig. 35.21 Longitudinal ultrasound images of a five-year-old female spayed Shih Tzu with a large nephrolith and secondary hydronephrosis. The urine in the renal pelvis is echogenic that may be secondary to hemorrhage or pyuria. In this case, pyelocentesis confirmed pyelonephritis.

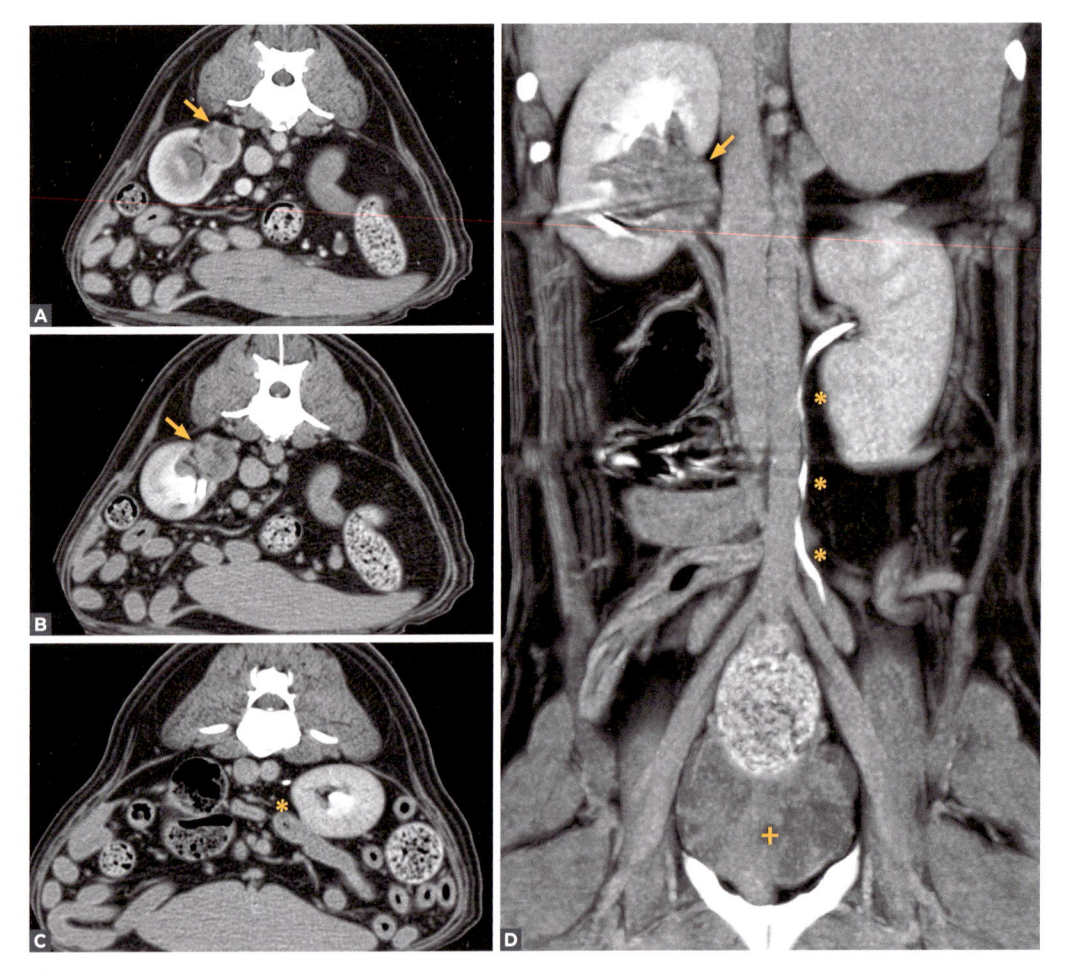

Fig. 35.22 (**A**, **B**, **C**) Transverse and (**D**) dorsal maximal intensity projection CT images in a soft tissue window of a 12-year-old intact male Old English Sheepdog presenting for hematuria. (**A**) A rounded mass (arrow) is seen in the one-minute post-contrast image at the level of the right kidney. (**B**, **D**) Following diuretic administration (furosemide), right ureteral obstruction is confirmed where contrast medium pools in the right renal pelvis but does not enter the right ureter. (**C**, **D**) Conversely, the left ureter (asterisk) remains patent and normal in size. In the dorsal plane image, prostatomegaly is visible (+). The prostate is bulbous, heterogeneous in enhancement, and occupies most of the pelvic canal. This patient was diagnosed with benign prostatic hyperplasia and urothelial cell carcinoma.

often find the cause. Ureteral tumors can also cause hydronephrosis (**fig. 35.22**). Tumors in the urinary bladder which impinge on the ureteral papillae can result in obstruction and hydronephrosis. Chronic, severe hydronephrosis can result in complete loss of the renal parenchyma with a residual thin rim of tissue surrounding a severely dilated balloon-like renal pelvis, which may eventually reduce in size (**fig. 35.23**).

A renal pelvis measuring over 1.3 cm is consistent with obstructive hydronephrosis.[20] However, recent work has shown that cats with ureteral obstruction can have small renal pelvises despite complete obstruction confirmed with pyelography.[21,22]

Polycystic kidney disease

Polycystic kidney disease is an autosomal dominant inherited disorder[27] that primarily affects Persian cats. However, other breeds are affected, including Exotic Shorthair, Himalayan, British Shorthair, American Shorthair, Burmilla, Ragdoll, Maine Coon, Neva Masquerade, and Chartreux.[28] The kidneys can be enlarged and have deformation of the renal borders or radiographs, but the kidneys usually retain a normal shape but may appear normal. Ultrasound[27] (**fig. 35.24**) or genetic markers are required for a diagnosis. Sonographically, a single cyst in a Persian cat <15 months of age is compatible with autosomal dominant polycystic kidney disease (AKPKD). Cysts progress over time and, in older cats, a greater number of cysts must be found to make a diagnosis of AKPKD. That is, two or more cysts should be present in Persian cats between 16-32 months, three or more cysts between 33-49

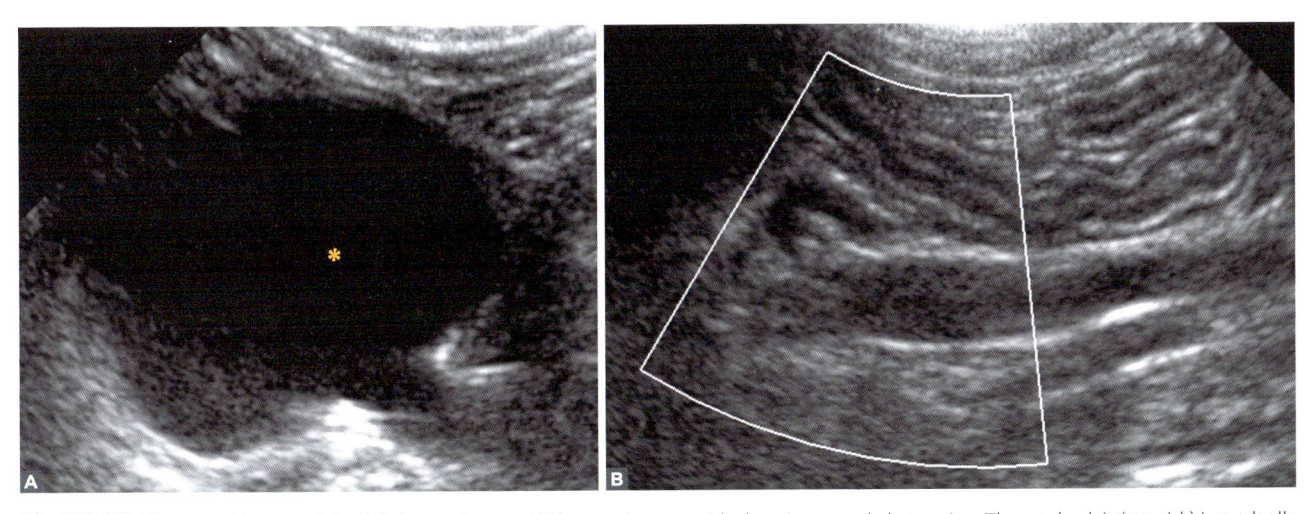

Fig. 35.23 Ultrasound images of the (**A**) right kidney and (**B**) ureter in a cat with chronic ureteral obstruction. The renal pelvis (asterisk) is markedly dilated, with only a thin rim of tissue remaining. Despite this, the kidney can be recognized based on its anatomic location and characteristic shape. (**B**) The right ureter can be distinguished from blood vessels with color Doppler interrogation as it does not demonstrate any flow.

Fig. 35.24 (**A**) Longitudinal and (**B**) transverse ultrasound images of a cat with polycystic kidney disease. There are numerous fluid-filled cystic lesions within the renal cortex that contain variably echogenic fluid. Overall, there is loss of corticomedullary definition, increased renal echogenicity, and mild plyelectasia (**B**).

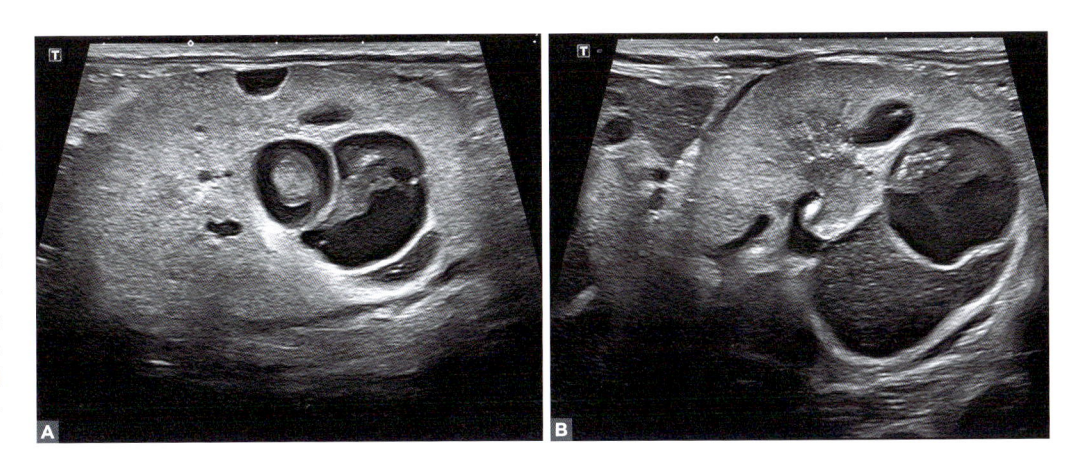

SECTION V ABDOMEN

months, and four or more cysts in Persian cats 50-66 months to warrant a diagnosis of AKPKD. Polycystic kidney disease should not be confused with degenerative renal cysts that occur commonly in dogs and cats. These are typically smaller and less often expand the renal margins. As with polycystic kidney disease, renal cysts are readily apparent on ultrasound (**figs. 35.25** and **35.26B**) and CT (**fig. 35.26A**, **35.26C**, and **35.26D**). Renal cysts range in size from a few millimeters in diameter, which do not expand cortical margins to larger expansile lesions that can disrupt a large portion of the kidney and sometimes lead to clinical signs such as abdominal pain.

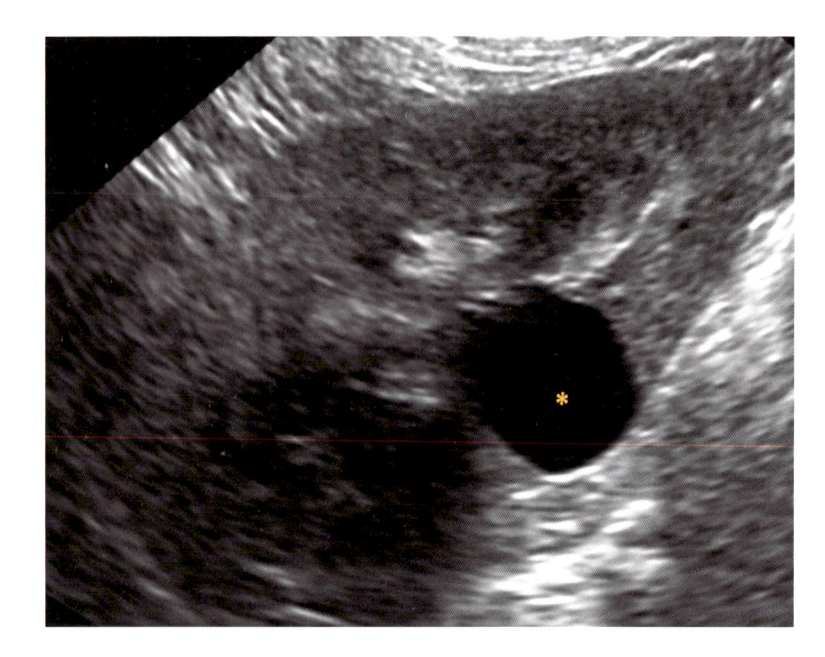

Fig. 35.25 Longitudinal ultrasound image of the right kidney in a Beagle with a simple cortical cyst (asterisk).

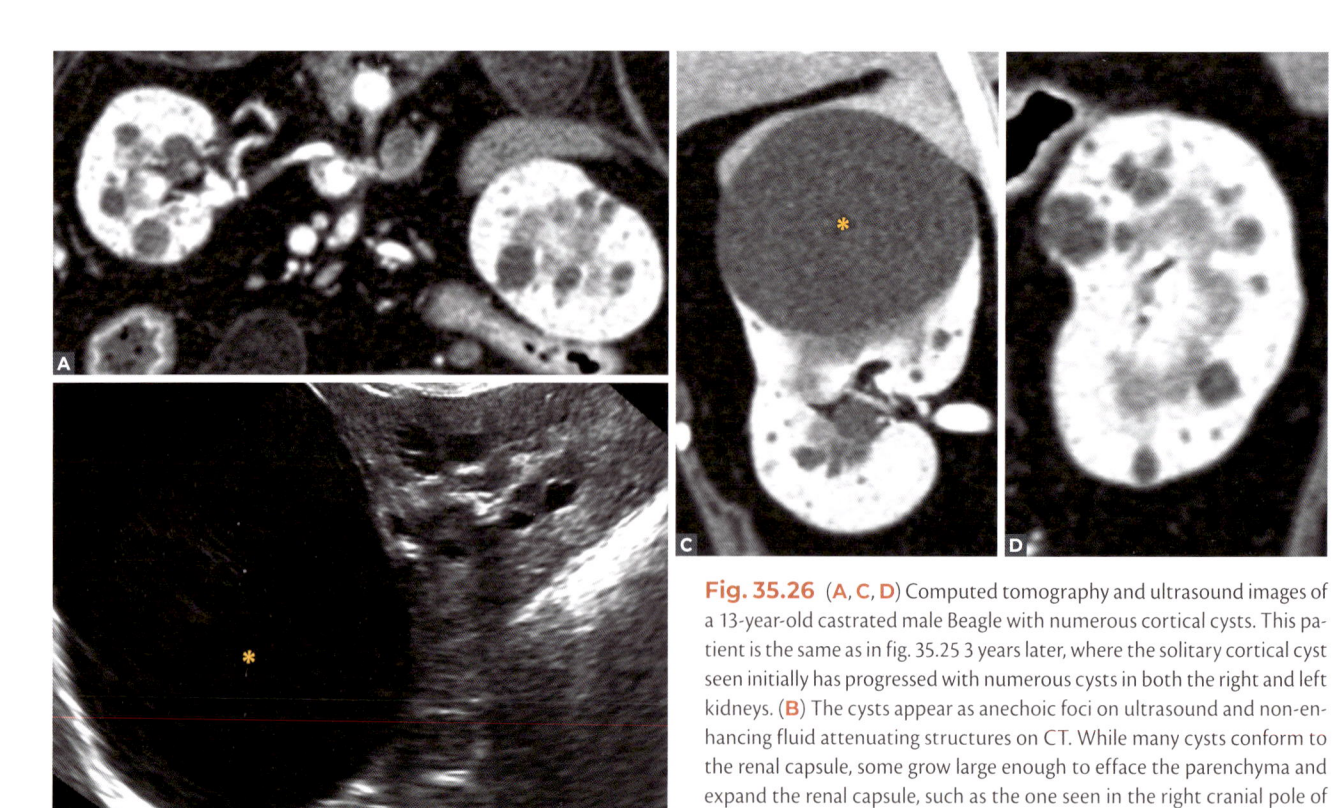

Fig. 35.26 (**A, C, D**) Computed tomography and ultrasound images of a 13-year-old castrated male Beagle with numerous cortical cysts. This patient is the same as in fig. 35.25 3 years later, where the solitary cortical cyst seen initially has progressed with numerous cysts in both the right and left kidneys. (**B**) The cysts appear as anechoic foci on ultrasound and non-enhancing fluid attenuating structures on CT. While many cysts conform to the renal capsule, some grow large enough to efface the parenchyma and expand the renal capsule, such as the one seen in the right cranial pole of the right kidney (asterisk).

Perinephric pseudocyst

Perinephric pseudocyst is uncommon and presents as fluid accumulation between the renal capsule and cortex. Perinephric pseudocysts occur most commonly in older cats, usually with concurrent CKD, and may be unilateral or bilateral.[33] To the author's knowledge, these are exceedingly rare in dogs and have only been reported twice.[34,35] The pseudocysts may be very large and are often palpable, and clinical signs are related to the large volume of the pseudocyst(s) and CKD. These cannot be differentiated by palpation or radiography (**figs. 35.27** and **35.27B**) from other causes of renomegaly. Ultrasound is the recommended imaging modality that can identify the normal or degenerative kidney surrounded by a fluid-filled sac (**fig. 35.27C**).

Acute toxic nephropathy

Toxic nephropathies may lead to mild renal enlargement with smooth margins and increase in echogenicity.[36] Acute nephropathy can occur secondary to toxins such as ethylene glycol (**fig. 35.28**), which has a near pathognomonic appearance of markedly increased cortical and medullary echogenicity.[37] Other acute nephropathies, either toxic or infectious, can have a variable appearance but often still include evidence of renal enlargement and increases in renal echogenicity (**fig. 35.29**). Acute toxic nephropathy may also cause perinephric effusion.

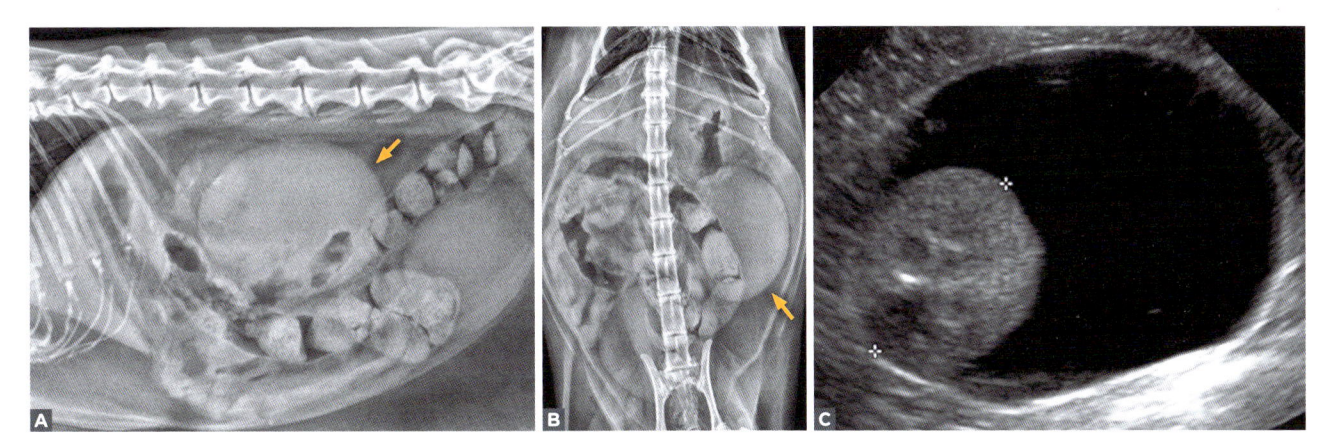

Fig. 35.27 (**A**) Lateral and (**B**) ventrodorsal radiographs and (**C**) corresponding ultrasound image of a cat with a perinephric pseudocyst. Note the severely enlarged left kidney radiographically (arrow) that corresponds with a small kidney sonographically surrounded (calipers) by a large anechoic fluid pocket. This case demonstrates the insensitivity of radiographs to the underlying cause of renomegaly in dogs and cats. The right kidney shows multiple calculi in the pelvic diverticula. Images courtesy of Dr. Alex zur Linden.

Fig. 35.28 Longitudinal image of a kidney acquired from point-of-care ultrasound in a patient presenting in anuric renal failure secondary to ethylene glycol toxicity. Notice the marked hyperechogenicity of the renal cortex and central aspect of the renal medulla. A linear hyperintensity is present at the level of the renal pelvis compatible with nephrolithiasis. Blood gas identified a high anion gap metabolic acidosis and a lactate value too high to read due to interaction with ethylene glycol on the radiometer. Calcium oxalate monohydrate crystals were identified on urinalysis. Image courtesy of Dr. Patricia Biello.

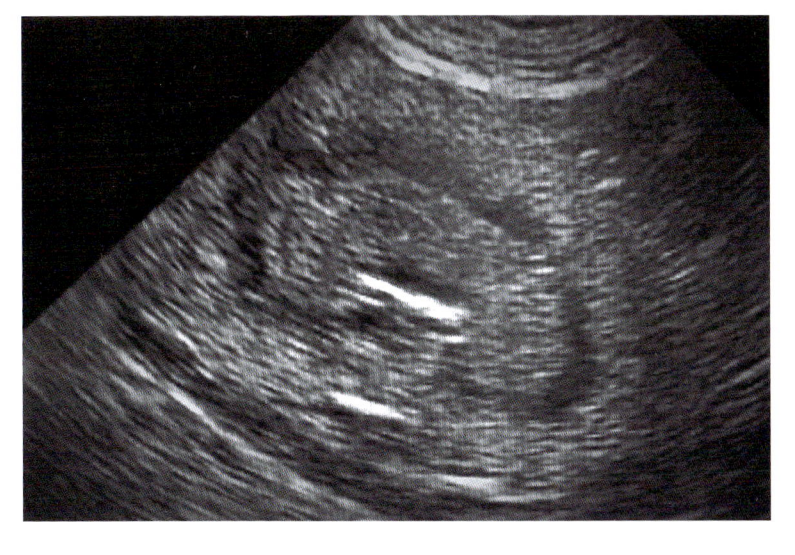

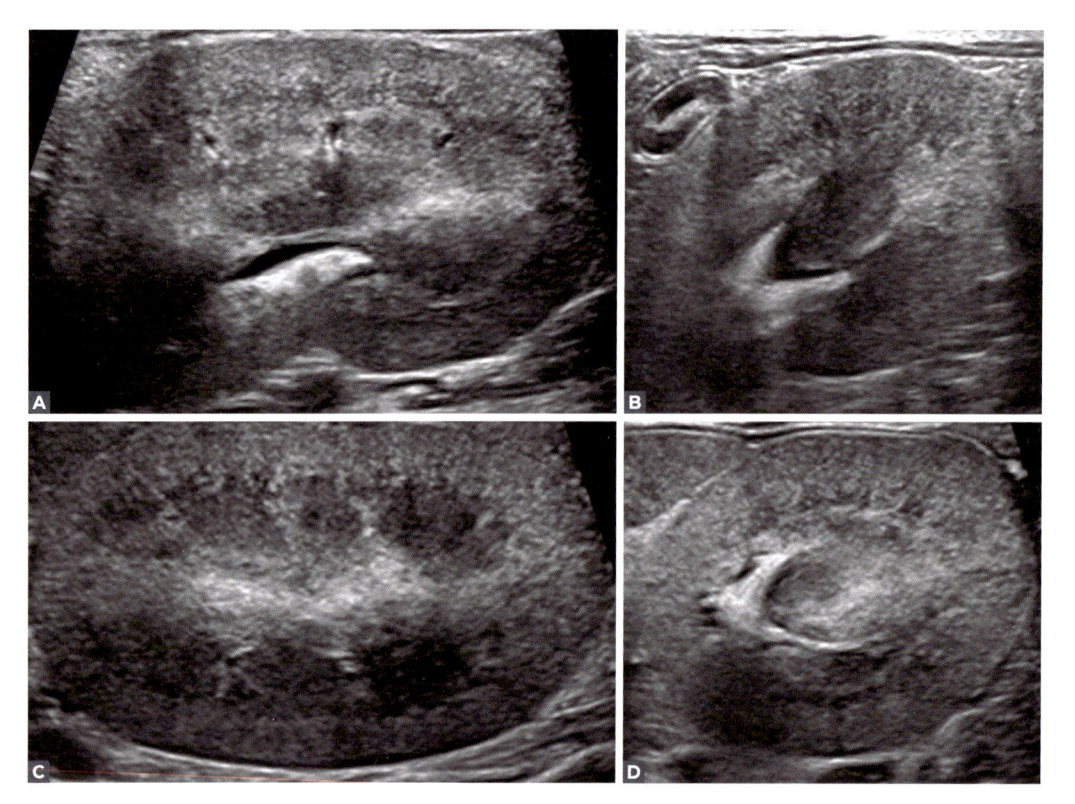

Fig. 35.29 Ultrasound images of the right (A, B) and left (C, D) kidneys in a one-year-old mixed breed dog presenting for acute onset of azotemia. The kidneys are large, with echogenicity of the cortex and medulla characterized by hyperechoic streaks and reduced corticomedullary definition. The patient was diagnosed with acute nephropathy of unknown etiology, with toxic or infectious etiologies being most likely. Mild right pyelectasia is present.

Renal infection

Infections of the kidneys are most commonly bacterial. However, both fungal[38] and parasitic etiologies have been reported. Bacterial infection of the kidney (figs. 35.21 and 35.30) is most often ascending and results in either pyelonephritis (inflammation of the renal pelvis and adjacent parenchyma) or pyonephrosis (sloughing or epithelium and inflammatory cells into a dilated renal pelvis). Sonographic features associated with pyelonephritis include pyelectasia, ureteral dilation, and decreased corticomedullary definition.[39,40] In dogs with pyonephrosis, ultrasound findings include increased echogenicity of the fluid in the renal pelvis, either entirely occupying the space or creating a fluid line.[41]

Parasitic infection of the kidney is typically associated with the giant kidney worm, *Dioctophyme renale* (fig. 35.31). This nematode has a worldwide distribution being endemic in South America[42-44] and having reports of cases reported in Canada[45] and Europe.[46] The infection typically occurs in the right kidney and can be identified as ring-like structures with an echogenic wall and anechoic center on ultrasound and a hyperdense wall and hypodense center on CT.[44] Parasites can also be free within the peritoneal cavity but are less commonly seen on ultrasound or CT.[44]

Calculi

Radiographs are often used as a screening tool for mineralization in the urinary tract. The presence of mineralization, while abnormal, does not always correlate with clinical signs. On ultrasound, nephroliths appear as hyperechoic foci in the renal pelvis that can cause distal acoustic shadowing (fig. 35.21). These foci can sometimes be confirmed as mineral by the use of color Doppler, which results in a twinkling artifact (fig. 35.32).

Mild mineralization in the kidneys can be seen as speckling (figs. 35.5 and 35.6) in either the cortex or peridiverticular tissues.

CHAPTER 35 Kidneys and ureters

Fig. 35.30 (**A**) Longitudinal and (**B**) transverse ultrasound images of a dog with left-sided hydronephrosis secondary to acute pyelonephritis. Echogenic material accumulates within a markedly distended renal pelvis (arrows).

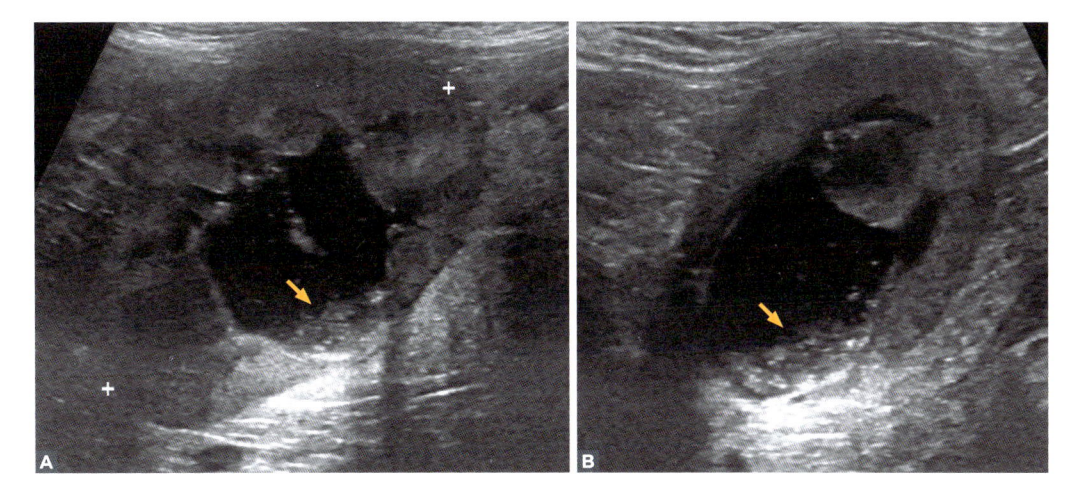

Fig. 35.31 (**A**) Longitudinal ultrasound images of an eight-month-old Golden Retriever with a right-sided infection of *Dioctophyme renale* (giant kidney worm) and a normal left kidney (**B**). Large tubular structures efface the right renal parenchyma that is compatible with the kidney worm *in situ* within the shell of the right kidney. (**C**, **D**) Computed tomography images of a seven-year-old mixed breed dog that also had a right-sided infection of *D. renale*. Similar to ultrasound images, the worm is visible as a peripherally hyperattenuating thin rim and central soft tissue attenuating material. The right kidney has lost the normal architecture compared to the normal left kidney.

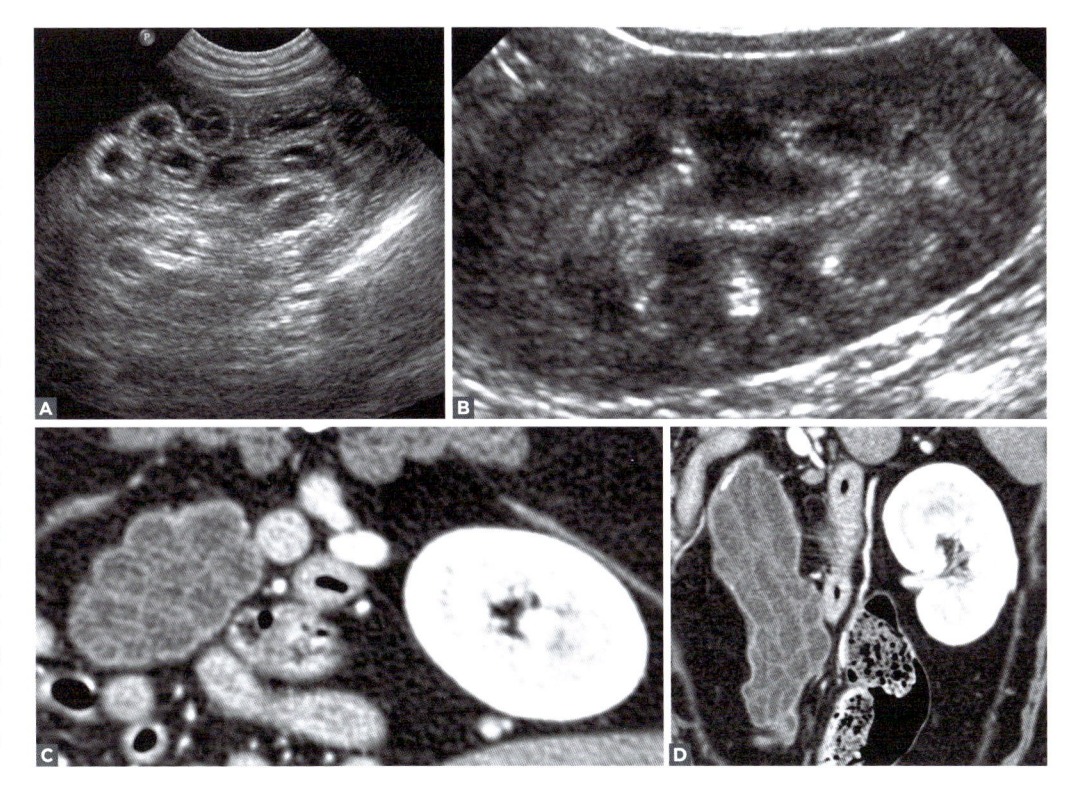

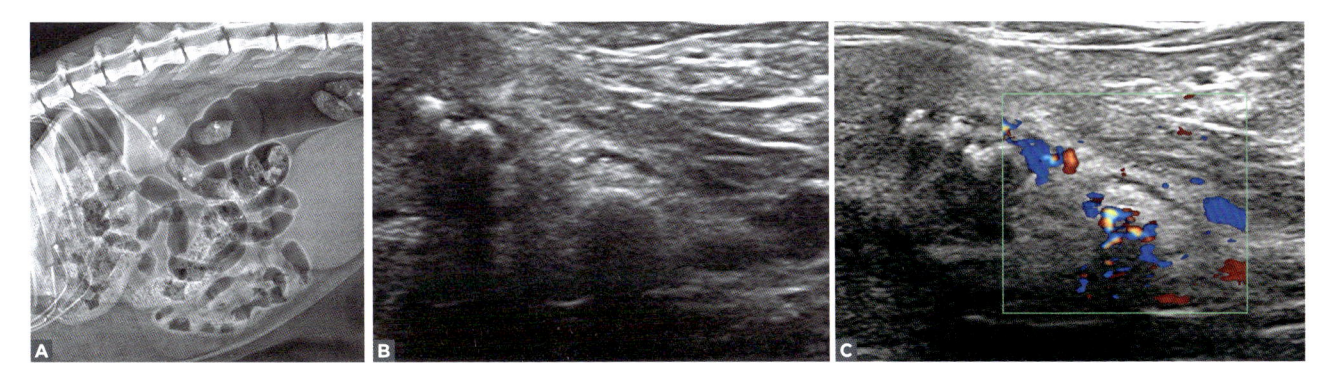

Fig. 35.32 Nephroliths and ureteroliths in an 11-year-old spayed female Domestic shorthair cat. (**A**) The calculi are visible on radiographs. While not clinically relevant in this case, Doppler interrogation can help to confirm the presence of mineralization if there is a clinical concern between mineralization and any other cause of hyperechogenicity on ultrasound. (**C**) A twinkle artifact appears as a consistent, intense Doppler signal over the hyperechoic focus where there should be no Doppler signal.

Ureters

Normal ureters are not visible on radiographs and are usually not visible with ultrasound. As with much of the urinary tract, a linear high-frequency ultrasound probe provides the most value in imaging ureters. The wall of the ureter can be identified with a linear high-frequency probe (**fig. 35.20F**), whereas it is not usually visible using lower frequency probes (**fig. 35.20E**). The ureters are normally very thin (~1 mm in external diameter) tubular structures that can occasionally be traced from the renal pelvis to the bladder in smaller patients. Peristaltic waves can sometimes be identified along the length of the ureters. The ureters can be traced more easily with CT following contrast medium administration. Many diseases of the ureter, which will be discussed, result in dilation of the ureter. Mild dilation is sometimes referred to as ureterectasia, and marked dilation known as hydroureter.

Ectopia

Ectopic ureters are a congenital malformation where one or both ureters do not open into the bladder in the correct position. This aberrant ureteral course can either be extramural, that is, the entire ureter is outside the bladder wall, or intramural, tunneling through the bladder wall and typically insert in the urethra or sometimes the vagina.[47] Ectopic ureters are more common in female dogs than males and exceedingly rare in cats.[48] Diagnosis is often challenging and usually requires a combination of excretory urography, CT urography,[49] or ultrasound.[50] The administration of furosemide (1 mg/kg) either intravenously or subcutaneously can aid in the sonographic identification of ureteral jets (**fig. 35.33** and **video 35.1**) in dogs.[51] Ureteral jets are visible if there is a difference in the specific gravity of urine in the bladder and urine delivered via the ureters. They may also be seen in patients receiving intravenous fluids, patients sedated with alpha-2 agonists, which cause diuresis, and if there is suspended echogenic material in the bladder lumen. If two ureteral jets can be identified in the bladder, an ectopic ureter is very unlikely. If only a single jet is identified, this increases suspicion of an ectopic ureter, but intravenous urography or CT urography are needed for confirmation.

Ectopic ureters can also occur in conjunction with ureteroceles, a cystic dilation of the distal ureter. These can be either intravesicular (within the bladder) or ectopic (any portion within the urethra).[52] Diagnosis is often made with sonography (**figs. 35. 34** and **35.35**), where a thin, soft tissue membrane often creates a rounded fluid-filled structure within the bladder or urethra.

VIDEO 35.1

Ureteral Jets. Transverse sonography at the level of the ureterovesicular junctions showing ureteral jets. In this patient jets are visible without Doppler applied and are more obvious after Doppler interrogation.

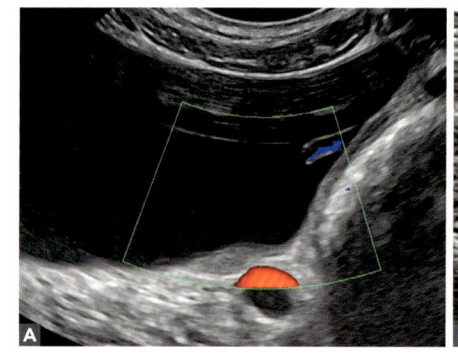

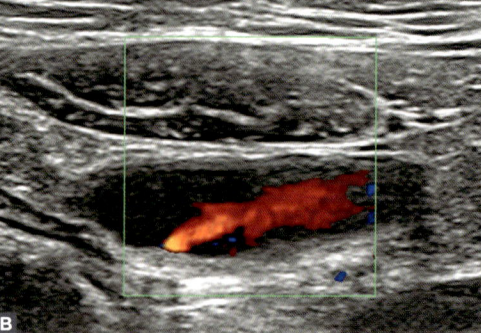

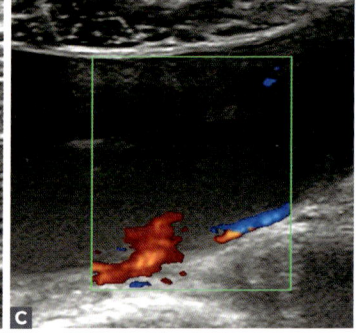

Fig. 35.33 Normal ureteral jets in three dogs following administration of 1 mg/kg of furosemide intravenously. Doppler interrogation can be used to identify urine flowing into the urinary bladder. Images acquired transverse to the urinary bladder at the level of the trigone with the right side of the patient towards the left of the image. (**A**, **B**) Often only one ureteral jet is seen at a time, and the region must be evaluated for a few minutes with slight variations in transducer positioning. The direction of the urine flow should be taken into account. In these examples, red is towards the transducer, and blue is away from the transducer. The ultrasound transducer is angled such that the left ureteral jet is oriented away from the transducer, and the left ureteral jet is seen as a pulsating blue streak. The right ureteral jet is a pulsing red streak. (**C**) Both ureteral jets can be seen at the same time.

CHAPTER 35 Kidneys and ureters

Trauma

External or penetrating trauma may cause ureteral transection or avulsion of the ureter from the kidney or bladder and results in retroperitoneal leakage of urine. Urine empties into the retroperitoneal space and causes inflammation (**fig. 35.36**). Radiographically this can appear as streaking or wispy soft tissue opacity in the retroperitoneal space, loss of retroperitoneal contrast, and expansion of the retroperitoneal space. Complete avulsion of the ureter from the bladder may allow urine to leak into the peritoneal space. The major differential diagnosis for traumatic ureteral avulsion and uroretroperitoneum is hemorrhage, which is more common. Ultrasound can be used for guided sampling to determine the type of fluid. Excretory urography can be performed to identify contrast medium leakage into the retroperitoneal space and retraction of an avulsed ureter. Contrast-enhanced CT can allow identification of the ureter and trace its course to confirm avulsion.

Neoplasia

Carcinoma is the most common tumor of the ureters and can either occur primarily in the ureter (**fig. 35.22**), extend proximally from the bladder, or into the ureter from the kidney (**fig. 35.37**). Imaging findings are non-specific and often show a small mass on either ultrasound or CT. Ureteral tumors are not typically identified on radiographs.

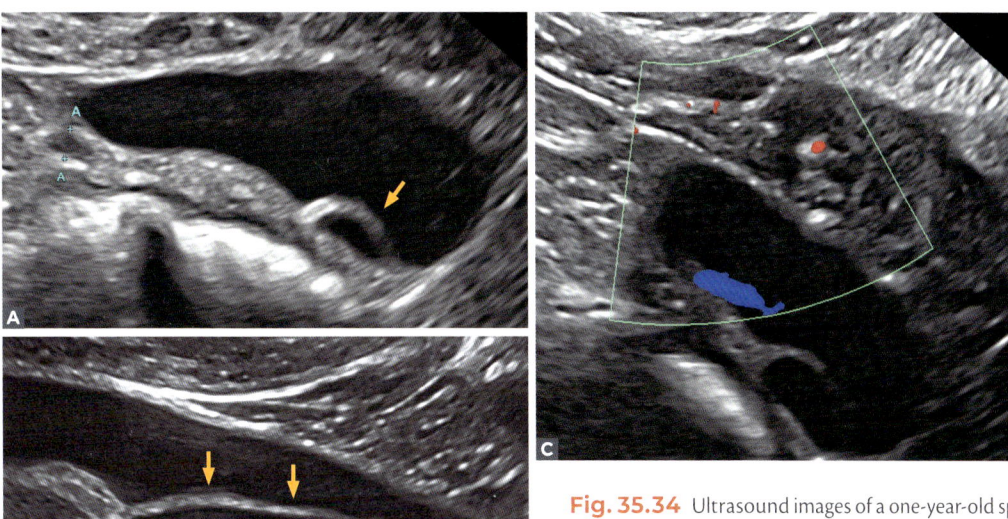

Fig. 35.34 Ultrasound images of a one-year-old spayed female Labrador Retriever with left ureteral ectopia. The right ureter has a normal insertion (calipers in **A**). The left ureter (arrows) is moderately, uniformly dilated and seen tunneling through the bladder wall. Its insertion was confirmed in the distal urethra via cystoscopy. (**C**) A normal right ureteral jet was seen following furosemide administration.

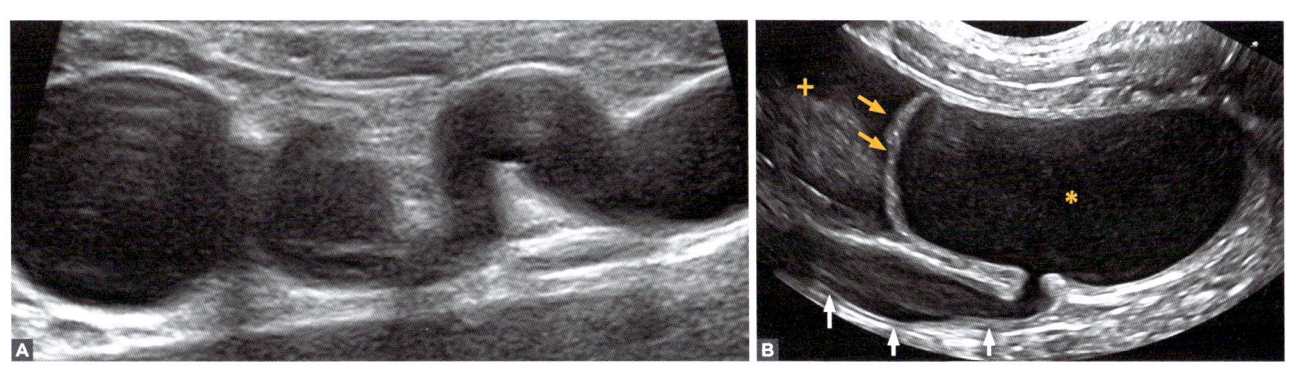

Fig. 35.35 Ultrasound images of a one-year-old female Labradoodle with an intravesicular ureterocele. (**A**) The left ureter is dilated and tortuous. (**B**) The dilated ureter is visible dorsal to the bladder (white arrows) and inserts into the bladder where a thin, soft tissue membrane (orange arrows) separates the ureterocele (asterisk) from the remainder of the bladder lumen (+).

SECTION V ABDOMEN

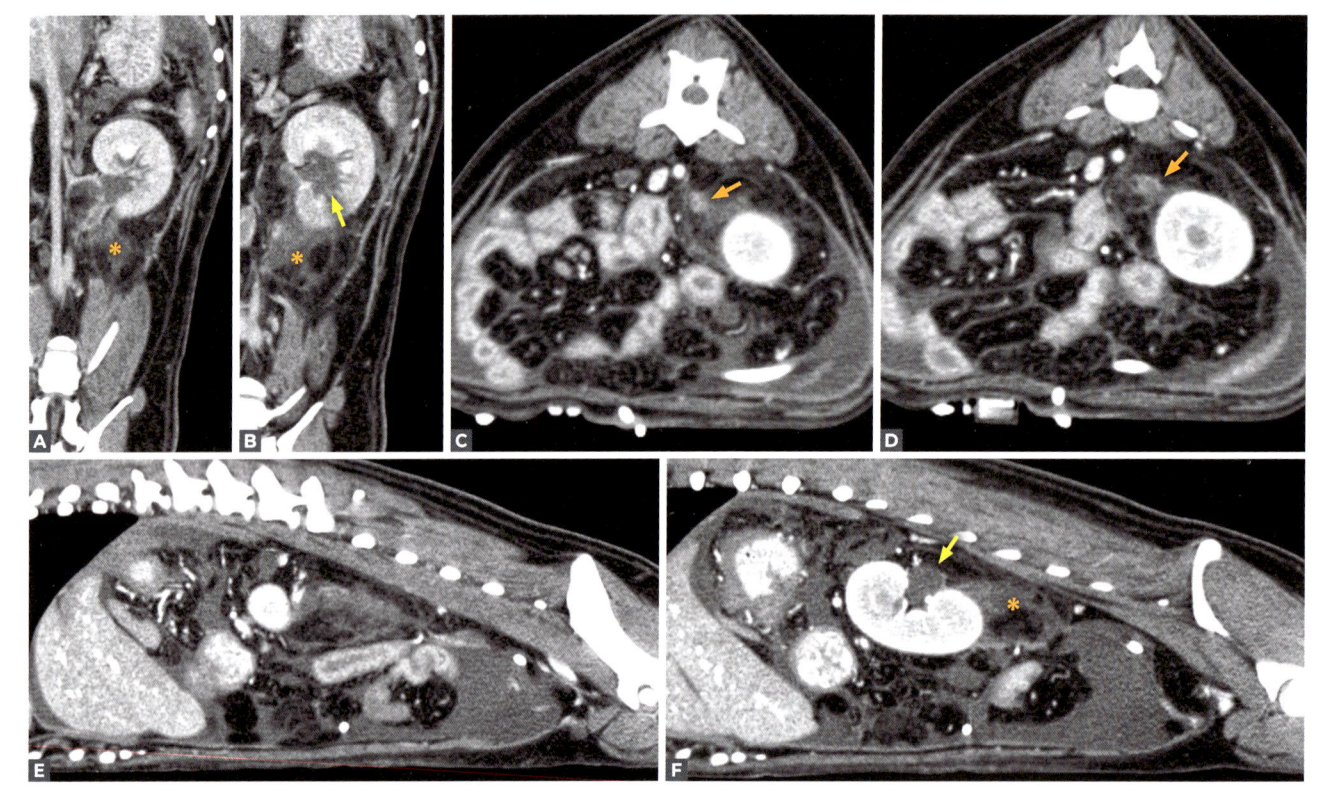

Fig. 35.36 Computed tomographic images of a three-year-old dog that presented following motor vehicle trauma. The left ureter is ruptured (orange arrows) and is causing retroperitoneal urine leakage. Peritoneal fluid is also present from hemorrhage and inflammation. (**A**, **B**) Dorsal plane images and (**E**, **F**) sagittal images demonstrate left hydronephrosis (yellow arrows) and perinephric fluid (asterisk).

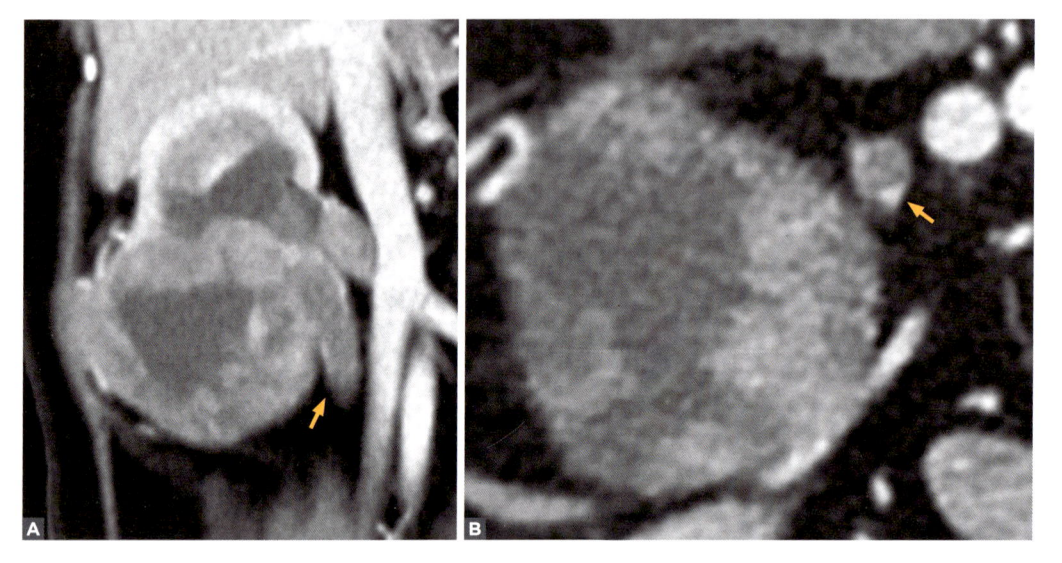

Fig. 35.37 (**A**) Dorsal and (**B**) transverse plane CT images post-contrast in a soft tissue window of a ten-year-old Cocker Spaniel with right renal carcinoma. The mass extends into the right ureter (arrows), which is mildly dilated and contains contrast-enhancing tissue similar to that of the mass.

Calculi

In cats and less often in dogs, nephroliths may dislodge and enter the ureter. These can either be non-obstructive, partially obstructive, or completely obstructive. Radiographs can sometimes identify radiopaque ureteroliths (**figs. 35.5**, **35.38**, and **35.39**). The deep circumflex iliac artery (**fig. 35.38**) should not be mistaken for a ureterolith. Its position is often more dorsal than the typical course of the ureter. Ultrasound or CT is required to determine if the ureterolith is obstructive or incidental. This is sometimes easier said than done. Ureteroliths appear as hyperechoic foci within the ureteral lumen on ultrasound. Sometimes, if sufficiently large, these will cause distal acoustic shadowing. In the author's experience, the size of the ureterolith is not always correlated with the degree of obstruction. That is, large calculi may be incomplete or non-obstructive, and small calculi may cause complete obstruction. Clinical determination of the degree of obstruction is often challenging. Some combination of clinical signs, degree of azotemia, amount of urine production, and imaging findings play a role in making this decision. As noted previously, the degree of renal pelvic dilation can indicate obstruction; however, minimal renal pelvic dilation can still be seen in patients with complete obstruction. In some instances, ultrasound-guided pyelography may be used to confirm obstruction.

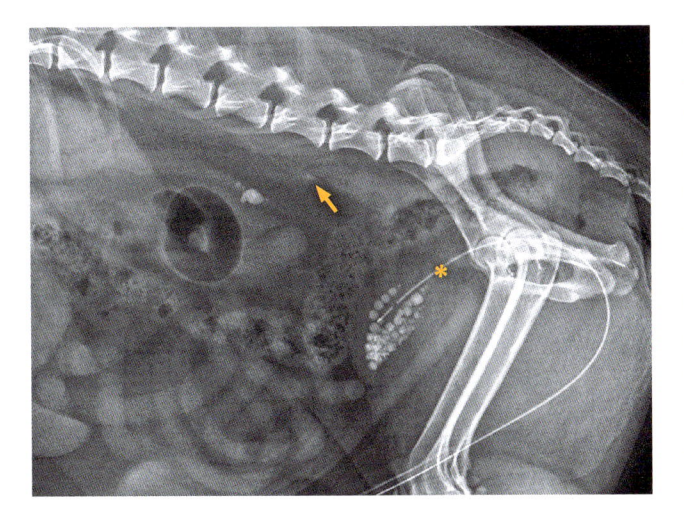

Fig. 35.38 Right lateral radiograph of a dog with ureterolithiasis and cystic calculi. Variably sized mineral opacity calculi in the mid-dorsal abdomen are consistent with the location in the ureter(s). End on projection of the deep circumflex iliac artery (arrow) in the retroperitoneal space can mimic ureterolithiasis and should not be confused on imaging. A urinary catheter and numerous calculi are present in the urinary bladder (asterisk).

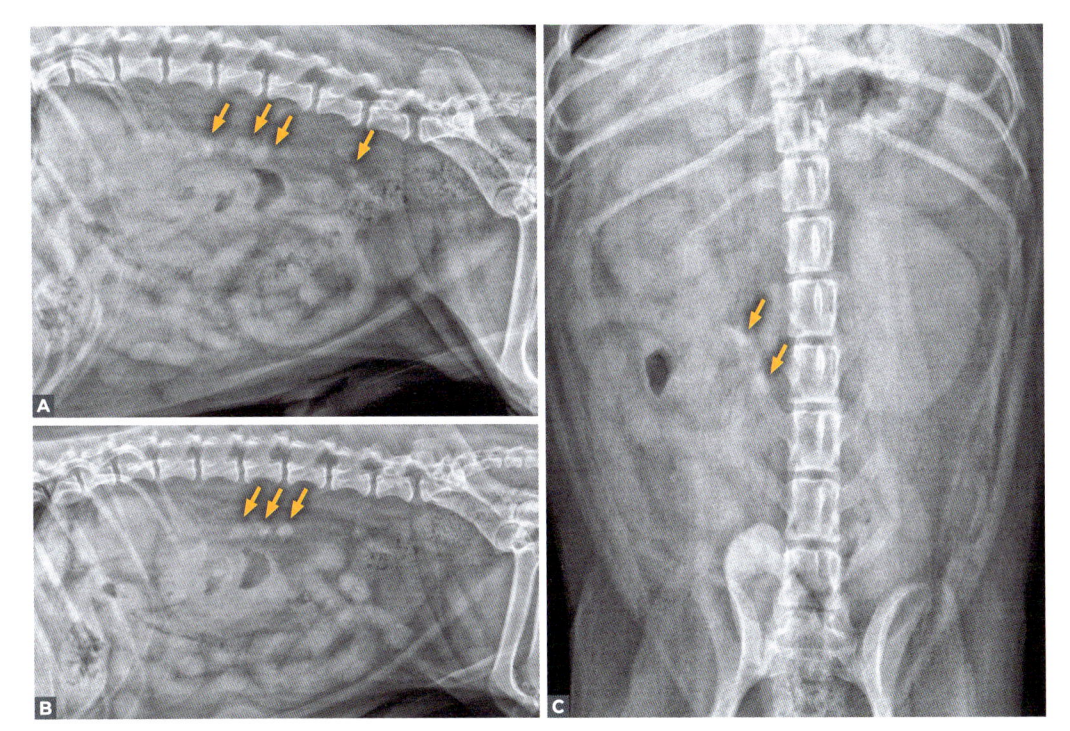

Fig. 35.39 (A, B) Lateral and (C) ventrodorsal radiographs of a dog with bilateral ureteroliths. Roughly oblong mineral opacity structures are seen in the plane of the ureters in the lateral projections (arrows) and right to the vertebral column in the ventrodorsal view.

References

1. Finco DR, Stiles NS, Kneller SK, Lewis RE, Barrett RB. Radiologic estimation of kidney size of the dog. *J Am Vet Med Assoc* 159:995-1002, 1971.
2. Lobacz MA, Sullivan M, Mellor D, Hammond G, Labruyère J, Dennis R. Effect of breed, age, weight and gender on radiographic renal size in the dog. *Vet Radiol Ultrasound* 53:437-441, 2012.
3. Shiroma JT, Gabriel JK, Carter RL, Scruggs SL, Stubbs PW. Effect of reproductive status on feline renal size. *Vet Radiol Ultrasound* 40:242-245, 1999.
4. Hart D Vander, Winter MD, Conway J, Berry CR. Ultrasound appearance of the outer medulla in dogs without renal dysfunction. *Vet Radiol Ultrasound* 54:652-658, 2013.
5. Mareschal A, D'Anjou MA, Moreau M, Alexander K, Beauregard G. Ultrasonographic measurement of kidney-to-aorta ratio as a method of estimating renal size in dogs. *Vet Radiol Ultrasound* 48:434-438, 2007.
6. Walter PA, Feeney DA, Johnston GR, Fletcher TF. Feline renal ultrasonography: quantitative analyses of imaged anatomy. *Am J Vet Res* 48:596-599, 1987.
7. Conroy M, Brodbelt DC, O'Neill D, Chang YM, Elliott J. Chronic kidney disease in cats attending primary care practice in the UK: A VetCompass TM study. *Vet Rec* 184:526, 2019.
8. O'Neill DG, Elliott J, Church DB, McGreevy PD, Thomson PC, Brodbelt DC. Chronic kidney disease in dogs in UK veterinary practices: prevalence, risk factors, and survival. *J Vet Intern Med* 27:814-821, 2013.

9. Marino CL, Lascelles BDX, Vaden SL, Gruen ME, Marks SL. Prevalence and classification of chronic kidney disease in cats randomly selected from four age groups and in cats recruited for degenerative joint disease studies. *J Feline Med Surg* 16:465-472, 2014.
10. Dickerson VM, Rissi DR, Brown CA, Brown SA, Schmiedt CW. Assessment of acute kidney injury and renal fibrosis after renal ischemia protocols in cats. *Comp Med* 67:56-66, 2017.
11. McLeland SM, Cianciolo RE, Duncan CG, Quimby JM. A comparison of biochemical and histopathologic staging in cats with chronic kidney disease. *Vet Pathol* 52:524-534, 2015.
12. Yan GY, Chen KY, Wang HC, Ma TY, Chen KS. Relationship between ultrasonographically determined renal dimensions and International Renal Interest Society stages in cats with chronic kidney disease. *J Vet Intern Med* 34:1464-1475, 2020.
13. Cordella A, Pey P, Dondi F, et al. The ultrasonographic medullary "rim sign" versus medullary "band sign" in cats and their association with renal disease. *J Vet Intern Med* 34:1932-1939, 2020.
14. Bryan JN, Henry CJ, Turnquist SE, et al. Primary renal neoplasia of dogs. *J Vet Intern Med* 20:1155-1160, 2018.
15. Henry CJ, Turnquist SE, Smith A, et al. Primary renal tumours in cats: 19 cases (1992-1998). *J Feline Med Surg* 1:165-170, 1999.
16. Moore A. Extranodal lymphoma in the cat: prognostic factors and treatment options. *J Feline Med Surg* 15:379-390, 2013.
17. Williams AG, Hohenhaus AE, Lamb KE. Incidence and treatment of feline renal lymphoma: 27 cases. *J Feline Med Surg* 23:936-944, 2021.
18. Klein MK, Cockerell G, Harris CK, et al. Canine primary renal neoplasms: a retrospective review of 54 cases. *J Am Anim Hosp Assoc*, 1988.
19. Moe L, Lium B. Computed tomography of hereditary multifocal renal cystadenocarcinomas in German shepherd dogs. *Vet Radiol Ultrasound* 38:335-343, 1997.
20. D'Anjou MA, Bédard A, Dunn ME. Clinical significance of renal pelvic dilation on ultrasound in dogs and cats. *Vet Radiol Ultrasound* 52:88-94, 2011.
21. Quimby JM, Dowers K, Herndon AK, Randall EK. Renal pelvic and ureteral ultrasonographic characteristics of cats with chronic kidney disease in comparison with normal cats, and cats with pyelonephritis or ureteral obstruction. *J Feline Med Surg* 19:784-790, 2017.
22. Lemieux C, Vachon C, Beauchamp G, Dunn ME. Minimal renal pelvis dilation in cats diagnosed with benign ureteral obstruction by antegrade pyelography: a retrospective study of 82 cases (2012-2018). *J Feline Med Surg* 23:892-899, 2021.
23. Chew DJ, DiBartola SP, Schenck PA. Familial renal diseases of dogs and cats. In Dennis J. Chew DJ, DiBartola SP, Schenck PA (editors). Canine and Feline Nephrology and Urology 2nd edition. St. Louis, Elsevier, 2011, pp 197-217.
24. Hoppe A, Karlstam E. Renal dysplasia in boxers and Finnish harriers. *J Small Anim Pract* 41:422-426, 2000.
25. Abraham L, Beck C, Slocombe R. Renal dysplasia and urinary tract infection in a Bull Mastiff puppy. *Aust Vet J* 81:336-339, 2003.
26. Seiler GS, Rhodes J, Cianciolo R, Casal ML. Ultrasonographic findings in cairn terriers with preclinical renal dysplasia. *Vet Radiol Ultrasound* 51:453-457, 2010.
27. Guerra JM, Freitas MF, Daniel AGT, et al. Age-based ultrasonographic criteria for diagnosis of autosomal dominant polycystic kidney disease in Persian cats. *J Feline Med Surg* 21:156-164, 2019.
28. Schirrer L, Marín-García PJ, Llobat L. Feline polycystic kidney disease: An update. *Vet Sci* 8, 2021.
29. Katic N, Bartolomaeus E, Böhler A, Dupré G. Traumatic diaphragmatic rupture in a cat with partial kidney displacement into the thorax. *J Small Anim Pract* 48:705-708, 2007.
30. Marolf A, Kraft S, Lowry J, Pelsue D, Veir J. Radiographic diagnosis-Right kidney herniation in a cat. *Vet Radiol Ultrasound* 43:237-240, 2002.
31. Marolf A, Kraft S, Lowry J. Radiographic diagnosis-Right kidney herniation in a cat. *Vet Radiol Ultrasound* 43:237-240, 2002.
32. Appleby R, Linden A Zur, Singh A, Finck C, Crawford E. Computed tomography diagnosis of a thoracic and abdominal penetrating foreign body in a dog. *Can Vet J* 56:1149-1152, 2015.
33. Ochoa VB, DiBartola SP, Chew DJ, Westropp J, Carothers M, Biller D. Perinephric pseudocysts in the cat: a retrospective study and review of the literature. *J Vet Intern Med* 13:47-55, 1999.
34. Orioles M, Di Bella A, Merlo M, Ter Haar G. Ascites resulting from a ruptured perinephric pseudocyst associated with a renal cyst in a dog. *Vet Rec Case Reports* 2:1-4, 2014.
35. Miles KG, Jergens AE. Unilateral perinephric pseudocyst of undetermined origin in a dog. *Vet Radiol Ultrasound* 33:277-281, 1992.
36. Cole LP, Mantis P, Humm K. Ultrasonographic findings in cats with acute kidney injury: a retrospective study. *J Feline Med Surg* 21:475-480, 2018.
37. Adams WH, Toal RL, Walker MA, Breider MA. Early renal ultrasonographic findings in dogs with experimentally induced ethylene glycol nephrosis. *Am J Vet Res* 50:1370-1376, 1989.
38. Day MJ, Holt PE. Unilateral fungal pyelonephritis in a dog. *Vet Pathol* 31:250-252, 1994.
39. Bouillon J, Snead E, Caswell J, Feng C, Hélie P, Lemetayer J. Pyelonephritis in dogs: retrospective study of 47 histologically diagnosed cases (2005-2015). *J Vet Intern Med* 32:249-259, 2018.
40. Dorsch R, Teichmann-Knorrn S, Sjetne Lund H. Urinary tract infection and subclinical bacteriuria in cats: a clinical update. *J Feline Med Surg* 21:1023-1038, 2019.
41. Choi J, Jang J, Choi H, Kim H, Yoon J. Ultrasonographic features of pyonephrosis in dogs. *Vet Radiol Ultrasound* 51:548-553, 2010.
42. Paras KL, Miller L, Verocai GG. Ectopic infection by *Dioctophyme renale* in a dog from Georgia, USA, and a review of cases of ectopic dioctophymosis in companion animals in the Americas. *Vet Parasitol Reg Stud Reports* 14:111-116, 2018.
43. Nakagawa TLDR, Bracarense APFRL, Reis ACF dos, Yamamura MH, Headley SA. Giant kidney worm (*Dioctophyme renale*) infections in dogs from Northern Paraná, Brazil. *Vet Parasitol* 145:366-370, 2007.
44. Rahal SC, Mamprim MJ, Oliveira HS, et al. Ultrasonographic, computed tomographic, and operative findings in dogs infested with giant kidney worms (*Dioctophyme renale*). *J Am Vet Med Assoc* 244:555-558, 2014.
45. Hart E, Singh A, Peregrine A, et al. Laparoscopic ureteronephrectomy for the treatment of giant kidney worm infection in 2 dogs. *Can Vet J* 61:1149-1154, 2020.
46. Angelou A, Tsakou K, Mprandiitsas K, Sioutas G, Moores DA, Papadopoulos E. Giant kidney worm: novel report of *Dioctophyme renale* in the kidney of a dog in Greece. *Helminthol* 57:43-48, 2020.
47. Reichler IM, Eckrich Specker C, Hubler M, Alois B, Haessig M, Arnold S. Ectopic ureters in dogs: clinical features, surgical techniques and outcome. *Vet Surg* 41:515-522, 2012.
48. Kuzma AB, Holmberg DL. Ectopic ureter in a cat. *Can Vet J* 29:59-61, 1988.
49. Fox AJ, Sharma A, Secrest SA. Computed tomographic excretory urography features of intramural ectopic ureters in 10 dogs. *J Small Anim Pract* 57:210-213, 2016.
50. Lamb CR, Gregory SP. Ultrasonographic findings in 14 dogs with ectopic ureter. *Vet Radiol Ultrasound* 39:218-223, 1998.
51. Gremillion C, Cohen EB, Vaden S, Seiler G. Optimization of ultrasonographic ureteral jet detection and normal ureteral jet morphology in dogs. *Vet Radiol Ultrasound* 62:583-590, 2021.
52. Stiffler KS, McCrackin Stevenson MA, Mahaffey MB, Howerth EW, Barsanti JA. Intravesical ureterocele with concurrent renal dysfunction in a dog: a case report and proposed classification system. *J Am Anim Hosp Assoc* 38:33-39, 2002.

CHAPTER 36

Urinary bladder and urethra

Ryan B. Appleby

> **KEY POINTS**
>
> ▎ Lower urinary tract disease is common in small animals.
> ▎ Pollakiuria, stranguria, urinary bladder obstruction, and urine discoloration are all common presenting complaints.
> ▎ Radiography is an important first-line diagnostic to rule out major abnormalities such as mineralization in the urinary tract.
> ▎ Normal radiographs do not exclude urinary bladder or urethral disease.
> ▎ Ultrasound is the recommended second-line imaging modality for the bladder due to its ease of use, accessibility, and greater sensitivity.
> ▎ Contrast urethrography is used to assess the patency and integrity of the urethra.
> ▎ Computed tomography is an excellent diagnostic tool that is valuable in evaluating complex cases and surgical planning.

Diseases of the lower urinary tract (bladder and urethra) are common in small animals. Acquired diseases are more common than congenital abnormalities, which can predispose to acquired disease. Similar to the upper urinary tract, while radiographs are an excellent baseline diagnostic tool, they are limited to detecting changes in opacity, namely screening for mineralization. Radiographic studies are often complemented by, or in some cases, replaced by ultrasound, contrast urethrography, and computed tomography (CT).

Normal anatomy

The bladder is a hollow organ in the caudal abdomen that stores urine. The ureters open into the caudodorsal aspect of the bladder, delivering urine from the kidneys. The trigone is defined as the region bounded by the ureteral papillae and vesicourethral junction. On radiographs, the urinary bladder is a well-defined, rounded soft tissue opacity structure, ventral to the colon and cranial to the pelvic inlet (**figs. 36.1** and **36.2**). Diseases of the urinary bladder often present with increased frequency of urination (pollakiuria), difficulty urinating (stranguria), or urinary blockage. In some instances, hemorrhage or, less often, pyuria may result in urine discoloration.

Radiographs are a useful primary screening tool but are insensitive. Radiography can only detect changes in bladder opacity, size, and, rarely, shape. As the bladder should be uniformly soft tissue, the presence of air or mineral in the bladder represents an abnormality. The normal bladder wall cannot be distinguished from the urine in the lumen, and radiography cannot detect changes within the bladder wall. The degree of bladder distention in dogs can affect the bladder location on radi-

SECTION V ABDOMEN

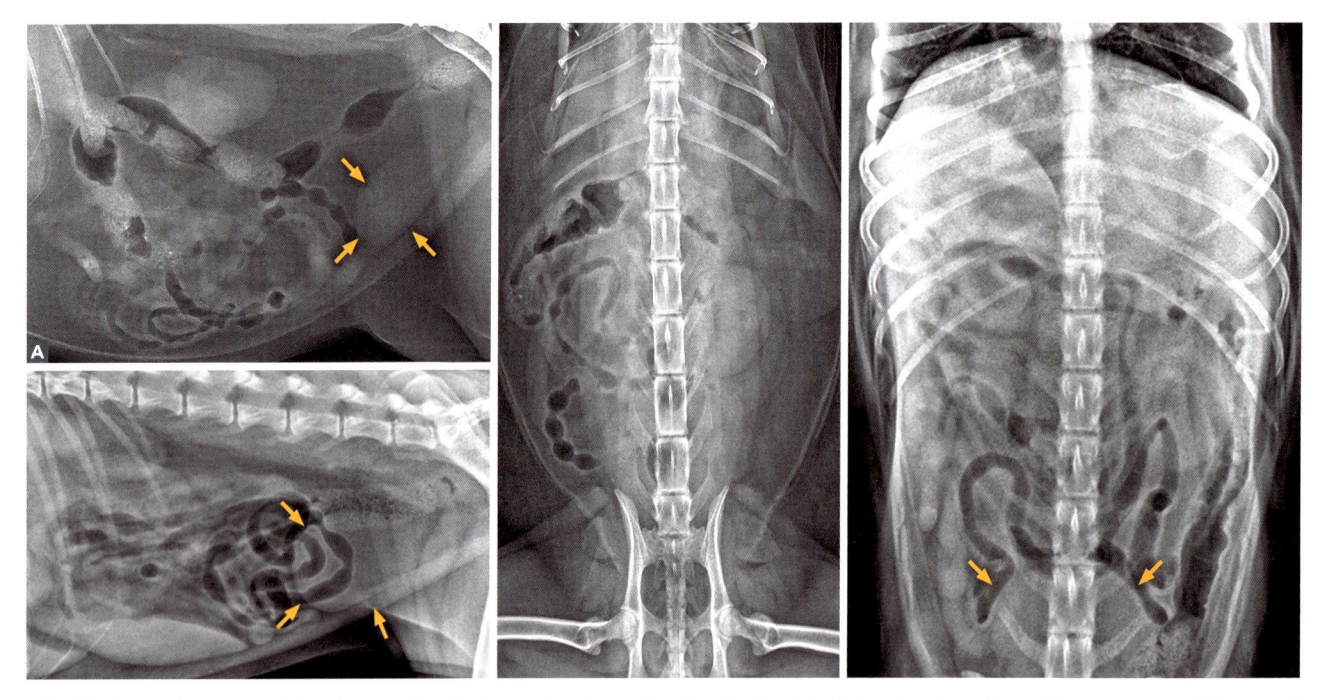

Fig. 36.1 (**A**, **B**) Lateral and (**C**, **D**) ventrodorsal radiographs of a cat (**A**, **C**) and a dog (**B**, **D**) showing the radiographic appearance of the normal urinary bladder. The bladder is sometimes seen in the ventrodorsal projections (**D**) but is often superimposed on the vertebrae and epaxial muscle (**C**).

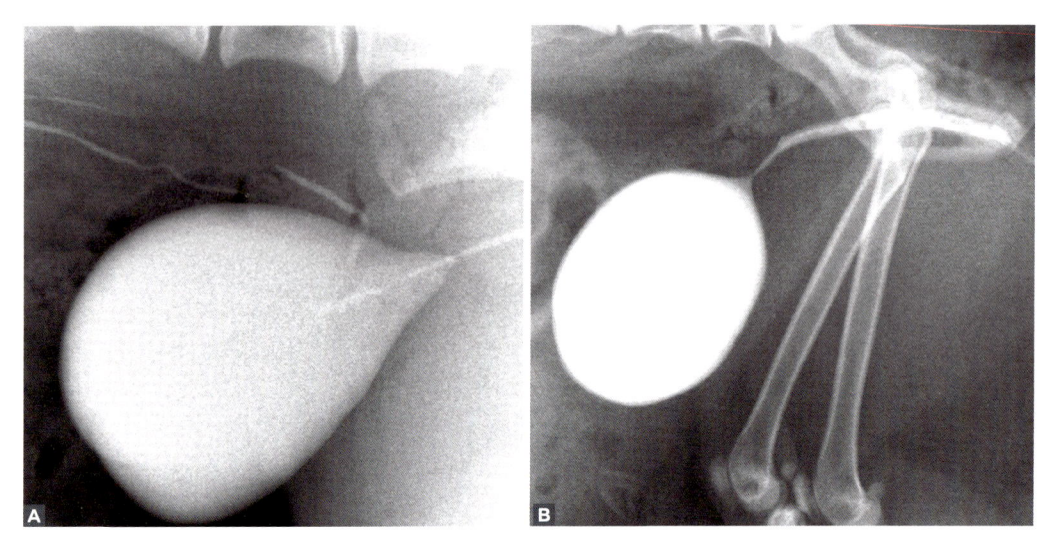

Fig. 36.2 Normal positioning of the bladder in the dog (**A**) and cat (**B**). Retrograde cystography performed in these patients highlights the normal positioning of the bladder. While bladder size is variable based on the volume of urine, the bladder size shown here represents a near full bladder in normal dogs and cats. (**A**) In the dog, a catheter has been placed into the urethra (catheter tip visible immediately cranial to the pelvic canal), and iodinated contrast medium has been administered into the urinary bladder. A small amount of contrast medium has refluxed into the ureters, a normal finding. (**B**) In the cat, the catheter is present in the distal urethra, caudal to the ischia, and contrast medium was administered. A gas bubble is present within the urethra and superimposes the pubis.

ographs. Minimally filled or empty bladders are sometimes not seen, obscured by the intestine, or entirely contained in the pelvis. Conversely, in cats, the bladder is almost always seen unless obscured by intestinal content, peritoneal fluid, or absence of fat, regardless of the degree of distention.[1] The upper extent of normal bladder size is variable, especially in house-trained dogs. In the author's experience, a distended bladder will often extend to the level of the cranial end plate of L5 (**fig. 36.2**). Pathologic urinary bladder distention should be diagnosed with care based on presenting signs and not on bladder size alone.

CHAPTER 36 Urinary bladder and urethra

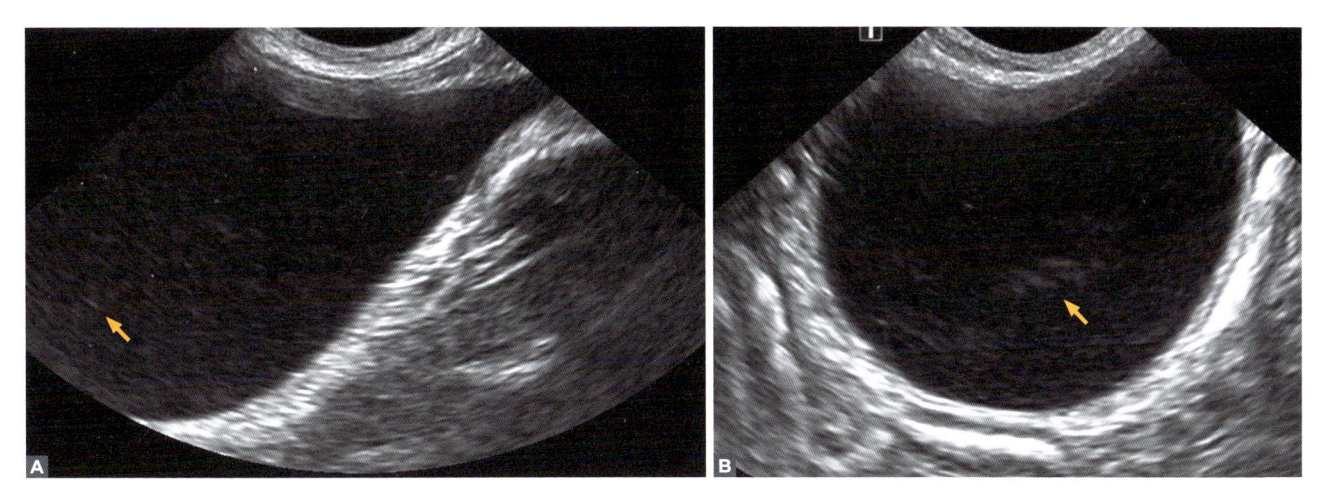

Fig. 36.3 Longitudinal and transverse ultrasound images of the normal bladder in a three-year-old Shih Tzu. While the urine is predominantly anechoic, faint echoes are present in the bladder lumen (arrow). The sonographer should take care not to confuse these artifactual echoes due to clutter with pathologic causes of increased echogenicity, as will be shown later in the chapter.

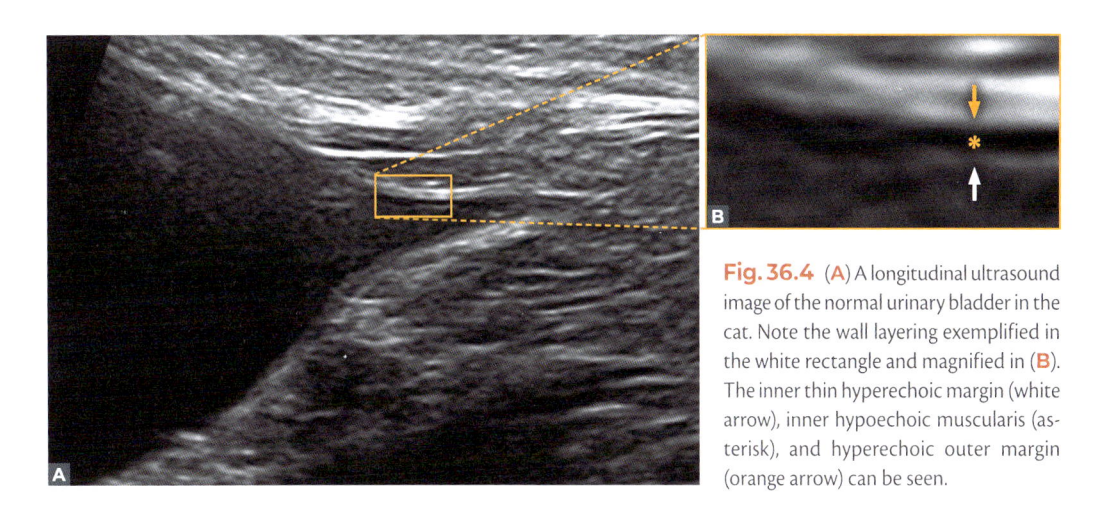

Fig. 36.4 (**A**) A longitudinal ultrasound image of the normal urinary bladder in the cat. Note the wall layering exemplified in the white rectangle and magnified in (**B**). The inner thin hyperechoic margin (white arrow), inner hypoechoic muscularis (asterisk), and hyperechoic outer margin (orange arrow) can be seen.

On ultrasound, the normal bladder is a thin-walled organ containing anechoic fluid (**fig. 36.3**). While normal urine is uniformly anechoic, sonographers should take care not to misdiagnose artifactual echoes from slice thickness/volume averaging or side lobes/grating lobes as luminal debris (**fig. 36.3**). The wall layers of the urinary bladder can be distinguished as an inner hyperechoic mucosal interface, a hypoechoic muscular layer and a peripheral hyperechoic layer[2] (**fig. 36.4**). With lower frequency probes, or with either marked distention or emptying of the bladder, the individual wall layers are sometimes not observed. The presence of material in the urinary bladder is commonly encountered in small animals. Material within the bladder may be incidental and benign, such as the presence of lipids in feline urine[3] (**fig. 36.5**).

The normal urethra is not visible on radiographs. In male dogs, an os penis partly surrounds the distal aspect of the urethra (**fig. 36.6**). An os penis is sometimes present in male cats[4] (**fig. 36.7**). Radiographing the male urethra in dogs requires that the pelvic limbs are pulled cranially, and the beam is centered on the perineum, just caudal to the base of the os penis (**fig. 36.6**). This projection should be performed in any male dog presenting for lower urinary signs. This allows evaluation of the membranous and penile urethral segments without superimposition of the pelvic limbs.

579

SECTION V ABDOMEN

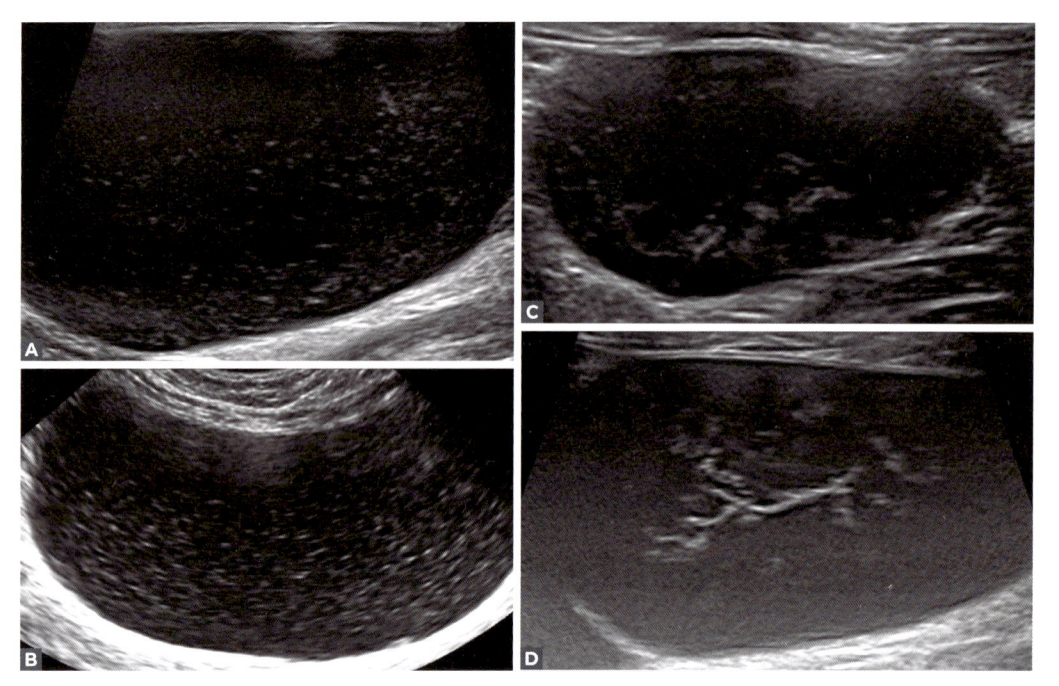

Fig. 36.5 Sonographic appearance of lipiduria in four cats. The volume, shape, and overall echogenicity of the material can vary. The hyperechoic material is suspended and appears as either numerous pinpoint foci or a conglomerate of central echogenic material.

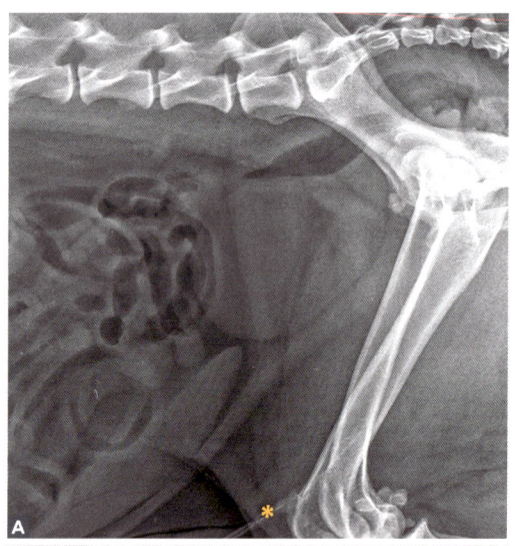

Fig. 36.6 Lateral radiographs of a 13-year-old castrated male Beagle with a normal bladder and urethra. (A) Note that in the standard lateral projection of the abdomen, the most caudal aspect of the urethra is collimated out of view, and the urethra at the level of the os penis (asterisk) is obscured by the pelvic limbs. The flexed leg lateral projection allows visualization of the entire urethra. In both images, mineralization is present along the margin of the pelvis, which can sometimes be confused with urethral calculi. Mineralization of either the prepubic tendon (as in this case) or the coxofemoral (hip) joints can superimpose this region. A ventrodorsal projection (not shown) can aid in distinguishing musculoskeletal mineralization from urinary origin.

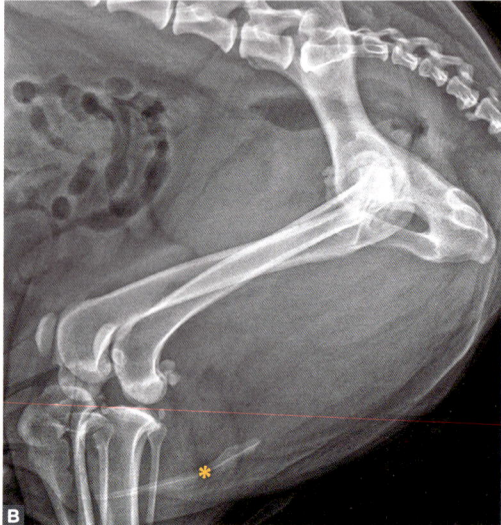

Fig. 36.7 Lateral radiograph of a nine-year-old Domestic longhair cat with a faintly visible os penis.

CHAPTER 36 Urinary bladder and urethra

Neoplasia

Bladder tumors are reported to comprise 2% of neoplasms in dogs,[5] and are very rare in cats.[6,7] The most common is urothelial carcinoma, also referred to as transitional cell carcinoma,[5] usually at the bladder trigone and vesicourethral junction. Dogs may present with increased frequency of urination, urinary obstruction, and both local and distant metastasis. Urothelial cell carcinoma is best imaged sonographically. Cytological assessment of urine sediment or sample obtained by traumatic catheterization may confirm a diagnosis but is sometimes inconclusive. PCR testing for the BRAF mutation in urine has good sensitivity and excellent specificity and is probably the best screening test.[8] Radiographs rarely identify intralesional mineralization, and the bladder usually appears normal. Visible metastatic enlargement of the sublumbar lymph node groups may be present in patients with long-standing signs. In such cases, periosteal proliferation from infiltrative metastasis may also be present on the last few lumbar vertebrae, sacrum, and iliac shafts. Diagnosis is best made with ultrasound (**figs. 36.8-36.11**) or CT. The ultrasound appearance of bladder wall masses is variable, with both heterogeneous and homogeneous appearances. The masses are occasionally mineralized. Masses often have an irregular mucosal margin and broad base, and less often are pedunculated (**fig. 36.9**). Ultrasound is much more sensitive for detection of lymph node enlargement, either from reactive inflammatory change or metastasis. There is overlap in the sonographic appearance of chronic polypoid cystitis and urothelial carcinoma, and a BRAF test, cytology, histology, or serial assessments should be used for confirmation.

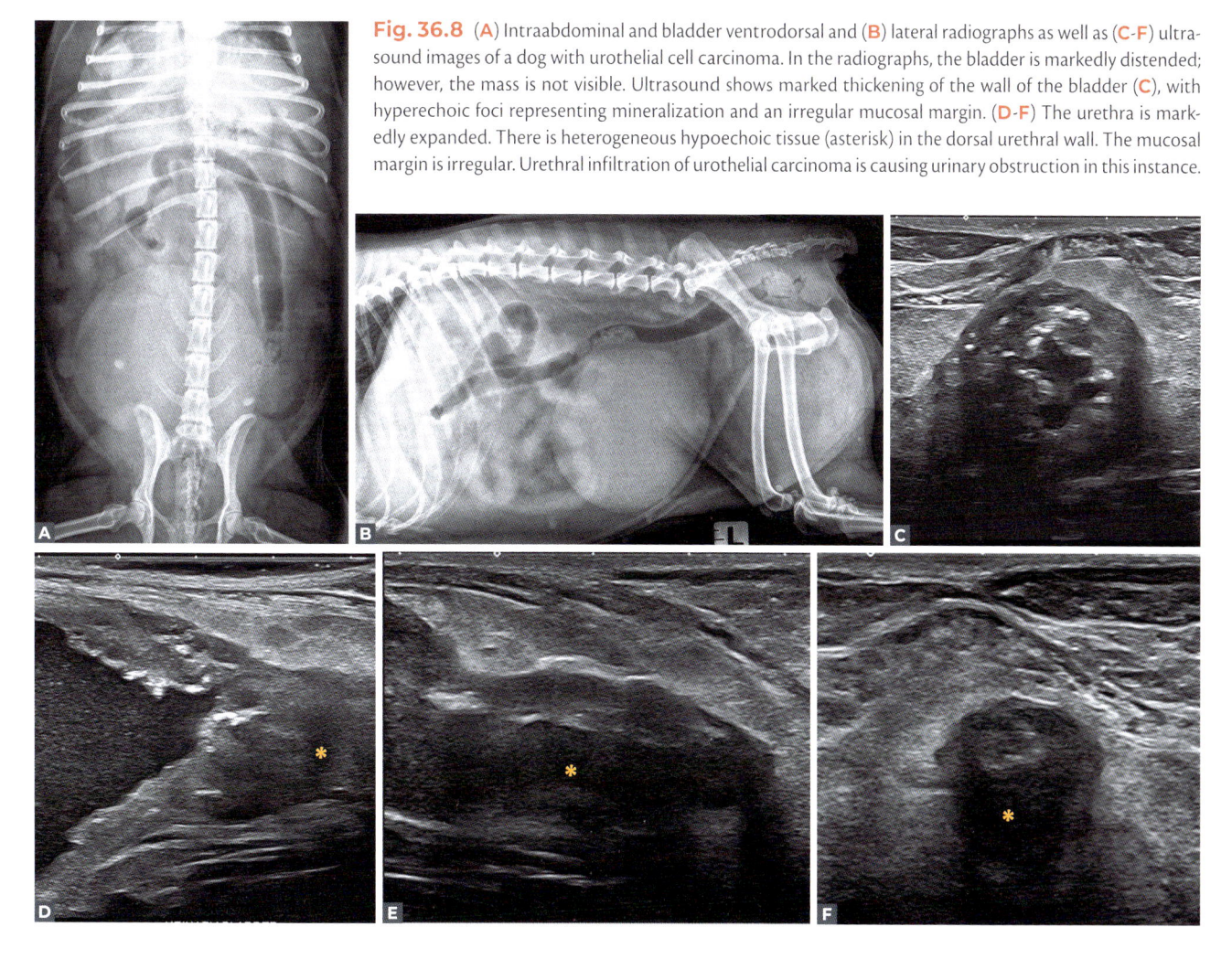

Fig. 36.8 (**A**) Intraabdominal and bladder ventrodorsal and (**B**) lateral radiographs as well as (**C-F**) ultrasound images of a dog with urothelial cell carcinoma. In the radiographs, the bladder is markedly distended; however, the mass is not visible. Ultrasound shows marked thickening of the wall of the bladder (**C**), with hyperechoic foci representing mineralization and an irregular mucosal margin. (**D-F**) The urethra is markedly expanded. There is heterogeneous hypoechoic tissue (asterisk) in the dorsal urethral wall. The mucosal margin is irregular. Urethral infiltration of urothelial carcinoma is causing urinary obstruction in this instance.

581

SECTION V ABDOMEN

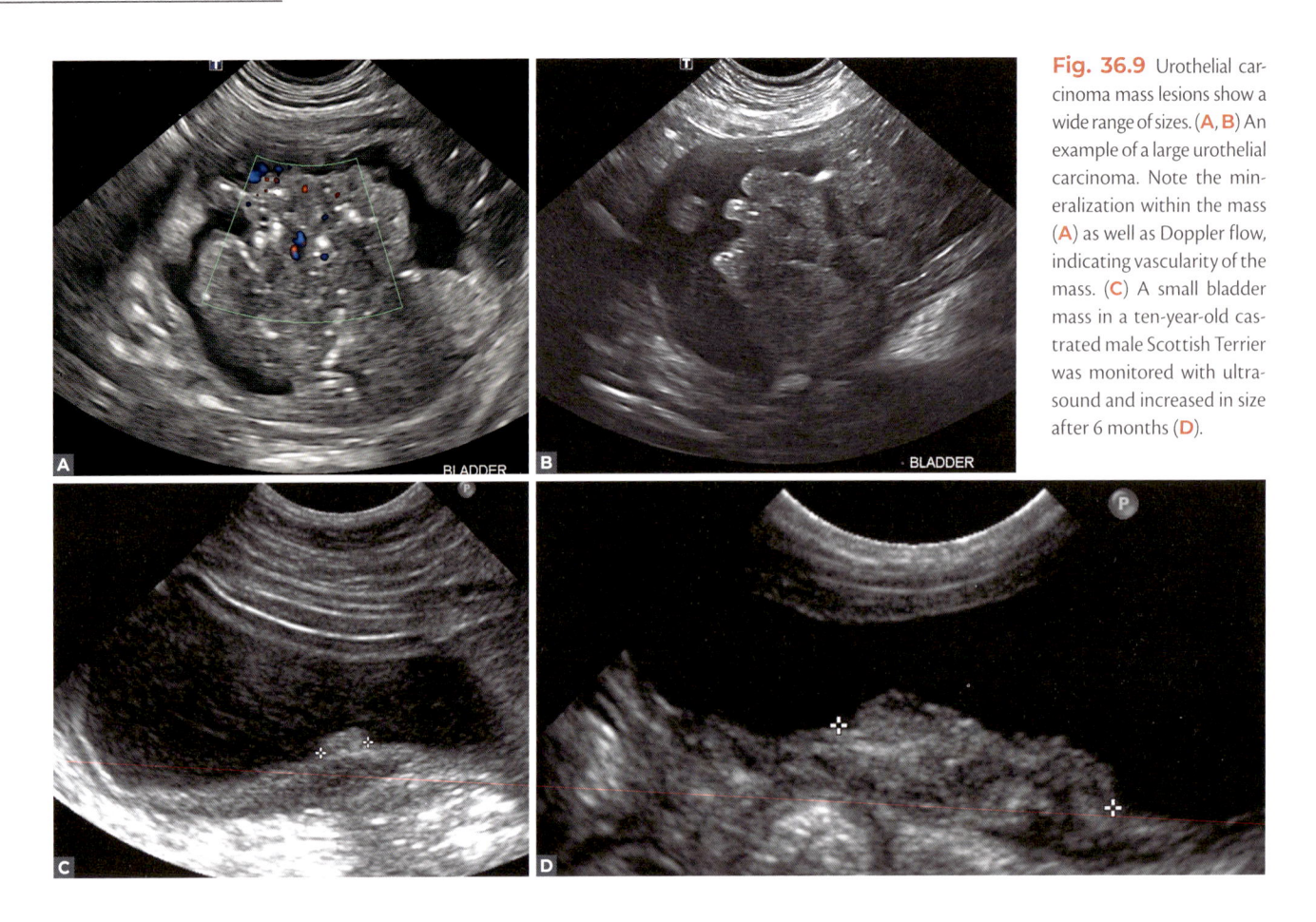

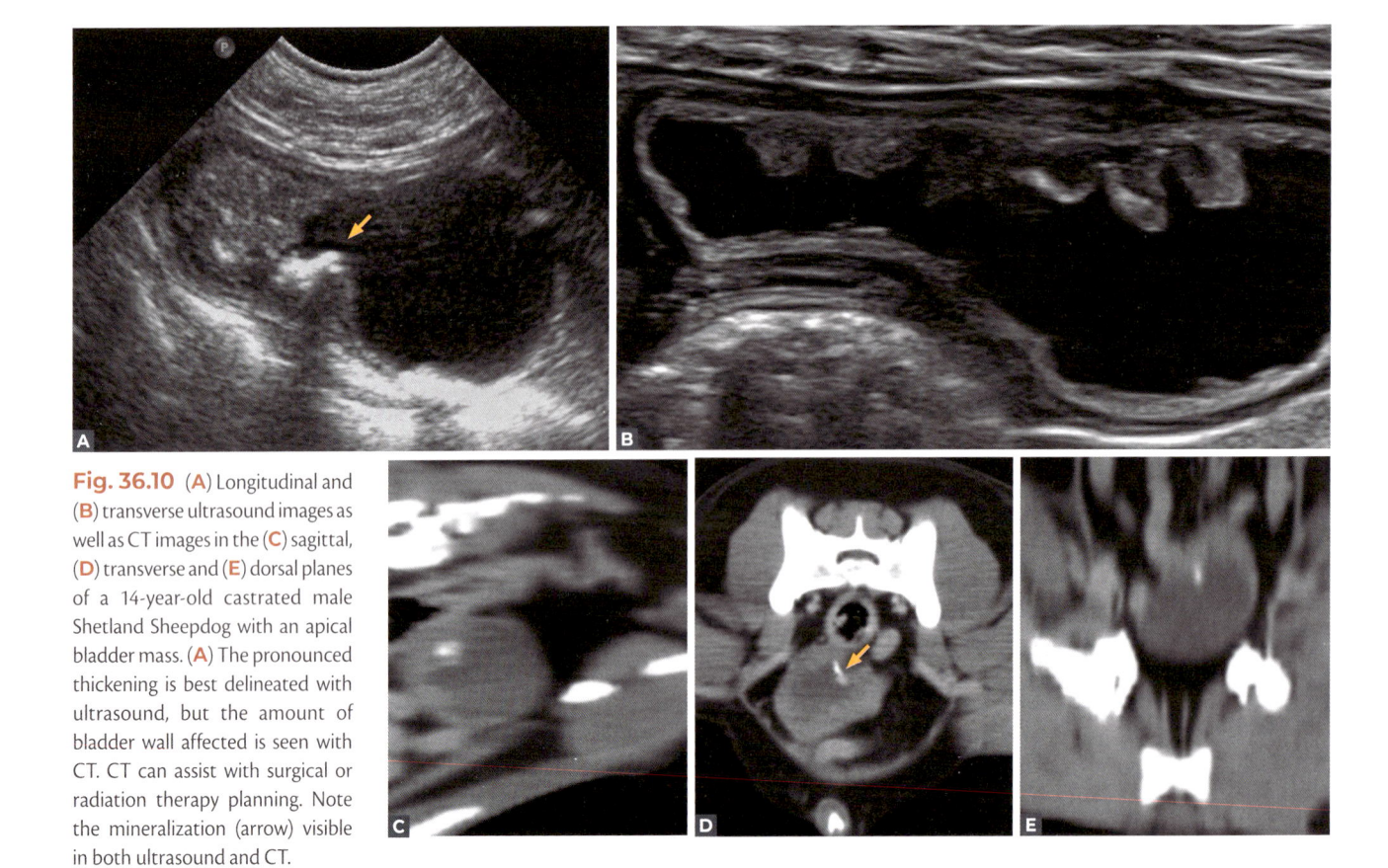

Fig. 36.9 Urothelial carcinoma mass lesions show a wide range of sizes. (**A**, **B**) An example of a large urothelial carcinoma. Note the mineralization within the mass (**A**) as well as Doppler flow, indicating vascularity of the mass. (**C**) A small bladder mass in a ten-year-old castrated male Scottish Terrier was monitored with ultrasound and increased in size after 6 months (**D**).

Fig. 36.10 (**A**) Longitudinal and (**B**) transverse ultrasound images as well as CT images in the (**C**) sagittal, (**D**) transverse and (**E**) dorsal planes of a 14-year-old castrated male Shetland Sheepdog with an apical bladder mass. (**A**) The pronounced thickening is best delineated with ultrasound, but the amount of bladder wall affected is seen with CT. CT can assist with surgical or radiation therapy planning. Note the mineralization (arrow) visible in both ultrasound and CT.

582

CHAPTER **36** Urinary bladder and urethra

Transitional cell carcinoma is the most common neoplasm of the urethra. Urethral neoplasia may arise in the bladder and extend into the urethra or arise from the urethra itself and extend to the bladder neck. Sonographic features of urethral tumors are similar to those of bladder tumors with expansion of the wall and loss of layering, and lymph node enlargement (**fig. 36.12**). Only the intraabdominal portion can be assessed with ultrasound and contrast urethrography, or CT of the pelvic canal is often required to confirm the lesion and assess the extent.

Fig. 36.11 (**A**, **B**) Higher resolution imaging of the urinary bladder with a linear probe can be of value to better define mucosal masses and confirm extension into the muscular layer. (**C**, **D**) While the mass can still be seen with a lower frequency sector probe, the structure and the degree of wall involvement are better delineated with higher frequency and better near-field resolution of a linear probe. (**A**) Color Doppler and (**C**) power Doppler confirm perfusion in this mass.

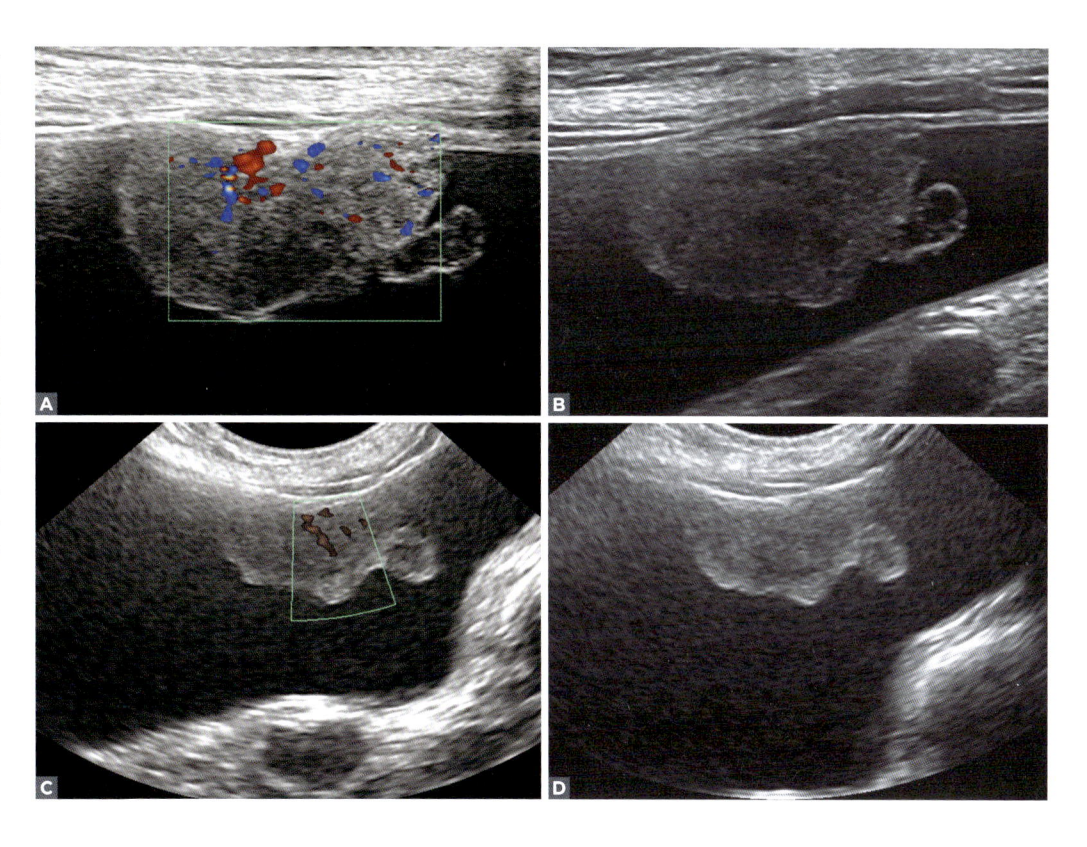

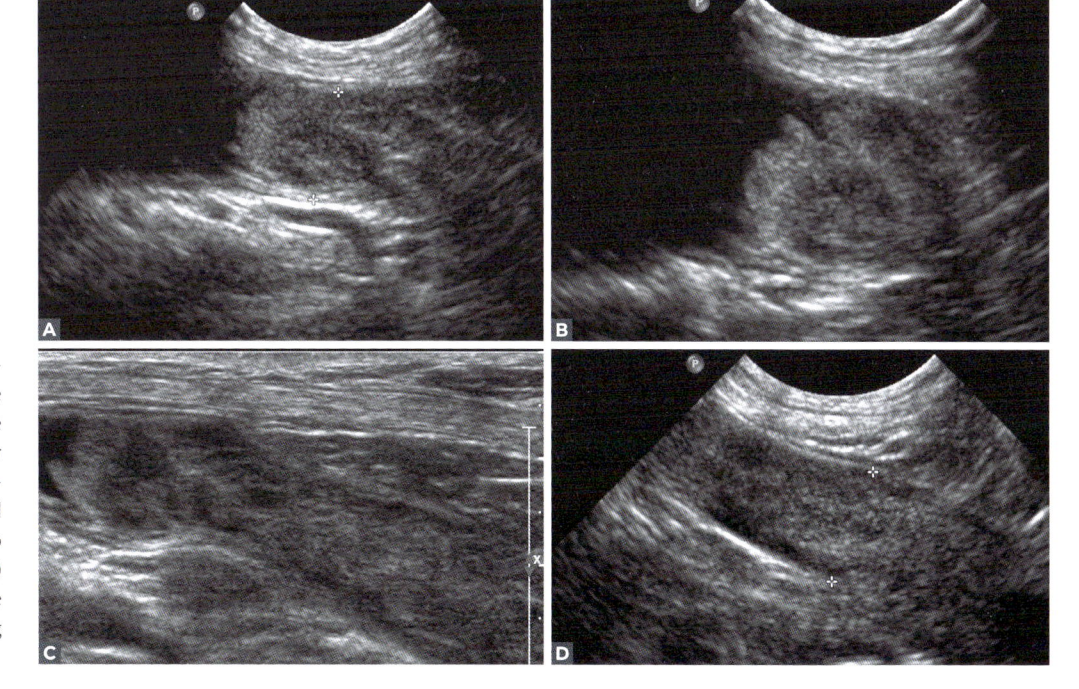

Fig. 36.12 (**A**) Longitudinal and (**B**) transverse ultrasound images at the level of the urinary bladder trigone showing a pedunculated mass (urothelial carcinoma) extending into the bladder lumen. (**C**, **D**) The tumor infiltrates the urethra, causing thickening and loss of wall layering.

583

SECTION V ABDOMEN

Cystitis

Cystitis is inflammation of the urinary bladder. Radiographs appear normal unless cystitis is secondary to radiopaque calculi. The diagnosis is commonly made with ultrasound in combination with clinical presentation, urinalysis, and culture. Affected patients usually show pollakiuria and often have an empty or almost empty bladder. Confining the patient to prevent urination or instillation of saline via a urethral catheter is usually required to assess the bladder wall. Acute cases often appear normal on ultrasound, but severe or chronic cases may show bladder wall thickening. The thickening usually affects the apical region and should be diagnosed with caution, giving consideration to the degree of distension. There may be visible suspended or gravity-dependent debris in the bladder lumen, representing mucosal or inflammatory cells and/or hemorrhage. There is overlap of the sonographic appearance of cystitis with other causes of bladder wall thickening such as hemorrhage or neoplasia.

In dogs, cystitis most commonly occurs secondary to bacterial infection. It is more common in female dogs compared to males as the long male urethra provides a protective mechanism against ascending infection. In cats, cystitis may be secondary to infection or be the result of a complex process known as feline idiopathic cystitis (FIC).[9] FIC is the most common cause of feline lower urinary tract disease (FLUTD), affecting up to 69% of cats with FLUTD.[10] FIC is defined as cystitis without other concurrent disorders such as bacterial infection, urolithiasis, or other diseases such as neoplasia.[10] Therefore, imaging is required to rule out concurrent diseases and support this diagnosis by exclusion.

Cystitis often occurs in combination with urolithiasis (**fig. 36.13**) due to either the predisposing nature of urease-producing bacterial infections (e.g., *Staphylococcus* spp.) to form struvite cystoliths[11] or mechanical irritation of the cystolith on the urinary bladder mucosa resulting in the breakdown of the mucosal barrier (**fig. 36.14**).

Emphysematous cystitis is an infection by gas-producing bacteria causing gas accumulation in the bladder lumen and wall, which may extend into the broad ligaments of the bladder. It most commonly occurs in diabetic patients with glucosuria[12] (**fig. 36.15**).

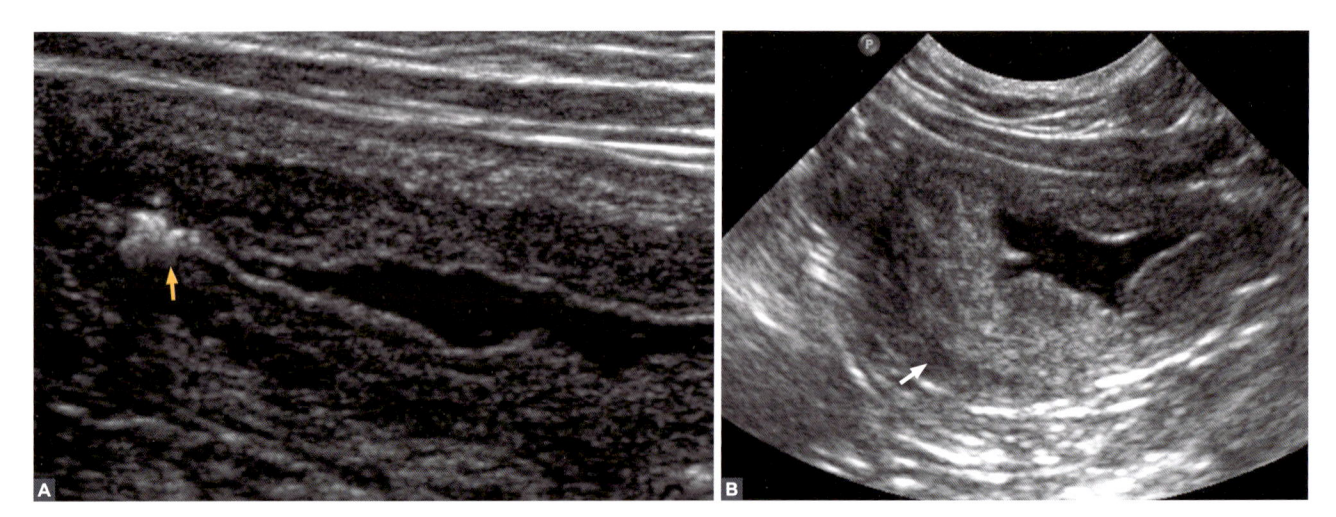

Fig. 36.13 (**A**) Longitudinal ultrasound image of the urinary bladder in a cat with small cystoliths (orange arrow) and thickened bladder wall. Thickening of the bladder wall may be partly due to limited distention; however, the clinical signs and cystoliths likely indicate concurrent cystitis in this patient. (**B**) A transverse ultrasound image of a dog shows marked thickening of the bladder wall. The asymmetry noted to the wall with a thicker portion at the right dorsal aspect (white arrow) indicates that there is more than just relative thickening from under the distention. In this case, the patient had lower urinary signs, pyuria with bacteria, and a diagnosis of bacterial cystitis.

CHAPTER 36 Urinary bladder and urethra

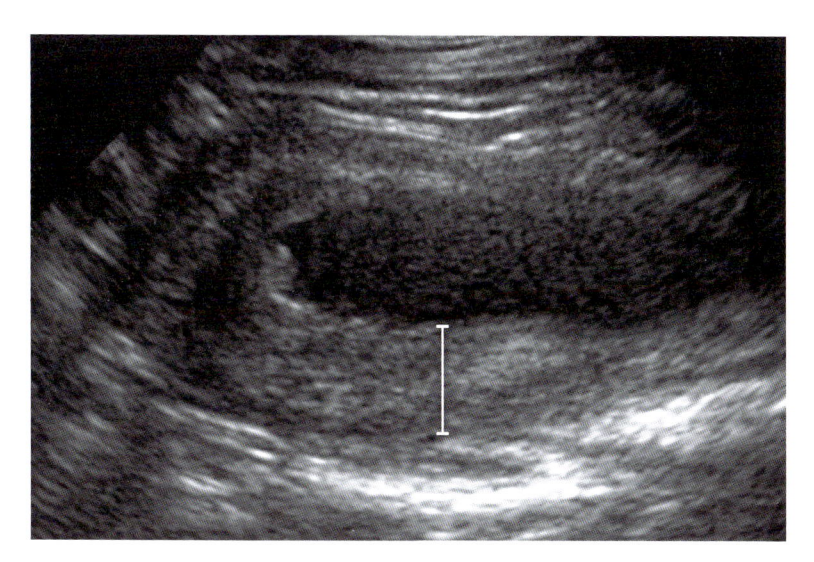

Fig. 36.14 Longitudinal ultrasound image of a dog with sterile hemorrhagic cystitis secondary to cyclophosphamide therapy. Note the uniform circumferential thickening of the bladder wall (bar). The wall is diffusely hyperechoic with blurring of the layering.

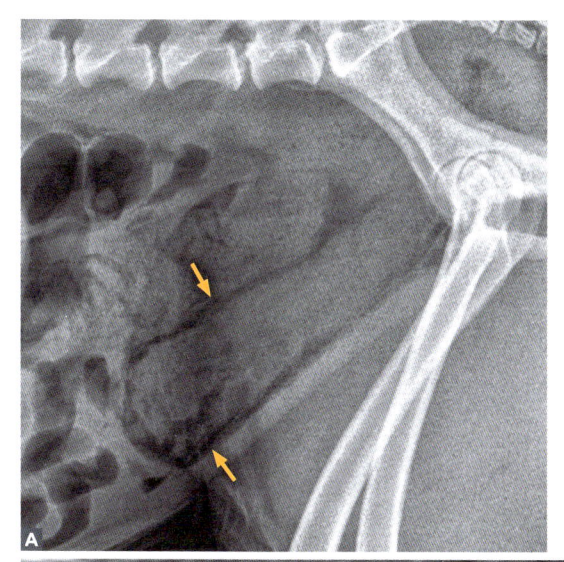

Fig. 36.15 (A) Lateral radiograph and (B) corresponding longitudinal ultrasound images of a nine-year-old female mixed breed dog with diabetes. Gas is present throughout the bladder wall (arrows) on both radiographs and ultrasound. On ultrasound, there are hyperechoic reverberating foci in the bladder wall, which partially obscure the lumen.

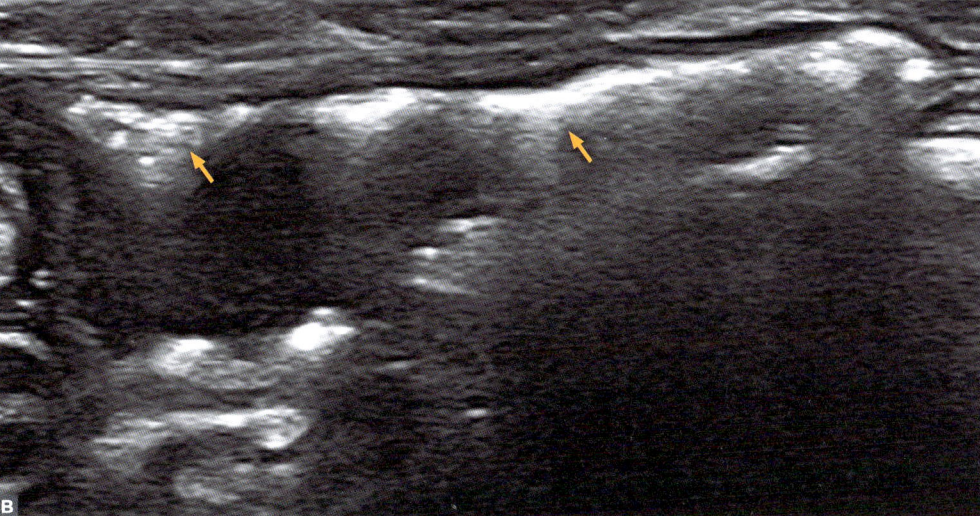

585

Calculi and sediment

Causes of small sonographic speckles aside from lipiduria include crystalluria (**fig. 36.16**), cellular material, and hemorrhage (**fig. 36.17**). Larger volumes of material settle to the dependent portion of the bladder. Agitation of the bladder under probe pressure or repositioning the patient can sometimes dislodge the material from the dependent portion and help delineate it from the bladder wall if there is concern that consistently dependent material is arising from the wall rather than intraluminal.

Urinary calculi are a common cause of lower urinary tract signs in both dogs and cats. Calculi can be identified radiographically, sonographically, and with CT. Urate and cysteine calculi are not radiopaque and therefore are only seen with contrast radiography, ultrasound, or CT. Calculi are quite variable in size and number, ranging from sand-like material to quite large calculi (**figs. 36.18** and **36.19**). Cystoliths typically settle to the dependent portion of the bladder and are visible as a hyperechoic structure with acoustic shadowing on ultrasound (**figs. 36.20** and **36.21**). Individual calculi can be resolved in some patients. In others, multiple calculi form a single irregular hyperechoic interface with a distal acoustic shadow. In most cases, it is not possible to accurately count calculi with ultrasound. Twinkle artifacts can be used to confirm the presence of minerals. This appears as a rapidly changing color during color Doppler interrogation of highly reflective structures such as minerals (**fig. 36.20B**).[13] Radiography cannot distinguish between types of calculi with a large degree of overlap between stone types.[14]

During urination, calculi can displace into the urethra (**figs. 36.22-36.24**). This may cause urethral obstruction (**fig. 36.23**) or pollakiuria. The flexed leg lateral projection is important for diagnosing urethral calculi in male dogs (**fig. 36.22**).

In cats, idiopathic cystitis may cause urethral spasm and lower urinary tract signs that mimic urethral obstruction.[9] Non-mineralized plugs and/or small calculi may lodge in the urethra, causing an obstruction (**fig. 36.25**). Small calculi may be visible on radiographs and should not be mistaken for the inconsistent feline os penis. Urethrography is especially important in cats to assess the integrity of the urethra and to assess strictures which are a common sequel to obstruction and predispose to re-obstruction.

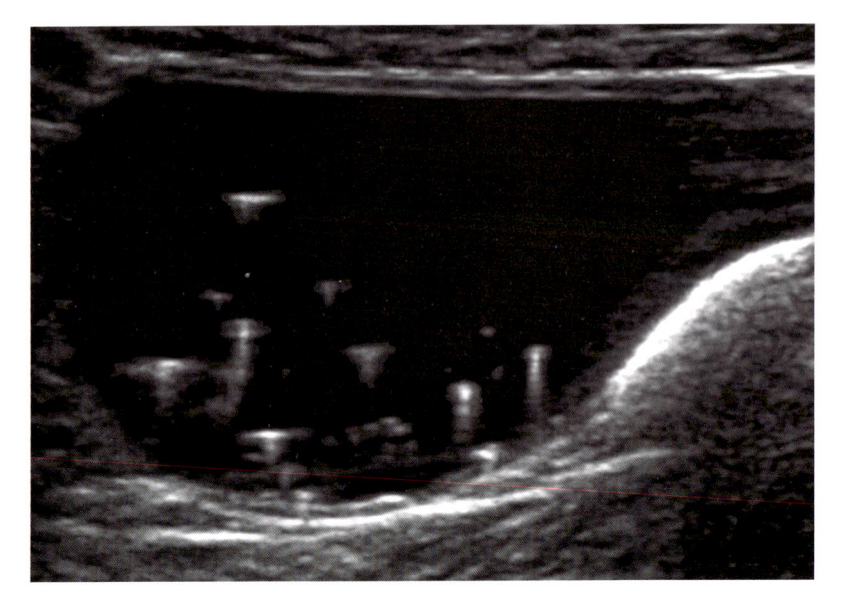

Fig. 36.16 Longitudinal ultrasound image of the bladder of an eight-year-old spayed female Boston Terrier with suspended echogenic foci in the bladder. Differential diagnoses for this include cellular material or crystalluria. This patient demonstrated calcium oxalate crystals on urinalysis.

CHAPTER 36 Urinary bladder and urethra

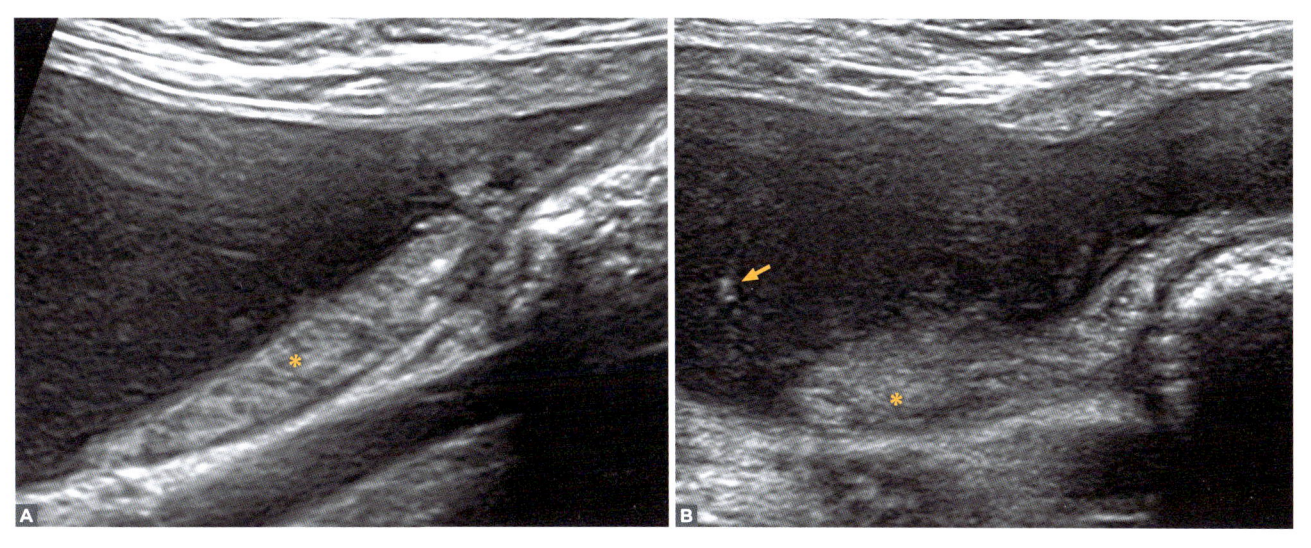

Fig. 36.17 (A) Longitudinal and (B) transverse ultrasound images of an 11-year-old spayed female Domestic shorthair cat with hematuria in association with feline lower urinary tract disease. There is a combination of suspended (arrow) and dependent (asterisk) material within the bladder lumen. (B) The altered distribution and suspension of some of the dependent material are due to ballottement. The bladder was agitated by applying pressure with the ultrasound probe and moving side to side, thus shaking the material in the bladder lumen. This technique is useful to distinguish free-floating but settled material from adherent material or a bladder wall mass.

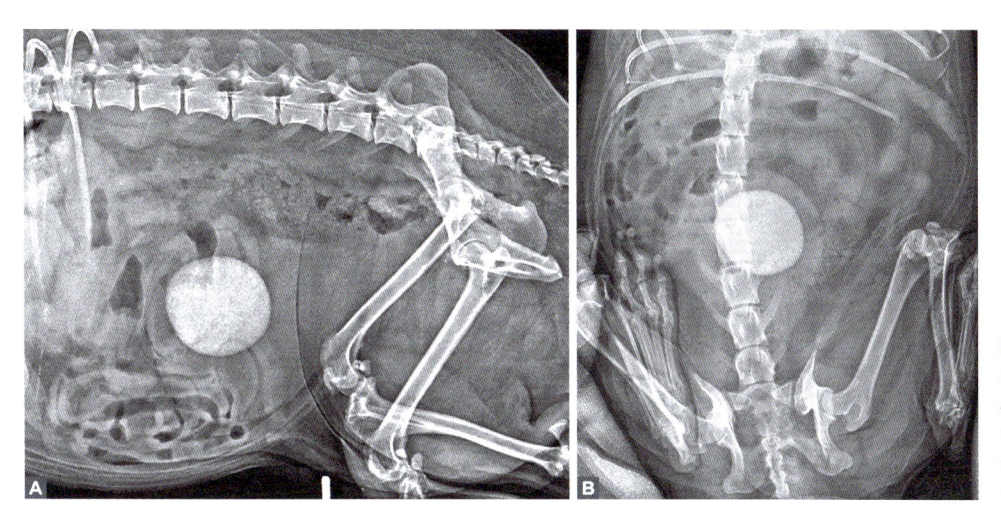

Fig. 36.18 (A) Left lateral and (B) dorsoventral projections of an eight-year-old dog presenting with hematuria. A single large calculus with slightly heterogeneous opacity is present in the urinary bladder.

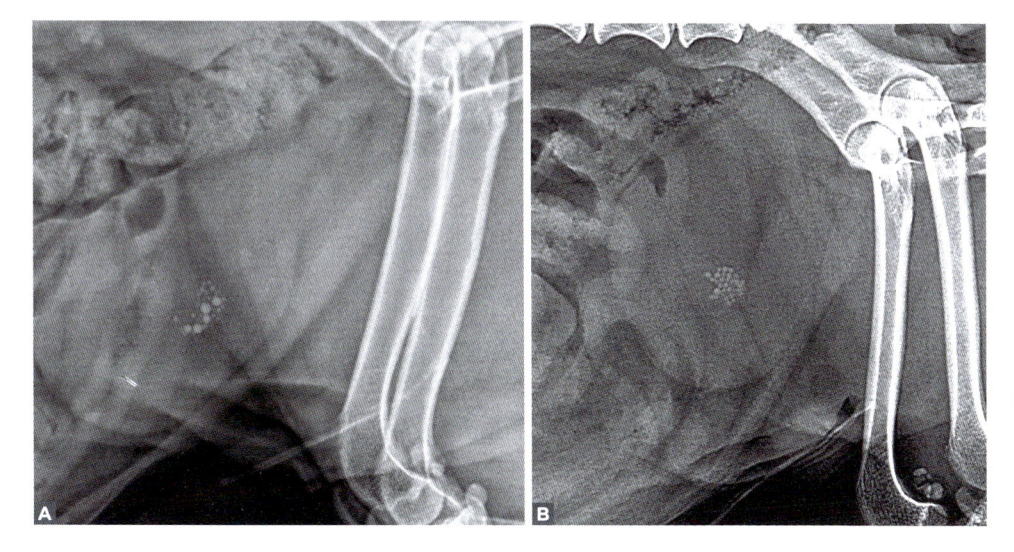

Fig. 36.19 Lateral radiographs of two dogs with cystic calculi. The calculi vary in size. Note that the larger calculi are more opaque and more readily identified.

587

SECTION V ABDOMEN

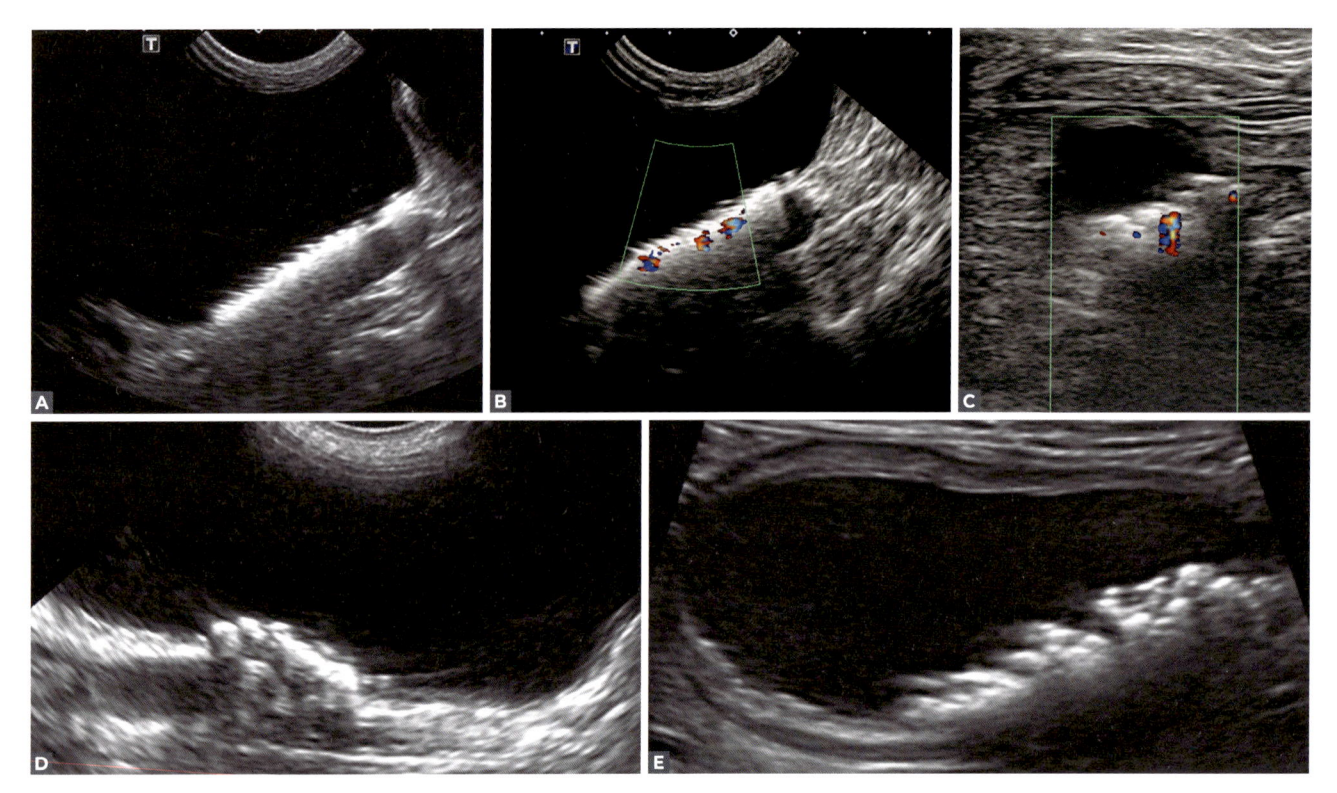

Fig. 36.20 The common sonographic appearance of small calculi in the dog. Hyperechoic foci that typically cast a distal acoustic shadow are present in the dependent portion of the bladder. (A, B) An 11-year-old spayed female mixed breed dog presenting for hematuria. (C, E) An eight-year-old castrated male Bichon Frisé presenting for straining to urinate. (D) A ten-month-old mixed breed with a portosystemic shunt and presumed urate calculi. (E) A five-year-old Chihuahua presenting for hematuria and stranguria. (B, C) Color Doppler has been applied to hyperechoic foci in the bladder, and a twinkling artifact is present. A twinkling artifact appears as an intense color Doppler signal where no blood flow is present, which changes in color and intensity in real-time examination. This artifact can help confirm the presence of mineralization.

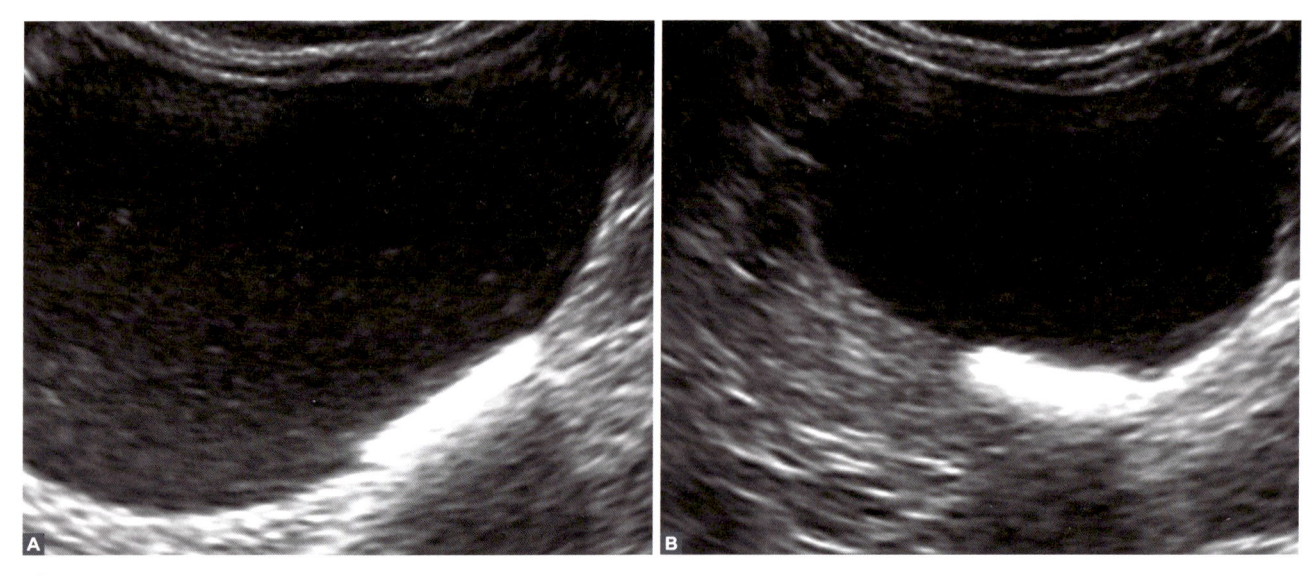

Fig. 36.21 (A) Longitudinal and (B) transverse ultrasound images of an accumulation of mineralized debris, commonly referred to as "sand" or "grit" in a cat. This material is often encountered in cats with FLUTD and can cause obstruction if dislodged to occupy the urethra. The material accumulates in the dependent portion of the bladder and can cause distal acoustic shadowing.

CHAPTER 36 Urinary bladder and urethra

Fig. 36.22 (**A**) Standard lateral and (**B**) flexed leg lateral radiograph of a 12-year-old castrated male mixed breed dog with a urethral calculus. Notice that the calculus (arrow) cannot be seen with the standard lateral projection and requires a flexed leg lateral projection for visualization.

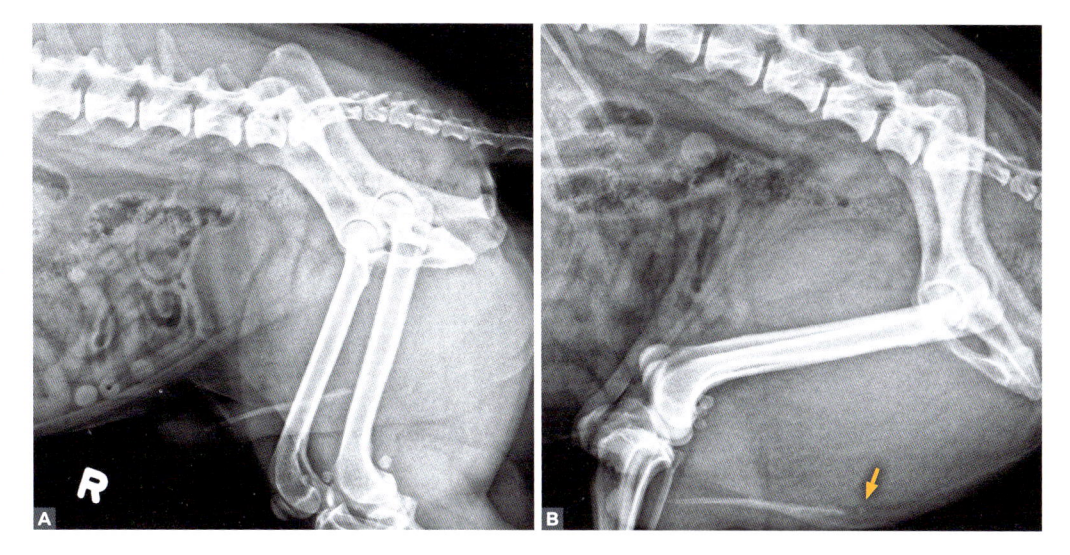

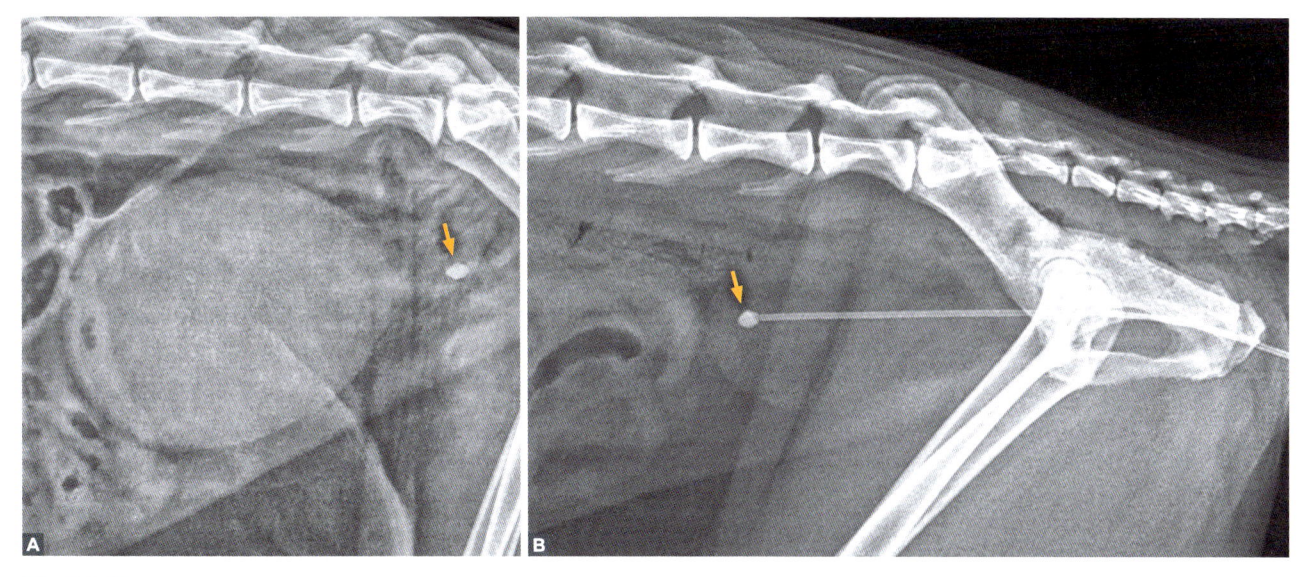

Fig. 36.23 Lateral radiographs of a 15-year-old castrated male Domestic shorthair cat with an obstructive urethral calculus. (**A**) The bladder is distended due to the presence of a large calculus (arrow) in the proximal urethra. There is streaky fluid opacity in the periurethral fat, representing urine extravasation from complete urethral obstruction. (**B**) The calculus was retropulsed into the bladder lumen, and after the placement of a catheter the bladder was smaller.

Fig. 36.24 Lateral radiograph of a five-year-old castrated male Domestic shorthair cat with numerous small calculi in the bladder and urethra (arrows). This patient presented for straining to urinate, and a cystocentesis was performed, resulting in a few gas bubbles in the urinary bladder (aasterisk).

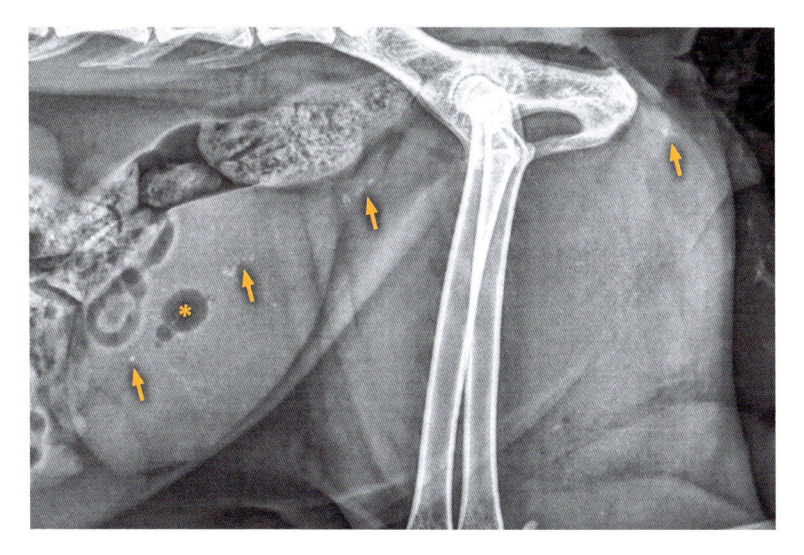

589

SECTION V ABDOMEN

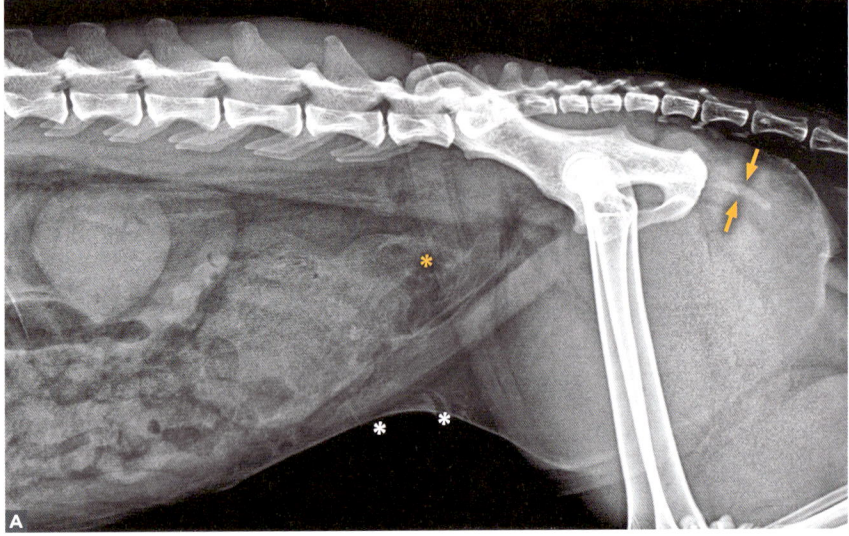

Fig. 36.25 (**A**) Lateral and (**B**) ventrodorsal radiographs of a cat with a urethral plug. The plug is best seen in the lateral projection (arrows) and requires adjustment of the image contrast to delineate. The plug cannot be seen in the ventrodorsal projection due to superimposition with the tail. The bladder is moderately distended, and a small amount of abdominal effusion is present (orange asterisk). Additionally, the patient has numerous wispy soft tissue opacities superimposing the caudal abdomen compatible with wet hair artifact (white asterisk).

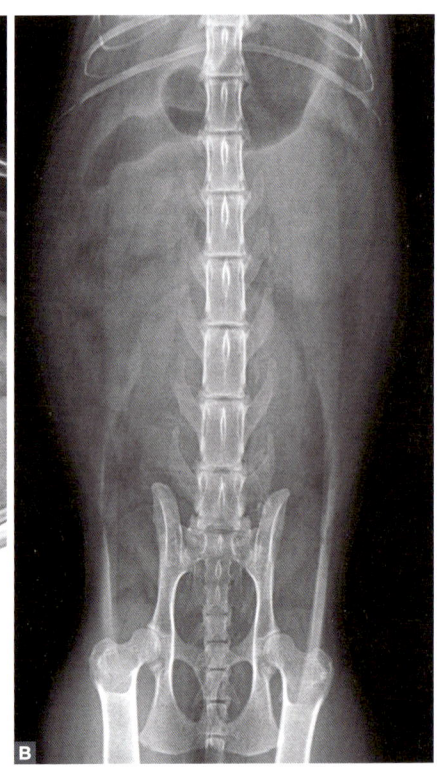

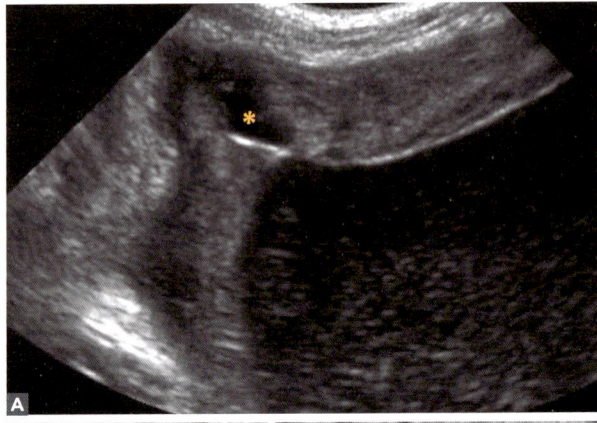

Fig. 36.26 (**A**) Longitudinal ultrasound, (**B**) sagittal, (**C**) dorsal, and (**D**) transverse CT images of a ten-month-old American Bulldog with an abscessed urachal diverticulum. The urachal diverticulum (asterisk) is a fluid-filled pocket at the ventral apex of the bladder (**A**). In CT, the following day the diverticulum was larger than that noted on ultrasound. In both ultrasound and CT, communication between the bladder lumen and diverticulum was seen. Echogenic and hyperattenuating material is present in the bladder lumen, compatible with a combination of hemorrhage and purulent material.

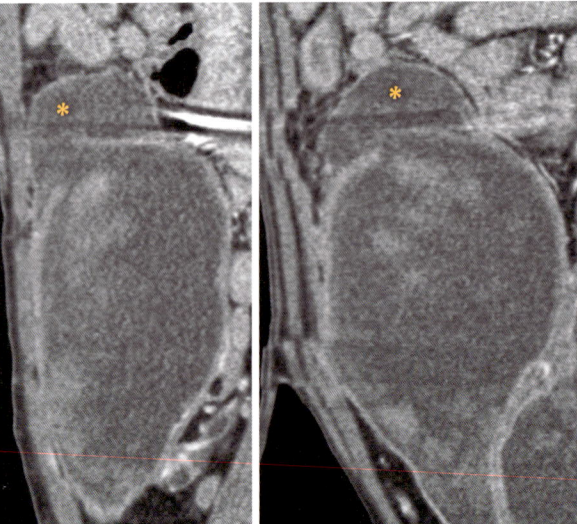

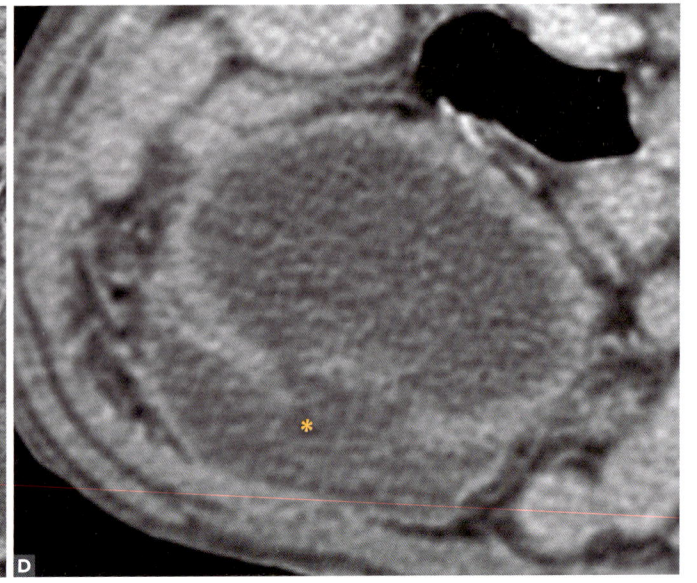

Congenital anomalies

Congenital anomalies of the urinary bladder include aberrant insertion of the ureters (discussed in the preceding chapter), urachal anomalies, and aberrant bladder positioning. Urachal anomalies such as urachal diverticuli, urachal sinus, urachal cyst, and patent urachus have been well described in dogs and cats and may be visible on ultrasound, CT (**fig. 36.26**), and occasionally radiographs (**fig. 36.27**). Vesiculourachal diverticula are the most common urachal anomaly, and both dogs and cats are typically asymptomatic.[15] Urachal anomalies can lead to urinary tract infections.

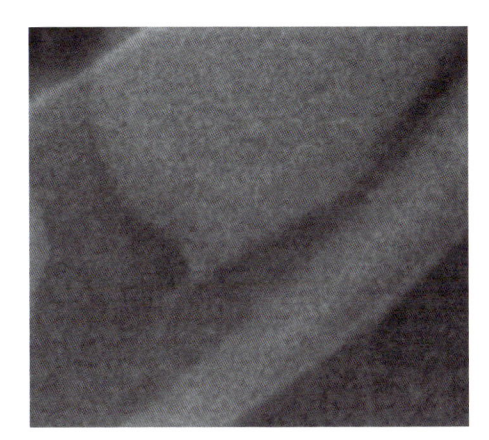

Caudal positioning of the urinary bladder has been reported and is sometimes associated with additional congenital anomalies.[16]

Urethral diverticula (**fig. 36.28**) have been reported in dogs and cats. Other congenital anomalies, such as urethral duplication, have been reported.[17]

Fig. 36.27 Lateral radiograph showing a urachal diverticulum in a cat. The appearance and location of the triangular soft tissue opacity protrusion arising from the apical bladder wall are consistent with a urachal diverticulum, but this was an incidental finding in this patient.

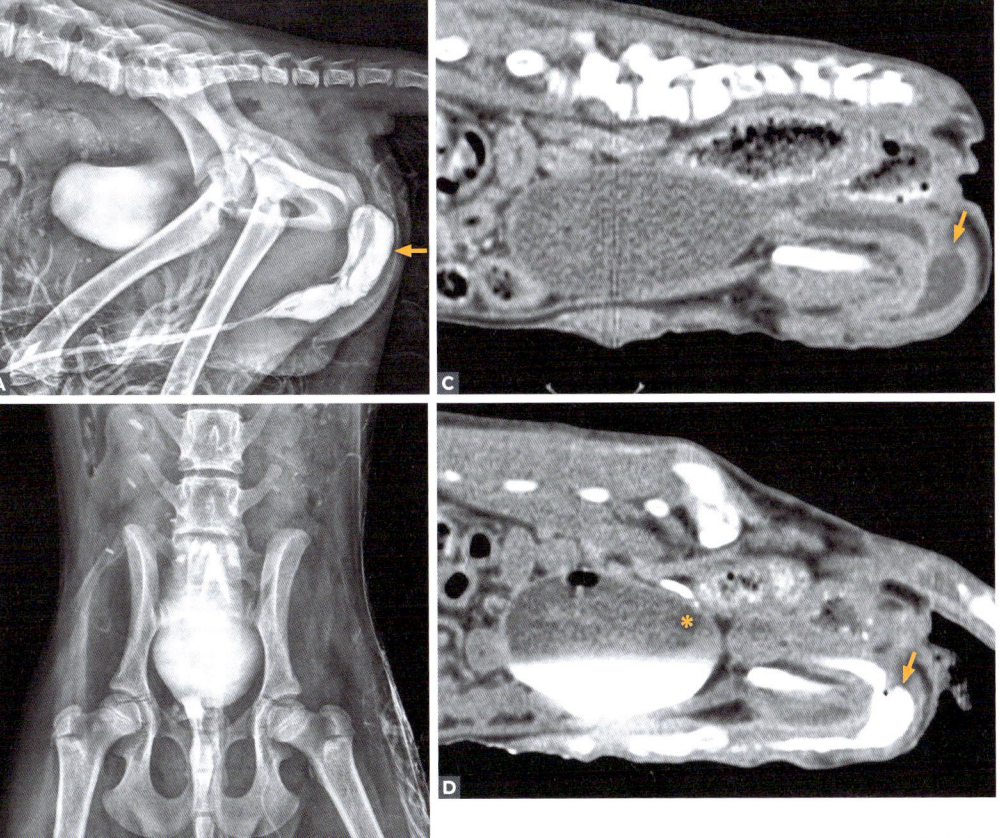

Fig. 36.28 (**A**) Lateral and (**B**) ventrodorsal retrograde urethrography, and (**C**) contrast-enhanced CT and (**D**) CT retrograde urethrography of a three-month-old male mixed breed dog with a urethral diverticulum. (**A**, **B**) The bladder is filled with contrast medium and a focal enlargement of the penile urethra is noted (arrow). (**C**) This finding is confirmed with CT, where there is a fluid-filled cavity (arrow) confluent with the urethra. Intravenous contrast medium highlights the margins of the bladder and urethra (**C**), while retrograde CT cystourethrography (**D**) can also help identify the affected portion of the urinary tract. (**D**) The expanded urethra noted in (**C**) is filled with positive contrast medium. While diagnosis can be made with radiographs, CT allows complete visualization and confirms whether the ureters enter the diverticulum. In this instance, the ureters are normally positioned (asterisk).

Bladder rupture

Rupture of the urinary bladder can occur either secondary to blunt force trauma, such as that from motor vehicle trauma, or from complete urethral obstruction. Rupture of the bladder will present as fluid in the peritoneal space (**fig. 36.29**). The bladder is usually small in these cases and is partly or completely obscured by fluid. Bladder rupture can be suspected based on history but must be confirmed with abdominocentesis confirming uroperitoneum and confirmation of site of rupture by cystogram and urethrogram (**fig. 36.30**).

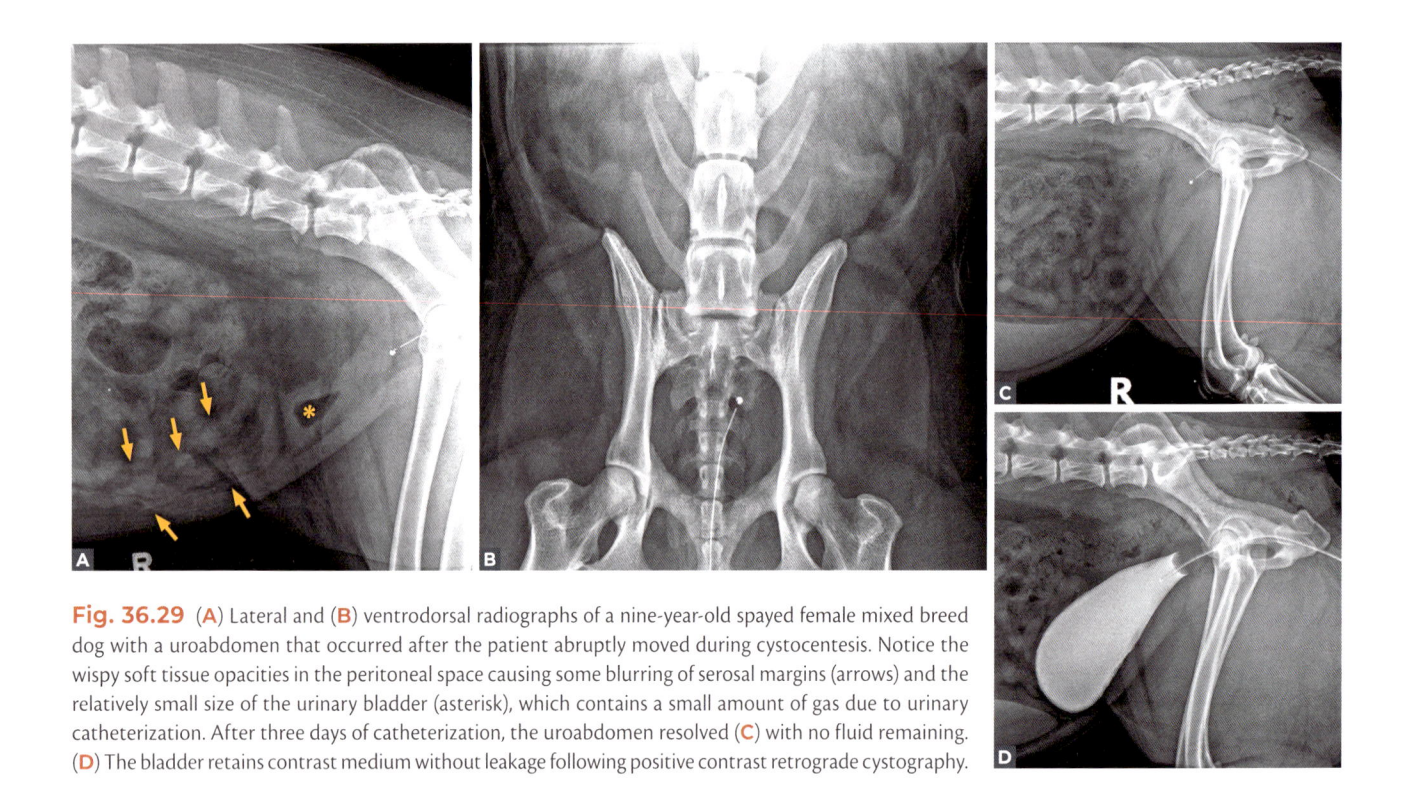

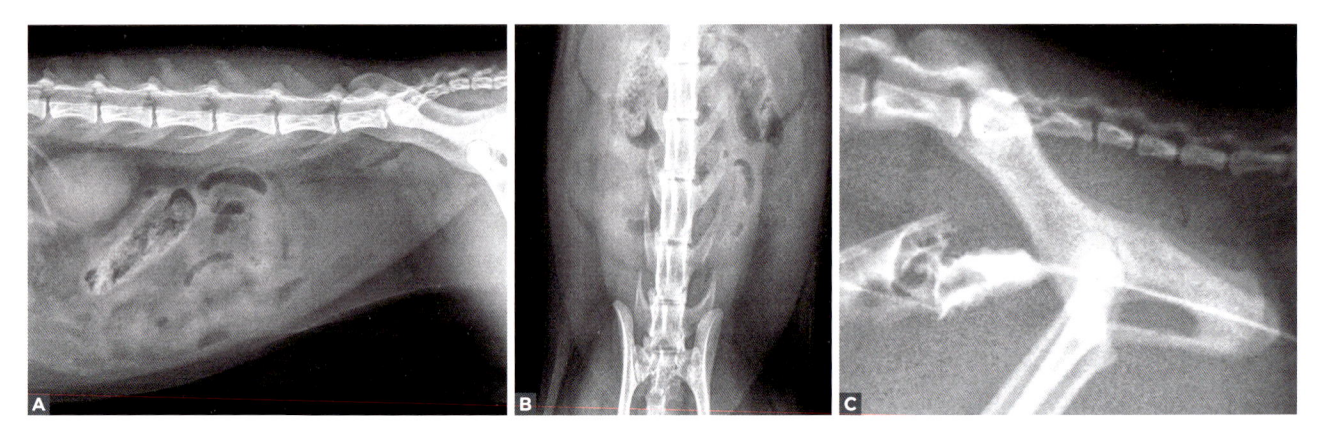

Fig. 36.29 (**A**) Lateral and (**B**) ventrodorsal radiographs of a nine-year-old spayed female mixed breed dog with a uroabdomen that occurred after the patient abruptly moved during cystocentesis. Notice the wispy soft tissue opacities in the peritoneal space causing some blurring of serosal margins (arrows) and the relatively small size of the urinary bladder (asterisk), which contains a small amount of gas due to urinary catheterization. After three days of catheterization, the uroabdomen resolved (**C**) with no fluid remaining. (**D**) The bladder retains contrast medium without leakage following positive contrast retrograde cystography.

Fig. 36.30 (**A**) Lateral and (**B**) ventrodorsal radiographs of a six-year-old spayed female Siamese cat with peritoneal effusion. The bladder is obscured due to silhouetting with abdominal fluid. (**C**) A retrograde cystogram confirms bladder rupture. The contrast medium leaks into the peritoneal cavity, and the bladder does not fill.

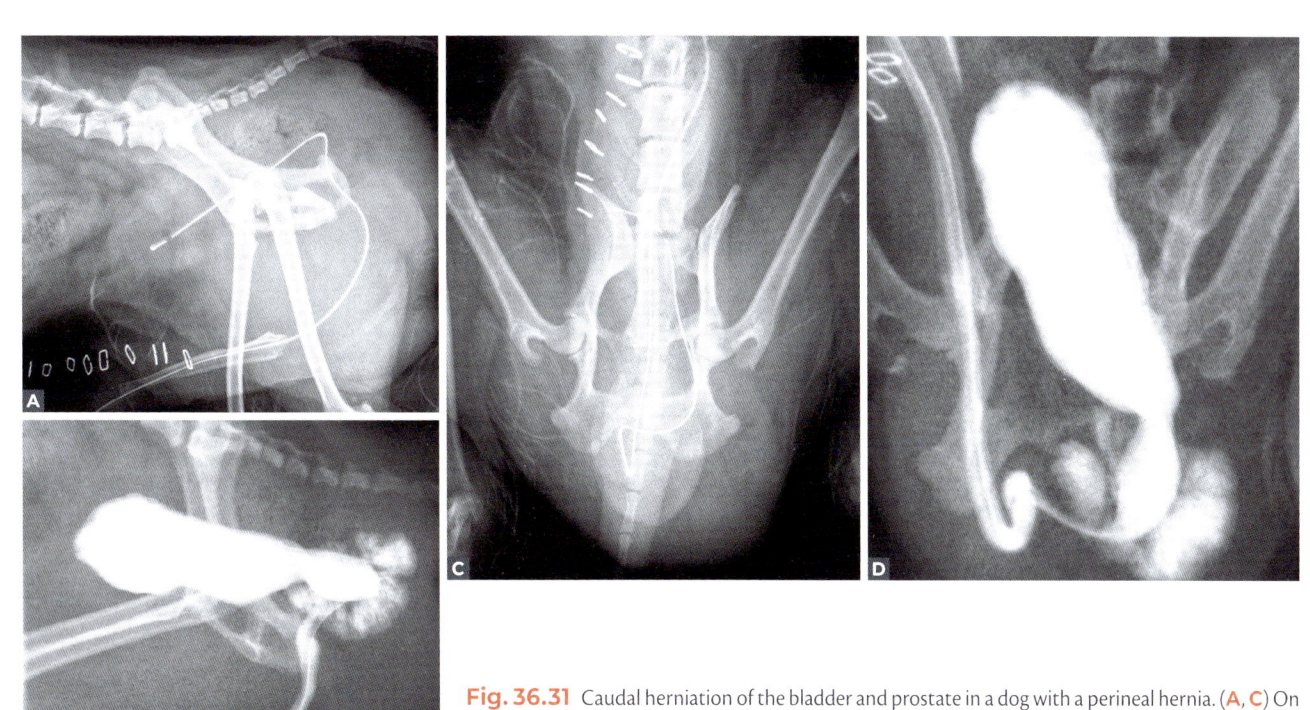

Fig. 36.31 Caudal herniation of the bladder and prostate in a dog with a perineal hernia. (**A, C**) On survey radiographs with a urinary catheter in place, the catheter kinks caudally, and there is swelling of the perineal region. (**B, D**) Retrograde cystourethrography shows the bladder is displaced caudally and largely intrapelvic, and the prostate is herniated into the perineal region. Normal contrast reflux into the prostatic ducts is present.

Bladder herniation

A common direction of bladder herniation is caudally in cases of perineal hernia. In these instances, there is often a clinically noted perineal swelling that is sometimes appreciated on radiographs. The hernia can be evaluated with ultrasound to determine its content, or a retrograde cystourethrogram can confirm the location of urinary structures within the hernia (**fig. 36.31**). Trauma can also result in bladder herniation which will occasionally occur ventrally through the abdominal wall. Survey radiographs may confirm a bladder herniation, though ultrasound or a contrast cystogram is often required to confirm body wall rupture and herniation.

Hemorrhage

Hemorrhage can occur in the urinary bladder either within the wall (intramurally) or into the lumen. Neither can be diagnosed with survey radiographs. Hemorrhage can occur either from trauma or coagulopathies.[18,19] Intramural hemorrhage appears as bladder wall thickening (**fig. 36.32**), typically diffusely hyperechoic.[18] The appearance may be similar to other causes of mural thickening (such as cystitis and neoplasia), and clinical correlation is helpful in confirming hemorrhage. Intraluminal hemorrhage (**fig. 36.33**) can form clots in the bladder lumen that can mimic mural mass lesions. Repositioning the patient to determine if the structure is fixed or mobile can help to distinguish between clots and mucosal lesions. Color Doppler imaging can also be used to determine if the structure is perfused, which would exclude a clot.

SECTION V ABDOMEN

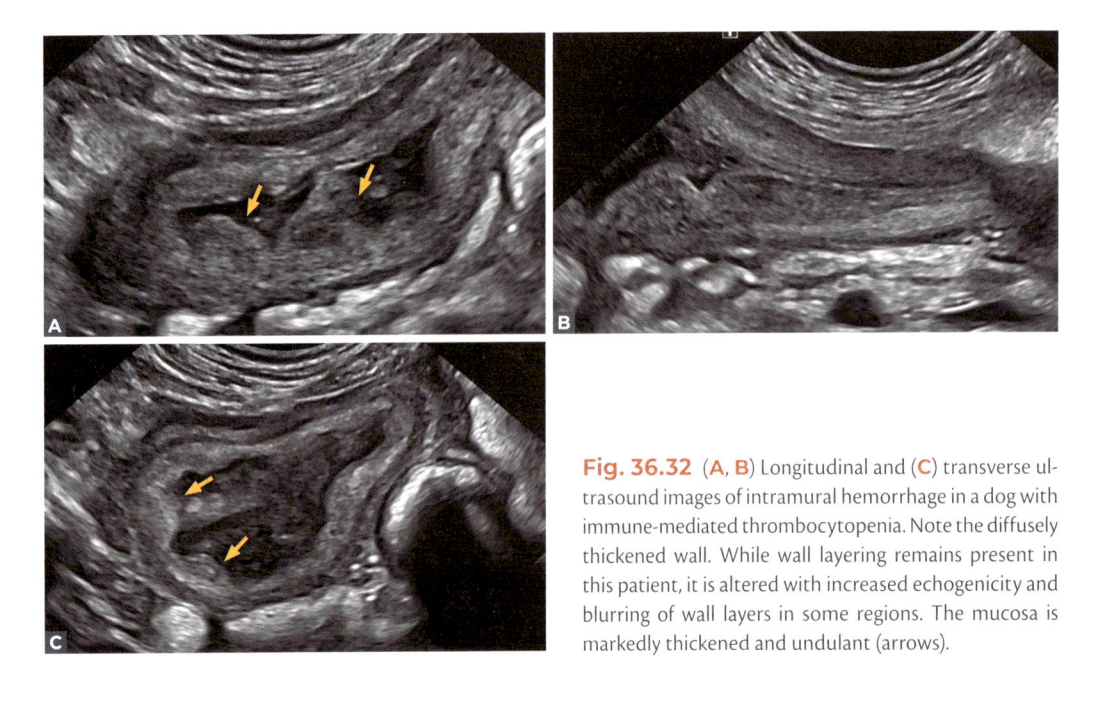

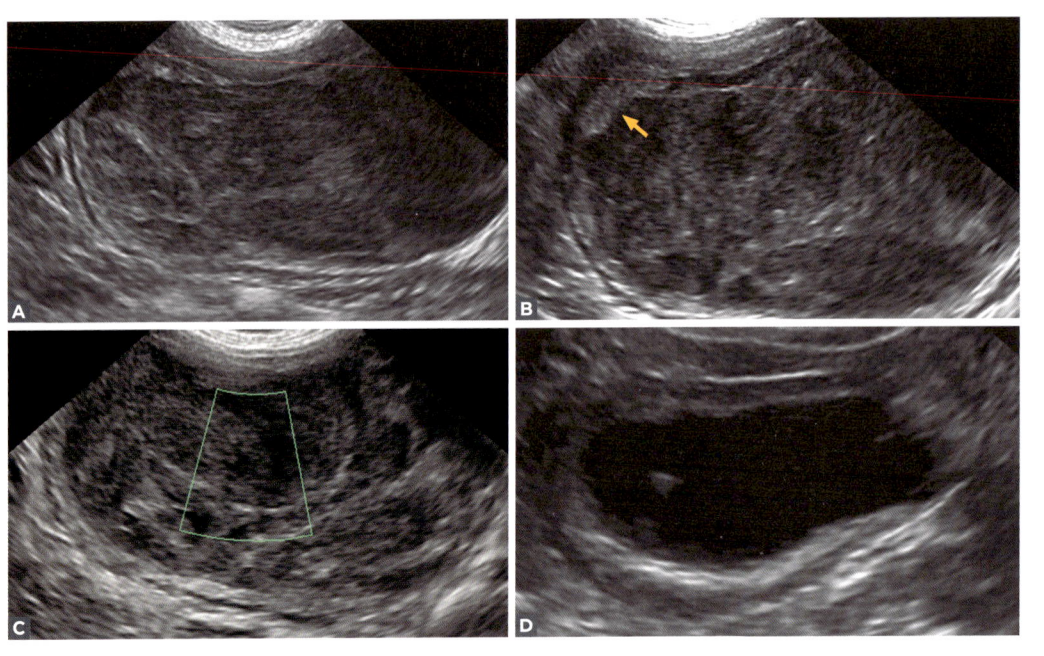

Fig. 36.32 (A, B) Longitudinal and (C) transverse ultrasound images of intramural hemorrhage in a dog with immune-mediated thrombocytopenia. Note the diffusely thickened wall. While wall layering remains present in this patient, it is altered with increased echogenicity and blurring of wall layers in some regions. The mucosa is markedly thickened and undulant (arrows).

Fig. 36.33 Ultrasound images of a six-year-old male Cocker Spaniel with intraluminal bladder hemorrhage. Note the amorphous echogenic content filling the bladder. This is a large clot in the bladder. (C) When color Doppler is applied, there is no evidence of perfusion in the structure. Mild wall thickening is noted along the ventral bladder apex (arrow). This patient was diagnosed with coagulopathy secondary to platelet dysfunction.

Canine prostate

In the neutered male dog, the prostate atrophies and is not seen on radiographs. In intact male dogs, the prostate may be intrapelvic, partly intraabdominal, or intraabdominal. The cranioventral margin of an enlarged prostate can be outlined by fat in the caudal abdomen (**fig. 36.34**) interposed between the caudoventral margin of the bladder, the body wall, and the prostate. An enlarged and mineralized prostate in a dog neutered as a juvenile is most often from prostatic or urethral neoplasia (**fig. 36.35**).[20] Sonographically, a neutered male has a small prostate visible as a fusiform hypoechoic structure surrounding the urethra. In intact male dogs, the prostate is relatively hyperechoic (**fig. 36.36B** and **36.36C**) compared to castrated dogs (**fig. 36.36A**). Enlargement of the prostate in intact dogs is most often from benign prostatic hyperplasia (BPH).

CHAPTER **36** Urinary bladder and urethra

Fig. 36.34 Lateral radiographs showing an enlarged prostate (asterisk) in (**A**) a 12-year-old male intact Old English Sheepdog and (**B**) a ten-year-old intact Bernese Mountain dog. (**A**) Note the triangle of fat created by the presence of the enlarged prostate (yellow lines). (**B**) The prostate is markedly enlarged with rounded and asymmetric margins (orange line). This patient was diagnosed with benign cystic prostatic hyperplasia.

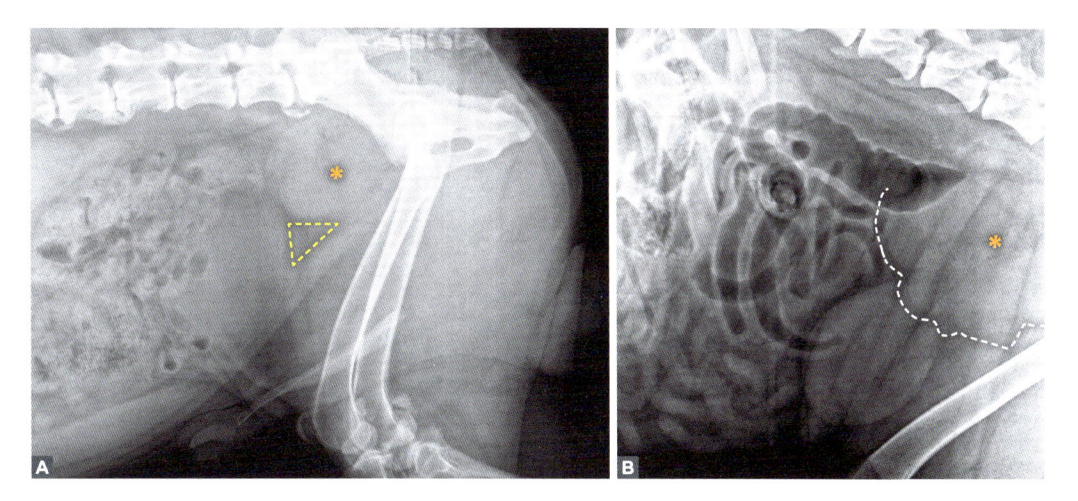

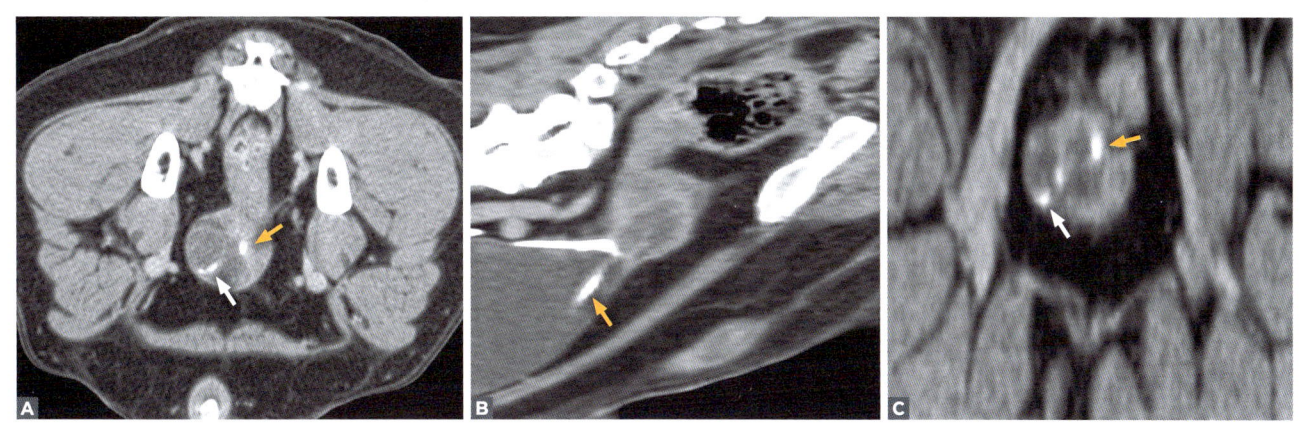

Fig. 36.35 (**A**) Transverse, (**B**) sagittal, and (**C**) dorsal computed tomographic images of an 11-year-old castrated male Weimaraner with prostatic carcinoma. The prostate is enlarged with cysts present and mineralization in the right ventral aspect (white arrows). A urinary catheter is in place (orange arrows), and contrast medium can be seen in the left ureter (**B**) at the caudodorsal margin of the bladder.

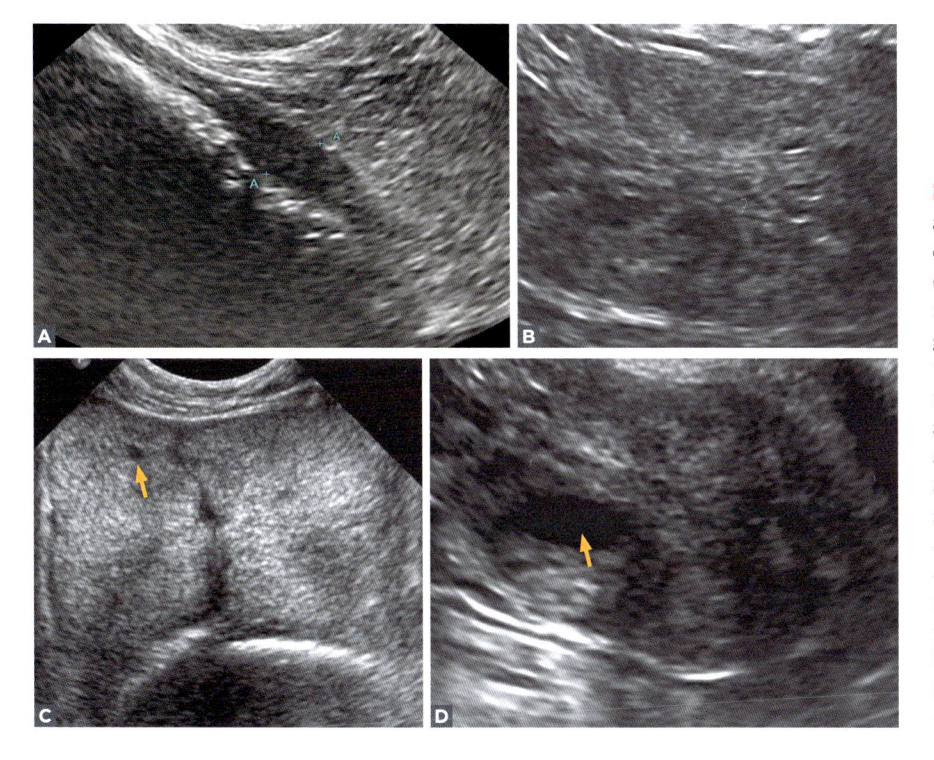

Fig. 36.36 Comparative sonographic image of the prostate in dogs. (**A**) A nine-year-old male castrated Havanese shows a small (5 mm) hypoechoic prostate with a smooth margin. (**B**) A six-year-old intact male Corgi showing a larger prostate (approximately 1 cm) with heterogeneously hyperechoic parenchyma. (**C**) Transverse ultrasound image of an eight-year-old German Shepherd showing a uniformly hyperechoic prostate, an appearance common in intact male dogs. Note the symmetry of the prostatic lobes in this plane. A small cyst is present in the ventral aspect of the right lobe (arrow). (**D**) Longitudinal ultrasound image of the prostate in a seven-year-old intact mixed breed dog identifying a larger cyst (approximately 5 mm) with a mildly heterogeneously hyperechoic remainder of the prostatic parenchyma.

595

SECTION V ABDOMEN

Infections of the prostate may occur as a sequel to BPH. Large fluid-filled lesions with echogenic material and evidence of inflammation of the peritoneal space around the enlarged prostate or mass are common imaging findings (**fig. 36.37**).

Paraprostatic cysts can be identified as rounded soft tissue masses in the caudal abdomen near the urinary bladder. These may be uniform soft tissue opacity, but some have a thin mineralized capsule (**fig. 36.38**).[21]

Urethral strictures

Strictures can occur secondary to prior urethral insult, such as that due to urethral calculi. Strictures require retrograde contrast urethrography to diagnose (**fig. 36.39**). Contrast medium must be administered under pressure, and multiple radiographs obtained to ensure that the narrowing is not due to inadequate filling or spasm.

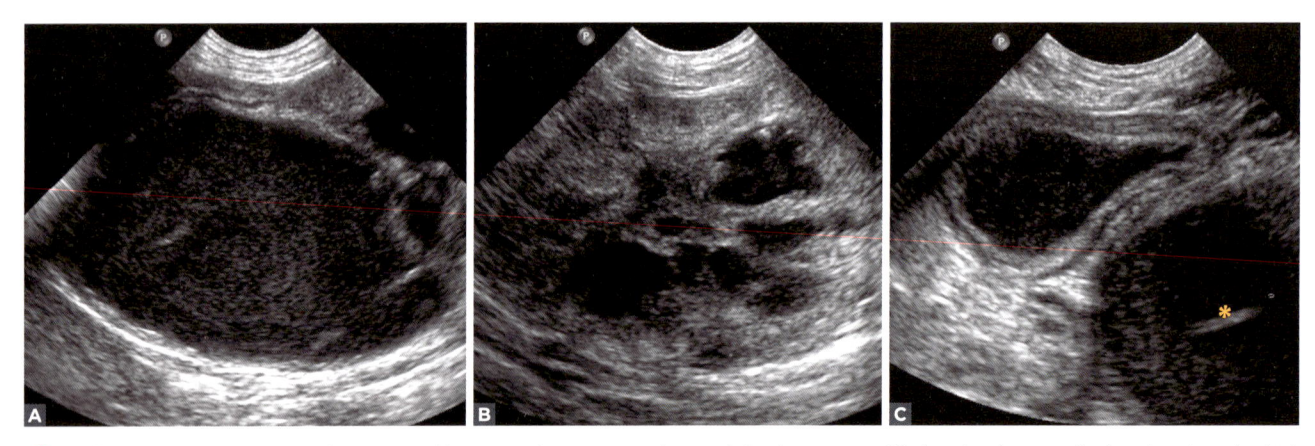

Fig. 36.37 Ultrasound images of a six-year-old Corgi with a prostatic abscess. (**A**) A large cavity filled with echogenic fluid and a relatively thick wall arises from the margin of the prostate. (**B**) The prostate is markedly enlarged with numerous variably sized fluid-filled cavities. (**C**) The bladder is displaced by the fluid-filled mass caudal to it but retains normal wall layering and size. The large fluid-filled cavity pictured in (**A**) can be seen displacing the bladder in (**C**) (asterisk).

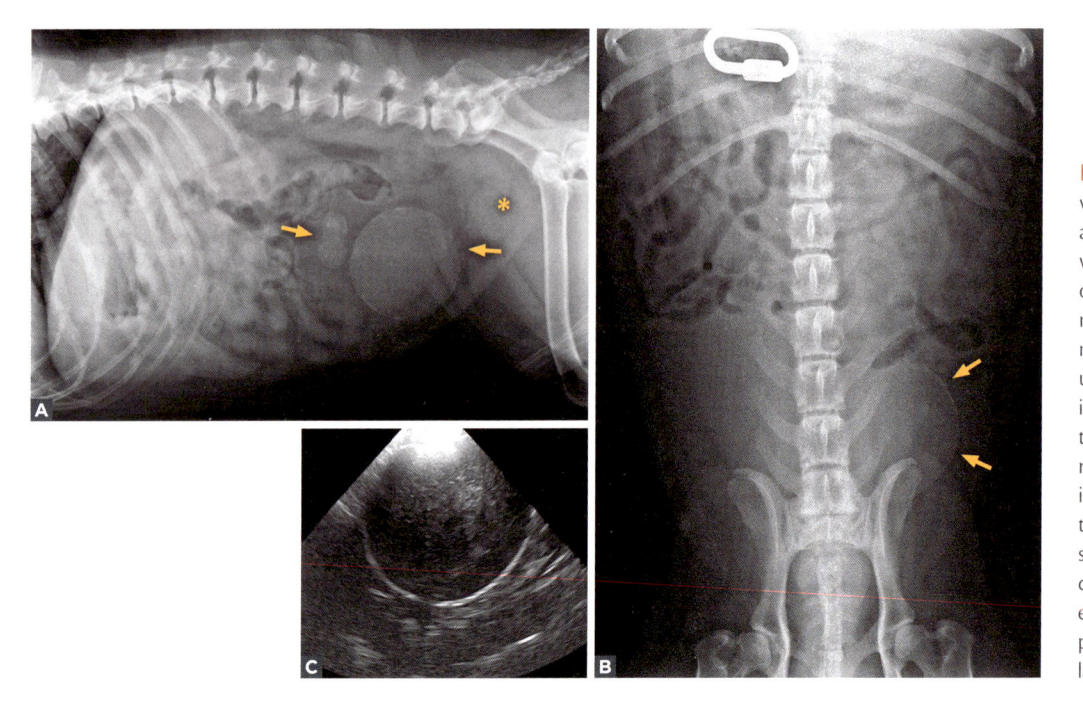

Fig. 36.38 Lateral and ventrodorsal radiographs and corresponding transverse ultrasound image of a seven-year-old intact mixed breed dog. A large mass and two smaller nodular lesions with mineralized shells are present in the left caudal abdomen representing paraprostatic cysts. Sonographically these appear as fluid-filled structures with a hyperechoic rim. A moderately enlarged intraabdominal prostate can be seen in the lateral projection (asterisk).

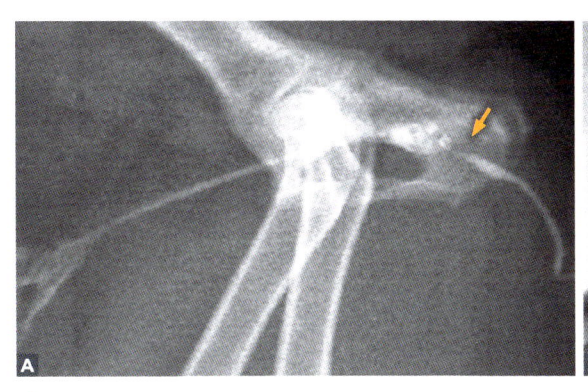

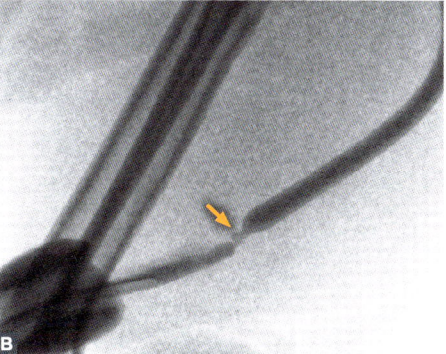

Fig. 36.39 Retrograde positive contrast urethrography in (**A**) a cat and (**B**) a dog with urethral strictures. Retrograde urethrography can be performed with (**A**) radiographs or (**B**) fluoroscopy. Strictures can be seen as focal regions of narrowing (arrows) that do not distend under pressure. (**A**) A retrograde cystourethrogram identifies a normal urethral diameter to the level of the ischium followed by marked narrowing denoted by the arrow. Cranial to the narrowing, there is moderate dilation of the urethra. A thin column of contrast medium extends cranially to this into the urinary bladder. (**B**) A retrograde urethrogram in a dog is performed by placing a catheter in the distal urethra, immediately proximal to the os penis. Contrast medium administered identifies a focal narrowing in the distal penile urethra a few centimeters proximal to the os penis (arrow). The urethra, both proximal and distal to this site, is of normal diameter.

References

1. Johnston GR, Osborne CA, Jessen CR, Feeney DA. Effects of urinary bladder distention on location of the urinary bladder and urethra of healthy dogs and cats. *Am J Vet Res* 47:404-415, 1986.
2. Geisse L, Lowry JE, Schaeffer DJ, Smith CW. Sonographic evaluation of urinary bladder wall thickness in normal dogs. *Vet Radiol Ultrasound* 38:132-137, 1995.
3. Sislak MD, Spaulding KA, Zoran DL, Bauer JE, Thompson JA. Ultrasonographic characteristics of lipiduria in clinically normal cats. *Vet Radiol Ultrasound* 55:195-201, 2014.
4. Piola V, Posch B, Aghte P, Caine A, Herrtage ME. Radiographic characterization of the os penis in the cat. *Vet Radiol Ultrasound* 52:270-272, 2011.
5. Fulkerson CM, Knapp DW. Management of transitional cell carcinoma of the urinary bladder in dogs: A review. *Vet J* 205:217-225, 2015.
6. Griffin MA, Culp WTN, Giuffrida MA, et al. Lower urinary tract transitional cell carcinoma in cats: clinical findings, treatments, and outcomes in 118 cases. *J Vet Intern Med* 34:274-282, 2020.
7. Wilson HM, Chun R, Larson VS, Kurzman ID, Vail DM. Clinical signs, treatments, and outcome in cats with transitional cell carcinoma of the urinary bladder: 20 Cases (1990-2004). *J Am Vet Med Assoc* 231:101-106, 2007.
8. Ostrander E, Decker B, Parker HG, et al. Homologous mutation to human BRAF V600E is common in naturally occurring canine bladder cancer—Evidence for a relevant model system and urine-based diagnostic test. *Mol Cancer Res* 17:1310-1314, 2012.
9. Forrester SD, Towell TL. Feline idiopathic cystitis. *Vet Clin North Am Small Anim Pract* 45:783-806, 2015.
10. Kaul E, Hartmann K, Reese S, Dorsch R. Recurrence rate and long-term course of cats with feline lower urinary tract disease. *J Feline Med Surg* 22:544-556, 2020.
11. Lulich JP, Berent AC, Adams LG, Westropp JL, Bartges JW, Osborne CA. ACVIM Small Animal Consensus Recommendations on the treatment and prevention of uroliths in dogs and cats. *J Vet Intern Med* 30:1564-1574, 2016.
12. Fumeo M, Manfredi S, Volta A. Emphysematous cystitis: review of current literature, diagnosis and management challenges. *Vet Med Res Reports* 10:77-83, 2019.
13. Jae Young Le, Seung Hyup Kim, Joeng Yeon Cho, Han D. Color and power doppler twinkling artifacts from urinary stones: clinical observations and phantom studies. *Am J Roentgenol* 176:1441-1445, 2001.
14. Weichselbaum RC, Feeney DA, Jessen CR, Osborne CA, Holte J. An integrated epidemiologic and radiographic algorithm for canine urocystolith mineral type prediction. *Vet Radiol Ultrasound* 42:311-319, 2001.
15. Perondi F, Puccinelli C, Lippi I, et al. Ultrasonographic diagnosis of urachal anomalies in cats and dogs: retrospective study of 98 cases (2009-2019). *Vet Sci* 7:1-12, 2020.
16. Adams WM, DiBartola SP. Radiographic and clinical features of pelvic bladder in the dog. *J Am Vet Med Assoc* 182:1212-1217, 1983.
17. Palm CA, Glaiberman CB, Culp WTN. Treatment of a urethral duplication in a dog using cyanoacrylate and coil embolization. *J Vet Intern Med* 29:727-731, 2015.
18. O'Brien RT, Wood EF. Urinary bladder mural hemorrhage associated with systemic bleeding disorders in three dogs. *Vet Radiol Ultrasound* 39:354-356, 1998.
19. Hooi KS, Lemetayer JD. The use of intravesicular alteplase for thrombolysis in a dog with urinary bladder thrombi. *J Vet Emerg Crit Care* 27:590-595, 2017.
20. Bradbury CA, Westropp JL, Pollard RE. Relationship between prostatomegaly, prostatic mineralization, and cytologic diagnosis. *Vet Radiol Ultrasound* 50:167-171, 2009.
21. Renfrew H, Barrett EL, Bradley KJ, Barr FJ. Radiographic and ultrasonographic features of canine paraprostatic cysts. *Vet Radiol Ultrasound* 49:444-448, 2008.

SECTION V ABDOMEN

There have been substantial developments in our knowledge about reproductive diagnostic imaging examination in carnivores over the last 20 years and these facilitate performance of a breeding soundness examination, routine monitoring of reproductive function, diagnosis and monitoring of pregnancy, and investigation of reproductive tract disease.

Males

Ultrasound is the imaging modality of choice to study the reproductive tract of the male dog. Imaging is best performed with the dog in the standing position, however lateral or dorsal recumbency is also frequently used in daily practice. The testis and the majority of the epididymis can be imaged scrotally and the prostate transabdominally.

Prostate

The prostate is an ovoid-shape bilobed gland positioned at the bladder neck which encircles the proximal urethra. The normal prostate is positioned within or immediately cranial to the pelvis and is bordered dorsally by the rectum.

Radiographs can be used to determine the size, shape, contour and location of the prostate, and is the examination of choice to evaluate vertebral complications (discospondylitis) in cases of prostatitis that cause hindlimb stiffness or lumbosacral pain. Radiography cannot differentiate prostatic diseases. In cases with suspicion of prostatic neoplasia, thoracic and abdominal radiographs should be performed to evaluate the presence of metastasis in regional lymph nodes, vertebral bodies and lungs. CT examination of the canine prostate can be useful as it provides information regarding location and morphological features of the gland, evaluation of the lymph nodes and assessment of metastatic lesions. CT is more sensitive than abdominal radiography to detect alterations of the parenchyma of the prostate gland, and allows more accurate staging of prostatic tumors.

On ultrasound the gland is smoothly marginated and the parenchyma in intact dogs has a moderate homogenous echogenicity, with a fine to medium coarse echotexture (**fig. 37.1**).

Prostatic size is assessed by measurement of the maximum prostatic width in the transverse plane or by calculation of the prostatic volume using the formula for volume of an ellipse: volume = length × width × height × 0.523.

Prostatic size varies depending on age, breed and sexual status. It is often possible to image the urethra; in the transverse plane the mucosal and muscular components may be identified, although more commonly the urethra is recognized simply as a hypoechoic region between the two prostatic lobes. In normal castrated dogs, the prostate is atrophied and smaller (**fig. 37.2**).

After castration the prostatic parenchyma becomes more hypoechoic. The combination of reduced size and reduced echogenicity often makes it difficult to differentiate the gland margins from the periprostatic fat. Prostatic size does not seem to relate to body mass in castrated dogs. It is noteworthy that while castration eliminates all but other prostatic disease, it does not protect completely from prostatic neoplasia. This diagnosis should be considered in older dogs which were neutered as juveniles and have prostatomegaly.

The two lobes of the dog's prostate gland each have an independent vascular supply. The prostatic artery has an anatomically variable origin, but commonly arises from the internal pudendal artery. For each lobe various vessels can be identified: (1) cranial, (2) dorsal and ventral subcapsular (also called lateral by some authors), (3) caudal, and (4) parenchymal. Blood flow from the prostate can be detected only in short segments of the relevant vein.

Color Doppler ultrasound is useful for identification of the location of the prostatic arterial supply and vessels may be imaged in the transverse or longitudinal plane. Flow characteristics vary according to the region of the prostate artery.

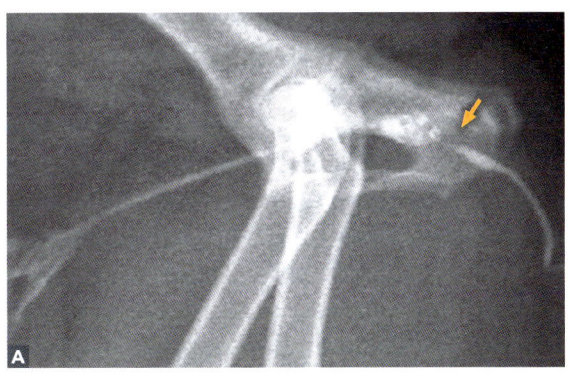

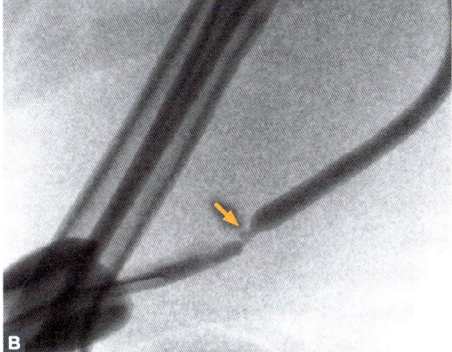

Fig. 36.39 Retrograde positive contrast urethrography in (**A**) a cat and (**B**) a dog with urethral strictures. Retrograde urethrography can be performed with (**A**) radiographs or (**B**) fluoroscopy. Strictures can be seen as focal regions of narrowing (arrows) that do not distend under pressure. (**A**) A retrograde cystourethrogram identifies a normal urethral diameter to the level of the ischium followed by marked narrowing denoted by the arrow. Cranial to the narrowing, there is moderate dilation of the urethra. A thin column of contrast medium extends cranially to this into the urinary bladder. (**B**) A retrograde urethrogram in a dog is performed by placing a catheter in the distal urethra, immediately proximal to the os penis. Contrast medium administered identifies a focal narrowing in the distal penile urethra a few centimeters proximal to the os penis (arrow). The urethra, both proximal and distal to this site, is of normal diameter.

References

1. Johnston GR, Osborne CA, Jessen CR, Feeney DA. Effects of urinary bladder distention on location of the urinary bladder and urethra of healthy dogs and cats. *Am J Vet Res* 47:404-415, 1986.
2. Geisse L, Lowry JE, Schaeffer DJ, Smith CW. Sonographic evaluation of urinary bladder wall thickness in normal dogs. *Vet Radiol Ultrasound* 38:132-137, 1995.
3. Sislak MD, Spaulding KA, Zoran DL, Bauer JE, Thompson JA. Ultrasonographic characteristics of lipiduria in clinically normal cats. *Vet Radiol Ultrasound* 55:195-201, 2014.
4. Piola V, Posch B, Aghte P, Caine A, Herrtage ME. Radiographic characterization of the os penis in the cat. *Vet Radiol Ultrasound* 52:270-272, 2011.
5. Fulkerson CM, Knapp DW. Management of transitional cell carcinoma of the urinary bladder in dogs: A review. *Vet J* 205:217-225, 2015.
6. Griffin MA, Culp WTN, Giuffrida MA, et al. Lower urinary tract transitional cell carcinoma in cats: clinical findings, treatments, and outcomes in 118 cases. *J Vet Intern Med* 34:274-282, 2020.
7. Wilson HM, Chun R, Larson VS, Kurzman ID, Vail DM. Clinical signs, treatments, and outcome in cats with transitional cell carcinoma of the urinary bladder: 20 Cases (1990-2004). *J Am Vet Med Assoc* 231:101-106, 2007.
8. Ostrander E, Decker B, Parker HG, et al. Homologous mutation to human BRAF V600E is common in naturally occurring canine bladder cancer—Evidence for a relevant model system and urine-based diagnostic test. *Mol Cancer Res* 17:1310-1314, 2012.
9. Forrester SD, Towell TL. Feline idiopathic cystitis. *Vet Clin North Am Small Anim Pract* 45:783-806, 2015.
10. Kaul E, Hartmann K, Reese S, Dorsch R. Recurrence rate and long-term course of cats with feline lower urinary tract disease. *J Feline Med Surg* 22:544-556, 2020.
11. Lulich JP, Berent AC, Adams LG, Westropp JL, Bartges JW, Osborne CA. ACVIM Small Animal Consensus Recommendations on the treatment and prevention of uroliths in dogs and cats. *J Vet Intern Med* 30:1564-1574, 2016.
12. Fumeo M, Manfredi S, Volta A. Emphysematous cystitis: review of current literature, diagnosis and management challenges. *Vet Med Res Reports* 10:77-83, 2019.
13. Jae Young Le, Seung Hyup Kim, Joeng Yeon Cho, Han D. Color and power doppler twinkling artifacts from urinary stones: clinical observations and phantom studies. *Am J Roentgenol* 176:1441-1445, 2001.
14. Weichselbaum RC, Feeney DA, Jessen CR, Osborne CA, Holte J. An integrated epidemiologic and radiographic algorithm for canine urocystolith mineral type prediction. *Vet Radiol Ultrasound* 42:311-319, 2001.
15. Perondi F, Puccinelli C, Lippi I, et al. Ultrasonographic diagnosis of urachal anomalies in cats and dogs: retrospective study of 98 cases (2009-2019). *Vet Sci* 7:1-12, 2020.
16. Adams WM, DiBartola SP. Radiographic and clinical features of pelvic bladder in the dog. *J Am Vet Med Assoc* 182:1212-1217, 1983.
17. Palm CA, Glaiberman CB, Culp WTN. Treatment of a urethral duplication in a dog using cyanoacrylate and coil embolization. *J Vet Intern Med* 29:727-731, 2015.
18. O'Brien RT, Wood EF. Urinary bladder mural hemorrhage associated with systemic bleeding disorders in three dogs. *Vet Radiol Ultrasound* 39:354-356, 1998.
19. Hooi KS, Lemetayer JD. The use of intravesicular alteplase for thrombolysis in a dog with urinary bladder thrombi. *J Vet Emerg Crit Care* 27:590-595, 2017.
20. Bradbury CA, Westropp JL, Pollard RE. Relationship between prostatomegaly, prostatic mineralization, and cytologic diagnosis. *Vet Radiol Ultrasound* 50:167-171, 2009.
21. Renfrew H, Barrett EL, Bradley KJ, Barr FJ. Radiographic and ultrasonographic features of canine paraprostatic cysts. *Vet Radiol Ultrasound* 49:444-448, 2008.

CHAPTER 37

Prostate, testicles, ovaries, and uterus

Marco Russo and Massimo Vignoli

KEY POINTS

- Diagnostic imaging evaluation of the reproductive tract is an important step in the evaluation of physiological changes as well for reproductive pathologic conditions.
- Benign prostatic hyperplasia is the most common canine prostatic disorder and appears on ultrasound as an increased echogenicity with uniform or coarse echotexture.
- Paraprostatic cysts will appear as a fluid-filled anechoic to mildly echogenic structure with variable wall thickness and usually a hypoechoic stalk connecting to the prostate is visible.
- Prostatic neoplasia has a variable ultrasonographic appearance in the early stage of the disease with focal, hypoechoic lesions, which are usually difficult to distinguish from other pathologies. Later in the course of the disease, heterogenous parenchyma is often detected, with frequent irregular anechoic regions and zones of calcification generating acoustic shadowing.
- Ultrasound examination is a sensitive method for evaluating testicular parenchymal diseases, allowing differentiation of testicular from extratesticular causes of scrotal enlargement.
- Testicular neoplasms are the second most common neoplasm affecting male dogs. Testicular tumors can range from circumscribed small nodules to large complex masses with heterogeneous echo-pattern and disruption of normal anatomy.
- Cryptorchidism predisposes to neoplasia and the most common tumors are Sertoli cell tumors and seminomas.
- Ultrasonography appears to be sensitive for the detection of ovarian masses, but there are no specific patterns that confirm the diagnosis of tumor type.
- Confirmation of the origin of large ovarian masses by ultrasound may not be possible and CT is more specific. CT is also superior for abdominal staging and assessment of surgical options.
- Radiographic diagnosis of pregnancy is first possible on the 42nd to 50th days after first mating. For the most accurate estimation of puppy numbers, radiographs should be taken at about day 52-55 post first breeding.
- Ultrasound at day 30 post breeding is a sensitive diagnostic tool to confirm pregnancy and to assess embryonic resorption.
- Cystic endometrial hyperplasia is generally seen on ultrasonographic examination as a diffuse thickening of the uterine wall, with multiple anechoic areas contained within the wall.
- Involution of the postpartum uterus is normally complete within four weeks in both the bitch and the queen. The uterine wall is initially thick and irregular, and there is some luminal content of variable echogenicity.

There have been substantial developments in our knowledge about reproductive diagnostic imaging examination in carnivores over the last 20 years and these facilitate performance of a breeding soundness examination, routine monitoring of reproductive function, diagnosis and monitoring of pregnancy, and investigation of reproductive tract disease.

Males

Ultrasound is the imaging modality of choice to study the reproductive tract of the male dog. Imaging is best performed with the dog in the standing position, however lateral or dorsal recumbency is also frequently used in daily practice. The testis and the majority of the epididymis can be imaged scrotally and the prostate transabdominally.

Prostate

The prostate is an ovoid-shape bilobed gland positioned at the bladder neck which encircles the proximal urethra. The normal prostate is positioned within or immediately cranial to the pelvis and is bordered dorsally by the rectum.

Radiographs can be used to determine the size, shape, contour and location of the prostate, and is the examination of choice to evaluate vertebral complications (discospondylitis) in cases of prostatitis that cause hindlimb stiffness or lumbosacral pain. Radiography cannot differentiate prostatic diseases. In cases with suspicion of prostatic neoplasia, thoracic and abdominal radiographs should be performed to evaluate the presence of metastasis in regional lymph nodes, vertebral bodies and lungs. CT examination of the canine prostate can be useful as it provides information regarding location and morphological features of the gland, evaluation of the lymph nodes and assessment of metastatic lesions. CT is more sensitive than abdominal radiography to detect alterations of the parenchyma of the prostate gland, and allows more accurate staging of prostatic tumors.

On ultrasound the gland is smoothly marginated and the parenchyma in intact dogs has a moderate homogenous echogenicity, with a fine to medium coarse echotexture (**fig. 37.1**).

Prostatic size is assessed by measurement of the maximum prostatic width in the transverse plane or by calculation of the prostatic volume using the formula for volume of an ellipse: volume = length × width × height × 0.523.

Prostatic size varies depending on age, breed and sexual status. It is often possible to image the urethra; in the transverse plane the mucosal and muscular components may be identified, although more commonly the urethra is recognized simply as a hypoechoic region between the two prostatic lobes. In normal castrated dogs, the prostate is atrophied and smaller (**fig. 37.2**).

After castration the prostatic parenchyma becomes more hypoechoic. The combination of reduced size and reduced echogenicity often makes it difficult to differentiate the gland margins from the periprostatic fat. Prostatic size does not seem to relate to body mass in castrated dogs. It is noteworthy that while castration eliminates all but other prostatic disease, it does not protect completely from prostatic neoplasia. This diagnosis should be considered in older dogs which were neutered as juveniles and have prostatomegaly.

The two lobes of the dog's prostate gland each have an independent vascular supply. The prostatic artery has an anatomically variable origin, but commonly arises from the internal pudendal artery. For each lobe various vessels can be identified: (1) cranial, (2) dorsal and ventral subcapsular (also called lateral by some authors), (3) caudal, and (4) parenchymal. Blood flow from the prostate can be detected only in short segments of the relevant vein.

Color Doppler ultrasound is useful for identification of the location of the prostatic arterial supply and vessels may be imaged in the transverse or longitudinal plane. Flow characteristics vary according to the region of the prostate artery.

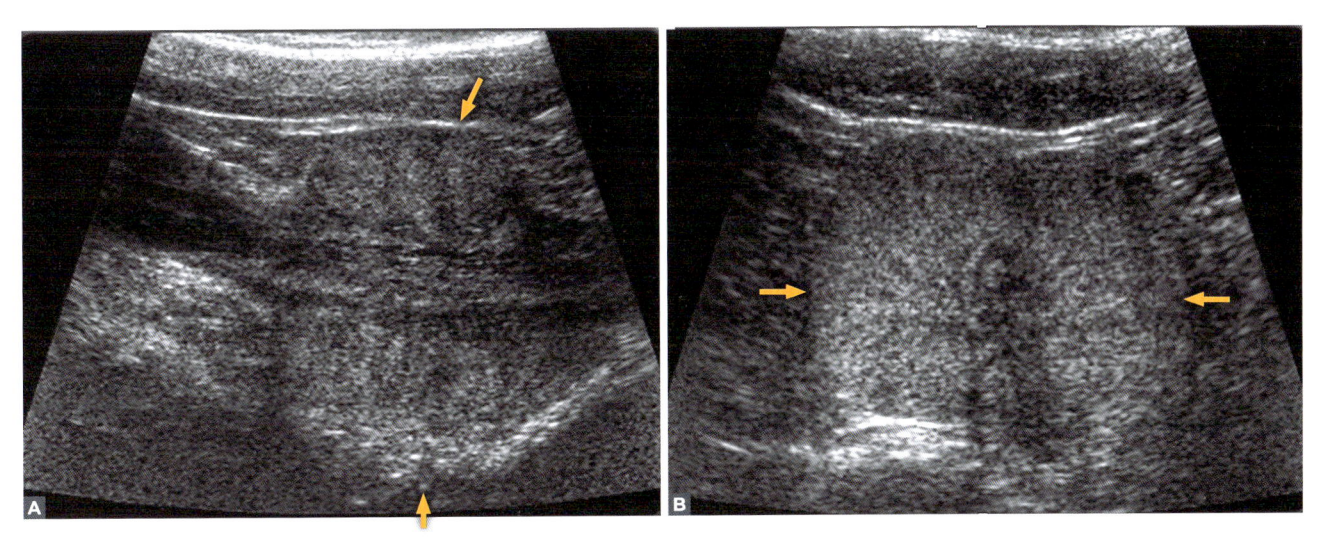

CHAPTER **37** Prostate, testicles, ovaries, and uterus

Fig. 37.1 Normal prostate: sagittal (**A**) and transverse (**B**) images of a three-year-old Pit Bull Terrier (arrows). The prostate gland appears homogeneous in echotexture, echogenic with smooth margins.

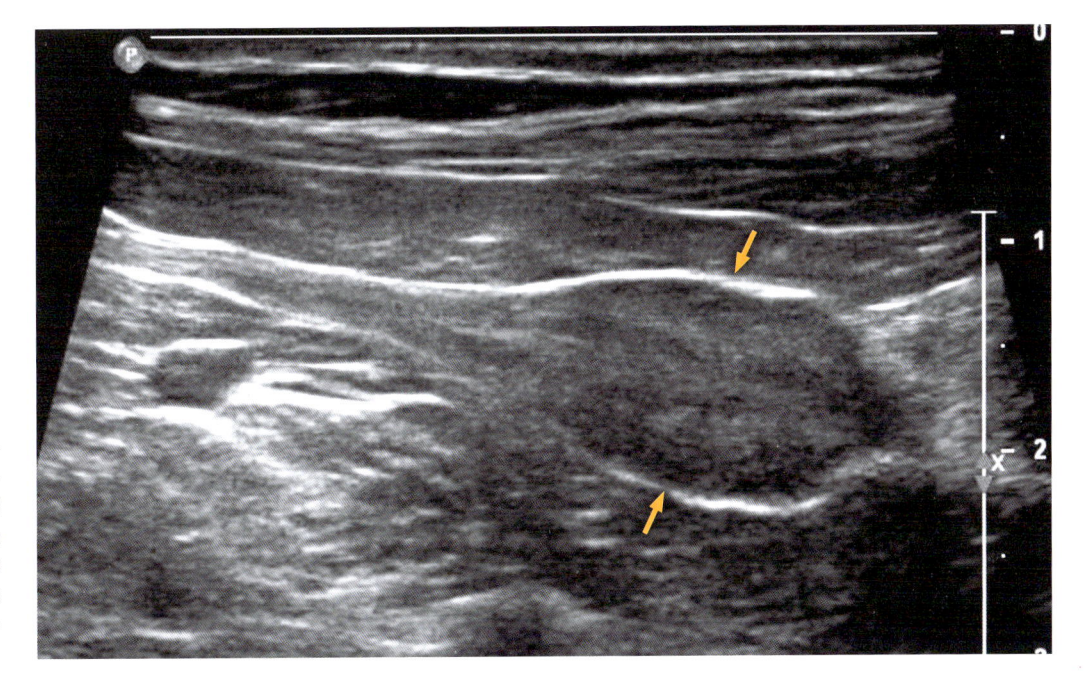

Fig. 37.2 Neutered prostate: a seven-year-old Cocker Spaniel. Longitudinal sonographic image of a normal prostate gland in a neutered dog, that appears oblong in shape and diffusely hypoechoic (arrows).

Abnormal prostate gland

Many diseases of the prostate gland may produce a similar appearance; further diagnostic tests including collection of prostatic fluid (ejaculation or urethral lavage), urinalysis, hematology, fine-needle aspiration or biopsy, and vertebral/thoracic radiographs are often required to confirm a diagnosis. A common but non-specific finding is prostatomegaly. Whilst ultrasound may be useful for measurement of prostatic size and calculation of prostatic volume, the substantial variation in prostatic size renders measurements unhelpful for diagnosis but these may be of some value to assess response to treatment. Asymmetrical enlargement is easier to detect if it alters the outline/margination of the gland. The prostate may develop both focal and diffuse parenchymal changes which may be hyperechoic, hypoechoic or of mixed echogenicity. These changes are non-specific and require further investigation that might include Doppler or contrast-enhanced ultrasound imaging. The presence of anechoic cystic structures which may be single or multiple, parenchymal and paraprostatic occur in a number of different pathologies.

601

▌**Benign prostatic hyperplasia** Benign prostatic hyperplasia (BPH) is a spontaneous and age-related condition of intact male dogs and a common incidental finding in older dogs. BPH does not occur in dogs that are castrated. In early cases there is symmetrical enlargement of the gland, increased echogenicity although there is often a patchy in-homogenous appearance with small 1-2 mm diameter anechoic cysts. Usually, the normal smooth outline of the prostate is maintained; however, if the enlargement is significant the gland may lose its bilobed appearance. Cysts from BPH appear as cavitated lesions filled with anechoic fluid ranging from a few millimeters up to 2 or 3 cm in size (**fig. 37.3**). The cysts may increase in size with the progression and severity of the disease, ultimately causing a honeycomb-like appearance.

▌**Cysts** When cysts become very large, they may have a similar appearance to a true paraprostatic cyst (fluid distention of a remnant *uterus masculinus*, Müllerian ducts), and can be difficult to differentiate, although the former is usually associated with other prostatic parenchymal changes typical of BPH, and in some cases the wide base of attachment/origin of the cyst within the prostate can be detected (in true paraprostatic cysts the cyst is attached only by a thin stalk-like structure). Large prostatic retention cysts or paraprostatic cysts have fluid that is anechoic but may become more echogenic and have obvious sediment. It is not uncommon for internal septation of the cyst cavity to be noted and for the cyst wall to become calcified, a similar appearance to some prostatic abscesses (**fig. 37.4**).

▌**Prostatitis** In cases of acute prostatitis, the gland may be enlarged, with a symmetrical or asymmetrical outline. The parenchyma is usually heterogenous and in acute prostatitis has a hypoechoic appearance, which is followed in more chronic cases by increased echogenicity, with focal echogenic regions. Prostatitis and BPH often coexist, and sampling is required to confirm the diagnosis. In chronic cases, patchy hypoechoic areas may appear and with time coalesce as microabscesses form; these are more irregularly marginated than the cysts seen with BPH, often contain particulate material or hypoechoic fluid (**fig. 37.5**). Abscess cavities may increase in size, and as a larger lumen forms calcification of the abscess wall may develop (**fig. 37.6**). Occasionally, prostatic abscesses contain gas. Anechoic or echogenic fluid may be present adjacent to the prostate (**fig. 37.7**). Steatitis or peritonitis affecting the periprostatic fat causes a hyperechoic and hyperattenuating appearance.

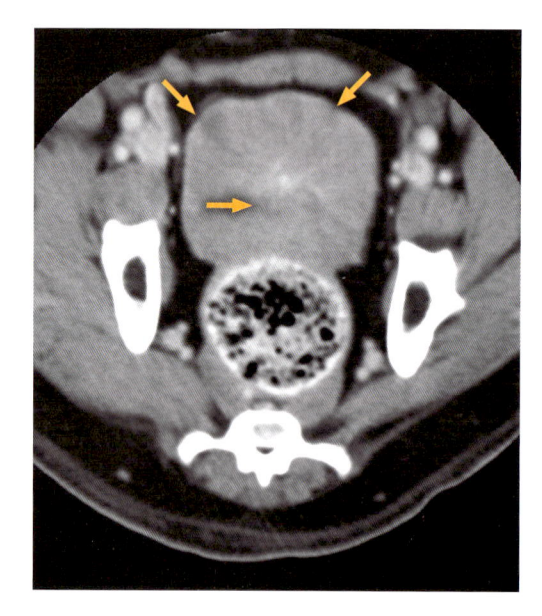

Fig. 37.3 CT: prostatomegaly and cysts. Transverse view of the prostate gland. An eight-year-old, mixed breed, intact male dog with a heterogenous prostate, increased in size with multiple cysts (arrows).

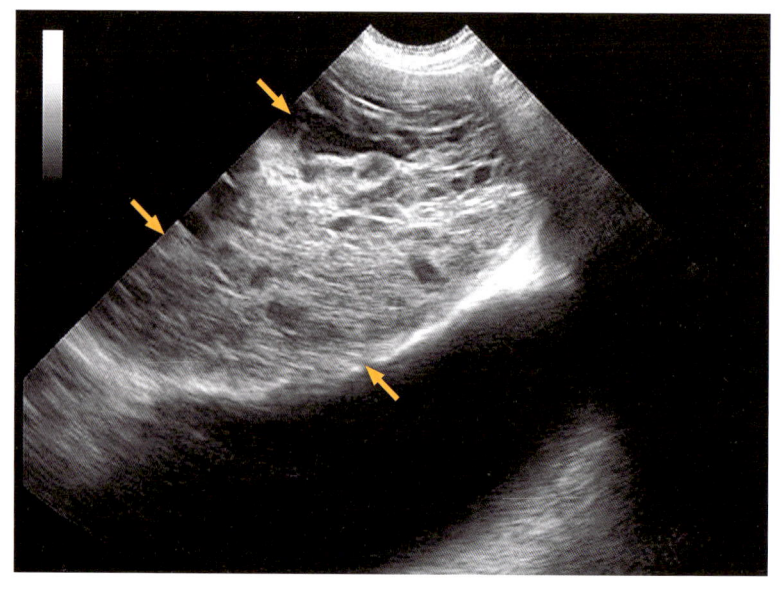

Fig. 37.4 Paraprostatic cyst. A ten-year-old German Shepherd dog with dysuria and constipation. Dorsal to the bladder there is t a smoothly marginated, complex mass (arrows), that displaces the bladder ventrally.

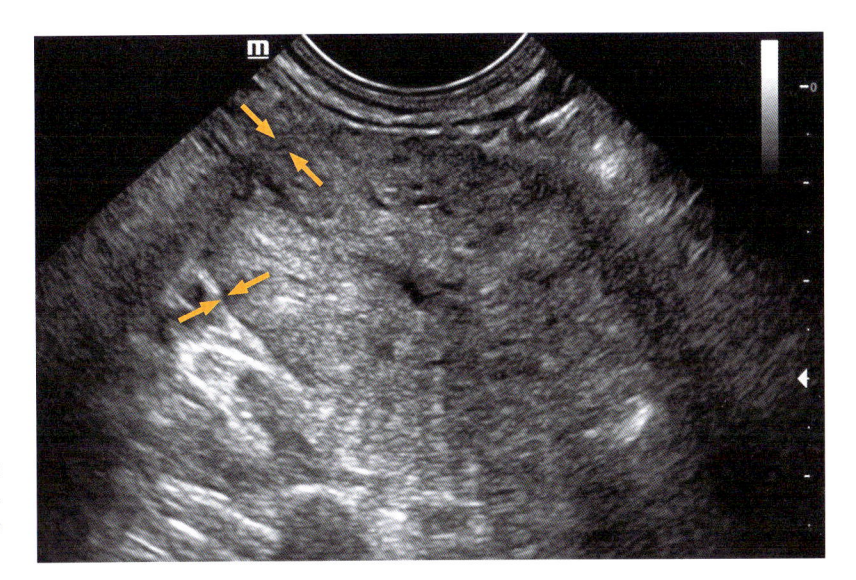

CHAPTER **37** Prostate, testicles, ovaries, and uterus

Fig. 37.5 Prostatitis. The transverse image shows an enlarged, irregularly marginated, heterogenous, hyperechoic prostate with a faint hypoechoic rim which may be edema or cellular infiltration (arrows).

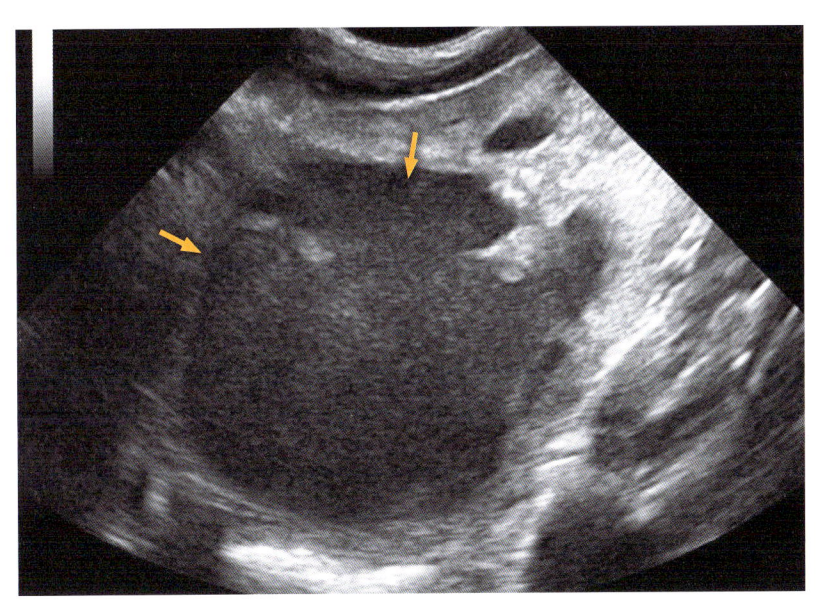

Fig. 37.6 Prostatic abscess. A nine-year-old Italian Bracco. Longitudinal plane of the prostate gland that appears enlarged and misshapen, with irregularly shaped cavities containing echogenic fluid (arrows) which, on aspiration, contained pus.

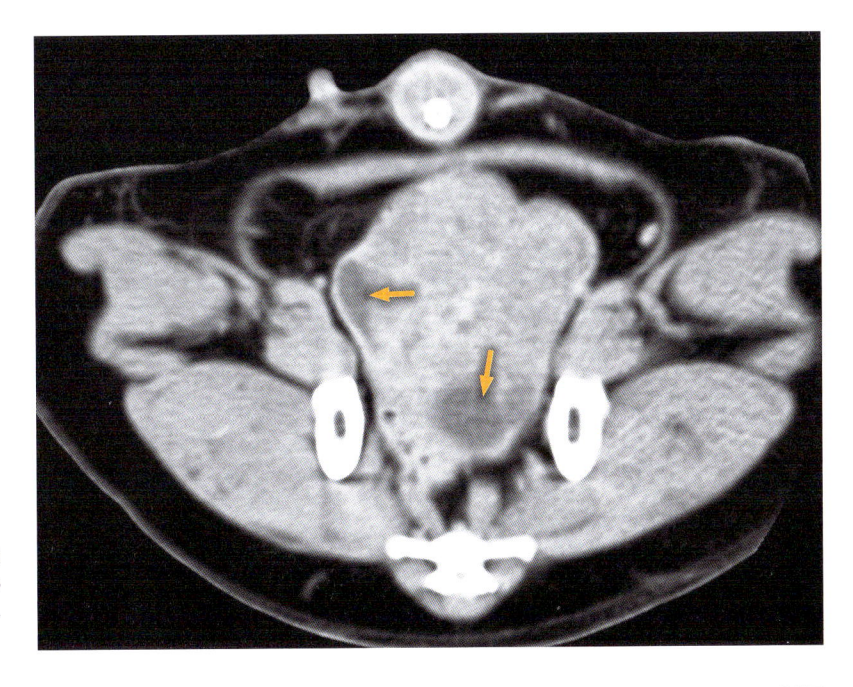

Fig. 37.7 CT: prostatic abscess. A nine-year-old German Shepherd dog with difficulty urinating. The prostate gland is asymmetrically enlarged with well-defined areas of low attenuation (arrows).

603

SECTION V ABDOMEN

Carcinoma Prostatic carcinoma has a variable ultrasonographic appearance in both intact and castrated dogs. Early cases of neoplasia are often focal hypoechoic lesions and can be difficult to differentiate from other conditions. Later in the disease the parenchymal changes are often diffuse, the gland is not symmetrical and the gland margin becomes irregular. There may be mixed hyperechoic heterogenous parenchyma, with irregular anechoic regions and foci of mineralization creating acoustic shadowing (**fig. 37.8**). In neutered patients, carcinoma may appear as a mildly enlarged hypoechoic gland, sometimes with mineralization. The medial iliac lymph node should be imaged to confirm or exclude enlargement from metastasis.

Testicles

The testicular parenchyma has uniform medium echogenicity with a fine echotexture with regular diffuse echogenic stippling scattered evenly throughout the organ (**fig. 37.9**). The stippling repre-

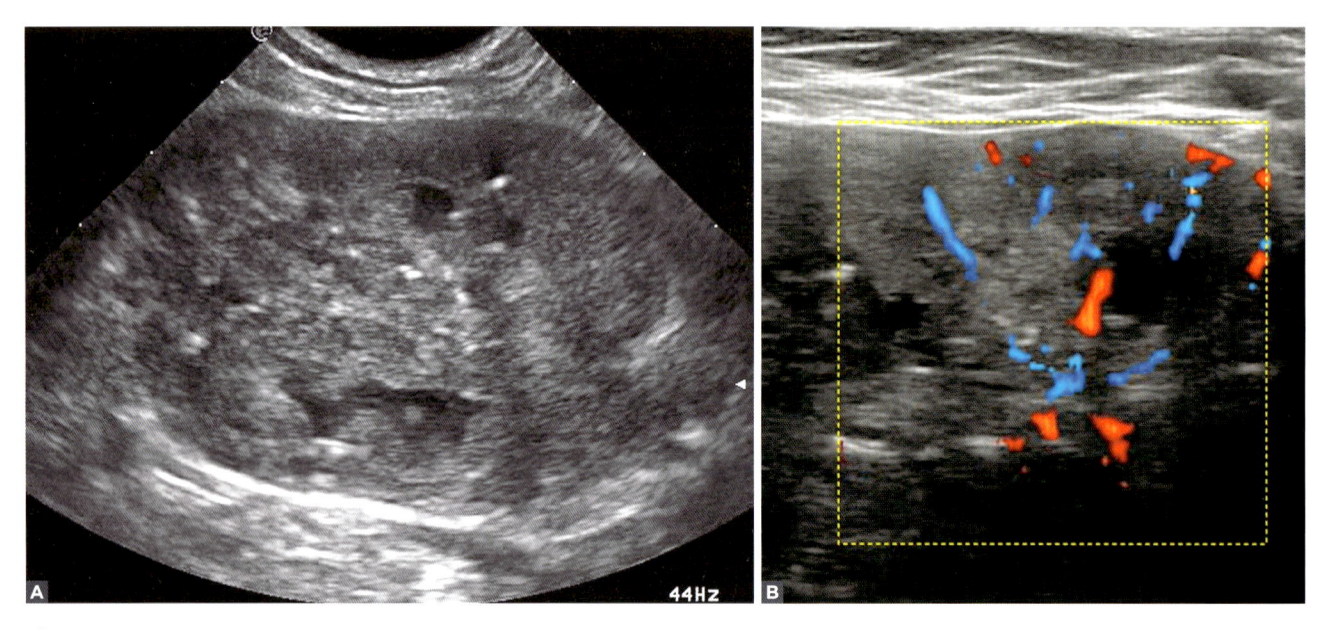

Fig. 37.8 Prostatic neoplasia. A nine-year-old Bolognese dog with stranguria, pollakiuria, and hematuria due to compression of the urethra by a prostatic adenocarcinoma. (**A**) The B-mode image shows that the prostate gland has irregular margins and heterogeneous echotexture with scattered echogenic foci and irregular hypoechoic cyst-like lesions. (**B**) The color Doppler shows irregular branching of arterial vessels throughout the prostatic parenchyma.

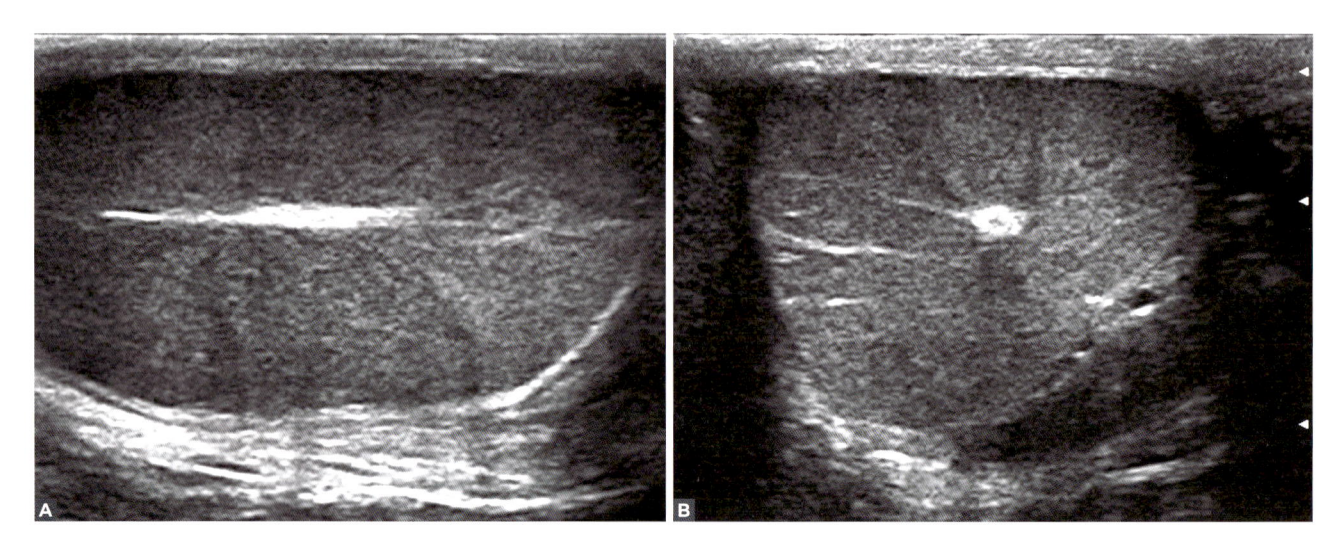

Fig. 37.9 Longitudinal (**A**) and transverse (**B**) ultrasound scan of the testis of a three-year-old Neapolitan Mastiff. Normal echotexture of the testis. Normal homogeneous, granular echotexture composed of uniformly medium-level echoes and linear hyperechoic mediastinum testis on longitudinal and circular hyperechoic structure on transverse scan.

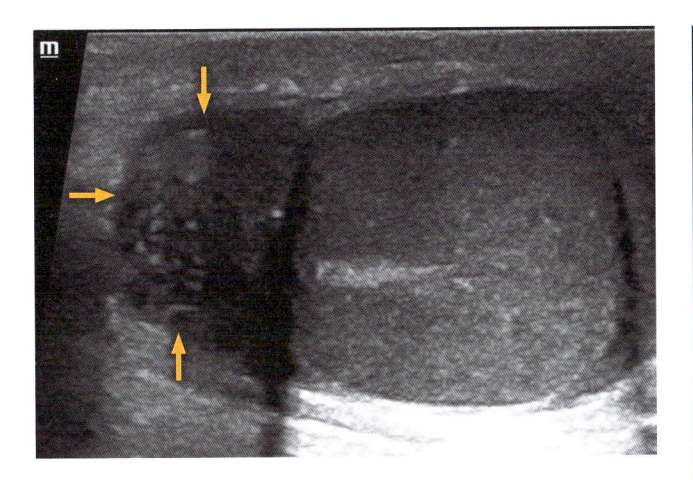

Fig. 37.10 An eight-year-old, mixed breed male with right testicular pain and swelling. Longitudinal gray-scale ultrasound image shows an enlarged heterogeneous epididymal head (arrows) and an edematous and enlarged right testicle.

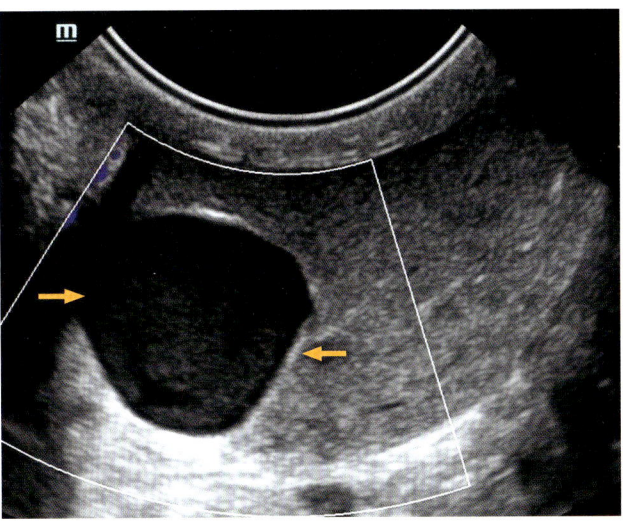

Fig. 37.11 Cyst associated with the cranial pole of the right testicle in a seven-year-old Yorkshire Terrier. A round anechoic structure (arrows) is associated with the testicular parenchyma.

sents an extension of the fibrous mediastinum, which is responsible for supporting the parenchymal tissue. The mediastinum testis, a fibrous invagination from the tunica albuginea, is located centrally within the testis. In a sagittal plane this structure appears as an echogenic line approximately 2 mm wide extending from the cranial to the caudal pole, whilst in the transverse plane it appears as a central echogenic circular structure.

The epididymis appears hypoechoic with respect to testicular parenchyma. Ultrasound is a useful method for measuring testicular volume (e.g., volume = length × width × height × 0.5236); sometimes the two testes do not have equal volumes. Gross changes in size may be predictive of infertility. While testicular and epididymal size increases in acute inflammation, it decreases in chronic cases (**fig. 37.10**).

Testicular or epididymal cysts are an occasional incident finding. They appear anechoic, well circumscribed, round areas, often with distal acoustic enhancement (**fig. 37.11**).

Focal testicular lesions are relatively simple to identify and usually there is a good relationship with gross pathology findings (**fig. 37.12**).

Microlithiases are commonly seen following testicular inflammation or in early-stage testicular degeneration, often associated with poor sperm morphology and poor sperm motility (**fig. 37.13**). Subtle generalized changes may be difficult to detect; dogs with testes that are more echogenic and less homogeneous have poorer semen quality. Simple classification schemes have been developed to evaluate testicular parenchyma. In dogs with generalized changes of the parenchyma, orchitis is a likely differential.

Cryptorchidism is the most common congenital testicular abnormality in dogs and cats. It predisposes to the development of testicular neoplasia. Cryptorchidism is defined as the non-descent of one or both testes to their normal anatomical location. Ultrasound scan is a valuable diagnostic tool to locate cryptorchid testes (**fig. 37.14**). However, retained testes atrophy and may be quite challenging to locate.

Cryptorchid testes have an approximately 13.6-fold higher risk of developing a tumor than scrotal testes, such as Sertoli cell tumors and seminomas (**fig. 37.15**). When the cryptorchid neoplastic testis exceeds 8 cm it may not be possible to confirm the origin with ultrasound, and CT is preferred. Testicular blood flow can be identified within the proximal suprastesticular artery, marginal artery and intratesticular arteries (**fig. 37.16**).

SECTION V ABDOMEN

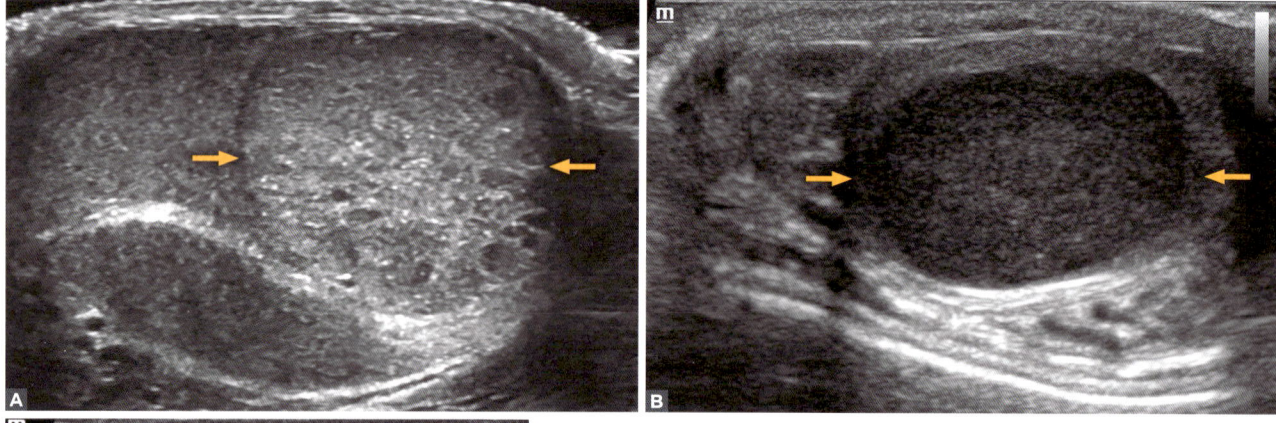

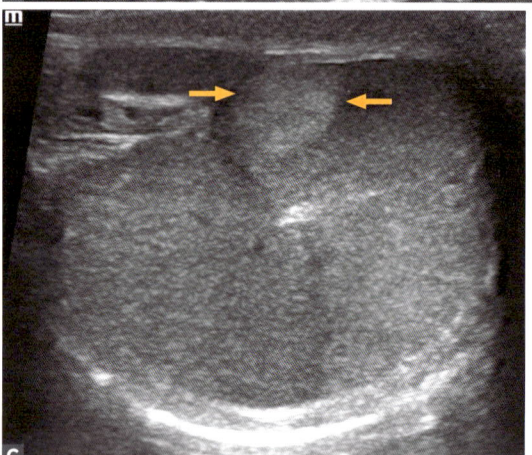

Fig. 37.12 (**A**) A six-year-old male Labrador Retriever with a painless right testicular mass. Longitudinal gray-scale ultrasound image of the right testicle shows a well-defined, heterogeneous nodule (arrows), affecting the caudal pole of the testicle. The patient subsequently underwent right orchiectomy. Histologically, the nodule was a seminoma. (**B**) A seven-year-old mongrel male with testicular tumor that presented with progressive pain and swelling in the right scrotum of one month duration. The ultrasound gray scale image shows a hypoechoic nodule occupying almost the entire testis with loss of visualization of the testicular mediastinum (arrows). (**C**) Single hyperechoic nodule (arrows) found as an incidental lesion, which was a Leydig tumor on histology.

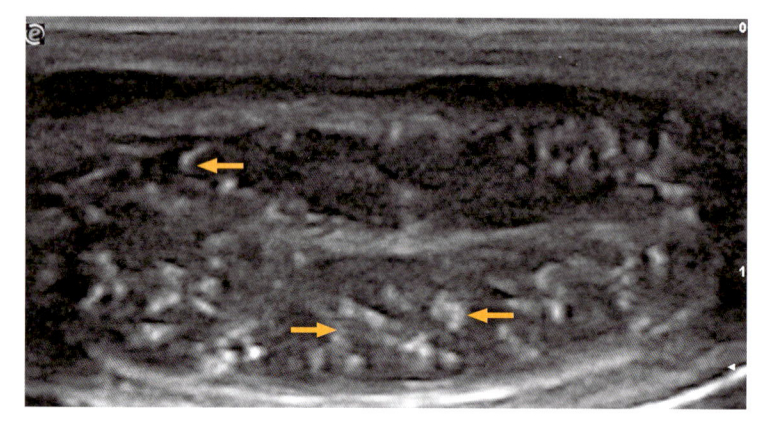

Fig. 37.13 A 12-year-old Bulldog with testicular microlithiasis. Multiple 2-3 mm shadowing non-shadowing echogenic foci scattered throughout the testicle (arrows).

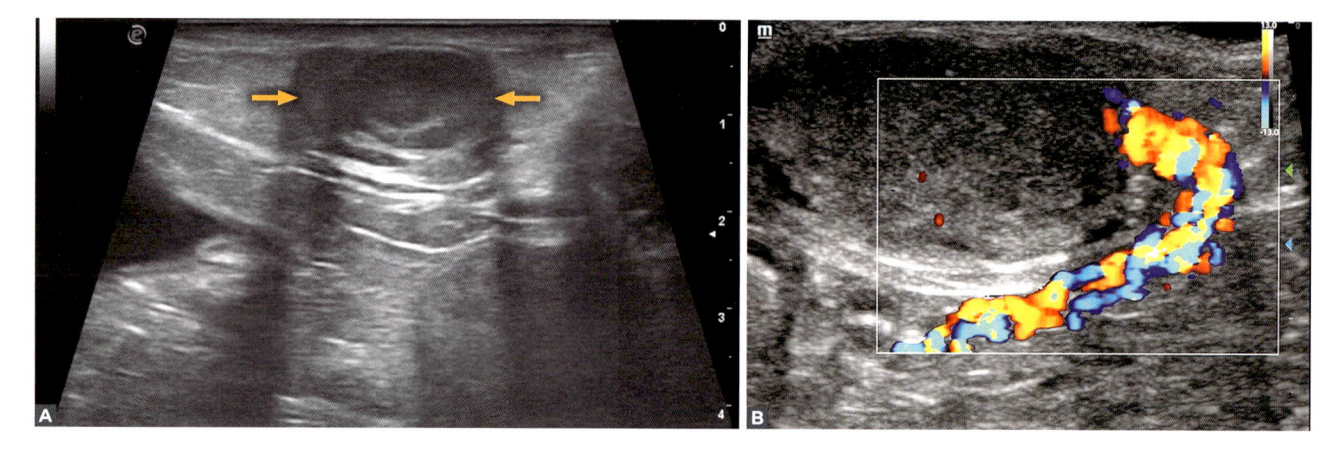

Fig. 37.14 (**A**) Right-sided cryptorchid inguinal testicle of a 1.5-year-old Shih Tzu. The testicle is diffusely hypoechoic (arrows) with an isoechoic nodule that obscures the linear mediastinum testis. (**B**) A nine-year-old Chihuahua with severe inguinal swelling shows that the right testicle is increased in size with loss of normal architecture and diffusely hypoechoic and no evidence of the linear mediastinum testis internally. On color Doppler the pampiniform plexus is displaced caudally and ventrally.

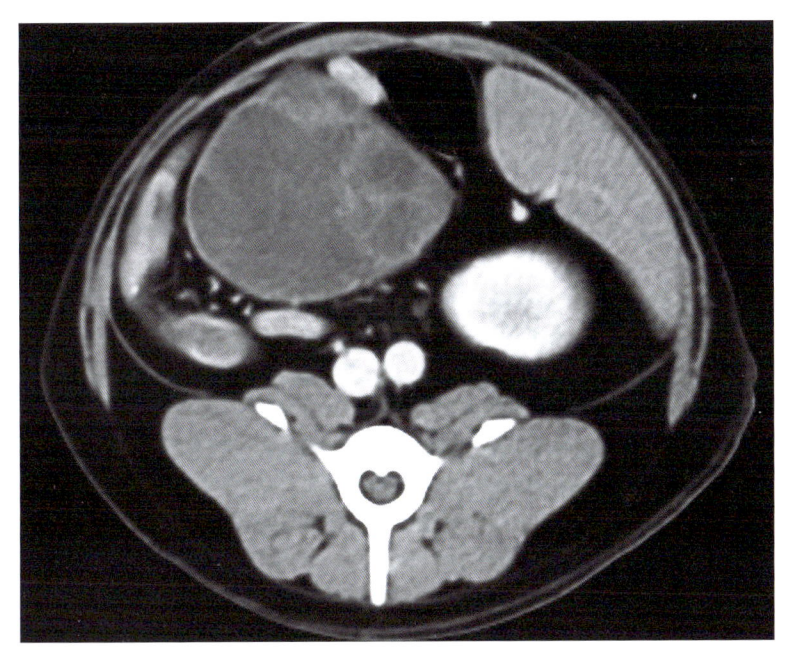

CHAPTER 37 Prostate, testicles, ovaries, and uterus

Fig. 37.15 Sertolioma. Post-contrast CT study of an eight-year-old English Setter. There is a rounded mass in the mid-abdomen, with sharp and well-defined borders, with peripheral contrast enhancement, and in some septa towards the center of the mass. Final diagnosis was sertolioma.

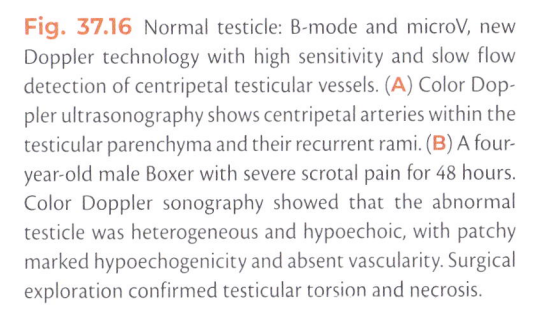

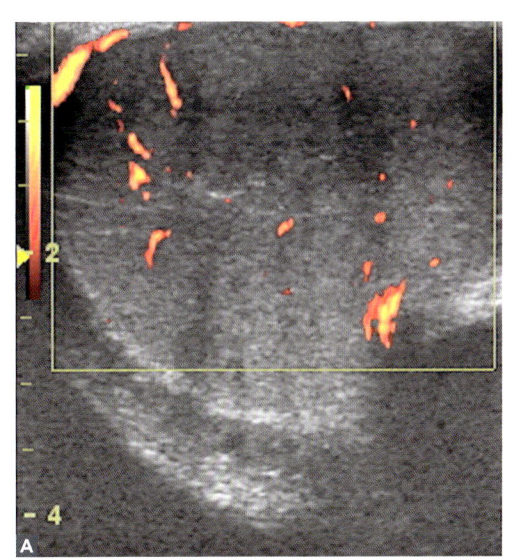

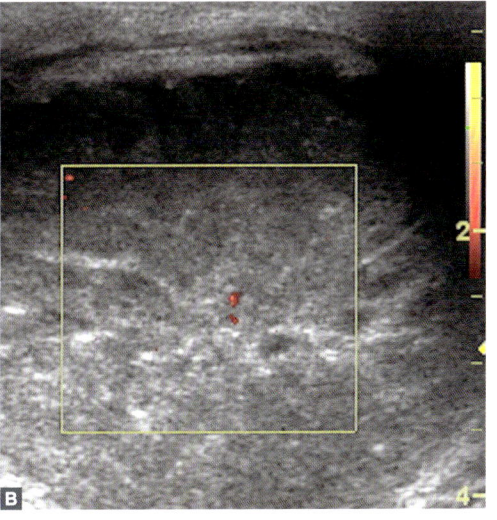

Fig. 37.16 Normal testicle: B-mode and microV, new Doppler technology with high sensitivity and slow flow detection of centripetal testicular vessels. (**A**) Color Doppler ultrasonography shows centripetal arteries within the testicular parenchyma and their recurrent rami. (**B**) A four-year-old male Boxer with severe scrotal pain for 48 hours. Color Doppler sonography showed that the abnormal testicle was heterogeneous and hypoechoic, with patchy marked hypoechogenicity and absent vascularity. Surgical exploration confirmed testicular torsion and necrosis.

Females

The uterus of the bitch and the queen is roughly "Y"-shaped and has relatively long uterine horns which run in the mid-abdomen to a relatively lateral position close to the abdominal wall. The ovaries are positioned caudal to the kidneys. The non-gravid uterus and the normal ovaries are not visible on survey radiographs. Ultrasonography is much more sensitive and is preferred for assessment of the uterus and ovaries.

Ovaries

Normal ovaries are not visible on radiographs. The ovarian appearance varies with the stage of the estrous cycle, when follicle growth can be readily detected in the thin animal.

Ultrasound (US) of the normal ovaries requires excellent scanning techniques and high-resolution transducers. The anestrus ovary can be difficult to image due to lack of follicles and surrounding bursal fat. In late anestrus small follicles are identifiable. Larger follicles of 4-8 mm diameter can be detected 8 days before ovulation (**fig. 37.17**). Ovulation can be difficult to detect unless there is frequent examination (perhaps twice daily). At the time of ovulation, the corpora lutea may become visible and this is the main criteria for identification of ovulation. The early corpora lutea are often cavitated and contain anechoic fluid and as such can be difficult to differentiate from a follicle (**fig. 37.18**). They do however have thick walls and the diameter of the lumen is smaller than the follicle that they replaced. Central cavities may persist for up to 25 days and do not compact until day 28.

SECTION V ABDOMEN

Fig. 37.17 Sagittal image of the left ovary in a six-year-old Labrador Retriever during the follicular phase of the ovarian cycle. Multiple thin-walled hypoechoic follicles are noted (arrows).

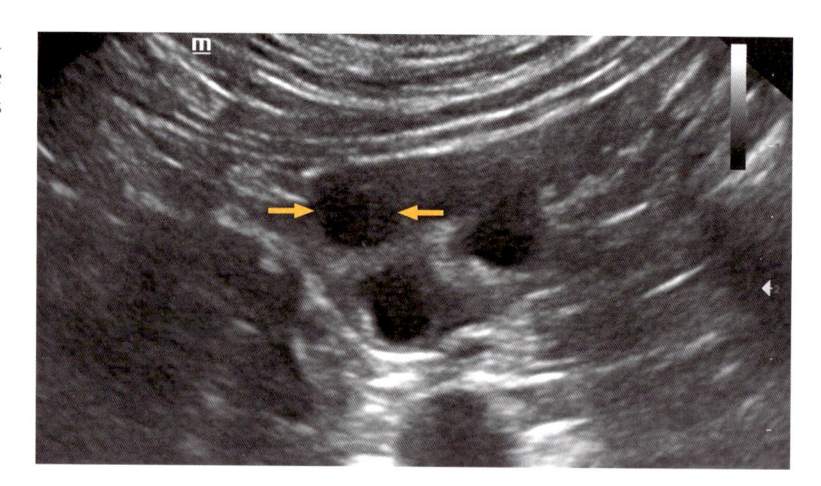

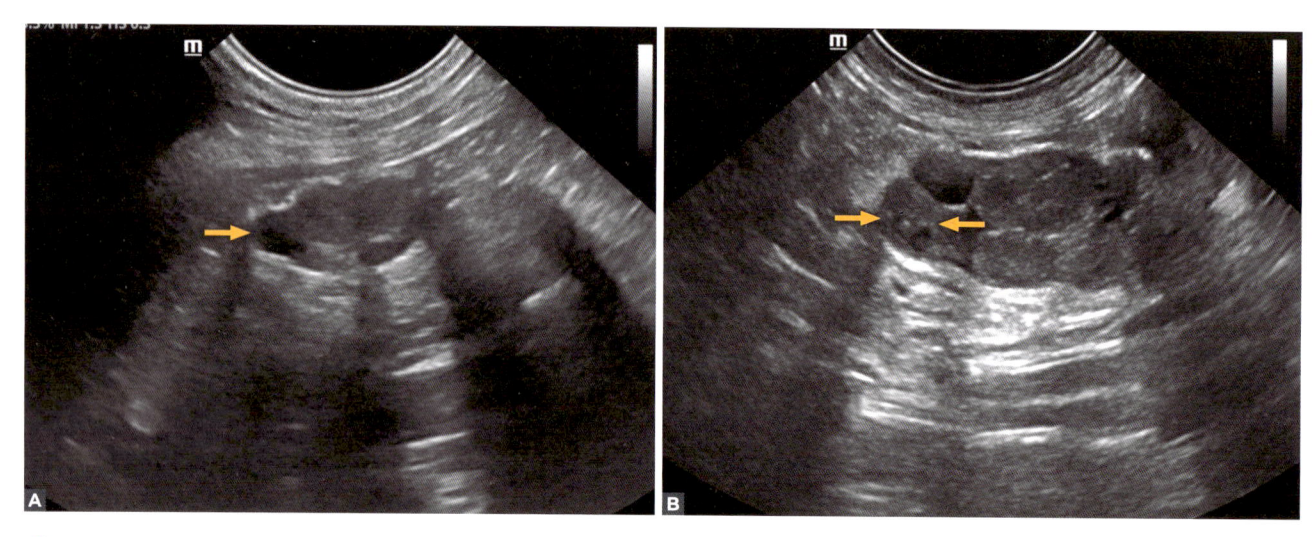

Fig. 37.18 (A) Sagittal image of an ovary (arrow) having recently undergone ovulation in a five-year-old Yorkshire Terrier. Small amount of periovarian fluid, indicating ovulation. The corpora hemorrhagica are isoechoic to the ovarian parenchyma as compared with the previous follicles. (B) Luteal phase of the ovarian cycle in a three-year-old Golden Retriever. Corpora lutea, when mature, have thicker walls and contain hypoechoic fluid (arrows).

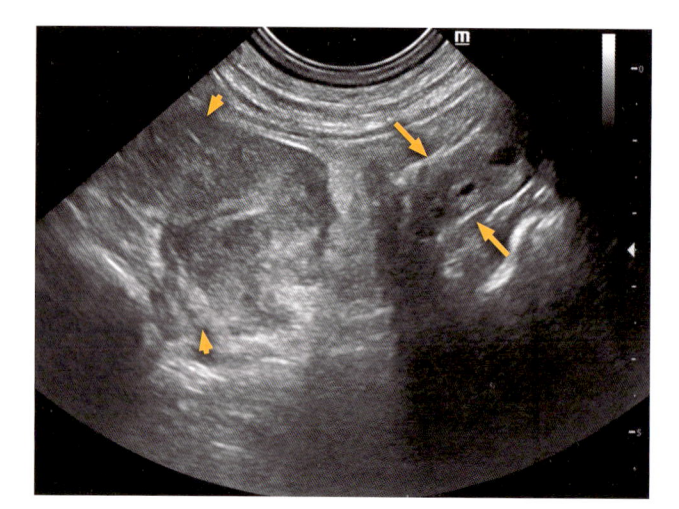

Fig. 37.19 Ovarian carcinoma in a nine-year mixed breed dog. A large, spherical, mixed echogenic mass (arrowheads) is located caudal to the left kidney. Caudal to the mass there is a segment of a uterine horn with multiple cysts (arrows).

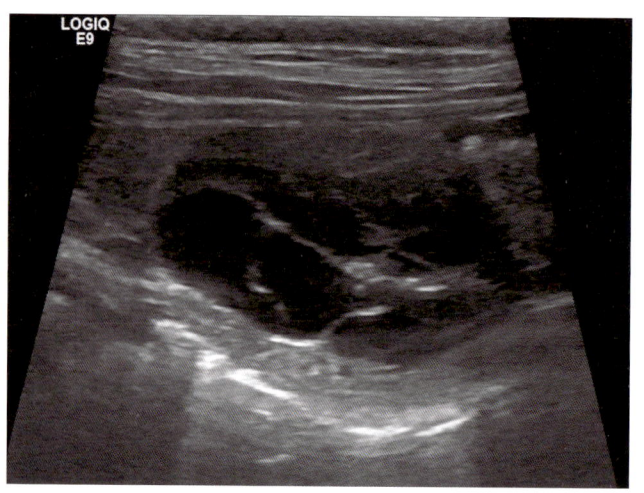

Fig. 37.20 Transverse image of a left ovary with multiple ovarian follicular cysts. Note the thin-walled appearance to the cysts and the anechoic cyst contents.

Abnormal ovaries

Ovarian neoplasms may be seen on survey radiographs. They usually descend to the ventral abdomen and cause ipsilateral intestinal displacement. A left ovarian mass may displace the descending colon ventrally and toward midline.

On ultrasound, bitches with ovarian tumors most commonly have increased size of the ovaries, with regional or focal lesions, that may be solid or cystic (**fig. 37.19**). The ovarian tumors can be unilateral or bilateral. If the lesion exceeds 10 cm in diameter it is very difficult to confirm an ovarian origin. The echogenicity and echotexture are extremely variable. Some lesions have internal cavitations filled with anechoic or echogenic fluid, from necrosis or hemorrhage. The presence of free fluid may be associated with peritoneal dissemination.

Ovarian cysts are not common, but may be identified as anechoic fluid-filled structures of variable size, several of which are commonly greater than 1 cm in diameter (**fig. 37.20**). Occasionally the follicular fluid has increased echogenicity.

Computed tomography (CT) can be helpful to confirm the origin of a primary ovarian tumor. Whole body CT may be used for tumor staging (**figs. 37.21** and **37.22**).

Uterus

The normal, non-gravid uterus is usually not visible on radiographs but is rarely visible on smaller obese patients.

On ultrasound, imaging of the uterus can be performed with the bitch in the standing position or in lateral or dorsal recumbency, after clipping the hair of the abdomen. Partial filling of the urinary bladder is helpful in identification of the body of the uterus and the larger diameter cervix, which are located dorsal to the urinary bladder and ventral to the descending colon. The uterine horns are surprisingly convoluted making it difficult to evaluate the entire horn. The distal portions of the two uterine horns can sometimes be imaged and traced laterally to the abdominal wall. The uterine body and uterine horn are composed of two distinct layers; a central homogeneous relatively hypoechoic region surrounded by a peripheral hyperechoic layer (**fig. 37.23**).

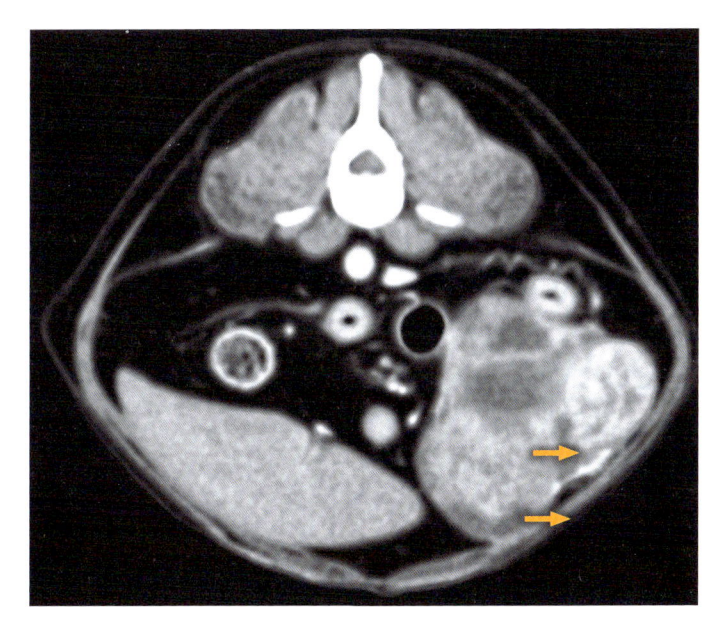

Fig. 37.21 CT image showing a large, multilobulated, hypoattenuating mass arising from the right ovary of a nine-year-old Bernese Mountain dog. The mass shows contrast enhancement of internal septa and the peripheral capsule (arrows).

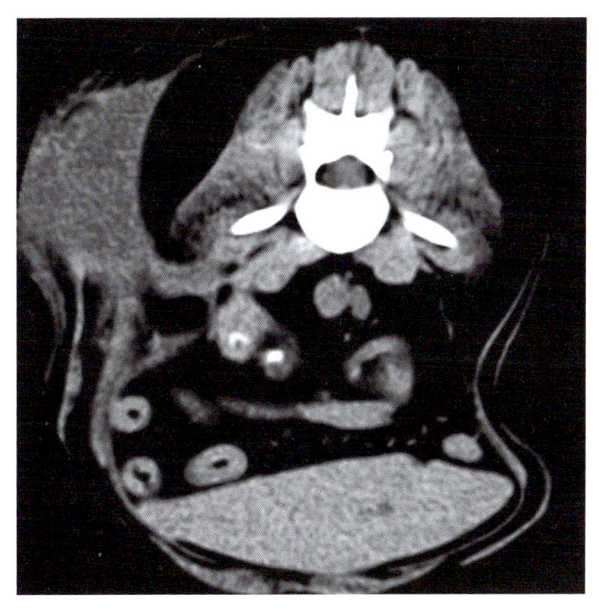

Fig. 37.22 The plain CT study shows two mineralized abdominal nodules in connection with the abdominal wall, where a mass with a soft tissue density is detected, slightly hypoattenuating compared to the neighboring muscles. The diagnosis of granuloma in ovarian ligament ligation and fistula with collection of pus and necrotic material in the subcutis was confirmed surgically.

The ability to differentiate these depends upon the stage of the cycle. During estrus the uterus becomes increasingly hypoechoic and is much larger in diameter.

▌ **Cystic endometrial hyperplasia (CEH) in clinically normal bitches** Ultrasound examination may demonstrate multiple small (up to 5 mm diameter) fluid-filled anechoic cysts scattered throughout the endometrium in otherwise clinically normal bitches (**fig. 37.24**). The incidence of these cystic lesions increases with age, with most bitches over seven years having some changes.

▌ **Cystic endometrial hyperplasia and pyometra** An enlarged uterus such as from pyometra may be visible on radiographs once it exceeds 2-3 times the diameter of the normal small intestine. It is easier to identify in patients with large amounts of intra-abdominal fat. With less severe enlargement, the uterine horns are more visible on the ventrodorsal projection, appearing as tubular soft tissue structures medial to the body wall in either or both caudal abdominal quadrants. Severe uterine enlargement causes a characteristic pattern of organ displacement. On the lateral projection, the uterus occupies the ventral mid and caudal abdomen causing dorsal and cranial displacement of the intestine. On the ventrodorsal projection the intestine is displaced towards midline and the uterine horns occupy the lateral abdomen (**fig. 37.25A**).

In cases of pyometra, ultrasonographically the uterus has an increased diameter, and may be folded upon itself so that two or more sections of each horn are imaged in a single plane. The diameter of the uterus may vary depending on whether the pyometra is "open" or "closed". The wall of the uterus is commonly increased in thickness, and may be up to 2 mm, and is relatively hypoechoic with respect to surrounding tissue. The uterine lumen is frequently grossly dilated with anechoic fluid, however, small echogenic particles and luminal echogenic bodies may be identified, which probably represent inflammatory debris or hemorrhage, although mucus may have a similar ultrasonographic appearance (**fig. 37.25B**).

▌ **Uterine mass lesions** A focal or generalized uterine enlargement may be seen on plain radiographs as a convoluted or spherical soft tissue opacity structure cranial to the bladder.

Uterine neoplasms can be diagnosed using ultrasound. These lesions are uncommon in the bitch and queen and since ultrasound cannot readily differentiate neoplastic from granulomatous tissue, it should not be relied upon as the sole diagnostic tool. The reported appearance of uterine neoplasia are homogeneous mass lesions attached to the uterine wall which project into the lumen with or

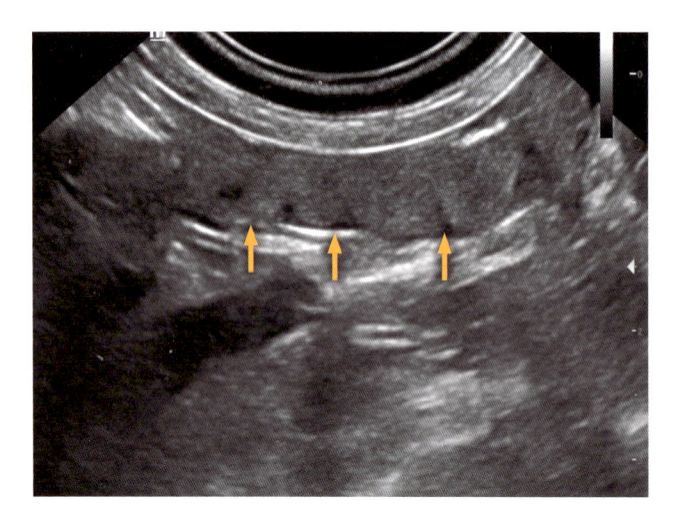

Fig. 37.23 Sagittal image of a four-year-old Pekinese dog in the late proestral phase of the reproductive cycle in which the uterine horn has a wavy appearance and echogenic content with smooth inner contour (arrows).

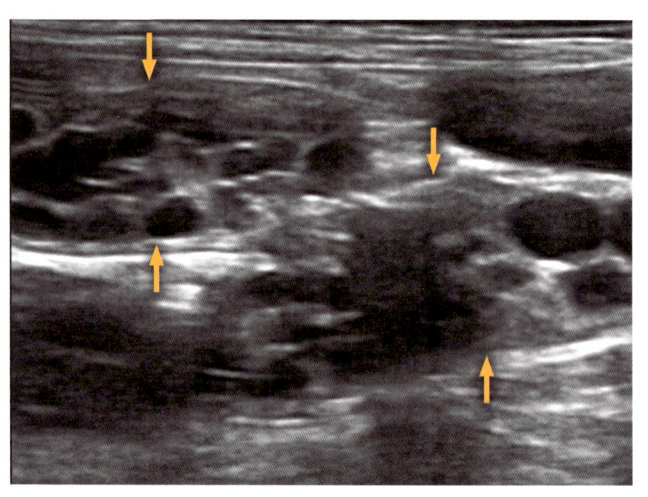

Fig. 37.24 Sagittal image of the left and right uterine horn of a seven-year-old Bolognese dog. The endometrium is irregular due to multiple cystic structures of varying size, just cranial to the urinary bladder (arrows).

without luminal fluid accumulation. Uterine neoplasms may also be echogenic or have a complex mixed echogenicity if they are necrotic of fibrotic (**fig. 37.26**).

Ultrasound examination may provide diagnostic information when investigating bitches with chronic draining flank fistulae, or chronic purulent vaginal discharges following ovariohysterectomy. Granulomata or abscesses usually comprise irregular mixed echogenicity tissue, which arises dorsal to the bladder and ventral to the colon (**fig. 37.27**).

The presence of discrete fluid filled zones within the mass may indicate uterine stump abscessation. Failure to identify a stump lesion does not eliminate this as a diagnosis. Infusion of saline into the vagina, using a Foley catheter, will allow a more accurate identification of the proximal portion of the stump. A CT study can be helpful to differentiate a large mass lesion of the uterus from other organs, and for tumoral staging.

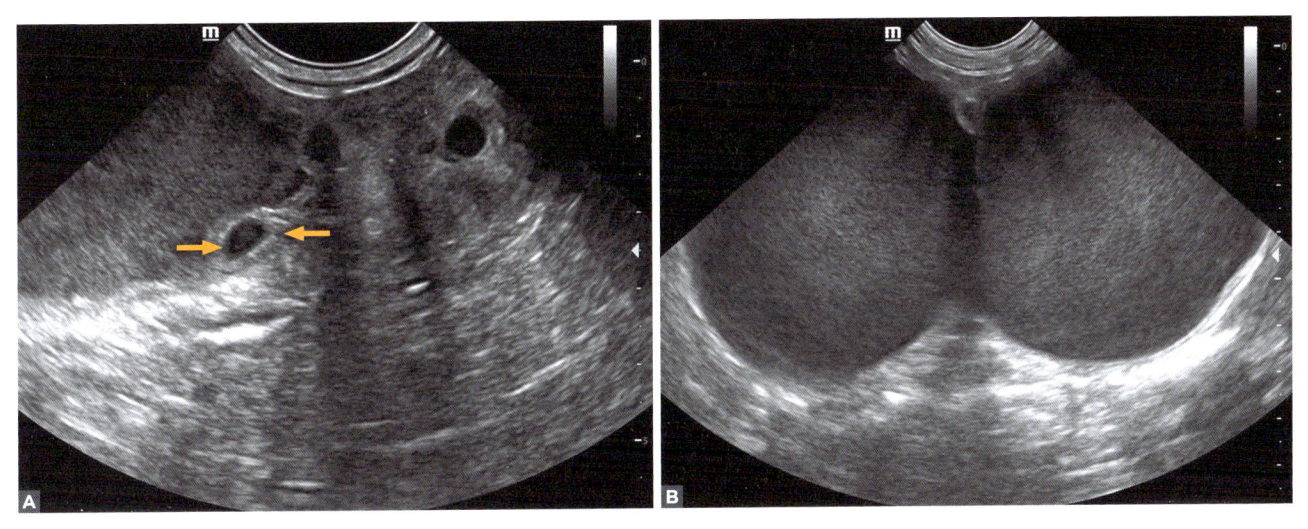

Fig. 37.25 (A) Cystic endometrial hyperplasia in an 11-year-old German Shepherd dog. Echogenic fluid is present in the left uterine horn lumen; the uterine wall is thick, irregular, and anechoic structures (arrows) are visible within the wall. (B) Closed pyometra. Marked dilation of the uterine horns segments is present, with abnormal echogenic fluid accumulation in a 12-year-old Beagle.

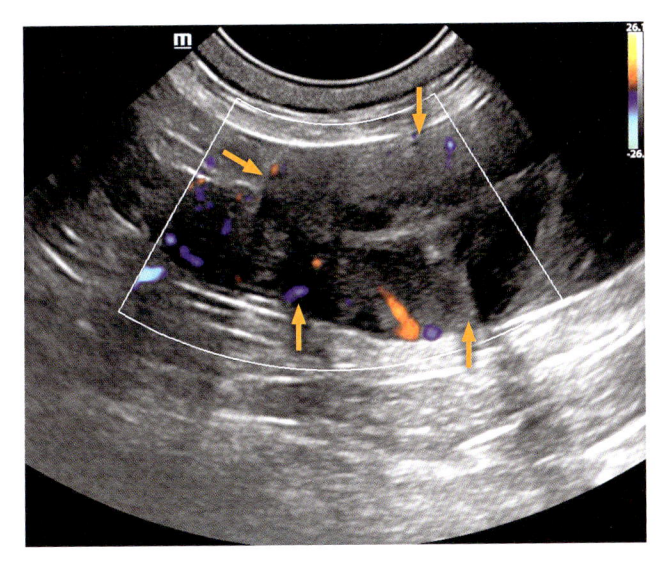

Fig. 37.26 Color Doppler longitudinal image of a 14-year-old intact Cocker Spaniel. Complex soft tissue masses occupying the uterine body. Fine-needle aspiration was obtained and the final diagnosis was leiomyosarcoma (arrows).

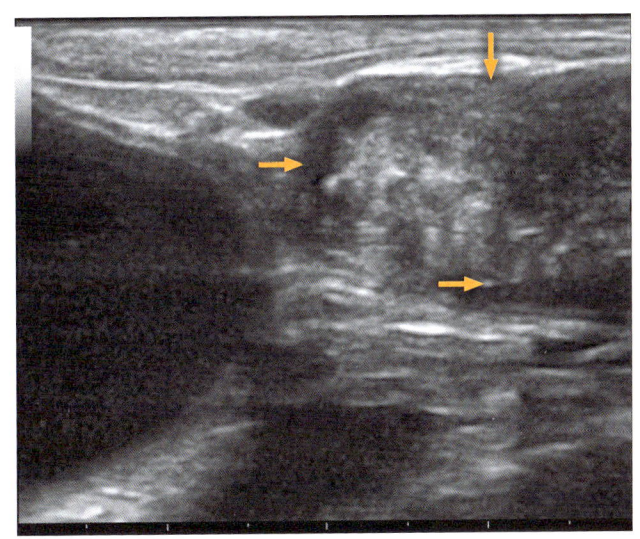

Fig. 37.27 Longitudinal ultrasound image of a nine-year-old spayed Italian Spinone. A uterine stump granuloma is visualized just cranial to the pubis, between the bladder and the colon as a complex mass lesion (arrows). Hyperechoic foci represent inflammation and ligature material.

Fig. 37.28 Early pregnancy in a 2.5-year-old Boxer dog. Transverse image of the gestational sac in which no embryo is yet visible. An echogenic inner placental layer is detected in the uterine wall.

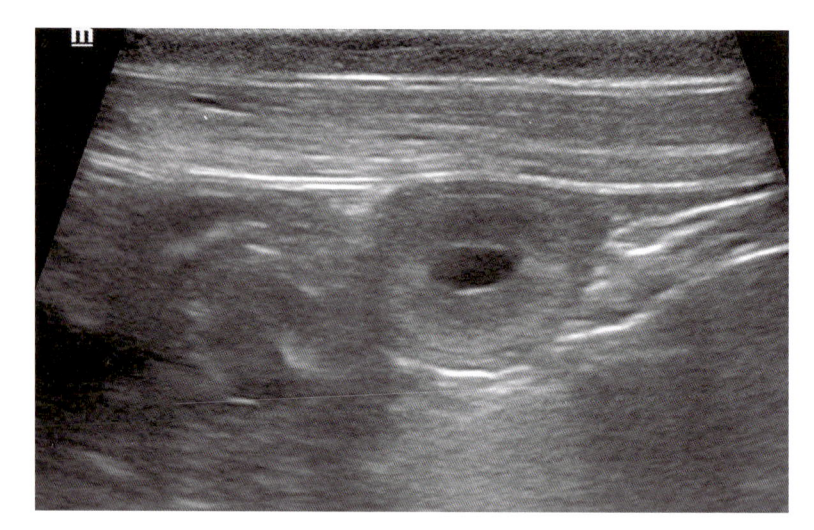

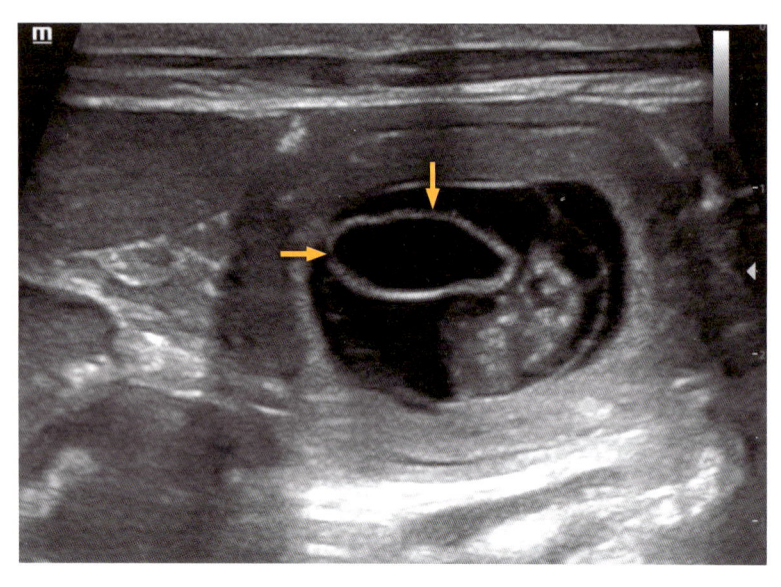

Fig. 37.29 Progression of normal pregnancy in a four-year-old Maltese dog. The fetus has recognizable morphology within the gestational sac (arrows). The yolk sac is the fluid-filled, echogenic, pear-shaped structure adjacent to the fetus.

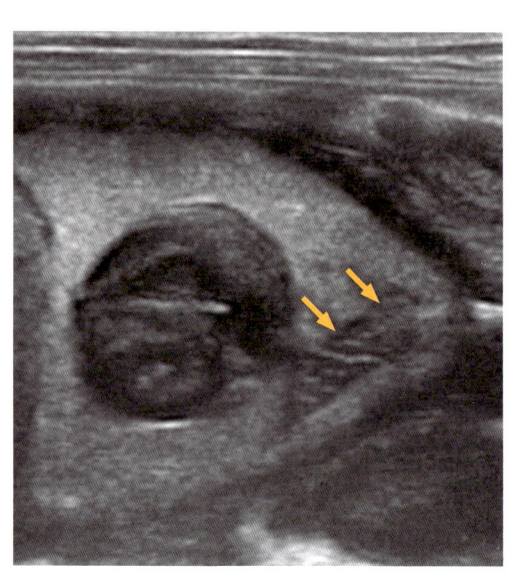

Fig. 37.30 Normal late-term pregnancy in a three-year-old Irish Setter. Sagittal image of the fetal thorax in which hyperechoic lungs surround the fetal heart. The trapezoidal hypoechoic band represents the fetal thymus.

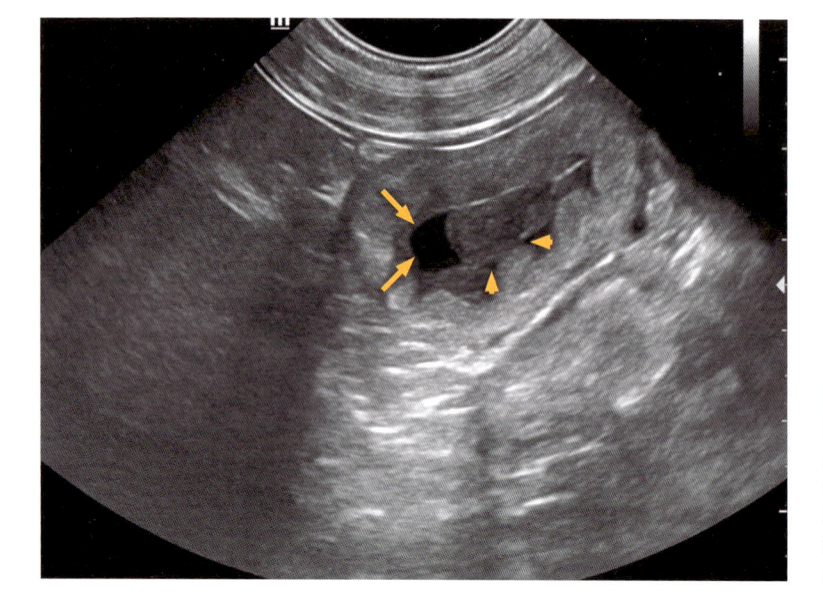

Fig. 37.31 Embryonic resorption in a two-year-old Weimaraner 28 days after the last breeding. Transverse image of a collapsed thick-walled gestational chamber (arrows), which contains a small amount of anechoic fluid. The embryo is no longer vital. Arrowhead indicates a hyperechoic forming placenta separated from the gestational chamber (arrowheads).

Pregnancy diagnosis

During pregnancy the uterus enlarges and can be seen on radiographs after 30 days of pregnancy, occasionally earlier, as a lobular soft tissue opacity structure, dorsal to the urinary bladder. Fetal mineralization can be detected as early as 35 days in cats and 41 days in dogs. Increasing bone opacity is visible in the last two weeks of pregnancy. Assessment of fetal numbers is best achieved by counting both fetal skulls and spines.

Uterine enlargement occurs during the luteal phase whether the bitch is pregnant or non-pregnant. During early pregnancy the embryo is located adjacent to the uterine wall and is not imaged (**fig. 37.28**). The conceptus rapidly increases in size and may lose its spherical outline, becoming oblate in appearance. From day 20 after ovulation the conceptus is approximately 7 mm in diameter and 15 mm in length and the embryo is visible with ultrasound (**fig. 37.29**).

The presence of the embryonic heart beat can be detected from approximately 22 days after ovulation. A fluid-filled sac, the amnion, may be noted later in pregnancy since it is surrounds, and initially is in close apposition to the fetus. The most rapid growth of the fetus occurs between days 32 and 55, and during this time the limb buds become apparent and there is clear differentiation of the head, trunk and abdomen. The zonary placenta can usually be easily identified from this stage of pregnancy onwards. The fetal skeleton becomes evident from 40 days onwards when fetal bone appears hyperechoic, and cast acoustic shadows. The heart can now be easily identified as the chambers and valves can be seen moving. Lung tissue surrounding the heart is hyperechoic with respect to the liver, and the region of the forming diaphragm can easily be identified.

From 45 days onwards it is possible to identify the fluid-filled (anechoic) stomach, kidneys and bladder. A few days later the intestines can be easily seen. In late pregnancy the head, vertebral column and ribs become more easily identifiable as discrete hyperechoic structures. Ultrasound may be used to estimate the gestational age (**fig. 37.30**). This may also be of value in bitches with multiple or uncertain mating times. Conventionally this is achieved using measures of fetal size; however, these have only been established for a few dog breeds. Therefore, an alternative approach is to use the time that specific organs can be identified using ultrasound. Monitoring fetal heart rate can be useful as part of examination of the prepartum bitch. Normal fetal heart rate at term is 170-230 bpm, or at least four times the maternal heart rate. Transient increases of heart rate occur with fetal movement. Fetal heart rates less than 150 bpm indicates stress (hypoxia). Fetal heart rates less than 130 bpm indicate poor survival if not delivered within 2 to 3 hours. Fetal heart rates less than 100 bpm require immediate (medical or surgical) intervention to hasten delivery before demise of the pups.

Abnormal pregnancy

Embryonic resorption occurs in up to 15% of otherwise normal pregnancies. In these cases, on ultrasound, fluid is present around the abnormal fetus and becomes increasingly echogenic (**fig. 37.31**). Then there is indentation of the uterine wall, and gradual loss of the embryo without affecting the littermates.

In many cases loss can be predicted by late identification of the embryo, late identification of the heartbeat, or abnormal growth rate. In later pregnancy fetal death may be noticed by absence of fetal heart beats an event that normally precedes fetal abortion. Radiography is sometimes used to assess fetal size to predict dystocia but this is imprecise. Radiography can be used to confirm malpresentation as a cause of dystocia (**fig. 37.32**). Radiographic signs of fetal death include hyperextension or hyperflexion of the fetus, collapse or overlapping of the skull bones and intrafetal gas. Mummified fetus appears as compact mineral opacity structures with densely packed overlapping distorted bones. These are sometimes chronic clinically silent incidental findings.

Accumulation of gas within the fetus and uterine lumen is termed physometra. The contrast from gas within the uterus may make the outline of the fetus distinctly visible (**fig. 37.33**).

SECTION V ABDOMEN

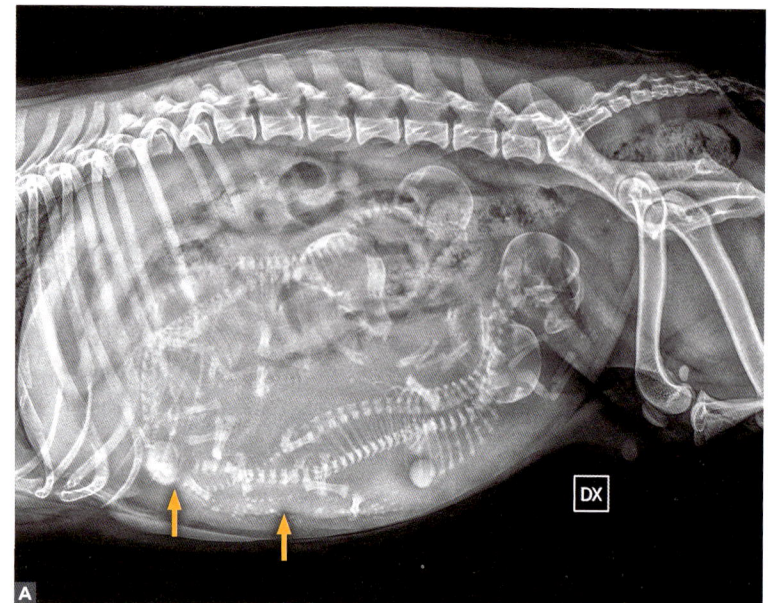

Fig. 37.32 Lateral and ventrodorsal abdominal radiographs of a pregnant bitch. Note that on the VD in close contact with the spleen, there is a small and irrregular, curled fetus, with loss of normal posture and overlapping of the cranium and collapse of the fetal skeleton (arrows).

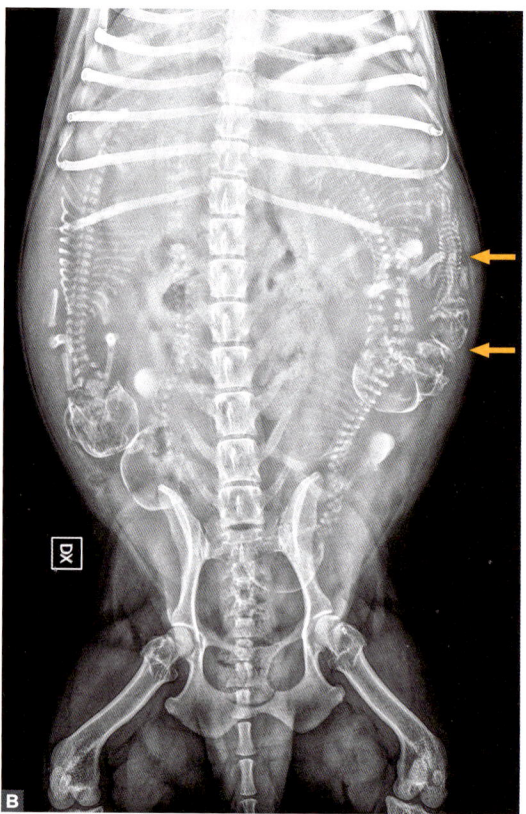

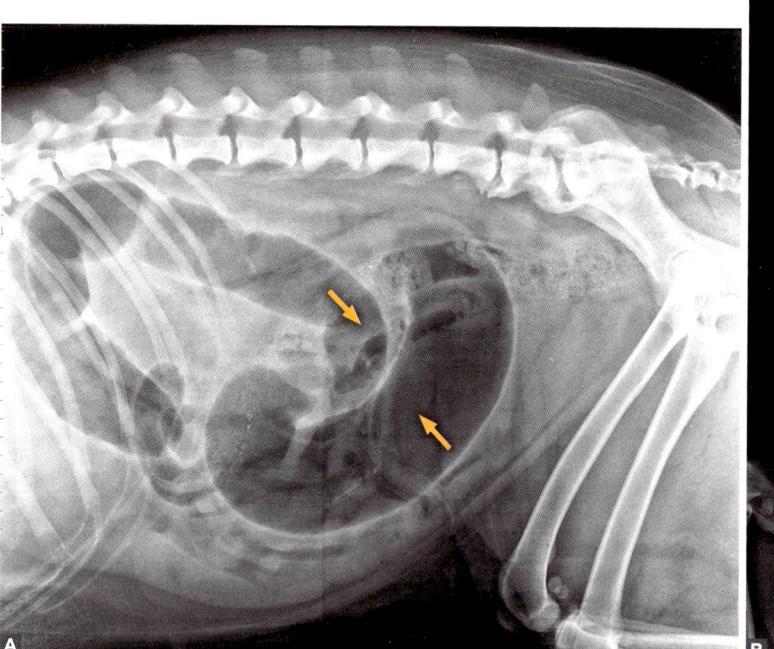

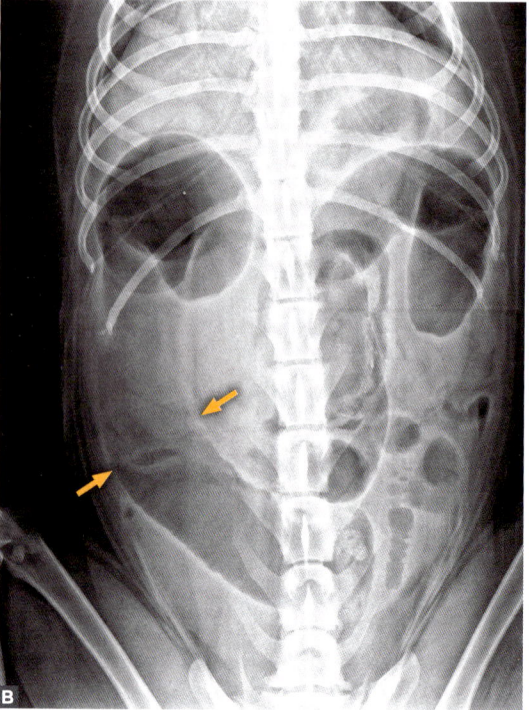

Fig. 37.33 Massive uterine distention associated with emphysematous pyometra in a four-year-old Jack Russel Terrier. There is a large amount of gas distended uterine horns (arrows).

614

Fig. 37.34 Normal uterine involution at 10 days postpartum. The left uterine horn is shown in longitudinal plane and is caudal to the spleen and in close contact of the left adrenal gland. The uterine wall is smooth with well-preserved wall layering and echogenic fluid is present (arrows).

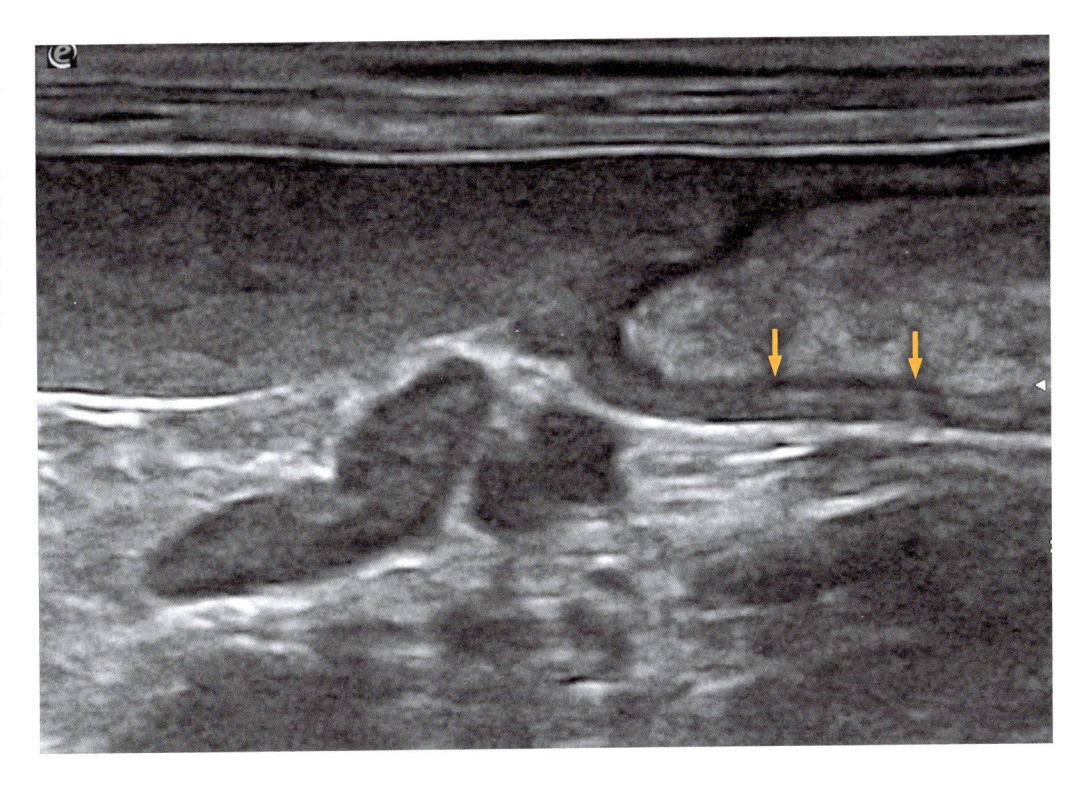

Postpartum uterus

Ultrasound is a particularly useful method for examining the postpartum bitch. In the very early phase, there may be luminal fluid which is often hypoechoic and contains echogenic material (**fig. 37.34**).

Uterine involution results in rapid expulsion of the fluid. The mucosa lumen interface appears as a central echogenic band in the uterus.

Cases of retained fetuses and placenta are not common, but echogenic fetal skeleton, or remnants of the zonary placenta may be identified in some cases.

Slow involution or subinvolution are relatively common and may be associated with a persistence of a muco-hemorrhagic vulval discharge.

References

1. England GCW, Allen WE. Real-time ultrasonic imaging of the canine ovary and uterus. *J Reprod Fertil Suppl* 39:91-100, 1989.
2. England GCW, Allen WE, Porter DJ. Studies on canine pregnancy using B-mode ultrasound; development of the conceptus and determination of gestational age. *J Small Anim Pract* 31:324-329, 1990.
3. England GCW. The relationship between ultrasonographic appearance, testicular size, spermatozoal output and testicular lesions in the dog. *J Small Anim Pract* 32:306-311, 1991.
4. England GCW, Russo M. Ultrasonographic characteristics of early pregnancy failure in bitches. *Theriogenol* 66:1694-1698, 2006.
5. England GCW, Russo M, Freeman SL. Follicular dynamics, ovulation and conception rates. *Reprod Dom Anim* 44:53-58, 2009.
6. Russo M, Vignoli M, Catone G, Rossi F, Attanasi G, England GCW. Prostatic perfusion in the dog using contrast-enhanced doppler ultrasound. *Reprod Dom Anim* 44:334-335, 2009.
7. Vignoli M, Russo M, Catone G, Rossi F, Attanasi G, Terragni R, Saunders JH, England GCW. () Assessment of vascular perfusion kinetics using contrast-enhanced ultrasound for the diagnosis of prostatic disease in dogs. *Reprod Dom Anim* 46:209-213, 2011.
8. England GC, Russo M, Freeman SL. The bitch uterine response to semen deposition and its modification by male accessory gland secretions. *Vet J* 195:179-184, 2012.
9. Russo M, Vignoli M, England GCW. B-mode and contrast-enhanced ultrasonographic findings in canine prostatic disorders. *Reprod Dom Anim* 6:238-242, 2012.
10. Freeman SL, Russo M, England GCW. Uterine artery blood flow character-

istics during oestrus in pregnant and non-pregnant bitches. *Vet J* 197:205-210, 2013.
11. Volta A, Manfredi S, Vignoli M, Russo M, England GCW, Rossi F, Bigliardi E, Di Ianni F, Parmigiani E, Bresciani C, Gnudi G. Use of contrast-enhanced ultrasonography in chronic pathologic canine testes. *Reprod Dom Anim* 49:202-209, 2014.
12. de Souza, MB, England GCW, Mota Filho AC, Ackermann CL, Sousa CV, de Carvalho GG, Silva HV, Pinto JN, Linhares JC, Oba E, da Silva LD. Semen quality, testicular B-mode and Doppler ultrasound, and serum testosterone concentrations in dogs with established infertility. *Theriogenol* 84:805-810, 2015.
13. Dimitrov R, Yonkova P, Vladova D, Kostrov D. Computed tomography imaging of the topographical anatomy of canine prostate. *Trakia J Sci* 8:78e82, 2010.
14. Pasikowska J, Hebel M, Nizanski W, Nowak M. Computed tomography of the prostate gland in healthy intact dogs and dogs with benign prostatic hyperplasia. *Reprod Domest Anim* 50:776e83, 2015.
15. Willmitzer F, Del Chicca F, Kircher PR, Wang-Leandro A, Kronen PW, Verdino D, Rüfenacht D, Porcellini B, Richter H. Diffusion-weighted and perfusion-weighted magnetic resonance imaging of the prostate gland of healthy adult dogs. *Am J Vet Res* 80:832e9, 2019.

SECTION VI

INTERVENTIONAL RADIOLOGY

CHAPTER 38

Diagnostic and therapeutic interventional radiology

Massimo Vignoli

> **KEY POINTS**
>
> - Biopsies or fine-needle aspiration are often required to reach a definitive diagnosis.
> - Image-guided imaging procedures can be employed for both diagnosis and treatment.
> - Most common procedures are performed using ultrasound, computed tomography, or fluoroscopic guidance.
> - Patient preparation and planning are extremely important.

Diagnostic imaging is an important tool for evaluating canine and feline patients, but it can seldom specifically diagnose inflammatory, infectious, metabolic, or neoplastic disorders.[1] Therefore, to obtain a definitive diagnosis, a better prognosis and assist therapeutic planning, biopsies for cytological or histopathological examinations are required.[2]

Ultrasound (US)-guided fine-needle aspiration (FNA) and tissue core biopsy (TCB) procedures are routine procedures in small animal medicine that allow precise needle placement with real-time monitoring. Computed tomography (CT) sampling biopsy is indicated mainly for intrathoracic and bone lesions or lesions located in areas that are not readily accessible with US.[3-4] Although magnetic resonance imaging (MRI) guidance is feasible, the expensive equipment and significant time requirement preclude its widespread use in veterinary medicine.

In veterinary medicine, ultrasonography is the method of choice in daily practice due to the wide availability of US equipment and the lower cost compared to CT, whereas CT is used more widely in specialist or referral clinics.[5]

Interventional radiology is broadly divided into diagnostic and therapeutic procedures. It allows the veterinarian to characterize better the pathological condition and to offer minimally invasive treatments as an alternative to conventional treatment. Novel interventional procedures also offer therapeutic options for some conditions where none existed previously. The use of imaging guidance by fluoroscopy, ultrasound, or computed tomography is of paramount importance for these procedures.

Patient assessment

Basic patient assessment is the same for both diagnostic or therapeutic procedures and is designed to identify significant abnormalities which might preclude the procedure:

- Physical examination.
- Laboratory testing.
- Thoracic radiographs.

SECTION VI INTERVENTIONAL RADIOLOGY

Especially in the case of biopsies of organs likely to bleed, a coagulation profile with a platelet count is necessary, specifically:

- Activated partial thromboplastin time (aPTT).
- One-stage prothrombine time (OSPT).
- Platelets (no biopsy if <80000/μL).
- Hematocrit (HCT).

Dogs with prolonged OSPT and cats with prolonged aPTT are more likely to have a hemorrhage. An increased risk of bleeding has been reported if the HCT is = or <30% in the dog and 23% in the cat.[6]

Patient preparation

- Intravenous catheter.
- Sedation/anesthesia.
- Clip hair.
- Preparation of skin as for surgical procedure.
- Sterile sleeve/cover for ultrasound probe or thorough disinfection of the probe with chlorhexidine.

Biopsy needles

A fine-needle aspiration (FNA) biopsy is considered when the needle has a diameter <20 G or 1.0 mm.[7] Hypodermic, spinal or Chiba needles of appropriate length can be used (**fig. 38.1**):

- 21-22 G (0.8-0.7 mm) for solid organs.
- 22-23 G (0.7-0.6 mm) for fluids.
- 18-20 G (1.2-1.0 mm) for viscous fluids (such as pus).

Larger core needles are used to obtain a specimen adequate for a histopathological examination, termed tissue core biopsies (TCB). In general, a needle with distance markings etched or printed on the needle shaft is preferred by the author to assist needle placement within the organ/lesion. They are several needle types, automatic, semi-automatic, or manual[1,8-9] (**fig. 38.2**). With an auto-

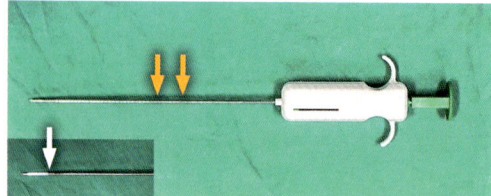

Fig. 38.2 A spring-loaded 1 cm graduated (arrows) semi-automatic Tru-cut needle utilized for image-guided biopsy. Once the needle has been loaded the trochar is pushed out and becomes visible the specimen notch (white arrow).

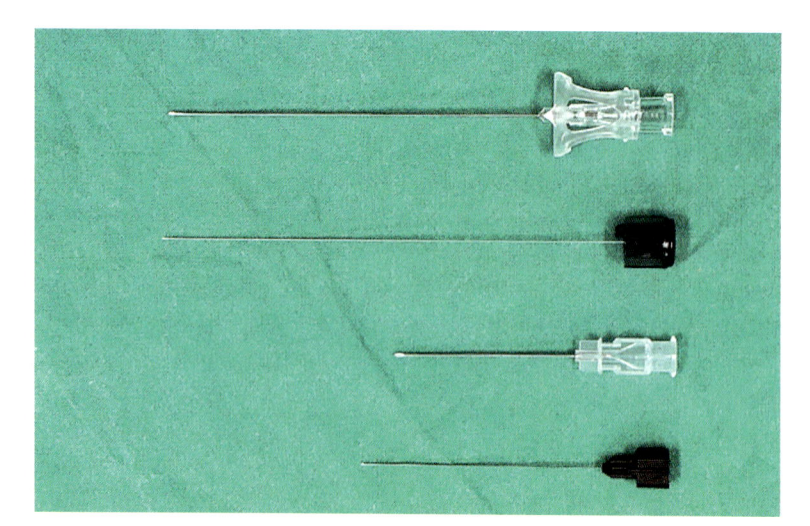

Fig. 38.1 Spinal needles of different lengths with the visible needle (transparent head) and the stylet (black head). This needle can be used for liquid collection or image-guided fine-needle aspiration biopsy.

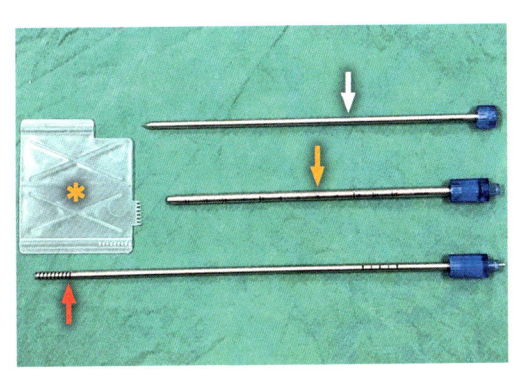

Fig. 38.3 The Spirotome® (Bioncise, Hasselt, Belgium) needle is a large core biopsy manual needle, graduated at 1 cm, composed of four parts: the 1 cm graduated cutting needle (orange arrow), the trochar (white arrow), the receiving needle or helix (red arrow), and the releasing device (asterisk).

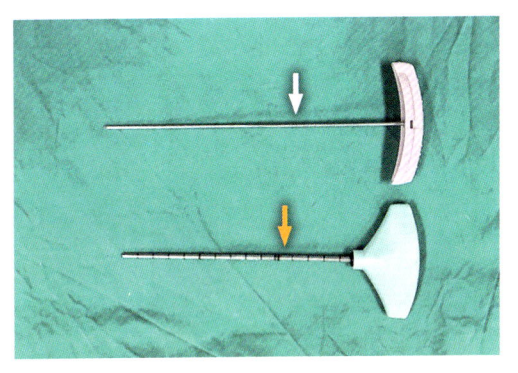

Fig. 38.4 A bone biopsy needle with a 1 cm scale is composed of a cutting needle (orange arrow) and a trochar (white arrow).

matic biopsy gun, the needle tip is inserted close to the lesion or target region. When the device is fired, the inner stylet is first advanced immediately followed by the outer cutting cannula transfixing the target. With such devices, it is of paramount importance to precisely know the needle excursion to avoid injury to blood vessels or other vital structures deep into the target. In some needles, it is possible to choose the excursion of the specimen notch between 8-23 mm.

With the semi-automatic biopsy needles, the inner stylet with a notch for sample collection is first advanced through the region to be sampled with US guidance. Once it is in the correct position the cutting cannula is fired to cut the sample. These devices are safer as the tip of the biopsy needle is placed under US guidance with no risk of overshooting, which is why the author prefers semi-automatic biopsy needles. As with automatic biopsy guns, some devices allow the user to select the sample length.

- Automatic or semi-automatic gun (keep in mind 8-23 mm of needle excursion).
- Manual.
- Menghini, Turner, Tru-cut.
- 14-18 G (2.0-1.2 mm).
- Needle marked at a minimum of 1 cm increments to assist in needle placement.
- Cut on a side or at the tip.
- Guide with stopper.

Manual biopsy needles can be used as well in more expert hands, such as the Spirotome™ (Bioncise, Hasselt, Belgium), which is a large core biopsy system, non-ferromagnetic also suitable for MRI-guided biopsy. It is composed of four elements: the cutting needle, the trochar, the receiving needle (helix), and the releasing device (**fig. 38.3**).[8]

For bone biopsy, a bone needle (Jamshidi) is utilized. There are numerous types of biopsy needles and the type of device used depends on user preference and experience, cost, and local availability. Bone needles can be of different types or diameters, 7-12 G (4.0-3.0 mm), calibrated or not (**fig. 38.4**).

Biopsy procedures

Freehand biopsy is the most common technique used in veterinary patients, for both cytology and histopathology. Needle guides can be obtained for most US machines and probes, and these direct the needle to the lesion at a fixed angle, which can sometimes be indicated by a line displayed on

SECTION VI INTERVENTIONAL RADIOLOGY

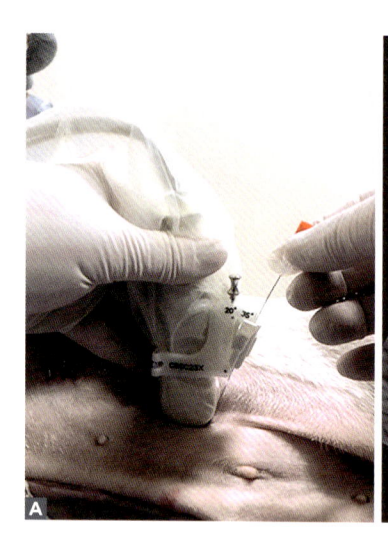

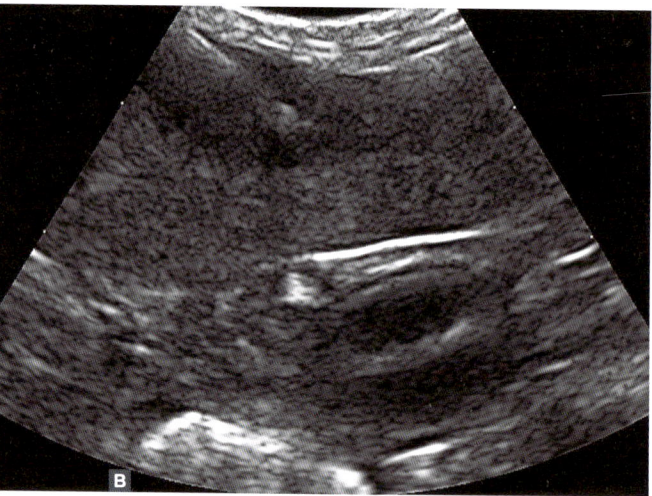

Fig. 38.5 (**A**) Ultrasound-guided FNA with the use of a needle guide (courtesy of Foschi, part of the Demas Group, Rome, Italy) of a splenic nodule (**B**). This guide dictates the angle of needle insertion. See video 38.1.

the screen (**fig. 38.5** and **video 38.1**). However, this technique is limited by the fixed angle of needle insertion which sometimes makes it difficult to avoid vital structures interposed between the skin and the target lesion. Biopsy guides are often unsuitable for biopsies of superficial lesions. It is the author's opinion that this technique can be useful for beginners, while for experts it is more convenient to use a freehand biopsy technique.

VIDEO 38.1
FNA of a splenic nodule

Ultrasound-guided biopsy
Before performing the procedure, the distance between the skin (needle entrance) and the target should be measured to plan the biopsy, especially if an indexed needle is used. The transducer is positioned over the area to be sampled and the needle is aligned with the center of the US beam so that the operator can monitor its passage into the lesion. Visualization of the needle tip can be improved by moving the needle back and forth gently as it is directed toward the target.

Fine-needle aspiration
The needle should be inserted as rapidly as is safe into the lesion since tissue trauma activates coagulation, which can plug the needle and affect the sample quality.[11] The biopsy material should be rapidly expelled onto glass slides using a syringe previously filled with air, and the smears should be made immediately to avoid blood clotting. The effects of operator experience, needle characteristics, number of needle passes, use of negative pressure aspiration or not, target tissue, and presence of a cytopathologist for immediate review of specimen adequacy on FNAs have been evaluated.[5] The operator's experience made no difference when a standard protocol was used. A larger gauge needle is easier to visualize and is less flexible, facilitating FNAs, but better samples are obtained with the smaller gauge needles (e.g., 25 G for FNA of the thyroid gland) since these decrease the chance of dilution with blood products.[5] A needle length that allows placement into the middle of the lesion should be chosen (plus approximately 5 mm for movement), since a few long passes are less traumatic than many short passes. The target tissue is important; for example, epithelial and round cell tumors will yield cells more readily than mesenchymal tumors. Good knowledge of the most common types of tumors in different organs and their imaging features allows the most appropriate technique to be used. Aspiration of fluid can be performed with a venous catheter or by placing a spinal needle into the cavity, removing the stylet, and aspirating with a syringe. A three-way valve with an extension tube is useful for aspirating large amounts of fluid.[12] Percutaneous drainage of abdominal abscesses can be achieved under US guidance and is of value in debilitated patients since it is less invasive than surgery. Fluid can be aspirated from cystic lesions for cytological analysis or to relieve mechanical pressure. US-guided drainage of true cysts is rarely therapeutic unless an irritant such as ethanol is injected.[12,13]

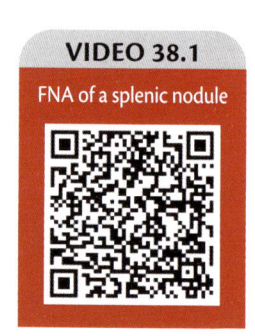

CHAPTER **38** Diagnostic and therapeutic interventional radiology

Tissue core biopsy

A small stab incision with a number 11 scalpel blade should be made to assist needle insertion for tissue core biopsy (TCB). Either a manual or automated needle type can be used for sampling from soft tissue lesions. If the biopsy is performed with a manual needle, an assistant places and steers the biopsy needle whilst the operator keeps the position of the transducer. If an automated needle is used, the operator can manipulate the transducer while collecting the biopsy. Needles with centimeter markings indicate to the operator the insertion depth, which is especially useful if the biopsy is not taken in real-time (i.e., under CT-guidance).

Most Tru-cut type biopsies are taken with 14 or 18 G needles (**fig. 38.6**). It has been reported that using a small needle decreases the risks of complications, but with a normal coagulation profile and a direct path from the transducer to the lesion, better diagnostic samples are obtained with larger needles in our hands. The percutaneous guided biopsy is a relatively safe procedure, although many cats have a subclinical decrease in PCV. A study reported that conventional coagulation tests did not predict complications or the magnitude of bleeding; therefore, more sensitive indicators are needed, such as fibrinogen, factor analysis, and thromboelastography. Cats with hepatic lipidosis tend to bleed more after biopsy and if this diagnosis is suspected, biopsy is contraindicated and FNA is preferred.[14] If there is a need to traverse other organs before reaching the lesion, needles with a smaller diameter are preferred.[5] Bone biopsies are usually performed with a Jamshidi needle.

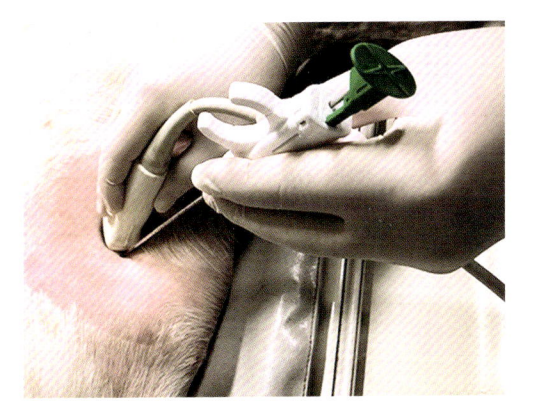

Fig. 38.6 Example of US-guided biopsy with a spring-loaded semi-automatic biopsy needle.

Ultrasound-guided biopsy of abdominal organs

Liver

Subcostal or intercostal approaches can be used for US-guided biopsy of the liver[2] (**fig. 38.7** and **video 38.2**). Biopsy of diffuse liver disease is routinely performed in the left medial or lateral lobe, away from the diaphragm, portal veins, caudal vena cava, hepatic artery, and gallbladder.[15]

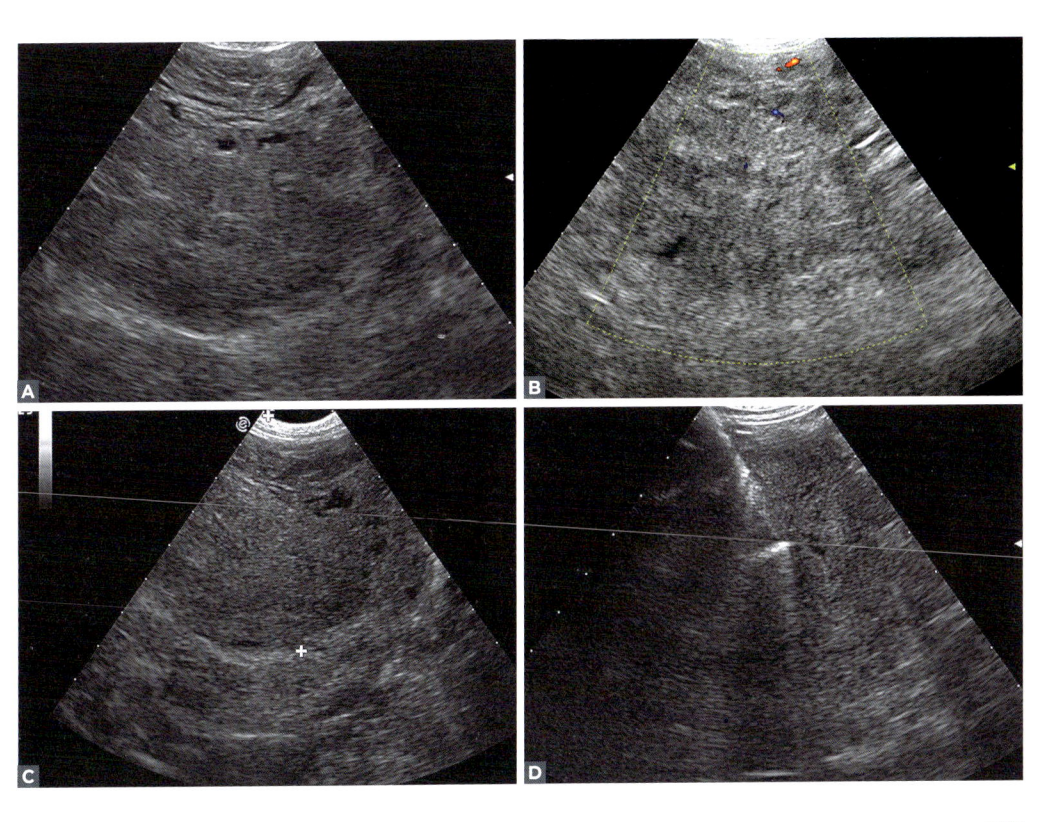

VIDEO 38.2
Ultrasound-guided biopsy of the liver

Fig. 38.7 (**A**) Ultrasound-guided biopsy of the liver. A heterogeneous mass lesion is visible. (**B**, **C**) Color Doppler to confirm or exclude the presence of large vessels in the needle path in the mass. The depth from the skin and the target region within the mass is measured to estimate the distance for safe needle insertion. Finally, the needle is placed within the lesion with US guidance before being "shot" to obtain the biopsy (**D**).

621

The patient's position can be decided according to the preferences of the operator. Usually, dorsal or right lateral recumbency are chosen, so that the left hepatic lobe can be biopsied with the needle directed craniodorsal or lateral to avoid the great vessels and porta hepatis. A subcostal approach is usually employed.

However, in the presence of lesions located quite cranial in the liver or in dogs with a deep-chested conformation, there may be a need to use an intercostal window. In this case, the lateral recumbency is necessary, with the part to be biopsied placed uppermost. While an FNA can usually be done with the patient conscious or lightly sedated, for TCB the patients are anesthetized or deeply sedated to eliminate risk of movement during the biopsy.

Aspiration of the gallbladder contents is a safe procedure that can be performed for culture of bacteria from bile, for gallbladder decompression in patients with extrahepatic biliary obstruction and pancreatitis. The gallbladder should be emptied to reduce bile leakage and subsequent peritonitis, although a small amount of bile leakage usually has no consequences.

Spleen

For US-guided splenic TCBs, 16 or 18 G cutting needles are recommended, whereas 22 G needles are recommended for FNAs, without suction to decrease blood contamination[2] (**fig. 38.5B** and **video 38.1**). FNAs and TCBs of complex splenic masses (e.g., hemangiosarcoma) are often non-diagnostic because of blood dilution.[15]

Pancreas

Biopsies of the pancreas can be used to differentiate between pancreatitis, pancreatic abscesses, pseudocysts, and neoplasia.[15] FNA or TCB of the pancreas can be performed safely under US guidance. If possible, the passage of the needle through normal pancreatic tissue should be avoided because this will likely provoke acute pancreatitis.[15]

Kidneys

US-guided FNA of the kidneys is frequently performed for diagnosis of lymphoma in dogs and cats, while TCB often can be used to establish a definitive diagnosis for other renal diseases but is seldom performed as it usually has no impact on treatment or prognosis.[16] US-guided biopsies for diffuse renal disease should be obtained from the cortex in the pole of the kidney or in a sagittal plane along the lateral cortex, avoiding the arcuate arteries and medulla.[2] The left kidney is usually more accessible and is preferred. Care should be taken with needle placement and direction to avoid laceration of the aorta, caudal vena cava, and renal vessels.

US-guided pyelocentesis can be performed to collect urine from the renal pelvis for bacterial culture and cytology. Iodinated water-soluble contrast medium can be injected for radiographic or CT imaging, with the significant advantage that the risk of contrast-induced hypotension or renal failure is obviated, and the study is not dependent on the ability of the kidney(s) to concentrate the contrast medium. Percutaneous pyelography is used to evaluate the size, shape, and patency of the renal pelvis and ureters, most often in older cats with ureteral calculi. A spinal needle (22-25 G) is inserted through the renal cortex into the renal pelvis under US guidance. Care should be taken to avoid the hilar and arcuate vessels. Urine is removed and, if a contrast study is to be performed, one half of the removed volume of iodinated contrast medium is slowly introduced. Potential complications include leakage of contrast medium, hemorrhage (subcapsular or into the renal pelvis), needle breakage, and seeding of infection. Complications of renal sampling are reported in 13.4% of dogs and 18.5% of cats.[16] The most common complication is mild to moderate hemorrhage and occasionally hydronephrosis. Death is uncommon.[16] Renal TCB also poses a risk of renal damage, leading to uremia and hypertension.

Urinary bladder

US-guided cystocentesis is the most commonly performed image-guided procedure. In most patients the procedure is simple and the anechoic urine in the bladder lumen makes seeing the needle easier than when it is placed in echogenic tissue. Percutaneous needle centesis may be difficult to perform due to the elasticity of the bladder when there is limited filling. Depending on the user's preference, the US probe may be placed in either a transverse or sagittal plane and swept slightly back and forth and side to side to ensure there is no intestine interposed between the body wall and bladder. The needled is advanced at an angle of approximately 45° to the skin and urine aspirated once the tip is seen in the lumen.

Tumoral seeding after percutaneous US-guided sampling of transitional cell carcinomas has been described and this technique should be avoided.[17] Ultrasound-guided catheter suction biopsy is a simple technique for sampling which does not have this risk. A urethral catheter is advanced into the urinary bladder with US guidance, when the tip or side port is apposed to the lesion, suction with a syringe is applied and maintained while the catheter is withdrawn. This usually retrieves a tissue fragment large enough to perform histological examination.[18]

Prostate gland
Prostatic samples can be obtained by aspiration or needle core biopsy. Care should be taken to avoid the urethra and the large vessels that lie close to the prostate gland. Mild hematuria may present for one or more days after a TCB is taken.[15]

Other indications
US-guided FNA of bone lesions may eliminate the need for TCB if conclusive,[19] and does not reach further weakening of lytic bone, especially if conservative treatment is elected. US-guided FNA of the gastrointestinal tract and central or peripheral nervous system has been described.[2] US-guided thoracic interventional procedures are also possible. Since the US beam is largely reflected or absorbed by bone and air, diagnostic ultrasonography of non-cardiac thoracic structures is generally limited to evaluation of structures within or adjacent to the thoracic wall using a parasternal, intercostal, or thoracic inlet imaging window. Pleural fluid creates an excellent acoustic window, allowing US visualization of intrathoracic anatomy, including pulmonary, chest wall, and mediastinal lesions not visible radiographically.

Computed-tomography guided biopsy
CT examination is the method of choice for staging dogs with masses. CT allows a more precise localization, evaluation of the primary mass, and the relationship with the surrounding tissues/organs. Moreover, in veterinary medicine, is the imaging modality of choice to assess the presence of metastases. However, often the lesions are not specific for malignancy and for the histotype of malignancy. Therefore, a biopsy is necessary to characterize the lesion. Patients can be positioned on the CT table in a manner offering easiest access to the lesion based on its location as seen on thoracic radiographs; however, it must be considered that lateral or dorsal recumbency lead the dependent part of the lung to collapse, and therefore some small nodular lesions can be missed. On the other hand, if the patient is positioned in sternal recumbency to avoid lung collapse, it could be possible that the lesion is not in an easy position to biopsy and there is the need to rescan the patient in a different recumbency. With experience, the operator can decide the recumbency before taking the whole study. Usually, surgical preparation is done before the CT study.

After the CT study (plain and contrast) is completed, an assessment of the location and extent of the lesion and the selection of the target plane are carried out. The target plane is chosen in an area with significant changes, especially contrast enhancement to obtain viable tissue samples. Areas suspected to be necrotic (with no contrast enhancement) and large vessels should be avoided.

Then the CT table is moved to the target plane, as indicated by the laser light in the gantry. In this plane, the site for insertion of the needle is subjectively chosen and marked with a sterile radiopaque metal marker or with a syringe needle. Subsequently, additional slices (5-10) in the marker area are acquired to measure the distance from the skin to the proximal and distal borders of the lesion

SECTION VI INTERVENTIONAL RADIOLOGY

and to the area to biopsy. Those measurements facilitate the choice of correct depth and angle of needle insertion. CT table is moved out of the gantry so that the needle (for FNA) or the Tru-cut or bone needle (for TCB) can be placed and advanced to the preset distance and angle following a skin incision. The position of the biopsy needle tip is evaluated with additional images and the needle placement can be corrected when necessary before the lesion is sampled. For FNA, once the needle is in a correct position, the stylet is retracted and suction is applied with a syringe. For TCB, when the needle is in the correct position, the biopsy can be performed.
Further images are taken in the biopsy area to check for complications.

Technique to biopsy the skeleton

The freehand technique can be performed as follows:

- Standard CT examination (pre- and post-contrast study with 600 mg/kg nonionic iodinated CM IV).
- Identification of the target lesion.
- Move the table so that positioning lasers are at the level of the target lesion.
- Localization of the area on the skin for needle placement with laser light.
- Confirmation of the penetration site with a sterile metal marker or placement of short hypodermic needle with 3-4 more scans.
- Stab skin incision, about 4-5 mm with n° 11 scalpel blade.
- Use calibrated bone needle (7-12 G) or spinal needle (22 G). In case muscular tissue is involved, a Tru-cut needle (14-18 G) can be used.
- Determine the position of the tip of the needle with 3-4 more scans.

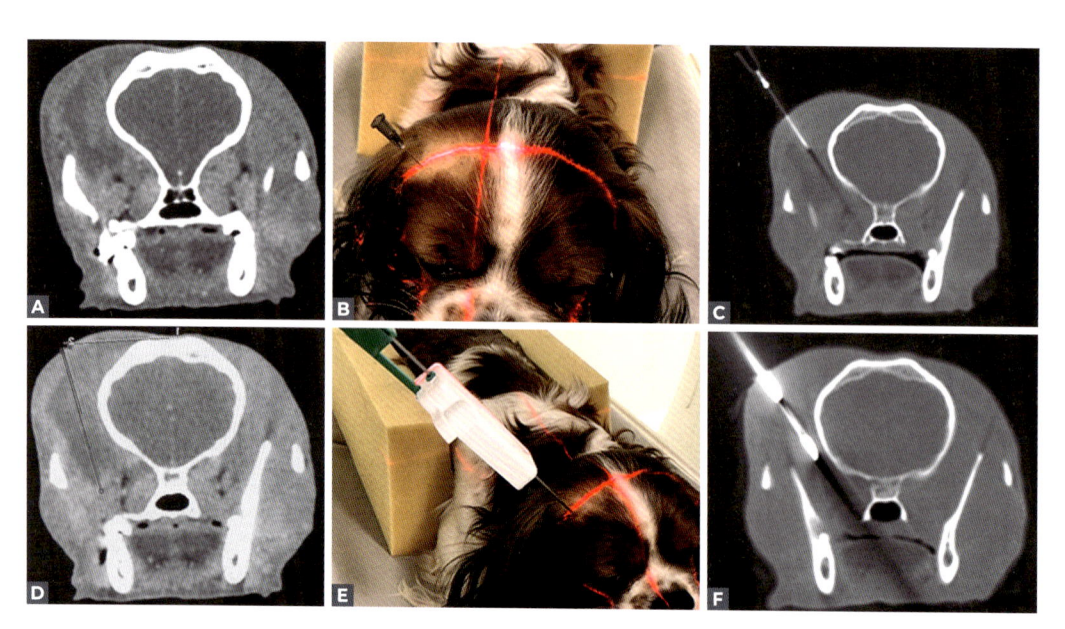

Fig. 38.8 A six-year-old old male Cavalier King Charles Spaniel with multifocal muscular lesions. The images show the sequence of the CT-guided biopsy. (**A**) First, the target is identified in a post contrast soft tissue window image, measurements from the skin to the deep margin of the lesion are obtained and the path for insertion is planned (**D**). After hair clipping and disinfection, the table is moved to the target, and localization of the area on the skin for needle placement is checked with laser marking lights (**B**). Confirmation of the penetration site with a hypodermic needle is done and checked with three/four more scans (**C**). At this point, a stab skin incision is performed, and a calibrated biopsy needle is inserted in the lesion (**E**). A few more scans are made to confirm satisfactory needle placement and the needle is redirected if needed. Once the needle is in the correct position the biopsy is done. Multifocal myositis was the final diagnosis.

CHAPTER **38** Diagnostic and therapeutic interventional radiology

One study on skeletal biopsies in 21 dogs and cats reported 100% of diagnosis 17/17 for TCB and 83% for FNA with an overall accuracy of 95.7%. Mild-to-moderate transient nasal bleeding was observed after biopsies of the nose. Two dogs had mild, transient worsening of the lameness during 3 days after the biopsy. Major complications were not noticed.[9] (**figs. 38.8-38.11**).

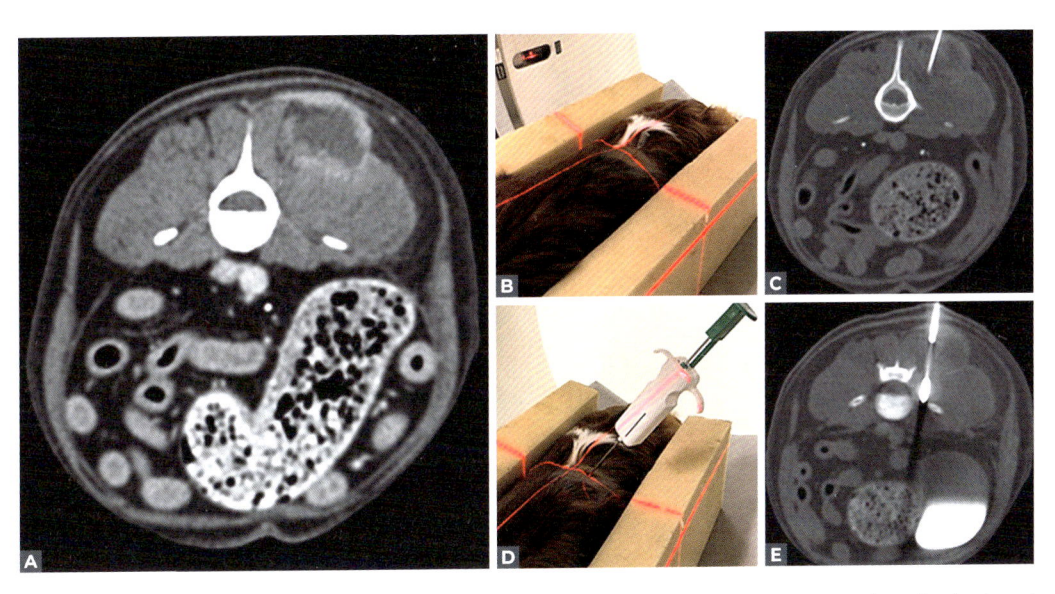

Fig. 38.9 Same dog as in fig. 38.8. This figure shows the sequence of the biopsy in a lumbar muscle, with selection of the target (**A**), localization of the biopsy site with the laser light markers (**B**), hypodermic needle insertion (**C**), insertion of the biopsy needle (**D**) and verification of satisfactory needle placement before biopsy (**E**).

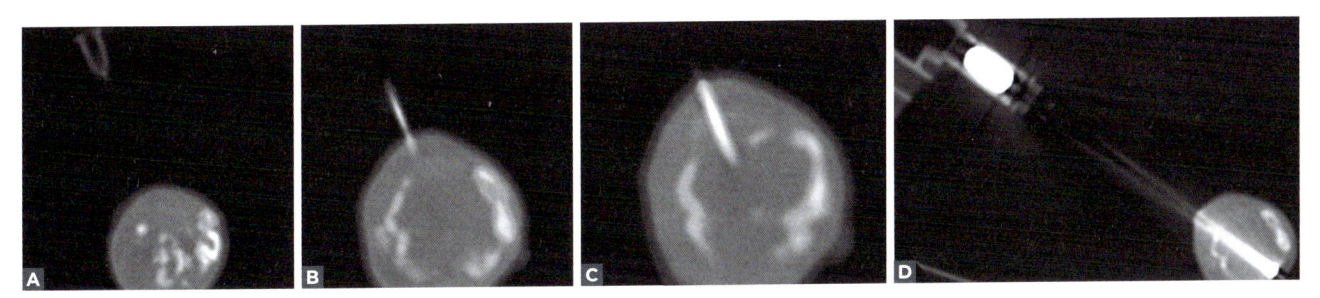

Fig. 38.10 CT-guided biopsy of a lytic lesion in the tarsus of a 15-year-old spayed female mixed breed dog. The phases of the procedure are shown, with hypodermic needle placement (**A-C**), erroneously obliqued inserted. This is necessary to identify the penetration site for the bone needle. (**D**) Bone needle within the lesion verified by CT. At this point, the needle can be retracted with a syringe suction to avoid losing the specimen. The final diagnosis was undifferentiated sarcoma.

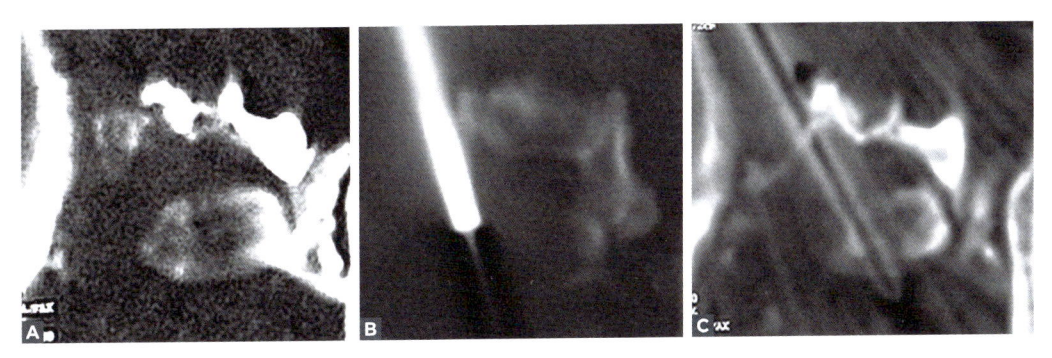

Fig. 38.11 A 12-year-old female mixed breed dog that developed a lytic vertebral lesion several months after mastectomy for mammary carcinoma. (**A**) Target selection, followed by a scan after needle insertion to check the position of the needle (**B**). Second check after needle placement using measurements taken at the beginning of the procedure. The CT-guided biopsy confirmed metastasis from the mammary carcinoma.

SECTION VI INTERVENTIONAL RADIOLOGY

Technique to biopsy the lung and mediastinum

It is similar to the one described for the skeleton (**figs. 38.12-38.16**). A study on the Clinical Value of CT-Guided Fine Needle Aspiration and Tissue-Core Biopsy of Thoracic Masses in the Dog and Cat[20] on 52 dogs and 10 cats reported to be diagnostic 43/62 FNA (69.4%) and 59/62 TCB (95.2%) with an accuracy of 67.7% and 95.2%. Combining the two techniques, the overall accuracy was 98.4%. Mild pneumothorax was seen in 16 cases, whereas mild hemorrhage occurred in three cases. No major complications were encountered. Mild to moderate bleeding after biopsies of the nose was seen.[21]

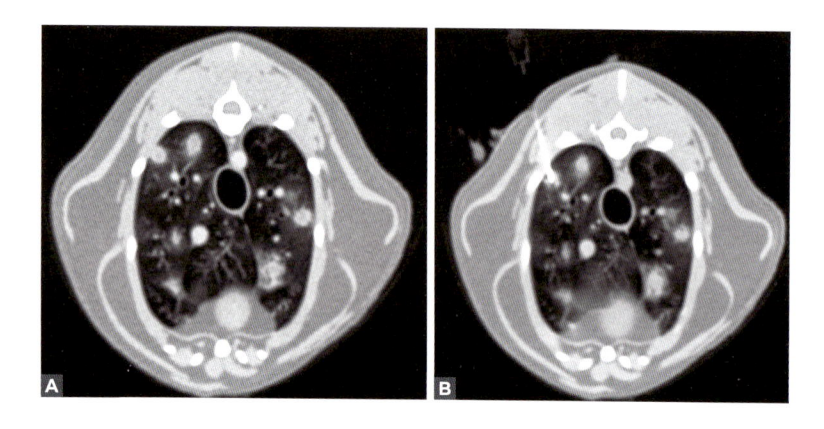

Fig. 38.12 (**A**) Patient with pulmonary nodules. (**B**) A FNA of a 5 mm diameter lung nodule is visible.

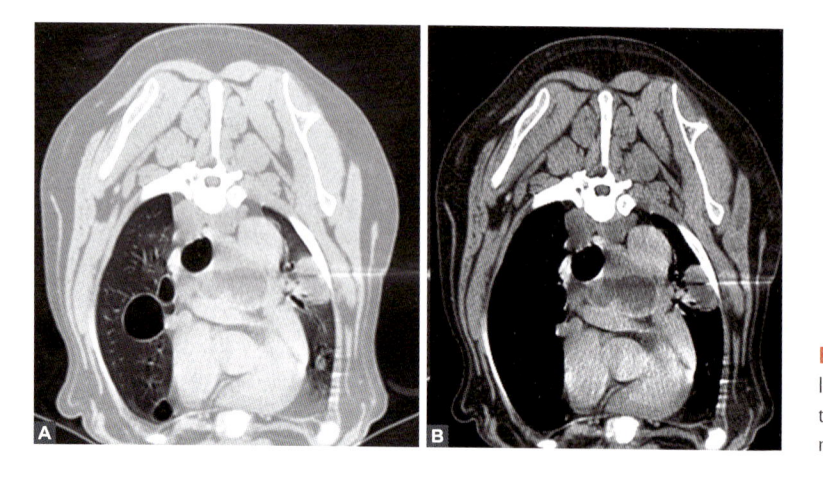

Fig. 38.13 A 12-year-old male mixed breed dog with a lung mass in the cranial lung lobe. (**A**) Lung and (**B**) soft tissue windows of a CT-guided FNA biopsy. The final diagnosis was carcinoma.

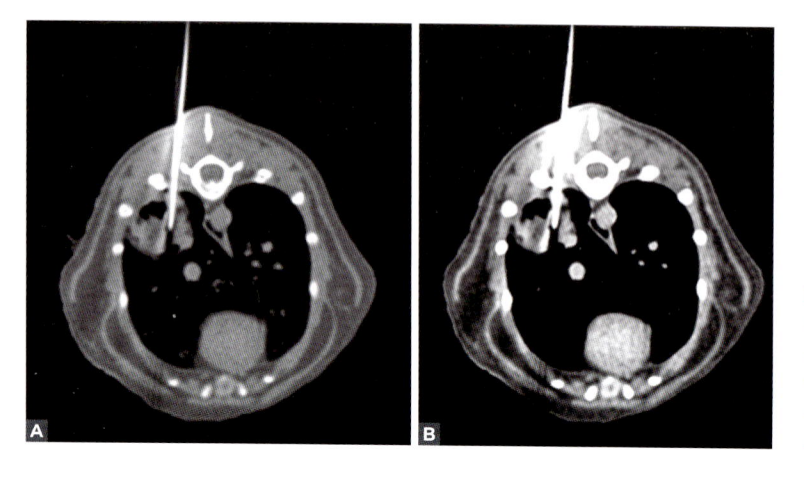

Fig. 38.14 A 13-year-old spayed female Domestic shorthair cat. The CT study shows a 2.5 cm cavitated mass in the right caudal lobe. The images show the placement of a biopsy needle in the bone (**A**) and soft tissue (**B**) window. CT-guided biopsy of the mass wall confirmed a diagnosis of squamous cell carcinoma.

Fig. 38.15 A nine-year-old neutered male cat with a history of over a month of malaise. Radiographs and CT showed pleural effusion and lung mass in the left caudal lung lobe. The lung window CT shows bilateral pneumothorax, secondary to previous thoracentesis. (A) There is also a thick-walled mass with a central gas-filled cavity in the left caudal lung lobe. (B) FNA of the cavitated mass resulted in a diagnosis of an abscess, confirmed by surgery and histopathological examination. The cat underwent surgical lobectomy and recovered completely.

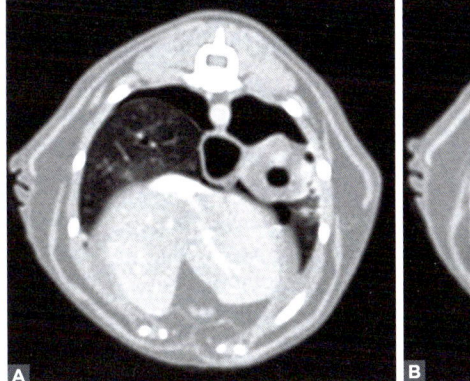

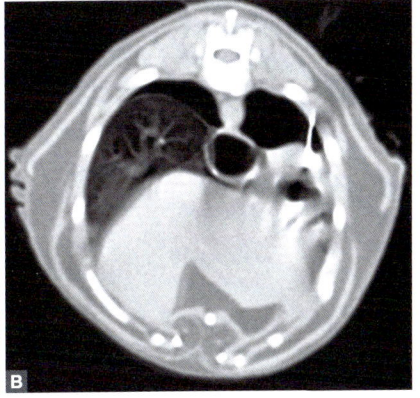

Fig. 38.16 An eight-year-old male mixed breed dog with a rib mass. Images in the bone window show different phases of a CT-guided biopsy of the rib mass, histologically diagnosed as chondrosarcoma.

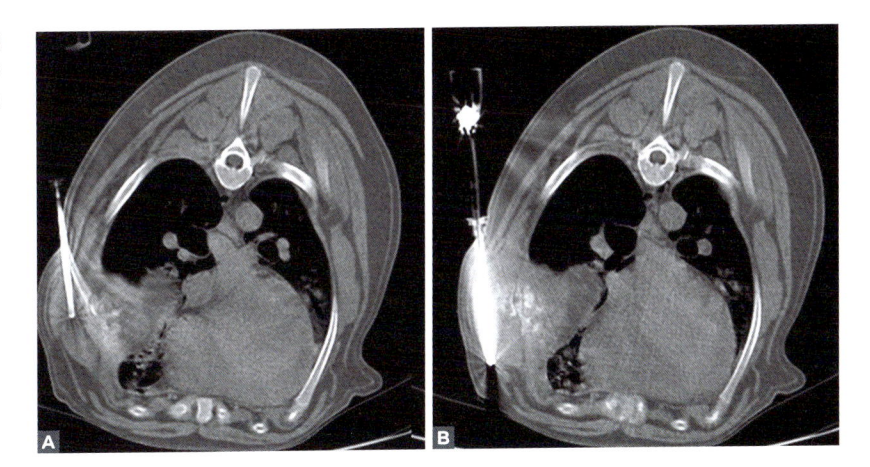

Fluoroscopic guided biopsy and treatment

Fluoroscopy is rarely used as biopsy guidance, mainly due to radiation hazards, low spatial and contrast resolution, and high cost of the unit. However, it can be used in selected cases as guidance for treatment with stent or chemoembolization of tumors.

In modern CT units, CT-fluoroscopy can be present, and they are two types of fluoro-CT: non-real-time and real-time. In the latter case, it is possible to biopsy or treat the patient with a real-time guidance as in US (**figs. 38.17-38.19**).

Other imaging modalities as US or CT are most commonly used as a guide for a treatment (**figs. 38.20-38.22**).

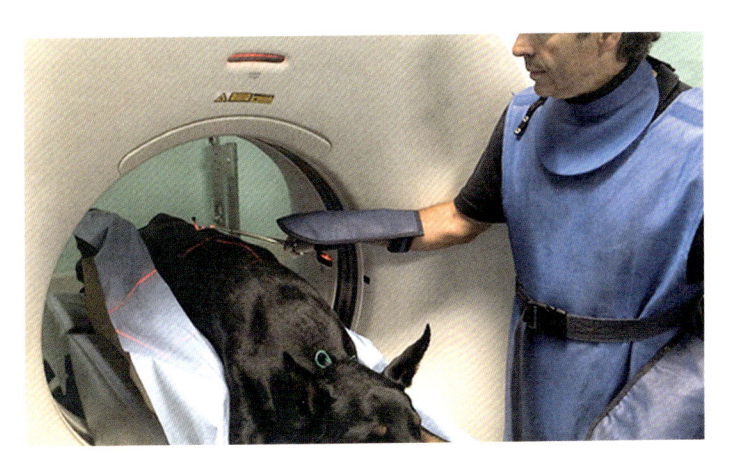

Fig. 38.17 The radiologist during the fluoroscopic CT-guided procedure. Despite the use of surgical forceps to avoid direct exposure from the primary beam and the protective lead equipment for protection from scatter radiation, radiation exposure remains the main limitation of this procedure. However, in some specific instances, especially when the biopsy site is close to a vital organ, or for therapeutic procedures, this technique may be very useful.

SECTION VI INTERVENTIONAL RADIOLOGY

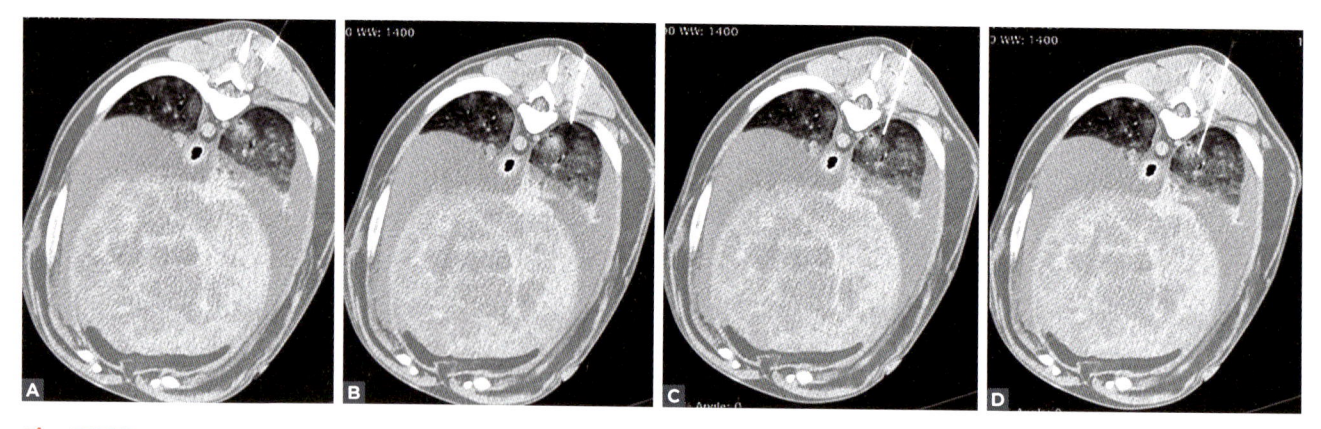

Fig. 38.18 An 11-year-old male mixed breed dog with a liver mass and lung nodules. Lung window images show the sequence of a fluoroscopic CT-guided FNA of a lung nodule.

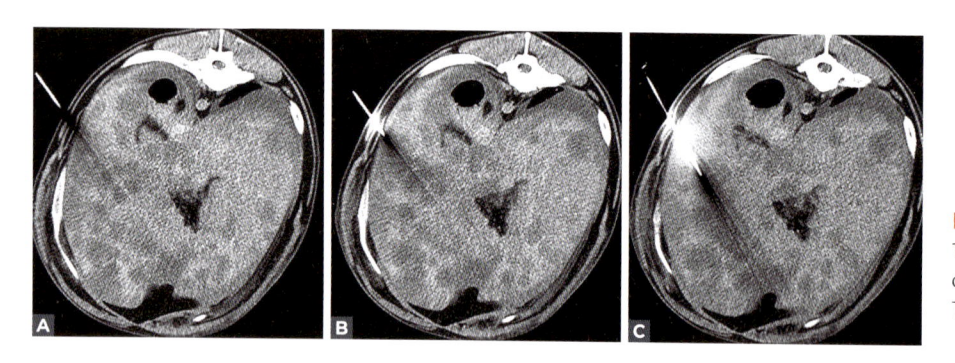

Fig. 38.19 Same dog as in fig. 38.18. These images show the sequence of a fluoroscopic CT-guided biopsy of the liver mass. The final diagnosis was hemangiosarcoma.

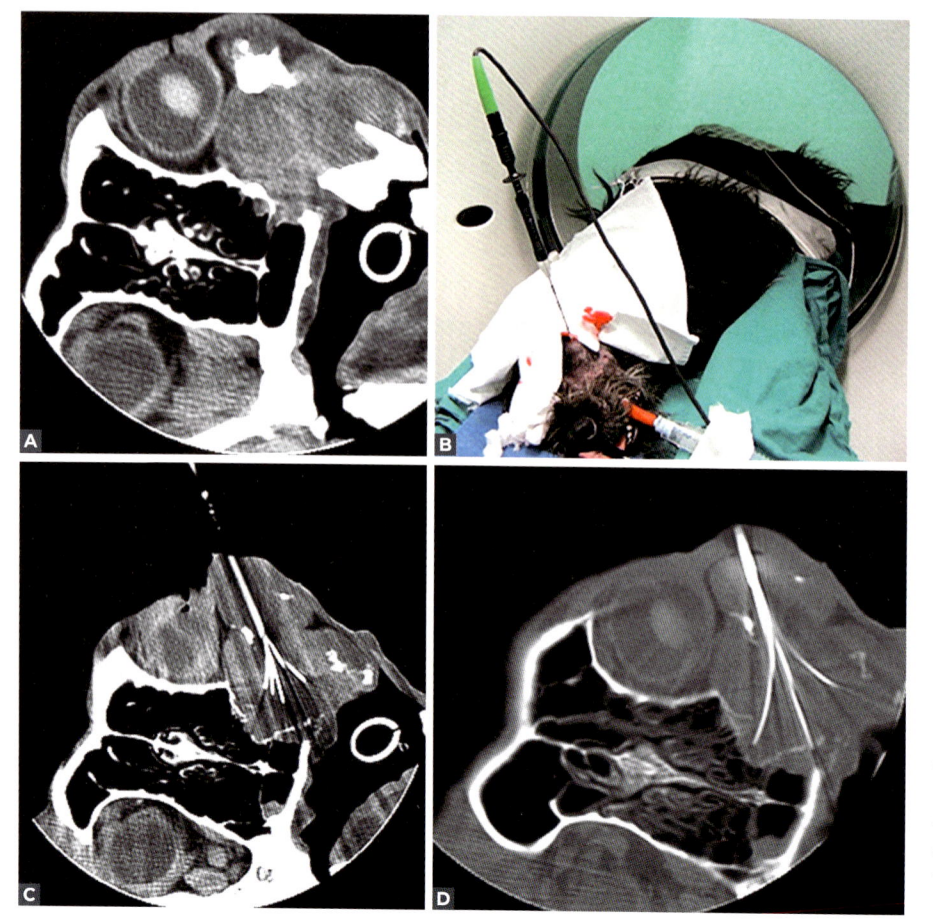

Fig. 38.20 (**A-B**) CT-guided tumor ablation with radiofrequency using a soft tissue (**C**) and a bone (**D**) window. The radiofrequency probe has been partially opened (**C**) with correct positioning; it can be opened completely (**D**), and treatment can be started. (Courtesy of Vignoli M and Saunders J. Image-guided interventional procedures in the dog and cat. *Vet J* 187:297-303, 2011).

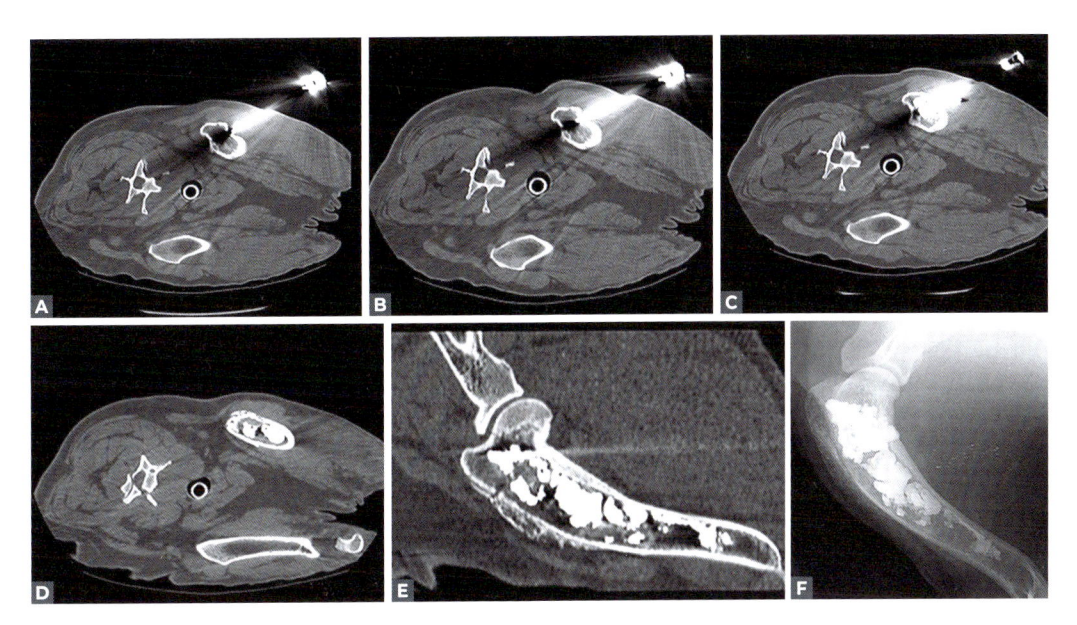

CHAPTER 38 Diagnostic and therapeutic interventional radiology

Fig. 38.21 An eight-year-old Newfoundland male dog with humeral osteosarcoma. After palliative radiation therapy the dog underwent a CT-guided cementoplasty. (**A-B**) CT-guided needle introduction (**C-D**) and cement injection are shown. A sagittal plane reconstruction (**E**) and a mediolateral radiographic projection show filling of the humerus with the cement. The dog did well but developed a pathological fracture 14 months later.

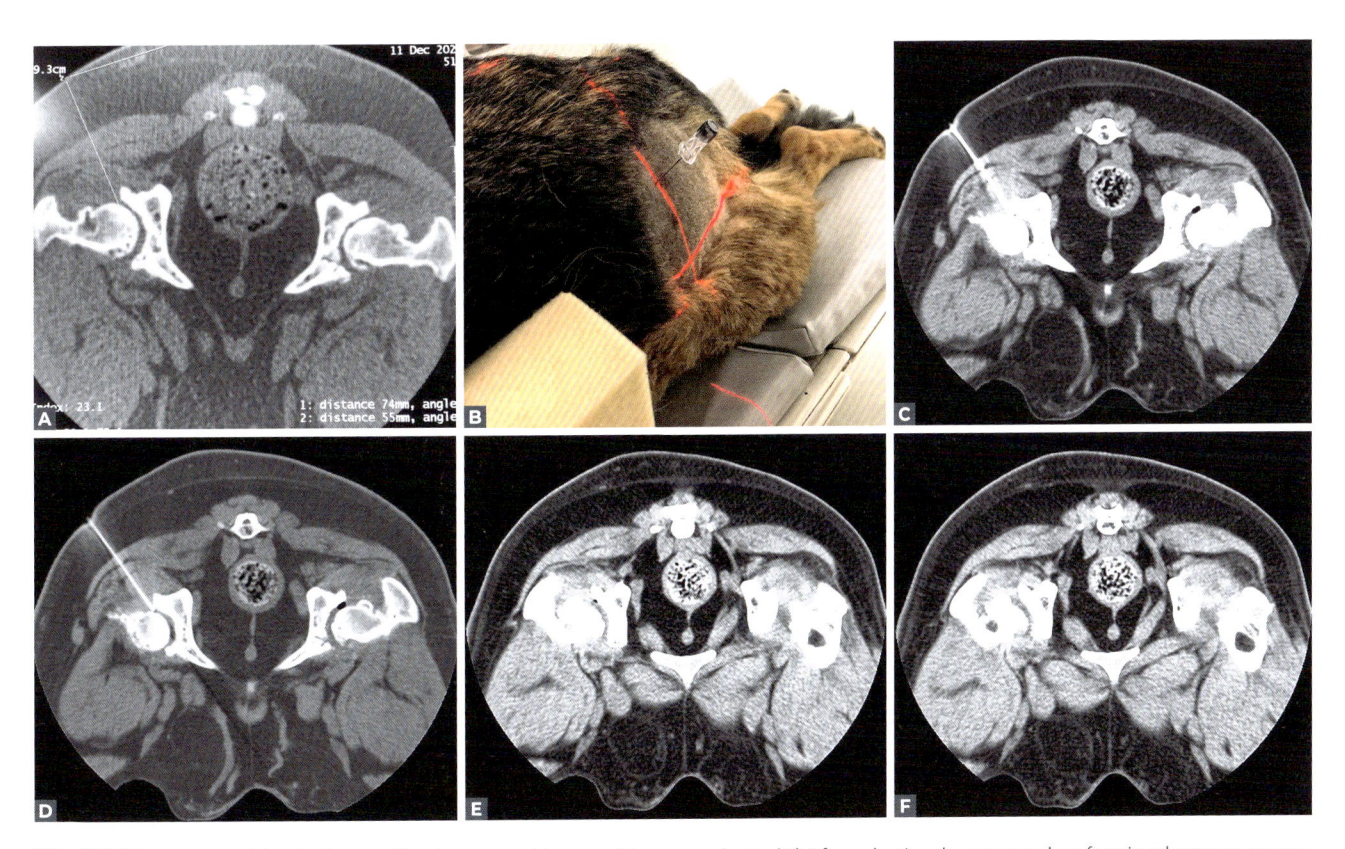

Fig. 38.22 A 14-year-old male German Shepherd dog with severe hip osteoarthritis. (**A**) After selecting the target and performing the measurement, the table is moved and the needle is inserted with the help of the laser light (**B**). A few slices are acquired to confirm needle positioning, and if correct in soft tissue and bone windows (**C-D**), injection of the therapeutic agent, in this case platelet-rich plasma (PRP), can be performed and delivery to the correct target region can be confirmed (**E-F**).

Complications

Biopsy complications can be broadly divided into minor and major. Minor complications are most commonly limited to hemorrhage and are reported to occur in 5.6-21.9% of cases. Major complications requiring intervention (e.g., fluid therapy, blood transfusion) are reported in 1.2-6% of cases. Significant hemorrhage has been observed in thrombocytopenic dogs, those with a prolonged OSPT, and cats with prolonged aPTT. In one study, the complication rate was organ-dependent (higher for the kidneys than for the liver) and all major complications occurred within 10 h of biopsy.[22] When there is a known potential risk, such as too low thrombocyte count (<80.000 μL)) or too high OSPT and aPTT, the biopsy should be avoided. Bleeding from unintended injury, patient movement, or poor operator technique is also possible.

Another common complication is pneumothorax in case of lung biopsy, or less common for aspirate. However, these are usually self-limiting pneumothorax; the author has never experienced the need of chest drainage.

If a proper procedure is conducted, the risk of infection and tumoral seeding is a rare event in veterinary medicine, if transitional cell carcinoma of the urogenital tract is excluded.

References

1. Vignoli M, Saunders JH. Image-guided interventional procedures in the dog and cat. *Vet J* 187:297-303, 2011.
2. Finn-Bodner ST, Hathcock JT. Image-guided percutaneous needle biopsy: ultrasound, computed tomography, and magnetic resonance imaging. *Semin Vet Med Surg Small Anim* 8:258-278, 1993.
3. Tidwell AS, Johnson KL. Computed tomography-guided percutaneous biopsy in the dog and cat: description of the technique and preliminary evaluation in 14 patients. *Vet Radiol Ultrasound* 35:445-456, 1994.
4. Zekas LJ, Crawford JT, O'Brien RT. Computed tomography-guided fine needle aspirate and tissue-core biopsy of intrathoracic lesions in thirty dogs and cats. *Vet Radiol Ultrasound* 46:200-204, 2005.
5. Winter TC, Lee FT, Hinshaw JL. Ultrasound-guided biopsies in the abdomen and pelvis. *Ultrasound Q* 24:45-68, 2008.
6. Bigge LA, Brown DJ, Penninck DG. Correlation between coagulation profile and bleeding complications after ultrasound-guided biopsies: 434 cases (1993-1996). *J Am Anim Hosp Assoc* 37:228-233, 2001.
7. Buscarini L, Di Stasi M. Ecografia interventistica e diagnostica: materiali e tecniche. In Buscarini L, Di Stasi M. (editors). Trattato Italiano di Ecografia. Poletto Editore srl, Gudo Visconti (MI), Italy 3:924-929, 1993.
8. Vignoli M, Barberet V, Chiers K, Duchateau L, et al. Evaluation of a manual biopsy device 'Spirotome' on fresh canine organs: liver, spleen, and kidneys, and first clinical experiences in animals. *Eur J Cancer Prev* 20:140-145, 2011.
9. Vignoli M, Ohlerth S, Rossi F, Pozzi L, et al. Computed tomography-guided fine-needle aspiration and tissue-core biopsy of bone lesions in small animals. *Vet Radiol Ultrasound* 45:125-130, 2004.
10. Charboneau JW, Reading CC, Welch TJ. CT and sonographically guided needle biopsy: current techniques and new innovations. *AJR Am J Roentgenol* 154:1-10, 1990.
11. Menard M, Papageorges M. Ultrasound corner. Technique for ultrasound guided fine needles biopsies. *Vet Radiol Ultrasound* 36:137-138, 1995.
12. Penninck DG, Finn-Bodner ST. Updates in interventional ultrasonography. *Vet Clin North Am Small Anim Pract* 28:1017-1040, 1998.
13. Zatelli A, Bonfanti U, Zini E, D'Ippolito P, Bussadori C. Percutaneous drainage and alcoholization of hepatic abscesses in five dogs and a cat. *J Am Anim Hosp Assoc* 41:34-38, 2005.
14. Pavlick M, Webster CR, Penninck DG. Bleeding risk and complications associated with percutaneous ultrasound-guided liver biopsy in cats. *J Feline Med Surg* 21:529-536, 2019.
15. Nyland TG, Mattoon JS, Herrgesell EJ, Wisner ER. Ultrasound-guided biopsy. In Nyland TG, Matton JS. (editors). Small Animal Diagnostic Ultrasound 2nd edition. W.B. Saunders Company, 2002, Philadelphia, Pennsylvania, pp 30-48.
16. Vaden SL, Levine JF, Lees GE, Groman RP, Grauer GF, Forrester SD. Renal biopsy: a retrospective study of methods and complications in 283 dogs and 65 cats. *J Vet Intern Med* 19:794-801, 2005.
17. Vignoli M, Rossi F, Chierici C, Terragni R, et al. Needle tract implantation after fine needle aspiration biopsy of transitional cell carcinoma of the urinary bladder and adenocarcinoma of the lung. *Schweiz Arch Tierheilkd* 149:314-318, 2007.
18. Lamb CR, Trower ND, Gregory SP. Ultrasound-guided catheter biopsy of the lower urinary tract: technique and results in 12 dogs. *J Small Anim Pract* 37:413-417, 1996.
19. Samii VF, Nyland TG, Werner L, Baker TW. Ultrasound-guided fine needle aspiration biopsy of bone lesions: a preliminary report. *Vet Radiol Ultrasound* 40:82-86, 1999.
20. Vignoli M, Tamburro R, Felici A, Del Signore F, et al. Clinical Value of CT-Guided Fine Needle Aspiration and Tissue-Core Biopsy of Thoracic Masses in the Dog and Cat. *Animals (Basel)* 11:883, 2021.
21. Tamburro R, Millanta F, Del Signore F, Terragni R, Magni T, Vignoli M. Evaluation of the Spirotome Device for Nasal Tumors Biopsy in Eleven Dogs. *Top Companion Anim Med* 40:100436, 2020.
22. Bigge LA, Brown DJ, Penninck DG. Correlation between coagulation profile and bleeding complications after ultrasound-guided biopsies: 434 cases (1993-1996). *J Am Anim Hospital Assoc* 37:228-233, 2001.